PATIENT SELF-ASSESSMENT FORMS

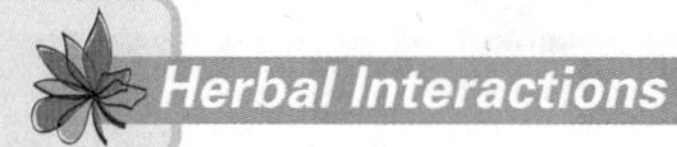

COMPANION CD-ROM RESOURCES

REVIEW QUESTIONS FOR THE NCLEX® EXAMINATION for each chapter

ANIMATIONS

Adenosine for Supraventricular Tachycardia
Anthrax Infection
Asthma
Atropine for Sinus Bradycardia
Cancer Treatment: Chemotherapy
Cancer Treatment: Radiation Therapy
Congestive Heart Failure
Diltiazem for Atrial Fibrillation
Epinephrine for Ventricular Fibrillation
Heparin for Acute Coronary Syndrome
Heparin for Atrial Fibrillation
Intravenous Antibiotic Therapy for Streptococcal Infection
Smallpox
Tuberculosis Infection
Vaccination

APPENDICES

A Prescription Abbreviations
B Medical Abbreviations
C Nomogram for Calculating the Body Surface Area of Adults and Children
D Commonly Used Laboratory Tests and Drug Values
E Recommended Childhood and Adolescent Immunization Schedule: United States, 2006
F MedWatch
G Dyskinesia Identification System: Condensed User Scale (DISCUS)
H A Simple Method to Determine Tardive Dyskinesia Symptoms: AIMS Examination Procedure
I Template for Developing a Written Record for Patients to Monitor Their Own Therapy

PATIENT SELF-ASSESSMENT FORMS

Sleeping Medication (Chapter 14)
Antiparkinson Agents (Chapter 15)
Antianxiety Medication (Chapter 16)
Antidepressants (Chapter 17)
Anticonvulsants (Chapter 19)
Analgesics (Chapter 20)
Anticoagulants (Chapter 27)
Cardiovascular Agents (Chapter 28)
Diuretics or Urinary Antibiotics (Chapter 29)
Respiratory Agents (Chapter 31)
Agents Affecting the Digestive System (Chapter 33)
Antidiabetic Agents (Chapter 36)
Thyroid Medications; Antithyroid Medications (Chapter 37)
Corticosteroids (Chapter 38)
Prenatal Care; Postpartum Care (Chapter 40)
Urinary Antibiotics (Chapter 42)
Eye Medications (Chapter 43)
Antineoplastic Agents (Chapter 44)
Muscle Relaxants (Chapter 45)
Antibiotics (Chapter 46)
Nutritional Therapy (Chapter 47)
Self-Monitoring Drug Therapy Record (Appendix I)

AUDIO GLOSSARY

DRUG DOSAGE CALCULATORS

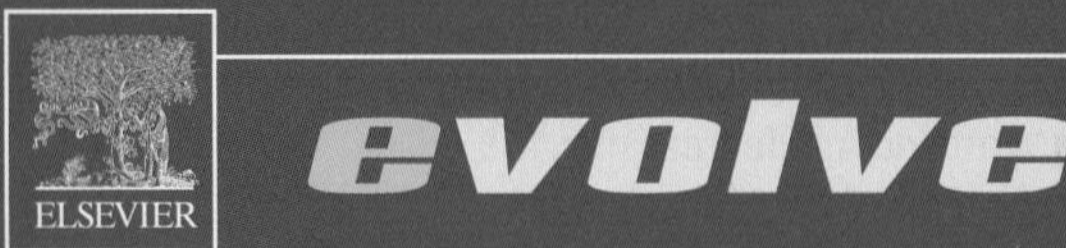

To access your Student Resources, visit:

http://evolve.elsevier.com/Clayton/

Evolve® Student Learning Resources for ***Clayton, Stock, & Harroun: Basic Pharmacology for Nurses, Fourteenth Edition,*** offer the following features:

Student Resources

- **WebLinks**
  A dynamic resource that lets you link to hundreds of websites carefully chosen to supplement the content of the textbook. The WebLinks are regularly updated, with new ones added as they develop.
- **Drugs @ FDA—A Catalog of FDA Approved Drug Products**
  A comprehensive and up-to-date database of drug approvals and withdrawals.
- **Elsevier ePharmacology Update Newsletter**
  An informative, full-color newsletter that provides current and well-documented information related to pharmacology.
- **Appendices**
  Appendices from the textbook are easily accessible on Evolve as well as on the Companion CD-ROM.

DRUG CLASSIFICATIONS

ACE inhibitors Prevent the synthesis of angiotensin II, a potent vasoconstrictor; used to treat hypertension and heart failure
acetylcholinesterase inhibitors Promote the accumulation of acetylcholine, resulting in prolonged cholinergic effects
adrenergic Produce effects similar to the neurotransmitter norepinephrine; see Chapter 13
adrenergic blocking agents Inhibit the adrenergic system, preventing stimulation of the adrenergic receptors
aldosterone receptor antagonists Block stimulation of mineralocorticoid receptors by aldosterone, thus reducing high blood pressure by preventing sodium reabsorption
aminoglycosides Gentamicin, tobramycin, and related antibiotics; particularly effective against gram-negative microorganisms; noted for potentially dangerous toxicity
amylinomimetic agents Used to reduce elevated postprandial hyperglycemia in patients with type 1 or type 2 diabetes mellitus
analgesics Narcotic and nonnarcotic; relieve pain without producing loss of consciousness or reflex activity
androgens These steroid hormones produce masculinizing effects
anesthetics For example, local anesthesia, general anesthesia; cause a loss of sensation with or without a loss of consciousness
angiotensin II receptor antagonists Also known as ARBs (angiotensin receptor blockers); act by binding to angiotensin II receptor sites, preventing angiotensin II (a very potent vasoconstrictor) from binding to receptor sites in vascular smooth muscle, brain, heart, kidneys, and adrenal gland, thus blocking the blood pressure–elevating and sodium-retaining effects of angiotensin II
antacids Reduce the acidity of the gastric contents
antianginals Used to prevent or treat attacks of angina pectoris; most common is nitroglycerin
antianxiety Used to treat anxiety symptoms or disorders; also known as minor tranquilizers or anxiolytics, although the term *tranquilizer* is avoided today to prevent the misperception that the patient is being tranquilized
antibiotics Used to treat infections caused by pathogenic microbes; the term is often used interchangeably with antimicrobial agents
anticholinergics Block the action of acetylcholine in the parasympathetic nervous system; also known as cholinergic blocking agents, antispasmodics, and parasympatholytic agents
anticoagulants Do NOT dissolve existing blood clots, but do prevent enlargement or extension of blood clots
anticonvulsants Suppress abnormal neuronal activity in the CNS, preventing seizures
antidepressants Relieve depression
antidiabetics Also known as hypoglycemics; include insulin (used to treat type 1 diabetes mellitus) and oral hypoglycemic agents (used in the treatment of type 2 diabetes mellitus)
antidiarrheals Relieve or control the symptoms of acute or chronic diarrhea
antidysrhythmics Used to correct cardiac dysrhythmias (any heart rate or rhythm other than normal sinus rhythm)
antiemetics Used to prevent or treat nausea and vomiting
antifungals Used to treat fungal infections
antiglaucoma Used to reduce intraocular pressure
antigout Used to treat active gout attacks or to prevent future attacks
antihistamines Used to treat allergy symptoms; may also be used to treat motion sickness, insomnia, and other nonallergic reactions
antihypertensives Used to treat elevated blood pressure (hypertension)
antilipemics Used to reduce serum cholesterol and/or triglycerides; most common are statins
antimicrobials Chemicals that eliminate living microorganisms pathogenic to the patient; also called antibiotics or antiinfectives
antineoplastics Also called chemotherapy agents; used alone or in combination with other treatment modalities such as radiation, surgery, or biologic response modifiers to treat cancer
antiparkinson's Used in the treatment of Parkinson's syndrome and other dyskinesias
antiplatelets Prevent platelet clumping (aggregation), thereby preventing an essential step in formation of a blood clot; most common are aspirin and clopidogrel
antipsychotics Used to treat severe mental illnesses; also known as major tranquilizers or neuroleptics, although the term *tranquilizer* is avoided today to prevent the misperception that the patient is being tranquilized
antipyretics Used to reduce fevers associated with a variety of conditions; most common are aspirin and acetaminophen
antispasmodics Actually anticholinergic agents
antithyroid Used to treat the symptoms of hyperthyroidism; also known as thyroid hormone antagonists
antituberculins Used to prevent or treat an infection caused by *Mycobacterium tuberculosis*
antitussive Used to suppress a cough by acting on the cough center of the brain
antiulcer agents These drugs, such as histamine (H2) antagonists, decrease the volume and increase the pH of gastric secretions
antivirals Used to treat infections caused by pathogenic viruses
beta blockers Inhibit the activity of sympathetic transmitters, norepinephrine, and epinephrine; used to treat angina, dysrhythmias, hypertension, and glaucoma
bronchodilators Stimulate receptors within the tracheobronchial tree to relax and dilate the airway passages, allowing a greater volume of air to be exchanged and improving oxygenation
calcium channel blockers Also called calcium ion antagonists, slow channel blockers, or calcium ion influx inhibitors; inhibit the movement of calcium ions across the cell membrane; used to decrease dysrhythmias, slow rate of contraction of the heart, and cause vasodilation
carbapenems Antibiotics (imipenem, ertapenem, meropenem) with a broad spectrum of activity against gram-positive and gram-negative bacteria; they act by inhibiting cell wall synthesis
carbonic anhydrase inhibitors Interfere with the production of aqueous humor, thereby reducing intraocular pressure associated with glaucoma
cell-stimulating agents Improve immune function by stimulating the activity of various immune cells
cholinergic Also known as parasympathomimetics; produce effects similar to those of acetylcholine
cholinesterase inhibitors These enzymes destroy acetylcholine, the cholinergic neurotransmitter
coating agent This drug, sucralfate, forms a complex that adheres to the crater of an ulcer, protecting it from aggravation from gastric secretions
colony-stimulating factors Stimulate progenitor cells in bone marrow to increase numbers of leukocytes, thereby improving immune function
corticosteroids These hormones are secreted by the adrenal cortex of the adrenal gland
cycloplegics Anticholinergic agents that paralyze accommodation of the iris of the eye
cytotoxics Agents that cause direct cell death; often used for cancer chemotherapy
decongestants Reduce swelling in the nasal passages caused by a common cold or allergic rhinitis, usually by vasoconstriction.
digestants Combination products containing digestive enzymes used to treat various digestive disorders and to supplement deficiencies of natural digestive enzymes
digitalis glycosides A class of drugs, also known as cardiac glycosides, that increase the force of contraction and slow the heart rate, thereby improving cardiac output; digoxin is the prototype
diuretics Act to increase the flow of urine
emetics Used to induce vomiting
estrogens Steroids that cause feminizing effects

Continued

expectorants Liquefy mucus by stimulating the natural lubricant fluids from the bronchial glands
fluoroquinolones Ciprofloxacin and related agents; widely used broad-spectrum antibiotics
gastric stimulants Used to increase stomach contractions, relax the pyloric valve, and increase peristalsis in the gastrointestinal tract; result in a decrease in gastric transit time and more rapid emptying of the intestinal tract
glucocorticoids Also known as adrenocorticosteroids; are used to regulate carbohydrate, fat, and protein metabolism
gonadal hormones Hormones produced by the testes in the male and ovaries in the female
herbals Plant products usually sold as food supplements; may have pharmacologic effects that are not evaluated or regulated by the FDA
histamine (H2) antagonists Decrease the volume and increase the pH of gastric secretions both during the day and the night
HMG-CoA reductase enzyme inhibitors Also known as the statins; antilipemic agents that inhibit hydroxymethyl-glutaryl coenzyme A (HMG-CoA) reductase enzyme, the enzyme that stimulates the conversion of HMG-CoA to mevalonic acid, a precursor in the biosynthesis of cholesterol, thus reducing the potential for atherosclerosis
hyperuricemics Used to decrease the production or increase the excretion of uric acid
hypnotics Used to produce sleep
incretin-mimetics Used to reduce basal glucose concentrations and elevate postprandial glucose concentrations; used to treat diabetes mellitus
insulins Hormone required for glucose transport to the cells
lactation suppressants Used to prevent physiologic lactation
laxatives Act by a variety of mechanisms to treat constipation
low molecular weight heparins Derivatives of heparin; anticoagulants for the prophylactic treatment of pulmonary thromboembolism and deep vein thrombosis
macrolides Erythromycin, azithromycin, and related antibiotics
MAO inhibitors Agents that block monoamine oxidase, thereby preventing the degradation and prolonging the action of norepinephrine and serotonin
mineralocorticoids Steroids that cause the kidneys to retain sodium and water
miotics Cause constriction of the iris
mucolytics Reduce the thickness and stickiness of pulmonary secretions by acting directly on the mucous plugs to dissolve them
muscle relaxants Relieve muscle spasms
mydriatics Cause dilation of the iris
neuromuscular blockers Skeletal muscle relaxants used to produce muscle relaxation during anesthesia; reduce the use and side effects of general anesthetics; used to ease endotracheal intubation and prevent laryngospasm
nitrates Metabolize to nitric oxide, a potent vasodilator used to treat angina
nonsteroidal antiinflammatory drugs (NSAIDs) These "aspirin-like" drugs are chemically unrelated to the salicylates but are prostaglandin inhibitors
opioids Centrally acting analgesic agents related to morphine
oral contraceptives Used for birth control; administered orally
oral hypoglycemics Used in type 2 diabetes mellitus to improve glucose metabolism and lower blood glucose levels
progestins Steroids regulating endometrial and myometrial function; used alone or in combination with estrogen for oral contraception
protease inhibitors Saquinavir, ritonavir, indinavir, and related drugs; block the maturation of human immunodeficiency virus; used to treat HIV infections
salicylates Effective as analgesics, antipyretics, and antiinflammatory agents
sedatives Given to an individual to produce relaxation and rest; do not necessarily produce sleep
selective serotonin reuptake inhibitors (SSRIs) Antidepressants that act by specifically blocking the reuptake of serotonin, thus prolonging its action
serotonin antagonists Used to block serotonin; prevent emesis induced by chemotherapy, radiation therapy, and surgery
statins (HMG-CoA reductase inhibitors) Block the synthesis of cholesterol
stool softeners or **fecal softeners** Draw water into the stool, thereby softening it
sympatholytics Interfere with the storage and release of norepinephrine
sympathomimetics Mimic the action of dopamine, norepinephrine, and epinephrine
thrombolytics A specific group of drugs (alteplase, anistreplase, streptokinase, urokinase) given to dissolve existing blood clots
thyroid hormone antagonists Used to counteract or block the action of excessive formation of thyroid hormones
thyroid hormones Used when thyroid hormones are not being produced or are not produced in sufficient quantities to meet the body's physiologic needs
tricyclic antidepressants Inhibit the reuptake of norepinephrine and serotonin (include doxepin, amitriptyline, and imipramine)
uricosuric agents Act on the tubules of the kidneys to enhance the excretion of uric acid
urinary analgesics Produce a local anesthetic effect on the mucosa of the ureters and bladder to relieve burning, pain, urgency, and frequency associated with urinary tract infections (UTIs)
urinary antimicrobials Substances excreted and concentrated in the urine in sufficient amounts to have an antiseptic effect on the urine and the urinary tract
uterine relaxants Used primarily to prevent preterm labor and delivery
uterine stimulants Increase the frequency or strength of uterine contractions
vaccines Suspensions of either live, attenuated, or killed bacteria or viruses administered to induce immunity against infection of specific bacteria or viruses
vasodilators Relax the arteriolar smooth muscle causing a dilation of the blood vessels

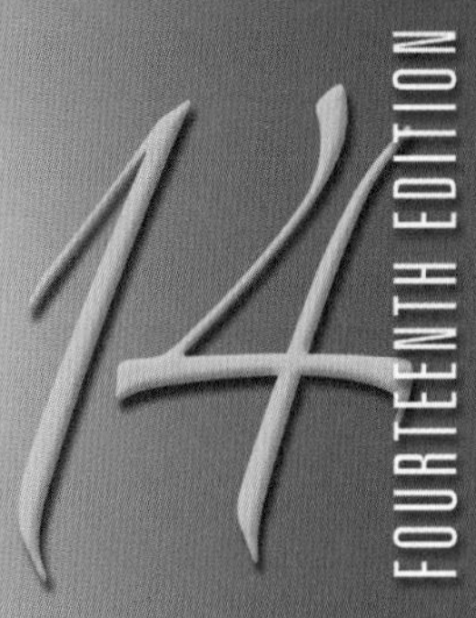

BASIC PHARMACOLOGY FOR NURSES

Bruce D. Clayton, BS, PharmD, RPh

Professor of Pharmacy Practice
College of Pharmacy & Health Sciences
Butler University
Indianapolis, Indiana

Yvonne N. Stock, MS, RN

Professor Emeritus, Nursing
Health Occupations Department
Iowa Western Community College
Council Bluffs, Iowa

Renae D. Harroun, MSN, RN

Assistant Professor
Trinity College of Nursing and Health Sciences
Rock Island, Illinois

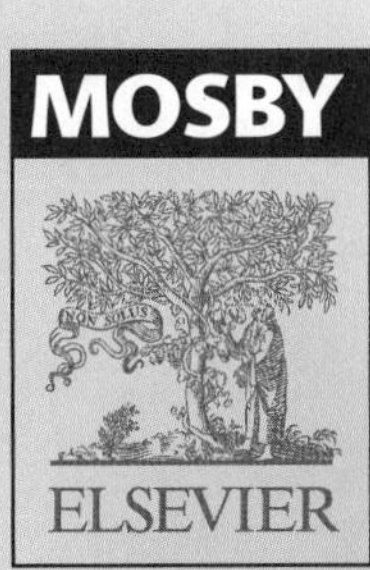

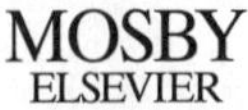

11830 Westline Industrial Drive
St. Louis, Missouri 63146

BASIC PHARMACOLOGY FOR NURSES

ISBN-13: 978-0-323-03559-0
ISBN-10: 0-323-03559-0

Notice

Knowledge and best practice in this field are constantly changing. As new research and experience broaden our knowledge, changes in practice, treatment and drug therapy may become necessary or appropriate. Readers are advised to check the most current information provided (i) on procedures featured or (ii) by the manufacturer of each product to be administered, to verify the recommended dose or formula, the method and duration of administration, and contraindications. It is the responsibility of the practitioner, relying on their own experience and knowledge of the patient, to make diagnoses, to determine dosages and the best treatment for each individual patient, and to take all appropriate safety precautions. To the fullest extent of the law, neither the Publisher nor the Authors assume any liability for any injury and/or damage to persons or property arising out or related to any use of the material contained in this book.

The Publisher

ISBN-13: 978-0-323-03559-0
ISBN-10: 0-323-03559-0

Acquisitions Editor: Lee Henderson
Senior Developmental Editor: Rae L. Robertson
Publishing Services Manager: Jeff Patterson
Senior Project Manager: Mary Stueck
Design Direction: Teresa McBryan

Printed in China
Last digit is the print number: 9 8 7 6 5 4 3 2 1

To ***Francine***
for her unfailing support and encouragement
and to
Sarah *and* ***Beth,***
the lights of our lives.

—BDC

To my family and close friends for
their continued encouragement
on a daily basis.

—YNS

To my husband ***Wade***
and our children ***Michael, Ashley, Levi,*** *and* ***Sarah***
Thank you for your support and always believing in me.
Also, a special thank you to my friend ***Sharon,***
who helped make this all possible.

—RDH

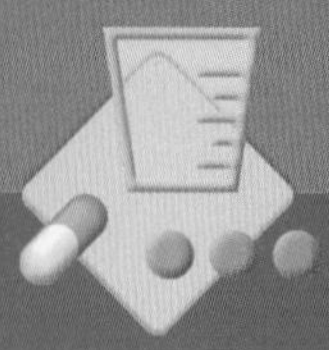

To the Instructor

The 50th anniversary, fourteenth edition of *Basic Pharmacology for Nurses*, in the tradition of the book's standards first established in 1957, advocates the administration of medication with safety and precision while focusing on health promotion through medication monitoring and patient education. In the practice setting, not only must the nurse demonstrate knowledge of the underlying disease process, but he or she must be able to perform an accurate assessment to identify individualized nursing diagnoses. The nurse must also plan and implement care in a manner that involves the patient as an active participant in decisions affecting care. Therefore, a primary concern throughout this book is the integration of patient teaching about drug therapy to enable the patient to reach therapeutic goals and attain an optimum level of health. The nurse must also validate patient understanding to ensure that the individual has the ability to provide safe self-care and monitoring of the prescribed treatment plan. User-friendly in content, structure, and layout, the text is concise and easy to read. With its emphasis on the Six Rights of Drug Administration *(right drug, right time, right dose, right patient, right route,* and *right documentation), Basic Pharmacology for Nurses* provides students with the information they will need to provide safe, effective nursing care for patients receiving drug therapy.

ORGANIZATION AND SPECIAL FEATURES

Table of Contents

Units One and Two teach nomenclature and legal considerations. They also guide the student toward appropriate nursing decisions based on monitoring of therapeutic and adverse drug effects. Unit One explores the *Foundations of Pharmacology, Principles of Drug Action and Drug Interactions, Drug Action Across the Life Span, The Nursing Process and Pharmacology,* and *Patient Education and Health Promotion.* Unit Two contains chapters on *Arithmetic Review* and the *Illustrated Atlas of Medication Administration.* The comprehensive arithmetic review (Chapter 6) includes fractions, percents, decimals, household measures, metric system, ratios and proportions, and calculation of drip rates. The unique *Illustrated Atlas of Medication Administration* in Unit Two provides extensive step-by-step illustrations that show primary routes of administration and proper administration techniques for all forms of medications. The atlas contains chapters on *Principles of Medication Administration; Percutaneous Administration; Enteral Administration; Parenteral Administration: Safe Preparation of Parenteral Medications; Parenteral Administration: Intradermal, Subcutaneous, and Intramuscular Routes;* and *Parenteral Administration: Intravenous Route.*

Units Three through Nine provide an overview of each drug class, followed by narrative discussions of the most common individual drugs. Units and chapters are organized by body system: Unit Three, *Drugs Affecting the Autonomic and Central Nervous Systems;* Unit Four, *Drugs Affecting the Cardiovascular System;* Unit Five, *Drugs Used to Treat Disorders of the Respiratory System;* Unit Six, *Drugs Affecting the Digestive System;* Unit Seven, *Drugs Affecting the Endocrine System;* Unit Eight, *Drugs Affecting the Reproductive System;* Unit Nine, *Drugs Affecting Other Body Systems.*

Chapter Organization

- Each drug chapter in Units Three through Nine begins with an **overview of the clinical problem** and its management.
- A **general application of the nursing process** for that problem follows, including clearly identified headings for *Assessment, Nursing Diagnosis, Planning, Implementation,* and *Evaluation.*
- This general nursing process section concludes with a **Patient Education and Health Promotion** section that helps the nurse to incorporate patient education and health promotion into the overall treatment plan.
- **Drug monographs** are provided for each major drug class. These monographs describe *Actions, Uses,* and *Therapeutic Outcomes* for each class.
- A **drug-class–specific nursing process section** is provided for each drug monograph, and these sections highlight *Side Effects to Expect, Side Effects to Report,* and *Drug Interactions.*

Special Features

Basic Pharmacology for Nurses includes special features designed to foster effective learning and comprehension.

- This edition incorporates Mosby/Elsevier's ***Content Threads*** design and learning elements. You are likely to be familiar with these shared features from other books in the curriculum (see also *Content Threads* overview):
  - Chapter-opening features include **Chapter Content** outlines, **Objectives,** and **Key Terms** lists.
  - **Clinical Landmine boxes** have been updated and expanded to highlight critically important

clinical considerations to help students practice safely and to reduce medication errors.
    - **Life Span Issues boxes** are positioned throughout the text and focus on the implications of drug therapy for children, pregnant and breastfeeding women, and older adults.
    - **Herbal Interactions boxes** highlight *well-documented* interactions among drugs, herbal therapies, and dietary supplements.
    - A handy bulleted list of **Key Points** at the end of most chapters facilitates review of essential chapter content.
- Reproducible **Patient Self-Assessment Forms** guide students to promote patient education by helping patients monitor their own drug therapy.

NEW TO THIS EDITION

- This edition includes the latest FDA approvals and withdrawals, including up-to-date clinical drug indications and **75 new drugs.**
- Unit Four (Chapters 21 to 29) has been revamped to more accurately reflect the clinical progression of cardiovascular disease. New diagrams illustrate pathogenesis and sites of action of drugs used to treat hypertension, dysrhythmias, and heart failure.
    - A **new chapter, Chapter 21, *Introduction to Cardiovascular Disease and Metabolic Syndrome,*** describes the emerging understanding of the role of type 2 diabetes mellitus, abdominal obesity, hypertriglyceridemia, low levels of high-density lipoproteins (HDLs), and hypertension in the development of cardiovascular disease.
    - Chapter 22, *Drugs Used to Treat Dyslipidemias,* incorporates **the latest National Cholesterol Education Program (NCEP) recommendations** on the recognition and treatment of dyslipidemias.
    - Chapter 23, *Drugs Used to Treat Hypertension,* incorporates **the latest (JNC 7) recommendations** for prevention, detection, evaluation, and treatment of hypertension.
    - Chapter 28, *Drugs Used to Treat Heart Failure,* includes the latest (2005) **American College of Cardiology/American Heart Association Guidelines** on the management of heart failure.
- Chapter 36, *Drugs Used to Treat Diabetes Mellitus,* has been extensively revised to include **new guidelines on exercise, diet, and medicines to treat types 1 and 2 diabetes mellitus.** A new diagram illustrates the locations of action of the variety of medicines used to treat type 2 diabetes. The new incretin-mimetic agent, amylinomimetic agent, and new dosage forms of insulin, including inhaled insulin, are described.
- **Chapter 47, *Nutrition,* has been extensively revised** to include a new discussion of *Dietary Guidelines for Americans, 2005;* Harvard University's *Healthy Eating Pyramid;* and Asian, Latin, Mediterranean, and vegetarian evidence-based food pyramids for healthy eating. The National Academy of Sciences 2005 guidelines for *Dietary Reference Intakes for Energy, Carbohydrate, Fiber, Fat, Fatty Acids, Cholesterol, Protein, and Amino Acids* are also discussed. The Estimated Energy Requirement (EER) with new equations for calculating energy requirements are included.
- **NANDA Taxonomy II (2005-2006) nursing diagnoses** have been incorporated throughout to help students apply the nursing process to drug therapy.
- A new **Medication Safety Review** section featuring **Critical Thinking Questions** (with answers provided in the Instructor's Electronic Resource), **Math Review Questions,** and **Content Review Questions** concludes most chapters. Answers to the Math and Content Review questions are printed inside the back cover. These sections serve as one more means of helping students to practice safely and reduce medication errors.
- An **updated, full-color design** now distinguishes, with improved clarity, the general nursing process sections from the drug-class–specific nursing process sections. It also provides special shading in tables that makes table rows easier to read than ever.
- **New illustrations,** most in full color, clarify difficult concepts and help to facilitate learning.

TEACHING AND LEARNING PACKAGE

For Students

- A media-rich **Companion CD-ROM** is included with every book. Helpful student-learning features include **15 new 3-D animations** that illustrate pharmacologic management of common conditions, an expanded searchable **Audio Glossary** with definitions and pronunciations, more fully **customizable *Patient Self-Assessment Forms*** provided as "completable" PDF documents, an expanded collection of **400 NCLEX-style *Review Questions,*** and 12 interactive ***Drug Dosage Calculators.*** The Companion CD also now houses all of the book's appendices.

- The **Study Guide** has been completely revamped for the fourteenth edition to provide additional learning resources that *complement* those in the textbook. The popular two-column question-and-answer ***Review Sheet*** has been retained, supplemented by a rich collection of ***Learning Activities. Practice Questions for the NCLEX Examination*** are included for each textbook chapter, with answers provided in the Instructor's Electronic Resource.
- An **Evolve website** provides free student resources, including a sign-up page for the quarterly *Elsevier ePharmacology Update* newsletter, a link to the FDA's "Catalog of FDA Approved Drug Products," and new WebLinks that supplement the textbook. The book's appendices are also available on the Evolve website.

For Instructors

- An **Instructor's Electronic Resource** (available on CD-ROM and online on Evolve) includes the following:
  - An updated **Instructor's Resource Manual** that has been thoroughly revised to include ***Teaching Strategies*** (strategies for the classroom, the clinical setting, and for incorporating technology), new ***Web Research Activities, Case Studies,*** and ***Quizzes*** for each chapter. The Instructor's Resource Manual also includes Answer Keys for the Study Guide.
  - A **Test Bank,** delivered in ExamView, that now provides an expanded collection of 850 multiple-choice and alternate-format NCLEX-style questions—750 revised and 100 new. Each question includes the *Correct Answer, Rationale, Step of the Nursing Process,* and *NCLEX Client Needs Category,* as well as corresponding text page numbers.
  - New printable **Drug Administration Checklists,** corresponding to the drug administration procedures provided in the text, that allow the instructor to ensure student mastery of these vital skills.
  - A new **Image Collection** that contains every reproducible image from the text. Images are suitable for incorporation into classroom lectures, PowerPoint presentations, or distance-learning applications.
  - A new collection of **PowerPoint Lecture Slides** specific to the text.
  - An updated **TEACH Lesson Plan Manual** that provides ready-to-use lesson plans that tie together all of the text and ancillary components provided for *Basic Pharmacology for Nurses.*

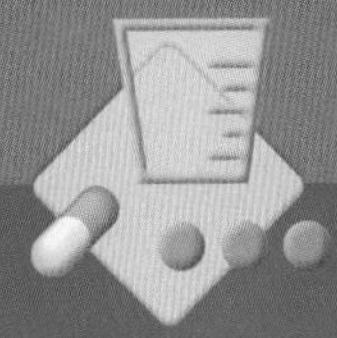

Acknowledgments

We would like to acknowledge the following reviewers:

Roy T. Dobson, PhD, MBA, BSc (Pharm), Saskatoon, Saskatchewan
Michael A. Vitale, Jr., PharmD, RPh, Philadelphia, Pennsylvania

Dr. Dobson reviewed and helped us to update the Canadian drug information in the fourteenth edition. Dr. Vitale reviewed every chapter to help us ensure content accuracy.

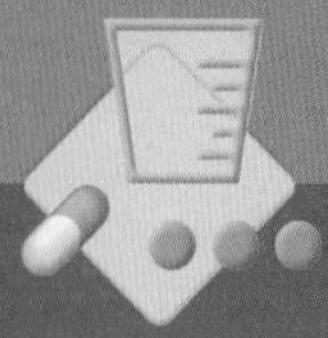

Content Threads

Basic Pharmacology for Nurses, fourteenth edition, shares some features and design elements with other Elsevier books that you may be using. The purpose of these *Content Threads* is to make it easier for students and instructors to use the variety of books required by a fast-paced and demanding curriculum.

The shared features in *Basic Pharmacology for Nurses,* fourteenth edition, include the following:

- Cover and internal **design similarities;** the colorful, student-friendly design encourages reading and learning of this core content.
- Numbered lists of **Objectives** that begin each chapter.
- **Key Terms** for selected terms at the beginning of each chapter; the key terms are in color when they are defined in the chapter.
- Bulleted lists of **Key Points** at the end of each chapter.
- **Critical Thinking Questions** in the chapter-ending Medication Safety Review feature.
- Multiple-choice **Content Review Questions** at the end of each chapter; answers inside the back cover for easy access.
- A complete **Bibliography** at the end of the book.

In addition to content and design threads, these textbooks benefit from the advice and input of the Elsevier Advisory Board.

Advisory Board

SHIRLEY ANDERSON, MSN
Kirkwood Community College
Cedar Rapids, Iowa

M. GIE ARCHER, MS, RN, C, WHCNP
Dean of Health Sciences
LVN Program Coordinator
North Central Texas College
Gainesville, Texas

MARY BROTHERS, MEd, RN
Coordinator, Garnet Career Center School of Practical Nursing
Charleston, West Virginia

PATRICIA A. CASTALDI, RN, BSN, MSN
Union County College
Plainfield, New Jersey

DOLORES ANN COTTON, RN, BSN, MS
Meridian Technology Center
Stillwater, Oklahoma

LORA LEE CRAWFORD, RN, BSN
Emanuel Turlock Vocational Nursing Program
Turlock, California

RUTH ANN ECKENSTEIN, RN, BS, MEd
Oklahoma Department of Career and Technology Education
Stillwater, Oklahoma

GAIL ANN HAMILTON FINNEY, RN, MSN
Nursing Education Specialist
Concorde Career Colleges, INC
Mission, Kansas

PAM HINCKLEY, RN, MSN
Redlands Adult School
Redlands, California

DEBORAH W. KELLER, RN, BSN, MSN
Erie Huron Ottawa Vocational Education School of Practical Nursing
Milan, Ohio

PATTY KNECHT, MSN, RN
Nursing Program Director
Center for Arts & Technology
Brandywine Campus
Coatesville, Pennsylvania

LT COL (RET) TERESA Y. McPHERSON, RN, BSN, MSN
Adjunct Instructor
St. Philip's College LVN/AND Nursing Program
San Antonio, Texas

FRANCES NEU SHULL, RN, MS, BSN
Miami Valley Career Technology Center
Clayton, Ohio

BEVERLEY TURNER, MA, RN
Director, Vocational Nursing Department
Maric College, San Diego Campus
San Diego, California

SISTER ANN WIESEN, RN, MRA
Erwin Technical Center
Tampa, Florida

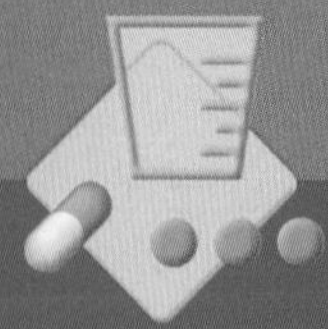

To the Student

Basic Pharmacology for Nurses focuses on health promotion through medication monitoring and patient education. Full-color art and new design features accompany detailed, understandable discussions of drugs organized by body system.

Reproducible **Patient Self-Assessment Forms** are a handy tool for patient teaching.

Chapters open with **Chapter Content Overviews, Objectives,** and **Key Terms.**

Step-by-step **full color art** showing proper medication administration techniques.

Chapters end with a handy bulleted list of **Key Points** for review of essential chapter content.

Herbal Interactions boxes describe possible side effects of alternative therapies.

Drug Tables that list generic name, brand name, availability, and dosage range.

Incorporates the most recent (2005-2006) NANDA-approved **nursing diagnoses** throughout.

Emphasizes **Patient Education and Health Promotion** in the overall treatment plan.

Medication Safety Review sections include **Math Review, Critical Thinking,** and **Content Review Questions** at the end of each chapter.

Life Span Issues boxes focus on implications of drug therapy for children, pregnant and nursing women, and older adults.

Comprehensive **Drug Class** discussions with clearly identified **Nursing Process** steps.

Clinical Landmines boxes highlight critically important clinical considerations.

STUDY GUIDE Includes a unique two-column question and answer *Review Sheet, Learning Activities,* and *Practice Questions for the NCLEX Examination* for each textbook chapter. Answers are available from your instructor.

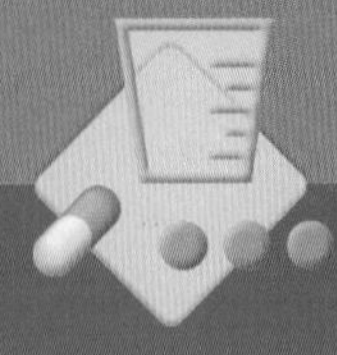

Contents

CHAPTER

1 Definitions, Names, Standards, and Information Sources

UNIT ONE FOUNDATIONS OF PHARMACOLOGY

evolve http://evolve.elsevier.com/Clayton

Chapter Content

DEFINITIONS

Objectives

1. State the origin and definition of pharmacology.
2. Explain the meaning of therapeutic methods.

Key Terms

pharmacology
therapeutic methods
drugs
medicines

Pharmacology

Pharmacology (Greek *pharmakon,* drugs, and *logos,* science) deals with the study of drugs and their actions on living organisms.

Therapeutic Methods

Diseases may be treated in several different ways. The approaches to therapy are called **therapeutic methods.** Most illnesses require a combination of therapeutic methods for successful treatment. Examples of therapeutic methods include the following:

- Drug therapy: treatment with drugs
- Diet therapy: treatment by diet, such as a low-salt diet for patients with cardiovascular disease
- Physiotherapy: treatment with natural physical forces such as water, light, and heat
- Psychological therapy: identification of stressors and methods to reduce or eliminate stress and/or the use of drugs

Drugs

Drugs (Dutch *droog,* meaning dry) are chemical substances that have an effect on living organisms. Therapeutic drugs, often called **medicines,** are those drugs used in the prevention or treatment of diseases. Up until a few decades ago, dried plants were the greatest source of medicines; thus the word *drug* was applied to them.

DRUG NAMES (UNITED STATES)

Objectives

1. Describe the process used to name drugs.
2. Differentiate among the chemical, generic, official, and brand names of medicines.

Key Terms

chemical name
generic name
official name
trademark
brand name
proprietary names
over-the-counter (OTC) drugs
illegal drugs

Many drugs have a variety of names. This may cause confusion to the patient, physician, and nurse, so care must be taken in obtaining the exact name and spelling of a particular drug. When administering the prescribed drug, the spelling on the drug package must correspond exactly to the spelling of the drug ordered to ensure that the proper medicine is administered.

Chemical Name

The **chemical name** is most meaningful to the chemist. By means of the chemical name, the chemist understands exactly the chemical constitution of the drug and the exact placing of its atoms or molecular groupings.

Generic Name (Nonproprietary Name)

Before a drug becomes official, it is given a **generic name,** or common name. A generic name is simpler than the chemical name. It may be used in any country and by any manufacturer. The first letter of the generic name is not capitalized. Students are strongly encouraged to learn and refer to drugs by their generic name because formularies are maintained by generic name. When a therapeutically equivalent drug is available in a generic form, a generic medicine is routinely substituted for the brand name medicine.

Generic names are provided by the United States Adopted Names (USAN) Council, which is an organization sponsored by the U.S. Pharmacopeial Convention, the American Medical Association, and the American Pharmaceutical Association.

Official Name

The **official name** is the name under which the drug is listed by the U.S. Food and Drug Administration (FDA). The FDA is empowered by federal law to name the drugs for human use in the United States.

Trademark (Brand Name)

A **trademark** or **brand name** or **proprietary name** is followed by the symbol ®. This indicates that the name is registered and that its use is restricted to the owner of the drug, who is usually the manufacturer. Most drug companies place their products on the market under trade names instead of official names. The trade names are deliberately made easier to pronounce, spell, and remember. The first letter of the trade name is capitalized.

EXAMPLE (Figure 1-1):
Chemical name: 4-Thia-1-azabicyclo[3.2.0]heptane-2-carboxylic acid, 6-[(aminophenylacetyl)amino]-3,3-dimethyl-7-oxo-, [2S-[2α,-5α,6β(S*)]]-
Generic name: ampicillin
Official name: ampicillin, USP
Brand names: Principen, Polycillin

Drug Classifications

Drugs may be classified according to which *body system* they affect (e.g., drugs affecting the central nervous system, drugs affecting the cardiovascular system, or drugs affecting the gastrointestinal system).

Drugs may be classified by their *therapeutic use* or *clinical indications* (e.g., antacids, antibiotics, antihypertensives, diuretics, or laxatives).

Drugs may be classified using the *physiologic* or *chemical action* (e.g., anticholinergics, beta adrenergic blockers, calcium channel blockers, and cholinergics).

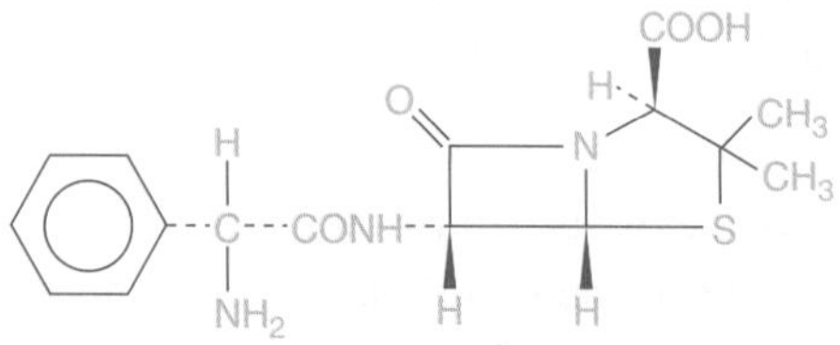

FIGURE 1-1 Ampicillin, an antibiotic.

Drugs may be further classified as *prescription* or *nonprescription*, also known as **over-the-counter (OTC) drugs.** Prescription drugs require an order by a health professional who is licensed to prescribe, such as a physician, nurse practitioner, physician assistant, pharmacist, or dentist. The manufacturer's label will identify prescription medicines with the phrases: "Rx only" or "Caution: Federal Law Prohibits Dispensing Without a Prescription." Nonprescription, or OTC, drugs are sold without a prescription in a pharmacy or the health section of department or grocery stores.

Illegal drugs, sometimes referred to as *recreational drugs,* are drugs or chemical substances used for nontherapeutic purposes. These substances are obtained illegally or have not received approval for use by the FDA. See Chapter 49 for further information on substance abuse.

DRUG NAMES (CANADA)

Objective

1. Differentiate between the *official drug* and the *proper name* of a medicine.

Key Term

Food and Drug Regulations

Official Drug

The term *official drug* pertains to any drug for which a standard is described either specifically in the **Food and Drug Regulations** or in any publication named in the Food and Drugs Act as satisfactory for officially describing the standards for drugs in Canada. The chemical and generic names of medicines are the same in both Canada and the United States, but there are some dissimilarities in brand names.

Proper Name

The *proper name* is the nonproprietary (generic) name used to describe an official drug in Canada.

SOURCES OF DRUG STANDARDS (UNITED STATES)

Objective

1. List official sources of American drug standards.

Key Term

The *United States Pharmacopeia (USP)/National Formulary (NF)*

Standardization is needed to ensure that drug products made by different manufacturers, or in different batches by the same manufacturer, will be uniformly pure and potent. The United States Pharmacopeial Convention, Inc. is a non-government organization that promotes the public health by establishing state-of-the-art standards to ensure the quality of medicines and other health care technologies. These standards are developed by a unique process of public involvement and are accepted worldwide. The United States Pharmacopeial Convention, Inc. operates as a nonprofit organization that achieves its goals through the contributions of volunteers representing pharmacy, medicine, and other health care professions, as well as science, academia, the U.S. government, the pharmaceutical industry, and consumer organizations. The organization's Internet address is www.usp.org.

The *United States Pharmacopeia (USP)/National Formulary (NF)*

Before 1820, many drugs were manufactured in different parts of the United States and had varying degrees of purity. This problem was solved by the establishment of two authoritative, science-based books, *United States Pharmacopeia* and *National Formulary,* which set forth required standards of purity for drugs, as well as laboratory tests to determine purity. The texts are now published as a single volume *(The United States Pharmacopeia [USP]/ National Formulary [NF])* by the United States Pharmacopeial Convention and are revised annually. Supplements are published semiannually to keep the reference current. The *USP* contains 4000 monographs and 180 General Tests and Assays for drug substances and products. It also contains monographs and general chapters pertaining specifically to nutritional supplements. The *NF* contains more than 380 monographs for excipients (inert substances used as a filler in phamaceutical manufacturing) and dietary supplements.

The primary purpose of this volume is to provide standards for identity, quality, strength, and purity of substances used in the practice of health care. The standards set forth in the *USP/NF* are enforced by the FDA as the official standards for the manufacture and quality control of medicines and nutritional supplements produced in the United States.

USP Dictionary of USAN and International Drug Names

The *USP Dictionary of USAN and International Drug Names*, published annually, is a compilation of more than 10,000 drug names. Each drug monograph contains the United States Adopted Name (USAN), a pronunciation guide, the molecular and graphic formula, chemical and brand names, manufacturer, and therapeutic category. It also contains the Chemical Abstracts Service registry numbers for drugs.

Manufacturers submit to the USAN Council a proposal for a name, in which they announce that a certain chemical compound has therapeutic potential and that they plan to investigate its use in humans. The council studies the chemical name, applies a series of nomenclature guidelines, and then selects the USAN (generic name). It is now customary for the FDA to accept the adopted generic name as the FDA official name for a chemical compound.

SOURCES OF DRUG STANDARDS (CANADA)

Objective

1. List official sources of Canadian drug standards.

Key Terms

The United States Pharmacopeia (USP)/National Formulary (NF)
European Pharmacopoeia

The Food and Drugs Act recognizes the standards described by international authoritative books to be acceptable as official drugs in Canada. The acceptable publications are *The United States Pharmacopeia (USP)/ National Formulary (NF), European Pharmacopoeia,* the *International Pharmacopoeia,* the *British Pharmacopoeia,* the *British Pharmaceutical Codex,* and the *Canadian Formulary.*

SOURCES OF DRUG INFORMATION (UNITED STATES)

Objectives

1. List and describe literature resources for researching prescription and nonprescription medications.
2. List and describe literature resources for researching drug interactions and drug incompatibilities.

Key Terms

American Drug Index
American Hospital Formulary Service, Drug Information
Drug Interaction Facts
Drug Facts and Comparisons
Handbook on Injectable Drugs
Handbook of Nonprescription Drugs
Martindale—The Complete Drug Reference
Natural Medicines Comprehensive Database
Physicians' Desk Reference (PDR)

American Drug Index

The *American Drug Index* is edited annually by Norman F. Billups, and is published by Facts and Comparisons. It is an index of all medicines available in the United States.

Drugs in the *Index* are listed alphabetically by generic name and brand name. The generic name monographs indicate that the drug is recognized in the *United States Pharmacopeia/National Formulary* or USAN Council listing and they provide the chemical name, phonetic pronunciation, use, and cross-references to brand names. Each brand name monograph lists the manufacturer, composition, strength, pharmaceutical forms available, package size, dosage, and use. Other features of this reference book include a list of common medical abbreviations; tables of weights, measures, and conversion factors; normal laboratory values; a list of drug names that look and sound alike; oral dosage forms that should not be crushed or chewed; FDA pregnancy categories; a glossary to aid in interpretation of the monographs; a labeler code index to identify drug products; and a list of manufacturers' addresses. The book is useful for quickly comparing brand names and generic names, and also for checking the availability of strengths and dosage forms.

American Hospital Formulary Service

The *American Hospital Formulary Service, Drug Information,* is a comprehensive reference book published annually by the American Society of Health-System Pharmacists in Bethesda, Maryland. This volume contains monographs on virtually every single-drug entity available in the United States. The monographs emphasize rational therapeutic use of drugs, including approved and unapproved uses. Each monograph is subdivided into sections on uses and drug dosage and administration, followed by cautionary information on adverse effects, precautions, contraindications, drug interactions, and acute and chronic toxicity. Less frequently used sections on pharmacology, pharmacokinetics, and chemistry and stability are at the end of the monographs. The index is cross-referenced by both generic and brand names. Supplements and updated cautionary information are available online throughout the year at www.ahfsdruginformation.com. The *American Hospital Formulary Service, Drug Information* is available as a printed text, on a networkable CD-ROM, and as an electronic version that can be downloaded into a personal digital assistant (PDA).

The *American Hospital Formulary Service, Drug Information,* has been adopted as an official reference by the U.S. Public Health Service and the Department of Veterans Affairs. It has also been approved for use by the American Health Care Association, the American Hospital Association, the Catholic Health Care Association of the United States, the National Association of Boards of Pharmacy, and the American Pharmaceutical Association. It is recognized by the U.S. Congress, the Centers for Medicare and Medicaid Services (formerly the Health Care Financing Administration), and various third-party health care insurance providers, and is included as a required or recommended standard reference in pharmacies in many states.

Drug Interaction Facts

Drug Interaction Facts is published by Facts and Comparisons. This three-ring, loose-leaf, nearly 800-page binder was first published in 1983 and is currently the most comprehensive book available on the subject of drug interactions. The format is somewhat different from that of most other books; the index is in the front, and the book is not subdivided into chapters, but grouped every 100 pages by a plastic tab sheet. Each page is a single monograph describing a drug interaction. Each monograph consists of a table that lists the onset and severity of the drug interaction, a statement on the expected effects, the proposed mechanism, and how to manage the interaction. A short discussion (with references) on the relevance of the interaction follows.

One of the most meaningful, although not obvious, benefits is the source of information used to develop *Drug Interaction Facts.* All of the information is reviewed by an internationally renowned group of physicians and pharmacists who have the clinical experience, scientific background, library, and computer resources to collect, collate, review, and evaluate the scientific accuracy of descriptions of drug interactions from world literature. Thus the book is an extremely reliable source of information. Subscribers receive a quarterly update supplement.

Drug Facts and Comparisons

Drug Facts and Comparisons is a large looseleaf compendium of more than 2000 pages published by Facts and Comparisons. The book is divided into 15 chapters, arranged by organ system. At the beginning of each chapter is a detailed table of contents. All drugs within each chapter are grouped by therapeutic classes. For each therapeutic class of drug, a monograph provides a brief description of indications for use, administration and dosage, actions, contraindications, warnings, precautions, drug interactions, adverse reactions, overdose, and patient information. The database for the monographs is the most current FDA-approved package insert and publications from official groups such as the Centers for Disease Control and Prevention (CDC) and the National Academy of Sciences. The editors have reformatted the material and included information from the medical literature on investigational uses of the drugs.

At the beginning of each monograph are tables of all drugs in that therapeutic class. The tables are particularly valuable because they are designed to allow comparison of similar products, brand names, manufacturers, cost indexes, and available dosage forms.

The index, located in the front of the book for easy access, is quite comprehensive and is updated both monthly and quarterly. Within each chapter is an excellent cross-referencing system that makes it easy to gain information on drugs that may be categorized by more than one therapeutic class. Updated supplements for the entire book are published monthly. *Drug Facts and Comparisons* is also available on CD-ROM and is updated monthly.

Handbook on Injectable Drugs

The *Handbook on Injectable Drugs,* the most comprehensive reference available on the topic of compatibility of injectable drugs, is written by Lawrence A. Trissel and published by the American Society of Health-System Pharmacists of Bethesda, Maryland. It is a collection of monographs on more than 300 injectable drugs that are listed alphabetically by generic name. Each well-referenced monograph is subdivided into sections on availability of concentrations, dosage and rate of administration, stability, pH, compatibility information, and other useful information about administration of the drug. Each of the drugs is cross-referenced with the American Hospital Formulary Service Drug Information category number for further information.

Handbook of Nonprescription Drugs

The *Handbook of Nonprescription Drugs* is prepared and published by the American Pharmaceutical Association in Washington, D.C. It is the most comprehensive text available on OTC medications that can be purchased in the United States.

The book is subdivided into units organized by body systems. Most chapters within the units begin with a discussion of the epidemiologic, etiologic, and pathophysiologic characteristics and the clinical manifestations of the disorder. This is followed by comprehensive discussions of nonprescription products, nondrug therapies, and preventive therapies. Methods for assessing the illness, such as detailed questions to ask the patient, follow the treatment section. The chapters conclude with a summary of counseling information to be imparted to the patient and an explanation of how to evaluate the therapeutic outcomes. This book has three particular advantages for the health professional: (1) a list of questions to ask the patient to determine whether treatment should be recommended, (2) product selection guidelines for determining the most appropriate products, and (3) instructions to the patient on proper use of the recommended product.

Martindale—The Complete Drug Reference

Martindale—The Complete Drug Reference is a 2700-page volume published by the Pharmaceutical Press, the publication division of the Royal Pharmaceutical Society of Great Britain. It is published every 3 years; however, the electronic versions are updated more frequently (www.pharmpress.com). It is one of the most comprehensive texts available for information on drugs in current use throughout the world. Part 1 contains extensive referenced monographs on the pharmacologic activity and side effects of more than 4418 medicinal agents. The drug monographs have been arranged in 51 chapters that bring together monographs on drugs and groups of drugs that have similar actions or uses. The chapter introductions describe diseases with reviews of the treatment options. Part 2 contains alphabetically listed short monographs on another 926 agents that are no longer considered standards of treatment or are too new for inclusion in Part 1. Many herbal medicines are described in this section. Part 3 gives the composition and manufacturers of almost 50,000 preparations or groups of preparations from 33 countries, including those in the United States of America, United Kingdom, Europe, Australia, South Africa, and Japan. The listings include the proprietary name, manufacturer, the active ingredients with cross-references to the drug monographs, and a summary of indications.

The index contains more than 130,000 entries. Medicinal agents are indexed by official names, chemical names, synonyms, and proprietary names.

Natural Medicines Comprehensive Database

The *Natural Medicines Comprehensive Database* is published by Therapeutic Research Faculty of Stockton, California. In the past few years, the *Natural Medicines Comprehensive Database* has become the scientific gold standard for evidence-based information on herbal medicines and combination products of herbal medicines. The text is subdivided into five major sections: herbal monographs, references, a brand name listing, charts section, and a general index. The monograph section uses a standardized, referenced format to discuss more than 1000 herbal medicines. The monographs are arranged alphabetically by most common name. Sections within each monograph include additional common names, scientific names, uses of the herbal medicine, safety, effectiveness, mechanism of action and active ingredients, adverse reactions, interactions, dosage, and administration. The safety and effectiveness sections are particularly valuable because of the scientific studies used to support safety and efficacy ratings. Every monograph includes a safety rating for use in pregnancy and lactation, and for pediatric safety if use in children is a concern. More than 8300 references are cited in the reference index. The brand names list contains several thousand brand name products, citing the manufacturer and all of the ingredients in the combination product. The charts section provides tables on use of herbal medicines in specific diseases, potential drug interactions, and drugs that may cause nutritional deficiencies. The general index is comprehensive; it cross-references the scientific name, common names, and botanical names of every listing in the monograph section. The general index does not include brand names because they are listed in the monograph and the brand name listing. *The Natural Medicines Comprehensive Database* is also available as an Internet subscription that is updated daily, at www.NaturalDatabase.com.

Physicians' Desk Reference (PDR)

The *Physicians' Desk Reference (PDR)* is published annually by Medical Economics, Inc., of Montvale, New Jersey. It discusses more than 4000 therapeutic agents. The book is divided into seven color-coded sections for easier access.

Section 1 (White): Manufacturers' Index

Section 1 is an alphabetic listing of each manufacturer whose products are listed in the *PDR,* their addresses, emergency phone numbers, and a partial list of available products.

Section 2 (Pink): Brand and Generic Name Index

Section 2 is a comprehensive alphabetic listing of the generic and brand name products discussed in the Product Information section of the book.

Section 3 (Blue): Product Category Index

In section 3, products are subdivided by therapeutic classes, such as analgesics, laxatives, oxytocics, and antibiotics. Following section 3 are white pages containing the definitions of controlled substances categories, the U.S. Food and Drug Administation telephone directory, poison control centers arranged alphabetically by state and city, and a Vaccine Adverse Event Reporting form.

Section 4 (Gray): Product Identification Guide

In section 4, manufacturers have provided actual-size color pictures of their tablets and capsules. These are invaluable aids in product identification.

Section 5 (White): Product Information Section

Section 5 contains reprints of the package inserts for the major products of manufacturers, with information on action, uses, administration, dosages, contraindications, composition, and how each drug is supplied.

Section 6 (White): Diagnostic Product Information

In the 2006 *PDR,* section 6 contains alphabetically arranged monographs on two diagnostic products.

The last (unlabeled) section of the book contains lists of drug information centers organized by states; Use-in-Pregnancy ratings with drugs in each category; the Drug Enforcement Administration (DEA) office directory; state aids drug-assistance programs; patient assistance programs offered by manufacturers; drugs that should not be crushed; dosing instructions in Spanish; and drugs excreted in breast milk. The last page of the book is a tear-out form for the MedWatch program, a voluntary reporting of adverse effects of drugs by health professionals (see Appendix F).

The *Physicians' Desk Reference* and other resources are also available as part of the *PDR Electronic Library* on CD-ROM. This provides a complete database of *PDR* prescribing information that is electronically searchable for quick retrieval.

Package Inserts

Before a new drug is marketed, the manufacturer develops a comprehensive but concise description of the drug, indications and precautions for clinical use, recommendations for dosage, known adverse reactions, contraindications, and other pharmacologic information relating to the drug. Federal law requires that this material be approved by the FDA before the product is released for marketing and that it be presented on an insert that accompanies each package of the product.

The Food and Drug Administration recently proposed a new format for package inserts in an effort to help reduce medical errors. The proposed new labeling is expected to reduce practitioners' time looking for information, decrease the number of preventable medical errors, and improve treatment effectiveness. Because these labeling revisions represent considerable effort and are most critical for newer and less familiar drugs, the proposal will apply only to relatively new prescription drug products. A new website sponsored by the National Library of Medicine will also provide a database for new package inserts that is searchable by product name, indications, dosage and administration, warnings, description of drug product, active and inactive ingredients, and how the drug is supplied. See the section below that discusses electronic databases.

Nursing Journals

Many specialty journals have articles on drug therapy relating to a specific field of interest (e.g., *Geriatric Nursing, Heart and Lung*). Nursing journals such as *RN, American Journal of Nursing (AJN),* and others provide drug update information as well as articles that discuss nursing considerations relating to the drug therapy and drugs.

The nurse must keep in mind the purpose of using resources and must be mindful of the accuracy of the information contained. Nurses should check the dates on articles to validate the currency of the information. Reliable sources to validate drug information are listed in the section, Sources of Drug Information (United States).

Electronic Databases

With exponential growth of information about medicines and health, it is almost impossible to make the information available without the use of electronic databases. The National Library of Medicine (NLM) provides Medline and other searchable databases (www.nlm.nih.gov) on the Internet at no cost. Most of the drug information sources listed above are available through electronic retrieval at libraries. Many college libraries subscribe via CD-ROM to CINHAL, a cumulative index of nursing and allied health literature. These sources give nurses access to a wealth of information from sources published in the United States and other countries.

A new website becoming available to health care providers and the public with a standard, comprehensive up-to-date look-up and download resource about medicines is DailyMed. The DailyMed system (http://dailymed.nlm.nih.gov) was developed in collaboration with federal agencies including the FDA, the National Library of Medicine (NLM), Agency for Healthcare Research and Quality (AHRQ), and the National Cancer Institute (NCI) in the Department of Health and Human Services, and the Department of Veteran Affairs (VA) to provide high quality information about marketed drugs. This information includes FDA-approved package inserts. Over time, DailyMed will also include information for biologics such as vaccines, medical devices, veterinary drugs, and some food products.

SOURCES OF DRUG INFORMATION (CANADA)

Objectives

1. Describe the organization of the *Compendium of Pharmaceuticals and Specialties* and the information contained in each colored section.
2. Describe the organization of the *Canadian Self-Medication.*

Key Terms

Compendium of Pharmaceuticals and Specialties (CPS)
Patient Self-Care: Helping Patients Make Therapeutic Choices
Compendium of Self-Care Products (CSCP)

Compendium of Pharmaceuticals and Specialties

The *Compendium of Pharmaceuticals and Specialties (CPS)* is published annually by the Canadian Pharmacists Association. It provides a comprehensive list of the pharmaceutical products distributed in Canada as well as other information of practical value to health care professionals. Manufacturers voluntarily submit information concerning their products for this text. The book is divided into sections.

Introductory Section

This untitled section contains a range of information including a glossary of abbreviated terms, a glossary of abbreviated Latin prescription terms, microorganism abbreviations, editors' message, how to use the *CPS*, editorial policy, erratum policy, and discontinued products.

Green Section: Brand and Generic Name Index

The green section is an alphabetic cross-reference that lists drugs by both generic and brand names; it also indicates whether the product was available in Canada at the time of publication. Brand names that are in boldface type have a product monograph in the *CPS* white section.

Pink Section: Therapeutic Guide

The Therapeutic Guide is a clinical guide for the use of single-entity drugs listed in the *CPS*. Most products listed are single entity, but there are some combination products (e.g., oral contraceptives, antacids). The guide uses the Canadian version of the World Health Organization's *Anatomical Therapeutic Chemical Classification.* Drugs are classified under 16 anatomical groups (e.g., gastrointestinal tract) and then grouped into therapeutic categories (e.g., antacids, antiemetics, digestive enzymes, laxatives). Drugs are then further subclassified under specific therapeutic, pharmacologic, or chemical subheadings within the therapeutic category (e.g., antacids—aluminum containing, calcium containing). Medicines may be classified under more than one section if used for more than one indication. Once a generic name has been identified, the corresponding brand name can be found in the Brand and Generic Name Index (green section).

Photograph Section: Product Identification

The photograph section contains color photographs of drug products arranged according to the size and color shadings of individual dosage forms (tablets, capsules, liquids). Products are cross-referenced to the monographs (white section). This section is also printed in French.

Yellow Section: Dirctory

I. Poison Control Centres: names and addresses
II. Health Organizations: addresses, phone numbers, websites
III. Manufacturers' Index: names, addresses, and telephone numbers of the manufacturers and distributors of pharmaceutical products in Canada, as well as product listings for many of the manufacturers

Lilac Section: Clin-Info

The lilac section contains tables and charts describing a wide range of information of interest to health care professionals that would otherwise rarely be easily accessible, particularly in a single reference book. Topics include the nonmedicinal ingredients of selected pharmaceuticals (e.g., sulfite, gluten, alcohol, tartrazine content), Systѐme International unit conversion factors, drugs and sports competition, clinical monitoring (e.g., anticoagulant drug monitoring, body surface area nomograms, serum drug concentration monitoring), clinical information on cardiac arrest, travel (e.g., drinking water purification, immunization schedules, malaria prevention and treatment), drug interactions, dietary recommendations, poison control centers in Canada and a summary of Canadian regulations for narcotics and controlled drugs, and the procedure to obtain on an emergency basis a drug not approved for use in Canada.

White Section: Monographs of Pharmaceuticals and Specialties

The white section contains an alphabetic arrangement of manufacturers' brand information and numerous general monographs for common multisource drugs; a few medical devices are described.

Two sections previously published in the book have been removed and placed on websites. "Product News" is published in e-CPS, available at www.e-cps.ca. It contains information on new and revised product monographs submitted by the pharmaceutical manufacturers. Entries include new products, updates about approval of new indications, and the availability of new dosage forms. "Information for the Patient" is now available at www.pharmacists.ca under "Healthcare Professionals, CPS Updates." This site lists the information to be conveyed to patients on more than 400 individual products. The information is arranged alphabetically by brand name.

Appendices

This section provides examples of Health Canada drug regulatory and monitoring programs' reporting and request forms. Forms include narcotic, controlled drugs, benzodiazepines and other targeted substances; special access program; vaccine-associated adverse events: surveillance and reporting; report of a vaccine-associated adverse event; adverse drug reactions: surveillance and reporting; and report of suspected adverse reaction due to drug products marketed in Canada (vaccines excluded).

Patient Self-Care: Helping Patients Make Therapeutic Choices

Patient Self-Care: Helping Patients Make Therapeutic Choices, formerly known as *Nonprescription Drug Reference for Health Professionals,* is published approximately every 4 years by the Canadian Pharmacists Association. The text provides comprehensive information for health professionals and consumers about the nonprescription drug products available in Canada. The chapters are organized by organ systems and then subdivided by disease states (e.g., the chapter on musculoskeletal conditions is subdivided into units on osteoporosis, low back pain, osteoarthritis, and sports injuries). Each chapter provides a review of anatomy and pathophysiology and the conditions suitable for self-medication as well as a section on assessment of patients with specific conditions, followed by a treatment algorithm. Treatment measures include both nonpharmacologic and pharmacologic management suggestions and a review of the nonprescription drug alternatives available. All chapters conclude with patient information on separate pages. Health care providers are encouraged to photocopy the patient information for their clients.

Compendium of Self-Care Products

The *Compendium of Self-Care Products (CSCP)* is a nonprescription companion of *CPS* and *Patient Self-Care.* It offers quick-glance, comparative tables on thousands of products and monographs on hundreds of commonly used nonprescription products. *CSCP* is composed of two major sections: product tables and product information. The product tables represent a comprehensive listing of nonprescription products available in Canada. The product tables are designed to be used for quick reference in the practice setting. Tables are arranged by therapeutic class and list the brand name alphabetically, the ingredients, and the dosage forms available. Those products highlighted in bold and identified by an asterisk are cross-referenced with additional information in the product information section.

The product information section contains monographs listed alphabetically by product brand names. The monographs are developed by the Canadian Pharmacists Association editorial staff and are reviewed by the manufacturers. The monographs may contain information somewhat different from the Health Canada–approved product monographs. The monographs follow a standard format of pharmacology: indications, contraindications, warnings, precautions, drug interactions, adverse effects, dosage, and dosage forms available on the market.

Between the two major sections are approximately 24 blue pages titled "Information for the Patient." The information is abbreviated from the corresponding chapters in the *Patient Self-Care: Helping Patients Make Therapeutic Choices.* These summaries provide brief overviews of the condition and the patient information that should be provided to the patients on the treatment of the condition. The patient information pages may be reprinted to send copies home with patients.

The compendium concludes with a manufacturers' index, printed on yellow paper, that includes names, addresses, phone and fax numbers, and products listed.

The book index, printed on green paper, provides an alphabetical cross-listing of all generic and brand names.

SOURCES OF PATIENT INFORMATION

Objective

1. Cite a literature resource for reviewing information to be given to the patient concerning a prescribed medication.

Key Terms

United States Pharmacopeia Dispensing Information (USPDI)
Therapeutic Choices

Over the past two decades it has become evident that health care providers must do a better job of helping patients assume responsibility for their own health care. The following material is an excellent source of information for teaching patients how to use their medications properly.

United States Pharmacopeia Dispensing Information

United States Pharmacopeia Dispensing Information (USPDI) is an annual publication of the United States Pharmacopeial Convention, Inc. *USPDI* is a three-volume set supplemented with bimonthly updates.

The first volume, *Drug Information for the Health Care Professional,* includes dispensing information arranged in alphabetically ordered monographs. Each monograph is subdivided into sections on the drug's use, mechanism of action, precautions, side effects, patient consultation information, general dosing information, and dosage forms available.

The second volume, *Advice for the Patient,* provides in nontechnical language the patient consultation guidelines found in the first volume. The second volume is designed to be used at the discretion of the health care provider as an aid to counseling the patient if written information is to be given to the patient. The publisher permits all health care providers to reproduce the pages of advice for their patients receiving the prescribed drug. Generic and brand names are cross-referenced in the index of *Advice for the Patient.*

The third volume, *Approved Drug Products and Legal Requirements,* is a reference source that provides a list of all drugs approved by the FDA that are proven to be safe and effective. It also lists which products are considered therapeutically equivalent when a drug is made by more than one manufacturer. This allows the prescriber and pharmacist to select the least expensive product, because it is therapeutically equivalent to the original product. Most insurance companies and state offices of health care only reimburse at the lowest cost for therapeutically equivalent medicines, so it is extremely important to have a resource for easy access to check therapeutic equivalence of medicines.

Therapeutic Choices

Therapeutic Choices (fourth edition), published by the Canadian Pharmacists Association, is a 1200-page handbook describing major diseases and their treatment. The discussions of medical conditions are very brief, but the text focuses on goals of therapy, management algorithms, and discussion of nonpharmacologic and pharmacologic therapy. Many of the chapters end with a pharmacoeconomic discussion of the different treatment options.

DRUG LEGISLATION (UNITED STATES)

Objectives

1. List legislative acts controlling drug use and abuse.
2. Differentiate among Schedule I, II, III, IV, and V medications, and describe nursing responsibilities associated with the administration of each type.

Key Terms

Federal Food, Drug, and Cosmetic Act
Controlled Substances Act
schedules

Drug legislation protects the consumer and the patient. The need for such protection is great because manufacturers and advertisers may make unfounded claims about the benefits of their products.

Federal Food, Drug, and Cosmetic Act, June 25, 1938 (Amended 1952, 1962)

The **Federal Food, Drug, and Cosmetic Act** of 1938 authorizes the FDA of the Department of Health and Human Services (HHS) to determine the safety of drugs before marketing and to ensure that certain labeling specifications and standards in advertising are met in the marketing of products. Manufacturers are required to submit new drug applications to the FDA for review of safety studies before products can be released for sale.

The Durham-Humphrey Amendment in 1952 tightened control by restricting the refilling of prescriptions.

The Kefauver-Harris Drug Amendment in 1962 was brought about by the thalidomide tragedy. Thalidomide was an incompletely tested drug approved for use as a sedative-hypnotic during pregnancy. Fetuses exposed to thalidomide were born with serious birth defects. This amendment provides greater control and surveillance of the distribution and clinical testing of investigational drugs and requires that a product be proven both safe and effective before release for sale.

Controlled Substances Act, 1970

The Comprehensive Drug Abuse Prevention and Control Act was passed by Congress in 1970. This statute, commonly referred to as the **Controlled Substances Act,** repealed almost 50 other laws written since 1914 that relate to the control of drugs. The new composite law is designed to improve the administration and regulation of manufacturing, distributing, and dispensing of drugs that have been found necessary to be controlled.

The Drug Enforcement Administration (DEA) was organized to enforce the Controlled Substances Act, gather intelligence, and train and conduct research in the area of dangerous drugs and drug abuse. The DEA is a bureau of the Department of Justice. The director of the DEA reports to the Attorney General of the United States.

The basic structure of the Controlled Substances Act consists of five classifications or **schedules** of controlled substances. The degree of control, the conditions of record-keeping, the particular order forms required, and other regulations depend on these classifications. The five schedules, their criteria, and examples of drugs in each schedule are listed below.

Schedule I Ⓒ Drugs

1. A high potential for abuse
2. No currently accepted medical use in the United States
3. A lack of accepted safety for use under medical supervision

EXAMPLES:
lysergic acid diethylamide (LSD), marijuana, peyote, STP, heroin, hashish

Schedule II Ⓒ Drugs

1. A high potential for abuse
2. A currently accepted medical use in the United States
3. An abuse potential that may lead to severe psychological or physical dependence

EXAMPLES:
secobarbital, pentobarbital, amphetamines, morphine, meperidine, methadone, Percodan, methylphenidate

Schedule III Ⓒ Drugs

1. A high potential for abuse, but less so than drugs in Schedules I and II
2. A currently accepted medical use in the United States
3. An abuse potential that may lead to moderate or low physical dependence or high psychological dependence

EXAMPLES:
Empirin with codeine, Lortab, Fiorinal, Tylenol with codeine

Schedule IV Ⓒ Drugs

1. A low potential for abuse, compared with those in Schedule III
2. A currently accepted medical use in the United States
3. An abuse potential that may lead to limited physical or psychological dependence, compared with drugs in Schedule III

EXAMPLES:
phenobarbital, propoxyphene, chloral hydrate, paraldehyde, chlordiazepoxide, diazepam, flurazepam, temazepam

Schedule V Ⓒ Drugs

1. A low potential for abuse, compared with those in Schedule IV
2. A currently accepted medical use in the United States
3. An abuse potential of limited physical or psychological dependence liability, compared with drugs in Schedule IV. Because abuse potential is low, a prescription may not be required.

EXAMPLES:
Lomotil, Robitussin A-C

The U.S. Attorney General, after public hearings, has authority to reschedule a drug, bring an unscheduled drug under control, or remove controls on scheduled drugs.

Every manufacturer, physician, nurse practitioner, physician assistant, dentist, pharmacy, and hospital that manufactures, prescribes, or dispenses any of the drugs listed in the five schedules must register biannually with the DEA.

A health care provider's prescription for substances named in this law must contain the health care provider's name, address, DEA registration number, and signature; the patient's name and address; and the date of issue. The pharmacist cannot refill such prescriptions without the approval of the health care provider.

All controlled substances for ward stock must be ordered on special hospital forms used to help maintain inventory and dispersion control records of the scheduled drugs. When a nurse administers a Schedule II drug under a health care provider's order, the following information must be entered on the controlled substances record: name of the patient, date of administration, drug administered, and drug dosage.

Possession of Controlled Substances

Federal and state laws make the possession of controlled substances a crime, except in specifically exempted cases. The law makes no distinction between professional and practical nurses in regard to possession of controlled drugs. Nurses may give controlled substances only under the direction of a physician or dentist who has been licensed to prescribe or dispense these agents. Nurses may not have controlled substances in their possession unless (1) they are giving them to a patient under a doctor's order, (2) the nurse is a patient for whom a doctor has prescribed schedule drugs, or (3) the nurse is the official custodian of a limited supply of controlled substances on a ward or department of the hospital. Controlled substances ordered but not used for patients must be returned to the source from which they were obtained (doctor or pharmacy). Violation or failure to comply with the Controlled Substances Act is punishable by fine, imprisonment, or both.

DRUG LEGISLATION (CANADA)

Objectives

1. List legislative acts controlling drug use and abuse.
2. Differentiate between Schedule F and Controlled Drugs, and describe nursing responsibilities with each.

Key Terms

Food and Drugs Act, 1927
Food and Drug Regulations, 1953, 1954, 1979
Controlled Drugs and Substance Act, 1997
nonprescription drugs

Food and Drugs Act 1927; Food and Drug Regulations 1953 and 1954, Revised 1979 and Periodic Amendments

The Food and Drugs Act and the Food and Drug Regulations empower Health Canada to protect the public from foreseeable risks relating to the manufacture and sale of drugs. The Therapeutic Products Directorate administers this legislation. The legislation provides for a review of the safety and efficacy of drugs before their clearance for marketing in Canada and determines whether the medicine is prescription or nonprescription. Also included in this legislation are requirements for good manufacturing practices, adequate labeling, and fair advertising. In Canada, as in the United States, an individual province (or individual state in the United States) may have its own legislation that is more restrictive than the national legislation. Over the years, there became wide variation among the provinces on which medicines were prescription and nonprescription and where medicines could be sold. In an effort to align the provincial drug schedules so that the conditions for the sale of medicines are consistent across Canada, the National Association of Pharmacy Regulatory Authorities proposed a new national drug scheduling model. This model is in various stages of implementation across the provinces of Canada. Under this model, all medicines in Canada are assigned to one of four categories:

- Schedule I: All prescription drugs, including narcotics
- Schedule II: Restricted Access Nonprescription Drugs (see Nonprescription Drugs, following)
- Schedule III: Pharmacy Only Nonprescription Drugs (see Nonprescription Drugs, following)
- Unscheduled Drugs: Those drugs not assigned to the above categories

Drugs requiring a prescription, except for controlled drugs, are listed on Schedule F of the Food and Drug Regulations.

Schedule F Prescription Drugs

Schedule F drugs may be prescribed only by qualified practitioners (e.g., physicians, dentists, or veterinarians) because they would normally be used most safely under supervision.

EXAMPLES:
Most antibiotics, antineoplastics, corticosteroids, cardiovascular drugs, antipsychotics

The Controlled Drugs and Substance Act, 1997

The Controlled Drugs and Substance Act establishes the requirements for the control and sale of narcotics and substances of abuse in Canada. The Controlled Drugs and Substance Act describes eight schedules of controlled substances. Assignment to a schedule is based on potential for abuse and the ease with which illicit substances can be manufactured in illegal laboratories. The degree of control, the conditions of record keeping, and other regulations depend on these classifications. Schedules I through IV are defined below; schedules V through VIII are not yet finalized.

- Schedule I: Opium poppy and its derivatives (e.g., heroin); coca and its derivatives (e.g., cocaine)
- Schedule II: Cannabis and its derivatives (e.g., marijuana, hashish)
- Schedule III: Amphetamines, methylphenidate, lysergic acid diethylamide (LSD), methaqualone, psilocybin, mescaline
- Schedule IV: Sedative/hypnotic agents (e.g., barbiturates, benzodiazepines); anabolic steroids

The Controlled Drugs and Substance Act also provides for the nonprescription sale of certain codeine preparations. The content must not exceed the equivalent of 8 mg codeine phosphate per solid dosage unit or 20 mg per 30 mL of a liquid, and the preparation must also contain two additional nonnarcotic medicinal ingredients. These preparations may not be advertised or displayed and may be sold only by pharmacists. In hospitals, the pharmacy usually requires strict inventory control of these products as well as other narcotics.

EXAMPLES:
Tylenol No. 1 with codeine, Benylin with codeine

Requirements for the legitimate administration of drugs to patients by nurses are generally similar in Canada and the United States. Individual hospital policy determines specific record-keeping requirements based on federal and provincial laws. Violations of these laws would be expected to result in fines or imprisonment in addition to the loss of professional license.

Nonprescription Drugs

The provincial health authorities acknowledge three categories of nonprescription drugs. Schedule II drugs are Restricted Access Nonprescription Drugs that are available for sale directly from the pharmacist and are "kept behind the counter." Examples include insulin, glucagon, ipecac, loperamide, and nitroglycerin. This restriction is to ensure that patients are not self-diagnosing medically serious diseases such as diabetes mellitus or angina and to help ensure proper use of the medicines through appropriate counseling by the pharmacist. Schedule III drugs are Pharmacy Only Nonprescription Drugs. These medicines can be sold only through pharmacies and include most antihistamines and the low-dose histamine-2 antagonists. It is expected that if clients have questions, they could easily consult with the pharmacist. Medicines that are not categorized in Schedules I, II, or III are considered to be "unscheduled" (examples: nicotine gum and patches, aspirin, ibuprofen, some lower-dosage "cough and cold" preparations), and can be sold at any retail outlet.

EFFECTIVENESS OF DRUG LEGISLATION

The effectiveness of drug legislation depends on the interest and determination used to enforce these laws, the appropriation by the government of adequate funds for enforcement, the vigor used by proper authorities in enforcement, the interest and cooperation of professional people and the public, and the education of the public concerning the dangers of unwise and indiscriminate use of drugs in general. Many organizations help in this education, including the National Coordinating Council on Patient Information and Education; the American Medical Association; the American Dental Association; the American Pharmaceutical Association; the American Society of Health-System Pharmacists; and local, state, and county health departments.

NEW DRUG DEVELOPMENT

Objective

1. Describe the procedure outlined by the FDA to develop and market new medicines.

Key Terms

preclinical research
clinical research
New Drug Application
postmarketing surveillance
health orphans

Health care professionals and consumers alike often ask why it takes so long from the time a drug is discovered to the time it is brought to the market. It now takes an average of 8 to 15 years and up to $1 billion in research and development costs to bring a single new drug to market. The Pharmaceutical Manufacturers Association estimates that only 1 out of 10,000 chemicals investigated is actually found to be "safe and effective" and brought to the pharmacist's shelf.

The Food, Drug, and Cosmetic Act of 1938 charged the FDA with the responsibility to regulate new drugs. Rules and regulations evolved by the FDA divide new drug development into four stages: (1) preclinical research and development; (2) clinical research and development; (3) New Drug Application (NDA) review; and (4) postmarketing surveillance (Figure 1-2).

Preclinical Research and Development Stage

The preclinical research phase of new drug development begins with discovery, synthesis, and purification of the drug. The goal at this stage is to use laboratory studies to determine whether the experimental drug has therapeutic value and whether the drug appears to be safe in animals. Enough data must be gained to justify testing the experimental drug in humans. The preclinical phase of data collection may require 1 to 3 years, although the average length of time is 18 months. Near the end of this phase, the investigator (often a pharmaceutical manufacturer) submits an Investigational New Drug (IND) application to the FDA, which describes all studies completed to date and the safety and testing planned for human subjects. The FDA must make a decision based on safety considerations, within 30 days, on whether to allow the study to proceed. Only about 20% of the chemicals tested in the preclinical phase advance to the clinical testing phase.

Clinical Research and Development Stage

The "testing in humans" stage (clinical research, or IND stage) is usually subdivided into three phases. Phase 1 studies determine an experimental drug's pharmacologic properties, such as its pharmacokinetics, metabolism, safe dosage range, potential for toxicity at a certain dosage and safe routes of administration. The study population is either normal volunteers or the intended treatment population, such as those patients who have failed standard treatments of certain cancers or dysrhythmias. Phase 1 studies usually require 20 to

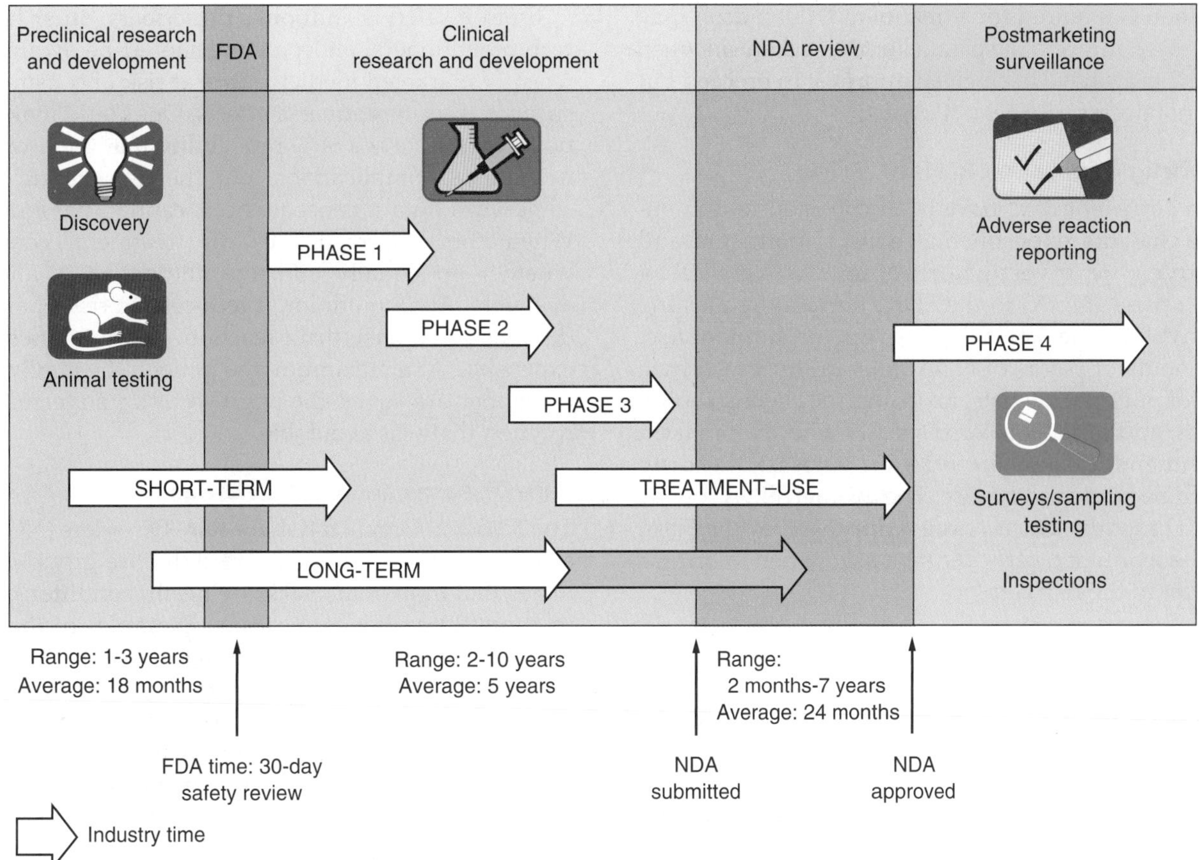

FIGURE 1-2 New drug review process.

100 subjects who are treated for 4 to 6 weeks. If phase 1 trials are successful, the drug is moved to phase 2, which uses a smaller population of patients who have the condition that the drug is designed to treat. Studies are conducted to determine the success rate of a drug for its intended use. If successful, the drug is advanced to phase 3 trials, in which larger patient populations are used to ensure statistical significance of the results. Phase 3 studies also provide additional information on proper dosing and safety. The entire clinical research phase may require 2 to 10 years, with the average experimental drug requiring 5 years. Each study completed is reviewed by the FDA to help ensure patient safety and efficacy. Only one out of five drugs that enter clinical trials makes it to the marketplace. The others fall out of the running because of efficacy or safety problems or lack of commercial interest.

To expedite drug development and approval for life-threatening illnesses such as acquired immunodeficiency syndrome (AIDS), the FDA has drafted rules that allow certain INDs to receive highest priority for review within the agency. This procedure is sometimes known as *fast tracking*. Additional rules allow INDs to be used for treatment of a life-threatening disease in a particular patient, even though the patient does not fit the study protocol for the drug, when there is no alternative therapy. These cases are known as *treatment INDs*. A potentially lifesaving drug may be allowed for treatment IND status late in phase 2 studies, during phase 3 studies, or after all clinical studies have been completed but before marketing approval.

Another mechanism to make INDs available to patients with life-threatening illnesses is known as *parallel tracking*. Under this procedure, an IND may be used for patients who cannot participate in controlled clinical trials and when there is no satisfactory standard therapeutic alternative. Parallel track studies are conducted along with the principal controlled clinical trials, but unlike controlled studies, the parallel track does not involve concurrent control groups. Investigators and patients must realize that there may be greater uncertainty regarding the risks and benefits of therapy with agents that are in relatively early stages of testing and development. Parallel tracking is similar to the treatment IND process, but it allows access to investigational agents when there is less accumulated evidence of efficacy than is required for a treatment IND. A drug may be released through the parallel track mechanism when phase 2 trials have been given approval to proceed but have not necessarily been started.

New Drug Application Review

When sufficient data have been collected to demonstrate that the experimental drug is both safe and effective, the investigator submits a **New Drug Application** (NDA) to the FDA, formally requesting approval to market a new drug for human use. Thousands of pages of NDA data are reviewed by a team of pharmacologists, toxicologists, chemists, physicians, and others (as appropriate) who then make a recommendation to the FDA on whether the drug should be approved for use. The average NDA review takes 17 months. Once a drug is approved by the FDA, it is the manufacturer's decision as to when to bring a product to the marketplace.

Postmarketing Surveillance

If the manufacturer decides to market the medicine, the **postmarketing surveillance** phase, or fourth phase of drug product development, starts. It consists of an ongoing review of adverse effects of the new drug, as well as periodic inspections of the manufacturing facilities and products. Other studies completed during the fourth phase include identifying other patient populations in whom the drug may be useful, refining dosing recommendations, or exploring potential drug interactions. Health care practitioners make a significant contribution to the knowledge of drug safety by reporting adverse effects of drugs to the FDA by using the MedWatch program for voluntary reporting of adverse event and product problems (see Appendix F).

Even though the FDA drug approval process is one of the most conservative in the world, a recent study demonstrated the value of ongoing safety review of medicines and the use of the MedWatch program. Of the 548 new chemical entities approved by the FDA from 1975 to 1999, a total of 56 drugs (10.2%) acquired a new "black box warning" (very serious, potentially life-threatening) or were withdrawn from the market because of serious or fatal complications.* The probability of acquiring a new black box warning or being withdrawn from the market over 25 years is estimated at 20%. Consequently, it is the responsibility of all health care professionals to constantly monitor for adverse effects of drugs and complete a MedWatch form when adverse effects are suspected.

From a safety standpoint, prescribers, other health care practitioners, and patients should be aware that recently marketed medicines are at risk of causing unsuspected serious adverse effects. One could make the point that there is a 90% probability that there will be no serious complications, but the devastating (and sometimes fatal) consequences cannot be ignored. When choosing medicines for treatment, consider whether an equally effective alternative is already available. At a minimum, it reduces the risk of an undiscovered adverse drug reaction, and it is often less expensive. At a maximum, the patient, the family, and prescriber are saved the anguish of an adverse drug reaction that was avoidable.

Rare Diseases and Orphan Drugs

The National Organization for Rare Disorders (NORD), a coalition of 140 voluntary rare-disease groups, estimates that more than 5000 rare health conditions exist in about 20 million Americans. Examples of the rare diseases are cystic fibrosis, Hansen's disease (leprosy), sickle cell anemia, blepharospasm, infant botulism, and *Pneumocystis jiroveci* (formerly *carinii*) pneumonia (PCP). Historically, pharmaceutical manufacturers have been reluctant to develop products that could be used to treat these illnesses because they have been unable to recover the costs of the research because there is a very limited use of the final product. Because no companies would "adopt" the disease to complete extensive research to develop products for treatment, the diseases became known as **health orphans.**

In 1983, the U.S. Congress passed the Orphan Drug Act to stimulate development and market availability of products used for the treatment of rare diseases. The act defines "rare disease" as conditions affecting fewer than 200,000 people in the United States. The law provides research grants, protocol development assistance by the FDA, special tax credits for the cost of clinical trials, and 7 years of exclusive marketing rights after the product has been approved. The act has been quite successful—more than 100 new drugs have been approved by the FDA for the treatment of rare diseases, benefiting several million people. Recent examples are the use of pentamidine and atovaquone for PCP, thalidomide for Hansen's disease, zidovudine for HIV, DNase (Pulmozyme) for cystic fibrosis, and Leustatin for hairy cell leukemia.

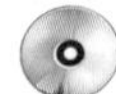

Go to your Companion CD-ROM for Appendices, an Audio Glossary, animations, Drug Dosage Calculators, customizable Patient Self-Assessment forms, and Review Questions for the NCLEX® Examination.

evolve Be sure to visit the companion Evolve site at http://evolve.elsevier.com/Clayton for WebLinks and additional online resources.

*Lasser KE, et al: Timing of black box warnings and withdrawal for prescription medications, *JAMA* 287:2215, 2002.

MEDICATION SAFETY REVIEW

CRITICAL THINKING QUESTIONS

1. Differentiate among generic, trade, brand, and proprietary names assigned to medicines.
2. Describe the different ways drugs may be classified.
3. Prepare a list of books used as drug resources.
4. Discuss implications of herbal product use and the importance of checking for drug-herbal interactions.
5. Describe the drug approval process in the United States.

CONTENT REVIEW QUESTIONS

1. Medicines are most commonly classified by:
   1. brand or generic name.
   2. chemical name.
   3. proprietary name.
   4. body systems, clinical use, or physiology.
2. The *Physicians' Desk Reference* is available:
   1. electronically and in book form.
   2. on every nursing unit.
   3. biannually.
   4. as a package insert with each drug.
3. According the Controlled Substances Act, morphine and Percodan fall into which schedule?
   1. Schedule I
   2. Schedule II
   3. Schedule III
   4. Schedule IV

CHAPTER

2 Principles of Drug Action and Drug Interactions

evolve http://evolve.elsevier.com/Clayton

Chapter Content

BASIC PRINCIPLES

Objectives

1. Identify five basic principles of drug action.
2. Explain nursing assessments necessary to evaluate potential problems associated with the absorption of medications.
3. Describe nursing interventions that can enhance drug absorption.
4. List three categories of drug administration and state the routes of administration for each category.
5. Differentiate between general and selective types of drug distribution mechanisms.
6. Name the process that inactivates drugs.
7. Identify the meaning and significance to the nurse of the term *half-life* when used in relation to drug therapy.

Key Terms

receptors	**parenteral**
pharmacodynamics	**percutaneous**
agonists	**distribution**
antagonists	**drug blood level**
partial agonists	**metabolism**
ADME	**biotransformation**
pharmacokinetics	**excretion**
absorption	**half-life**
enteral	

How do drugs act in the body? The following are a few key facts to remember:

1. Drugs do not create new responses, but alter existing physiologic activity. Drug response must be stated in relation to what the physiologic activity was before the response to drug therapy (e.g., an antihypertensive agent is successful if the patient's blood pressure is lower during therapy than before therapy). Therefore it is important to perform a thorough nursing assessment to identify the baseline data. Once that is done, results from regular assessments can be compared with the baseline data by the physician, nurse, and pharmacist to evaluate the effectiveness of the drug therapy.
2. Drugs interact with the body in several different ways. Usually the drug forms chemical bonds with specific sites, called **receptors,** within the body. This bond forms only if the drug and its receptor have similar shapes. The relationship between a drug and a receptor is similar to that between a key and a lock (Figure 2-1, *A*). The study of the interactions between drugs and their receptors and the series of events that result in a pharmacologic response is called **pharmacodynamics.**
3. Most drugs have several different atoms within each molecule that interlock into various locations on a receptor. The better the fit between the receptor and the drug molecule, the better the response. The intensity of a drug response is related to how well the drug molecule fits into the receptor and to the number of receptor sites that are occupied.
4. Drugs that interact with a receptor to stimulate a response are known as **agonists** (Figure 2-1, *B*). Drugs that attach to a receptor but do not stimulate a response are called **antagonists** (Figure 2-1, C). Drugs that interact with a receptor to stimulate a response but inhibit other responses are called **partial agonists** (Figure 2-1, *D*).
5. Once administered, all drugs go through four stages: ***a***bsorption, ***d***istribution, ***m***etabolism, and ***e***xcretion **(ADME).** Each drug has its own unique ADME characteristics. The study of the

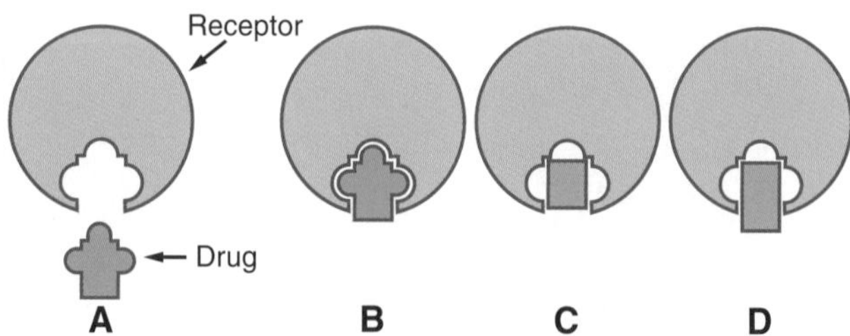

FIGURE **2-1** **A,** Drugs act by forming a chemical bond with specific receptor sites, similar to a key and lock. **B,** The better the "fit," the better the response. Those with complete attachment and response are called *agonists.* **C,** Drugs that attach but do not elicit a response are called *antagonists.* **D,** Drugs that attach and elicit a small response, but also block other responses are called *partial agonists.*

mathematical relationships among the absorption, distribution, metabolism, and excretion of individual medicines over time is called pharmacokinetics.

Absorption

Absorption is the process by which a drug is transferred from its site of entry into the body to the circulating fluids of the body (i.e., blood and lymph) for distribution. The rate at which this occurs depends on the route of administration, the blood flow through the tissue where the drug is administered, and the solubility of the drug. It is therefore important to (1) administer oral drugs with an adequate amount of fluid, usually a large (8 oz) glass of water; (2) give parenteral forms properly so that they are deposited in the correct tissue for enhanced absorption; and (3) reconstitute and dilute drugs only with the diluent recommended by the manufacturer in the package literature so that drug solubility is not impaired. Equally important are nursing assessments that reveal poor absorption (e.g., if insulin is administered subcutaneously and a lump remains at the site of injection 2 to 3 hours later, absorption from that site may be impaired).

The three categories of drug administration are enteral, parenteral, and percutaneous routes. In the enteral route, the drug is administered directly into the gastrointestinal (GI) tract by oral, rectal, or nasogastric routes. The parenteral routes bypass the GI tract by using subcutaneous (subQ), intramuscular (IM), or intravenous (IV) injection. Methods of percutaneous administration include inhalation, sublingual (under the tongue), or topical (on the skin) administration.

Regardless of the route of administration, a drug must be dissolved in body fluids before it can be absorbed into body tissues. For example, before a solid drug taken orally can be absorbed into the bloodstream for transport to the site of action, it must disintegrate and dissolve in the GI fluids and be transported across the stomach or intestinal lining into the blood. The process of converting the drug into a soluble form can be partially controlled by the pharmaceutical dosage form used (e.g., solution, suspension, capsule, and tablets with various coatings). This conversion process can also be influenced by administering the drug with or without food in the patient's stomach.

The rate of absorption when a drug is administered by a parenteral route depends on the rate of blood flow through the tissues. Circulatory insufficiency and respiratory distress may lead to hypoxia and further complicate this situation by resulting in vasoconstriction. For that reason, the nurse should not give an injection when circulation is known to be impaired. Another site on the rotation schedule should be used. Subcutaneous injections have the slowest absorption rate, especially if peripheral circulation is impaired. IM injections are more rapidly absorbed because of greater blood flow per unit weight of muscle compared with subcutaneous tissue. (Depositing the medication into the muscle belly is important. The nurse must carefully assess the individual patient for the correct length of needle to ensure that this occurs.) Cooling the area of injection slows the rate of absorption, whereas heat or massage hastens the rate of absorption. The drug is dispersed throughout the body most rapidly when administered by IV injection. (The nurse must be thoroughly educated regarding the responsibilities and techniques associated with administering IV medications. Once the drug enters the patient's bloodstream, it cannot be retrieved.)

Absorption of topical drugs applied to the skin can be influenced by the drug concentration, length of contact time, size of affected area, thickness of skin surface, hydration of tissue, and degree of skin disruption. Percutaneous absorption is greatly increased in newborns and young infants, who have thin, well-hydrated skin. When drugs are inhaled, their absorption can be influenced by depth of respirations, fineness of the droplet particles, available surface area of mucous membranes, contact time, hydration state, blood supply to the area, and concentration of the drug itself.

Distribution

Distribution refers to the ways in which drugs are transported by the circulating body fluids to the sites of action (receptors), metabolism, and excretion. Drug distribution includes transport throughout the entire body by the blood and lymphatic systems, and transport from the circulating fluids into and out of the fluids that bathe the receptor sites. Organs with the most extensive blood supplies, such as the heart, liver, kidneys, and brain, receive the distributing drug most rapidly. Areas with less extensive blood supplies, such as the muscle, skin, and fat, receive the drug more slowly.

Once a drug has been dissolved and absorbed into the circulating blood, its distribution is determined by the chemical properties of the drug and how it is affected by the blood and tissues it contacts. Two of the factors that influence drug distribution are protein binding and lipid (fat) solubility. Most drugs are transported in combination with plasma proteins, especially albumin, which act as carriers for relatively insoluble drugs. Drugs bound to plasma proteins are pharmacologically inactive because the large size of the complex keeps them in the bloodstream and prevents them from reaching the sites of action, metabolism, and excretion. Only the free or unbound portion of a drug is able to diffuse into tissues, interact with receptors, and produce physiologic effects or be metabolized and excreted. The same proportion of bound and free drug is maintained in the blood at all times. Thus as the free drug acts on receptor sites or is metabolized, the decrease in the serum drug level causes some of the bound drug to be released from protein to maintain the ratio between bound and free drug.

When a drug is circulating in the blood, a blood sample may be drawn and assayed to determine the amount of drug present. This is known as a **drug blood level.** It is important for certain drugs (e.g., anticonvulsants and aminoglycoside antibiotics) to be measured to ensure that the drug blood level is within the therapeutic range. If the drug blood level is low, the dosage must be either increased or the medicine must be administered more frequently. If the drug blood level is too high, the patient may develop signs of toxicity; either the dosage must be reduced or the medicine administered less frequently. See Appendix D for therapeutic blood levels for selected medicines.

Once a drug leaves the bloodstream, it may become bound to tissues other than those with active receptor sites. The more lipid-soluble drugs have a high affinity for adipose tissue, which serves as a repository site for these agents. Because there is relatively low blood circulation to fat tissues, the more lipid-soluble drugs tend to stay in the body much longer. An equilibrium is established between the repository site (lipid tissue) and circulation so that as the drug blood level drops as a result of binding at the sites of physiologic activity, metabolism, or excretion, more drug is released from the lipid tissue. By contrast, if more drug is given, a new equilibrium is established among the blood, receptor sites, lipid tissue repository sites, and metabolic and excretory sites.

Distribution may be general or selective. Some drugs cannot pass through certain types of cell membranes, such as the blood-brain barrier (central nervous system) or the placental barrier (placenta), whereas other types of drugs readily pass into these tissues. The distribution process is very important because the amount of drug that actually gets to the receptor sites determines the extent of pharmacologic activity. If little of the drug actually reaches and binds to the receptor sites, the response will be minimal.

Metabolism

Metabolism, also called **biotransformation,** is the process by which the body inactivates drugs. The enzyme systems of the liver are the primary site for metabolism of drugs, but other tissues and organs (e.g., white blood cells, GI tract, and lungs) metabolize certain drugs to a minor extent. Genetic, environmental, and physiologic factors are involved in the regulation of drug metabolism reactions. The most important factors for conversion of drugs to their metabolites are genetic variations of enzyme systems, concurrent use of other drugs, exposure to environmental pollutants, concurrent illnesses, and age (see Variable Factors Influencing Drug Action, p. 20).

Excretion

Elimination of drug metabolites and, in some cases, the active drug itself from the body is called **excretion.** The two primary routes of excretion are through the GI tract to the feces and through the renal tubules into the urine. Other routes of excretion include evaporation through the skin, exhalation from the lungs, and secretion into saliva and breast milk.

Because the kidneys are a major organ of drug excretion, the nurse should review the patient's chart for the results of urinalysis and renal function tests. A patient with renal failure often has an increase in the action and duration of a drug if the dosage and frequency of administration are not adjusted to allow for the patient's reduced renal function.

Figure 2-2 shows a schematic review of the ADME process of an oral medication. It is important to note how little of the active ingredient actually reaches the receptor sites for action.

Half-Life

Drugs are eliminated from the body by means of metabolism and excretion. A measure of the time required for elimination is the half-life. The **half-life** is defined as the amount of time required for 50% of the drug to be

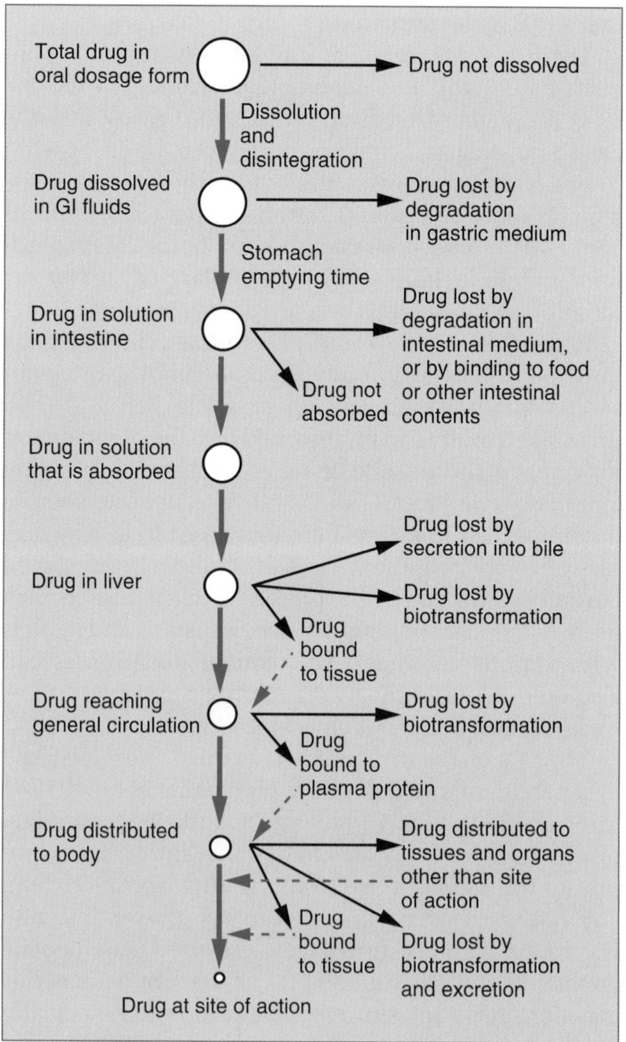

FIGURE 2-2 Factors modifying the quantity of drug reaching a site of action after a single oral dose.

eliminated from the body. For example, if a patient is given 100 mg of a drug that has a half-life of 12 hours, the following would be observed:

TIME (HOURS)	HALF-LIFE	DRUG REMAINING IN BODY
0	—	100 mg (100%)
12	1	50 mg (50%)
24	2	25 mg (25%)
36	3	12.5 mg (12.5%)
48	4	6.25 mg (6.25%)
60	5	3.12 mg (3.12%)

Note that as each 12-hour period (one half-life) passes, the amount remaining is 50% of what was there 12 hours earlier. After six half-lives, more than 98% of the drug is eliminated from the body.

The half-life is determined by an individual's ability to metabolize and excrete a particular drug. Because most patients metabolize and excrete a particular drug at approximately the same rate, the approximate half-lives of most drugs are now known. When the half-life of a drug is known, dosages and frequency of administration can be calculated. Drugs with a long half-life, such as digoxin at 36 hours, need to be administered only once daily, whereas drugs with a short half-life, such as aspirin at 5 hours, need to be administered every 4 to 6 hours to maintain therapeutic activity. In patients who have impaired hepatic or renal function, the half-life may become considerably longer because of their reduced ability to metabolize or excrete the drug. An example is digoxin, which has a half-life of about 36 hours in a patient with normal renal function, but a half-life of about 105 hours in a patient in complete renal failure. Monitoring diagnostic tests that measure renal or hepatic function is important. Whenever laboratory data reflect impairment of either function, the nurse should notify the physician.

DRUG ACTION

Objective

1. Compare and contrast the following terms used in relationship to medications: desired action, side effects, adverse effects, allergic reactions, and idiosyncratic reactions.

Key Terms

desired action	allergic reactions
side effects	urticaria
adverse effects	hives
toxicity	carcinogenicity
parameters	teratogen
idiosyncratic reaction	

No drug has a single action. When a drug enters a patient and is absorbed and distributed, the **desired action** (i.e., expected response) usually occurs. All drugs, however, have the potential to affect more than one body system simultaneously, producing responses known as **side effects** or **adverse effects.** When adverse effects are severe, the reaction is sometimes referred to as a **toxicity.** The World Health Organization's definition of an adverse drug reaction (ADR) is "any noxious, unintended, and undesired effect of a drug, which occurs at doses used in humans for prophylaxis, diagnosis, or therapy." A more common definition is: "Right drug, right dose, right patient, bad effect." ADRs should not be confused with medication errors, or adverse drug events (ADEs), which are defined as "an injury resulting from medical intervention related to a drug"; this is discussed in Chapter 7.

Recent studies indicate the following:

- ADRs may be responsible for more than 100,000 deaths among hospitalized patients per year, making them one of the top six leading causes of death in the United States.
- An average of 6% of hospitalized patients suffer a significant ADR sometime during their hospitalization.
- Between 5% and 9% of the cost of hospitalizations are attributable to adverse drug reactions.
- The most commonly seen ADRs are rash, nausea, itching, thrombocytopenia, vomiting, hyperglycemia, and diarrhea.
- The classes of medicines that account for the largest number of ADRs are antibiotics, cardiovascular medicines, cancer chemotherapy agents, and analgesics/antiinflammatory agents.
- Among the 1.6 million residents of nursing homes in the United States, drug-related injuries are estimated to occur at a rate of 350,000 events per year, and more than half may be preventable. There may be as many as 20,000 life-threatening or fatal ADEs per year among nursing home residents; of these, 80% may be preventable.

Most adverse drug effects are predictable, and patients should be monitored so that dosages can be adjusted to allow the maximum therapeutic benefits with a minimum of side effects. As described in Part Two of this text, each drug has a series of **parameters** (e.g., therapeutic actions to expect, side effects to expect, adverse effects to report, and probable drug interactions) that should be monitored by the nurse, physician, pharmacist, and patient to optimize therapy while reducing the possibility of serious adverse effects.

All hospitals have internal mechanisms for reporting suspected ADRs, and health professionals should not hesitate to report possible reactions. By monitoring and tracking the occurrences of ADRs, clinical protocols and improved patient screening will reduce the frequency of recurrences. The FDA's MedWatch program is also available for voluntary reporting of adverse events (see Appendix F).

Two other types of drug action are much more unpredictable. These are idiosyncratic reactions and allergic reactions. An **idiosyncratic reaction** occurs when something unusual or abnormal happens when a drug is first administered. The patient usually shows an *overresponse* to the action of the drug. This type of reaction is usually the result of a patient's inability to metabolize a drug because of a genetic deficiency of certain enzymes. Fortunately, this type of reaction is rare.

Allergic reactions, also known as hypersensitivity reactions, occur in about 6% to 10% of patients taking medications. Allergic reactions occur in patients who have previously been exposed to a drug and have developed antibodies to it from their immune systems. On reexposure, the antibodies cause a reaction, most commonly seen as raised, irregularly shaped patches on the skin and severe itching, known as **urticaria** or **hives.** Occasionally, a patient has a severe, life-threatening reaction that causes respiratory distress and cardiovascular collapse, known as an *anaphylactic reaction.* This condition is a medical emergency and must be treated immediately. Fortunately, anaphylactic reactions occur much less often than the more mild urticarial reactions. If a patient has a mild reaction, it should be understood as a warning not to take the medication again. The patient is much more likely to have an anaphylactic reaction at the next exposure to the drug. Patients should receive information regarding the drug name and be instructed to tell health care professionals such as nurses, physicians, pharmacists, and dentists that they have had a reaction and must not receive the drug again. In addition, patients should wear a medical-alert bracelet or necklace that explains the allergy.

Carcinogenicity is the ability of a drug to induce living cells to mutate and become cancerous. Many drugs have this potential, so all drugs are tested in several animal species before human investigation to eliminate this potential.

A drug that induces birth defects is known as a **teratogen.** Fetal organs of the body are particularly susceptible to malformation if they are exposed to a drug while in the uterus. Because most organ systems are formed during the first trimester of pregnancy, the greatest potential for birth defects caused by drugs occurs during this period.

VARIABLE FACTORS INFLUENCING DRUG ACTION

Objective

1. List factors that cause variations in the absorption, distribution, metabolism, and excretion of drugs.

Key Terms

placebo effect	**tolerance**
nocebo effect	**drug dependence**
placebo	**drug accumulation**

Patients often state, "That drug really knocked me out!" or "That drug didn't touch the pain!" The effects of drugs are unexpectedly potent in some patients, whereas other patients show little response at the same dosage. In addition, some patients react differently to the same dosage of a drug administered at different times. Because of individual patient variation, exact responses to drug therapy are difficult to predict (see Chapter 3, p. 29; see also Chapter 4, Table 4-3, pp. 50 to 55). The following factors have been identified as contributors to a variable response to drugs.

Age

Infants and the very elderly tend to be the most sensitive to the effects of drugs. There are important differences in the absorption, distribution, metabolism, and excretion of drugs in premature neonates, full-term newborns, and children. The aging process brings about changes in body composition and organ function that can affect the elderly patient's response to drug therapy. See Chapter 3 for a more complete discussion of age-related variables influencing drug action.

Body Weight

Considerably overweight patients may require an increase in dosage to attain the same therapeutic response as the general population. Conversely, patients who are underweight (compared with the general population) tend to require lower dosages for the same therapeutic response. It is extremely important to obtain accurate heights and weights of patients because the dosage of medicine may be calculated using these parameters. Most pediatric dosages are calculated by milligrams of drug per kilogram (mg/kg) of body weight to adjust for growth rate. The dosages of other medicines, particularly the chemotherapeutic agents, are ordered based on body surface area (BSA) (see Appendix C). To ensure accurate measurements, weights should be taken at the same time, with similar clothing, at admission, and at intervals ordered by the physician throughout the provision of care.

Metabolic Rate

Patients with a higher than average metabolic rate tend to metabolize drugs more rapidly, thus requiring either larger doses or more frequent administration. The converse is true for those with lower than average metabolic rates. Chronic smoking enhances the metabolism of some drugs (e.g., theophylline), thus requiring larger doses to be administered more frequently for a therapeutic effect.

Illness

Pathologic conditions may alter the rate of absorption, distribution, metabolism, and excretion. For example, patients in shock have reduced peripheral vascular circulation and will absorb intramuscularly or subcutaneously injected drugs slowly. Patients who are vomiting may not be able to retain a medication in the stomach long enough for dissolution and absorption. Patients with diseases such as nephrotic syndrome or malnutrition may have reduced amounts of serum proteins in the blood necessary for adequate distribution of drugs. Patients with kidney failure must have significant reductions in the dosages of medications that are excreted by the kidneys.

Psychological Aspects

Attitudes and expectations play a major role in a patient's response to therapy and the willingness to take the medication as prescribed. Patients with diseases that have relatively rapid consequences if therapy is ignored, such as type 1 (insulin dependent) diabetes, usually have a good rate of compliance. Patients with "silent" illnesses, such as hypertension, tend to be much less compliant with the treatment regimen.

Another psychological consideration is the "placebo effect" and the "nocebo effect." It is well documented that a patient's positive expectations about treatment and the care received can positively affect the outcome of therapy, a phenomenon known as the placebo effect (Latin, *I will please*). Although more difficult to prove because of ethical considerations, it is also felt that negative expectations about therapy and the care received can have a nocebo effect (Latin, *I will harm*), resulting in less than optimal outcomes of therapy. It is thought that the nocebo effect plays a major role in psychogenic illness, especially in stress-related problems, by worrying about it. Caregivers can help diminish the nocebo effect by having a positive mental attitude and emphasizing the positive aspects of therapy.

A placebo is a drug dosage form, such as a tablet or capsule, that has no pharmacologic activity because the dosage form has no active ingredients. When taken, the patient may report a therapeutic response. This response can be beneficial in patients being treated for such illnesses as anxiety, because the patient tends to take fewer potentially habit-forming drugs. Placebos are frequently used in studies of new medicines to measure the pharmacologic effects of a new medicine compared with the inert placebo. The American Pain Society and the Agency for Health Care Policy and Research recommend the avoidance of deceitful use of placebos in current clinical practice guidelines for pain management. It is felt that the deceitful use of placebos in pain management violates a patient's rights to the highest quality of care possible.

Tolerance

Tolerance occurs when a person begins to require a higher dosage to produce the same effects that a lower dosage once provided. An example is the person who is addicted to heroin. After a few weeks of use, larger doses are required to provide the same "high." Tolerance can be caused by psychological dependence, or the body may metabolize a particular drug more rapidly than before, causing the effects of the drug to diminish more rapidly.

Dependence

Drug dependence, also known as *addiction* or *habituation,* occurs when a person is unable to control the ingestion of drugs. The dependence may be *physical,* in which the person develops withdrawal symptoms if the drug is withdrawn for a certain period, or *psychological,* in which the patient is emotionally attached to the drug. Drug dependence occurs most commonly with the use of the scheduled, or controlled, medications listed in Chapter 1 such as opiates and benzodiazepines. Many people, especially elderly, worry about becoming addicted to pain medication and therefore may not take pain medication even when it is needed. The nurse needs to assure them that studies have shown that less than 1% of patients using opioids for pain relief become addicted, and that it is important for their overall well-being to be as pain-free as possible (see Chapter 49).

Cumulative Effect

A drug may accumulate in the body if the next dose is administered before the previously administered dose has been metabolized or excreted. Excessive drug accumulation may result in drug toxicity. An example of drug accumulation is the excessive ingestion of alcoholic beverages. A person becomes "drunk" or "inebriated" when the rate of consumption exceeds the rate of metabolism and excretion of the alcohol.

DRUG INTERACTIONS

Objectives

1. State the mechanisms by which drug interactions may occur.
2. Differentiate among the following terms used in relationship to medications: additive effect, synergistic effect, antagonistic effect, displacement, interference, and incompatibility.

Key Terms

drug interaction	antagonistic effect
unbound drug	displacement
additive effect	interference
synergistic effect	incompatibility

A drug interaction is said to occur when the action of one drug is altered by the action of another drug. Drug interactions are elicited in two ways: (1) agents that when combined *increase* the actions of one or both drugs; and (2) agents that when combined, *decrease* the effectiveness of one or both of the drugs. Some drug interactions are beneficial, such as the use of caffeine, a central nervous system (CNS) stimulant, with an antihistamine, a CNS depressant. The stimulatory effects of the caffeine counteract the drowsiness caused by the antihistamine without eliminating the antihistaminic effects.

The mechanisms of drug interactions can be categorized as those that alter the absorption, distribution, metabolism, and/or excretion of a drug, and those that enhance the pharmacologic effect of a drug. Most drug interactions that alter absorption take place in the GI tract, usually the stomach. Examples of this type of interaction include the following:

- Antacids inhibit the dissolution of ketoconazole tablets by increasing the gastric pH. The interaction is managed by giving antacids at least 2 hours after ketoconazole administration.
- Aluminum-containing antacids inhibit the absorption of tetracycline. Aluminum salts form an insoluble chemical complex with tetracycline. The interaction is managed by separating the administration of tetracycline and antacids by 3 to 4 hours.

Drug interactions that cause an alteration in distribution usually affect the binding of a drug to an inactive site, such as circulating plasma albumin or muscle protein. Once a drug is absorbed into the blood, it is usually transported throughout the body bound to plasma proteins. It often binds to other proteins such as those in the muscle. A drug that is highly bound (e.g., >90% bound) to a protein-binding site may be displaced by another drug that has a higher affinity for the binding site. Significant interactions can take place this way because little displacement is required to have a major impact. Remember that only the **unbound drug** is pharmacologically active. If a drug is 90% bound to a protein, then 10% of the drug is providing the physiologic effect. If another drug is administered with a stronger affinity for the protein-binding site and displaces just 5% of the bound drug, there is now 15% unbound for physiologic activity. This is the equivalent of a 50% increase in dosage, from 10% to 15% active drug. For example, the anticoagulant action of warfarin is increased by administration with furosemide, which is a loop diuretic. Furosemide displaces warfarin from albumin-binding sites, increasing the amount of unbound anticoagulant. This interaction is managed by decreasing the warfarin dosage.

Drug interactions usually result from an alteration in metabolism by either inhibiting or inducing (stimulating) the enzymes that metabolize a drug. Medicines known to bind to enzymes and slow the metabolism of other drugs include verapamil, chloramphenicol, ketoconazole, amiodarone, cimetidine, and erythromycin. Serum drug levels usually increase as a result of inhibited metabolism when these drugs are given concurrently, and the dosages usually must be reduced to prevent toxicity. For example, erythromycin inhibits the metabolism of theophylline; therefore the dose of theophylline must be reduced based on theophylline serum levels and signs of toxicity. Because erythromycin (an antibiotic) is usually administered only in short courses, the theophylline dosage usually needs to be increased when the erythromycin is discontinued.

Common enzyme inducers are phenobarbital, carbamazepine, rifampin, and phenytoin. Drugs whose metabolism is stimulated include disopyramide, doxycycline, griseofulvin, warfarin, metronidazole, mexiletine, quinidine, theophylline, and verapamil. When administered with enzyme inducers, the dosage of the more rapidly metabolized drug usually should be increased to provide therapeutic activity. The patient must be monitored closely for adverse effects, especially if the enzyme inducer is discontinued. The metabolism of the induced drug decelerates, leading to accumulation and toxicity if the dosage is not reduced. For example, if a woman taking oral contraceptives (e.g., Ortho-Novum, Lo/Ovral) requires a course of rifampin antimicrobial therapy, the rifampin will induce the enzymes that metabolize both the progesterone and estrogen components of the contraceptive, causing an increased incidence of menstrual abnormalities and reduced effectiveness of conception control. This interaction is managed by advising the patient to use an additional form of contraception while receiving rifampin therapy.

Drugs that interact by altering excretion usually act in the kidney tubules by altering the pH to enhance or inhibit excretion. The classic example of altered urine pH is with acetazolamide, a drug that elevates urine pH, and quinidine. The alkaline urine produced by acetazolamide causes quinidine to be reabsorbed in the renal tubules, potentially increasing the physiologic and toxic effects of quinidine. Frequent monitoring of quinidine serum levels and assessment for signs of quinidine toxicity are used as guides for reducing quinidine dosages.

Major drug interactions also occur with drugs that enhance the physiologic effect of another drug, for example, those that cause CNS depression, such as a sedative-hypnotic and alcohol, or the potentiation of neuromuscular blockade between an aminoglycoside antibiotic and a neuromuscular blocking agent such as tubocurarine.

The following terminology is used in describing drug interactions:

Additive effect: Two drugs with similar actions are taken for a doubled effect.

EXAMPLE:
propoxyphene + aspirin = added analgesic effect

Synergistic effect: The combined effect of two drugs is greater than the sum of the effect of each drug given alone.

EXAMPLE:
aspirin + codeine = much greater analgesic effect

Antagonistic effect: One drug interferes with the action of another.

EXAMPLE:
tetracycline + antacid = decreased absorption of the tetracycline

Displacement: The displacement of the first drug by a second drug increases the activity of the first drug.

EXAMPLE:
warfarin + valproic acid = increased anticoagulant effect

Interference: The first drug inhibits the metabolism or excretion of the second drug, causing increased activity of the second drug.

EXAMPLE:
probenecid + spectinomycin = prolonged antibacterial activity from spectinomycin due to blocking renal excretion by probenecid

Incompatibility: The first drug is chemically incompatible with the second drug, causing deterioration when both drugs are mixed in the same syringe or solution; incompatible drugs should not be mixed together or administered together at the same site; signs of incompatibility are haziness, a precipitate, or a change in color of the solution when the drugs are mixed.

EXAMPLE:
ampicillin + gentamicin = ampicillin inactivates gentamicin

The side effects of medicines are perhaps better tolerated by younger people than elderly individuals. Dizziness in the elderly may cause a decrease in activity for fear of falling; a dry mouth can initiate poor tolerance of dentures, along with alterations in taste and chewing, thus reducing nutritional intake. Even a minor, subtle alteration in mental or behavioral functioning deserves to be investigated for the possibility of a drug-induced change before any additional medicines are prescribed for the symptoms. Drug-induced side effects are commonly mistaken for disease symptoms. Many medicines (e.g., reserpine, beta blockers, antiparkinsonian drugs, and corticosteroids) cause depression. Confusion may be the first and only symptom of drug accumulation. Because confusion and delirium are often observed in the elderly population, such as residents of a nursing home, what actually may be a drug-induced symptom is often treated with yet another agent.

Because it is impossible to memorize all possible drug interactions, the nurse must check for drug interactions when suspected. The nurse must take the time to consult drug resource books and pharmacists to ensure that a patient receiving multiple medications does not suffer from unplanned drug interactions.

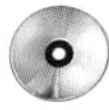

Go to your Companion CD-ROM for Appendices, an Audio Glossary, animations, Drug Dosage Calculators, customizable Patient Self-Assessment forms, and Review Questions for the NCLEX® Examination.

evolve Be sure to visit the companion Evolve site at http://evolve.elsevier.com/Clayton for WebLinks and additional online resources.

MEDICATION SAFETY REVIEW

CRITICAL THINKING QUESTIONS

1. How do drugs interact with receptor sites in the body?
2. Explain the differences among a drug agonist, partial agonist, and antagonist, and give examples of each.
3. How do you calculate a drug's half-life?
4. What stages does a drug go through in the process of pharmacokinetics?
5. Discuss the effects of ADRs on individual patients and on the costs of health care.
6. Investigate mechanisms used at your clinical site to report drug errors and adverse drug effects.
7. What effect do body weight, body surface area, metabolic rate, and illness have on drug therapy?
8. Discuss the difference between bound and unbound drugs and the resultant effects on drug action.

Continued

CONTENT REVIEW QUESTIONS

1. A patient takes 50 mg of a drug that has a half-life of 12 hours. What percentage of the dose remains in the body 36 hours after the drug is administered?
   1. 50 mg (100%)
   2. 25 mg (50%)
   3. 12.5 mg (25%)
   4. 6.25 mg (12.5%)
2. The portion of a drug that is pharmacologically active is known as the:
   1. protein-bound drug.
   2. unbound drug.
   3. drug tolerance level.
   4. incompatibility factor.
3. A person who has an increased metabolic rate (e.g., hyperthyroidism) would generally require a dosage that is:
   1. normal.
   2. lower than normal.
   3. higher than normal.
   4. based on thyroid function levels.

CHAPTER

3 Drug Action Across the Life Span

evolve http://evolve.elsevier.com/Clayton

Chapter Content

Objectives

1. Discuss the effects of patient age on drug action.
2. Cite major factors associated with drug absorption, distribution, metabolism, and excretion in the pediatric and geriatric populations.
3. Cite major factors associated with drug absorption, distribution, metabolism, and excretion in men and women.

Key Terms

gender-specific medicine
pharmacogenetics
polymorphisms
passive diffusion
hydrolysis
intestinal transit
protein binding
drug metabolism
metabolites
polypharmacy
therapeutic drug monitoring

CHANGING DRUG ACTION ACROSS THE LIFE SPAN

The age of the patient can have a significant impact on drug therapy. When discussing the effect of age on drug therapy, it is helpful to subdivide the population into the following categories:

AGE	TITLE OF STAGE
<38 weeks' gestation	Premature
0-1 month	Newborn, neonate
1-24 months	Infant, baby
1-5 years	Young child
6-12 years	Older child
13-18 years	Adolescent
19-54 years	Adult
55-64 years	Older adult
65-74 years	Elderly
75-84 years	The aged
85+ years	The very old

Gender also affects drug therapy. Men and women respond to medications differently. **Gender-specific medicine** is a developing science that studies the differences in the normal function of men and women and how people of each sex perceive and experience disease. Unfortunately, few scientific data exist to document differences in the pharmacokinetics of most drugs in men and women. In 1993, the U.S. Food and Drug Administration (FDA) issued guidelines stating that drug development must evaluate the effects on both genders. Testing is also needed to assess differences in pharmacokinetic parameters between men and women. Within the women's studies, the research must distinguish among pre- and postmenopausal women, as well as women in different phases of the menstrual cycle. Substantial new information has been gained over the past few years, teaching us the following:

- In nearly every body system, men and women function differently.
- Men and women perceive and experience disease differently.
- Fundamental questions remain about how humans normally function and the effect of disease on function.

Another unfolding science is **pharmacogenetics,** which is the study of how drug response may vary according to inherited differences in drug metabolism. **Polymorphisms** are naturally occurring variations in the structures of genes and the products they make for the body. Research has shown significant differences among racial and ethnic groups in the metabolism, clinical effectiveness, and side effect profiles of medications. Most studies to date have concentrated on cardiovascular and psychiatric drugs, analgesics, antihistamines, and ethanol. Most of the research applies to African Americans, whites, and Asians, but more research is now focusing on Hispanics because they represent the largest racial or ethnic group after whites in the United States.

As described in Chapter 2, drug action depends on four factors: *a*bsorption, *d*istribution, *m*etabolism, and *e*xcretion (ADME). Each of these factors varies depending on age, gender, and polymorphisms. Polymorphisms may influence a drug's action by altering these pharmacokinetic or pharmacodynamic (effect on the body) properties.

Drug Absorption

Age Considerations

Before a medicine can be absorbed, it must be administered. Pediatric and geriatric patients each require special considerations for medication administration. For example, the absorption of medicines given intramuscularly (IM) may be affected by differences in muscle mass, blood flow to muscles, and muscle inactivity in patients who are bedridden.

Topical administration with percutaneous absorption is usually effective in infants because the outer layer of skin (stratum corneum) is not fully developed. Because the skin is more fully hydrated at this age, water-soluble drugs are absorbed more readily. Infants wearing plastic-coated diapers are also more susceptible to skin absorption because the plastic acts as an occlusive dressing that increases hydration of the skin. Inflammation (e.g., diaper rash) also increases the amount of drug absorbed.

Transdermal administration in geriatric patients is often difficult to predict. Although dermal thickness decreases with aging and may enhance absorption, factors that may diminish absorption occur, such as drying, wrinkling, and a decrease in hair follicles. With aging, decreased cardiac output and diminishing tissue perfusion may also affect transdermal drug absorption.

In most cases, medicines are administered orally. However, tablet and capsule forms are often too large for either pediatric or geriatric patients to swallow. It is often necessary to crush a tablet for administration with food or use a liquid formulation for easier administration. Taste also becomes a factor when administering oral liquids because the liquid comes into contact with the taste buds. Timed-release tablets (p. 130), enteric-coated tablets (p. 131), and sublingual tablets (p. 118) should not be crushed because of the effect on the absorption rate and the potential for toxicity.

Infants and older adults often lack a sufficient number of teeth for chewable medicines. Chewable tablets should not be given to children with loose teeth (pp. 30 to 31). Geriatric patients often have reduced salivary flow (pp. 31 to 32), making chewing and swallowing more difficult.

Gastrointestinal (GI) absorption of medicines is influenced by a variety of factors, including gastric pH, gastric emptying time, motility of the GI tract, enzymatic activity, blood flow of the mucous lining of the stomach and intestines, permeability and maturation of the mucosal membrane, and concurrent disease processes. Absorption by **passive diffusion** across the membranes and gastric emptying time depend on the pH of the environment. Newborns and geriatric patients have reduced gastric acidity and transit time when compared with adults. Premature infants have a high gastric pH (6 to 8) because of immature acid-secreting cells in the stomach. In a full-term newborn, the gastric pH is also 6 to 8, but within 24 hours the pH decreases to 2 to 4 because of gastric acid secretion. At 1 year of age, the child's stomach pH approximates that of an adult (1 to 3). Geriatric patients often have a higher gastric pH because of loss of acid-secreting cells. Drugs destroyed by gastric acid (e.g., ampicillin, penicillin) are more readily absorbed and have higher serum concentrations in older adults because of the lack of acid destruction. In contrast, drugs that depend on an acidic environment for absorption (e.g., phenobarbital, acetaminophen, phenytoin, aspirin) are more poorly absorbed and have lower serum concentrations in older adults. Premature infants and geriatric patients also have a slower gastric emptying time, partly because of the reduced acid secretion. A slower gastric emptying time may allow the drug to stay in contact with the absorptive tissue longer, allowing increased absorption with a higher serum concentration. There is also the potential for toxicity caused by extended contact time in the stomach for ulcerogenic drugs (e.g., nonsteroidal antiinflammatory agents).

Another factor affecting drug absorption in the newborn is the absence of enzymes needed for **hydrolysis.** Infants cannot metabolize palmitic acid from chloramphenicol palmitate (an antibiotic), thus preventing absorption of the chloramphenicol. Oral phenytoin dosages are also greater in infants less than 6 months of age because of poor absorption (neonates: 15 to 20 mg/kg/24 hr as compared with infants and children: 4 to 7 mg/kg/24 hr).

The **intestinal transit** rate also varies with age. As the newborn matures into infancy, the GI transit rate increases, causing some medicines to be poorly absorbed. Sustained-release capsules (e.g., theophylline [Theo-24]) move through the intestines so rapidly at this age that only about 50% of a dose is absorbed, compared with dose absorption in children more than 5 years of age. The elderly develop decreased GI motility and intestinal blood flow. This has the potential for altered absorption of medicines, as well as either constipation or diarrhea, depending on the medicine.

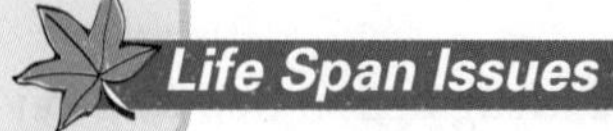

Life Span Issues

Pediatric and geriatric patients each require special considerations for medication administration. Medicines given IM are usually erratically absorbed in both neonates and older adults. Differences in muscle mass, blood flow to muscles, and muscle inactivity in patients who are bedridden make absorption unpredictable.

Gender Considerations

Generally, women's stomachs empty solids more slowly than men's do and may have greater gastric acidity, thus slowing the absorption of certain types of medicines, such as aspirin. A slower gastric emptying time may allow the drug to stay in contact with the absorptive tissue longer, allowing more absorption with a higher serum concentration. There is also an increased potential for toxicity, caused by more contact time in the stomach for potentially ulcerogenic drugs (e.g., nonsteroidal antiinflammatory agents). Women also have lower gastric levels of an enzyme, alcohol dehydrogenase, needed to metabolize ingested alcohol. Thus larger amounts of ingested alcohol may be absorbed instead of metabolized in the stomach, leading to a higher blood alcohol level in a woman than in a man for equal amounts of ingested alcohol. Other factors such as body weight and drug distribution (see following) may aggravate the higher blood alcohol level and state of intoxication in women when compared with men.

Drug Distribution

Distribution refers to the ways in which drugs are transported by the circulating body fluids to the sites of action (receptors), metabolism, and excretion. Distribution is dependent on pH, body water concentrations (intracellular, extracellular, and total body water), presence and quantity of fat tissue, protein binding, cardiac output, and regional blood flow.

Age and Gender Considerations

Most medicines are transported either dissolved in the circulating water (in blood) of the body or bound to plasma proteins within the blood. Body water composition as a percentage of weight changes substantially with age (Table 3-1). Note that the total body water content of a preterm infant is 83%, whereas that of an adult man is 60%. The significance of this is that infants have a larger volume of distribution for water-soluble drugs and require a higher dose on a milligram per kilogram (mg/kg) basis than an older child or adult.

As we age, lean body mass and total body water decrease while total fat content increases. The body weight of a preterm infant may be composed of 1% to 2% fat, whereas a full-term newborn may have 15% fat. Adult total body fat ranges from 18% to 36% for men and 33% to 48% for women between ages 18 and 35. Drugs that are highly fat soluble (e.g., antidepressants, phenothiazines, benzodiazepines, calcium channel blockers) require a longer onset of action and accumulate in fat tissues, prolonging their action and increasing the potential for toxicity. For water-soluble drugs such as ethanol and aminoglycoside antibiotics, a woman's greater proportion of body fat produces a higher blood level compared with that of a man when given as an equal dose per kilogram of body weight. In the case of ethanol, this effect tends to cause a higher level of ethanol in brain cells, resulting in greater intoxication. Highly fat-soluble medicines (e.g., diazepam) must be given in smaller mg/kg dosages to low-birthweight infants because there is less fat tissue to bind the drug, leaving more drug to be active at receptor sites.

Drugs that are relatively insoluble are transported in the circulation by being bound to plasma proteins (albumin and globulins), especially albumin. **Protein binding** is reduced in preterm infants because of decreased plasma protein concentrations, lower binding capacity of protein, and decreased affinity of proteins for drug binding. Drugs known to have lower protein binding in neonates than in adults include phenobarbital, phenytoin, theophylline, propranolol, lidocaine, penicillin, and chloramphenicol. Because serum protein binding is diminished, the drugs are distributed over a wider area of the neonate's body, and a larger loading dose is required than in older children to achieve therapeutic serum concentrations. Several drugs used to treat neonatal conditions may compete for binding sites. Sulfisoxazole is well known for displacing bilirubin from protein-binding sites, thus allowing the bilirubin to accumulate and pass into the brain, causing kernicterus (degeneration of brain nerve cells caused by binding of bilirubin to cells).

Little difference exists between albumin protein in men and women, although there are some differences between the globulin proteins (corticosteroid-binding and sex-hormone–binding globulins). In adults older than 40 years of age, the composition of body proteins begins to change. Although the total body protein concentration is unaffected, albumin concentrations gradually decrease, and other proteins (e.g., globulins) increase. As albumin levels diminish, the level of unbound, active drug increases. Increased levels of naproxen, diflunisal, salicylate, and valproate have been found in older adults, presumably as a result of decreased albumin levels. Disease states such as cirrhosis, renal failure, and

Table 3-1 ***Percentages of Body Water****

AGE (WEIGHT)	EXTRACELLULAR WATER (%)	INTRACELLULAR WATER (%)	TOTAL BODY WATER (%)
Premature (1.5 kg)	60	40	83
Full-term (3.5 kg)	56	44	74
5 months (7 kg)	50	50	60
1 year (10 kg)	40	60	59
Adult male	40	60	60

*Developmental changes from birth to adulthood. Extracellular and intracellular water is expressed as a percentage of total body weight. (Data from Friis-Hansen B: Body composition during growth, *Pediatrics* 47:264, 1971.)

malnutrition can lower albumin levels. Initial doses of highly protein-bound drugs (e.g., warfarin, phenytoin, tolbutamide, propranolol, digitoxin, or diazepam) should be reduced and then increased slowly if there is evidence of decreased serum albumin. Lower protein binding may also lead to greater immediate pharmacologic effect because more active drug is available, but the duration of action may be reduced because more of the unbound drug is available for metabolism and excretion.

Drug Metabolism

Age Considerations

Drug metabolism is the process by which the body inactivates medicines. It is controlled by factors such as genes, diet, age, and maturity of enzyme systems. Enzyme systems, primarily in the liver, are the major pathway of drug metabolism. All enzyme systems are present at birth, but they mature at different rates, taking several weeks to a year to fully develop.

Liver weight, the number of functioning hepatic cells, and hepatic blood flow decrease with age. This results in slower metabolism of drugs in older adults. Reduced metabolism can be seriously aggravated by the presence of liver disease or heart failure. Drugs that are extensively metabolized by the liver (e.g., morphine, lidocaine, propranolol) can have substantially prolonged duration of action if hepatic blood flow is reduced. Dosages usually must be reduced or the time interval between doses extended to prevent accumulation of active medicine and potential toxicity. Drug metabolism also can be affected at all ages by genetics, smoking, diet, gender, other medicines (Table 3-2), and diseases (e.g., hepatitis, cirrhosis). Unfortunately, no specific laboratory tests are available for measuring liver function; renal function must be assessed to adjust dosages.

Gender Considerations

It is now recognized that males and females differ in the concentrations of some of these enzyme systems throughout life. The CYP3A4 component of the cytochrome P-450 system of enzymes metabolizes more than 50% of all drugs, and is 40% more active in women. Drugs such as erythromycin, prednisolone, verapamil, and diazepam are metabolized faster in women than in men. In the future, the effect on metabolism by these differences in enzyme systems will likely be identified by the FDA guidelines on new drug development.

Drug Excretion

Metabolites of drugs and, in some cases, the active drug itself, are eventually excreted from the body. The primary routes are through the renal tubules into the urine and the GI tract to the feces. Other generally minor routes of excretion include evaporation through the skin, exhalation from the lungs, and secretion into the saliva and breast milk.

Age Considerations

At birth, a preterm infant has up to 15% of the renal capacity of an adult, whereas a full-term newborn has approximately 35%. The filtration capacity of an infant increases to about 50% of adult capacity at 4 weeks of age and is equivalent to full adult function at 9 to 12 months. Drugs that are excreted primarily by the kidneys (e.g., penicillin, gentamicin, tobramycin) must be administered in increased dosages or given more often to maintain adequate therapeutic serum concentrations as renal function matures.

As the body ages, important physiologic changes take place in the kidneys, including decreased renal blood flow caused by atherosclerosis and reduced cardiac output, a loss of glomeruli, and decreased tubular

Table 3-2 ***Medications that Require Hepatic Monitoring*†***

GENERIC NAME	BRAND NAME
amiodarone	Cordarone
atorvastatin	Lipitor
azathioprine	Imuran
carbamazepine	Tegretol
diclofenac	Voltaren
efavirenz	Sustiva
felbamate	Felbatol
fluvastatin	Lescol
gemfibrozil	Lopid
griseofulvin	Gris-PEG
indinavir	Crixivan
isoniazid	Nydrazid
ketoconazole	Nizoral
lamivudine	Epivir
leflunomide	Arava
lovastatin	Mevacor
meloxicam	Mobic
methotrexate	Rheumatrex
nevirapine	Viramune
niacin	Niaspan
oxcarbazepine	Rileptal
pentamidine	Pentam
pioglitazone	Actos
pravastatin	Pravachol
rifampin	Rifadin
ritonavir	Norvir
rosiglitazone	Avandia
rosuvastatin	Crestor
simvastatin	Zocor
tacrine	Ognex
terbinafine	Lamisil
tolcapone	Tasmar
valproic acid	Depakote

Adapted from: Tice AA, Parry D: Medications that require hepatic monitoring, *Hosp Pharm* 38(4):456, 2001.
*A list of the more common drugs requiring periodic liver function tests, usually at the beginning of therapy and then every few weeks to months thereafter. See individual monographs.
†Liver function tests routinely monitored are alkaline phosphatase (Alk-P), alanine aminotransferase (ALT), and aspartate aminotransferase (AST). If liver function tests become elevated, the physician should be notified for individualized treatment.

function and concentrating ability. There is, however, a great degree of individual variation in changes in renal function, and no prediction of renal function can be made solely on the basis of a person's age. Renal function of older adult patients should be, at a minimum, estimated using mathematic equations that factor in the patient's age. More optimally, renal function should be calculated by measuring urine creatinine specimens over time. Serum creatinine can give a general estimate of renal function, but in older adult patients these methods tend to exaggerate actual functional capability. This happens because the production of creatinine depends on muscle mass, which is diminished in older adults. Significant elevations occur only when there has been major deterioration of renal function. Blood urea nitrogen (BUN) concentration is also a poor predictor of renal function because it is significantly altered by diet, status of hydration, and blood loss either externally or into the GI tract (Table 3-3).

Therapeutic Drug Monitoring

Therapeutic drug monitoring is the measurement of a drug's concentration in biologic fluids to correlate the dosage administered and the level of medicine in the body with the pharmacologic response. Assay of blood (serum) samples for drug concentrations are most commonly used, but assays using saliva are being perfected for some medicines. Saliva samples have the advantage of easy collection of specimens without pain or the loss of blood that may require replacement by transfusion at a later date. Therapeutic drug monitoring is essential in neonates, infants, and children to ensure that drugs are within an appropriate therapeutic range, given the major physiologic changes that affect drug absorption, distribution, metabolism, and excretion. Dosage and frequency of administration must often be adjusted to help maintain therapeutic serum concentrations. Therapeutic drug monitoring is also routine in conditions such as epilepsy (e.g., phenytoin, carbamazepine, valproic acid, phenobarbital), arrhythmias (e.g., lidocaine, quinidine, procainamide), heart failure (e.g., digoxin), and antimicrobial therapy (e.g., gentamicin, tobramycin, isoniazid) to prevent toxicities and ensure that dosages are adequate to provide appropriate therapeutic levels. Blood levels of drugs can also be measured if toxicity is suspected. The extent to which a serum drug level is elevated may dictate how the toxicity should be treated (e.g., acetaminophen, digoxin). Blood and urine samples can also be obtained for legal purposes if it is suspected that drugs (e.g., ethanol, amphetamines, marijuana, benzodiazepines, cocaine) have been consumed illicitly. Appendix D lists medicines that are commonly monitored using serum assays to attain appropriate therapeutic effect.

The timing of the drug's administration and the collection of the specimen is crucial to the accurate interpretation of the data obtained after assay. Certain medicines (e.g., aminoglycosides: gentamicin, tobramycin) require that blood be drawn twice to assess

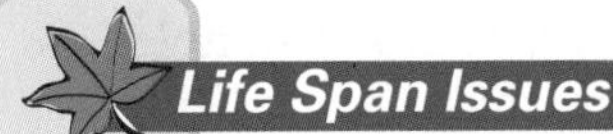

Life Span Issues

At birth, a preterm infant has up to 15% of the renal capacity of an adult, whereas a full-term newborn has approximately 35%. The filtration capacity of an infant increases to about 50% of adult capacity at 4 weeks of age and is equivalent to adult function at 9 to 12 months. Drugs excreted primarily by the kidneys (e.g., penicillin, gentamicin, tobramycin) must be given in increased doses or more often to maintain adequate therapeutic serum concentrations as renal function matures.

Table 3-3 ***Selected Medications that Require Dosage Adjustment In Renal Failure****

THERAPEUTIC CATEGORY	DRUG CLASS	EXAMPLES
Antibiotics	Aminoglycosides	amikacin, gentamicin, tobramycin
	Cephalosporins	cefotaxime, cefotetan, ceftazidime, ceftriaxone, cefuroxime, cefpodoxime
	Penicillins	ampicillin, piperacillin, ticarcillin
	Quinolones	ciprofloxacin, norfloxacin
	Others	vancomycin, minocycline, aztreonam, imipenem, cotrimoxazole, ethambutol
Antifungal agents		amphotericin B, fluconazole
Antiviral agents		acyclovir, ganciclovir, stavudine
Cardiovascular agents	ACE Inhibitors	benazapril, captopril, ramipril
	Antiarrhythmic agents	quinidine, flecainide, procainamide
	Beta-adrenergic blocking agents	atenolol, labetalol, pindolol
		metoprolol, nadolol, propranolol
	Digitalis glycoside	digoxin
Gastrointestinal agents	Histamine-2 antagonists	cimetidine, ranitidine
Other		lithium, allopurinol, meperidine, methotrexate

*Medicines are representative examples only. See the *Physicians' Desk Reference*, Montvale, NJ, 2006, or the *American Hospital Formulary Service—Drug Information*, Bethesda, Md, 2006, for appropriate dosing and monitoring parameters.

subtherapeutic levels and the potential for toxicity. One of the levels is drawn at 30 minutes before the next dose is to be administered to obtain the *trough* or lowest blood level of medicine, and another is drawn at 20 minutes after the medicine has been administered intravenously to obtain the *peak* or highest blood level. All institutions have policies that prescribe the best approach to therapeutic drug monitoring with specific medicines to ensure accuracy and usefulness of results. To coordinate blood draws with the timing of drug administration, check institutional policies on the handling of laboratory requests.

NURSING IMPLICATIONS WHEN MONITORING DRUG THERAPY

Chapter 4 discusses in detail how nursing actions are applied to pharmacology. In this chapter on drug action across the life span, it is appropriate to discuss nursing actions relating to high-risk populations, such as pediatric patients, elderly patients, pregnant patients, and breast-feeding patients.

Use of Monitoring Parameters

As described in Chapter 4 and Part Two of this text, all medicines have a series of parameters (e.g., expected therapeutic actions, expected side effects, reportable adverse effects, and probable drug interactions) that a nurse must be knowledgeable about before taking on the responsibility of administering medications to patients. When peak and trough levels for a medication have been ordered, it is important that the nurse check the laboratory results in a timely manner and make sure the physician is notified of the laboratory results. The next dosage of the medication should not be given until the dosage has been clarified based on the blood levels measured.

Although many of the same monitoring parameters (e.g., vital signs, urine output, and renal function tests) are used to plan dosages and monitor the effects of drug therapy in patients of all ages, it is absolutely crucial that the normal values for these monitoring parameters and laboratory tests be related to the age of the patient being monitored. For example, neonates have a greater respiratory and heart rate and lower normal blood pressure than adults. It is also important that measuring devices be suited to the individual patient (e.g., appropriately sized blood pressure cuff). Using a cuff that is too narrow yields a falsely high blood pressure because it takes extra pressure to compress the artery.

As with all medications, health teaching is important. Involving the appropriate family members, babysitters, and school nurse in the overall health teaching plan is essential (see Chapter 5). Identify those people who will be directly involved in the provision of care and provide instructions at an appropriate pace, keeping in mind that the patient's cultural beliefs and practices may differ from those of the caregiver.

Pediatric Patients

Children are not smaller versions of adults and therefore the principles of drug therapy cannot be extrapolated to infants and children only on the basis of size. Infants and children are at greater risk for complications from drug therapy because their body and organ functions are in an ongoing state of development.

General principles that a nurse can apply to the care of a pediatric patient include the following:

- Although infants and young children have a higher total body water content, they are more susceptible to dehydration from fever, vomiting, or diarrhea.
- Weight variations and growth spurts are expected in pediatric patients during normal maturation. Dosage adjustments are frequently necessary in patients who are taking medicine on a regular basis (e.g., seizure medicines, allergy medicines) because they "outgrow" their dosages. (See Appendix C for a nomogram to estimate body surface area.) Therefore it is important to obtain accurate height and weight measurements on a regular basis.
- Therapeutic drug monitoring is essential in neonates, infants, and children to ensure that drugs are within an appropriate therapeutic range. Document the precise times that blood samples are drawn and the time over which the medicine was infused for accurate interpretation of the results.
- It is often difficult to assess the therapeutic response to the medicines administered to neonates, infants, and young children because these patients are often nonverbal or cannot tell us "where it hurts." The nurse must rely more on laboratory values and assessment parameters such as temperature, pulse, respirations, heart sounds, lung sounds, bowel sounds, intake and output data, appetite, general appearance, and responsiveness.
- Nurses may find it difficult to accurately measure and administer doses of oral medicines to pediatric patients. The volume delivered by a household teaspoon ranges from 2.5 to 7.5 mL and may vary when the same spoon is used by different caregivers. The American Academy of Pediatrics recommends the use of appropriate devices for liquid administration, such as a medication cup, oral dropper, and oral syringe (see p. 132). Tablets and capsules can usually be swallowed by a child 5 years or older. Tablets that are not sustained-release or enteric-coated formulations may be crushed. Most capsules may be opened and the contents sprinkled on small amounts of food (e.g., applesauce, jelly, or pudding). Table 3-4 provides selected pediatric administration guidelines for oral administration.
- Oral and parenteral medicines available in powder form must be diluted properly according to

Table 3-4 ***Selected Guidelines for Administration of Oral Medicine to Pediatric Patients****

INFANTS
Use a calibrated dropper or oral syringe.
Support the infant's head while holding the infant in the lap.
Give small amounts of medicine to prevent choking.
If desired, crush nonenteric-coated or slow-release tablets to a powder and sprinkle on small amounts of food.
Provide physical comforting while administering medications to help calm the infant.
TODDLERS
Allow the toddler to choose a position in which to take the medication.
If necessary, disguise the taste of the medication with a small volume of flavored drink or small amounts of food (a rinse with a flavored drink or water will help remove an unpleasant aftertaste).
Use simple commands in the toddler's jargon to obtain cooperation.
Allow the toddler to choose which medications (if multiple) to take first.
Provide verbal and tactile responses to promote cooperation taking of medication.
Allow the toddler to become familiar with the oral dosing device.
PRESCHOOL CHILDREN
If possible, place a tablet or capsule near the back of the tongue, then provide water or a flavored liquid to aid in swallowing the medication.
If the child's teeth are loose, do not use chewable tablets.
Use a straw to administer medications that could stain teeth.
Use a follow-up rinse with a flavored drink to help minimize any unpleasant medication aftertaste.
Allow the child to help make decisions about dosage formulation, place of administration, medication to take first, and type of flavored drink to use.

Adapted from Isetts BJ, Brown LM: Patient assessment and consultation. In RR Berardi, editor: *Handbook of Non-Prescription Drugs,* ed 14, American Pharmaceutical Association, Washington, D.C., 2004.
*NOTE: For all age-groups listed, use a liquid dosage form if available.

manufacturers' directions to allow accurate measurement of doses and to prevent hyperosmolar solutions from being administered. When taken orally, hyperosmolar solutions may cause diarrhea and dehydration.

- Many medicines are not approved by the FDA for use in children. Physicians may still legally prescribe medicines for what is called *off-label use,* but it is important for the nurse to question a specific dose of medicine if it is not readily available for cross-checking in reference texts or the drug information service in the pharmacy. Document in the nurse's notes that the drug order was verified before administering the prescribed medicine. Be well versed in the monitoring parameters of the drug and report adverse effects to the physician.
- In general, salicylates (aspirin) should not be administered to pediatric patients from infancy through their teenage years. Children in this age-group are susceptible to a life-threatening illness known as Reye's syndrome if they ingest aspirin at the time of or shortly after a viral infection of chickenpox or influenza.
- Medicines routinely used for analgesia and antipyresis (fever reduction) in pediatric patients are ibuprofen and acetaminophen.
- Allergic reactions can occur quite rapidly in children, particularly if the medicine is administered intravenously. Reactions occur most commonly to antibiotics, especially penicillins. The nurse needs to be observant for response to medication administration and, if an event should occur, intervene promptly. The first symptoms may be intense anxiety, weakness, sweating, and shortness of breath. Other symptoms may include hypotension, shock, arrhythmia, respiratory congestion, laryngeal edema, nausea, and defecation. Summon assistance (call a "code" if severity warrants), stay with the child to provide comfort, facilitate breathing (administer oxygen, as needed), and if the child stops breathing, initiate cardiopulmonary resuscitation.

Geriatric Patients

Geriatric patients represent an ever-increasing portion of the population. Although people older than the age of 65 years in the United States represent about 14% of the population, they consume more than 25% of all prescription medicines and 33% of all nonprescription medicines sold. It is important that health care professionals understand the physiologic and pathologic changes that develop with advancing age and adjust drug therapy for the individual patient. Factors that place the older adult at greater risk for drug interactions or drug toxicity are reduced renal and hepatic function, chronic illnesses that require multiple drug therapy **(polypharmacy),** and a greater likelihood of malnourishment. Unfortunately, our lack of complete understanding of the effects of medicines in older

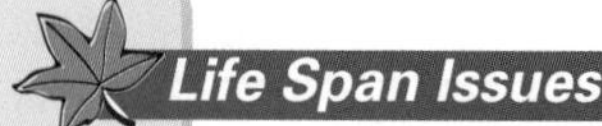

Life Span Issues

It is important that health care professionals understand the physiologic and pathologic changes that develop with advancing age and adjust drug therapy for the individual patient. Factors that place older adults at greater risk for drug interactions or drug toxicity include reduced renal and hepatic function, chronic illnesses that require multiple drug therapy (polypharmacy), and a greater likelihood of malnourishment.

adults also leads to the opposite problem of overuse, that of underuse. Caregivers walk a fine line between polypharmacy and undertreatment because of the complexity of chronic illnesses, changes in physiology and nutrition, compliance with multiple-drug regimens, and the pharmacokinetic factors associated with drug therapy during the later decades of a person's life. Although medicines may impair a geriatric patient's quality of life, medicines are also the most cost-effective treatment in preventing illness and disability in the geriatric population.

General principles that a nurse can apply to the care of a geriatric patient include the following:

- It is important to complete a thorough drug history, including use of nonprescription and herbal medicines (especially laxatives and antacids), nutritional supplements, and alternative therapy (e.g., aromatherapy, heat therapy, cold therapy).
- Likewise, a thorough nutrition history should be completed for the patient. Determine whether the patient's diet is balanced in carbohydrate, fat, protein, and vitamins. Assess whether a loss of teeth could interfere with chewing, or if loose-fitting dentures could make it difficult to chew.
- When evaluating a new symptom in a geriatric patient, determine first whether it was induced by medicines being taken. Adjustment of dosages or elimination of medicines is often the easiest, quickest, and most cost-effective therapy available.
- When discontinuing drug therapy, taper the dosage when appropriate (e.g., beta blockers, antidepressants) to prevent symptoms that can occur from sudden discontinuation.

When initiating therapy with a geriatric patient:

- Start at one third to one half the normal adult recommended dosage and gradually increase at appropriate intervals to assess for therapeutic effect and the development of adverse effects.
- Keep multidrug regimens simple; use aids such as a calendar or a pillbox with time slots to prevent confusion.
- Use therapeutic drug monitoring when serum drug level data are available for a particular medicine.
- Offer assistance in destroying old prescriptions to minimize confusion with the current medication regimen.
- Periodically review the regimen to see if any medications can be discontinued, such as allergy medicines in nonallergy season. Ask whether new prescriptions from other health care providers or nonprescription or herbal medicines have been started.
- Be alert to prescriptions for medications listed in Table 3-5. These medicines are considered to be potentially inappropriate (but not contraindicated) for elderly patients. Their use should be documented as the best alternative for a patient's particular needs.
- Geriatric patients may have difficulty with swallowing large tablets or capsules. Tablets may

Table 3-5 ***Potentially Inappropriate Medications for Geriatric Patients****

GENERIC NAME	BRAND NAME
AVOID	
barbiturates	Seconal, Nembutal
belladonna alkaloids	Donnatal
chlorpropamide	Diabinese
dicyclomine	Bentyl
flurazepam	Dalmane
hyoscyamine	Levsin, Levsinex
meprobamate	Equanil, Miltown
meperidine	Demerol
pentazocine	Talwin
propantheline	Pro-Banthine
trimethobenzamide	Tigan
RARELY APPROPRIATE	
carisoprodol	Soma
chlordiazepoxide	Librium, Librax
chlorzoxazone	Paraflex
cyclobenzaprine	Flexeril
diazepam	Valium
metaxalone	Skelaxin
methocarbamol	Robaxin
propoxyphene	Darvon
SOME INDICATIONS	
amitriptyline	Elavil
chlorpheniramine	ChlorTrimeton
cyproheptadine	Periactin
diphenhydramine	Benadryl
disopyramide	Norpace, Norpace CR
doxepin	Sinequan
hydroxyzine	Vistaril, Atarax
methyldopa	Aldomet
promethazine	Phenergan
reserpine	Serpasil
ticlopidine	Ticlid

Adapted from Zhan C, Sangl J, Bierman AS, et al: Potentially inappropriate medication use in the community-dwelling elderly, *JAMA* 286(22):2823, 2001; and Beers H: Explicit criteria for determining potentially inappropriate medication use by the elderly, *Arch Intern Med* 57:1531-1536, 1997.

*These medicines are still approved for use; however, it is felt that the adverse effects are generally more common and should be avoided in geriatric patients unless treatment has failed with other medicines.

need to be broken in half or crushed if there is a score mark on the tablet. Remember that timed-release tablets, enteric-coated tablets, and sublingual tablets should never be crushed because of the effect on the absorption rate and the potential for toxicity. Applesauce, ice cream, and jelly are good foods for administering crushed medications.

- It is extremely important that patients understand the purpose of the medication they are taking, and any complications that could occur if they discontinue the drug.
- When handing patients new prescriptions to be filled, inquire about their ability to pay for the new medicines. Do not let an inability to pay be a barrier to therapy; refer the patient to social services, as needed.

Pregnant Patients

Because of the potential for injury to the developing fetus, drug therapy during pregnancy should be avoided if at all possible. Studies indicate, however, that about two thirds of women take at least one drug while pregnant, and that about two thirds of the medicines are nonprescription self-care remedies. Medicines most commonly taken include acetaminophen, antacids, and cold and allergy products. Because few data are available for determining the safety of medicines in humans during pregnancy, very few medicines can be considered completely safe for use in pregnancy. Drugs that are known teratogens (causing birth defects) and thus contraindicated during pregnancy are listed in Table 3-6.

General principles that a nurse can apply to the care of a pregnant patient include the following:

- When taking a history, be alert to the possibility of pregnancy in any woman of childbearing age, especially those showing symptoms of early pregnancy, including nausea, vomiting (especially in the morning), and frequent urination.
- Complete a thorough drug history, including use of nonprescription and herbal medicines and nutritional supplements.
- Complete a thorough nutrition history; assess for a diet balanced in carbohydrates, fats, proteins, and vitamins. Good nutrition with appropriate ingestion of vitamins (especially folic acid) and minerals (calcium and phosphorus) are particularly important in preventing birth defects.
- Instruct the patient to avoid drugs, in general, at any stage of pregnancy, unless such use is recommended by the patient's physician.
- Advise against the consumption of alcohol during pregnancy. Excessive use may cause the child to be born with fetal alcohol syndrome, a lifelong condition that can be avoided by eliminating use of alcohol during pregnancy. If the woman is planning to become pregnant, it is recommended that she stop using alcohol 2 to 3 months before planned conception.
- Advise against the use of tobacco. Mothers who smoke have a higher frequency of miscarriage, stillbirths, premature births, and low-birthweight infants.
- Before using medicines, try nonpharmacologic treatments. For morning sickness the patient can try lying down when feeling nauseated; ingesting crackers or sipping small quantities of liquids before arising; eating small, frequent meals high in carbohydrates; or lowering fat content of meals. Avoid spicy foods, dairy products, and smells or situations that may cause vomiting.
- Herbal medicines have not been scientifically tested on humans during pregnancy and should be avoided.
- See also Chapter 41.

Table 3-6 Drugs Known to Be Teratogens

Drugs Known to Be Teratogens
ANDROGENIC AND ESTROGENIC HORMONES
oral contraceptives; diethylstilbestrol; chlorotrianisene; estrogens, conjugated; clomiphene
ANGIOTENSIN-CONVERTING ENZYME (ACE) INHIBITORS
benazepril, captopril, enalapril, fosinopril, lisinopril, moexipril, perindopril, ramipril, trandolapril
ANGIOTENSIN II RECEPTOR ANTAGONISTS
candesartan, eprosartan, irbesartan, losartan, olmesartan, telmisartan, valsartan
ANTICONVULSANTS
carbamazepine, phenytoin, trimethadione, valproic acid
ANTIMANIC AGENT
lithium
ANTITHYROID
propylthiouracil, methimazole
CHEMOTHERAPY
busulfan, cyclophosphamide, methotrexate
HYDROXYMETHYLGLUTARYL COENZYME A (HMG-CoA) REDUCTASE INHIBITORS (STATINS)
atorvastatin, fluvastatin, lovastatin, pravastatin, rosuvastatin
OTHER TERATOGENS
cocaine, ethanol (high dose, frequent use), isotretinoin, tetracycline, thalidomide, vitamin A (>18,000 international units/day), warfarin

Breast-Feeding Patients

Many drugs are known to enter breast milk of nursing mothers and have the potential to harm the infant. The American Academy of Pediatrics provides a list of medicines and their potential effects on nursing infants (Table 3-7).

General principles that a nurse can apply to the care of a patient who is breast-feeding include the following:

Table 3-7 ***Drugs and Nursing Infants***

DRUGS THAT MAY INTERFERE WITH METABOLISM OF A NURSING INFANT cyclophosphamide cyclosporine doxorubicin methotrexate **DRUGS OF ABUSE REPORTED TO HAVE ADVERSE EFFECTS ON NURSING INFANTS** amphetamine cocaine heroin marijuana phencyclidine **DRUGS FOR WHICH THE EFFECT ON NURSING INFANTS IS UNKNOWN, BUT MAY BE OF CONCERN** **Antianxiety Medicines** benzodiazepines (alprazolam, diazepam, prazepam, quazepam)	**Antidepressants** Cyclic antidepressants: amitriptyline, clomipramine, nortriptyline, desipramine, imipramine, doxepin, bupropion, nortriptyline, trazodone Serotonin reuptake inhibitors (SSRIs): fluoxetine, fluvoxamine, paroxetine, sertraline Antipsychotic drugs: chlorpromazine, clozapine, haloperidol, mesoridazine, trifluoperazine Others: amiodarone, chloramphenicol, lamotrigine, metronidazole **DRUGS ASSOCIATED WITH SIGNIFICANT EFFECTS ON NURSING INFANTS (GIVE TO NURSING MOTHERS WITH CAUTION)** aspirin beta-adrenergic blocking agents (acebutolol, atenolol) clemastine lithium phenobarbital primadone

Adapted from American Academy of Pediatrics: The transfer of drugs and other chemicals into human milk, *Pediatrics* 108(3):776-789, 2001.

- Although the levels of drug in breast milk may be safe, it is always best to discuss all medications, including prescription, nonprescription, and herbal products with the physician before taking the medicine.
- If medicine is being taken, encourage the mother to take her medicine immediately after the infant finishes breast-feeding or just before the infant's longer sleep periods. Educate the mother on what adverse effects might occur in the infant so that other therapy can be considered if necessary.

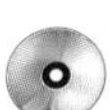

Go to your Companion CD-ROM for Appendices, an Audio Glossary, animations, Drug Dosage Calculators, customizable Patient Self-Assessment forms, and Review Questions for the NCLEX® Examination.

evolve Be sure to visit the companion Evolve site at http://evolve.elsevier.com/Clayton for WebLinks and additional online resources.

MEDICATION SAFETY REVIEW

CRITICAL THINKING QUESTIONS

1. What terms are used to describe people at different points of the life cycle?
2. Discuss what is meant by gender-specific medicine and reflect on possible implications for the future.
3. Cite conditions affecting the absorption of drugs applied to the skin.
4. Summarize the effects of gastric pH on drug absorption.
5. Describe the effect of enzyme systems on drug metabolism.
6. Discuss renal function levels in newborns, infants, adults, and the elderly. What are the possible effects on drug therapy?

CONTENT REVIEW QUESTIONS

1. Protein binding is _____ in preterm infants; therefore _____ dosage adjustments on a mg/kg basis would be required.
   1. the same in an adult as; no
   2. the same in the elderly as; no
   3. increased; lower
   4. reduced; higher loading

2. Enzyme systems are primarily found in the _____; therefore laboratory values to assess functioning of this organ may be a required premedication assessment.
   1. kidney
   2. liver
   3. lungs
   4. blood

3. Pediatric renal function is equivalent to that of an adult at:
   1. full-term birth.
   2. an infant at 4 weeks.
   3. an infant at 9 to 12 months.
   4. a young child at 2 years.

CHAPTER

4 The Nursing Process and Pharmacology

evolve http://evolve.elsevier.com/Clayton

Chapter Content

Objectives

1. Explain the purpose of the nursing process and methodology used to apply to the study of pharmacology.
2. State the five steps in the nursing process and describe them in terms of a problem-solving method used in nursing practice.

Key Terms

nursing process
nursing classification systems

THE NURSING PROCESS

The practice of nursing is an art and science that uses a systematic approach to identify and solve the potential problems individuals may experience as they strive to maintain basic human function along the wellness-illness continuum. The focus of all nursing care is to help individuals maximize their potential for maintaining the highest possible level of independence in meeting self-care needs. Conceptual frameworks for the basis of nursing practice, such as Henderson's Complementary-Supplement Model (1980), Roger's Life Process Theory (1979, 1980), Roy's Adaptation Model (1976), and the Canadian Nurses Association Testing Service (1980), are examples of models used today.

The **nursing process** is the foundation for the clinical practice of nursing. It provides the framework for consistent nursing actions, using a problem-solving approach rather than an intuitive approach. When implemented properly, the nursing process also provides a method to evaluate the outcomes of the therapy delivered. In addition to quality of care, the nursing process provides a scientific, transferable method for health care planners to assign nursing staff to patients and to determine and justify the cost of providing nursing care in this age of soaring health care costs.

The capabilities of electronic information systems and the need to control health care costs have led to the development of software that integrates the computer systems of large health care networks. These computer systems can be used to download information into regional and national databases, enabling evaluation of the quality of care provided and comparison of the costs associated with providing care. **Nursing classification systems** such as Nursing Minimum Data Set (NMDS), Nursing Interventions Classification (NIC), and Nursing Outcomes Classification (NOC) are designed to provide a standardized language for reporting and analyzing nursing care delivery that has been individualized for the patient. These information systems can measure and validate the impact of actual nursing diagnoses and interventions on outcomes for patients, families, and communities.

Many nursing education programs and health care facilities use a five-step model (i.e., assessment, nursing diagnosis, planning, implementation, and evaluation) that we will use for purposes of discussion (Table 4-1). These five steps are actually an overlapping process (Figure 4-1). Information from each step is used to formulate and develop the next step in the process. Table 4-1 illustrates the process used to assemble data and organize information into categories that help the learner identify the patient's strengths and problem areas. Thereafter, nursing diagnosis statement(s) can be developed and focused nursing assessments can be initiated. Planning can be individualized, and measurable goals and anticipated therapeutic outcomes can be identified. Concurrently, individualized nursing interventions can be developed to coincide with the individual's abilities, resources, and the disease processes being treated. During the implementation process the individual's physical, psychosocial, and cultural needs must be considered. The assessment process should continue to focus not only on the evolving changes in the presenting symptoms and problems, but also on the detection of potential complications that may occur (see p. 39 for the definitions of nursing diagnoses).

Nurses should familiarize themselves with the nurse practice act in the state where they practice, to identify the educational and experiential qualifications necessary to perform physical assessment and develop nursing diagnoses. Formulation of nursing diagnoses requires a broad knowledge base to make the discriminating judgments needed to identify the individual patient's care needs. All members of the health care

Table 4-1 Principles of the Nursing Process

ASSESSMENT	NURSING DIAGNOSES* STATEMENT(S)	PLANNING	INTERVENTION	EVALUATION
Collect all relevant data associated with the individual patient's diagnosis to detect actual, risk/high-risk, or possible problems needing intervention. Primary data sources Secondary data sources Tertiary data sources Based on the data collected, formulate a statement of the behaviors or problems of concern and the cause. This is referred to as an "actual" nursing diagnosis when the defining characteristics are present; as a "risk/high-risk" nursing diagnosis when there is a likelihood of the diagnosis developing or being prevented; or a "possible" nursing diagnosis when more data are required to substantiate or refute the problem. A "wellness" nursing diagnosis is a one-part diagnosis statement used for persons desiring and capable of attaining a higher level of wellness who currently have an effective health status. A "syndrome" nursing diagnosis is a cluster of actual and high-risk diagnoses likely to be present in certain situations. (Check hospital policy for the nursing personnel who are to assume responsibility for performing the assessment process.)	Formulate nursing diagnosis statements for problems amenable to nursing actions. Identify and seek orders/direction from appropriate health team members for *collaborative problems.*	Prioritize the problems identified from the assessment data, with the most severe or life-threatening first. Other problems are arranged in descending order of importance. (Maslow's hierarchy is frequently used as a basis for prioritizing; other approaches may be equally valid.) Develop short- and long-term patient goals/outcomes in measurable statements appropriate to the clinical setting and length of stay. Identify the monitoring parameters to be used to detect possible complications of the disease process or treatments being used. Plan nursing approaches to correlate with each identified patient goal/outcome. Integrate outcomes/ classification systems into critical pathways and/or standardized care plans utilized in clinical settings.	Perform the nursing intervention planned to achieve the established goals/outcomes. Monitor the patient's response to treatments, and monitor for complications related to existing pathophysiology. Provide for patient safety. Perform ongoing assessments on a continuum. Document care given and additional findings on the patient chart.†	Evaluation is an ongoing process that occurs at every phase of the nursing process. Establish target data to review and analyze at intervals prescribed by guidelines in the practice setting. Review and analyze the data regarding the patient and modify the care plan so that goals/outcomes of care (used to return the patient to the highest level of functioning) are attained. Evaluate outcomes using the classification system and critical pathways and/or standardized care plans utilized in the clinical setting. Unrealistic goals/ outcomes may require revision or discontinuation. Follow a systematic approach to recording progress, depending on the setting and charting methodology. Continue the nursing process, initiate referral to a community-based health agency, or execute discharge procedures as ordered by the health care provider.

*Nursing diagnosis: Because not all patient problems are amenable to resolution by nursing actions, those complications or problems associated with medical diagnosis or from treatment-related complications are placed in a category known as *collaborative problems* that the nurse monitors.

†Integrate classification system currently in use in the clinical setting when charting (e.g., NMDS [Nursing Minimum Data Set], NIC [Nursing Interventions Classification], NOC [Nursing Outcomes Classification]) or others (e.g., The Omaha System, Home Health Care Classification).

team need to contribute data regarding the patient's care needs and response to the prescribed treatment regimen.

Just as body functions are constantly undergoing adjustments to maintain homeostasis in the internal and external environment, the nursing process is an ongoing, cyclic process that must respond to the changing requirements of the patient. The nurse must continually interact with people in a variety of settings to creatively and cooperatively establish and execute nursing functions to meet the holistic care needs of patients (see Figure 4-1).

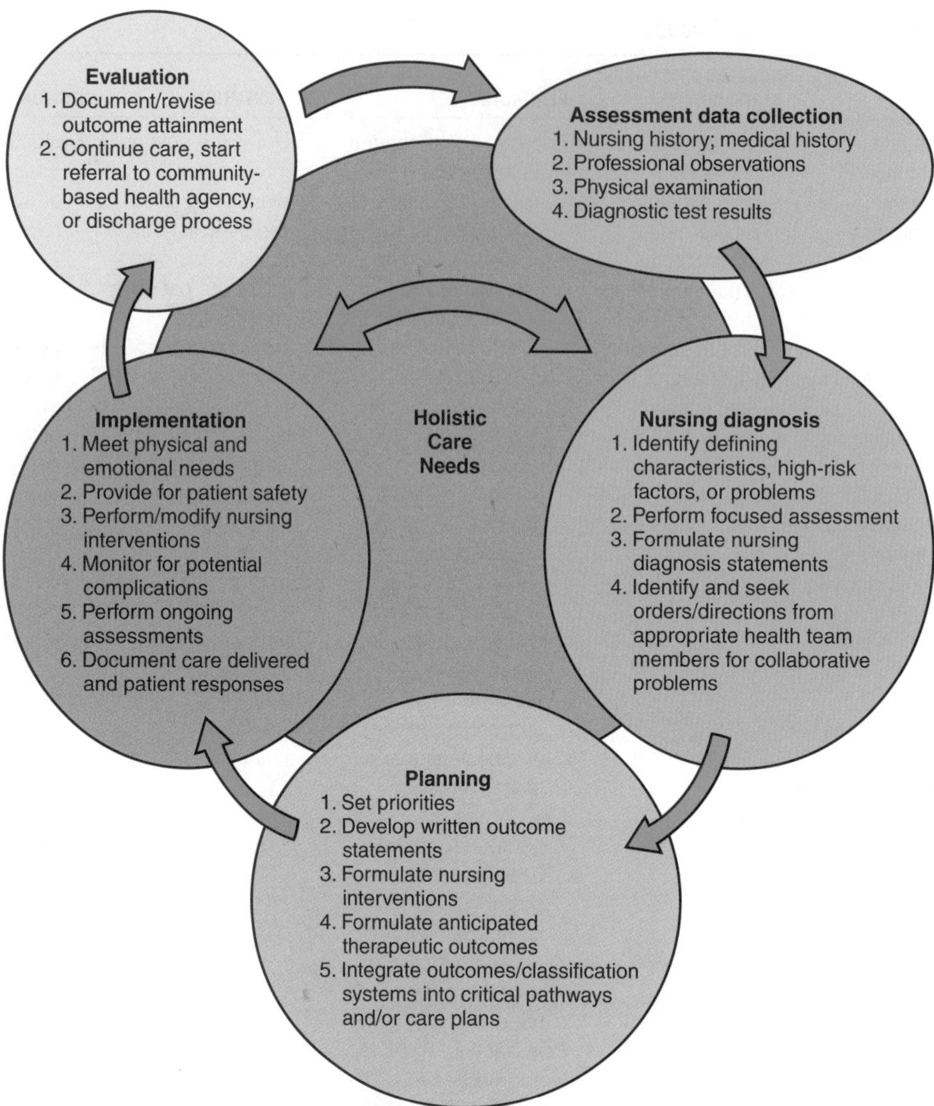

FIGURE **4-1** The nursing process and the holistic needs of the patient.

Assessment

Objectives

1. Describe the components of the assessment process.
2. Compare current methods used to collect, organize, and analyze information about the health care needs of patients and their significant others.

Key Term

assessment

Assessment is an ongoing process that starts with the admission of the patient and continues until the patient is discharged from care. It is the problem-identifying phase of the nursing process. The initial assessment must be performed by a registered nurse who has the necessary assessment skills to complete the physical examination and the knowledge base to analyze the data assembled and identify patient problems based on defining characteristics (i.e., signs, symptoms, and clinical evidence). In addition, the nurse should identify risk factors that cause an individual or group of people to be more vulnerable to the development of certain problems in response to a disease process or to the prescribed therapeutic interventions when used (e.g., side effects to drugs that may require modification of the regimen).

During the assessment phase, the nurse collects a comprehensive information base about the patient from the physical examination, nursing history, medication history, and professional observation. Formats commonly used for data collection, organization, and analysis are the head-to-toe assessment, body systems assessment, or Gordon's Functional Health Patterns Model. Both the head-to-toe and body systems approaches focus on physiology and thereby limit the nurse's knowledge of sociocultural, psychological, spiritual, and developmental factors affecting the individual's needs. Box 4-1 shows Gordon's Functional Health Patterns Model.

Box 4-1 Gordon's Functional Health Patterns Model

1. Health Perception–Health Management Pattern
2. Nutrition-Metabolic Pattern
3. Elimination Pattern
4. Activity-Exercise Pattern
5. Cognitive-Perceptual Pattern
6. Sleep-Rest Pattern
7. Self-Perception–Self-Concept Pattern
8. Role-Relationship Patterns
9. Sexuality-Reproductive Patterns
10. Coping–Stress Tolerance Pattern
11. Value-Belief Pattern

From Gordon M: *Nursing diagnosis: process and application*, ed 3, St Louis, 1994, Mosby.

Nursing Diagnosis

Objectives

1. Define the term *nursing diagnosis* and discuss the wording used in formulating nursing diagnosis statements.
2. Define the term *collaborative problem.*
3. Differentiate between a nursing diagnosis and a medical diagnosis.
4. Differentiate between problems that require formulation of a nursing diagnosis and those categorized as collaborative problems, which may not require nursing diagnosis statements.

Key Terms

nursing diagnosis
actual nursing diagnosis
risk/high-risk nursing diagnosis
possible nursing diagnosis
wellness nursing diagnosis
syndrome nursing diagnosis
defining characteristics
medical diagnosis
collaborative problem
focused assessment

Nursing diagnosis is the second phase of the five-step nursing process. The North American Nursing Diagnosis Association International (NANDA-I) approved the following official definition relating to nursing diagnosis: *A clinical judgment about individual, family, or community responses to actual or potential health problems/life processes.* Nursing diagnoses provide the basis for the selection of nursing interventions to achieve outcomes for which the nurse is accountable (Figure 4-2, *A* and *B*).

A systematic method of working with patients is used to identify five types of nursing diagnoses: (1) actual, (2) risk/high-risk, (3) possible, (4) wellness, and (5) syndrome nursing (patient problems). This text will focus on actual, risk/high-risk, and possible nursing diagnoses, particularly those related to drug therapy that influence the actions the nurse must initiate to correct the problems encountered.

Actual nursing diagnosis: Based on human responses to health conditions and life processes that exist in an individual, family, or community. It is supported by defining characteristics (manifestations or signs and symptoms) that cluster in patterns of related cues or inferences.

Risk/high-risk nursing diagnosis: A clinical judgment that an individual, family, or community is more susceptible to the problem than others in the same or similar situation. It is supported by risk factors that contribute to increased vulnerability. In some instances when an individual is more likely to develop a particular problem the phrase *high risk for* is added.

Possible nursing diagnosis: Suspected patient problems requiring additional data for confirmation.

Wellness nursing diagnosis: A clinical judgment about an individual, group, or community in transition from a specific level of wellness to a higher level of wellness.

Syndrome nursing diagnosis: These nursing diagnoses cluster actual or high-risk signs and symptoms that are predictive of certain circumstances/events. The etiologic (causative) or contributing factors for the diagnosis are contained in the diagnostic label. The five currently approved syndrome diagnoses are (1) Rape-Trauma Syndrome, (2) Disuse Syndrome, (3) Post-Trauma Syndrome, (4) Relocation Stress Syndrome, and (5) Impaired Environmental Interpretation Syndrome.

Using knowledge and skill in anatomy, physiology, nutrition, psychology, pharmacology, microbiology, nursing practice skills, and communication techniques, the nurse analyzes the data collected to identify whether certain major and minor **defining characteristics** (manifestations or signs and symptoms) relate to a particular patient problem. If so, the nurse may conclude that certain actual problems are present. These patient-related problems are referred to as a *nursing diagnosis.* See Figure 4-2, *A* for steps in determining an actual nursing diagnosis and Figure 4-2, *B* for differentiating between a risk nursing diagnosis and possible nursing diagnoses.

It should be noted that not all patient problems identified during an assessment are treated by the nurse alone. Many of the identified problems require a multidisciplinary approach. When the nurse cannot legally order the definitive interventions required under the presenting circumstances, a collaborative problem exists (Figure 4-3).

As nursing care has gained recognition as a cognitive process in planning patient care, national conferences have been held to identify the diagnostic terms that describe areas of potential health problems nurses should anticipate and may treat. NANDA International has revised the listing, and NANDA-I's Taxonomy 2005 is included in Box 4-2.

A **medical diagnosis** is a statement of the patient's alterations in structure and function and results in a diagnosis of a disease or disorder that impairs normal physiologic function. A *nursing diagnosis* usually refers

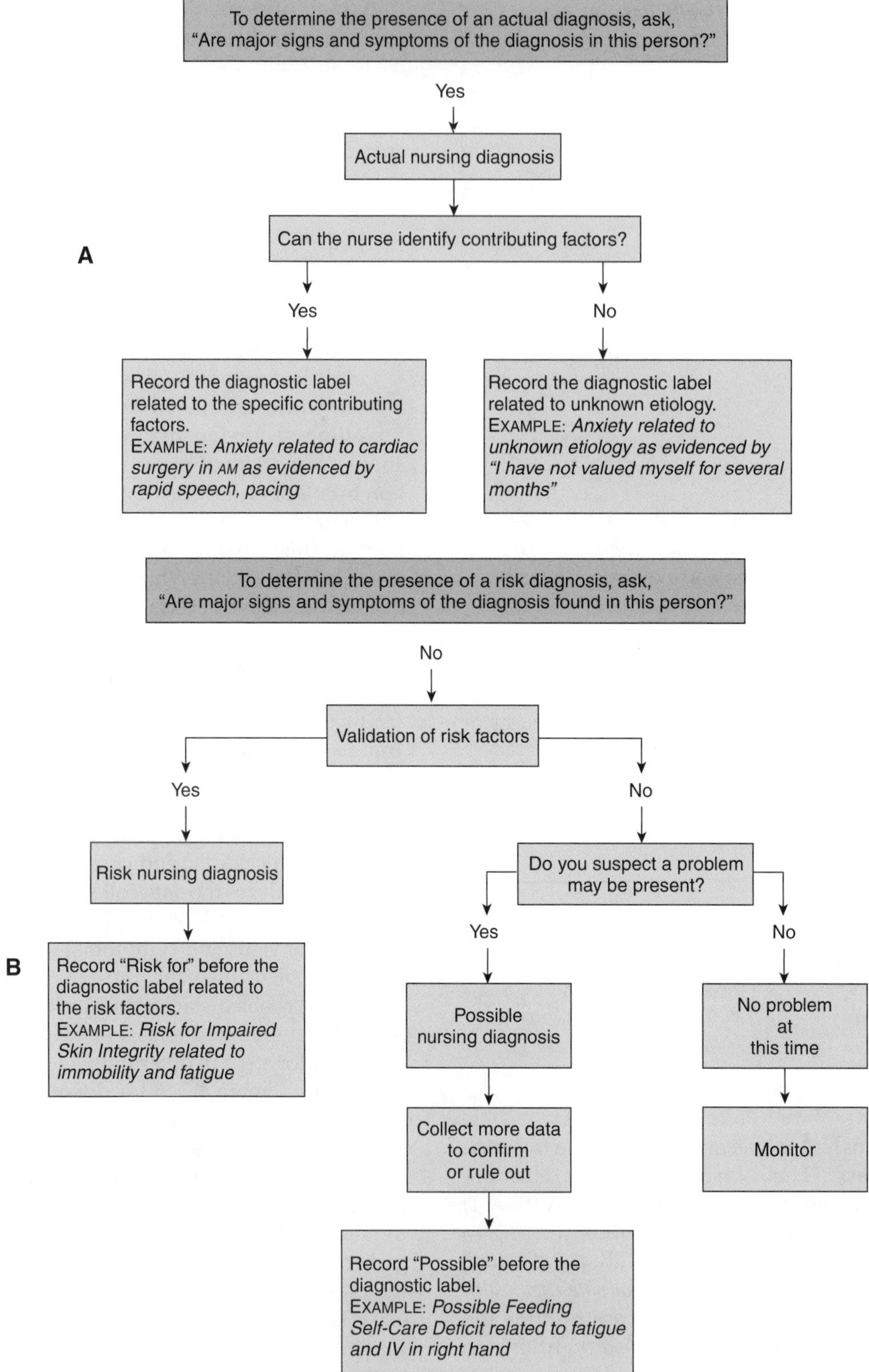

FIGURE **4-2** **A,** Decision tree for actual nursing diagnosis. **B,** Decision tree for differentiating between a risk and possible nursing diagnosis.

to the patient's ability to function in activities of daily living (ADLs) in relation to the impairment induced by the medical diagnosis; it identifies the individual's or group's response to the illness. A medical diagnosis also tends to remain unchanged throughout the illness, whereas nursing diagnoses may vary depending on the patient's state of recovery. Concepts that help distinguish a nursing diagnosis from a medical diagnosis include the following.

1. Conditions described by nursing diagnoses can be accurately identified by nursing assessment methods.

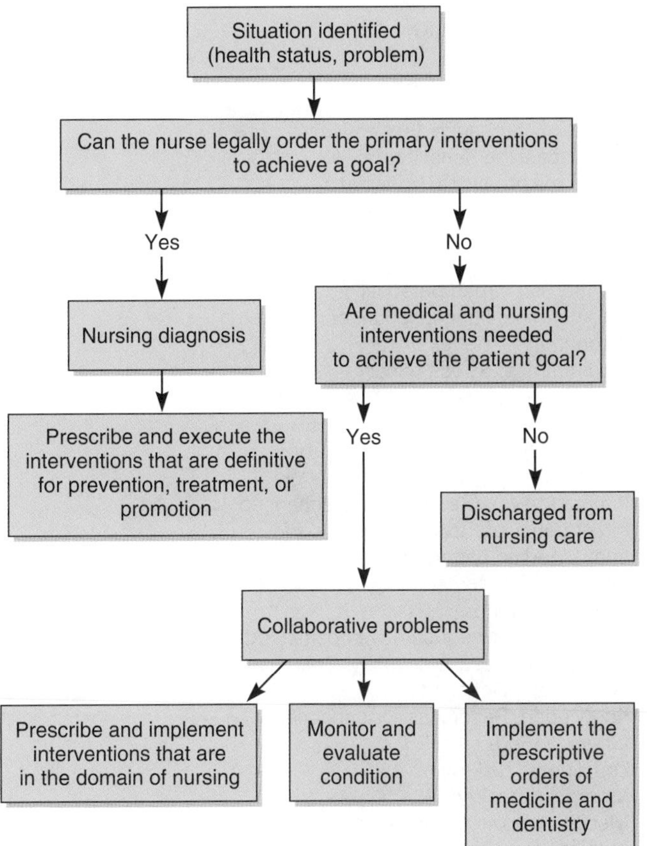

FIGURE **4-3** Differentiation of nursing diagnosis from collaborative problems.

2. Nursing treatments, or methods of risk factor reduction, can resolve the condition described by a nursing diagnosis.
3. Because the necessary treatment to resolve a nursing diagnosis is within the scope of nursing practice, nurses assume accountability for outcomes.
4. Nurses assume responsibility for the research required to clearly identify the defining characteristics and etiologic factors, and to improve methods of treatment and treatment outcomes for conditions described by nursing diagnoses (Gordon, 1987).

The wording of an *actual nursing diagnosis* takes the form of a three-part statement. These statements consist of (1) a diagnostic label from the NANDA-I–approved list, (2) the contributing factors or cause if known or, if not known, stated as *etiology unknown*, and (3) the defining characteristics (manifestations or signs and symptoms).

The *risk/high-risk nursing diagnosis* statement consists of two parts: (1) the diagnostic label from the NANDA-I–approved list, and (2) the risk factors that make the individual or group more susceptible to the development of the problem. A risk diagnosis is validated by the presence of risk factors that would contribute to the individual or group developing the stated problem. High-risk diagnoses are used for patients who are particularly vulnerable to a problem.

Possible nursing diagnosis identifies a problem that may occur, but the assembled data are insufficient to confirm it. Possible nursing diagnoses are worded as two-part statements that include the diagnostic label and the suspected, unconfirmed etiology or unconfirmed defining characteristics (see Figure 4-2).

A *wellness nursing diagnosis* statement has only a one-part label. It is initiated by *potential for enhanced,* followed by the nursing diagnosis being applied to the situation or group. The individual or group must understand that the higher level of functioning is feasible. This diagnosis can be applied only to individuals or groups when the potential for a higher level of wellness is realistic.

Further discussion of the philosophy and clinical use of nursing diagnoses; the specifics regarding the wording of *actual, risk/high-risk,* and *possible* nursing diagnoses; and the new categories of *wellness* and *syndrome* nursing diagnoses can be found in other primary texts and reference works, especially those developed solely for the purpose of explaining nursing diagnoses.

Collaborative Problems

Not all patient problems identified by the nurse can be resolved by nursing actions. The nurse is, however, responsible for monitoring the patient on a continuum for potential complications that are associated with the medical diagnosis, diagnostic procedures, or treatments prescribed. To differentiate between a problem requiring a nursing diagnosis and a **collaborative problem,** the nurse must decide whether the definitive interventions can be ordered to prevent or treat the problem to maintain the health status of the patient (Carpenito, 1985, 1987, 1990, 1995, 2002, 2005). See Figure 4-3 for an illustration of this decision-making process. Collaborative problem statements are worded with *potential complication* (PC). An example would be: PC: Hypokalemia. Outcome criteria for collaborative problems are found on critical pathways or multidisciplinary plans.

Focused Assessment

A **focused assessment** is the process of collecting additional data specific to a patient or family that validates a suggested problem or nursing diagnosis. The questions asked or data collected are used to confirm or rule out the defining characteristics associated with a specific nursing diagnosis statement. During the focused assessment collaborative problems requiring prescriptive orders can be identified and differentiated from problems the nurse can prescribe and implement nursing actions for within the nurse's scope of practice.

Box 4-2 ***Nursing Diagnoses Approved by NANDA International (2005-2006)****

Activity intolerance
Activity intolerance, Risk for
Adjustment, Impaired
Airway clearance, Ineffective
Allergy response, Latex
Allergy response, Risk for latex
Anxiety
Anxiety, Death
Aspiration, Risk for
Attachment, Risk for impaired parent/infant/child
Autonomic dysreflexia
Autonomic dysreflexia, Risk for
Body image, Disturbed
Body temperature, Risk for imbalanced
Bowel incontinence
Breastfeeding, Effective
Breastfeeding, Ineffective
Breastfeeding, Interrupted
Breathing pattern, Ineffective
Cardiac output, Decreased
Caregiver role strain
Caregiver role strain, Risk for
Communication, Impaired verbal
Communication, Readiness for enhanced
Conflict, Decisional
Conflict, Parental role
Confusion, Acute
Confusion, Chronic
Constipation
Constipation, Perceived
Constipation, Risk for
Coping, Compromised family
Coping, Defensive
Coping, Disabled family
Coping, Ineffective
Coping, Ineffective community
Coping, Readiness for enhanced
Coping, Readiness for enhanced community
Coping, Readiness for enhanced family
Denial, Ineffective
Dentition, Impaired
Development, Risk for delayed
Diarrhea
Disuse syndrome, Risk for
Diversional activity, Deficient
Energy field, Disturbed
Environmental interpretation syndrome, Impaired
Failure to thrive, Adult
Falls, Risk for
Family processes: Alcoholism, Dysfunctional
Family processes, Interrupted
Family processes, Readiness for enhanced
Fatigue
Fear
Fluid balance, Readiness for enhanced
Fluid volume, Deficient
Fluid volume, Excess
Fluid volume, Risk for deficient
Fluid volume, Risk for imbalanced
Gas exchange, Impaired
Grieving, Anticipatory
Grieving, Dysfunctional
Grieving, Risk for dysfunctional
Growth, Risk for disproportionate
Growth and development, Delayed
Health maintenance, Ineffective
Health-seeking behaviors
Home maintenance, Impaired
Hopelessness
Hyperthermia
Hypothermia
Identity, Disturbed personal
Incontinence, Functional urinary
Incontinence, Reflex urinary
Incontinence, Stress urinary
Incontinence, Total urinary
Incontinence, Urge urinary
Incontinence, Risk for urge urinary
Infant behavior, Disorganized
Infant behavior, Readiness for enhanced organized
Infant behavior, Risk for disorganized
Infant feeding pattern, Ineffective
Infection, Risk for
Injury, Risk for
Injury, Risk for perioperative-positioning
Intracranial adaptive capacity, Decreased
Knowledge, Deficient
Knowledge, Readiness for enhanced
Lifestyle, Sedentary
Loneliness, Risk for
Memory, Impaired
Mobility, Impaired bed
Mobility, Impaired physical
Mobility, Impaired wheelchair
Nausea
Neglect, Unilateral
Noncompliance
Nutrition, Readiness for enhanced
Nutrition: less than body requirements, Imbalanced
Nutrition: more than body requirements, Imbalanced
Nutrition: more than body requirements, Risk for imbalanced
Oral mucous membrane, Impaired
Pain, Acute
Pain, Chronic
Parenting, Impaired
Parenting, Readiness for enhanced
Parenting, Risk for impaired
Peripheral neurovascular dysfunction, Risk for
Poisoning, Risk for
Post-trauma syndrome
Post-trauma syndrome, Risk for
Powerlessness
Powerlessness, Risk for
Protection, Ineffective
Rape-trauma syndrome
Rape-trauma syndrome, compound reaction
Rape-trauma syndrome, silent reaction
Religiosity, Impaired
Religiosity, Readiness for enhanced
Religiosity, Risk for Impaired
Relocation stress syndrome
Relocation stress syndrome, Risk for
Role performance, Ineffective
Self-care deficit, Bathing/hygiene
Self-care deficit, Dressing/grooming
Self-care deficit, Feeding

Modified from North American Nursing Diagnosis Association International: *Nursing diagnoses: definitions and classification 2005-2006,* Philadelphia, 2005, NANDA International.

**New diagnoses appear in italics.*

Box 4-2 Nursing Diagnoses Approved by NANDA International (2005-2006)—cont'd

Self-care deficit, Toileting
Self-concept, Readiness for enhanced
Self-esteem, Chronic low
Self-esteem, Situational low
Self-esteem, Risk for situational low
Self-mutilation
Self-mutilation, Risk for
Sensory perception, Disturbed
Sexual dysfunction
Sexuality pattern, Ineffective
Skin integrity, Impaired
Skin integrity, Risk for impaired
Sleep, Readiness for enhanced
Sleep deprivation
Sleep pattern, Disturbed
Social interaction, Impaired
Social isolation
Sorrow, Chronic
Spiritual distress
Spiritual distress, Risk for
Spiritual well-being, Readiness for enhanced
Sudden Infant Death Syndrome, Risk for
Suffocation, Risk for
Suicide, Risk for
Surgical recovery, Delayed
Swallowing, Impaired
Therapeutic regimen management, Effective
Therapeutic regimen management, Ineffective
Therapeutic regimen management, Ineffective community
Therapeutic regimen management, Ineffective family
Therapeutic regimen management, Readiness for enhanced
Thermoregulation, Ineffective
Thought processes, Disturbed
Tissue integrity, Impaired
Tissue perfusion, Ineffective
Transfer ability, Impaired
Trauma, Risk for
Urinary elimination, Impaired
Urinary elimination, Readiness for enhanced
Urinary retention
Ventilation, Impaired spontaneous
Ventilatory weaning response, Dysfunctional
Violence, Risk for other-directed
Violence, Risk for self-directed
Walking, Impaired
Wandering

Planning

Objectives

1. Identify the steps in the planning of nursing care.
2. Explain the process of prioritizing individual patient needs using Maslow's hierarchy of needs.
3. Formulate measurable goal statements for assigned patients in the clinical practice setting.
4. State the behavioral responses around which goal statements revolve when the discharge of a patient is planned.
5. Identify the purposes and uses of a patient care plan.
6. Integrate outcome/classification system(s) and critical pathways into care plans.
7. Differentiate between nursing interventions and therapeutic outcomes.

Key Terms

nursing care plan
critical care pathway
priority setting
measurable goal statements
patient goals
nursing action
nursing intervention
nursing orders
anticipated therapeutic statements
expected outcome statements

Once the patient has been assessed and problems have been diagnosed, plans should be formulated to meet the patient's needs. Planning usually encompasses four phases: (1) priority setting, (2) development of measurable goal/outcome statements, (3) formulation of nursing interventions, and (4) formulation of anticipated therapeutic outcomes that can be used to evaluate the patient's status. The written or computer-generated document that evolves from this planning process is called the **nursing care plan.** Handwritten care plans are being replaced by critical pathways, which use standardized, automated care plans that integrate standards, interventions, and goals/outcomes within electronic medical records (EMRs).

A **critical care pathway** is a standardized care plan derived from "best practice" patterns, enabling the nurse to develop a treatment plan that sequences detailed clinical interventions to be performed over a projected amount of time for a specific case type or disease process. One type of critical care pathway, the CareMap, is used to document patient progress toward established outcomes needed for discharge. The clinical interventions are integrated into the care plan and are evaluated on a continuum to achieve the patient outcomes desired and to provide for delivery of quality care in an efficient, economical manner.

When the care plan is completed using the format adopted in a particular health care setting, it is placed in the patient's Kardex, chart, or the EMR, where it serves as a communication system for all health care providers. Because care needs are constantly changing, the care plan and priorities also must be evaluated and modified on a continuing basis to meet the patient's needs.

Priority Setting

After the nursing diagnoses and collaborative problems have been identified, they must be prioritized. Maslow's hierarchy of needs is a model often used to establish priorities. Maslow identified five levels of needs, beginning with physiologic needs at the lowest point on the hierarchy and ending with self-actualization needs at the highest point. Nurses can use Maslow's hierarchy to perform **priority setting** of an individual patient's needs by organizing them in relation to their direct effects on the maintenance of homeostasis. Usually, physiologic needs such as oxygenation, temperature maintenance, or nutritional and fluid requirements take precedence over psychological needs. Table 4-2 lists the priority ranking of Maslow's subcategories of human needs.

Measurable Goal/Outcome Statements

After the patient's needs have been prioritized, goals must be established and statements written. Goals are usually divided into short-term and long-term plans, depending on the length of stay and clinical site. The **measurable goal statements** start with an action word (verb), followed by the behavior(s) to be performed by the patient or family, with a specific amount of time allocated for attainment.

NOC is a comprehensive standardized classification system of patient/client outcomes developed to evaluate the effect of nursing interventions on patient care. These outcomes have been linked to NANDA International diagnoses, Gordon's functional patterns, the Taxonomy of Nursing Practice, Omaha System problems, resident admission protocols (RAPs) used in nursing homes, the Outcome and Assessment Information Set (OASIS) System used in home care, and NIC (see following) interventions. Each outcome has a definition, a list of indicators used to evaluate patient status in relation to the outcome, a target outcome rating, a place to identify the source of data, a five-point Likert scale to measure patient status, and a short list of references used in the development of the outcome. Standardized outcomes are necessary for documentation in electronic records, for use in clinical information systems, for the development of nursing knowledge, and the education of professional nurses. NOC is one of the standardized languages recognized by the American Nurses Association (ANA).

All goal/outcome statements must be individualized and based on the patient's abilities. The nurse must also refer to critical care pathways when establishing the parameters. Statements must take into consideration the degree of rehabilitation that is realistic

Table 4-2 ***Priority Ranking of Maslow's Subcategories of Human Needs***

PHYSIOLOGIC NEEDS	**SELF-ESTEEM NEEDS**
Oxygen, circulation	Recognition
Water-salt balance	Dignity
Food balance	Appreciation from others
Acid-base balance	Importance, influence
Waste elimination	Reputation of good character
Normal temperature	Attention
Sleep, rest, relaxation	Status
Activity, exercise	Dominance over others
Energy	**SELF-ACTUALIZATION NEEDS**
Comfort	Personal growth and maturity
Stimulation	Awareness of potential
Cleanliness	Increased learning
Sexuality	Full development of potential
SAFETY NEEDS	Improved values
Protection from physical harm	Religious, philosophic satisfaction
Protection from psychological threat	Increased creativity
Freedom from pain	Increased reality perception and problem-solving abilities
Stability	Less rigid conventionality
Dependence	Less of the familiar, more of the novel
Predictable, orderly world	Greater satisfaction in beauty
BELONGING NEEDS	Increased pleasantness
Love and affection	Less of the simple, more of the complex
Acceptance	
Warm, communicating relationship	
Approval from others	
Unity with loved ones	
Group companionship	

From Campbell C: *Nursing diagnosis and intervention in nursing practice,* New York, 1978, John Wiley & Sons.

for the patient in the amount of time during which the care will be delivered. It is sometimes difficult to accept that not everyone can return to their preillness health status; therefore the nurse must be realistic in setting a measurable goal, and strive to assist the individual to an optimal degree of functioning that is consistent with personal capabilities.

When goals are being established, it is important to include the patient and appropriate significant others in decision making, because the patient and his or her support systems will be responsible for accomplishing the goals. Involvement of the patient is essential to promote cooperation and compliance with the therapeutic regimen and a sense of control over the disease process and course of treatment. The goals established should be **patient goals,** not nursing goals for the patient.

With the advent of shorter hospital stays, most of the goal statements will be short-term goals. The nurse must keep in mind the usual length of hospitalization and be realistic about the number and types of goals/outcomes being established. Short-term goals should serve as a bridge to meet the long-term goals established in a care plan. Long-term goals can be established with assistance from referral agencies as appropriate to the individual's needs and circumstances. The long-term goals are then implemented in long-term care settings, rehabilitation centers, mental health facilities and community-based home health care delivery settings.

The planning process may be scheduled with all significant others present at one or more meetings. Today, the case manager plays an important role in this process. It is important to convey a willingness to consider each person's input into the final plan. The strengths and weaknesses of each participant in the final care plan must be analyzed, and the patient goal statements must be realistically achievable for the group. Most goal statements are based on the patient's need to do the following:

1. Reduce or resolve the symptoms (usually the chief complaint) of the disease that caused the person to seek medical attention.
2. Understand the disease process and its effect on lifestyle and ADLs.
3. Gain knowledge and skills associated with the treatment procedures so as to attain the highest level of function possible (e.g., nutrition, comfort measures, medication regimen, and physical therapy).
4. Understand reasonable expectations of the therapy, including signs and symptoms of improvement versus complications requiring health care provider consultation.
5. Identify monitoring parameters that should be maintained on a written record that reflects the response to the prescribed therapy.
6. Establish a schedule for follow-up evaluation.

The beginning practitioner should consult a text on nursing diagnosis for further information on the correct wording of measurable goal statements associated with nursing diagnosis and collaborative problems.

Nursing Actions or Nursing Interventions

Nursing action or **intervention** statements list in a concise form exactly what the nurse will do to achieve each goal developed for each nursing diagnosis. A nursing action is a statement that describes nursing interventions applicable to any patient (e.g., promote adequate respiratory ventilation). **Nursing orders** describe how specific actions will be implemented for an individual patient.

EXAMPLES:

(date): Cough, turn, deep breathe: 0800, 1000, 1200, 1600, 1800, 2000, 2200

(date): Educate patient re: abdominal breathing, splinting the abdomen, pursed-lip breathing, and assuming correct position to facilitate breathing

(date): Auscultate breath sounds: 0800, 1200, 1600, 2000

(date): Increase patient's fluid intake to at least 2000 mL/24 hr:
0700-1500: 1000 mL
1500-2300: 800 mL
2300-0700: 200 mL

(date): Assess respiratory depth and rate: 0800, 1200, 1600, 2000, 2400

NIC is a comprehensive, research-based, standardized classification of interventions that nurses perform. This is useful for clinical documentation, communication of care across settings, integration of data across systems and settings, effectiveness research, productivity measurement, competency evaluation, reimbursement, and curricular design. This system includes the interventions that nurses do on behalf of patients/clients, both independent and collaborative interventions, both direct and indirect care. NIC can be used in all settings and all specialties.

Anticipated Therapeutic and Expected Outcome Statements

Measurable **anticipated therapeutic** and **expected outcome statements** are also developed to document the effectiveness of the care delivered. In the previous example, the patient will do the following:

- Improve the ability to perform coughing technique.
- Maintain an adequate fluid intake as evidenced by achieving a mutually set goal of 2000 mL within 24 hours.
- Attain a respiratory rate between 18 and 24 breaths per minute.
- Perform ADLs without feeling fatigued.

Therapeutic and expected outcomes have been developed throughout this book for each drug classification. These can be used by the student to identify the outcomes anticipated from the use of the drugs listed in a particular classification.

EXAMPLE:
The primary therapeutic outcome expected from the benzodiazepine antianxiety agents is a decrease in the level of anxiety to a manageable level for the patient (e.g., coping is improved, physical signs of anxiety such as look of anxiety, tremor, and pacing are reduced).

Nursing Intervention or Implementation

Objective

1. Compare the types of nursing functions classified as dependent, interdependent, and independent and give examples of each.

Key Terms

nursing intervention or implementation
nursing actions
dependent actions
interdependent actions
independent actions

Nursing intervention or implementation is the actual process of carrying out the established plan of care. Nursing care is directed at meeting the physical and emotional needs of the patient, providing for patient safety, monitoring for potential complications, and performing ongoing assessments as a part of the continual process of data collection and evaluation to identify changes in the patient's care needs. **Nursing actions** are suggested by the etiologies of the problems identified in the nursing diagnoses and are used to implement plans. They may include activities such as counseling, teaching, providing comfort measures, coordinating, referring, using communication skills, and performing a health care provider's orders. Documentation of all care given, including patient education and the patient's apparent response, should be performed regularly, both to assist in evaluation and reassessment and to make other health care professionals aware of the patient's changing needs.

Nursing Actions

Within the nursing process are three types of nursing actions: (1) dependent, (2) interdependent, and (3) independent. **Dependent actions** are those performed by the nurse based on the health care provider's orders, such as the administration of prescribed medications and treatments. It is important to note that even though this is a dependent function, the nurse is still responsible for exercising professional judgment in performing the action. **Interdependent actions** are those nursing actions the nurse implements cooperatively with other members of the health care team for restoring or maintaining the patient's health. This allows the nurse to coordinate his or her interventions with those of other health professionals to maximize knowledge and skills from various disciplines for the well-being of the patient. **Independent actions** are those nursing actions not prescribed by a health care provider that a nurse can provide by virtue of the education and licensure attained. These actions are usually written in the nursing care plan and originate from the nursing diagnosis.

Evaluating and Recording Therapeutic and Expected Outcomes

Objective

1. Describe the evaluation process used to establish whether patient behaviors are consistent with the identified short-term or long-term goals.

The final step of the nursing process is evaluation of the expected outcomes of the patient's behavior. All care is evaluated against the established nursing diagnoses (goal statements), planned nursing actions, and anticipated therapeutic outcomes. For the evaluation process to be successful, the participants (patient, family, significant others, and nurse) must be willing to receive feedback. Therefore plans for evaluation must involve the patient, family, and significant others from the beginning and should recognize the needs of a culturally diverse population with varying beliefs about health care.

Although the evaluation phase is the last step in the nursing process, it is not an end in itself. Evaluation recognizes successful completion of previously established goals, but it also provides a means for input of new, significant data indicating the development of additional problems or a lack of therapeutic responsiveness that may require additional nursing diagnoses or collaboration with the health care provider or other professionals on the health care team as plans for therapy are revised.

RELATING THE NURSING PROCESS TO PHARMACOLOGY

Assessment

Objectives

1. State the information that should be obtained as a part of a medication history.
2. Identify primary, secondary, and tertiary sources of information used to build a patient information base.

Key Terms

drug history
primary source
subjective data
objective data
secondary sources
tertiary sources

Assessment is an ongoing process that starts with the admission of the patient and is completed at the time of discharge. In relating the nursing process to the nursing functions associated with medications, assessment includes taking a **drug history** for three reasons: (1) to evaluate the patient's need for medication; (2) to obtain his or her current and past use of over-the-counter (OTC) medication(s), prescription medication(s), herbal products, and street drugs; and (3) to identify problems related to drug therapy. Nurses will also want to identify risk factors such as allergy to certain medications (e.g., penicillins), or the presence of other diseases (e.g., hypertension) that may limit the use of certain types of drugs (e.g., sympathomimetic agents).

The nurse draws on three sources to build the medication-related information base. Whenever the patient is able to provide reliable information, the patient should be used as the **primary source** of information. Subjective and objective data serve as the baseline for the formulation of drug-related nursing diagnoses. **Subjective data** are information provided by the patient (e.g., "Whenever I take this medicine I feel sick to my stomach"). **Objective data** are gained from observations that the nurse makes using physiologic parameters (e.g., skin pale, cold, and moist; temperature 99.2° F orally). Other required objective information is the patient's height and weight, which may be needed to select drug regimens and a monitoring parameter for drug therapy later.

In some cases it is necessary to obtain information from **secondary sources** (e.g., relatives, significant others, medical records, laboratory reports, nursing notes, or other health care professionals). Secondary sources of information are subject to interpretation by someone other than the patient. Data collected from secondary sources should be analyzed using other portions of the database to validate the conclusions reached.

Tertiary sources of information, such as a literature search, provide an accurate depiction of the characteristics of a disease, nursing interventions, diagnostic tests used, pharmacologic treatment prescribed, diets, physical therapy, and other factors pertinent to the patient's care requirements. When using these sources, the nurse should be aware that the patient has individual needs and that the plan of care must be adapted to the patient's identified needs.

Assessment related to drug therapy continues throughout the hospitalization period. Examples of ongoing assessment activities include visiting with the patient; the need for as needed (PRN) medication; monitoring vital signs; and observation for therapeutic effects, side effects to expect, side effects to report, and potential drug interactions.

In preparation for the patient's eventual discharge and need for education about new health-related responsibilities, the assessment process should include collection of data related to the patient's health beliefs, existing health problems, prior compliance with prescribed regimens, readiness for learning both emotionally and experientially, and ability to learn and execute the skills required for self-care.

Nursing Diagnoses

Objectives

1. Define the problem.
2. Describe the process that is used to identify factors that could result in patient problems when medications are prescribed.
3. Review the content of several drug monographs to identify information that may result in patient problems from the medication therapy.

Key Terms

drug monographs
side effects

To deal effectively with identified problems (diagnoses), the nurse must recognize the etiologic and contributing factors.

The etiologic and contributing factors are those clinical and personal situations that can cause the problem or influence its development. Situations can be organized into five categories: (1) pathophysiologic, (2) treatment related, (3) personal, (4) environmental, or (5) maturational (Carpenito, 2002).

When identifying problems related to medication therapy, the nurse should review the **drug monographs** given later in this text for each prescribed drug. Several nursing diagnoses can be formulated based on the patient's drug therapy. Although the most commonly observed are those associated with drug treatment of a disease or the **side effects** from drug therapy, nursing diagnoses can also originate from pathophysiology caused by drug interactions.

EXAMPLES:

Drugs prescribed for Parkinson's disease are administered to provide relief of symptoms (e.g., muscle tremors, slowness of movement, muscle weakness with rigidity, and alterations in posture and equilibrium). An actual nursing diagnosis of *Mobility, impaired physical: related to neuromuscular impairment (Parkinson's disease)* would be formulated based on the defining characteristics established for this nursing diagnosis. These nursing diagnoses are labeled as (indications) in the nursing diagnosis subsection of the nursing process related to drug therapy sections throughout the textbook, meaning that the diagnosis is associated with the medical diagnosis or signs and symptoms of the disease process for which the medications are being prescribed. Evaluation of the therapeutic and expected outcomes from the prescribed medications is based on the degree of improvement noted in the symptoms present.

A second nursing diagnosis would be *Injury, risk for: related to amantadine side effects (confusion, disorientation, dizziness, light-headedness)*. Nursing diagnoses of this type are labeled as side effects in the nursing diagnosis subsection of the nursing process related to drug therapy sections throughout the book.

In this example, side effects of the drug amantadine, prescribed to treat the symptoms of the disease, is also the basis of the first nursing diagnosis. The second nursing diagnosis is a collaborative problem that requires the nurse to monitor the development of these side effects. In other words, a patient with Parkinson's disease is at risk of developing the defining characteristics needed to have this occur. When the defining characteristics are observed, notification of the health care provider is required, and the nurse would need to intervene to provide for the patient's safety.

Two nursing diagnoses that apply to all types of medications prescribed are as follows:

- Deficient knowledge (actual, risk, or possible) related to: the medication regimen (patient education).
- Noncompliance (actual, risk, or possible) related to: the patient's value system, cognitive ability, cultural factors, or economic resources.

Planning

Objectives

1. Identify steps used to plan nursing care in relation to a medication regimen prescribed for a patient.
2. Describe an acceptable method of organizing, implementing, and evaluating the patient education delivered.
3. Practice developing short- and long-term patient education objectives and have them critiqued by the instructor.

Key Terms

therapeutic intent
side effects to expect
side effects to report

Planning, with reference to the prescribed medications, must include the following steps:

1. Identification of the **therapeutic intent** for each prescribed medication. Why was the drug prescribed? What symptoms should be relieved?
2. Review of the drug monograph in this text to identify the **side effects to expect** (symptoms that can be alleviated or prevented by actions of the nurse or patient will require immediate planning for patient education).
3. Review of the drug monograph in this text to identify the **side effects to report** (a collaborative problem in which the nurse has a responsibility to monitor the patient for adverse effects of drug therapy and report suspected adverse effects to the health care provider).
4. Identification of the recommended dosage and route of administration (compare the recommended dosage with the dosage ordered; confirm that the route of administration is correct and that the dosage form ordered can be tolerated by the patient).
5. Scheduling of the administration of the medication based on the health care provider's orders and the policies of the health care facility (medications prescribed must be reviewed for drug-drug interactions and drug-food interactions; laboratory tests may also need to be scheduled if serum levels of the drug have been ordered).
6. Teaching the patient to keep written records of his or her responses to the prescribed medications (see Appendix I).
7. Additional education as needed on techniques of self-administration, such as injection, topical patches, or instillation of drops.
8. Information as needed on proper storage, how to refill a medication, or how to fill out an insurance claim for reimbursement.

Priority ranking in preparation for health education may encompass several factors: (1) the patient's concerns and health belief system and the patient's priorities; (2) the urgency or time available for the learning to take place; (3) a sequence that allows the patient to move from the simple to the more complex concepts; and (4) a review of the overall needs of the individual. The content taught to the patient should be well planned and delivered in increments that the patient is capable of mastering. The complete teaching plan should be in the Kardex, on the patient's chart, or in the EMR.

EXAMPLE:
Mr. Jones will be able to state the following for each prescribed medication by (date) and will show retention of this information by repeating it on (date):

1. Drug name
2. Dosage
3. Route and administration times
4. Anticipated therapeutic response
5. Side effects to expect
6. Side effects to report
7. What to do if a dosage is missed
8. When, how, or if to refill the medication

To attain this goal, the patient's ability to name all these factors would need to be checked at the initial time of exposure and on subsequent meetings to validate retention. Once the goals have been formulated, they should not be considered final but should be reevaluated as needed throughout the course of treatment.

Possible NOC labels that could be used for the previously mentioned nursing diagnosis are:

- Deficient knowledge (actual, risk, or possible) related to: the medication regimen (patient education).
  NOC—Knowledge: Medication
- Noncompliance (actual, risk, or possible) related to: the patient's value system, cognitive ability, cultural factors, or economic resources.
  NOC—Compliance Behavior

Nursing Intervention or Implementation

Objective

1. Differentiate among dependent, interdependent, and independent nursing actions and give an example of each.

Nursing actions applied to pharmacology may be categorized as dependent, interdependent, or independent.

Dependent Nursing Actions

The health care provider admits the patient, states the admitting diagnosis, and orders diagnostic procedures and medications for the immediate well-being of the patient. The health care provider reviews data on a continuing basis to determine the risks and benefits of maintaining or modifying the medication orders. Maintenance or modification of the medication orders is the health care provider's responsibility; however, the data collected and recorded by the nurse on the patient's chart are essential for evaluation of the effectiveness of the medications prescribed.

Interdependent Nursing Actions

The nurse performs baseline and subsequent assessments that are valuable in establishing therapeutic goals, duration of therapy, detection of drug toxicity, and frequency of reevaluation.

The nurse should approach any problems related to the medication prescribed collaboratively with appropriate members of the health care team. Whenever the nurse is in doubt about medication calculations, monitoring for therapeutic efficacy and side effects, or the establishment of nursing interventions or patient education, another qualified professional should be consulted.

The pharmacist reviews all aspects of the drug order, then prepares the medications and sends them to the unit for storage in a medication room or a unit dose medication cart. If any portion of the drug order or the rationale for therapy is unclear, the nurse and pharmacist may consult with each other or the health care provider for clarification.

The frequency of medication administration is defined by the health care provider in the original order. The nurse and pharmacist establish the schedule of the medication based on the standardized administration times used at the practice setting. The nurse, and occasionally the pharmacist, also coordinates the schedule of the medication administration and the collection of blood samples with the laboratory phlebotomist to monitor drug serum levels.

The nurse completes laboratory test requisitions based on the health care provider's orders to monitor drug therapy, establish dosages, and identify the most effective medication for pathogenic microorganisms.

As soon as laboratory and diagnostic test results are available, the nurse and pharmacist review them to identify values that could have an influence on drug therapy. The results of the tests are conveyed to the health care provider. The nurse should also have current assessment data available for collaborative discussion of signs and symptoms that may relate to the medications prescribed, dosage, therapeutic efficacy, or adverse effects.

Patient education, including discharge medications, requires that an established plan be developed, written in the patient's medical record, implemented, documented, and reinforced by all persons delivering care to the patient (see the sample teaching plan on p. 65).

Independent Nursing Actions

The nurse visits with the patient and obtains the nursing history, which includes a medication history. The history of current and past medications, including prescription, OTC, herbal products, and street drugs, is reviewed to identify treatment-related problems.

The nurse verifies the drug order and assumes responsibility for correct transcription of the drug order to the nurse's Kardex, medication administration record (MAR), or computer. As part of the transcribing process, the nurse makes professional judgments concerning the class of drug, therapeutic intent, usual dosage, and the patient's ability to tolerate the drug dosage form ordered. If all aspects of the verification and transcription procedure are considered to be correct, a copy of the original order is sent to the pharmacy.

The nurse formulates appropriate nursing diagnoses and actions to monitor for therapeutic effects and side effects of medications. To do this, the nurse may need to review drug monographs to formulate the diagnoses and goal statements. Criteria for therapeutic responses should describe the improvement expected in symptoms of the disease for which the medication was prescribed.

The nurse prepares the prescribed medications using procedures to ensure patient safety. As part of this process, nursing professional judgments must include the following:

1. Selection of the correct supplies (e.g., needle gauge, length, type of syringe) for administration of the medications.
2. Verification of all aspects of the medication order before preparing the medication; the order should be verified again immediately following preparation and again before actual patient administration (patients should always be identified immediately before administration of the medication, and each time a medication is to be administered). One of the National Patient Safety Goals established by the Joint Commission on Accreditation of Healthcare Organizations (JCAHO) is to improve the accuracy of patient identification. It is now recommended that two patient identifiers, neither of which is the room number, be used when administering medications. For example,

Text continued on p. 56

Table 4-3 The Nursing Process Applied to the Patient's Pharmacologic Needs

ASSESSMENT	NURSING DIAGNOSIS	PLANNING	INTERVENTION	EVALUATION
DATA COLLECTION				
Collect data on patient symptoms Disease process is based on the history and physical examination, patient and/or family information, nursing assessments, and interview	Analyze data collected during assessment process and develop actual, risk/high-risk, or possible nursing diagnosis statement(s) appropriate for individual patient Identify/seek orders from appropriate health team members for collaborative problems.	Identify and prioritize: • Patient problems • Baseline assessment data to be monitored to evaluate the patient's symptoms • Anticipated drug side effects and those to report • Examine drug monograph and data to determine the therapeutic outcomes	Perform the identified baseline patient assessments on a regularly scheduled basis (e.g., blood pressure, pulse, respirations, pain level [frequency, duration, activity associated with onset], presence of leg pain)	Analyze data collected on a continuum; chart and report *changes* of significance in the baseline data and/or patient's status; report escalation of symptoms or ineffective response to drug therapy
DRUG HISTORY				
Ask questions in a simple, direct manner to elicit information about drugs currently being taken, or those taken during the preceding year; ask about over-the-counter drugs, including herbal products used on a regular basis		Plan to monitor patient's total drug needs; develop goals to deal with any drug interactions, incompatibilities, or diagnostic tests potentially affected by drugs being administered Examine drug monograph to identify premedication data needed	Perform drug preparation, scheduling, and administration to coincide with specific patient needs or problems	Analyze data collected on a continuum
Ask about any prior drug "allergies" and specifics of the "reaction" and treatment used		Plan to monitor patient at risk for the development of an allergic reaction	Perform premedication assessment, and implement monitoring parameters Implement monitoring parameters	Analyze observed symptoms for potential drug reaction or interactions; report alterations to the prescribing health care provider
Age and disease process present		Plan modifications in dosage, administration technique, and observations if the individual's age and physiologic status indicate problem with drug absorption, distribution, metabolism, or excretion; confirm drug doses BEFORE administering any drug in question	Implement the proper administration of confirmed drug doses	As therapy continues, analyze the patient's weight, mental status, and disease processes that may be indicative of a problem with drug absorption, distribution, metabolism, or excretion; report abnormal laboratory values or *changes* from the patient's baseline assessment data
Body weight		Plan to weigh the patient daily or as needed	Perform the procedure of weighing the patient at the same time, in the same weight clothing, and on the same scale at the intervals ordered	Report weight gains or losses (this is of particular importance with drugs such as digitalis glycosides, corticosteroids, thyroid medications, and chemotherapy)

Metabolic rate		Plan nursing intervention to correlate with diseases that alter metabolic rate (e.g., hyperthyroidism, hypothyroidism, heart failure)	Institute nursing measures directed at nutritional status, activity/exercise needs, environmental alterations needed	Analyze effectiveness of approaches utilized; observe closely for an increase or decrease in therapeutic effect
MONITORING PARAMETERS				
Laboratory data (see Appendix D for normal values): review data to determine potential problems in absorption, distribution, metabolism, and elimination of prescribed drug	Analyze data collected during assessment process and develop actual, risk/high-risk, or possible nursing diagnosis statement(s) appropriate for the individual patient	Follow hospital policies for ordering and assisting with laboratory/diagnostic test; always check for drugs that may interact with scheduled laboratory tests		
Hepatic function		AST, ALT, alkaline phosphatase, LDH, GGT, bilirubin (total and direct); A/G ratio	Complete appropriate forms to order tests; assist in drawing blood samples and providing patient support during procedure	As soon as results are received on the unit, report any abnormal diagnostic value to the health care provider
Renal function		Serum creatinine, creatinine clearance, BUN, urinalysis, protein (total and 24-hr urine)	Same as above Collect urine sample by clean catch or, if ordered, by catheterization Check for drugs being given and record on urinalysis slip Send urine sample to laboratory promptly after collection; make certain it is refrigerated/iced as appropriate Always record the exact start date/time and end date/time on laboratory slip for 12 hr/24 hr urine collection (e.g., urine creatinine)	Elevated serum creatinine levels generally indicate renal disease Elevated BUN levels occur in renal disease, dehydration, a high-protein diet, or a catabolic state Depressed BUN levels are found in severe hepatic damage, overhydration, and malnutrition In a urinalysis, always report RBCs, casts, crystals, proteinuria, glycosuria, high or low pH, or specific gravity outside the normal range (1.000-1.017)
In addition to the previous test, the following tests may be used to monitor disease and drug				
• Infectious disease • Assessment for site/source of the infection		Culture and sensitivity (C&S)	Collect specimen properly to maintain sterility of the culture tip so that the source examined is the only surface touched Label appropriately; take to laboratory immediately	Report results of a C&S promptly; particularly important are results that indicate that the drug being administered is not effective against the organism cultured

ALT, Alanine aminotransferase; *AST*, aspartate aminotransferase; *BUN*, blood urea nitrogen; *GGT*, gamma-glutamyltransferase; *LDH*, lactic dehydrogenase; *RBCs*, red blood cells.

Continued

Table 4-3 The Nursing Process Applied to the Patient's Pharmacologic Needs—cont'd

ASSESSMENT	NURSING DIAGNOSIS	PLANNING	INTERVENTION	EVALUATION
MONITORING PARAMETERS—cont'd				
• Complete blood count (CBC)		Plan intervention based on the organism, the site of the infection, fever, hematuria, and drainage	Implement nursing measures to deal effectively with the patient's needs—fever, pain, drainage, and degree of precautions appropriate to the organism	Elevated WBCs, bands, segs, lymphocytes need to be reported to the health care provider Analyze subsequent CBC reports for significant changes; continue performing baseline assessments to detect degree of responsiveness to therapy
Assessment of drug therapy		Minimum inhibitory concentration (MIC) and minimum effective concentration (MEC)	MIC measures sensitivity of a particular organism to various antimicrobial agents, (expressed as mcg/ml); this is minimum amount of drug needed to inhibit an organism growth in a laboratory The MEC is the minimum concentration level of a drug in the blood plasma required to achieve a therapeutic response; toxic concentrations occur when the drug level is too high Record drug name, dosage, and time and route of administration on requisition	The MIC test is one of several factors considered by the health care provider when selecting an antibiotic; there is an increased drug sensitivity in infants due largely to the immaturity of their body systems and pharmacokinetic processes (absorption, metabolism, excretion, drug protein binding, and blood brain barrier to the CNS)
MONITORING OF DRUG LEVELS				
Routinely monitored: digoxin theophylline, aminoglycosides, lithium, lidocaine, phenytoin, procainamide, quinidine, vancomycin, cyclosporine, chloramphenicol (see Chapter 49, Appendix D)	Analyze data collected during the assessment process and develop actual, risk/high-risk, or possible nursing diagnosis statement(s) appropriate for the individual patient	Plan to requisition the laboratory tests ordered by the health care provider to monitor serum blood levels at the scheduled times; ensure that the patient will be available at the required times Therapeutic monitoring is usually accomplished through the use of peak level (highest concentration of drug in blood serum) and trough level (lowest concentration of drug in blood serum)		Therapeutic doses of certain drugs can be established through a combination of monitoring of serum levels and patient assessments of essential data *Example:* Aminoglycosides (e.g., gentamicin)—Patient's age and disease factors modify dosage needs; therefore patients with cardiac, pulmonary, or renal dysfunction may require serum concentration as a guide to dosage amounts. *The current clinical status of the patient is always important; therefore regular assessments specifically planned to detect therapeutic and toxic activity are imperative to effective patient management*

				Check specific drug monographs for other drugs that may alter laboratory results; report results promptly for the health care provider's evaluation
Other laboratory tests		Prothrombin time (PT) expressed as International Normalized Ratio (INR) (for warfarin) Partial thromboplastin time (PTT) (for heparin)	Requisition the prescribed laboratory test so that the drug dosage can be ordered by the health care provider; perform nursing assessments associated with anticoagulant therapy and the disease process specifically being treated	Be certain the correct date and patient data are relayed to the health care provider when seeking or confirming the anticoagulant drug order; always double check the date, time, and specific dosage of the anticoagulant drug order; anticoagulants should be checked with a second qualified nurse at the time of preparation and administration
		Blood glucose	Withhold daily insulin until blood sample is drawn; test blood for glucose as ordered or ac and hs; check for daily and sliding scale insulin orders	Correlate the results of the laboratory reports to the patient's status and degree of response to drug therapy; carefully evaluate patient symptoms for hyper- and hypoglycemia Report laboratory data and patient status changes to the health care provider
		Glycosylated hemoglobin	Measures average blood glucose control for past 120 days No food or fluid restriction	
		Fructosamine	Measures average blood glucose control for previous 1 to 3 wk	
NURSE'S RESEARCH OF PRESCRIBED DRUGS				
Drug action: review introductory nursing assessments in specific drug monographs to correlate drug action and monitoring parameters to the patient's presenting symptoms and disease process	Analyze data collected during the assessment process and develop actual, risk/high-risk, or possible nursing diagnosis statement(s) appropriate for the individual patient	Develop goal statements for monitoring presence or absence of response Plan the administration schedule to correlate with known information about time of administration in relation to food, tests, and planned sleep Plan interventions to minimize or alleviate drug-related complications (side effects)	Assess the patient for baseline data before administering the drug; assess at regular intervals to evaluate therapeutic response to the drug Administer the prescribed drug: RIGHT patient RIGHT drug RIGHT dose RIGHT route RIGHT time RIGHT documentation	Document all assessments by carefully recording all pertinent observations in the patient's chart Analyze the collected data and compare to the baseline data gathered before initiation of drug therapy; report significant changes in the patient's status

ac, Before meals; *CNS*, central nervous system; *hs*, at bedtime; *WBCs*, white blood cells.

Continued

Table 4-3 The Nursing Process Applied to the Patient's Pharmacologic Needs—cont'd

ASSESSMENT	NURSING DIAGNOSIS	PLANNING	INTERVENTION	EVALUATION
NURSE'S RESEARCH OF PRESCRIBED DRUGS—cont'd				
Side effects to expect		Consult specific drug monographs for side effects to expect; plan assessments to detect and the intervention to manage these as they occur	Monitor the patient for development of expected side effects; implement measures designed to effectively manage or minimize effects; assist patient to understand and cope with specific symptoms as developed	Once expected side effects develop, evaluate the nursing measures designed to minimize or reproduce the effects; report lack of responsiveness; modify intervention appropriately; analyze the patient's level of tolerance of the side effects
		Plan specific teaching that incorporates side effects to expect	Teach which side effects to expect and how to alleviate discomfort Encourage the patient to discuss relevant symptoms with the health care provider and to adhere to the medication prescribed; suggest discussion of symptoms and encourage cooperative planning for modifications in the medications taken; discourage discontinuance or self-adjusted dosages	Document specific teaching performed and the degree of understanding observed through direct questioning and return demonstrations Analyze verbal and nonverbal behaviors observed to detect patient response to suggestion of cooperative goal-setting between the health care provider and patient
Side effects to report		Plan nursing assessments and intervention for side effects that are serious and require reporting Develop a specific teaching plan that incorporates teaching of side effects to report Plan teaching of necessary monitoring parameters (e.g., blood pressure, pulse, respirations, daily weights)	Perform regularly scheduled nursing assessments to detect any side effects from drug therapy that should be reported Perform health teaching of the observations the patient should make and the findings that require reporting Teach and repeat at appropriate intervals to achieve patient/family mastery	Analyze data collected on a continuum; report deviations appropriately Carefully evaluate the patient's attitude toward adherence with drug therapy and intent to report problems for discussion and needed modifications Evaluate the degree of accuracy attained by the patient or family members; refer to social services or community agencies if assistance is needed at time of discharge

Patient understanding of drug therapy	Analyze data collected during the assessment process and develop actual, risk/high-risk, or possible nursing diagnosis statement(s) appropriate for the individual patient	Plan teaching of drug name, dosage, route of administration, and exact time schedule; record overall teaching plan on the Kardex or chart Plan teaching of medications taken on a PRN basis (e.g., nitroglycerin) and establish goals to evaluate understanding of frequency of dose, repeating of dose, and lack of response Plan teaching of any self-administration techniques (oral, inhalation, injection, rectal, etc.)	Throughout the hospitalization, discuss medication information and how it will benefit the course of treatment; seek cooperation and understanding of the following points so that medication adherence may be enhanced: 1. Name 2. Dosage 3. Route and administration times 4. Anticipated therapeutic response 5. Side effects to expect 6. Side effects to report 7. What to do if a dose is missed 8. When, how, or if to refill the medication prescription Teach name of drug being taken, symptoms that can be relieved by the PRN drug, when to take it, amount to take, what to do if not effective Teach administration techniques to be used at home; give simple written instructions to follow at home	Document teaching performed and the individual's understanding; try role-playing a situation or, when appropriate during hospitalization, have the patient describe what needs to be done Validate the patient/significant other's understanding by return demonstration; document teaching of administration techniques and degree of understanding in nurse's notes
Patient understanding of entire treatment plan		Develop goal statements for teaching the individual's care that will assist the patient in gaining knowledge of all aspects of self-care for the disease process present (nutritional status, activity or exercise modifications, psychologic, medication, physical therapy, etc.) Incorporate assessments to determine the individual's readiness and capability to learn, degree of understanding, and tolerance for needed alterations	Implement planned nursing measures appropriate to the specific disease process affecting the individual Incorporate teaching techniques (e.g., visual aids, demonstrations and return demonstrations, role playing)	Analyze the patient's response to *each* component of the entire treatment plan Throughout the courses of teaching, establish target dates to evaluate the degree of understanding by having the patient perform appropriate activities (e.g., choose the therapeutic diet from the hospital menu) Evaluate the tolerance exhibited to restrictions and modifications implemented or to drug side effects expected and present; document all facets of health teaching performed, degree of understanding attained, or intolerances observed or experienced

best practice would be to look at the patient's name band for identity, but also request that the patient state his or her name and birth date.
3. Collection of appropriate data, also known as premedication assessment(s) to serve as a baseline for later assessments of therapeutic effectiveness and to detect adverse effects of drugs.
4. Administration of the medication by the correct route at the correct site. The selection and rotation of sites for medication should be based on established practices for rotation of sites and on principles of drug absorption, which in turn may be affected by the presence of pathophysiologic characteristics, such as poor tissue perfusion.
5. Documentation in the chart of all aspects of medication administration; subsequent assessments should be documented to identify the drug efficacy, the development of expected side effects, or any adverse effects.
6. Implementation of nursing actions to minimize expected side effects and to identify side effects to be reported promptly.
7. Education of patients as appropriate for the medications prescribed, in addition to other facets of the therapeutic regimen; when noncompliance is identified, the nurse should attempt to ascertain the patient's reasons for not following the regimen and collaboratively discuss approaches to the problems viewed by the patient as hindrances to following the prescribed regimen. The nurse needs to be cognizant of the belief systems of a culturally diverse population regarding medications, illness, and aging among patients and their families, along with language and other barriers that may impede communication with the health care providers.

Possible NIC labels that could be used for the previously discussed nursing diagnosis are:

- Deficient knowledge (actual, risk, or possible) related to: the medication regimen (patient education).
  NOC—Knowledge: Medication
  NIC—Teaching: Prescribed Medication
- Noncompliance (actual, risk, or possible) related to: the patient's value system, cognitive ability, cultural factors, or economic resources.
  NOC—Compliance Behavior
  NIC—Learning Readiness Enhancement or Financial Resource Assistance

Evaluating Therapeutic Outcomes

Objective

1. Describe the procedure for evaluating the therapeutic outcomes obtained from prescribed therapy.

Evaluation associated with drug therapy is an ongoing process that assesses response to the medications prescribed, observes for signs and symptoms of recurring illness or the development of adverse effects of the medication, determines the patient's ability to receive patient education and self-administer medications, and notes potential for compliance. Table 4-3 on pp. 50 to 55 show how the nursing process is applied to the nursing responsibilities associated with drug therapy.

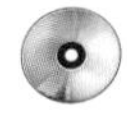

Go to your Companion CD-ROM for Appendices, an Audio Glossary, animations, Drug Dosage Calculators, customizable Patient Self-Assessment forms, and Review Questions for the NCLEX® Examination.

evolve Be sure to visit the companion Evolve site at http://evolve.elsevier.com/Clayton for WebLinks and additional online resources.

MEDICATION SAFETY REVIEW

CRITICAL THINKING QUESTIONS

1. Practice writing nursing diagnosis statements specific to drug therapy prescribed for patients with (1) sleep disorder, (2) advanced heart failure, and (3) dyslipidemia.
2. Explain the components for performing a focused assessment on patients with each of the three conditions identified in question 1.
3. Use Table 4-3 to identify common drugs requiring monitoring of drug levels.
4. Explain the rationale for performing a premedication assessment before administering a prescribed medicine.

CONTENT REVIEW QUESTIONS

1. A patient develops edema as a side effect to report to a prescribed medication. A gain of 5 pounds has occurred in 24 hours and 2+ edema is present in the legs. An appropriate nursing diagnosis statement would be:
   1. Fluid volume, Excess, related to calcium ion antagonist therapy (nifedipine) as evidenced by dependent edema (2+) and weight gain of 5 pounds in 24 hours.
   2. Fluid volume, Excess, related to drug therapy, manifested by 5-pound weight gain and leg edema.
   3. Fluid volume, Excess, related to drug side effects evidenced by unknown etiology.
   4. Fluid volume, Risk for imbalance, related to drug side effects.

2. The nursing diagnosis developed in question 1 is known as a/an:
   1. risk diagnosis.
   2. actual nursing diagnosis.
   3. collaborative nursing diagnosis.
   4. possible nursing diagnosis.

3. Which of the following is an example of a primary source of information?
   1. Subjective data provided by the patient
   2. Information from relatives
   3. Medical records
   4. Literature search

4. Which of the following is an example of an independent nursing action?
   1. Maintaining and modifying the medication orders
   2. Collaborating with qualified professionals about medication calculations
   3. Reviewing the laboratory results
   4. Obtaining the patient's medication history

CHAPTER 5

Patient Education and Health Promotion

evolve http://evolve.elsevier.com/Clayton

Chapter Content

Objectives

1. Differentiate among cognitive, affective, and psychomotor learning domains.
2. Identify the main principles of learning applied when teaching a patient, family, or group.
3. Apply the principles of learning to the content taught in pharmacology.

Key Terms

cognitive domain
affective domain
psychomotor domain
objectives
ethnocentrism
scientific biomedical paradigm
magicoreligious paradigm
holistic paradigm
ethnography
health teaching

THE THREE DOMAINS OF LEARNING

Cognitive Domain

The cognitive domain is the level at which basic knowledge is learned and stored. It is the thinking portion of the learning process and incorporates a person's previous experiences and perceptions.

Previous experiences with health and wellness influence the learning of new materials. Prior knowledge and experience are the foundation for adding new concepts. Thus the learning process begins by identifying what experiences the person has had with the subject.

Yet thinking involves more than the delivery of new information or concepts. A person must build relationships between prior experiences and the new concepts to formulate new meanings. At a higher level in the thinking process, the new information is used to question something that is uncertain, to recognize when to seek additional information, and to make decisions during real-life situations.

Affective Domain

Affective behavior is conduct that expresses feelings, needs, beliefs, values, and opinions. The affective domain is the most intangible portion of the learning process. It is well known that individuals view events from different perspectives. People often choose to internalize feelings rather than express them. The nurse must be willing to approach patients in a nonjudgmental fashion, listen to their concerns, recognize the nonverbal messages being given, and assess their needs with an open mind.

Developing a sense of trust and confidence in health care providers can have a powerful effect on the attitude of the patient and family members. This can influence the learner's response to the new information being taught. The nurse should be positive and accepting, and should involve the learner in a discussion to draw out his or her views toward the solution to problems.

Psychomotor Domain

The psychomotor domain involves the learning of a new procedure or skill. It is often referred to as the *doing domain.* Learning is usually done by demonstration of the procedure or task using a step-by-step approach, with reciprocal demonstrations by the learner to validate the degree of mastery obtained.

PRINCIPLES OF LEARNING

Focus the Learning

The patient must be allowed to focus on the material or task to be learned. The environment must be conducive to learning; it must be quiet and well lit and have the essential equipment needed to complete the lesson.

The learner needs repetition of new information to master it. Nurses may feel obligated to teach the patient or family members everything they know about a disease or procedure, overwhelming them with information. Instead, first glean what information is essential. Then consider what the patient wants to know. It is best to begin with the patient's questions and proceed from there, otherwise you may be explaining things the patient is not interested in knowing, and the individual may not be focused on the presentation. By beginning with the patient's needs, you give the person some control over the learning and increase participation in the process. Active participation in the learning process increases the learning that takes place.

Learning Styles

Learning styles vary. Some people can read and readily comprehend directions, whereas others need to see, feel, hear, touch, and think to master a task. To be effective, the nurse must fit the teaching techniques to the learner's style. Therefore, a variety of materials should be made available for health education. The nurse can select the instructional approach to be used from written materials such as pamphlets, video recordings, motion pictures, models, slides, filmstrips, audiocassettes, photographs, charts, transparencies, and computer-aided instruction. A variety of these materials supplies the audiovisual component that may be essential to the person's learning style.

Organization Fosters Learning

In most clinical settings today, patient education materials are developed by the staff and then reviewed by a committee for adoption. Specific objectives should be formulated for the patient education sessions. The **objectives** should state the purpose of the activities and the expected outcomes. Objectives may be developed in conjunction with a nursing diagnosis statement (e.g., *Nutrition, Imbalanced: Less than body requirements*), or they can be developed for common conditions requiring care delivery (e.g., care of the patient receiving chemotherapy). Regardless of the format used, these instructional materials have an established content given in outline form and are arranged so that one nurse can initiate the teaching and document the degree of understanding, and another nurse can continue the teaching on a different shift or day. The first nurse should check off what has been accomplished so that the next nurse knows where to resume the lesson. At the start of each subsequent teaching session it is important to review what has been covered previously and to affirm the retention of information from the previous lessons. Organizing materials this way standardizes the content, allows for more than one nurse to be able to teach the same patient, allows for the material to be covered in increments the patient can handle, and makes documentation easier. This information is then readily available for review before the patient is discharged and can support the necessity for additional home care when a patient has not mastered self-care needs.

When psychomotor skills are being taught, reciprocal demonstrations are particularly useful for ensuring mastery. It helps to allow the learner to practice a task several times. Giving the person immediate feedback on skills mastered and then giving time to practice those skills that are more difficult allows the learner to improve in manual dexterity and mastery of the sequencing of the procedure. If appropriate, the equipment may be left with the learner for practice before the next session. Sometimes it is particularly useful to set up a videotape player for the learner to view skill demonstrations alone at a convenient time. At the next meeting, the videotape can be reviewed together and important points discussed and clarified should the patient express confusion or uncertainty. This technique reinforces what has been said, reviews what has been learned, and provides the learner with repetition, which may be necessary for learning.

Motivating the Individual to Learn

Before initiating a teaching plan, the nurse should be certain that the patient is able to focus and concentrate on the tasks and materials to be learned. The patient's basic needs (e.g., food, oxygen, pain relief) must be met before he or she is able to focus on the learning. The nurse must recognize the individual's health beliefs when trying to motivate the learner. Because health teaching requires the integration of the patient's beliefs, attitudes, values, opinions, and needs, an individualized teaching plan must be developed, or a standardized teaching plan must be adapted to the individual's beliefs and needs.

Teaching does not require a formal setting. Some of the most effective teaching can be done while care is being delivered. The patient can be exposed to a skill, a treatment, or facts that must be comprehended in small increments. The nurse who explains a procedure and informs the patient why certain procedures are being done reinforces the need for it and motivates the individual to learn. When the patient understands the personal benefits of performing a task, his or her willingness to do it is strengthened. As the patient practices using the new skill or procedure, the nurse can reinforce the benefits and the technique for mastery.

Readiness to Learn

A patient's perception of health and health status may differ from the nurse's judgment; therefore the values of health to each individual may differ greatly. The patient may not realize that a healthy lifestyle will provide significant benefits. A person who commonly indulges in alcohol, smoking, high-fat diets, and leads a sedentary lifestyle may not consider the consequences of these practices in relation to health. Not everyone is interested in the concept of healthy living. The nurse must respect the individuality of the patient, family, or group, and should accept that not everyone is motivated by the possibility of a higher level of wellness.

The nurse can positively influence the learning process by being enthusiastic about the content to be taught. A patient's response to the new information will vary and depends on several influences, for example, the need to know, life experiences, self-concept, the effect of the illness on lifestyle, experience with learning new materials, and readiness to learn. In research by Kaluger and Kaluger (1984) it was discovered that readiness or the ability to engage in learning depends on motive, relevant preparatory training, and physiologic maturation. In other words, is the learner motivated? Is the learner willing to make behavioral changes? Is the patient's illness or wellness at a point when learning will be beneficial and appropriate? Consideration must be given to the patient's psychosocial adaptation to illness and ability to focus on learning. During the denial, anger, or bargaining stages of grieving, the patient usually is neither prepared nor willing to accept the limitations imposed by the disease process. In the resolution and acceptance stages of the grieving process, the patient moves toward accepting responsibility and willingness to learn what is necessary to attain an optimal level of health.

In teaching activities conducted with children, psychosocial, cognitive, and language abilities must be considered. Cognitive and motor development, as well as the learner's language usage and understanding must be assessed. Age definitely influences the types and amount of self-care activities the child is capable of learning and executing independently. The nurse should consult a text on developmental theory for further information.

Adult education is usually oriented toward learning what is necessary to maintain a particular lifestyle. In general, adults need to understand why they must learn something before they undertake the effort to learn it. When planning the educational needs of the patient, the nurse must assess what the patient already knows and what additional information is desired. It is imperative that the nurse make the content relevant to the individual and that his or her health beliefs be incorporated into the overall plan.

The older adult needs additional assessments before implementation of health teaching. Assess vision, hearing, and short- and long-term memory. If a task is to be taught, fine and gross motor abilities need to be evaluated as well. An elderly patient may also have major concerns regarding the cost of the proposed treatments in relation to available resources. A patient will often evaluate the benefits of planned medical interventions and their overall effect on the quality of life. Any of these situations can affect the ability to focus on the new information to be taught, influencing responses and the overall outcome of the teaching. The elderly have often experienced losses, and may be facing social isolation as well as physical (functional) losses and financial constraints. Because the elderly often have more chronic health problems, a new diagnosis, exacerbation of a disease, or a new crisis may be physically and emotionally overwhelming. Therefore timing of patient instruction is of great significance.

When teaching an elderly patient, it is prudent to slow the pace of the presentation and limit the length of each session to prevent overtiring. Older adults can learn the material, but often they process things more slowly than younger people because their short-term memory may be more limited. The nurse must work with the learner to develop ways to remember what is being taught. The more the older person is involved in forming the associations to remember new ideas and to connect these ideas with past experiences, the better the outcome. Many learners are embarrassed by the inability to master a task. Asking them if they understand is useless because they will not reveal embarrassment. The nurse should provide information in small increments; allow for practice, review, practice, review, and practice until success is achieved. The nurse can stop at appropriate intervals and reschedule sessions to meet the learning needs.

When the learner becomes anxious, the presentation of new information can be slowed down, repeated, or stopped and the session rescheduled. The nurse should compliment positive aspects of the session before ending it. Fear and anxiety often impair the ability to focus on the task or content being presented, creating an environment that is conducive to learning is important. Consider the lighting so there is no glare on reading materials, face the learner for better eye contact, and speak directly in a clear tone without shouting. Be calm; use tact and diplomacy if frustrations develop, and try to instill confidence in the learner's ability to surmount any problems.

Spacing the Content

Spacing or staggering the amount of material given in one session should be considered, regardless of the age of who is being taught. People tend to remember what is learned first. Based on this principle, multiple short sessions are usually better than a few longer sessions that may overwhelm the learner. New teachers tend to focus on giving all the materials to the individual and indicating on checklists that the materials were taught. *Providing* information is not synonymous with *learning* the information.

The patient's learning style should be assessed to determine if he or she likes to read materials and then discuss them or whether the person prefers other methods of study such as audiovisual sessions. After this is determined, the spacing of the content can be tailored to the types of learning materials available to teach the content.

Repetition Enhances Learning

Repetition is known to enhance learning. Making a plan that incorporates multiple practice sessions reinforces this principle. Because of limited duration of hospitalization, multiple practice sessions may not be feasible. Therefore, it is important to validate in the charting those aspects of the patient's educational needs that have been mastered and those that still require assistance from home health care providers.

Education Level

Vocabulary and reading level used during the teaching sessions must be tailored to the patient's ability to understand the information. The information must be presented at an appropriate educational level. Medical terms may not be understood, and written instructions left at the bedside may be misinterpreted or not read at all. Some people may be illiterate, whereas others may read at a first-grade, seventh-grade, or collegiate level. Therefore if written materials are used, it is important to consider these wide variations in literacy.

Culture and Ethnic Diversity

Many health care providers have limited understanding of what other cultures believe and the importance of these benefits to the learning process. **Ethnocentrism** is the assumption that one's culture provides the right way, the best way, and the only way to live. In short, people who believe in the theory of ethnocentrism assume that their way of viewing the world is superior to that of others (Leininger, 1978). As understanding of cultural diversity increases, health care providers must expand their knowledge of the basic tenets of belief systems they may encounter among their patients.

Albers Herberg (1989) described scientific, magicoreligious, and holistic paradigms as three ways people explain life events. Table 5-1 is a summary of belief systems about health and illness. The **scientific biomedical paradigm** is the one most familiar to health care providers educated in the United States. The basic tenet of this health care system is that all disease has a cause. Even when the causative factors are unknown, scientific research can be directed toward finding a cure.

The **magicoreligious paradigm** views the world and its inhabitants as being under the control of supernatural mystical forces. People who attribute their illnesses to this model believe in evil spirits and gods, witchcraft, spells, and other forces that impose illness on a person. Health can be a gift or a blessing from God, and an illness may be punishment from God. Conversely, it can be a way in which the individual has been chosen to carry out God's will. Illnesses are natural and intended by God, or unnatural and not a part of God's plan.

Table 5-1 ***Summary of Belief Systems About Health and Illness***

MAGICORELIGIOUS	SCIENTIFIC-BIOMEDICAL	HOLISTIC
WORLD VIEW		
Fate of world is under control of supernatural forces. God(s) or other supernatural forces for good or evil are in control; humans are at the mercy of these forces.	Life is controlled by physical and biochemical processes that can be studied and manipulated by humans.	Harmony, natural balance. Human life is only one aspect of nature and part of the general order of the cosmos. Everything in the universe has a place and role according to laws that maintain order.
ILLNESS/DISEASE		
Initiated by supernatural agent with or without justification, via sorcery. Cause of health or illness is not organic, it is mystical. Causes: possession by evil spirits, breaching a taboo, supernatural forces (sorcery, witchcraft).	Wear and tear, accident, injury, pathogens, and fluid and chemical imbalance. Cause-effect relationship exists for natural events. Life related to structure and functions similar to machines. Life can be reduced or divided into smaller parts. Mind and body are two distinct entities. Cause exists, if only it were known.	Disease, imbalance, and chaos result when these laws are disturbed.
HEALTH		
Gift or reward is given as a sign of God's blessing and good will.	Illness prevention activities, restoration through exercise, medication, treatments, and other means.	Environment, behavior, and sociocultural factors are influential in maintenance of health and prevention of disease. Maintaining and restoring balance are important to health.
ETHNIC GROUP		
Hispanic Americans, African Americans; components found in other groups	White Americans	Native Americans, Asian Americans; components found in other groups
OTHER CONCEPTS		
		Yin/yang Hot/cold Harmony/disharmony

Modified from Albers cited in Herberg P: Theoretical foundations of transcultural nursing. In Boyle JS, Andrews MM: *Transcultural concepts in nursing care,* Boston, 1989, Scott, Foresman. Data from Babcock DE, Miller MH: *Client education: theory and practice,* St Louis, 1994, Mosby.

The **holistic paradigm** recognizes harmony among the body, mind, and spirit. This model identifies disease as a direct result of an imbalance among these natural components. Health is restored by bringing these three components—body, mind, and spirit—into balance.

Because there are differing beliefs, it is important that the nurse explore the meaning of an illness with the patient. Members of other cultures do not always express themselves when their views are in conflict with another culture. Unless a careful assessment of psychosocial needs is done, the true meaning of an illness or the proposed intervention may never be uncovered. Even the assessment process has obstacles attached. People in some cultures do not believe that family information should be shared outside the family. For example, some Eastern European cultures prefer not to reveal any history of psychiatric illness or treatment and are usually reluctant to share any sexual history. Others, such as the Native American culture, believe that only the affected individual may reveal information.

Communication is vitally important within any cultural group, yet verbal and nonverbal communication means different things to different cultures. For example, whites tend to value eye contact, but in other cultures (e.g., Native Americans, Asians) direct eye contact is a sign of disrespect or rudeness. As a part of communication, knowing how to address the patient is also important. African American patients prefer to have their formal name used rather than their first name, especially when addressing older family members. Chinese people tend to be more formal than Americans, and husbands and wives do not necessarily have the same last name. The simple gesture of asking an individual how he or she prefers to be addressed is both helpful and respectful.

Apparent aggressiveness, paranoia, and other behaviors experienced when conversing with some ethnic groups may be a result of defensiveness arising from conditioning during life experiences and from perceptions of racial prejudice. When these behaviors are exhibited, the nurse must remain calm and nonjudgmental and intervene only to clarify the cause of the miscommunication.

Working with an interpreter when a language barrier exists presents several additional challenges to understanding. Does the interpreter have experience with medical terminology to understand what you are saying? Are there comparable words in the patient's language that can be used to translate what you are saying? Is the interpreter explaining what the learner is saying? Any time a third person enters into the communication cycle, lack of clarity and misinterpretation can occur. The nurse should keep questions brief, asking them one at a time to give the interpreter an opportunity to rephrase the question and obtain a response. Sometimes supplementing questions with pictures and pantomime may be helpful. When using an interpreter, the nurse should look directly at the patient, not at the interpreter, while conversing.

The health team members should always try to ascertain the patient's beliefs regarding illness. For instance: Is "good health" defined as the ability to work or to fulfill family roles, or is it a reward from God or a balance with nature? Does the patient believe that health care can improve health outcomes, or does fate determine the outcome? Are any cultural or religious disease prevention approaches used in the household? Do family members wear talismans or charms for protection against illness? Are cultural healers important (e.g., Chinese herbalist, Native American medicine man)?

As part of the *cultural assessment* the nurse should determine factors relating to the cultural beliefs for the family. Inquire as to whether other family members should be included in the discussion of the patient's medical care. Does the individual require the continued presence of the family in the immediate clinical setting? Should the family be involved in the direct delivery of care such as bathing and feeding? Who is the decision maker or family spokesperson? Be sure to include the decision makers in the teaching session so that the teaching will not be wasted. Always remain sensitive to the patient and family cultural beliefs and practices. Nurses can demonstrate understanding, empathy, respect, and patience for the patient's cultural values through their communication and actual delivery of health care. Consult assessment textbooks for more extensive coverage of ethnic and cultural issues.

As cultural mixes become more common, educational materials are being adapted to meet a variety of cultural considerations. Unfortunately this does not solve all problems. Interpreting written materials still leaves the chance for misunderstanding because many people cannot read or do not read at the level of the provided materials.

Adherence

Health care providers and educators tend to think that a patient should change behaviors and adhere to a new therapeutic regimen simply because the educator said so. However, patients do have the right to make their own life choices and they often do. Unfortunately there is no way to ensure adherence unless the patient recognizes the value of it.

Success with a health regimen is enhanced when the educator conveys an enthusiastic attitude, appears positive about the subject matter, and shows confidence in the abilities of the participants to understand the lesson. Reinforcing positive accomplishments fosters successful achievement.

The patient's response to the therapeutic regimen (including medications) and degree of compliance is influenced by several variables, including the following:

- Beliefs about the seriousness of the illness
- Perception of the benefits of the proposed treatment plans

- Personal beliefs, values, and attitudes toward health, the provider of the medication, and the health care system, including prior experience within the system
- The effect of the proposed changes on personal lifestyle
- Acceptance (or denial) of the illness and its associated problems. Other psychological issues such as anger about the illness, apathy, depression, forgetfulness, or confusion
- High stress or day-to-day stresses such as dysfunctional families, difficult living situations, poverty, long working hours in a tense environment, or problematic parenting issues
- Comprehension and understanding of the health regimen or frequent changes in the regimen; inability to read written instructions
- Multiple physicians or health care providers prescribing medication
- Cost of treatment in relation to resources and possible difficulty is getting medications filled
- Support of significant others or problems with assistance that is needed in the home
- Amount of control the individual experiences over the disease or condition and ultimately, over life as a result of the changes
- Side effects from the treatment and degree of inconvenience, annoyance, or impairment in functioning that they produce
- The degree of positive response achieved
- Physical difficulties limiting access or use of medication such as swallowing tablets, difficulty in opening the containers or handling small tablets, or the inability to distinguish colors or identifying markings on a medication
- Concerns about taking drugs and the fear of addiction

Evaluating the ability of a patient to comply with a proposed health regimen is a complex process that involves using established criteria to reach a conclusion. The ultimate goal is to assist patients in achieving the greatest degree of control possible within the context of their beliefs, values, and needs. Health care professionals can offer support and encouragement, be complimentary about positive achievements, and encourage examination of the available options and benefits of a healthy lifestyle. It is vital to assist patients in exploring options when a problem or complication arises rather than giving up the treatment because information about the alternatives is lacking. Financial considerations may affect the patient's decisions.

Needs are constantly changing; the learning objectives must be modified on a continuum and the plan of care adapted to the individual's current needs. The plan of care should evolve as a result of the nurse and patient discussing the available options and then establishing outcomes with which the patient is willing and able to live.

New Strategies to Increase Adherence

The challenge for nursing is to increase the adherence of patients to their health care regimen, and to minimize hospital readmission and suffering from complications. It is estimated that poor adherence to medical therapy accounts for about $300 billion in unnecessary health care expenses each year. One model used to induce behavioral change in patients is called the Case Management Adherence Guidelines, version 1 (CMAG-1). This project, developed by Pfizer and the Case Management Society of America, is a series of tools used by case managers (many of whom are nurses) to assess the patient's motivation level and knowledge of prescribed medications and other therapies. It also assesses a patient's social support system. The tools help identify those who are more at risk for nonadherence so interventions can be initiated early in care. A key principle of this model is that the caregiver must recognize the patient will make the final decisions. The caregiver must negotiate with (not dictate to) the patient to implement actions that may result in positive change. This approach gives the caregiver and the patient ownership of the goals to be achieved.

Another type of research technique used to study adherence is **ethnography.** When a patient is not meeting expected outcomes, an ethnographer may visit the patient at home to observe how the patient administers his or her health care regimen. Observations are made on how and what procedures are accomplished and what errors are being made. Industry has used these methods for many years to help design workflow in production, and it has been discovered that this is also a valuable tool in health care for improving patient outcomes. It is important to remember that the patient may not be purposefully nonadherent, but that the home environment may not allow for adherence to the proper treatment regimen.

PATIENT EDUCATION ASSOCIATED WITH MEDICATION THERAPY

Objectives

1. Describe essential elements of patient education in relation to the prescribed medications.
2. Describe the nurse's role in fostering patient responsibility for maintaining well-being and adhering to the therapeutic regimen.
3. Identify the types of information that should be discussed with the patient or significant others to establish reasonable expectations for the prescribed therapy.
4. Discuss specific techniques used in the practice setting to document the patient education performed and degree of achievement attained.

Health Teaching

During the past two decades, **health teaching** has evolved from an abstract form of intervention that occurred only if a specific need existed at discharge (and if the health care provider approved of providing the information to the patient) to its current formalized development of learning objectives that direct patients toward achieving goals based on their needs. Today health teaching is an important nursing responsibility that carries legal implications for failure to provide and document education.

NURSING PROCESS

The nursing process can be adapted to the health teaching process.

Assessment

Data should be gathered and critical information that requires patient learning should be identified. The patient's current level of knowledge and understanding of the content should be assessed. The individual's learning style, motivating factors, readiness to learn, education level, cultural and ethnic considerations, stage in the grieving process, developmental needs, and interest in self-responsibility should also be identified.

Nursing Diagnosis

The nursing diagnosis statement(s) based on the assessment data that incorporate the three learning domains (cognitive, affective, and psychomotor) should be formulated.

Planning

A teaching plan and associated nursing interventions that incorporate the patient's desires, needs, and values should be formulated. Mutual realistic and measurable learning goals or expected outcomes should be set and prioritized with the patient. The teaching methodologies to be used and resource materials available should be identified. A setting conducive to learning and a time that can allow for incorporation of family or significant others should be selected.

Implementation

The patient's physiologic and emotional needs should be met before initiating teaching. A language should be chosen in which the patient and significant others can readily understand and be able to incorporate cultural variables and developmental abilities into the delivery process. Behavior should be reinforced as appropriate, with time provided to ask questions and discuss concerns. The teaching plan can be adapted to the learner's needs throughout the teaching session(s). The degree of comprehension should be verified throughout the process, and the content, written materials provided, and patient understanding of the content should be documented.

Evaluation

The completed teaching plan and degree of mastery and attainment of the established measurable learning goals or expected outcomes should be reviewed, and the plan revised as needed. Referrals to community agencies should be arranged as necessary.

As illustrated in the teaching process, the content taught to the patient should be thoroughly planned (Box 5-1) and delivered in increments that the patient is capable of mastering. The complete teaching plan should be in the Kardex or patient chart. Each segment should be expressed in measurable behavioral terms. Once the goals have been formulated, they should be considered tentative and reevaluated on target dates throughout the course of treatment and modified if necessary. All teaching should be documented in the nurse's notes or on the health teaching record, along with observations that verify the patient's degree of understanding or proficiency of skill mastered. When an item is mastered, it should be checked off on the Kardex or health teaching form in the patient's chart.

Assessing the patient's readiness for learning is crucial to success. When anxiety is high, the ability to focus on details is reduced. The nurse should anticipate periods during the hospitalization when teaching can be more effective. Some teaching is most successful when done spontaneously, such as when the patient asks direct questions regarding progress toward discharge. The nurse also must learn to anticipate inopportune times to initiate teaching, such as during withdrawal after learning of a diagnosis with a poor prognosis. With reduced hospital stays, the ability to time patient education ideally and to perform actual teaching is a challenge. It is imperative that the nurse document those aspects of health teaching that have been mastered, and of equal importance, what has not been accomplished, and request referral to an appropriate agency for follow-up teaching and assistance.

During the process of patient education, the nurse should address the areas of communication and responsibility, expectations of therapy, changes in expectation, and changes in therapy through cooperative goal setting. ■

Communication and Responsibility

Nurses tend to think that patients will do what is suggested simply because they have been told it is beneficial. In the hospital, the nurse and other health team members reinforce the basic therapeutic regimen; at discharge, however, the patient leaves the controlled environment and is free to choose to follow the prescribed treatment or to alter it as deemed appropriate, based on personal values and beliefs. For learning to take place, the patient must perceive the information as relevant. Whenever possible, start with simple, attainable goals to build the patient's confidence. It is important to correlate the teaching with the patient's perspective on the illness and ability to control the signs and symptoms or course of the disease process.

Box 5-1 ***Sample Teaching Plan for a Patient with Diabetes Mellitus Taking One Type of Insulin****

Understanding of Health Condition

- Assess the patient's family's understanding of diabetes mellitus.
- Clarify the meaning of the disease in terms the patient is able to understand.
- Establish learning goals through mutual discussion. Arrange to teach most important data first. Set dates for teaching of content after discussion with patient.

Food and Fluids

- Arrange for the patient, family members, and significant others to attend nutrition lectures and demonstrations on food preparation.
- Reinforce knowledge of exchange lists (or other dietary method) by tactful questioning and by giving the patient a chance to practice food selections for daily meals from menus provided.
- Explain management of the diabetic diet during illness (e.g., nausea and vomiting, need for increase in fluid) and when to contact the health care provider.
- Stress interrelationship of food and onset, peak, and duration of the prescribed insulin.

Monitoring Tests

- Demonstrate the collection and testing of blood glucose samples and, as appropriate, urine testing.
- Validate understanding by having the patient collect, test, and record results of the testing for the remainder of the hospitalization.
- Stress performing serum glucose testing and urine tests (e.g., ketones) before meals and at bedtime.
- Explain the importance of regular follow-up laboratory studies (e.g., fasting plasma glucose testing or postprandial, glycosylated hemoglobin) to monitor the patient's degree of control.

Medications and Treatments

- Teach the name, dose, route of administration, desired action, storage, and refilling of the type of insulin prescribed.
- Explain the principles of insulin action, onset, peak, and duration (see Chapter 36).
- Demonstrate preparation and administration of the prescribed dose of insulin.
- Teach site location and self-administration of insulin.
- Give specific instructions on reading the syringe to be used at home.
- Teach how to obtain supplies (e.g., disposable syringes, needles, glucometer, glucose monitoring strips, insulin pen).
- Cite usual times for "reactions," signs and symptoms of hypoglycemia or hyperglycemia, and management of each complication.
- Validate the patient's understanding of the side effects to expect and those that require reporting.
- Teach and validate family members' and significant others' understanding of the signs and symptoms of hypoglycemia and hyperglycemia and management of each complication.
- Teach general approach to management of illnesses (e.g., if nausea and vomiting or fever occur—actions required; stress glucose monitoring before meals and at hour of sleep; and need to call health care provider).

Personal Hygiene

Discuss the management of personal hygiene measures of great importance to the patient with diabetes mellitus:

- Regular foot care.
- Meticulous oral hygiene and dental care.
- Care of cuts, scratches, minor and major injuries.
- Stress the management and needed alterations in insulin dosage during an illness; emphasize the need to consult the health care provider for guidance and discussion.

Activities

- Help the patient develop a detailed time schedule for usual activities of daily living. Incorporate diabetic care needs into the schedule.
- Encourage maintenance of all usual activities of daily living; discuss anticipated problems and possible interventions.
- Correlate personal care needs not only in the home environment, but also in the work setting as appropriate. (Consider involvement of the industrial nurse if available in the work setting.)
- Discuss effects of an increase or decrease in activity level on the management of the diabetes mellitus.

Home or Follow-Up Care

- Arrange for outpatient or health care provider follow-up appointments and for scheduling ordered laboratory tests.
- Tell the individual to seek assistance from the health care provider or from the nearest emergency room service for problems that may develop.
- Arrange appropriate referral to community health agencies if needed.
- Complete a Diabetic Alert card or other means of alerting people to the individual's needs (such as an identification necklace or bracelet).
- Discuss exercise program with the health care provider.

Special Equipment and Instructional Material

- Develop a list of equipment and supplies to be purchased; have a family member purchase and bring to the hospital for use during teaching sessions (e.g., ketone testing and blood glucose monitoring supplies, syringes, needles, alcohol, cotton balls).
- Show audiovisual materials available on insulin preparation, storage, administration; and on serum glucose and urine testing.
- Develop a written record (see Chapter 36) and assist the patient to maintain data during hospitalization.

Other

- Teach measures to make travel easier.
- Tell the patient of the American Diabetes Association and material available through this resource.

*Each item listed must be assessed for the individual's current knowledge base and level of understanding throughout the course of teaching. The process is reassessed and the teaching continued until the patient masters all facets of self-care needs. With the advent of shorter hospitalizations, inpatient and outpatient teaching may be necessary with referral to community-based health care agencies as necessary. Discharge charting and referral should carefully document those facets of the teaching plan mastered and those to be taught. The health care provider should be notified of deficits in learning ability or mastery of needed elements in the teaching plan.

Expectations of Therapy

Before discharge, reasonable responses to the planned therapy should be discussed. The patient should know what signs and symptoms may be altered by the prescribed medications. The precautions necessary when taking a medication must be explained by the nurse and understood by the patient (e.g., to use caution in operating power equipment or a motor vehicle, to avoid direct sunlight, or to ensure that follow-up laboratory studies are obtained).

Changes in Expectations

Changes should be assessed in the patient's expectations as therapy progresses and as the patient gains understanding and skill in managing the diagnosis. The expectations about therapy for patients with acute illnesses may vary widely from those of patients with chronic illnesses.

Changes in Therapy through Cooperative Goal Setting

An attitude of shared input into the goals and outcomes can encourage the patient into a therapeutic alliance. Therefore the patient should be taught to help monitor the parameters used to evaluate therapy. It is imperative that the nurse nurture a cooperative environment that encourages the patient to (1) keep records of the essential data needed to evaluate the prescribed therapy and (2) contact the health care provider for advice rather than alter the medication regimen or discontinue the medication entirely. For each major class of drugs in this book, written records are provided to help the nurse identify essential data that the patient needs to understand and record on a regular basis to assist the health care provider in monitoring therapy. (See the template in Appendix I; see also Box 5-1 for a plan for a patient with diabetes mellitus receiving one type of insulin.) In the event that the patient, family, or significant others do not understand all aspects of the continuing therapy prescribed, they may be referred to a community-based agency for the achievement of long-term health care requirements.

At Discharge

A summary statement of the patient's unmet needs must be written and placed in the medical chart. The health care provider should be consulted concerning the possibility of a referral to a community-based agency for continued monitoring or treatment. The nurse's discharge notes must identify the nursing diagnoses that are unmet and potential collaborative problems that require continued monitoring and intervention. All counseling information should be carefully written out in a manner that the patient can read and understand.

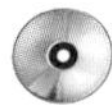

Go to your Companion CD-ROM for Appendices, an Audio Glossary, animations, Drug Dosage Calculators, customizable Patient Self-Assessment forms, and Review Questions for the NCLEX® Examination.

evolve Be sure to visit the companion Evolve site at http://evolve.elsevier.com/Clayton for WebLinks and additional online resources.

MEDICATION SAFETY REVIEW

CRITICAL THINKING QUESTIONS

1. Discuss differences in health belief systems and how these differences may affect patient education.
2. Describe what effect short hospitalization stays have on patient education delivery.

CONTENT REVIEW QUESTIONS

1. According to the magicoreligious belief system, health is:
   1. a supernatural agent with or without justification via sorcery.
   2. a gift as a sign of God's blessing.
   3. the fate of the world.
   4. based on mystical causes.
2. Short hospitalization stays have influenced patient education delivery by making it difficult to: *(Select all that apply.)*
   1. assess readiness to learn.
   2. assess learning that has occurred.
   3. have time to motivate the patient.
   4. request referral to home health.
3. The client who is most ready to begin a client teaching session is the client who has:
   1. had nausea and vomiting for the past 24 hours.
   2. just been told that he needs to have major surgery.
   3. voiced a concern about how insulin injections will affect her lifestyle.
   4. complained bitterly about the low-fat, low-cholesterol diet following his heart attack.

6 A Review of Arithmetic

evolve http://evolve.elsevier.com/Clayton

Chapter Content

Although many hospitals are using the *unit dose* system in dispensing medicines, it continues to be the nurse's responsibility to ascertain that the medication administered is exactly as prescribed by the health care provider. To give an accurate dose, the nurse must have a working knowledge of basic mathematics. This review is offered so that individuals may determine areas in which improvement is needed.

ROMAN NUMERALS

Objective

1. Read and write selected numerical values using Roman numerals.

Toward the end of the sixteenth century two systems of numbers emerged, Roman and Arabic. They are the basis for our communications in mathematics today, are used interchangeably, and are occasionally used by the health care provider in prescribing drugs. Roman numerals 1 through 100 are used more frequently in medicine. Key symbols are as follows:

I = 1	V = 5	X = 10	L = 50
C = 100	D = 500	M = 1000	

Whenever a Roman numeral is repeated, or when a smaller numeral follows, the numerals are added.

EXAMPLES:

I = 1	II = 2	III = 3	VI = 6
1 + 0 = 1	1 + 1 = 2	1 + 1 + 1 = 3	5 + 1 = 6
VII = 7	XI = 11	XII = 12	
5 + 1 + 1 = 7	10 + 1 = 11	10 + 1 + 1 = 12	

Whenever a smaller Roman numeral appears before a larger Roman numeral, subtract the smaller numeral.

EXAMPLES:

IV = 4	IX = 9	XC = 90
5 − 1 = 4	10 − 1 = 9	100 − 10 = 90

Whenever a smaller Roman numeral appears between two larger Roman numerals, subtract the smaller number from the numeral following it.

EXAMPLES:

XIX = 19	XIV = 14	XCIX = 99
10 + 10 − 1 = 19	10 + 5 − 1 = 14	100 − 10 + 10 − 1 = 99

The most common Roman numerals associated with medication administration are as follows:

ṡṡ = ½, i = 1, ii = 2, iii = 3, iv = 4, v = 5, vi = 6, vii = 7, viiṡṡ = 7½, viii = 8, ix = 9, x = 10, and xv = 15

Express the following in Roman numerals:

3 ______	20 ______	101 ______
9 ______	18 ______	499 ______
10 ______	49 ______	1979 ______

Express the following in Arabic numerals:

iv ______	xxxix ______	xix ______
vi ______	ix ______	xv ______

FRACTIONS

Objective

1. Demonstrate proficiency in mathematic problems using addition, subtraction, multiplication, and division of fractions.

Key Terms

numerator
denominator

Fractions are one or more of the separate parts of a substance, or less than a whole number or amount.

EXAMPLE:
1 − ½ = ½

Common Fractions

A common fraction is part of a whole number. The **numerator** (dividend) is the number above the line. The **denominator** (divisor) is the number below the line.

The line separating the numerator and denominator tells us to divide.

$$\frac{\text{Numerator (names how many parts are used)}}{\text{Denominator (tells how many pieces into which the whole is divided)}}$$

EXAMPLES:

The denominator represents the number of parts or pieces the whole is divided into.

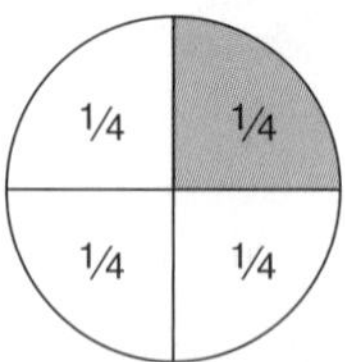

¼ means graphically that the whole circle is divided into four (4) parts; one (1) of the parts is being used.

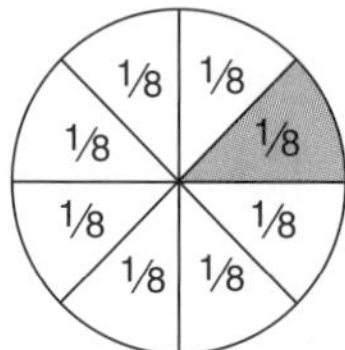

⅛ means graphically that the whole circle is divided into eight (8) parts; one (1) of the parts is being used.

From these two examples, ¼ and ⅛, you can see that the *larger* the *denominator* number, the *smaller* the *portion* is. (Each section in the ⅛ circle is smaller than each section in the ¼ circle.) This is an important concept to understand for people who will calculate medicine doses. The medicine ordered may be ¼ g and the drug source available on the shelf ½ g. Before proceeding to do any formal calculations, you should first decide if the dose you need to give is smaller or larger than the drug source available on the shelf.

EXAMPLES:

Visualize:

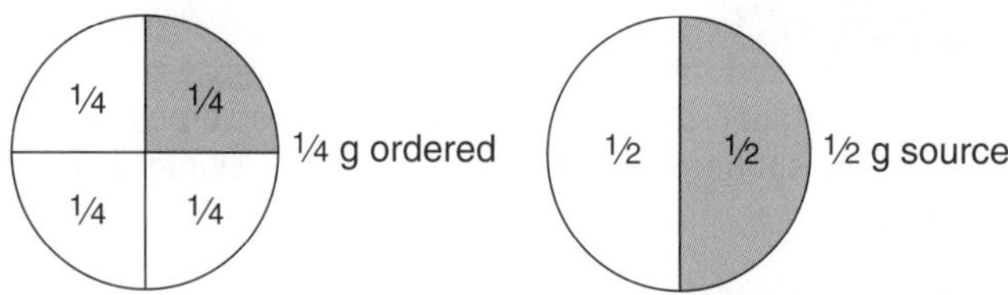

Decide: "Is what I need to administer to the patient a larger or smaller portion than the drug available on the shelf?"

Answer: ¼ g is smaller; thus it would be less than one tablet.

Try a second example: ⅛ g is ordered; the drug source on the shelf is ½ g.

Visualize:

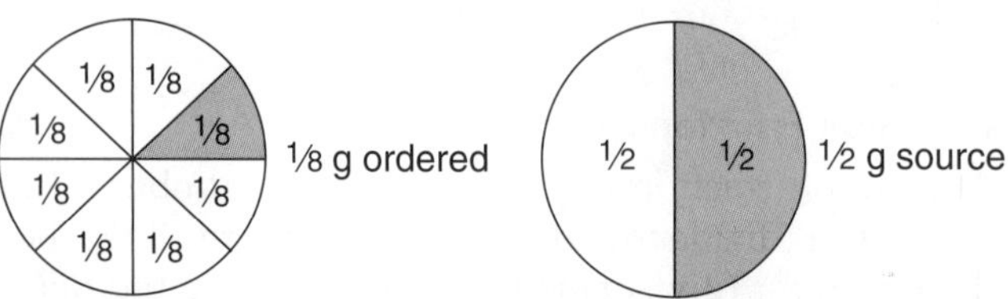

Decide: "Is what I need to administer to the patient a larger or smaller portion than the drug available on the shelf?"

Answer: ⅛ g is smaller than the drug source; thus it would be less than one tablet.

Types of Common Fractions

1. *Simple:* Contains *one* numerator and *one* denominator: $\frac{1}{4}$, $\frac{1}{20}$, $\frac{1}{60}$, $\frac{1}{100}$
2. *Complex:* May have a simple fraction in the numerator or denominator:

$$\tfrac{1}{2} \text{ over } 4 = \frac{\tfrac{1}{2}}{4}$$

or

$$\tfrac{1}{2} \div 4 =$$

$$\tfrac{1}{2} \div 4/1 =$$

$$\tfrac{1}{2} \div \tfrac{1}{4} = \tfrac{1}{8}$$

3. *Proper:* Numerator is smaller than denominator: $\frac{1}{8}$, $\frac{2}{5}$, $\frac{1}{100}$
4. *Improper:* Numerator is larger than denominator: $\frac{4}{3}$, $\frac{6}{4}$, $\frac{100}{10}$
5. *Mixed number:* A whole number and a fraction: $4\frac{5}{8}$, $6\frac{2}{3}$, $1\frac{5}{100}$
6. *Decimal:* Fractions written on the basis of a multiple of 10: $0.5 = \frac{5}{10}$, $0.05 = \frac{5}{100}$, $0.005 = \frac{5}{1000}$
7. *Equivalent:* Fractions that have the same value: $\frac{1}{3}$ and $\frac{2}{6}$

Working with Fractions

Reducing to Lowest Terms

Divide the numerator and the denominator by a number that will divide into both evenly (a common denominator).

EXAMPLE:

$$\frac{25}{125} \div \frac{25}{25} = \frac{1}{5}$$

Reduce the following:

$\frac{5}{100} =$ _____ $\frac{3}{21} =$ _____

$\frac{6}{36} =$ _____ $\frac{12}{44} =$ _____

$\frac{2}{4} =$ _____

Finding the lowest common denominator of a series of fractions is not always easy. The following are some points to remember:

- If the numerator and denominator are even numbers, 2 will work as a common denominator but may not be the smallest one.
- If the numerator and denominator end with 0 or 5, 5 will work as a common denominator but may not be the smallest one.
- Check to see if the numerator divides evenly into the denominator; this will be the smallest term. When all else fails, use the prime number method to find the lowest common denominator. A prime

number is a whole number, greater than 1, that can be divided only by itself and 1 (2, 3, 5, 7, 11, 19, 23, etc.).

Steps

1. Write down all the denominators in a row; divide each denominator by the lowest prime number until you can no longer use that number. Proceed to the next higher prime number and divide, using it until it can no longer be used. Continue this procedure until all number 1s are obtained.
2. Multiply all the prime numbers used to divide and you will have the lowest common denominator.

EXAMPLE:

Fractions: $\frac{7}{16}$ $\frac{5}{9}$ $\frac{13}{30}$ $\frac{7}{22}$

Write down all denominators:

Prime numbers:	16	9	30	22
2	8	9	15	11
2	4	9	15	11
2	2	9	15	11
2	1	9	15	11
3	1	3	5	11
3	1	1	5	11
5	1	1	1	11
11	1	1	1	1

Note that 2 is the smallest prime number. Keep dividing by this number until it no longer will divide into the denominators evenly. Proceed to the next higher prime and reuse if possible. Go to the next higher prime that will divide in evenly; continue until all 1s are obtained.

The lowest common denominator is as follows:

$2 \times 2 \times 2 \times 2 \times 3 \times 3 \times 5 \times 11 = 7920$

Addition

Adding Common Fractions. When denominators are the same figure, add the numerators.

EXAMPLE:

$$\frac{1}{4} + \frac{2}{4} + \frac{3}{4} = \frac{6}{4} = 1\frac{1}{2}$$

Add the following:

$$\frac{2}{6} + \frac{3}{6} + \frac{4}{6} = \frac{9}{6} = 1\frac{1}{2}$$

$$\frac{1}{100} + \frac{3}{100} + \frac{5}{100} = \frac{9}{100}$$

When the denominators are unlike, change the fractions to equivalent fractions by finding the lowest common denominator.

EXAMPLE:

$$\frac{2}{5} + \frac{3}{10} + \frac{1}{2} = \_\_\_\_$$

1. Determine the lowest common denominator. (Use 10 as the common denominator.)
2. Divide the denominator of the fraction being changed into the common denominator and multiply the product (answer) by the numerator.

$\frac{2}{5} = \frac{4}{10}$ (Divide 5 into 10 and multiply the answer [2] by 2.)

$\frac{3}{10} = \frac{3}{10}$ (Divide 10 into 10 and multiply the answer [1] by 3.)

$\frac{1}{2} = \frac{5}{10}$ (Divide 2 into 10 and multiply the answer [5] by 1)

$\frac{12}{10} = 1\frac{1}{5}$ (Add the numerators and place the total over the denominator [10]; then convert the improper fraction to a mixed number and reduce to lowest terms.)

Add the following:

a. $\frac{2}{8} = \frac{\_\_}{64}$

$+ \frac{4}{64} = \frac{\_\_}{64}$

$+ \frac{5}{16} = \frac{\_\_}{64}$

$\frac{\_\_}{64}$ *Answer:* $\frac{5}{8}$

b. $\frac{3}{7} = \frac{\_\_}{28}$

$+ \frac{9}{14} = \frac{\_\_}{28}$

$+ \frac{1}{28} = \frac{\_\_}{28}$

$\frac{\_\_}{28}$ *Answer:* $1\frac{3}{28}$

Adding Mixed Numbers. Add the fractions first; then add the whole numbers.

EXAMPLE:

$$2\frac{3}{4} + 2\frac{1}{2} + 3\frac{3}{8} = \_\_\_\_\_\_$$

1. Determine the lowest common denominator. (Use 8 as the common denominator.)
2. Divide the denominator of the fraction being changed into the common denominator and multiply the product (answer) by the numerator.

$2\frac{3}{4} = \frac{6}{8}$ (Divide 4 into 8 and multiply the answer [2] by 3.)

$2\frac{1}{2} = \frac{4}{8}$ (Divide 2 into 8 and multiply the answer [4] by 1.)

$+ 3\frac{3}{8} = \frac{3}{8}$ (Divide 8 into 8 and multiply the answer [1] by 3.)

$\frac{13}{8}$ (Add the numerators and place the total over the denominator [8].)

$7 + 1\frac{5}{8} = 8\frac{5}{8}$ (Convert the improper fraction $\left[\frac{13}{8}\right]$ to a mixed number $\left[1\frac{5}{8}\right]$ and add it to the whole numbers.)

Add the following:

a. $$\frac{1}{4} + \frac{3}{4} = \frac{\quad}{4}$$ *Answer:* $\frac{4}{4} = 1$

b. $$\frac{1}{2} = \frac{\quad}{6}$$
$$+\ \frac{1}{3} = \frac{\quad}{6}$$
$$+\ \frac{1}{6} = \frac{\quad}{6}$$
$$= \frac{\quad}{6}$$ *Answer:* $\frac{6}{6} = 1$

c. $$\frac{3}{5} = \frac{\quad}{50}$$
$$+\ \frac{4}{50} = \frac{\quad}{50}$$ *Answer:* $\frac{34}{50} = \frac{17}{25}$
$$= \frac{\quad}{50}$$ (Reduced to lowest term)

Subtraction

Subtracting Fractions. When the denominators are unlike, change the fractions to an equivalent fraction by finding the lowest common denominator.

EXAMPLE:

$\frac{1}{4} - \frac{3}{16} =$ ______

1. Determine the lowest common denominator. (Use 16 as the common denominator.)
2. Divide the denominator of the fraction being changed into the common denominator and multiply the product (answer) by the numerator.

$\frac{1}{4} = \frac{4}{16}$ (Divide 4 into 16 and multiply the answer [4] by 1.)

$-\ \frac{3}{16} = \frac{3}{16}$

$\frac{1}{16}$ (Subtract the numerators and place the total [1] over the denominator [16].)

Subtract the following:

a. $$\frac{3}{8} - \frac{2}{8} = \frac{\quad}{8}$$ *Answer:* $\frac{1}{8}$

b. $$\frac{1}{100} = \frac{\quad}{300}$$
$$-\ \frac{1}{150} = \frac{\quad}{300}$$
$$\frac{\quad}{300}$$ *Answer:* $\frac{1}{300}$

Subtracting Mixed Numbers. Subtract the fractions first; then subtract the whole numbers.

EXAMPLE:

$4\frac{1}{4} - 1\frac{3}{4} =$ ______

(Note: You cannot subtract $\frac{3}{4}$ from $\frac{1}{4}$; therefore borrow 1 [which equals $\frac{4}{4}$] from the whole numbers and add $\frac{4}{4} + \frac{1}{4} = \frac{5}{4}$.)

$4\frac{1}{4} = 3\frac{5}{4}$

$-\ 1\frac{3}{4} = 1\frac{3}{4}$

$2\frac{2}{4} = 2\frac{1}{2}$ (Subtract the numerators, place answer over the denominator [4]; reduce to lowest terms; subtract the whole numbers.)

When the denominators are unlike, change the fractions to equivalent fractions by finding the lowest common denominator.

EXAMPLE:

$2\frac{5}{8} - 1\frac{1}{4} =$ ______

1. Determine the lowest common denominator. (Use 8 as the common denominator.)
2. Divide the denominator of the fraction being changed into the common denominator and multiply the product (answer) by the numerator.

$2\frac{5}{8} = 2\frac{5}{8}$ (Divide 8 into 8 and multiply the answer [1] by 5.)

$-\ 1\frac{1}{4} = 1\frac{2}{8}$ (Divide 4 into 8 and multiply the answer [2] by 1.)

$1\frac{3}{8}$ (Subtract the numerators and place the total [3] over the denominator [8]; reduce to lowest terms; subtract the whole numbers.)

Subtract the following:

a. $$\frac{7}{8} = \frac{\quad}{24}$$
$$-\ \frac{3}{6} = \frac{\quad}{24}$$
$$\frac{\quad}{24}$$ *Answer:* $\frac{9}{24} = \frac{3}{8}$

b. $6\frac{7}{8} = \frac{}{16}$

$-\ 3\frac{1}{16} = \frac{}{16}$

$\frac{}{16}$ *Answer:* $3\frac{13}{16}$

Multiplication

Multiplying a Whole Number by a Fraction

EXAMPLE:

$3 \times \frac{5}{8} =$ ______

1. Place the whole number over 1 ($\frac{3}{1}$).
2. Multiply the numerators (top numbers) and multiply the denominators (bottom numbers).

$\frac{3}{1} \times \frac{5}{8} = \frac{15}{8}$

3. Change the improper fraction to a mixed number.

$\frac{15}{8} = 1\frac{7}{8}$

Multiply the following:

a. $2 \times \frac{3}{4} =$ ______ *Answer:* $\frac{3}{2} = 1\frac{1}{2}$

b. $15 \times \frac{3}{5} =$ ______ *Answer:* $\frac{9}{1} = 9$

Multiplying Two Fractions

EXAMPLE:

$\frac{1}{4} \times \frac{2}{3} =$ ______

1. Use cancellation to speed the process.

$\frac{1}{\cancel{4}_{2}} \times \frac{\cancel{2}^{1}}{3} = \frac{1}{6}$

2. Multiply the numerators (top numbers); multiply the denominators.

$\frac{1}{2} \times \frac{1}{3} = \frac{1}{6}$

Multiplying Mixed Numbers

EXAMPLE:

$3\frac{1}{2} \times 2\frac{1}{5} =$ ______

1. Change the mixed numbers (a whole number and a fraction) to an improper fraction (numerator is larger than denominator).

$3\frac{1}{2} \times 2\frac{1}{5} =$ ______ (Multiply the denominator times the whole number and add the numerator.)

$\frac{7}{2} \times \frac{11}{5} =$ ______

2. Multiply the numerators; multiply the denominators.

$\frac{7}{2} \times \frac{11}{5} = \frac{77}{10}$

3. Change the product (answer), an improper fraction, to a mixed number by dividing the denominator into the numerator; reduce to lowest terms.

$\frac{7}{2} \times \frac{11}{5} = \frac{77}{10} = 7\frac{7}{10}$

Multiply the following:

a. $1\frac{2}{3} \times \frac{3}{6} =$ ______ *Answer:* $\frac{5}{6}$

b. $1\frac{7}{8} \times 1\frac{1}{4} =$ ______ *Answer:* $\frac{75}{32} = 2\frac{11}{32}$

Division

Dividing Fractions

EXAMPLE:

$4 \div \frac{1}{2} =$ ______

1. Change the division sign to a multiplication sign.
2. Invert the divisor, the number after the division sign.
3. Reduce the fractions using cancellation.
4. Multiply the numerators and the denominators.

$4 \div \frac{1}{2} = \frac{4}{1} \times \frac{2}{1} = \frac{8}{1} = 8$

Dividing with a Mixed Number

1. Change the mixed number to an improper fraction.
2. Change the division sign to a multiplication sign.
3. Invert the divisor.
4. Reduce whenever possible.

EXAMPLES:

$4\frac{1}{2} \div \frac{3}{4} = \frac{9}{2} \div \frac{3}{4} = \frac{\cancel{9}^{3}}{\cancel{2}_{1}} \times \frac{\cancel{4}^{2}}{\cancel{3}_{1}} = \frac{6}{1}$ or 6

$6\frac{1}{4} \div 1\frac{1}{4} = \frac{25}{4} \div \frac{5}{4} = \frac{\cancel{25}^{5}}{\cancel{4}_{1}} \times \frac{\cancel{4}^{1}}{\cancel{5}_{1}} = \frac{5}{1}$ or 5

Fractions as Decimals

Fractions can be changed to a decimal form by dividing the numerator by the denominator.

EXAMPLE:

$\frac{1}{2} = 2\overline{)1.0}$ = 0.5

Change the following fractions to decimals:

$\frac{1}{100} =$ ______ *Answer:* 0.01

$\frac{5}{8} =$ ______ *Answer:* 0.625

$\frac{1}{2} =$ ______ *Answer:* 0.5

Using Cancellation to Speed Your Work

1. Determine a number that will divide evenly into both a numerator and a denominator.
2. Continue the process of dividing both a numerator and denominator by the same number until all numbers are reduced to the lowest terms.
3. Complete the multiplication of the problem.

EXAMPLE:

$$\frac{\overset{1}{\cancel{5}}}{\underset{2}{\cancel{6}}} \times \frac{\overset{3}{\cancel{9}}}{\underset{2}{\cancel{10}}} = \_\_\_\_\_$$

$$\frac{1}{2} \times \frac{3}{2} = \frac{3}{4}$$

4. Complete the division of the problem.

EXAMPLE:

$$\frac{6}{9} \div \frac{5}{8} = \_\_\_\_\_$$

$$\frac{2}{3} \times \frac{8}{5} = \frac{16}{15} = 1\frac{1}{15}$$

(Change the division sign to a multiplication sign; invert the number after the division sign; reduce and complete the multiplication of the problem.)

DECIMAL FRACTIONS

Objectives

1. Demonstrate proficiency in calculating mathematic problems using addition, subtraction, multiplication, and division of decimals.
2. Convert decimals to fractions and fractions to decimals.

When fractions are written to decimal form, the denominators are not written. The word *decimal* means "10."

When reading decimals, the numbers to the left of the decimal point are whole numbers. It helps to think of them as whole dollars. Numbers to the right of the decimal are fractions of the whole number and may be thought of as "cents."

EXAMPLES:

1.0 = one
11.0 = eleven
111.0 = one hundred eleven
1111.0 = one thousand one hundred eleven

Numbers to the right of the decimal point are read as follows:

EXAMPLES:

Decimal(s):	Fraction(s):
0.1 = one tenth	1/10
0.01 = one hundredth	1/100
0.465 = four hundred sixty-five thousandths	465/1000
0.0007 = seven ten thousandths	7/10,000

Here is another way to view reading decimals:

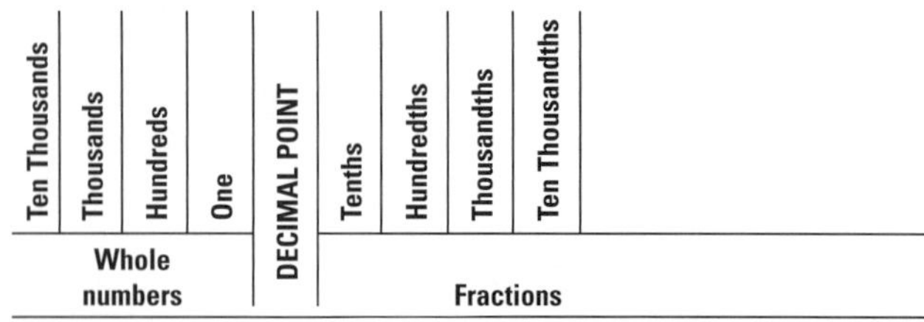

. 1 equals one-tenth (1/10)
. 2 2 equals twenty-two hundredths (22/100)
. 1 1 2 equals one hundred twelve thousandths (112/1000)
. 0 1 1 2 equals one hundred twelve ten thousandths (112/10,000)
1 . equals number one
1 0 . equals number ten
1 0 0 . equals number one hundred
1 0 0 0 . equals number one thousand

On prescriptions another way of expressing the decimal is by using a slanted line.

EXAMPLES:

1 mg = 0.001 g = 0/001 g
0.1 mg = 0.0001 g = 0/0001 g
30 mg = 0.030 g = 0/030 g
100 mg = 0.100 g = 0/100 g
1000 mg = 1.000 g = 1 g

(Note: Hospital policy now recommends that 1.000 g or 1/0 be written as "1 g" to avoid error. Often the decimal point is not recognized and very large doses have been accidentally administered. The rule is: Don't use trailing 0s to the right of decimal points.)

250 mg = 0.250 g = 0/250 g

Multiplying Decimals

Multiplying Whole Numbers and Decimals

1. Count as many places in the answer, starting from the right, as there are places in the decimal involved in the multiplication.
2. The multiplier is the bottom number with the ×, or multiplication sign, before it.
3. The multiplicand is the top number.

EXAMPLES:

500	1000	1000
× 0.02	× 0.04	× 0.009
10.00 (10)	40.00 (40)	9.000 (9)

7.25	500
× 4	× 0.009
29.00 (29)	4.500 (or 5)

Rounding the Answer

Note in the last example that the first number after the decimal point in the answer is 5. Instead of the answer remaining 4.5 it becomes the next whole number, 5. This would be true if the answer were 4.5, 4.6, 4.7, 4.8, or 4.9. In each case the answer would become 5. If the answer were 4.1, 4.2, 4.3, or 4.4 the answer would remain 4.

When the first number after the decimal point is 5 or above, the answer becomes the next whole number. When the first number after the decimal point is less than 5, the answer becomes the whole number in the answer.

Multiply the following:

1200	575	515	510
× 0.009	× 0.02	× 0.02	× 0.04

Multiplying a Decimal by a Decimal

1. Multiply the problem as if the numbers were both whole numbers.
2. Count decimal places in the answer, starting from the right, as many decimal places as there are in both of the numbers that were to be multiplied.

EXAMPLE:

$$\begin{array}{r} 3.75 \\ \times \quad 0.5 \\ \hline 1.875 = 2 \end{array}$$

There are two decimal places in 3.75 and one decimal place in 0.5, making three decimal places. Count three decimal places from the right. Round off the answer to 2.

Multiplying Numbers with Zero

EXAMPLES:

1. Multiply 223 by 40.
   a. Multiply 223 by 0. Write the answer, 0, in the unit column of the answer.
   b. Then multiply 223 by 4. Write this answer in front of the 0 in the product.

$$\begin{array}{r} 223 \\ \times \ 40 \\ \hline 8920 \end{array}$$

2. Multiply 124 by 304.
   a. First multiply 124 by 4. The answer is 496.
   b. Now multiply 124 by 0. Write the answer, 0, under the 9 in 496.
   c. Multiply 124 by 3. Write this answer in front of the 0 in the product.

$$\begin{array}{r} 124 \\ \times \ 304 \\ \hline 496 \\ 37\,20 \\ \hline 37{,}696 \end{array}$$

Dividing Decimals

1. If the divisor (number by which you divide) is a decimal, make it a whole number by moving the decimal point to the right of the last figure.
2. Move the decimal point in the dividend (the number inside the bracket) as many places to the right as you move the decimal point in the divisor.
3. Place the decimal point for the quotient (answer) directly above the new decimal point of the dividend.

EXAMPLES:

$0.25\overline{)10} = 25\overline{)1000.}$ (quotient 40.) $0.3\overline{)99.3} = 3\overline{)993.}$ (quotient 331.)

$0.4\overline{)1.68} = 4\overline{)16.8}$ (quotient 4.2)

Changing Decimals to Common Fractions

1. Remove the decimal point.
2. Place the appropriate denominator under the number.
3. Reduce to lowest terms.

EXAMPLES:

$0.2 = \frac{2}{10} = \frac{1}{5}$ $0.2 = \frac{20}{100} = \frac{1}{5}$

Change the following:

0.3 = ______   0.25 = ______

0.4 = ______   0.50 = ______

0.5 = ______   0.75 = ______

0.05 = ______   0.002 = ______

Changing Common Fractions to Decimal Fractions

Divide the numerator of the fraction by the denominator.

EXAMPLE:

$\frac{1}{4}$ means $1 \div 4$ or $4\overline{)1.00}$ (quotient 0.25)

Change the following:

$\frac{1}{2}$ means ______ $\frac{3}{4}$ means ______

$\frac{1}{6}$ means ______ $\frac{1}{50}$ means ______

$\frac{2}{3}$ means ______

PERCENTS

Objectives

1. Demonstrate proficiency in calculating mathematic problems using percentages.
2. Convert percents to fractions, percents to decimals, decimal fractions to percents, and common fractions to percents.

Determining Percent One Number Is of Another

1. Divide the smaller number by the larger number.
2. Multiply the quotient by 100 and add the percent sign.

EXAMPLE:
A certain 1000-part solution is 10 parts drug. What percent of the solution is drug?

$$1000\overline{)10.00} = 0.01$$

$0.01 \times 100 = 1.$ or 1%

Changing Percents to Fractions

1. Omit the percent sign to form the numerator.
2. Use 100 for the denominator.
3. Reduce the fraction.

EXAMPLES:

$5\% = \frac{5}{100} = \frac{1}{20}$ $\qquad 75\% = \frac{75}{100} = \frac{3}{4}$

Change the following:

$25\% = \frac{25}{100} =$ ______ $\qquad 2\% = \frac{2}{100} =$ ______

$15\% = \frac{15}{100} =$ ______ $\qquad 12\frac{1}{2}\% = \frac{12.5}{100} =$ ______

$10\% = \frac{10}{100} =$ ______ $\qquad \frac{1}{4}\% = \frac{\frac{1}{4}}{100} =$ ______

$20\% = \frac{20}{100} =$ ______ $\qquad 150\% = \frac{150}{100} =$ ______

$50\% = \frac{50}{100} =$ ______ $\qquad 4\% = \frac{4}{100} =$ ______

Changing Percents to Decimal Fractions

1. Omit the percent signs.
2. Insert a decimal point *two places to the left* of the last number, or express as hundredths, decimally.

EXAMPLES:
5% = .05 15% = .15

Change the following:

4% = ______ 25% = ______

1% = ______ 50% = ______

2% = ______ 10% = ______

Note in these examples that those numbers that were already hundredths, such as 10%, 15%, 25%, 50%, merely need to have the decimal point placed in front of the first number, because they are already expressed in hundredths; whereas 1%, 2%, 4%, 5% needed to have a zero placed in front of the number to express them as hundredths.

Change these percents to decimal fractions:

$12\frac{1}{2}\% =$ ______ $\qquad \frac{1}{4}\% =$ ______

If the percent is a mixed number, it should have the fraction expressed as a decimal. Then change the percent to a decimal by moving the decimal point two places to the left.

EXAMPLES:

$12\frac{1}{2}\% = 12.5\%$ or 0.125 $\qquad \frac{1}{4}\% = 0.25\%$ or 0.0025

Changing Common Fractions to Percents

1. Divide the numerator by the denominator.
2. Multiply the quotient by 100 and add the percent sign.

EXAMPLE:

$\frac{1}{50} = 50\overline{)1.00} = 0.02$; $0.02 \times 100 = 2\%$

Change the following:

$\frac{1}{400} =$ ______

$\frac{1}{8} =$ ______

Changing Decimal Fractions to Percents

1. Move the decimal point two places to the right.
2. Omit the decimal point if a whole number results.
3. Add the percent signs. (This is the same as multiplying the decimal fraction by 100 and adding the percent sign.)

EXAMPLE:

$0.01 = 1.00 = 1\%$ (or $\frac{1}{100}$)

Change the following:

0.05 = ______

0.25 = ______

0.15 = ______

0.125 = ______

0.0025 = ______

Points to Remember in Reading Decimals

1. 1. is the whole number 1. When it is written 1.0, it is still one or 1.
2. The whole number is usually written like this: 1 or 2 or 3 or 4, and so on. (Remember, do not use trailing 0s.)
3. Can you read this one? 0.1. This is one tenth. There is one number after the decimal point.
4. Can you read this one? .1. This is also one tenth. The zero in front of the decimal point does not change its value. One tenth can be written, then, in two ways: 0.1 and .1. (The leading 0 to the left of the decimal should be used to help prevent errors.)

RATIOS

Objective

1. Demonstrate proficiency in converting ratios to percentages and percentages to ratios, in simplifying ratios, and in use of the proportion method for solving problems.

A ratio expresses the relationship that one quantity bears to another.

EXAMPLES:
1:5 means 1 part of a drug to 5 parts of a solution.
1:100 means 1 part of a drug to 100 parts of a solution.
1:500 means 1 part of a drug to 500 parts of a solution.

A common fraction can be expressed as a ratio.

EXAMPLE:

$\frac{1}{5}$ is the same as 1:5

The ratio of one amount to an amount expressed in terms of the same unit is the number of units in the first divided by the number of units in the second. The ratio of 2 ounces of a disinfectant to 10 ounces of water is 2 to 10 or 1 to 5 or ⅕. This ratio may be written ⅕ or 1:5.

The two numbers compared are referred to by using the term *ratio*. The first term of a true ratio is always one, or 1. This is the simplest form of a ratio.

Changing Ratio to Percent

1. Make the first term of the ratio the numerator of a fraction; the denominator is the second term of the ratio.
2. Divide the numerator by the denominator.
3. Multiply by 100 and add the percent sign.

Change the following:

1:5 = ____

Changing Percent to Ratio

1. Change the percent to a fraction and reduce the fraction to lowest terms.
2. The numerator of the fraction is the first term of the ratio, and the denominator is the second term of the ratio.

EXAMPLE:

$$\frac{1}{2}\% = \frac{\frac{1}{2}}{100} = \frac{1}{2} \div \frac{100}{1}$$

$$= \frac{1}{2} \times \frac{1}{100} = \frac{1}{200} = 1{:}200$$

Change the following:

2% = ______

50% = ______

75% = ______

Simplifying Ratios

Ratios can be simplified as ratios or as fractions.

EXAMPLE:

$25 : 100 = 1 : 4$ or $\frac{25}{100} = \frac{1}{4}$

Simplify the following:

4:12 = ______	¼:100 = ______
5:10 = ______	15:20 = ______
10:5 = ______	3:9 = ______
75:100 = ______	

Proportions

A proportion shows how two *equal* ratios are related. This method is good because it is possible to prove that your answer is correct, and it is especially useful in working with solution concentrations.

1. Three factors are known. The fourth *unknown* (what you are looking for) is represented by x.
2. The first and fourth terms of a proportion are called extremes. The second and third are the means. The product of the means equals the product of the extremes, or multiplying the first and fourth equals the second and third.

EXAMPLE:

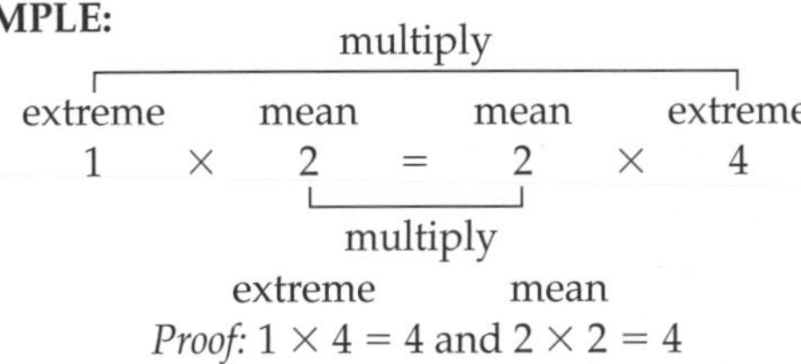

Proof: 1 × 4 = 4 and 2 × 2 = 4

If you did not know one number, you could solve for it as follows:

EXAMPLE:

$1 : 2 = 2 : x$
$1x = 4$
$x = 4 \times 1 = 4$
$x = 4$
Proof: 1 × 4 = 4 and 2 × 2 = 4

Solve the following:

a. $9 : x :: 5 : 300$ = ______
b. $x : 60 :: 4 : 120$ = ______
c. $5 : 3000 :: 15 : x$ = ______
d. $0.7 : 70 :: x : 1000$ = ______
e. $\frac{1}{400} : x :: 2 : 1600$ = ______
f. $0.2 : 8 :: x : 20$ = ______
g. $100{,}000 : 3 :: 1{,}000{,}000 : x$ = ______
h. $\frac{1}{4} : x :: 20 : 400$ = ______

Note: x is the unknown factor. It may be a mean or an extreme in any of the four positions in any problem.

SYSTEMS OF WEIGHTS AND MEASURES

Objectives

1. Memorize the basic equivalents of the household and metric systems.
2. Demonstrate proficiency in performing conversion of medication problems using the household and metric systems.

Key Terms

household measurements	liter
apothecary system	gram
metric system	milligram
meter	kilogram

Two systems of measurement are used during the calculation, preparation, and administration of medicines: household and metric.

Household Measurements

Household measurements are often the way pharmacologic agents are administered at home; however, they are the least accurate. The patient has grown up using this system of measurement and therefore understands it best. Household measurements include drops, teaspoons, tablespoons, teacups, cups, glasses, pints, quarts, and gallons. The first three measurements: drops, teaspoons, and tablespoons are used for medications, depending on the amount prescribed.

COMMON HOUSEHOLD EQUIVALENTS

1 quart = 4 cups
1 pint = 2 cups
1 cup = 8 ounces
1 teacup = 6 ounces
1 tablespoon = 3 teaspoons
1 teaspoon = approximately 5 mL

Apothecary Measurements

The apothecary system of measurement is an ancient system; the word *apothecary* means "pharmacist" or "druggist." Health care providers rarely order medicine using the apothecary system, and it is no longer recommended for use in the health care system. The metric system is the preferred system of measurement because it is more accurate.

Metric System

The metric system was invented by the French in the late eighteenth century. A committee of the Academy of Sciences, working under government authority, recommended a standard unit of linear measure. For a basis of measurement they chose a quarter of the earth's circumference measured across the poles. One ten-millionth of this distance was accepted as the standard unit of linear measure. The committee calculated the distance from the equator to the North Pole from surveys that had been made along the meridian that passes through Paris. The distance divided by 10,000,000 was chosen as the unit of length, or the meter.

Metric standards were adopted in France in 1799. The International Metric Convention met in Paris in 1875, and as a result of this meeting the International Bureau of Weights and Measures was formed. The bureau's first task was to construct an international standard meter bar and an international standard kilogram weight. Duplicates of these were made for all countries participating in the convention.

A measurement line was selected on the international standard meter bar. The distance between the two lines of measurement on the bar is the official unit of the metric system. The standards given to the United States are preserved at the National Institute of Standards and Technology, Gaithersburg, Maryland. There are 25.4 millimeters in 1 inch (2.5 centimeters).

The metric system uses the meter as the unit of length, the liter as the unit of volume (Figure 6-1), and the gram as the measurement of weight.

UNITS OF LENGTH (METER)

1 millimeter = 0.001	meaning 1/1000
1 centimeter = 0.01	meaning 1/100
1 decimeter = 0.1	meaning 1/10
1 meter = 1	meter

UNITS OF VOLUME (LITER)

1 milliliter = 0.001	meaning 1/1000
1 centiliter = 0.01	meaning 1/100
1 deciliter = 0.1	meaning 1/10
1 liter = 1	liter

UNITS OF WEIGHT (GRAM)

1 microgram = 0.000001	meaning 1/1,000,000
1 milligram = 0.001	meaning 1/1000
1 centigram = 0.01	meaning 1/100
1 decigram = 0.1	meaning 1/10
1 gram = 1	gram

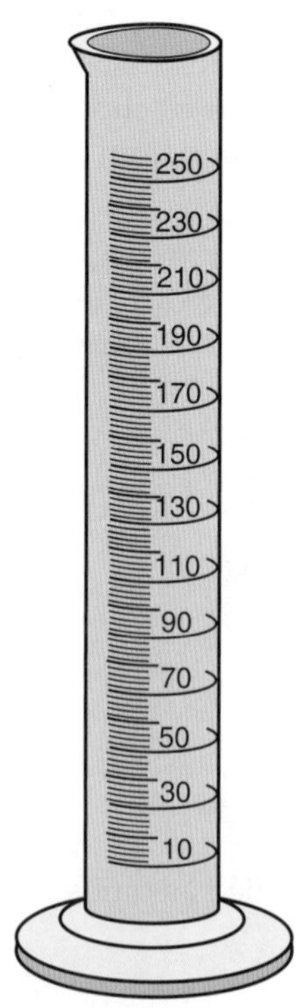

FIGURE **6-1** A graduated cylinder is used to measure the volume of liquids.

Other Prefixes

Deca means ten or 10 times as much. *Hecto* means one hundred or 100 times as much. *Kilo* means one thousand or 1000 times as much. These three prefixes can be combined with the words *meter, gram,* or *liter.*

EXAMPLES:

1 decaliter = 10 liters
1 hectometer = 100 meters
1 kilogram = 1000 grams

Arabic numbers are used to write metric doses.

EXAMPLES:

500 milligrams, 5 grams, 15 milliliters

Prefixes added to the units (meter, liter, or gram) indicate smaller or larger units. All units are derived by dividing or multiplying by 10, 100, or 1000.

COMMON METRIC EQUIVALENTS

1 milliliter (mL) = 1 cubic centimeter (cc)
1000 milliliters (mL) = 1 liter (L)
= 1000 cubic centimeters (cc)
1000 milligrams (mg) = 1 gram (g)
1000 micrograms (mcg) = 1 milligram (mg)
1,000,000 micrograms (mcg) = 1 gram (g)
1000 grams (g) = 1 kilogram (kg)

Differentiate among metric weight and metric volume. Mark each of the following MW for metric weight or MV for metric volume.

1. microgram = ______
2. milliliter = ______
3. liter = ______
4. gram = ______

Conversion of Metric Units

The first step in calculating the drug dosage is to make sure that the drug ordered and the drug source on hand are *both* in the same *system of measurement* (preferably in the metric system) and in the *same unit of weight* for example, both **milligrams** or both grams).

Converting Milligrams (Metric) to Grams (Metric) (1000 mg = 1 g)

Divide the number of milligrams by 1000 or move the decimal point of the milligrams three places to the left.

EXAMPLES:

200 mg = 0.2 g
0.6 mg = 0.0006 g

Convert the following milligrams to grams:

0.4 mg = ______ g
0.12 mg = ______ g
0.2 mg = ______ g
0.1 mg = ______ g
500 mg = ______ g
125 mg = ______ g
100 mg = ______ g
200 mg = ______ g
50 mg = ______ g
400 mg = ______ g

Can you take the gram dosages in these answers and convert them to milligrams?

Convert the following grams (g) to milligrams (mg):

0.2 g = ______ mg
0.250 g = ______ mg
0.125 g = ______ mg
0.0006 g = ______ mg
0.004 g = ______ mg

In the following example, both the health care provider's order and the medication available are in the metric system. They are *not* both in the *same unit of weight* within the metric system.

EXAMPLE:

The health care provider orders that the patient receive 0.25 g of a drug. The label on the bottle of medicine says 250 mg, meaning that each capsule contains 250 mg of the drug.

To change the gram dose into milligrams, multiply 0.25 by 1000 and move the decimal point three places to the right (a milligram is one thousandth of a gram); 0.250 g = 250 mg, so you would give one tablet of this drug.

TRY THIS ONE: The health care provider orders the patient to have 0.1 g of a drug. The label on the bottle states that the strength of the drug is 100 mg/capsule.

To change the gram dose into milligrams, move the decimal point three places to the right: 0.1 g = 100 mg, exactly what the bottle label strength states.

Solid Dosage for Oral Administration

If the dosage on hand and dosage ordered are both in the same system and in the same unit of weight, proceed to calculate the dosage using one of these methods.

EXAMPLE:

A health care provider orders that a patient receive 1 g of ampicillin. The ampicillin bottle states that each tablet in the bottle contains 0.5 g.

PROBLEM:

You do not have the 1 g as ordered. How many tablets will you give? (Both the amount ordered and the amount available are in the same system of measurement [metric] and the same unit of weight [grams]).

SOLUTION:

You may use two methods.

Method 1:

$$\frac{\text{Dose desired}}{\text{Dose on hand}} = \frac{1.0\text{ g}}{0.5\text{ g}} = 2$$

You will give two 0.5 g capsules to give the 1.0 g ordered.

Method 2 (Proportional):

Metric dosage ordered: Drug form
Metric dosage available: Drug form

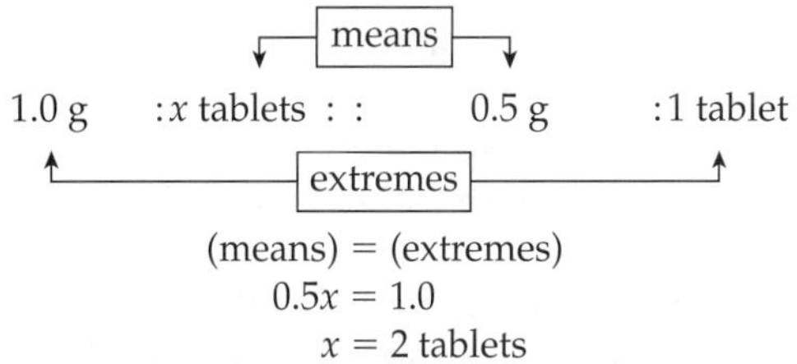

(means) = (extremes)
$0.5x = 1.0$
$x = 2$ tablets

Proof: Product of means: 2 (value of x) × 0.5 = 1
Product of extremes: 1 × 1 = 1

If the dosage on hand and dosage ordered are both in the same system of measurement, but they are *not* in the same unit of weight within the system, the units of weight must first be converted.

EXAMPLE:

The health care provider orders 1000 milligrams (metric) of ampicillin. On hand: 0.25 gram (metric) per tablet.

Rule: Converting grams (metric) to milligrams (metric) (1 g = 1000 mg)
Multiply the number of grams by 1000; move the decimal point of the grams three places to the right. 0.25 g = 250 mg

SOLUTION:

$$\frac{\text{Dose desired}}{\text{Dose on hand}} = \frac{1000\text{ mg}}{250\text{ mg}} = 4 \quad \text{Give four 0.25 g tablets.}$$

$$\frac{\text{mg}}{250} : \frac{\text{tablet}}{1} :: \frac{\text{mg}}{1000} : \frac{\text{tablet}}{x}$$

$$x = \frac{1000}{250} = 4 \text{ tablets}$$

Proof: Product of means: 1 × 1000 = 1000
Product of extremes: 250 × 4 = (value of *x*) = 1000

Conversion Problems

Some students understand problems in tablet or capsule dosage for oral administration if presented with their fractional equivalents as follows:

1. A health care provider orders that a patient receive 2 g of a drug in oral tablet form. The medicine bottle label states that the strength on hand is 0.5 g. This means each tablet in the bottle is the strength 0.5 g.
   How many tablets would be given to the patient? 1, 2, 3, 4, or 5? *Answer:* 4
   What strength is ordered? 2 g
   What strength is on the bottle label? 0.5 g
   What is the fractional equivalent of 0.5 g? ½ g
   How many ½ g (0.5 g) tablets would equal 2 g? 4

   $$2 \div \frac{1}{2} = \frac{2}{1} \times \frac{2}{1} = 4 \text{ tablets}$$

2. A health care provider orders that a patient receive 0.2 mg of a drug in oral tablet form. The medicine bottle label states that the strength on hand is 0.1 mg. This means each tablet in the bottle is the strength 0.1 mg.
   How many tablets would be given to the patient? 1, 2, 3, or 4? *Answer:* 2 tablets
   What strength is ordered? 0.2 mg
   What is the fractional equivalent of 0.2 mg? ²⁄₁₀
   What strength is on the bottle label (on hand)? 0.1 mg
   What is the fractional equivalent of 0.1 mg? ¹⁄₁₀
   How many ¹⁄₁₀ mg (0.1 mg) tablets would equal ²⁄₁₀ mg (0.2 mg)? 2

   0.1 mg = ¹⁄₁₀ mg or 1 tablet
   +0.1 mg = ¹⁄₁₀ mg or 1 tablet
   0.2 mg = ²⁄₁₀ mg or 2 tablets

   Dosage desired ÷ dosage on hand =

   $$\text{or } \frac{2}{10} \div \frac{1}{10} = \frac{2}{\cancel{10}_1} \times \frac{\cancel{10}^1}{1} = 2 \text{ tablets}$$

3. A health care provider orders a patient to receive 0.5 mg of a drug in oral capsule form. The medicine bottle label states that the strength on hand is 0.25 mg. This means each capsule in the bottle is the strength 0.25 mg.
   How many tablets would be given to the patient? 1, 2, 3, 4, or 5? *Answer:* 2 tablets
   What strength is ordered? 0.5 mg
   What fractional equivalent equals 0.5 mg? ½ mg
   What strength is on the bottle label? 0.25 mg
   What fractional equivalent equals the strength on hand? ¼ mg
   How many ¼ mg (0.25 mg) tablets would equal ½ mg (0.5 mg)? 2

   0.25 mg = ¼ mg or 1 tablet
   +0.25 mg = ¼ mg or 1 tablet
   0.50 mg = ½ mg or 2 tablets

   Dosage desired ÷ dosage on hand =

   $$\text{or } \frac{1}{2} \div \frac{1}{4} = \frac{1}{2} \times \frac{4}{1} = 2 \text{ tablets}$$

4. A health care provider orders a patient to receive 0.25 mg of a drug in oral capsule form. The medicine bottle label states that the strength on hand is 0.5 mg. This means that every capsule in the bottle is the strength 0.5 mg.
   How many tablets would be given? ½, 1, 1½, 2, 2½, 3, 4, or 5? *Answer:* ½ tablet
   What strength did the health care provider order? 0.25 mg
   What is the fractional equivalent of the strength the health care provider ordered? ¼ mg
   What strength is on the bottle label? 0.5 mg
   What is the fractional equivalent of the strength on the bottle label (on hand)? ½ mg
   Which is less: 0.5 mg (½ mg) or 0.25 mg (¼ mg)? *Answer:* 0.25 mg (¼ mg)
   Was the amount ordered less than the strength on hand or more? *Answer:* Less

   $$0.5\text{ mg} = \frac{1}{2}\text{ mg or 1 tablet}$$

   $$0.25\text{ mg} = \frac{1}{4}\text{ mg or half as much or } \frac{1}{2} \text{ tablet}$$

   $$\text{or } \frac{1}{4} \div \frac{1}{2} = \frac{1}{4} \times \frac{2}{1} = \frac{1}{2} \text{ tablet}$$

If the medication is also available in 0.25 mg tablets, request that size from the pharmacy. A tablet should be divided only when scored; even then the practice is not advised because the tablet often fragments into unequal pieces.

Converting Weight to Kilograms (1 kg = 2.2 lb)

Many health care providers request that the metric measure be used to record the body weight of the patient. Because the scales used in many hospitals are calibrated in pounds, conversion from pounds to kilograms is required.

1. To convert weight in kilograms to pounds, multiply the kilogram weight by 2.2.

   EXAMPLE:
   25 kg × 2.2 lb/kg = 55 lb

   Convert the following:

   35 kg = _______ lb
   16 kg = _______ lb
   65 kg = _______ lb

2. To convert weight in pounds to kilograms, divide the weight in pounds by 2.2.

   EXAMPLE:
   140 lb ÷ 2.2 kg/lb = 63.6 kg

   Convert the following:

   125 lb = _______ kg
   9 lb = _______ kg
   180 lb = _______ kg

   The weight of a liter of water at 40° C is 2.2 pounds.

Calculations with Other Forms of Measure That Do Not Require Conversions

Other forms of measure often used in medicine are the "unit" and the "milliequivalent." There are no conversions used with units or milliequivalent (mEq) because the medication ordered and the medication available are expressed in the same system of measurement. Units and milliequivalent quantities are stated in Arabic numbers, with "units" or "mEq" following. Some medications, such as insulin, heparin, and penicillin, are measured in units and are available in a standardized quantity of drug per volume (e.g., 100 units/mL of insulin, 1000 units/mL of heparin). It is important to read each medication label carefully because the term "unit" can vary between drugs measured in this manner.

EXAMPLE 1:
Heparin sodium injection, USP can be supplied as 10 units, 100 units, 1000 units, 2500 units, 5000 units, 7500 units, 10,000 units, 20,000 units, 40,000 units/mL, and 25,000 units/500 mL.

MEDICATION PROBLEM:
Health care provider order: Heparin sodium 8000 units subcut q12h

Available: Heparin sodium 10,000 units/mL

What volume of heparin will you administer? (Remember to have all heparin dosages checked by a second qualified individual according to clinic policy.)

Formula: Desired amount : x (desired volume) = Drug strength available : volume

8000 units : x (desired volume) = 10,000 units : 1 mL
Multiply means: (10,000 units)(x) = 10,000 units-x
Multiply extremes: (8000 units)(1 mL) = 8000 units-mL
10,000 units-x = 8000 units-mL

$$\text{Reduce: } x = \frac{80\cancel{00}\ \cancel{\text{units}}\text{-mL}}{10,\cancel{000}\ \cancel{\text{units}}} = \frac{8\text{ mL}}{10} = 0.8\text{ mL}$$

EXAMPLE 2:
Insulins: Insulins (e.g., aspart, lispro, regular, NPH, 70/30, 50/50, Lente) are supplied as 100 units/mL.

MEDICATION PROBLEM:
Health care provider order: Regular insulin 7 units subcut at 7 AM and 12 noon + regular insulin by sliding scale based on 6:45 AM and 11:45 blood glucose.

Sliding Scale Insulin Dosage

Blood glucose <60 = give 2 glasses of orange juice; call health care provider; repeat glucose monitoring 30 minutes after giving juice.

Blood glucose >100-150 = no insulin

Blood glucose >151-200 = 1 unit regular insulin

Blood glucose >201-250 = 2 units regular insulin

Blood glucose >251-300 = 3 units regular insulin

Blood glucose >301-350 = 4 units regular insulin

Blood glucose >350 = 5 units regular insulin, subcut; call health care provider; order blood glucose to be drawn.

If the blood glucose level at 6:45 AM is 258 mg/dL, how much sliding scale insulin would be required in addition to the prescribed dose of regular insulin of 7 units daily at 7 AM?

Answer: At 7 AM the patient would receive 7 units (daily dose) plus 3 units (sliding scale) for a total of 11 units of regular insulin.

What volume of insulin will you administer? (Remember to have all insulin dosages checked by a second qualified individual according to clinical policy.)

Available: Regular insulin 100 units/mL; calculate the dose:

Formula: Desired amount : x (desired volume) = Drug strength available : volume 11 units : x (desired volume) = 100 units : 1 mL

Multiply means: (100 units)(x) = 100 units-x
Multiply extremes: (11 units)(1 mL) = 11 units-mL
100 units-x = 11 units-mL

$$\text{Reduce: } x = \frac{11\ \cancel{\text{units}}\text{-mL}}{100\ \cancel{\text{units}}} = 0.11\text{ mL regular insulin}$$

At 11:30 AM, before lunch, the patient's glucose meter reading is 321 mg/dL. Using the sliding scale above, how much regular insulin should be administered?

Answer: 15 units regular insulin (7 units ordered + 8 units from sliding scale)

What volume of insulin will you administer? (Remember to have all insulin dosages checked by a second qualified individual according to clinical policy.)

Available: Regular insulin 100 units/mL; calculate the dose:

Formula: Desired amount : x (desired volume) = Drug strength available : volume 15 units : x (desired volume) = 100 units : 1 mL

Multiply means: (100 units)(x) = 100 units-x

Multiply extremes: (15 units)(1 mL) = 15 units-mL

100 units-x = 15 units-mL

Reduce: $x = \frac{15\ \cancel{\text{units}}\text{-mL}}{100\ \cancel{\text{units}}} = 0.15$ mL regular insulin

EXAMPLE 3:

Procaine penicillin is supplied as 300,000 units, 500,000 units, and 600,000 units/mL.

MEDICATION PROBLEM:

Health care provider order: Procaine penicillin 400,000 units IM q12h

Available: Procaine penicillin 600,000 units/mL

How many mL will you administer?

Formula: Desired amount : x (desired volume) = Drug strength available : volume 400,000 units : x (desired volume) = 600,000 units : 1 mL

Multiply means: (600,000 units)(x) = 600,000 units-x

Multiply extremes: (400,000 units)(1 mL) = 400,000 units-mL

600,000x = 400,000 units-mL

Reduce: $x = \frac{\cancel{400{,}000\ \text{units}}\text{-mL}}{\cancel{600{,}000\ \text{units}}} = 0.75$ mL procaine penicillin

EXAMPLE 4:

Potassium chloride is supplied: 6.7, 8, 10, and 20 mEq per tablet.

MEDICATION PROBLEM:

Health care provider order: Potassium chloride 40 mEq PO bid

Available: Potassium chloride 20 mEq/tablet

How many tablets will you administer per dose?

Formula: Desired amount : x (desired quantity) = Drug strength available : 1 tablet

40 mEq : x (desired quantity) = 20 mEq : 1 tablet

Multiply means: (20 mEq)(x) = 20 mEq-x

Multiply extremes: (40 mEq)(1 tablet) = 40 mEq-tablet

20 mEq-x = 40 mEq-tablet

Reduce: $x = \frac{40\ \cancel{\text{mEq}}/\text{tablet}}{20\ \cancel{\text{mEq}}/\text{tablet}} = 2$ tablets potassium chloride

(Note: Potassium chloride is best given with or after meals with a full glass of water to decrease gastric upset. Remind patient not to chew or crush tablets; swallow whole.)

CALCULATION OF INTRAVENOUS FLUID AND MEDICATION ADMINISTRATION RATES

Objective

1. Use formulas to calculate intravenous fluid and medicine administration rates.

Key Terms

administration sets
drip chamber
macrodrip
microdrip
drop factor (DF)
round

Intravenous Fluid Orders, Drip Rates, Pumps, and Rounding

Intravenous (IV) solutions (fluids) consist of a liquid (solvent) containing one or more dissolved substances (solutes). The health care provider orders a specific type and volume of solution to be infused over a specific time span. (See Chapter 12 for methods of IV administration, and Table 12-1 for a listing of common IV solutions and abbreviations.)

The order can be written in any of the following three ways:

1. 1000 mL 5% dextrose and water (D5W) to infuse intravenously over the next 8 hours
2. 1 L D5W IV over next 8 hours
3. Infuse 5% dextrose intravenously at 125 mL/hr

Administration sets used to deliver a specified volume of solution are different depending on the company manufacturing the set. The administration set can vary in different lengths and diameters of tubing, the presence or absence of inline filters, and a differing number of Y-ports (sites). (See Figure 12-1 in Chapter 12.)

The **drip chamber** of the administration set is either a **macrodrip,** a chamber that delivers large drops, or a **microdrip,** a chamber that delivers small drops.

All microdrip chambers deliver 60 drops (gtt) per mL. The microdrip administration set is used whenever a small volume of IV solution is ordered to be infused over a specified time (e.g., neonatal, pediatric units). In some clinical settings a microdrip administration set is used whenever the volume of solution to infuse is less than 100 mL per hour (Figure 6-2).

The manufacturer of the macrodrip administration set has standardized the *drops* per milliliter, called the **drop factor (DF),** for the specific brand of administration set as follows:

COMPANY NAME	DROP FACTOR (gtt/mL)
Abbott	15
Baxter International	10
B. Braun	15
IVAC	20

The box containing the administration set always has the drop factor printed on the label.

Rounding

Not all calculations used to compute IV fluid administration rates divide out evenly; it is necessary to have a uniform way to **round** the answers to whole numbers. One method commonly used is to divide the numbers, carry the calculations to hundredths, and round to tenths. If the tenth is 0.5 or more, increase the answer to

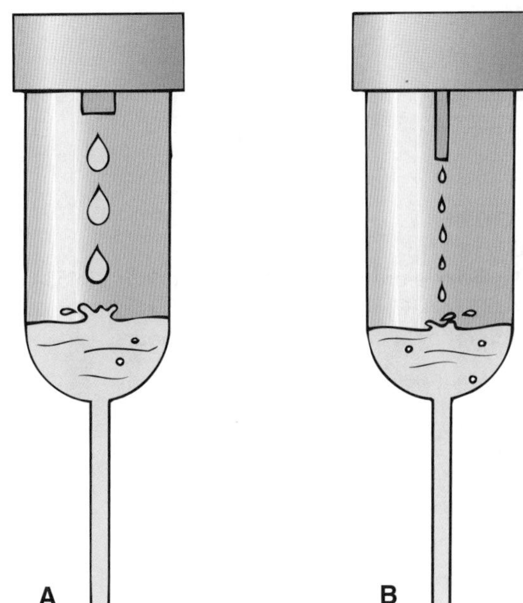

FIGURE 6-2 **A,** Macrodrip chamber. **B,** Microdrip chamber.

the next whole number. If the tenth is less than 0.5, leave the whole number at the current value.

EXAMPLES:

167.57 = 167.6 = 168
167.44 = 167.4 = 167
32.15 = 32.2 = 32
32.45 = 32.5 = 33

The nurse must be able to calculate the rate for the prescribed infusion, whether it is being given as an additive in the primary IV fluid (using a secondary set called a piggyback or rider setup [see Chapter 12] with calibrated regulators) or infused by means of an electronic infusion pump.

Volumetric and Nonvolumetric Pumps

When determining the flow rate for infusion pumps, the type of infusion pump must first be determined. Pumps are categorized as either volumetric or nonvolumetric. Volumetric pumps are set to measure the volume being infused in milliliters per hour, whereas nonvolumetric pumps are set in drops per minute. (Check the individual pump being used to see the type of calibration [mL/hr or gtt/min] printed on the display window of the pump.) (See Chapter 12 for a discussion on types of infusion control devices.)

Calculation of Flow Rates

Milliliters per Hour (mL/hr)

To calculate flow rates, divide the total volume in milliliters (number of mL) of fluid ordered for infusion by the total number of *hours* the infusion is to run. This will equal the milliliters per hour (mL/hr) the infusion is to run.

$$\frac{\text{Number of mL}}{\text{Number of hours}} = \text{mL/hr}$$

EXAMPLE:

Infuse 1000 mL lactated Ringer's (LR) solution over 10 hours

$$\frac{\text{Number of mL} = 1000 \text{ mL}}{\text{Number of hours} = 10 \text{ hr}} = 100 \text{ mL/hr}$$

Calculate the following problems:

HEALTH CARE PROVIDER'S ORDER	DURATION OF INFUSION	RATE (mL/hr)
1000 mL 5% dextrose in water	12 hr	= _____ mL/hr
1000 mL lactated Ringer's	6 hr	= _____ mL/hr
500 mL 0.9% sodium chloride	4 hr	= _____ mL/hr

Calculating Rates of Infusion for Other Than 1 Hour

The nurse must be able to convert infusion rates given in minutes to milliliters per hour because volumetric pumps are calibrated in milliliters. The formula is as follows: the volume of solution ordered times 60 minutes per hour divided by time (in minutes) to administer.

$$\frac{\text{Total volume (milliliters) to infuse} \times 60 \text{ min/hr}}{\text{Time}} = \text{mL/hr}$$

$$\frac{\text{Total volume (milliliters) to infuse} \times 60 \cancel{\text{min}}\text{/hr}}{\text{Time}} = \text{mL/hr}$$

Calculate the following problems:

HEALTH CARE PROVIDER'S ORDER	DURATION OF INFUSION	RATE (mL/hr)
50 mL 0.9% NaCl with ampicillin 1 g	20 min	= _____ mL/hr
150 mL D5W with gentamicin 80 mg	30 min	= _____ mL/hr
50 mL 0.9% NaCl with ondansetron 32 mg	15 min	= _____ mL/hr

Drops per Minute (gtt/min)

The nurse must calculate drops per minute whenever a drug infusion is given with the use of a secondary administration set, a nonvolumetric infusion pump, or a calibrated cylinder. The formula is as follows:

$$\frac{\text{Total volume (milliliters) to infuse} \times \text{Drop factor}}{\text{Time (min)}} = \text{gtt/min}$$

$$\frac{\text{Total volume (milliliters) to infuse} \times \text{Drop factor (gtt/mL)}}{\text{Time (min)}} = \text{gtt/min}$$

$$\frac{\text{Total volume (}\cancel{\text{milliliters}}\text{) to infuse} \times \text{Drop factor (gtt/}\cancel{\text{mL}}\text{)}}{\text{Time (min)}} = \text{gtt/min}$$

Remember that the answer, *drops,* cannot be given as a fraction; as previously discussed, the answer must be rounded to a whole number.

EXAMPLE:

31.4 gtt = 31 gtt; 31.5 gtt = 32 gtt

Calculate the following problems.

Directions: Use a drop factor of 15 gtt/mL for volumes of *100 mL or greater* per hour; use a microdrip (60 gtt/hr) for volumes below 100/hr. (Note: Whenever a microdrip is used, milliliters per hour equals drops per minute, so no calculations are needed.)

HEALTH CARE PROVIDER'S ORDER	DURATION OF INFUSION	RATE (mL/hr)
125 mL D5W	60 min	= _____ mL/hr
100 mL lactated Ringer's	60 min	= _____ mL/hr
50 mL 0.9% NaCl	20 min	= _____ mL/hr

Drugs Ordered in Units per Hour or Milligrams per Hour

Health care providers may order certain medicines to be administered in units per hour (units/hr) or in milligrams per hour (mg/hr). Drugs ordered in this way are administered by means of an electronic infusion pump. The formula is as follows:

Set up a proportion:

Total units or milligrams of drug added: Total volume of solution : ordered amount of drugs in units or mg/hr : x (volume of solution)

EXAMPLE:

Administered as units/hr

Health care provider's order: Mix 10,000 units of heparin in 1000 mL D5W; infuse 80 units per hour. What volume of solution should be administered?

10,000 units : 1000 mL : 80 units/hr : x mL

Multiply the means: 1000 mL × 80 units/hr = 80,000 mL − units/hr

Multiply the extremes: 10,000 units × x = 10,000 units-x.

10,000 units-x = 80,000 mL − units/hr

Divide both sides of equation by number with x.

$$\frac{10{,}000\text{ units-}x}{10{,}000\text{ units}} = \frac{80{,}000\text{ mL} - \text{units/hr}}{10{,}000\text{ units}}$$

$$\frac{\cancel{10{,}000\text{ units}}\text{-}x}{\cancel{10{,}000\text{ units}}} = \frac{\cancel{80{,}000}\text{ mL} - \cancel{\text{units}}\text{/hr}}{\cancel{10{,}000\text{ units}}}$$

x = 8 mL/hr

Set infusion pump at 8 mL per hour to deliver 80 units of heparin per hour.

EXAMPLE:

Administered as mL/hr.

The health care provider could order the number of milliliters of heparin per hour rather than specifying the order in units per hour.

Mix 10,000 units heparin in 1000 mL D5W; infuse at 15 mL/hr. How many units of heparin are being delivered per hour?

10,000 units: 1000 mL = x units: 15 mL/hr

Multiply the means: 1000 mL × x = 1000 mL-x

Multiply the extremes: 10,000 units × 15 mL/hr = 150,000 units-mL/hr.

1000 mL-x = 150,000 units-mL/hr

Divide both sides of equation by number with x.

$$\frac{1000\text{ mL-}x}{1000\text{ mL}} = \frac{150{,}000\text{ units-mL/hr}}{1000\text{ mL}}$$

$$\frac{\cancel{1{,}000\text{ mL}}\text{-}x}{\cancel{1{,}000\text{ mL}}} = \frac{150\cancel{,000}\text{ units-}\cancel{\text{mL}}\text{/hr}}{\cancel{1{,}000\text{ mL}}}$$

Reduce: x = 150 units

EXAMPLE:

milligrams/hr

Physician's order: Mix 500 mg dopamine in 500 mL of D5/0.45% NaCl to infuse at 30 mg/hr. What volume of solution should be administered per hour?

500 mg : 500 mL = 30 mg/hr : x volume

Multiply the means: 500 mL × 30 mg/hr = 15,000 mL-mg/hr

Multiply the extremes: 500 mg × x = 500 mg-x

500 mg-x = 15,000 mL-mg/hr

Divide both sides of equation by the number with x.

$$\frac{500\text{ mg-}x}{500\text{ mg}} = \frac{15{,}000\text{ mL-mg/hr}}{500\text{ mg}}$$

$$\frac{\cancel{500\text{ mg}}\text{-}x}{\cancel{500\text{ mg}}} = \frac{\overset{30}{\cancel{15{,}000}}\text{ mL-}\cancel{\text{mg}}\text{/hr}}{\cancel{500\text{ mg}}}$$

Reduce: x = 30 mL/hr

Set infusion pump at 30 mL/hr

Calculate the following problems:

Health care provider's order:

Heparin 20,000 units in 1 L lactated Ringer's solution infuse at 120 units/hr	= _____	mL/hr
Regular insulin 100 units in 100 mL normal saline (NS) infuse at 15 units/hr	= _____	mL/hr

FAHRENHEIT AND CENTIGRADE (CELSIUS) TEMPERATURES

Objective

1. Demonstrate proficiency in performing conversions between the centigrade and Fahrenheit systems of temperature measurement.

Key Terms

centigrade
Fahrenheit
Celsius

It is necessary for the nurse to be familiar with both the centigrade and the Fahrenheit scales of temperature measurement.

1. The centrigrade and Fahrenheit scales differ from each other in the way they are graduated.
   a. On the **centigrade (Celsius)** scale the point at which water freezes is marked "0°."

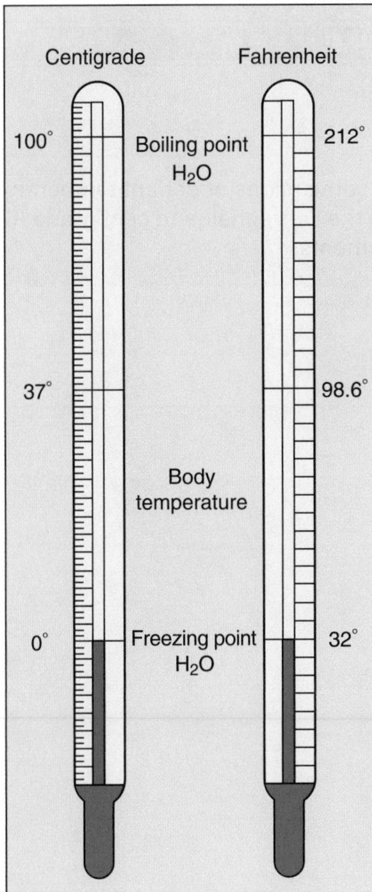

FIGURE 6-3 Clinical thermometers.

b. On the Fahrenheit scale the point at which water freezes is marked "32°."
c. The boiling point for water in centigrade is 100°.
d. The boiling point for water in Fahrenheit is 212°.

2. The value of graduations (degrees) on the centigrade thermometer differs from the value of degrees on the Fahrenheit thermometer.
   a. Using the centigrade scale, there are 100 increments (degrees) between the 0° point (freezing point) and the 100° point (boiling point of water).
   b. Using the Fahrenheit scale, there are 180 spaces (degrees) between the freezing and boiling points.
3. To convert readings from a centigrade scale to the Fahrenheit scale, the centigrade reading is multiplied by 180/100 or 9/5 and then added to 32.
4. To convert a Fahrenheit reading to centigrade scale, subtract 32 from the Fahrenheit reading and multiply by 5/9 (100/180).

Formula for Converting Fahrenheit Temperature to Centigrade Temperature

$$(\text{Fahrenheit} - 32) \times \frac{5}{9} = \text{Centrigrade}$$

$$(F - 32) \times \frac{5}{9} = C$$

EXAMPLE:
Change 212° F to C.

$$(F - 32) \times \frac{5}{9} = C$$

$$212 - 32 = 180$$

$$180 \times \frac{5}{9} = \frac{900}{9} = 100° \text{ C}$$

Convert the following Fahrenheit temperatures to centigrade:

98.6° F = ______° C
102.4° F = ______° C
95.2° F = ______° C

Formula for Converting Centigrade Temperature to Fahrenheit Temperature

$$(\text{Centigrade} \times \frac{9}{5}) + 32 = \text{Fahrenheit}$$

$$(C \times \frac{9}{5}) + 32 = F$$

EXAMPLE:
Change 100° C to F.

$$(C \times \frac{9}{5}) + 32 = F$$

$$(100 \times \frac{9}{5}) = \frac{900}{5} = 180$$

$$180 + 32 = 212° \text{ F}$$

Convert the following centigrade temperatures to Fahrenheit:

37° C = ______° F
35° C = ______° F
41° C = ______° F

Try these problems in converting centigrade to Fahrenheit and Fahrenheit to centigrade.

1. The nurse takes the following temperatures with Fahrenheit clinical thermometers: patient A, 104° F; patient B, 99° F; patient C, 101° F. The health care provider asks what the centigrade temperature is for each patient. Work your problems to convert Fahrenheit temperatures to centigrade. Check your answers. (*Answers:* patient A, 40° C; patient B, 37.2° C; patient C, 38.3° C.)
2. The nurse takes the following temperatures with centigrade clinical thermometers: patient D, 37° C; patient E, 37.8° C; patient F, 38° C. The health care provider asks what the Fahrenheit temperature is for each patient. Work your problems to convert centigrade to Fahrenheit. Check your answers. (*Answers:* patient D, 98.6° F; patient E, 100° F; patient F, 100.4° F.)

Most larger hospitals currently use electronic thermometers that give direct centigrade or Fahrenheit readings.

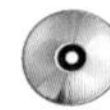
Go to your Companion CD-ROM for Appendices, an Audio Glossary, animations, Drug Dosage Calculators, customizable Patient Self-Assessment forms, and Review Questions for the NCLEX® Examination.

evolve Be sure to visit the companion Evolve site at http://evolve.elsevier.com/Clayton for WebLinks and additional online resources.

MEDICATION SAFETY REVIEW

CRITICAL THINKING QUESTIONS

1. State the formulas for converting dosages within the metric system.
2. State the formulas associated with performing IV infusion rate calculations.
3. Perform conversions of patient temperatures between the Fahrenheit and centigrade (Celsius) measurements.

CONTENT REVIEW QUESTIONS

Perform questions throughout the chapter.

CHAPTER

7 Principles of Medication Administration

evolve http://evolve.elsevier.com/Clayton

Chapter Content

Before medications are administered, the nurse must understand the professional responsibilities associated with medication administration, drug orders, medication delivery systems, and the nursing process as it relates to drug therapy. Ignorance of the nurse's overall responsibilities in the system may result in delays in receiving and administering medications, and serious administration errors. In either case, care is compromised and the patient may suffer unnecessarily.

LEGAL AND ETHICAL CONSIDERATIONS

Objectives

1. Identify the limitations relating to medication administration placed on licensed practical nurses, vocational nurses, registered nurses, and nurse clinicians by the nurse practice act in the state where you will be practicing.
2. Study the policies and procedures of the practice setting to identify specific regulations concerning medication administration by licensed practical nurses, vocational nurses, registered nurses, and nurse clinicians.

Key Terms

nurse practice act
standards of care

The practice of nursing under a professional license is a privilege, not a right. In accepting the privilege, the nurse must understand that this responsibility includes accountability for one's actions and judgments during the execution of professional duties. An understanding of the **nurse practice act** and the rules and regulations established by the state boards of nursing for the various levels of entry (practical nurse, registered nurse, and nurse practitioner) is a solid foundation for beginning practice. Many state boards have developed specific guidelines for the registered nurse to use when delegating medication duties to assistive personnel.

Standards of care are guidelines developed for the practice of nursing. These guidelines are defined by the nurse practice act of each state, by state and federal laws regulating health care facilities, by the Joint Commission on Accreditation of Healthcare Organizations (JCAHO), and by professional organizations such as the American Nurses Association (ANA), and other specialty nursing organizations such as the Intravenous Nurses Society, Inc. Nurses must also be familiar with the established policies of the employing health care agency. Policies developed by the health care agency must adhere to the minimum standards of state regulatory authorities; however, agency policies may be more stringent than those recognized by the state. Employment within the agency implies the willingness of the nurse to adhere to established standards and to work within established guidelines to make necessary changes in the standards. Examples of policy statements relating to medication administration include the following:

1. Educational requirements of professionals authorized to administer medications. Many health care facilities require passage of a written test to confirm the knowledge and skills needed for medication calculation, preparation, and administration before granting approval to administer any medications.
2. Approved lists of intravenous solutions and medications that the nurse can start or add to an existing infusion.
3. Lists of restricted medications (e.g., antineoplastic agents, magnesium sulfate, allergy extracts, lidocaine, RhoGAM, and heparin) that may be administered only by certain staff members.
4. Lists of abbreviations that are not to be used in documentation to avoid medication errors (see Appendix A).

Before administering any medication, the nurse must have a current license to practice, a clear policy statement that authorizes the act, and a medication order signed by a practitioner licensed with prescriptive privileges. The nurse must understand the individual patient's diagnosis and symptoms that correlate with the rationale for drug use. The nurse should also know why a medication is ordered, the expected actions, usual dosing, proper dilution, route and rate of administration, minor side effects to expect, adverse effects to report, and contraindications for the use of a particular drug. If drugs are to be administered using the same syringe or at the same intravenous (IV) site, drug compatibility should be confirmed before administration. If unsure of any of these key medication points, the nurse must consult an authoritative resource or the hospital pharmacist before administering a medication. The nurse must be accurate in calculating, preparing, and administering medications. The nurse must assess the patient to be certain that therapeutic and adverse effects associated with the medication regimen are reported. Nurses must be able to collect patient data at regularly scheduled intervals and record observations in the patient's chart for evaluating a treatment's effectiveness. Claiming unfamiliarity with any of these nursing responsibilities, when an avoidable complication arises, is unacceptable; in fact, it is considered negligence of nursing responsibility.

Nurses must take an active role in educating the patient, family, and significant others in preparation for discharge from the health care environment. (A person's health will improve only to the extent that the patient understands how to care for himself or herself.) Specific teaching goals should be developed and implemented. Nursing observations and progress toward mastery of skills should be charted to document the learner's degree of understanding.

PATIENT CHARTS

Objectives

1. Identify the basic categories of information available in a patient's chart.
2. Study patient charts at different practice settings to identify the various formats used to chart patient data.
3. Cite the information contained in a Kardex and describe the purpose of this file.

Key Terms

summary sheet
consent form
physician's order form
history and physical examination form
progress notes
critical pathways
nurses' notes
nursing history
nursing care plan
laboratory tests record
graphic record
flow sheets
consultation reports
other diagnostic reports
medication administration record (MAR)
medication profile
PRN
unscheduled medication orders
case management
patient education record
Kardex

The patient's chart is a primary source of information that is necessary in patient assessment for the nurse to create and implement plans for patient care. It is also where the nurse provides documentation of nursing assessments performed, observations reported to the physician for further verification, basic nursing measures implemented (e.g., daily bath and treatments), patient teaching performed, and observed responses to therapy.

This document serves as the communication link among all members of the health care team regarding the patient's status, care provided, and progress. The chart is a legal document that describes the patient's health, lists diagnostic and therapeutic procedures initiated, and describes the patient's response to these measures. The chart must be kept current as long as the patient is in the hospital. After the patient's discharge, it is stored in the medical records department until needed. While stored in medical records, the chart may be used for research to compare responses to selected therapy in a sampling of patients with similar diagnoses.

Contents of Patient Charts

Although each health care facility uses a slightly different format, the basic patient chart consists of the following elements.

Summary Sheet

The **summary sheet** gives the patient's name, address, date of birth, attending physician, gender, marital status, allergies, nearest relative, occupation and employer, insurance carrier and other payment arrangements, religious preference, date and time of admission to the hospital, previous hospital admissions, and admitting problem or diagnosis. The date and time of discharge is added when appropriate.

Consent Forms

The admission **consent form** grants permission to the health care facility and physician to provide treatment. Other types of consent forms are used during the course of a hospitalization, such as an operative procedure permit/consent, invasive procedure consent, and blood product consent.

Physician's Order Form

All procedures and treatments are ordered by the health care provider on the **physician's order form** (Figure 7-1). These orders include general care (activity, diet, frequency of vital signs), laboratory tests to be completed, other diagnostic procedures (e.g., radiographs, electrocardiogram [ECG], computed tomography [CT] scans), and all medications and treatments such as physical therapy or occupational therapy.

History and Physical Examination Form

On admission to the hospital, the patient is interviewed by the physician and given a physical examination. The physician records the findings on the **history and physical examination form** and lists the problems to be corrected (e.g., the diagnoses). The history and physical examination form is often referred to as *the H&P.*

Progress Notes

The physician records frequent observations of the patient's health status in the **progress notes.** In some hospitals, other health professionals such as

PHYSICIAN'S ORDER FORM

Addressogram here:

016-28-3978
Joseph Lorenzo
18 Bush Ave.
Hometown, USA

Dr. M. Martin
Unit-6W, Rm. 621

Martindale Hometown Hospital
Hometown, USA

Please Indicate Allergies

None	Codeine	Penicillin	Sulfa	Aspirin	Others

Date	Time	Prob. No.	Physician's Orders	Physician	Progress Record
1/6/yr	3:00 p.m.	6	Erythromycin 250 mg, po		
			q6h × 8 days	M. Martin	

FIGURE 7-1 Physician's order form and progress record.

pharmacists, dietitians, and physical and respiratory therapists may record observations and suggestions.

Critical Pathways

Critical pathways are also referred to as integrated care plans, care or clinical maps (Figure 7-2), and clinical trajectories. This document is a comprehensive standardized plan of care that is individualized at admission by the physician and nurse case manager. Critical pathways describe a multidisciplinary plan used by all caregivers to track the individual's progress toward expected outcomes within a specified period. Standardized outcomes and timetables require health care providers to make assessments regarding the patient's progress toward the goals of discharge while maintaining quality care. Revisions are made as necessary and communicated to

SEPSIS WITH NEUTROPENIA

DRG #416
Target LOS 9 days

	DATE	DATE	DATE
Hosp day	**HOSPITAL DAY 1**	**HOSPITAL DAY 2**	**HOSPITAL DAY 3**
CONSULTS	Notify Radiation Therapy if applicable	Dr. Clements if ordered Social Service Dietician	
TESTS	CBC, SMA 18, magnesium, creatinine Blood cultures × 2 sites before antibiotics started Chest x-ray Type and screen	CBC Blood cultures for chills or temp >101 No more than 3 sets in 24 hours	CBC ------------------> ------------------>
SPECIMENS	U/A for c&s before antibiotics started Sputum for c&s and Gram stain if productive cough	------------------>	------------------>
TREATMENTS	O_2 at 2L by NC if Hgb <8 Mouth care q4h per protocol	------------------> ------------------>	------------------> ------------------>
VITAL SIGNS	q4h	------------------>	------------------>
I & O	q8h	------------------>	------------------>
DIET	Neutropenic DAT until WBC >1.5	------------------>	------------------>
IVs	Fluids as ordered Antibiotics as ordered	Check w/MD re: fluid changes Continue antibiotics as ordered until d/c'd	Continue until d/c'd ------------------>
MEDS	ID home meds and check with MD Check those that are ordered: ___Tylenol gr × po temp >101 ___Pain PRN ___Sleeper ___Antidiarrhea ___Antiemetic ___Antianxiety	Check those that are ordered: ___Tylenol gr × po temp >101 ___Pain PRN ___Sleeper ___Antidiarrhea ___Antiemetic ___Antianxiety	Check those that are ordered: ___Tylenol gr × po temp >101 ___Pain PRN ___Sleeper ___Antidiarrhea ___Antiemetic ___Antianxiety
ACTIVITY	Up as tolerated	------------------>	------------------>
MISC	Restrict ill visitors and staff	------------------>	Continue until WBC >1.5
TEACHING	Instruct pt to report any: bleeding, diarrhea, N&V, pain	Dietitian to teach re: neutropenic diet Mouth care	Instruct re: personal hygiene
DISCHARGE PLANNING	Evaluate need for d/c planning	Social services called if appropriate	Determine d/c destination

	Shift	Shift	Shift
Nurse signature	______/___	______/___	______/___
Nurse signature	______/___	______/___	______/___
Nurse signature	______/___	______/___	______/___

Authored by Janie Barnett, RN; Lucy Wallace, LPN

FIGURE 7-2 First 3 days of 9-day CareMap for sepsis with neutropenia.

all members so the patient continues uninterrupted toward the discharge goals. Critical pathway programs are developed to monitor the care delivered at a specific clinical setting but are based on data gathered from many clinical sites. The use of standardized outcomes is designed to improve the quality of care provided, reduce the costs of care, and document the effect on patient outcomes influenced by the nursing care.

Nurses' Notes

Although format varies among institutions, the nurses' notes generally start with the nursing history. On admission, the nurse performs a complete health assessment of the patient. This process not only includes a head-to-toe physical assessment but also incorporates a patient and family history that provides insights into the individual and family needs, life patterns, psychosocial and

SUMMARY
PATIENT PROBLEMS/OUTCOME CRITERIA

Sepsis with neutropenia

Target LOS 9 days

Date	Initial	Nsg Diagnosis/Problem	Outcome Criteria/Goal	Date d/c	Initial
		1. Activity intolerance re: disease process	1. Pt. will be able to perform own hygiene care by d/c.		
		2. Imbalanced nutrition re: less than body requirements re: anorexia, illness, dehydration	2a. Pt. will be able to eat at least 1/3 of their ordered diets by d/c 2b. Pt. will identify at least three food items that they find appealing 2c. 1500 mL po flds q 24 h by d/c		
		3. Hyperthermia re: increase in metabolic rate and illness	3. Pt. will be afebrile by day 5.		
		4. Possible knowledge deficit re: s/s to report neutropenic diet, personal hygiene, activity restrictions	4. Prior to d/c, the pt/s.o. will be able to demonstrate competency and/or verbalize understanding of instructions provided.		

Signature

Title

FIGURE **7-2, cont'd** First 3 days of 9-day CareMap for sepsis with neutropenia.

cultural data, and spiritual needs. This assessment will serve as the basis for the development of the individualized care plan and as a baseline for comparison when ongoing assessment data are gathered.

Nurses record in their notes ongoing assessments of the patient's condition; responses to nursing interventions ordered by the physician (e.g., treatments or medications) or those initiated by the nurse (e.g., skin care or patient education); evaluations of the effectiveness of nursing interventions; procedures completed by other health professionals (e.g., wound cleaning by a physician or fitting for a prosthesis by a fitter); and other pertinent information such as physician or family visits and the patient's responses after these visits. Entries may be made on the nurses' notes throughout a shift, but general guidelines include the following: (1) completing records, including vital signs, immediately after making contact with and assessing of the patient, that is, when first admitted or returning from a diagnostic procedure or therapy; (2) recording all PRN medications immediately after administration and the effectiveness of the medication; (3) change in a client's status and who was notified (e.g., physician, manager, client's family); (4) treatment for a sudden change in client's status; and (5) transfer, discharge, or death of a client. In addition to accurately charting the observations in a clear, concise form, the nurse should report significant changes in a patient's status to the charge nurse. The charge nurse then makes a nursing judgment regarding notification of the attending physician. Nurses' notes are quickly being replaced by computerized charting methods that allow the nurse to document findings and basic care delivered using multiple screens of data and checklist-type formats.

Nursing Care Plans

After initial data collection, the nurse develops an individualized **nursing care plan.** Care plans incorporate nursing diagnoses, critical pathway information, and physician-ordered and nursing-ordered care (Figure 7-3).

NURSING CARE PLAN *Risk for Infection*

Assessment

Mrs. Spicer was admitted to the medical nursing unit 3 days ago with a diagnosis of lymphoma. She received her first dose of multiagent chemotherapy yesterday. Jess Ralston is the student nurse caring for Mrs. Spicer. He begins his shift of care by conducting a focused assessment.

Assessment Activities	*Findings/Defining Characteristics*
Reviews client's chart for laboratory data reflecting immune function.	Data show a reduction in number of white blood cells (leukopenia).
Ask client to describe appetite and review food intake for last 24 hours. Weigh client. Measure height.	Client reports she has not had an interest in eating for a couple of weeks. She has lost approximately 6 pounds. Her current weight is 125 lb, height 5′7″. Her food intake yesterday consisted of a small cup of applesauce, ½ bowl of soup, some crackers, and two glasses of juice. Client states, "I get full easily and lose interest in food."
Palpate client's cervical and clavicular lymph nodes.	Lymph nodes are enlarged and painless.
Review effects of chemotherapy in drug reference.	Multi agent chemotherapy causes drug-induced pancytopenia.

Nursing Diagnosis

- **Risk for infection** related to immunosuppression and reduced food intake.

Planning

Goal	*Expected Outcomes**
	Risk Detection
Client will remain free of infection.	Client will remain afebrile.
	Client will develop no signs or symptoms of local infection (e.g., remains free of cough, cloudy or foul-smelling urine, or purulent drainage from open wound or normal body opening).
	Knowledge: Infection Control
Client will become knowledgeable of infection risks.	Client will identify routines to follow in the home that reduce transmission of microorganisms.
	Client will identify signs and symptoms to report to health care provider indicating infection.

FIGURE 7-3 Standard care plan for Risk for Infection. (*Outcome classification labels from: Moorhead S, Johnson M, Maas M: *Nursing Outcomes Classification (NOC)*, ed 3, St. Louis, 2004, Mosby.)

Interventions*	Rationale
Fall Prevention	
Monitor client's body temperature routinely, inspect oral cavity for lesions, inspect urethral and vaginal orifices for drainage or discharge, inspect IV access site for drainage, and observe client for evidence of cough.	Interventions are designed to prevent and ensure early detection of infection in a client at risk (Dochterman and Bulechek, 2004).
Practice hand hygiene routinely before caring for client, between clients, and before any invasive procedures.	Rigorous hand hygiene reduces bacterial counts on the hands (Boyce and Pittet, 2002).
Teach client how to perform hand hygiene correctly.	Client can easily come in contact with infectious agents that can cause infection.
Consult with dietitian in providing a high-calorie, high-protein, low-bacteria diet. Minimize intake of salads, raw fruits and vegetables and undercooked meat, pepper, and paprika. Offer small frequent meals.	Maintaining calorie and protein intake will prevent weight loss. Foods high in bacteria should be avoided because they increase risk for gastrointestinal infection (Ignatavicius and Workman, 2006).
Infection Control	
Instruct client to report the following to physician: temperature greater than 100° F (38° C), persistent cough with or without sputum, pus or foul-smelling drainage from body site, presence of abscess, urine that is cloudy or foul smelling, or burning on urination.	Signs and symptoms are indicative of local or systemic infection.
Teach client to follow these activities at home: • Avoid crowds and large gatherings of people. • Bath daily. • Do not share personal toilet items (toothbrush, washcloth, deodorant stick) with family. • Take temperature twice daily. • Do not drink water that has been standing for longer than 15 minutes. • Do not reuse cups or glasses without washing.	These measures are designed to prevent infection in those clients with impaired immune function (Ignatavicius and Workman, 2006).

Evaluation

Nursing Actions	*Client Response/Finding*	*Achievement of Outcome*
Compare client's body temperature and other physical findings with baseline data.	Client remains afebrile and denies having cough or burning on urination. No signs of drainage or discharge from body site.	Client has no active infection at this time.
Ask client to describe signs and symptoms to report to health care provider.	Client able to identify temperature range to report. Was able to describe cough. Unable to identify signs of urinary infection or local discharge.	Client has partial understanding of signs and symptoms to report. Will require additional instruction. Offer information sheet.
Ask client to explain the measures to take at home to reduce exposure to infectious agents.	Client able to discuss need to avoid sharing personal hygiene articles. Asked for a listing of other precautions and requested that husband be included in discussion.	Client has partial understanding of restrictions. Will obtain printed guidelines and include husband in discussion this evening.

FIGURE **7-3, cont'd** Standard care plan for Risk for Infection. (Intervention classification labels from Dochterman JM, Bulechek GM: *Nursing Interventions Classification (NIC)*, ed 4, St. Louis, 2004, Mosby.)

Most acute care facilities require the nurse to chart against each identified nursing diagnosis stated in the care plan every 8 hours. Care plans are evaluated and modified on a continuum throughout the course of treatment. The plan should be shared with the health care team to ensure an interdisciplinary approach to care. Many institutions have developed standardized care plans for the various nursing diagnoses. It is the nurse's responsibility to identify those diagnoses, outcomes, and interventions that are appropriate for the patient.

Laboratory Tests Record

All laboratory test results are kept in one section of the chart (**laboratory tests record**). Hospitals using computerized reports may list consecutive values of the same test once that test has been repeated several times (e.g., electrolytes). Computerized laboratory data access provides online laboratory results as soon as the tests are completed. Other hospitals may attach small report forms to a full-size backing sheet as each report returns from the laboratory. Because some medication doses are

Martindale Hometown Hospital
Laboratory Summary Report

PATIENT NAME: Joseph Lorenzo — Rm. 621-2 — ADM: January 21
ID NO. 016-28-3978
DIAGNOSIS: Myocardial Infarction
PHYSICIAN: M. Martin, M.D.

TIME: 12:13 a.m.
DATE: 1/28

DATE	1/27	1/26	1/25	1/24	1/23	Normal
TIME	07:00	07:00	07:00	07:00	07:00	range
INR	1.5	1.4	2	1.4	1.3	2-3
aPTT	34	33	38	34	31	25-35 sec

FIGURE **7-4** Laboratory test reports. Example of the International Normalized Ratio (INR) for a patient receiving warfarin.

based on daily blood studies, it is important to be able to locate these data within the patient's chart. Figure 7-4 illustrates a series of International Normalized Ratio (INR) and partial thromboplastin time (PTT) results for a patient receiving warfarin.

Graphic Record

The graphic record, Figure 7-5, *A*, is an example of manual recording of temperature, pulse, respiration, and blood pressure. Figure 7-5, *B* is a computer database–generated example of the vital signs, fluid intake and output, glucose, dietary intake, and other information to be used for ongoing assessment of the patient's status.

Pain assessment, now known as the fifth vital sign, can also be recorded in a graphic form. In addition to the graphic recording of pain, other flow sheets within the chart will record the details of the pain events. Figure 7-6 illustrates preintervention and postintervention ratings as well as pain descriptors, pain interventions, medications administered, and patient teaching completed.

Flow Sheets

Flow sheets are a condensed form for recording information for quick comparison of the data. Examples of flow sheets in common use are diabetic, pain (see Figure 7-6), and neurologic flow sheets. The graphic record used for recording vital signs is another type of a flow sheet.

Consultation Reports

When other physicians or health professionals are asked to consult on a patient, the specialist's summary of findings, diagnoses, and recommendations for treatment are recorded in the consultation reports section.

Other Diagnostic Reports

Reports of surgery, electroencephalogram (EEG), ECG, pulmonary function tests, radioactive scans, and radiograph reports are usually recorded in the other diagnostic reports section of the patient's chart.

Medication Administration Record (MAR) or Medication Profile

The medication administration record (MAR) or medication profile is printed from the computerized patient database, ensuring that the pharmacist and the nurse have identical medication profiles for the patient. The MAR lists all medications to be administered. The medications are usually grouped according to the following categories: those *scheduled* on a regular basis (e.g., every 6 hours or twice a day), *parenteral, stat,* (from the Latin term *statim,* meaning "immediately"), and *preoperative* orders; *PRN medications* are usually listed at the bottom of the MAR or are found on a separate page as unscheduled medication orders.

The MAR provides a space for recording the time the medication is administered and who gives it. Generally, the nurse records and initials the time when the medication is given. The nurse also places his or her initials, name, and title in a designated place provided within the record for documentation.

MARs are kept in a notebook or clipboard file on the medication cart for the 24-hour period they are in use and then they become a permanent part of the patient's chart. In the acute care setting, a new MAR is generated every 24 hours at the same time the unit dose cart is refilled (Figure 7-7, *A*). Figure 7-7, *B* is an example of an electronic database–generated medication sheet listing all scheduled medications for an 8-hour shift. By clicking the cursor on the highlighted area (regular

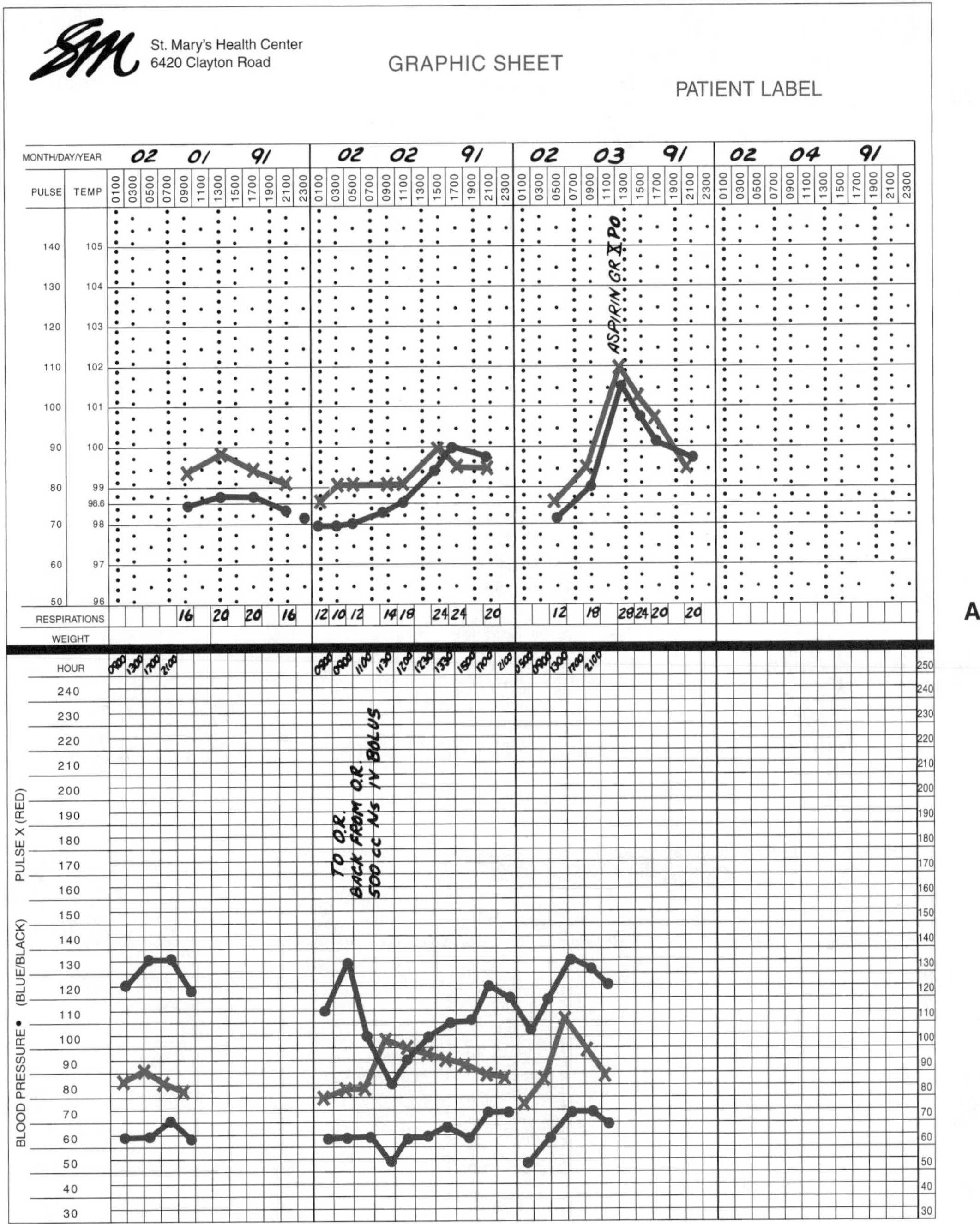

FIGURE 7-5 **A,** Manual vital signs record. *Continued*

insulin in this illustration), a window opens, revealing details of the order.

In the long-term care setting the MAR uses the same principles; however, it generally provides a space for medications to be recorded for up to 1 month (Figure 7-8). The medication record also shows the name of the pharmacy dispensing the prescribed medications and the assigned prescription number. Medications prescribed for residents in the long-term care setting are required to be reviewed on a scheduled basis; therefore the MAR identifies the reviewer and date (see Figure 7-8).

PRN or Unscheduled Medication Record

Some clinical settings use a PRN (Latin for *pro re nata,* meaning "as circumstances require") medication record rather than nurses' notes to record the date, time, PRN medication administered and dose, reason for administering the PRN medication, and patient's response to the drug given. In most clinical settings using MAR methods of charting, the PRN medications are recorded on a separate MAR sheet, sometimes referred to as **unscheduled medication orders** (see Figure 7-7, *A*). Figure 7-8 is an example of an MAR used in the long-term care setting.

B

Flowsheet - VS/ I&O Combined Report

	11/07/02 21:49	11/08/02 00:02	03:25	04:00	05:30	05:58	07:32
TEMP #1		99.2F Oral		98.6F Oral			99F Oral
PULSE #1		80		82			79
PULSE #2							
RESPIRATIONS		20		20			20
NIBP #1		96/56		106/64			103/61
5th VS/Pain Scor		0					6&
Accucheck BS							181
Pulse Equipment							Dyn
BP Equipment							Dyn
Dinner							
Oral	780				50		
Shift Total	780				50		
0.9% NS w/20 KCL			342			240	
Shift Total			342			582	
Intake Total	780		342		50	240	
Shift Total	1438		342		392	632	
Urine	0				850		
Shift Total	0				850		
Urine (O)	1				1		
Shift Total	1				1		
Stool (O)	0				0		

FIGURE **7-5, cont'd** **B,** Electronic charting of vital signs and intake and output.

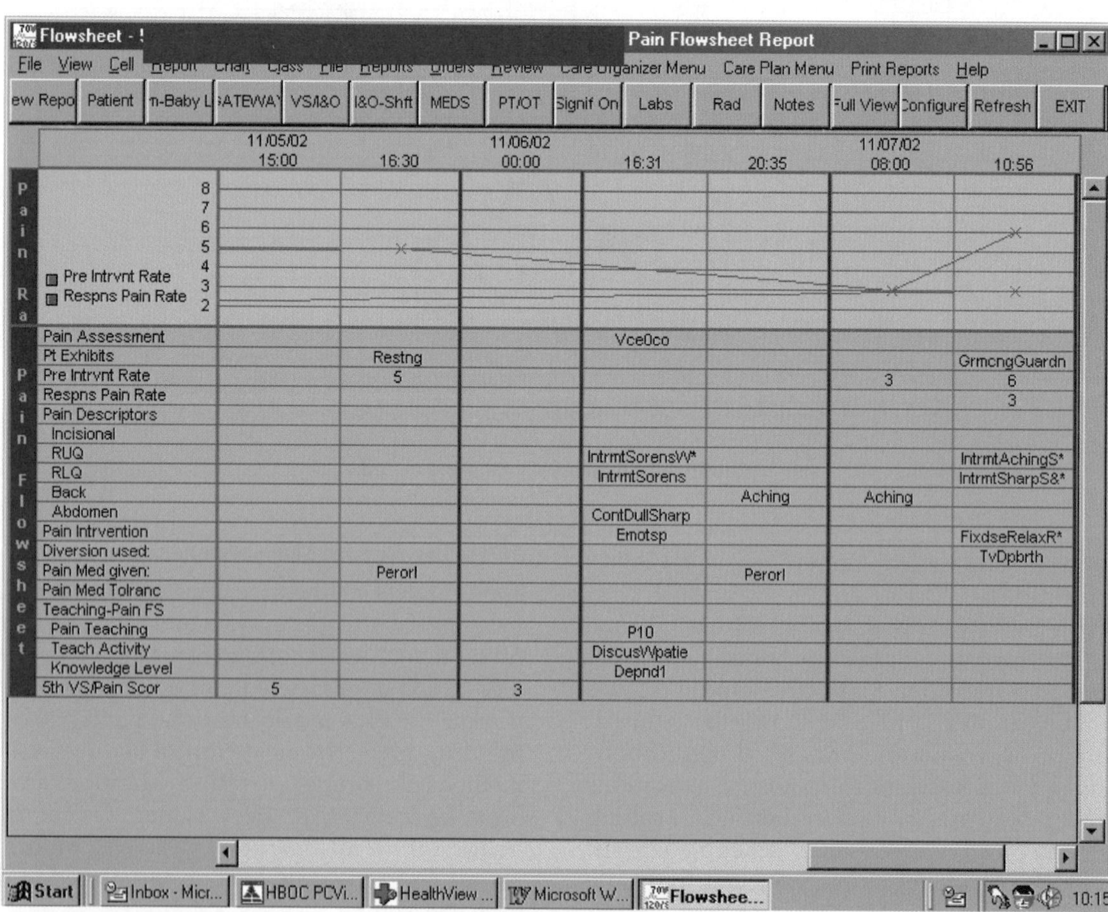

Flowsheet - Pain Flowsheet Report

	11/05/02 15:00	16:30	11/06/02 00:00	16:31	20:35	11/07/02 08:00	10:56
Pain Assessment				Vce0co			
Pt Exhibits		Restng					GrmcngGuardn
Pre Intrvnt Rate		5				3	6
Respns Pain Rate							3
Pain Descriptors							
Incisional							
RUQ				IntrmtSorensW*			IntrmtAchingS*
RLQ				IntrmtSorens			IntrmtSharpS&*
Back					Aching	Aching	
Abdomen				ContDullSharp			
Pain Intrvention				Emotsp			FixdseRelaxR*
Diversion used:							TvDpbrth
Pain Med given:		Perorl			Perorl		
Pain Med Tolranc							
Teaching-Pain FS							
Pain Teaching				P10			
Teach Activity				DiscusWpatie			
Knowledge Level				Depnd1			
5th VS/Pain Scor	5		3				

FIGURE **7-6** Pain flow sheet illustrates preintervention and postintervention ratings, as well as pain descriptors, interventions, teaching, and medications given.

MARTINDALE HOMETOWN HOSPITAL

MEDICATION ADMINISTRATION RECORD

				Init	Signature	Title
NAME:	Joseph Lorenzo		RM-BD: 621-2			
ID NO.	016-28-3978		AGE: 62			
DIAGNOSIS	Myocardial Infarction	SEX: M				
PHYSICIAN	M. Martin, M.D.	Ht: 6'	Wt:			

	SCHEDULED MEDICATIONS			
DATES:	MEDICATION—STRENGTH—FORM—ROUTE	0030-0729	0730-1529	1530-0029
1/25/yr	RANITIDINE ZANTAC 150 MG TABLET ORAL TWICE A DAY		0900	1800
1/25/yr	DILTIAZEM HYDROCHLORIDE CARDIZEM 90 MG TABLET ORAL 4 TIMES DAILY		0900 1300	1800 2100
1/25/yr	WARFARIN SODIUM COUMADIN 1 MG TABLET ORAL EVERY OTHER DAY	NOT GIVEN	TODAY	
	IV AND PIGGYBACK ORDERS			
1/25/yr	CEFTAZIDIME (FORTAZ) 1 G IV SODIUM CHLORIDE 0.9% 50 ML EVERY 8 HOURS INFUSE: 20 MIN	0200	1000	1800
1/25/yr	GENTAMICIN PREMIX 80 MG IV ISO-OSMOTIC SOLN 100 ML BY IV PUMP EVERY 12 HOURS INFUSE: 30 MIN	0200	1400	
1/25/yr	BY IV PUMP 1 IV DSW-5/0.2 NACI 1000 ML RATE: 100 ML/HR			
	PRN MEDICATIONS			
1/25/yr	ACETAMINOPHEN TYLENOL 650 MG (23325) TABLET ORAL EVERY 4 HOURS AS NEEDED PRN			
1/25/yr	MAGNESIUM HYDROXIDE MILK OF MAGNESIA 60 ML (CONC) ORAL CONC AS NEEDED PRN			
1/25/yr	ALBUTEROL PROVENTIL INHALER 90 MCG/INH AEROSOL INH AS NEEDED PRN SEE RESPIRATORY THERAPY NOTES AT BEDSIDE			

Age/Sex	HT	WT	Date	ALLERGIES CODEINE
62/ M	6'0"	200 lbs	1/25/yr	
Room-Bd	Name			
621 2	Joseph Lorenzo			

A

FIGURE 7-7 **A,** Example of medication administration record (MAR). (Note: separation of scheduled orders, IVs, and PRN medications.)

Continued

B

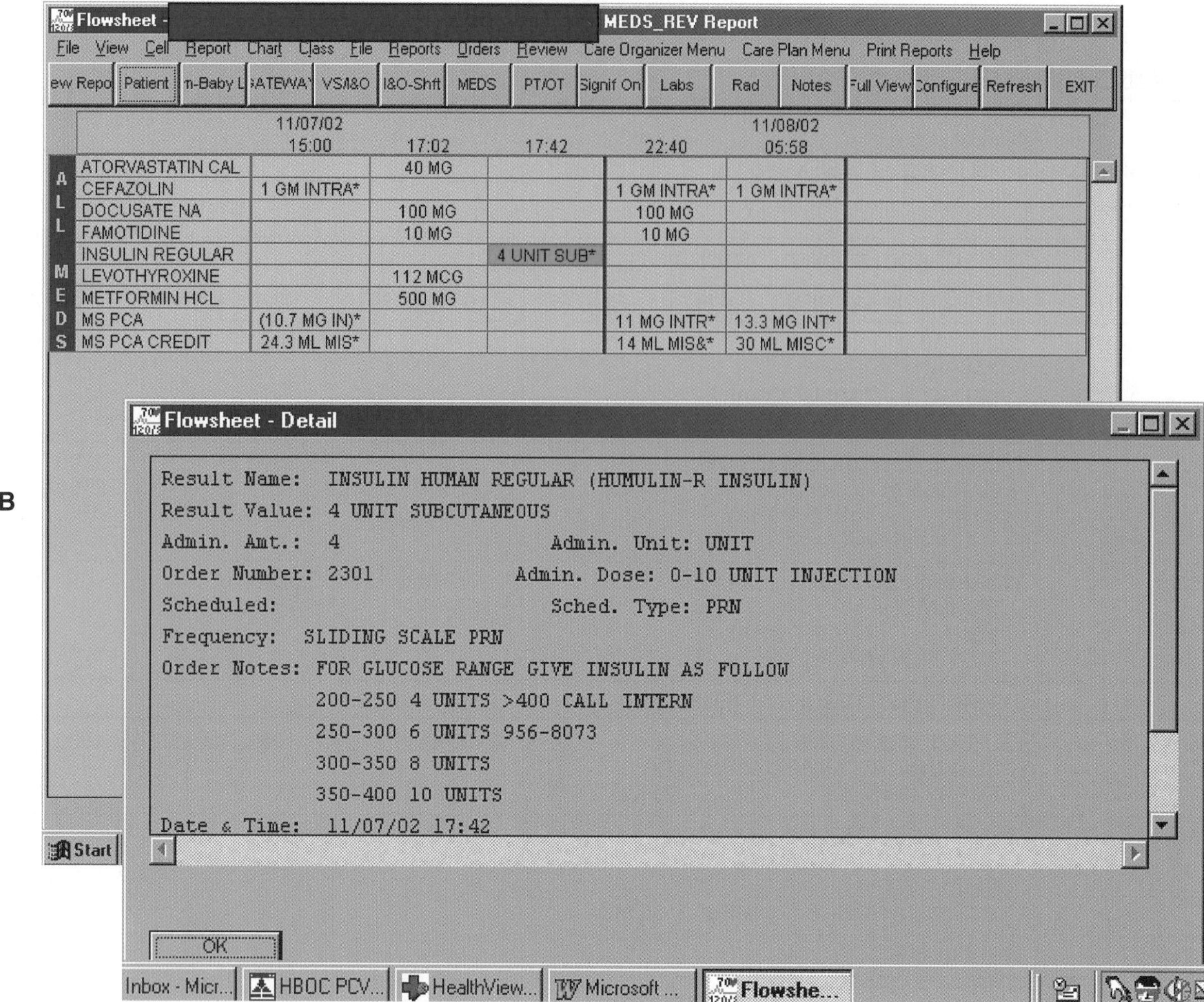

FIGURE **7-7, cont'd B,** Electronically generated medication sheet listing all scheduled medications for an 8-hour shift. By clicking the cursor on the highlighted area (4 UNIT SUB in this illustration), a window opens, revealing details of the order.

Case Management

The goal of case management is to coordinate patient care provided to individuals, their families, and significant others on a continuum, providing efficient transitions to services that may be needed after discharge at home, in clinics or in other health care facilities such as rehabilitation units or nursing homes. Success in case management requires minimizing costs while achieving high-quality care.

Patient Education Record

The patient education record provides a means of documenting the health teaching provided to the patient, family, or significant others and includes statements regarding the learner's mastery of the content presented.

Additional forms included in a patient's chart depend on the therapy prescribed. These may include separate medication administration reports; health teaching records; operative and anesthesiology records; recovery room records; physical, occupational, or speech therapy records; inhalation therapy reports; or a diabetic's daily record of insulin dosage and urine and blood sugar test results. Each page placed in the patient's chart is imprinted with the patient's name, registration number, and unit or room number. Nurses often use data from all of these sections to formulate a plan of nursing care.

Kardex Records

The Kardex (Figure 7-9) is a large index-type card usually kept in a flip-file or separate holder that contains pertinent information such as the patient's name, diagnosis, allergies, schedules of current medications with stop dates, treatments, and the nursing care plan. When all ordered medications are listed in the Kardex, the nurse can assemble the medication cards (Figure 7-9) for all assigned patients and verify each medication card against the Kardex. When the unit dose system is used, all medications are still

MEDICATION ADMINISTRATION RECORD

Nursing Home Name	PHARMACY PROVIDER	INIT.=GIVEN R=REFUSED V=VOMITED H=HELD O=HOME	INIT.	SIGNATURE	INIT.	SIGNATURE	INIT.	SIGNATURE
______________								
______ Mo. ______ Yr.								

RX#—DATE ORDERED	MEDICATION—DOSE—ROUTE	TIME	1	2	3	4	5	6	7	8	9	10	11	12	13	14	15	16	17	18	19	20	21	22	23	24	25	26	27	28	29	30	31

ALLERGIES	DIAGNOSIS

LAST NAME	FIRST	INIT.	LEVEL OF CARE	ROOM-BED	SEX	BIRTHDATE	DIET	IDENTIFICATION #	PHYSICIAN
					DATE OF MED. REVIEW______________ REVIEWED BY______________ (RPh) (RN)				

FIGURE **7-8** Example of medication administration record used in long-term care setting.

Name: Lorenzo, Joseph	
Room & bed: 621^2	Date started 1/25/06
Dr.: Martin	
Noted by: S. Over, RN	
Medication & route: ERYTHROMYCIN 250 mg	
po q 6 h	
Time: 0000, 0600, 1200, 1800	

FIGURE **7-9** Transcription of a medication order onto the Kardex or a medication card or ticket.

listed on the Kardex or separately on the medication profile so that individual medication cards are not necessary. Although used primarily by nurses, the Kardex makes patient data quickly accessible to all members of the health team. The Kardex is often completed in pencil and updated regularly. Because it is not a legal document, it is destroyed when the patient is discharged from the institution. Traditional Kardex information is evolving into an electronic database format that is continually updated through each shift. The latest information is printed at start of the next shift.

Evolving Charting Methodologies

Regardless of the method of charting used, the documentation process needs to adhere to JCAHO standards that incorporate established standards of care. JCAHO requires that all charting methodologies incorporate nursing process criteria, as well as evidence of teaching and discharge planning. When more than one health discipline is providing patient care, a multidisciplinary care plan must be completed.

The format and the extent of use of electronic database charting vary widely among institutions, yet each method incorporates the standards of care and JCAHO requirements. Some clinical sites have extensive online electronic charting developed, whereas others have little or none. As an example, one hospital may elect to combine all the elements formerly found in the Kardex, the care plan, the MAR and critical pathways into one printable document known as a patient profile that the nurse can access for each 8-hour shift. The nurse can also print out a summary of the laboratory test results and a summary of the nursing assessment data from past shifts. Regardless of the methodology used, the adage "If you didn't chart it, it didn't happen" holds true.

DRUG DISTRIBUTION SYSTEMS

Objectives

1. Cite the advantages and disadvantages of the ward stock system, computer-controlled ordering and dispensing system, the individual prescription order system, and the unit dose system.
2. Study the narcotic control system used at your assigned clinical practice setting and compare it with the requirements of the Controlled Substances Act of 1970.

Key Terms

floor or ward stock system
individual prescription order system
computer-controlled dispensing system
unit dose drug distribution system
long-term care unit dose system

Before administering medications, it is important that the nurse understand the overall medication delivery system used at the employing health care agency. Although no two drug distribution systems function exactly alike, the following general types are used.

Floor or Ward Stock System

In the floor or ward stock system all but the most dangerous or rarely used medications are stocked at the nursing station in stock containers. This system has been used most often in very small hospitals and hospitals where there are no charges directly to the patient for medications, such as in some government hospitals. Some advantages of this system are ready availability of most drugs, fewer inpatient prescription orders, and minimal return of medications. The disadvantages are as follows:

- Increased potential for medication errors because of the large array of stock medications from which to choose and the lack of review by the pharmacist of a patient's medication order
- Increased danger of unnoticed passing of expiration dates and drug deterioration
- Jeopardizing of patient safety
- Economic loss caused by misplaced or forgotten charges and misappropriation of medication by hospital personnel
- Increased amounts of expired drugs to be discarded
- Need for larger stocks and frequent total drug inventories
- Storage problems on the nursing units in many hospitals

Individual Prescription Order System

In the individual prescription order system, medications are dispensed from the pharmacy upon receipt of a prescription or drug order for an individual patient. The pharmacist usually sends a 3- to 5-day supply of medication in a bottle labeled for a specific patient. Once received at the nurses' station, medications are placed in the medication cabinet in accordance with institutional practices. Generally, the medication containers are arranged alphabetically by the patient's name, but they may be arranged numerically by the patient's room or bed number. This system provides greater patient safety due to the review of prescription orders by both the pharmacist and the nurse before administration, less danger of drug deterioration, easier inventory control, smaller total inventories, and reduced revenue loss due to improved charging systems and less pilferage. Although dispensing medication to individual patients is better than the floor or ward stock system, the major disadvantages of this system are the time-consuming procedures used to schedule, prepare, administer, control, and record the drug distribution and administration process.

Computer-Controlled Dispensing System

A newer system for medication ordering and administration is a **computer-controlled dispensing system** that is supplied by the pharmacy daily, stocked with single-unit packages of medicines. When a drug order is received in the pharmacy for a patient, it is entered into the computerized system. The nurse, using a security code and password, and for newer systems, a thumb print, accesses the system and selects the patient's name, medication profile, and drugs due for administration. The drug order appears on the screen, and a specific section of the cart automatically opens so the nurse can take the single dose of medicine out of the cart. This process continues until all drugs ordered for a specific time of administration are retrieved. During the actual administration process at the bedside, the nurse uses a handheld scanner that reads the barcodes on the nurse's identification badge, the patient's wristband, and the unit-dose medication packet, linking this information with the patient database. If there is an error such as the wrong dose, wrong time of administration, or wrong patient, an alarm sounds to stop the administration process. If the process is correct and the medicine is administered, there is automatic documentation in the patient's MAR of the administration.

Controlled drugs are also kept in this automated dispensing cart. The system provides a detailed record of the controlled substance dispensed including the date, time, and by whom it was accessed. A second qualified nurse must witness the disposal of a portion of a dose of a controlled substance or the return to the automated dispensing cart of any controlled substance not used. The automated dispensing system is the safest and most economical method of drug distribution in hospitals and long-term care facilities today (Figure 7-10).

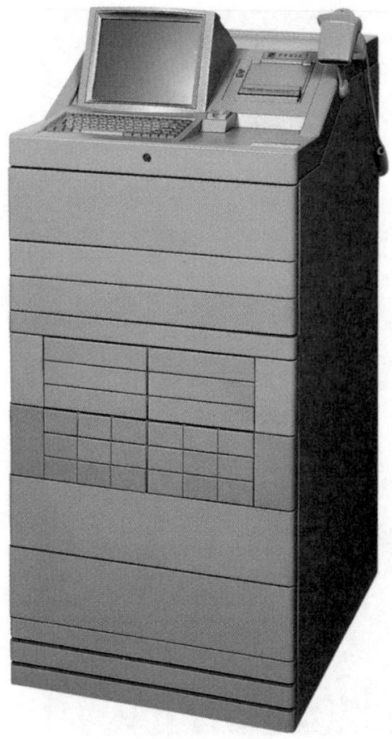

FIGURE **7-10** Electronic dispensing system—the Pyxis system.

Unit Dose System

Unit dose drug distribution systems use single-unit packages of drugs, dispensed to fill each dose requirement as it is ordered. Each package is labeled with generic and brand name, manufacturer, lot number, and expiration date. When dispensed by the pharmacy, the individual packages are placed in labeled drawers assigned to individual patients. The drawers are kept in a large unit dose cabinet (Figure 7-11) that is kept at the nurses' station. Under most unit dose systems, the pharmacist refills the drawers every 24 hours. In long-term care facilities, they are usually exchanged on 3- or 7-day schedules. The system was developed in the 1960s to overcome problems with inefficient use of nursing personnel, underuse by pharmacists, excessively high rates of medication errors, poor drug control, waste of medications, and large inventories.

Advantages of the system include the following:

- The time normally spent by nursing personnel in preparation of drugs for administration is drastically reduced.
- The pharmacist has a profile of all medications for each patient and is therefore able to analyze the prescribed medications for drug interactions or contraindications. This method increases the pharmacist's involvement and better utilizes his or her extensive drug knowledge.
- No dose calculations are necessary because of unit-of-use packaging, thus reducing errors.
- The nurse may double-check drugs and doses because each dose is individually packaged and labeled.
- There is less waste and misappropriation because single units are dispensed.
- Credit is given to the patient for unused medications because each dose is individually packaged.

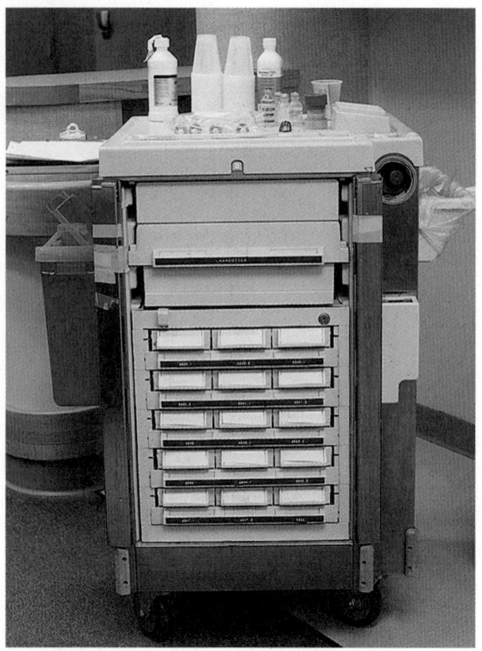

FIGURE **7-11** Unit dose cabinet.

(Under the individual prescription order system, returned bottles of unused medications are destroyed because of fear of contamination.)

An argument occasionally used by nurses against the unit or single-dose system is that someone else prepares the medications for the nurse to administer. Nurses have been taught to never administer anything they have not prepared themselves. In principle, this is certainly true. A nurse should not administer any drug mixed and left unlabeled by another individual. However, for decades, nurses have administered medications that a pharmacist has prepared and labeled. The unit dose medication is prepared under rigid controls and is dispensed only after pharmacists have completed quality control procedures. Nurses should always continue to check medications before administration. If there is a discrepancy between the Kardex (medication profile) and the medication in the cart, the pharmacist and the original physician's order should be consulted.

At the time of administration, the nurse should check all aspects of the medication order as stated on the medication profile against the medication container removed from the patient's drawer for administration. The number of doses remaining in the drawer for the shift also should be checked. If the number of remaining doses is incorrect, the medication order should be checked before continuing with the drug administration. It is always possible that the drug has been discontinued or that someone else has given the dose, omitted a dose, or given the wrong patient the wrong medication. In the event that an error has been made, it should be reported in accordance with hospital policies.

Long-Term Care Unit Dose System

The long-term care unit dose system is an adaptation of the system used in the acute care setting. The unit dose cart is designed with individual drawers to hold one resident's medication containers for 1 week. The drawer is labeled with the resident's name, room number, pharmacy name and telephone number, and name of the health care facility. The pharmacist fills the medication container with the prescribed drug. Each container has enough compartments to contain the prescribed number of doses of the drug for each day of the week. The individual compartments may be labeled with the days of the week. The medication cart has other compartments to store bottles of medication that cannot be placed in patient drawers. The cart has a storage area for medication cups, a medicine crusher, drinking cups, straws, alcohol sponges, syringes, and other necessities for the preparation and administration of the medications prescribed. The entire cart has a locking system that should be secured when the medication cart is not in use or is unattended while medications are being dispensed.

The unit dose systems may use a color-coding system to simplify finding the medication holder for a specific time of day; for example, purple = 6 AM (0600); pink = 8 AM (0800); yellow = noon (1200); green = 2 PM (1400) or 4 PM (1600); orange = early evening; and red = PRN. Using this method to organize the medications allows the nurse or medication aide to remove all the pink holders for administering the prescribed 8 AM (0800) tablets or capsules. Each medication holder is also labeled with the resident's name, physician's name, prescription number, generic/brand name of the drug, dose, frequency of drug order (e.g., four times a day), and the actual time the drug within this holder is to be administered (e.g., 8 AM, or 0800). This system is easy to use unless the user is colorblind. By using military time to mark the individual containers, the individual who is colorblind can use the military time as the guideline.

At the time of administration, the nurse or medication aide checks all aspects of the medication order (as stated on the medication profile) against the medication container that has been removed from one of the drawers. The number of doses remaining within the holder is checked against the days of the week that remain for the medication to be administered. If the resident refuses the medication, it must be charted on the record with the reason the medication was refused. In a long-term care setting, residents seldom wear identification bands; therefore, third-party identification of the resident must be relied on until the nurse or medication aide is able to identify the residents. Medications should be charted as soon as administered. The medication aide has specific limitations on the types of medications he or she can administer; therefore nurses should be thoroughly familiar with the law and guidelines of their state. The nurse is ultimately responsible for verifying the qualifications of the individual being supervised in the medication aide capacity and for the medications he or she is administering.

Narcotic Control Systems

As described in Chapter 1, laws regulating the use of controlled substances have been enacted and are rigidly enforced. Within hospitals and long-term care facilities, it is a standard policy that controlled substances are issued in single-unit packages and are kept in a locked cabinet. If the automated dispensing system is not available, the head nurse or a designated individual is responsible for the key to the cabinet. When controlled substances are issued to a nursing unit, they are accompanied by an inventory sheet (Figure 7-12) that lists each type of controlled substance being supplied. This record is used to account for the disposition of each type of medication issued. At the time the controlled substance supply is dispensed to the nursing unit by the pharmacist, the nurse receiving the drug supply is responsible for counting and verifying the number and types of controlled substances received. The nurse then signs a record attesting to the accuracy and receipt of the controlled substances, and locks them in the controlled substances (narcotic) cabinet.

When a controlled substance is ordered for a particular patient, the nurse caring for the patient uses a key to the cabinet to obtain and prepare the medication for administration. At the time of removal from the cabinet, the inventory control record (Figure 7-13) must be completed indicating the time, patient's name, drug, dose, and the signature of the nurse responsible for checking out the controlled substance. If a portion of the medication is to be discarded due to a smaller prescribed dose, two nurses must check the dose, preparation, and the portion discarded. Both nurses must then cosign the inventory control record to verify the transaction. The cabinet is relocked, the medicine is administered, and documentation is completed.

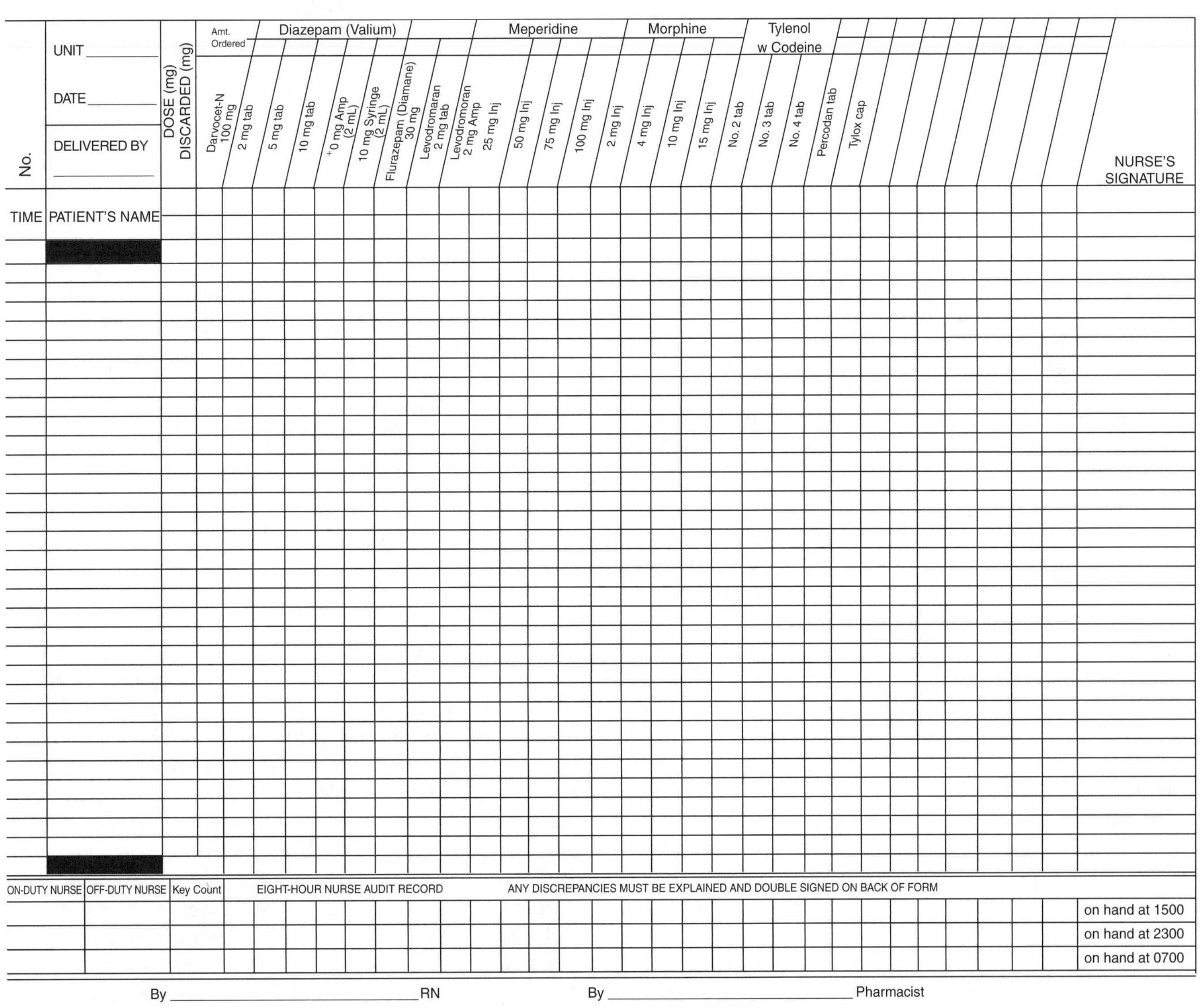

No. | UNIT ______ | DATE ______ | DELIVERED BY ______

TIME	PATIENT'S NAME	DOSE (mg) DISCARDED (mg)	Amt. Ordered: Darvocet-N 100 mg	Diazepam (Valium) 2 mg tab	5 mg tab	10 mg tab	+0 mg Amp (2 mL)	10 mg Syringe (2 mL)	Flurazepam (Diamane) 30 mg	Levodromaran 2 mg tab	Levodromoran 2 mg Amp	Meperidine 25 mg Inj	50 mg Inj	75 mg Inj	100 mg Inj	Morphine 2 mg Inj	4 mg Inj	10 mg Inj	15 mg Inj	Tylenol w Codeine No. 2 tab	No. 3 tab	No. 4 tab	Percodan tab	Tylox cap									NURSE'S SIGNATURE

ON-DUTY NURSE	OFF-DUTY NURSE	Key Count	EIGHT-HOUR NURSE AUDIT RECORD	ANY DISCREPANCIES MUST BE EXPLAINED AND DOUBLE SIGNED ON BACK OF FORM
				on hand at 1500
				on hand at 2300
				on hand at 0700

By ______________ RN   By ______________ Pharmacist

Approved By   Approved By

FIGURE 7-12 Controlled substances inventory form.

CLAYTON'S PHARMACY
213 West Third Street   Grand Island, Nebraska

NAME Joseph Lorenzo   AGE Adult
ADDRESS 18 Bush Ave., Hometown, USA DATE 3/18/06
Rx
ERYTHROMYCIN TABS 250 mg ENTERIC
#40   COATED
sig: TAB i q 6 h

Marilyn Wells, MD

DISPENSE AS WRITTEN   SUBSTITUTION PERMISSIBLE
THIS PRESCRIPTION WILL BE FILLED GENERICALLY UNLESS PHYSICIAN SIGNS ON THE LINE STATING "DISPENSE AS WRITTEN"

FIGURE **7-13** A prescription showing patient name, patient address, date, drug and strength, number of tablets, directions for use, and the health care provider's signature.

Before administration of any controlled substance, the patient's chart should be checked to verify that the time interval since the last use of the drug has elapsed, as specified in the physician's orders. (See Chapter 20 for details of monitoring pain and the use of analgesics.) Immediately after the administration of a controlled substance, the nurse administering the medication should complete the chart. At appropriate intervals following administration of a controlled substance, the degree and duration of effectiveness should be recorded in the nurses' notes or pain flow sheet.

At the end of each shift, the contents of the controlled substances cabinet or controlled substances cart are counted (inventoried) by two nurses, one from the shift that is about to end and the other from the oncoming shift. Each container is counted and the remaining number of tablets, ampules, and prefilled syringes is added to the amount used, according to the inventory control record. The amount of each drug remaining, plus the amount recorded as administered to individual patients, should equal the total number issued. During the counting procedure, packages of unopened prefilled syringes are visually inspected to verify that the seal and the cellophane coverings are intact. Once the package seal is broken, closer scrutiny of the package is required. These observations should include tilting the package of prefilled syringes to observe the rate of air bubble movement inside the barrel, uniformity of color of the solutions in each of the barrels, and the similarity in fluid level in each of the barrels. The same medication in the same type of syringe should be the same color and travel within the barrel at the same rate, and all fluid levels should be similar.

Discrepancies in the number of remaining doses are checked with nursing personnel on the unit to see if all controlled substances used have been charted. If this does not reveal the source of the inaccuracy, each patient's chart is checked to be certain that all controlled substances recorded on the individual patient's charts for the shift coincide with the controlled substances inventory record. If the error still is not found, the pharmacy and the nursing service office should be contacted in accordance with the policy of the institution. In the event that the count appears to be accurate but tampering with the contents of the containers is suspected, a report should be made to the pharmacy and the nursing service office. When the controlled substances inventory is complete, the two nurses who are counting sign the inventory control shift record to verify that the records and inventory are accurate at that time. With the controlled substance cart, the computer generates an end-of-shift report that also identifies discrepancies so that the staff involved can account for the use of controlled substances.

If an automated dispensing cart is used, all nurses that administered controlled substances must check the automated dispensing system printout for any discrepancies at the end of each shift. The pharmacy also checks for discrepancies when controlled substances are restocked in the automated dispensing system. Reconciliation sheets must be completed if there are inaccuracies in the count.

THE DRUG ORDER

Objectives

1. Define the four categories of medication orders used.
2. Describe the procedure used in the assigned clinical setting for taking, recording, transcribing, and verifying verbal medication orders.

Key Terms

stat order
single order
standing order
renewal order
PRN order

Medications for patient use must be ordered by licensed physicians or dentists (or in some states, by nurse practitioners and physician assistants) acting within their areas of professional training. Placing an order for a medication or treatment is known as issuing a *prescription.* Initially it may be issued verbally or in written form. Prescriptions issued for nonhospitalized patients use a form similar to that shown in Figure 7-13, whereas prescriptions for hospitalized patients are written on the physician's order form (see Figure 7-1). All prescriptions must contain the following elements: the patient's full name, date, drug name, route of administration, dose, duration of the order, and signature of the prescriber. Additional information may be required for certain types of medications (e.g., for IV administration, the concentration, dilution, and rate of flow should be specified in addition to the method—"IV push" or "continuous infusion").

Types of Medication Orders

Medication orders fall into four categories: stat, single, standing, and PRN orders.

The **stat order** is generally used on an emergency basis. It means that the drug is to be administered as soon as possible but only once. For example, if a patient is having a seizure, the physician may order *diazepam 10 mg IV stat*, which is meant to be given immediately, and one time only.

The **single order** means administration at a certain time but only one time. For example, a one-time order may be written for *furosemide 20 mg IV to be given one time at 7 AM*. Furosemide would then be administered at that time, but once only.

The **standing order** indicates that a medication is to be given for a specified number of doses, for example, *cefazolin 1 g q6h × 4 doses*. A standing order may also indicate that a drug is to be administered until discontinued at a later date, for example, *ampicillin 500 mg PO q6h*. In the interest of patient safety, however, all accredited health agencies have policies that automatically cancel an order after a certain number of doses are administered or a certain number of days of therapy have passed (e.g., surgery, after 72 hours for narcotics, after one dose only for anticoagulants, after 7 days for antibiotics). A **renewal order** must be written and signed by the physician before the nurse can continue to administer the medication.

A **PRN order** means *administer if needed*. This order allows a nurse to judge when a medication should be administered based on the patient's need and when it can be safely administered.

Verbal Orders

Health care agencies have policies regarding who may accept verbal orders and under what circumstances they should be accepted. The practice should be avoided whenever possible to prevent medication errors, but when a verbal order is accepted, the person who took the order is responsible for accurately entering it on the order sheet and signing it. The physician must cosign and date the order, usually within 24 hours.

Electronic Transmission of Patient Orders

With the advent of fax machines, many physicians' offices fax new orders to the area where the patient is admitted or transferred. These fax transmissions must have an original signature within a specified time, often 24 hours. Hospital units also find it useful to fax orders to the nursing home where the individual is being transferred. This allows the receiving agency to prepare for the patient or resident, and the original orders, signed by the physician, then accompany the individual at time of transfer.

MEDICATION ERRORS

Objective

1. Identify common types of drug errors and actions for their prevention.

Key Terms

adverse drug events (ADEs)
computerized prescriber order entry (CPOE)
clinical decision-making support systems (CDSS)
verification
transcription

Medication errors can result in serious complications known as **adverse drug events (ADEs)**. The National Academy of Science's Institute of Medicine (IOM) estimates the number of lives lost due to preventable medication errors accounts for more than 7000 deaths in hospitals annually. The IOM further estimates that the additional costs of ADEs annually are $2 billion in hospitals and more than $3 billion in extended-care facilities. Medication errors are defined as any errors in the medication process, including prescribing errors, transcription/order communication, dispensing errors, administration errors, and errors of monitoring or education for proper use (Table 7-1).

ADEs occur most commonly during the ordering and at the administration stage. Therefore preventive measures are being implemented that include substan-

Table 7-1 *Examples of Medication Errors*

PRESCRIBING ERRORS
Suboptimal drug therapy decisions
Drug for patient with known allergy or intolerability
Incorrect dose for diagnosis
Unauthorized drug prescribed
TRANSCRIPTION ERRORS
Misinterpretation/misunderstanding of drug ordered or directions
Illegible handwriting
Unapproved abbreviations
Omission of orders
DISPENSING
Wrong drug or dose sent to nursing unit
Wrong formulation or dosage form
ADMINISTRATION
Incorrect strength (dose) given
Extra dose given or missed dose
Wrong administration time
Incorrect administration technique
MONITORING
Suboptimal monitoring
Suboptimal assessments of drug response/revision of regimen
Suboptimal patient education

tial changes in the ordering system used for medications and laboratory studies. Software has been developed that allows computerized prescriber order entry (CPOE) that is supported by clinical decision-making support systems (CDSS). The computerized system integrates the ordering system with the pharmacy, laboratory, and nurses' station, thereby providing access instantly to online information that may affect a patient's care needs. This technology checks for potential drug interactions and appropriateness of drug dosages ordered, as well as for laboratory studies such as therapeutic drug levels at the time of order entry. Automated ordering and dispensing systems (previously described) are also being developed to minimize medication errors. Automated systems use robots and bar-coding technology to fill the orders entered by the physician. Robotics in the pharmacy can free some of the pharmacists for deployment to the clinical units where they can make patient rounds, check for medication response, review current laboratory data, and work with the prescriber in selecting, dosing, and monitoring drug therapy.

When a medication error does occur, an incident report is completed to describe the circumstances of the event. An incident report related to a medication error should include the following data: date, time the drug was ordered, drug name, dose, and route of administration. Information regarding these items should be given, and the therapeutic response or adverse clinical observations present should be noted. Also, the date, time, prescriber notified of the error, and any prescriber's orders given should be recorded. It is important to be *factual* and not state opinions on the incident report. Current practices for reporting medication errors are under scrutiny and facilities are being encouraged to adopt nonpunitive actions when a medication error occurs. It is much more important to determine why the error occurred and to educate all personnel on how to prevent repeat errors.

Nurse's Responsibilities

The importance of accuracy at every step during ordering, transcribing, administering, and monitoring drug therapy cannot be overemphasized.

Verification

With the nonautomated order and distribution systems, once a prescription order has been written for a hospitalized patient, the nurse interprets it and makes a professional judgment on its acceptability. Judgments must be made regarding the type of drug, therapeutic intent, usual dose, and mathematical and physical preparation of the dose. The nurse must also evaluate the method of administration in relation to the patient's physical condition, as well as any allergies and the patient's ability to tolerate the dose form. If any part of an order is vague, the prescriber who wrote the order should be consulted for clarification. Patient safety is of primary importance, and the nurse assumes responsibility for verification and safety of the medication order. If, after gathering all possible information, it is concluded that it is inappropriate to administer the medication as ordered, the prescriber should be notified immediately. An explanation should be given as to why the order should not be executed. If the prescriber cannot be contacted or does not change the order, the nurse should notify the director of nurses, the nursing supervisor on duty, or both. The reasons for refusal to administer the drug should be recorded in accordance with the policies of the employing institution.

Transcription

Transcription of the prescriber's order is necessary to put it into action. After verification of an order, a nurse or another designated person transcribes the order from the physician's order sheet onto the Kardex or onto an MAR. These data may also be entered into a computerized patient database that produces a Kardex or MAR. When this process is delegated to a ward clerk or unit secretary, the nurse is still responsible for verifying all aspects of the medication order. The nurse must sign the original medication order indicating that he/she received, interpreted, and verified the order. The nurse then sends a carbon copy of the original order to the pharmacy, often by fax. A small supply is issued either in unit dose or in a container containing a daily supply. The container is labeled with the date, patient's name, room number, and drug name and strength/dose. When the supply arrives from the pharmacy it is stored in the medication room or in the patient's medication drawer of a medication cart.

In the long-term care setting, carbon copies of new medication orders are sent to the local pharmacy to be filled. If a stat dose is needed or the medication must be started very soon, the pharmacy is notified via telephone or fax, and written verification of the medicine(s) ordered is also supplied to the pharmacy. Because the local pharmacy generates the medication administration record only on a monthly basis, new orders must be added to the current medication record by the nurse transcribing the order. Nurses also send requests to the pharmacy via the fax for drug reorders such as PRN orders.

The nurse, using standard drug administration methodology, prepares and administers a drug by following the order on the medication administration record or drug profile according to the six rights of drug administration. With the new CPOE that is supported by CDSSs, both the verification and transcription of the medication orders are built into the system. It should be emphasized that bar coding and handheld devices do not eliminate the need for the nurse to use standard administration procedures for medications such as checking all aspects of the drug order, right patient, right drug, right time, right dose, and right route, and for documentation of drug response.

THE SIX RIGHTS OF DRUG ADMINISTRATION

Objectives

1. Identify specific precautions needed to ensure that the *right drug* is prepared for the patient.
2. Memorize and recite standard abbreviations associated with the scheduling of medications.
3. Identify data found in the patient's chart used to determine if the patient has abnormal renal or hepatic function.
4. Describe specific safety precautions the nurse should follow to ensure that correct drug calculations are made.
5. Review the policies and procedures of the practice setting to identify drugs for which doses must be checked by two qualified people.
6. Describe the methods that should be used to ensure that the correct patient receives the correct medication, by the correct route, in the correct amount, at the correct time.
7. Compare each safety measure described to ensure safe preparation and administration of medications with those procedures used at the clinical practice setting.
8. Identify appropriate nursing actions to document the administration and therapeutic effectiveness of each medication administered.

Right Drug

See the Clinical Landmine box below.

Right Time

When scheduling the administration time of a medication, factors such as timing abbreviations, standardized times, consistency of blood levels, absorption, diagnostic testing, and the use of PRN medications must be considered.

Standard Abbreviations

The drug order specifies the frequency of drug administration. Standard abbreviations used as part of the drug order specify the times of administration. The nurse should also check institutional policy concerning medication administration. Hospitals often have standardized interpretations for abbreviations (e.g., "q6h" may mean 0600, 1200, 1800, and 2400; "qid" may mean 0800, 1200, 1600, and 2000). The nurse must memorize and use standard abbreviations in interpreting, transcribing, and administering medications accurately.

Standardized Administration Times

For patient safety, certain medications are administered at specific times. This allows laboratory work or electrocardiograms (ECGs) to be completed first, so that the size of the next dose to be administered can be determined. For example, warfarin or digoxin may be administered at 1300, if ordered by the physician. The medication administration times need to be standardized throughout a clinical facility, with all units using the same time schedule to help prevent medication errors.

Maintenance of Consistent Blood Levels

The schedule for the administration of a drug should be planned to maintain consistent blood levels of the drug to maximize the therapeutic effectiveness. If blood draws to establish the current serum blood level of a specific drug are ordered, the nurse should follow the guidelines stated in the drug monograph for the specific time when the blood sample should be drawn in relation to the drug dose administration schedule.

Maximum Drug Absorption

The schedule for oral administration of drugs must be planned to prevent incompatibilities and maximize absorption. Certain drugs require administration on an empty stomach. Thus they are given 1 hour before or 2 hours after meals. Other medications should be given with food to enhance absorption or reduce irritations. Still other drugs are not given with dairy products or antacids. It is important to maintain the recommended schedule of administration for maximum therapeutic effectiveness.

Diagnostic Testing

It is necessary to determine whether any diagnostic tests have been ordered for completion before initiating or continuing therapy. Before beginning antimicrobial therapy, all culture specimens (e.g., blood, urine, or wound) need to be collected. If a physician has ordered serum levels of the drug, the administration time of the medication should be coordinated with the time the phlebotomist is going to draw the blood sample. When completing the requisition for a serum level of a medication, a notation should be made of the date and time that the drug was last administered. Timing is important; if tests are not conducted at the same time intervals in the same patient, the data gained are of little value.

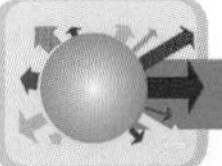

Clinical Landmine

Many drugs have similar spellings and variable concentrations. A significant number of medication errors occur as a result of look-alike packaging and similar drug names. Therefore before administering a medication, it is imperative to compare the exact spelling and concentration of the prescribed drug with the medication card or drug profile and the medication container. Regardless of the drug distribution system used, the drug label should be read at least three times:

1. Before removing the drug from the shelf or unit dose cart
2. Before preparing or measuring the actual prescribed dose
3. Before replacing the drug on the shelf or before opening a unit dose container (just before administering the drug to the patient)

PRN Medications

Before the administration of any PRN medication, the patient's chart should be checked to ensure that someone else has not administered the drug, and that the specified time interval has passed since the medication was last administered. When a PRN medication is given, it should be charted immediately. Record the response to the medication.

Right Dose

Check the drug dose ordered against the range specified in the reference books available at the nurses' station.

Abnormal Hepatic or Renal Function

The hepatic and renal function of the specific patient who will receive the drug should always be considered. Depending on the rate of drug metabolism and route of excretion from the body, certain drugs require a reduction in dose to prevent toxicity. Conversely, patients being dialyzed may require higher than normal doses. Whenever a dose is outside the normal range for that drug, it should be verified *before* administration. Once verification has been obtained, a brief explanation should be recorded in the nurses' notes and on the Kardex (or drug profile) so that others administering the medication will have the information and the physician will not be repeatedly contacted with the same questions. The following laboratory tests are used to monitor liver function: aspartate aminotransferase (AST), alanine aminotransferase (ALT), gamma glutamyl transferase (GGT), alkaline phosphatase, and lactic dehydrogenase (LDH). The blood urea nitrogen (BUN), serum creatinine (Cr_s), and creatinine clearance (C_{cr}) are used to monitor renal function.

Pediatric and Geriatric Patients

Specific doses for some drugs are not yet firmly established for the older adult or pediatric patient. The nurse should question any order outside the normal range *before* administration. For pediatric patients, the most reliable method is by proportional amount of body surface area or body weight (see Appendix C).

Nausea and Vomiting

If a patient is vomiting, oral medications should be withheld, and the prescriber should be contacted for alternate medication orders, because the parenteral or rectal route may be preferred. Investigate the onset of the nausea and vomiting. If it began after the start of the medication regimen, consideration should be given to rescheduling the oral medication. Administration with food usually decreases gastric irritation. Consult with the prescriber for changes in orders.

Accurate Dose Forms

Do not break a tablet unless it is scored. Better yet, consult with the pharmacist about other available dosage forms.

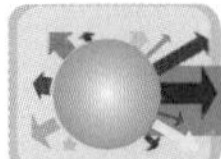

Clinical Landmine

Whenever a dose is questionable or when fractional doses are calculated, check the dose with another qualified individual. Most hospital policies require that certain medications (e.g., insulin, heparin, IV digitalis preparations) are checked by two qualified nurses before administration.

Accurate Calculations

Safety should always be maintained when calculating a drug dose.

Correct Measuring Devices

Accurate measurement of the volume of medication prescribed is essential. Fractional doses require the use of a tuberculin syringe, whereas insulin is generally measured in an insulin syringe that corresponds to the number of units in 1 mL (U-100 insulin is measured in a U-100 syringe).

There are numerous types of infusion pumps available and the nurse needs to be familiar with operation of the units used at the clinical setting. If in doubt, have another care provider with expertise in the device's use check all settings before administering a medication.

Right Patient

When using the medication card system, the name of the patient on the medication card should be compared with the patient's identification bracelet. With the unit dose system, the name on the drug profile should be compared with the individual's identification bracelet. When checking the bracelet under either system, always check for allergies. Some institutional policies require that the individual be called by name as a means of identification. This practice must take into consideration the patient's mental alertness and orientation. It is *always* much safer to check the identification bracelet. JCAHO recommends that at least two patient identifiers be used, such as the patient stating his or her name and birth date.

Pediatric Patients

Children should never be asked their names as a means of positive identification. They may change beds, try to avoid the staff, or seek attention by identifying themselves as someone else. Identification bracelets should be checked *every time.*

Geriatric Patients

It is important to not only check identification bracelets but also confirm names verbally. In a long-term care setting, residents usually do not wear identification bracelets. In these instances, only a person who is

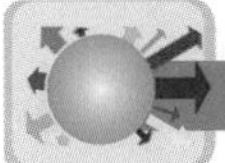

Clinical Landmine

It is important to check the identification bracelet *every time* a medication is administered. The adverse effects of administration of the wrong medication to the wrong patient and the potential for a lawsuit can thus be avoided. Even though automated technology will help reduce the frequency of medication errors, the technology does not eliminate the nurse's responsibility for checking the patient's identity as well as all other aspects of the drug order.

familiar with the residents should confirm his or her identity for administration of the medications.

Many errors may be avoided by carefully following the practices just presented.

Right Route

The drug order should specify the route to be used for the administration of the medication. One dosage form of medication should never be substituted for another unless the physician is specifically consulted and an order for the change is obtained. There can be a great variation in the absorption rate of the medication through different routes of administration. The IV route delivers the drug directly into the bloodstream. This route provides not only the fastest onset but also the greatest danger of potential adverse effects such as tachycardia and hypotension. The intramuscular (IM) route provides the next fastest absorption rate, based on availability of blood supply. This route can be quite painful, as is the case with many antibiotics. The subcutaneous route is next fastest, based on blood supply. In some instances the oral route may be as fast as the IM route, depending on the medication being given, the dose form (liquids are absorbed faster than tablets), and whether there is food in the stomach. The oral route is usually safe if the patient is conscious and able to swallow. The rectal route should be avoided, if possible, due to irritation of mucosal tissues and erratic absorption rates. In case of error, the oral and rectal routes have the advantage of recoverability for a short time after administration.

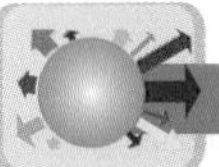

Clinical Landmine

To ensure that the right drug is prepared at the right time for the right patient using the right route, it is important to maintain the highest standards of drug preparation and administration. Attention should be focused on the calculation, preparation, and administration of the ordered medication. A drug reconstituted by a nurse should be clearly labeled with the patient's name, the dose or strength per unit of volume, the date and time the drug was reconstituted, the amount and type of diluent used, the expiration date and/or time, and the initials or name of the nurse who prepared it. Once reconstituted, the drug should be stored according to the manufacturer's recommendation.

Right Documentation

Documentation of nursing actions and patient observations has always been an important ethical responsibility, but now it is becoming a major medicolegal consideration as well. Indeed, it is becoming known as the sixth right. The chart should always have the following information: date and time of administration, name of medication, dose, route, and site of administration. Documentation of drug action should be made in the regularly scheduled assessments for changes in the disease symptoms the patient is exhibiting. Adverse symptoms observed should be promptly recorded and reported. Health teaching performed should be documented, and the degree of understanding exhibited by the patient should be evaluated and recorded.

- DO record when a drug is *not* administered and why.
- Under some circumstances a patient may refuse a medication. If this occurs, it is important for the nurse to try to obtain information about the reason for the refusal and to integrate these reasons into the care plan. In some instances it may be because of drug side effects and the lack of understanding about how to alleviate them. Other causes could include the cost of the medicine, inability to self-administer a drug, or the belief that the drug is ineffective. Health care providers must be sensitive to instances when the cause may be because of cultural belief. When a drug is refused, all information pertaining to the incident should be recorded in the nurses' notes, and the physician needs to be notified of the facts involved.
- DO NOT record a medication until after it has been given.
- DO NOT record in the nurses' notes that an incident report has been completed when a medication error has occurred. However, data regarding clinical observations of the patient related to the occurrence should be charted to serve as a baseline for future comparisons.

When a medication error does occur, an incident report is completed to describe the circumstances of the event. An incident report related to a medication error should include the following data: date, time the drug was ordered, drug name, dose, and route of administration. Information regarding the date, time, drug administered, dose, and route of administration should be given, and the therapeutic response or adverse clinical observations present should be noted. Finally, the date, time, physician notified of the error, and any physician's orders given should be recorded. It is important to be factual and avoid stating opinions

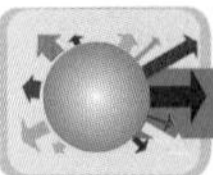

Clinical Landmine

CHECK the label of the container for the drug name, concentration, and route of appropriate administration.

CHECK the patient's chart, Kardex, MAR, or identification bracelet for allergies. If no information is found, ask the patient, before administering the medication, if he or she has any allergies.

CHECK the patient's chart, Kardex, or MAR for rotation schedules of injectable or topically applied medications.

CHECK medications to be mixed in one syringe with a list approved by the hospital or the pharmacy for compatibility. Normally, all drugs mixed in a single syringe should be administered within 15 minutes after mixing. Immediately before administration, *always check* the contents of the syringe for clarity and the absence of any precipitate; if either is present, *do not* administer the contents of the syringe.

CHECK the patient's identity using the two identifiers *every time* a medication is administered.

DO approach the patient in a firm but kind manner that conveys the feeling that cooperation is expected.

DO adjust the patient to the most appropriate position for the route of administration. For example, for oral medications, sit the patient upright to facilitate swallowing. Have appropriate fluids ready before administration.

DO remain with the patient to be certain that all medications have been swallowed.

DO use every opportunity to teach the patient and family about the drug being administered.

DO give simple and honest answers or explanations to the patient regarding the medication and treatment plan.

DO use a plastic container, medicine cup, medicine dropper, oral syringe, or nipple to administer oral medications to an infant or small child.

DO reward the child who has been cooperative by giving praise; comfort and hold the uncooperative child after completing the medication administration.

DO NOT prepare or administer a drug from a container that is not properly labeled or from a container in which the label is not fully legible.

DO NOT give any medication prepared by an individual other than the pharmacist. *Always* check the drug name, dose, frequency, and route of administration against the order. Student nurses must know the practice limitations instituted by the hospital or school and which medications can be administered under what level of supervision.

DO NOT return an unused portion or dose of medication to a stock supply bottle.

DO NOT attempt to administer any drug orally to a comatose patient.

DO NOT leave a medication at the patient's bedside to be taken "later"; remain with the individual until the drug is taken and swallowed. (Note: Few exceptions to this rule are available. One is that nitroglycerin may be left at the bedside for the patient's use. Second, in a long-term care setting certain patients are allowed to take their own medications. In both instances, a specific physician's order is required for *self-medication* and the nurse must still chart the medications taken and the therapeutic response achieved.)

DO NOT dilute a liquid medication form unless there are specific written orders to do so.

Before Discharge

1. Explain the proper method of taking prescribed medications to the patient (e.g., do not crush or chew enteric-coated tablets or any capsules; sublingual medication is placed under the tongue and is not taken with water).
2. Stress the need for punctuality in the administration of medications, and what to do if a dose is missed.
3. Teach the patient to store medications separately from other containers and personal hygiene items.
4. Provide the patient with written instructions reiterating the medication names, schedules, and how to obtain refills. Write the instructions in a language understood by the patient, and use LARGE, BOLD LETTERS when necessary.
5. Identify the anticipated therapeutic response.
6. Instruct the patient, family members, or significant others on how to collect and record data for use by the physician to monitor the patient's response to drug and other treatment modalities.
7. Give the patient, or another responsible individual, a list of signs and symptoms that should be reported to the physician.
8. Stress measures that can be initiated to minimize or prevent anticipated side effects to the prescribed medication. It is important to do this to further encourage the patient to be compliant with the prescribed regimen.

on the incident report. Current practices for reporting medication errors are under scrutiny and facilities are being encouraged to adopt nonpunitive actions when a medication error occurs. It is much more important to determine why the error occurred and to educate all personnel on how to prevent repeat errors.

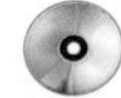

Go to your Companion CD-ROM for Appendices, an Audio Glossary, animations, Drug Dosage Calculators, customizable Patient Self-Assessment forms, and Review Questions for the NCLEX® Examination.

evolve Be sure to visit the companion Evolve site at http://evolve.elsevier.com/Clayton for WebLinks and additional online resources.

MEDICATION SAFETY REVIEW

CRITICAL THINKING QUESTIONS

1. Why are standards of care essential to nursing practice?
2. Explore components of a patient chart and its design in the clinical site where assigned.
3. Examine the different types of MARs used within a hospital and nursing home site where assigned.
4. Research computer-controlled medication systems on the Internet.
5. Compare the methodology used to record narcotics in a hospital and home setting.

CONTENT REVIEW QUESTIONS

1. A patient refuses an essential heart medication that has been prescribed. The nurse should first:
   1. call the physician.
   2. report it to the head nurse.
   3. seek patient reasons.
   4. document refusal on the MAR.
2. General guidelines for entering nurses' notes include completing nursing entries whenever:
   1. the patient complains.
   2. the head nurse requests.
   3. on admission, after PRN medications, before leaving area.
   4. periodically throughout the shift as care needs dictate.
3. Computerized prescriber order entry (CPOE) that is supported by clinical decision-making support systems (CDSS), when researched on the Internet, are found to be advantageous in preventing medication errors by:
   1. checking for potential drug interactions, associated laboratory values, and appropriateness of drug dosages ordered.
   2. providing the physician with the option of inputting orders in written format.
   3. using unit secretary to transcribe orders with registered nurse approval.
   4. freeing pharmacists from filling orders and allowing them to input all orders directly from the hospital units.
4. A telephone order:
   1. involves a physician giving any health care worker an order via the phone.
   2. carries no liability on the part of the nurse taking a phone order.
   3. is used in only an acute emergency.
   4. is best for accuracy and verification.
5. Which of the following rights has been added to the traditional five rights of medication administration?
   1. Right documentation
   2. Right route
   3. Right medication
   4. Right time
6. A nurse is having difficulty reading a physician's order for a medication. The nurse knows the physician is very busy and does not like to be called. The nurse should:
   1. call a pharmacist to interpret the order.
   2. call the physician to have the order clarified.
   3. consult the unit manager to help interpret the order.
   4. ask the unit secretary to interpret the physician's handwriting.
7. Most medication errors occur when the nurse:
   1. fails to follow routine procedures.
   2. is responsible for administering numerous medications.
   3. is caring for too many clients.
   4. is administering unfamiliar medications.

CHAPTER

8 Percutaneous Administration

evolve http://evolve.elsevier.com/Clayton

Chapter Content

ADMINISTRATION OF TOPICAL MEDICATIONS TO THE SKIN

Absorption of topical medications can be influenced by drug concentration, length of time the medication is in contact with the skin, size of the affected area, thickness of the skin, the hydration of tissues, and degree of skin disruption.

Percutaneous administration refers to application of medications to the skin or mucous membranes for absorption. Methods of percutaneous administration include the following: topical application of ointments, creams, powders, or lotions to the skin; instillation of solutions onto the mucous membranes of the mouth, eye, ear, nose, or vagina; and inhalation of aerosolized liquids or gases for absorption through the lungs. The primary advantage of the percutaneous route is that the action of the drug, in general, is localized to the site of application, which reduces the incidence of systemic side effects. Unfortunately, the medications are sometimes messy and difficult to apply. In addition, they usually have a short duration of action and thus require more frequent reapplication.

Topical preparations can be used to:

1. Cleanse and debride a wound.
2. Rehydrate the skin.
3. Reduce inflammation.
4. Relieve localized signs or symptoms, such as itching or rash.
5. Provide a protective barrier.
6. Reduce thickening of the skin, such as callus formation.

ADMINISTRATION OF CREAMS, LOTIONS, AND OINTMENTS

Objectives

1. Describe the topical forms of medications used on the skin.
2. Cite the equipment needed and techniques used to apply each of the topical forms of medications to the skin surface.

Key Terms

creams
lotions
ointments
dressings

Dose Forms

Creams

Creams are semisolid emulsions containing medicinal agents for external application. The cream base is generally nongreasy and can be removed with water. Many over-the-counter (OTC) creams are used as moisturizing agents.

Lotions

Lotions are usually aqueous preparations that contain suspended materials. They are commonly used as soothing agents to protect the skin and relieve rashes and itching. Some lotions have a cleansing action, whereas others have an astringent or drawing effect. To prevent increased circulation and itching, lotions should be gently but firmly patted on the skin, rather than rubbed in. Shake all lotions thoroughly immediately before application and use sparingly to avoid waste.

Ointments

Ointments are semisolid preparations of medicinal substances in an oily base such as lanolin or petrolatum. This type of preparation can be applied directly to the skin or mucous membrane and generally cannot be removed easily with water. The base helps keep the medicinal substance in prolonged contact with the skin.

Dressings

There are several types of **dressings** used to treat wounds, such as dry gauze sponges, nonadherent gauze dressings such as Telfa, self-adhesive transparent films that act as a second skin such as OpSite, and hydrocolloid dressings such as DuoDerm. Hydrogel dressings are used on partial-thickness and full-thickness wounds and on skin damaged by burns. There are also exudate absorbers such as calcium alginate dressings (e.g., AlgiDERM, Kaltostat, Sorbsan) manufactured from seaweed to be used on infected wounds.

Wound care products and wound care have become a complex science; specific chapters are devoted to these principles in fundamentals of nursing, medical-surgical nursing, or geriatric nursing textbooks. See one of these resources for a full discussion of dressing materials available and their correct use. Dressing recommendations for treatment of pressure ulcers are available from the Agency for Health Care Policy and Research, Public Health Service, U.S. Department of Health and Human Services. In the past, attempts were made to dry the wound surface, but it is now recognized that a major principle in wound healing is the need for a moist environment to propagate epithelialization of the wound.

Perform premedication assessments. See individual drug monographs.

Equipment

Prescribed cream, lotion, or ointment
2 × 2-inch gauze sponges
Cotton-tipped applicators
Tongue blade
Gloves
Medication administration record (MAR) or medication profile

Sites

Skin surfaces are affected by the disorder being treated.

Techniques

1. Wash your hands and assemble the equipment.
2. Use the five RIGHTS of medication preparation and administration throughout the procedure.
   RIGHT PATIENT
   RIGHT DRUG
   RIGHT ROUTE OF ADMINISTRATION
   RIGHT DOSE
   RIGHT TIME OF ADMINISTRATION
3. Provide privacy for the patient and give a thorough explanation of the procedure.
4. Position the patient so that the surface where the topical materials are to be applied is exposed. Assess current status of symptoms. Provide for patient comfort before starting therapy.
5. *Cleansing:* Follow the specific orders of the health care provider or clinical site policies for cleansing the site of application. Once the area is exposed and cleansed, perform a wound assessment.
6. *Application:* Wear gloves during the application process. Many of the agents used may be absorbed through the skin of both the patient and the person applying the medication.
   Lotions: Shake well until a uniform appearance of the suspension is obtained.
   Ointments or creams: Use a tongue blade to remove the desired amount from a wide-mouth container; squeeze the amount needed onto a tongue blade or cotton-tipped applicator from a tube-type container. Apply lotions firmly, but gently, by dabbing the surface. Apply ointments and creams with a gloved hand using firm but gentle strokes. Creams are gently rubbed into the area.
7. *Dressings:* Check specific orders regarding the type of dressing to be used. If a dressing is to be applied, spread the prescribed amount of ointment directly onto the dressing material with a tongue blade; the impregnated dressing material can then be applied to the affected skin surface. Secure the dressing in place.
8. *Wet dressings:* Always completely remove previous dressing. Wring out wet dressings to prevent dripping and apply the gauze in a single layer directly to the wound surface. For deeper wounds, pack the wound loosely with moist gauze sponges so that all surfaces are in contact with the moisture. Apply a layer of dry gauze sponges and an absorbent pad to the area. To secure a dressing requiring repeated changes, apply a binder or use Montgomery tapes.
9. Clean up the area and equipment used and make sure the patient is comfortable after the application procedure.
   Note: Sterile supplies, gloves, and equipment are used for some wounds; however, clean rather than sterile gauze, gloves, and so on may be used when applying some types of dressings such as to a pressure ulcer. Always check institutional policies and use clinical judgment.
10. Wash your hands.

Patient Teaching

1. If appropriate, teach the patient to apply the medication and dressings.
2. Teach personal hygiene measures appropriate to the underlying cause of the skin condition (e.g., acne, contact dermatitis, infection).
3. When dressings are ordered, discuss materials readily available at home, such as clean old muslin sheets or cloth diapers with no cotton filling. You may also suggest the purchase of gauze and other necessary supplies.
4. Stress gentleness and moderation in the amount of medication to be applied.
5. Emphasize that the patient must avoid touching or scratching the affected area.

6. Tell the patient to wash hands before and after touching the affected area or applying the medication. Stress the prevention of spread of infection, when present.

Documentation

Provide the RIGHT DOCUMENTATION of the medication administration and responses to drug therapy.

1. Chart the date, time, drug name, dosage, and route of administration.
2. Perform and record regular patient assessments for the evaluation of the therapeutic effectiveness (e.g., change in size of affected area, reduced drainage, decreased itching, lowered temperature with an infection).
3. Chart and report any signs and symptoms of adverse drug effects, as well as a narrative description of the area being treated.
4. Develop a written record for the patient to use in charting progress for evaluation of the effectiveness of the treatments being used. List the patient's symptoms (e.g., rash on lower leg with redness and vesicles present, decubitus ulcer on the sacrum). List the data to be collected regarding the medication prescribed and the effectiveness (e.g., vesicles now crusted, weeping, or appear to be drying; redness in lower leg is lessening; area of decubitus is extending, remaining the same, or shrinking).
5. Perform and validate essential patient education about the drug therapy and other important aspects of intervention for the disease process affecting the individual.

PATCH TESTING FOR ALLERGENS

Objectives

1. Describe the procedure used and purpose of performing patch testing.
2. Describe specific charting methods used with allergy testing.

Key Terms

patch testing
allergens
antigens

Patch testing is a method used to identify a patient's sensitivity to contact materials (e.g., soaps, pollens, dyes). The suspected allergens (antigens) are placed in direct contact with the skin surface and covered with nonsensitizing, nonabsorbent tape. Unless pronounced irritation appears, the patch is usually left in place for 48 hours, then removed. The site is left open to air for 15 minutes, and then "read." A positive reaction is noted by the presence of redness and swelling, which indicates allergy to the specific antigen. It may be necessary to read the areas in 3 days and again in 7 days to detect delayed reactions.

Intradermal tests may also be used to determine allergenicity to specific antigens. See Chapter 11 for further information on intradermal administration of allergens.

Perform premedication assessments. See individual drug monographs.

Equipment

Alcohol for cleansing the area
Solutions of suspected antigens
2 × 2-inch pieces of typewriter paper
1 × 1-inch gauze pads
Droppers
Mineral or olive oil
Water
Hypoallergenic tape
Record for charting data on substances applied and responses
MAR, computer profile, or doctor's order sheet

Sites

The back, arms, or thighs are commonly used. (DO NOT use the face or areas receiving friction from clothing.) Selected areas are spaced 2 to 3 inches apart. The type of allergen applied and the site of application are documented on the patient's chart (Figure 8-1). Hair is shaved from sites to ensure that the antigen is kept in close contact with the skin surface, thereby preventing a false-negative reaction.

Technique

CAUTION: DO NOT begin any type of allergy testing unless emergency equipment is available in the immediate area in case of an anaphylactic response. Personnel should be familiar with the procedure to follow if an emergency does arise.

1. Check with the patient before starting the testing to ensure that no antihistamines or antiinflammatory agents (e.g., aspirin, ibuprofen, corticosteroids) have been taken for 24 to 48 hours preceding the tests. If the patient has taken an antihistamine or antiinflammatory agent, consult the health care provider before proceeding with the testing. Review the chart to ensure that the patient is not in an immunocompromised state as a result of disease or treatments such as chemotherapy or radiation therapy.
2. Wash your hands and assemble the equipment.
3. Use the five RIGHTS of medication preparation and administration throughout the procedure.
   RIGHT PATIENT
   RIGHT DRUG
   RIGHT ROUTE OF ADMINISTRATION
   RIGHT DOSE
   RIGHT TIME OF ADMINISTRATION
4. Provide privacy for the patient and give a thorough explanation of the procedure.

5. Position the patient so that the surface where the test materials are to be applied is horizontal. Provide for patient comfort before starting testing.
6. Cleanse the selected area thoroughly using an alcohol pledget. Use circular motions starting at the planned site of application, continuing outward in circular motions to the periphery. Allow the area to air dry.
7. Prepare the designated solutions using aseptic technique.
8. Follow specific directions of the employing health care agency for the application of liquid and solid forms of suspected allergens. Usually, a dropper is used to apply suspected liquid contact-type materials; solid materials are applied directly to the skin surface and then moistened with mineral or olive oil.
9. The following methods may be used:
   - After application, each area used should be covered first with a 1 × 1-inch gauze followed by a 2 × 2-inch piece of typewriter paper; secure with hypoallergenic tape. (If the patient is known to be allergic to all types of tape, consider using a binder.)
   - Designated amounts of standardized-strength chemical solutions are arranged in metal receptacles that are backed with hypoallergenic adhesive. These are applied to the selected site. It is important to identify the contents of each receptacle correctly.
   - Patches impregnated with designated antigens are available for direct application to the prepared sites.
   - A patch test series kit is available, containing nonirritating concentrations of allergens packaged in syringes for dispersal. Although the kit contains 20 allergens, any number of them may be applied to individual patches or holding devices then applied to the patient's skin.
10. Chart the times, agents, concentrations, and amounts applied. Make a diagram in the patient's chart numbering each location. Record what agent and concentration was placed at each site. Subsequent readings of each area are then performed and charted on this record.

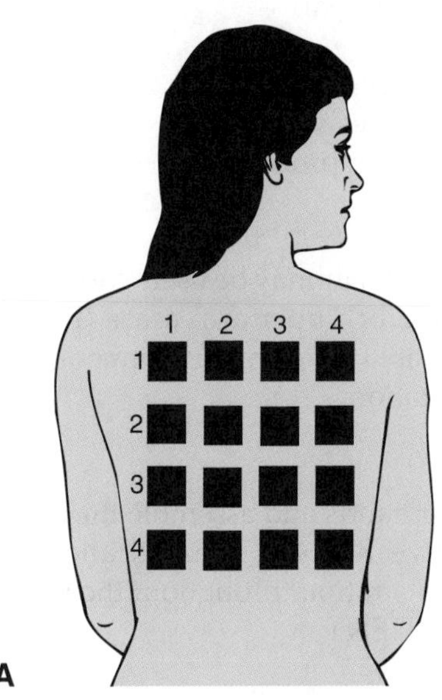

Reading Chart for Intradermal Testing

Patient Name: ______________________

Identification Number: ______________________

Physician Name: ______________________

B

DATE:	TIME:	AGENT	CONCENTRATION	DOSAGE	SITE NUMBER*	Reading Time in Hours or Minutes, 30 min or 24, 48, or 72 hr		

*Refer to diagram of sites, Figure 8-1, *A*

- Follow directions for the "reading" of the skin testing performed.
- Inspect sites in a good light
- Record reaction in upper half of box using the following guidelines, e.g., 2+

+	(1+) No wheal, 3 mm flare
++	(2+) 2 to 3 mm wheal with flare
+++	(3+) 3 to 5 mm wheal with flare
++++	(4+) >5 mm wheal

- Record measurement of induration (process of hardening) in mm in lower half of box, e.g., 5 mm

FIGURE **8-1** Patch test for contact dermatitis. **A,** Patch testing sites. **B,** Reading chart, patch testing.

11. Follow directions for the time of the reading of the skin testing being performed. Inspection of the testing sites should be performed in good light. Generally, a positive reaction (development of a wheal) to a dilute strength of a suspected allergen is considered clinically significant. Measure the diameter of erythema in millimeters and palpate and measure the size of any induration. Record this information in the patient's chart. No reaction should be noted at the control site. The following is a list of commonly used readings of reactions and appropriate symbols:

+ (1+)	No wheal, 3-mm flare
++ (2+)	2- to 3-mm wheal with flare
+++ (3+)	3- to 5-mm wheal with flare
++++ (4+)	>5-mm wheal

Patient Teaching

1. Tell the patient the time, date, and place of the return visit to have the test sites read.
2. Tell the patient not to bathe or shower until the patches are read and removed. Explain the need to avoid activities that could cause excessive perspiration.
3. If the patient develops an area of severe burning or itching, lift the patch and gently wash the area. Tell the patient to report immediately the development of any breathing difficulty, severe hives, or rashes. The patient should be told to go to the nearest emergency department if unable to reach the health care provider who prescribed the skin tests.

Documentation

Provide the RIGHT DOCUMENTATION of the allergen testing sites and responses to allergens applied.

1. Chart the date, time, drug name, dose, and site of administration (see Figure 8-1).
2. Read each site at 24, 48, and 72 hours after the application, as directed by the health care provider or policy of the health care agency. Additional readings may be required up to 7 days after application.
3. Chart and report any signs and symptoms of adverse drug effects.
4. Perform and validate essential patient education about the testing and other essential aspects of intervention for the disease process affecting the individual.

ADMINISTRATION OF NITROGLYCERIN OINTMENT

Objectives

1. Identify the equipment needed, sites and techniques used, and patient education required when nitroglycerin ointment is prescribed.
2. Describe specific documentation methods used to record the therapeutic effectiveness of nitroglycerin ointment therapy.

Dose Form

Nitroglycerin ointment (Nitro-Bid, Nitrol) provides relief of anginal pain for several hours longer than sublingual preparations. When properly applied, nitroglycerin ointment is particularly effective against nocturnal attacks of anginal pain. Specific instructions for nitroglycerin ointment are reviewed in this text because it is the only ointment currently available for which dosage is critical to the success of use (see Chapter 25).

Perform premedication assessments. See individual drug monographs.

Equipment

Gloves
Nitroglycerin ointment
Applicator paper
Clear plastic wrap
Nonallergenic adhesive tape
MAR or medication profile

Sites

Any area without hair may be used. Most people prefer the chest, flank, or upper arm areas (Figure 8-2). Do NOT shave an area to apply the ointment; shaving may cause skin irritation.

Techniques

1. Wash your hands and assemble the equipment.
2. Use the five RIGHTS of medication preparation and administration throughout the procedure
   RIGHT PATIENT
   RIGHT DRUG

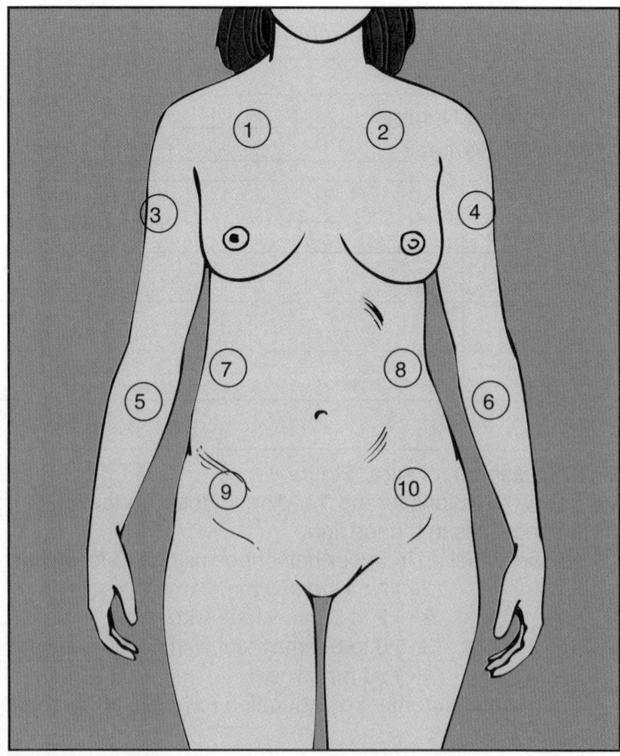

FIGURE 8-2 Sites for nitroglycerin application.

RIGHT ROUTE OF ADMINISTRATION
RIGHT DOSE
RIGHT TIME OF ADMINISTRATION

3. Provide privacy for the patient and give a thorough explanation of the procedure.
4. Don gloves.
5. Position the patient so that the surface where the topical materials are to be applied is exposed. Provide for patient comfort before starting therapy. Note: When reapplying ointment, remove plastic wrap, remove dose-measuring applicator paper from previous dose, and cleanse the area of remaining ointment on the skin surface. Select a new site for application of the medication, then proceed with steps 5 through 9.
6. Lay the dose-measuring applicator paper with the print side DOWN on the site (Figure 8-3, *A*). The ointment will smear the print.
7. Squeeze a ribbon of ointment of the proper length onto the applicator paper.
8. Place the measuring applicator on the skin surface at the site chosen on the rotation schedule, ointment side DOWN. Spread in a thin, uniform layer under the applicator. DO NOT RUB IN. Leave the paper in place. Note: Use of the applicator paper allows you to measure the prescribed dose and prevents absorption through the fingertips as you apply the medication (Figure 8-3, *B*).
9. Cover the area where the paper is placed with plastic wrap and tape it in place.
10. Remove gloves and dispose of them according to policy.
11. Wash your hands after applying the ointment.

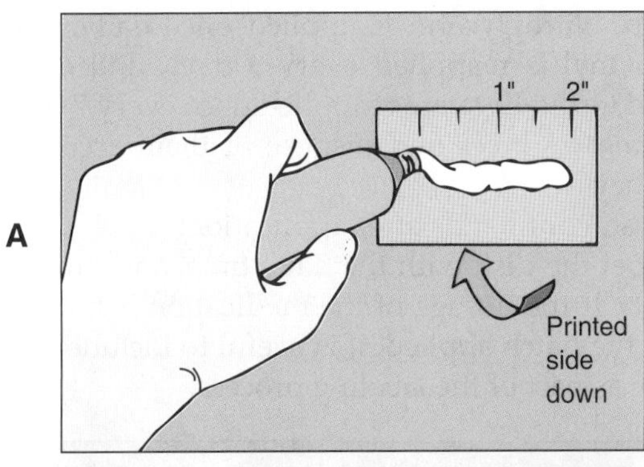

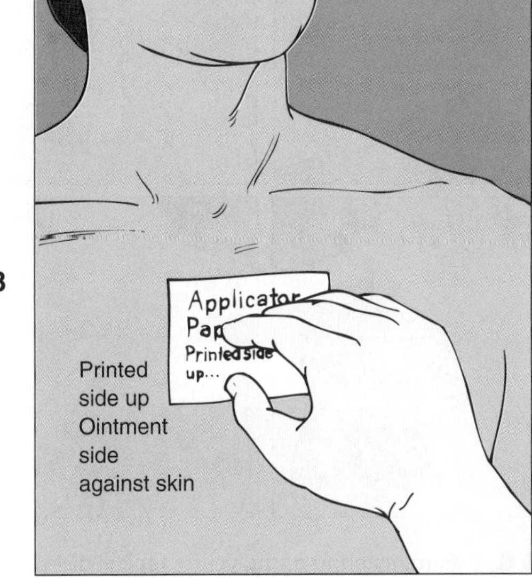

FIGURE **8-3** Administering nitroglycerin topical ointment. **A,** Lay applicator paper print side down, and measure ribbon of ointment. **B,** Apply applicator to skin site, ointment side down. Spread in a uniform layer under applicator; leave paper in place.

Patient Teaching

1. Guide the patient in learning how to apply the ointment.
2. Tell the patient that the medication may discolor clothing. Use of clear plastic wrap protects clothing.
3. When the dosage is regulated properly, the ointment may be used every 3 to 4 hours and at bedtime. Remind the patient that there should be a drug-free period, usually 10 to 12 hours, every 24 hours, as recommended by the health care provider.
4. Tell the patient to wash hands after application to remove any nitroglycerin that came in contact with the fingers.
5. When terminating the use of this topical ointment, the dosage and frequency of application should be gradually reduced over a 4- to 6-week period. Tell the patient to contact the health care provider if adjustment is felt to be necessary. Encourage the patient not to discontinue the medication abruptly (see Chapter 25).

Documentation

Provide the RIGHT DOCUMENTATION of the medication administration and responses to drug therapy.

1. Chart the date, time, drug name, dosage, site, and route of administration.

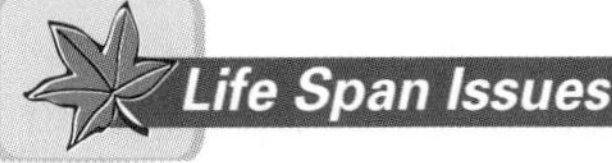

Life Span Issues

Applying Nitroglycerin

To promote personal safety, the nurse should always wear gloves, whether applying nitroglycerin ointment paper or handling transdermal patches. When nitroglycerin transdermal patches are applied, chart the specific site of the application. Occasionally, patients move the transdermal patch themselves because of convenience, skin irritation, or confusion. If the patch is not found at the original location at the scheduled time of removal, examine other areas of the body to find it; do not assume that the patch fell off or was removed. Tolerance and loss of antianginal response could develop if another patch is placed on the patient while the first patch is on at the new location.

Always dispose of used nitroglycerin paper or transdermal patches in a receptacle to which the patient, children, and pets will not have access. A substantial amount of nitroglycerin remains on the patch and can be toxic.

2. Perform and record regular patient assessment for the evaluation of therapeutic effectiveness (e.g., blood pressure, pulse, output, degree and duration of pain relief).
3. Chart and report any signs and symptoms of adverse drug effects.
4. Perform and validate essential patient education about the drug therapy and other important aspects of intervention for the disease process affecting the individual.

ADMINISTRATION OF TRANSDERMAL DRUG DELIVERY SYSTEMS

Objectives

1. Identify the equipment needed, sites used, techniques employed, and patient education required when transdermal medication systems are prescribed.
2. Describe specific documentation methods used to record the therapeutic effectiveness of medications administered using a transdermal delivery system.

Key Term

transdermal disk

Dose Form

The **transdermal disk** or patch provides controlled release of a prescribed medication (e.g., nitroglycerin, clonidine, estrogen, nicotine, scopolamine, fentanyl, Ortho Evra) through a semipermeable membrane for several hours to 3 weeks when applied to intact skin. The dose released depends on the surface area of the disk in contact with the skin surface and the individual drug. See specific monographs for onset and duration of action of drugs using this delivery system.

Perform premedication assessments. See individual drug monographs.

Equipment

Gloves
Transdermal disk or patch
Shaving equipment as appropriate for the site and skin condition
MAR or medication profile

Sites

Any area without hair may be used. Most people prefer the chest, flank, or upper arm areas. Develop a rotation schedule for use (see Figure 8-2).

Techniques

1. Wash your hands and assemble the equipment.
2. Use the five RIGHTS of medication preparation and administration throughout the procedure.
   RIGHT PATIENT
   RIGHT DRUG
   RIGHT ROUTE OF ADMINISTRATION
   RIGHT DOSE
   RIGHT TIME OF ADMINISTRATION
3. Provide for patient privacy and give a thorough explanation of what is to be done.
4. Don gloves.
5. Position the patient so that the surface on which the topical materials are to be applied is exposed. Provide for patient comfort. Note: When reapplying a transdermal disk or patch, remove the old disk or patch and cleanse the skin thoroughly. Select a new site for application. It is especially important in the older adult or confused patient to look for the old disk if it is not where the prior application is charted. The confused patient may have moved it elsewhere on the body or removed it. The old disk can be encased in the glove as the nurse removes it and should be disposed of in a receptacle on the medication cart, not in the patient's room.
6. Apply the small adhesive topical disk. Figure 8-4 illustrates nitroglycerin being applied to one of the sites recommended by the rotation schedule. The frequency of application depends on the specific medication being applied in the transdermal disk and the duration of action of the prescribed medication. Nitroglycerin is applied once daily, whereas fentanyl is reapplied every 3 days, and clonidine and Ortho Evra are reapplied once every 7 days.
7. Remove gloves and dispose of them according to policy.
8. Wash your hands after application.
9. Label the disk with the date, time, and nurse's initials. If the dosage of the medication is not printed on the patch applied, it is useful to include the dosage as part of the labeling process.

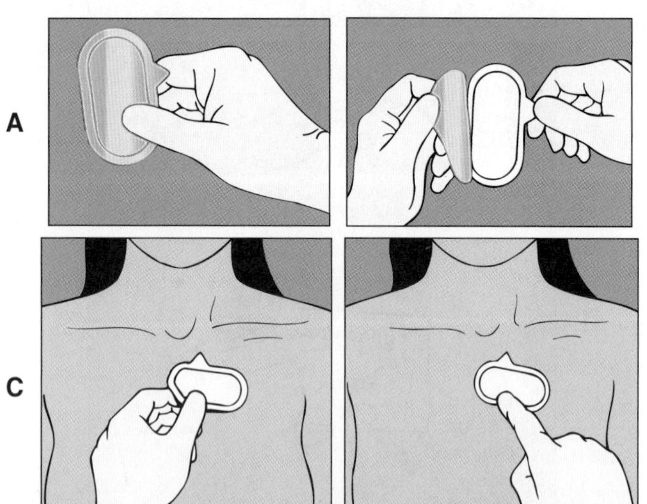

FIGURE 8-4 Administering nitroglycerin topical disks (Transderm Nitro). **A,** Carefully pick up the system lengthwise, with the tab up. **B,** Remove clear plastic backing from system at the tab. Do not touch inside of exposed system. **C,** Place the exposed adhesive side of the system on the chosen skin site; press firmly with the palm of the hand. **D,** Circle the outside edge of the system with one or two fingers.

Patient Teaching

1. Guide the patient in learning how and when to apply the disks. Note: Certain products may be worn while showering; others should be replaced after bathing or showering. Check the patient education instructions for specific application instructions. Scopolamine, used for motion sickness, must be applied at least 4 hours before travel. Clonidine transdermal systems are applied once every 7 days. Estrogen transdermal systems are designed to be worn continuously for 3 weeks, followed by a 1-week interval without a patch before applying the next patch. Ortho Evra is a contraceptive patch that is reapplied weekly for 3 weeks. The fourth week is patch free. A new patch and cycle of three patches starts the following week.
2. If a disk becomes partially dislodged, the recommendations of the product should be followed. Nitroglycerin disks are removed and a new one is applied. Clonidine transdermal disks, on the other hand, come with a protective adhesive overlay to be applied over the patch to ensure skin contact of the transdermal system should the disk become loosened. See Chapter 41 for further information on the OrthoEvra patch.
3. Patients receiving nitroglycerin transdermally may require sublingual nitroglycerin for anginal attacks, especially while the dose is being adjusted. In general, nitroglycerin patches are worn for 10 to 14 hours, followed by a drug-free period of 10 to 12 hours so that the nitroglycerin will maintain its effectiveness.
4. Fentanyl (Duragesic) may take up to 12 hours after application to be effective in the management of stable, chronic pain. Therefore it should be combined with a short-acting pain medication until a sufficient blood level of the fentanyl is achieved. Fentanyl patches are changed every 3 days. Breakthrough pain should be reported promptly to the health care provider. It may be necessary to increase the dosage to achieve a satisfactory level of pain relief.

Documentation

Provide the RIGHT DOCUMENTATION of the medication administration and the responses to drug therapy.

1. Chart the date, time, drug name, dosage, and route of administration.
2. Perform and record regular patient assessments for the evaluation of therapeutic effectiveness (e.g., blood pressure, pulse, degree and duration of pain relief).
3. Chart and report any signs and symptoms of adverse drug effects.
4. Perform and validate essential patient education about the drug therapy and other essential aspects of intervention for the disease process affecting the individual.

ADMINISTRATION OF TOPICAL POWDERS

Objective

1. Describe the dose form, sites used, and techniques employed to administer medications in topical powder form.

Dose Form

Powders are finely ground particles of medication contained in a talc base. They generally produce a cooling, drying, or protective effect where applied.

Perform premedication assessments. See individual drug monographs.

Equipment

Gloves
Prescribed powder
MAR or medication profile

Site

Apply to the skin surface of the body, as prescribed.

Technique

1. Wash your hands.
2. Use the five RIGHTS of medication preparation and administration throughout the procedure.
   RIGHT PATIENT
   RIGHT DRUG
   RIGHT ROUTE OF ADMINISTRATION
   RIGHT DOSE
   RIGHT TIME OF ADMINISTRATION
3. Don gloves.
4. Provide privacy for the patient and give a thorough explanation of the procedure.
5. Position the patient so that the surface on which the topical materials are to be applied is exposed. Provide patient comfort before starting therapy.
6. Wash and thoroughly dry the affected area before applying the powder.
7. Apply powder by gently shaking the container, distributing the powder evenly over the area. Gently smooth over the area for even coverage.
8. Remove gloves and dispose of them according to policy.
9. Wash your hands.

Patient Teaching

Tell the patient to cleanse the area of administration and reapply the powder to the external surface as directed by the physician. The patient should avoid inhaling the powder during application.

Documentation

Provide the RIGHT DOCUMENTATION of the medication administration and the responses to drug therapy.

1. Chart the date, time, drug name, dosage, site, and route of administration.

2. Perform and record regular patient assessments for the evaluation of therapeutic effectiveness.
3. Chart and report any signs and symptoms of adverse drug effects.
4. Perform and validate essential patient education about the drug therapy and other essential aspects of intervention for the disease process affecting the individual.

ADMINISTRATION OF MEDICATIONS TO MUCOUS MEMBRANES

Objectives

1. Describe the dose forms, sites, equipment used, and techniques for administration of medications to the mucous membranes.
2. Identify the dose forms safe for administration to the eye.
3. Describe patient education necessary for patients requiring ophthalmic medications.
4. Compare the techniques used to administer ear drops in patients younger than age 3 with those older than age 3.
5. Describe the purpose, precautions necessary, and patient education required for people requiring medications by inhalation.
6. Describe the dose forms available for vaginal administration of medications.
7. Identify the equipment needed, site, and specific techniques required to administer vaginal medications or douches.
8. State the rationale and procedure used for cleansing vaginal applicators or douche tips following use.
9. Develop a plan for patient education of people taking medications via percutaneous routes.

Key Terms

buccal
ophthalmic
otic
nebulae
aerosols
metered-dose inhaler
dry powder inhaler

Drugs are well absorbed across mucosal surfaces and therapeutic effects are easily obtained. However, mucous membranes are highly selective in absorptive activity and differ in sensitivity. In general, aqueous solutions are quickly absorbed from mucous membranes, whereas oily liquids are not. Drugs in suppository form can be used for local effects on the mucous membranes of the vagina, urethra, or rectum. A drug may be inhaled and absorbed through the mucous membranes of the nose and lungs. It may be dissolved and absorbed by the mucous membranes of the mouth, or applied to the eyes or ears for local action. It may be painted, swabbed, or irrigated on a mucosal surface.

ADMINISTRATION OF SUBLINGUAL AND BUCCAL TABLETS

Dose Forms

Sublingual tablets are designed to be placed under the tongue for dissolution and absorption through the vast network of blood vessels in this area. Buccal tablets are designed to be held in the **buccal** cavity (between the cheek and molar teeth) for absorption from the blood vessels of the cheek. The primary advantage of these routes of administration is the rapid absorption and onset of action because the drug passes directly into systemic circulation with no immediate pass through the liver, where extensive metabolism usually takes place. Contrary to most other forms of administration to mucous membranes, the action from these dose forms is usually systemic, rather than localized to the mouth.

Perform premedication assessments. See individual drug monographs.

Equipment

Prescribed medication

Note: The medications available to be administered by this route are forms of nitroglycerin. Once the self-administration technique is taught, the patient should carry the medication or keep it readily available at bedside for use as needed.

MAR or medication profile

Site

Administer at the sublingual area (under tongue) (Figure 8-5, *A*) or buccal pouch (between molar teeth and cheek) (see Figure 8-5, *B*).

Technique

See Chapter 9 for correct technique with either the medication card system or the unit dose system.

1. Wash your hands and assemble the equipment.
2. Use the five RIGHTS of medication preparation and administration throughout the procedure.
   RIGHT PATIENT
   RIGHT DRUG
   RIGHT ROUTE OF ADMINISTRATION

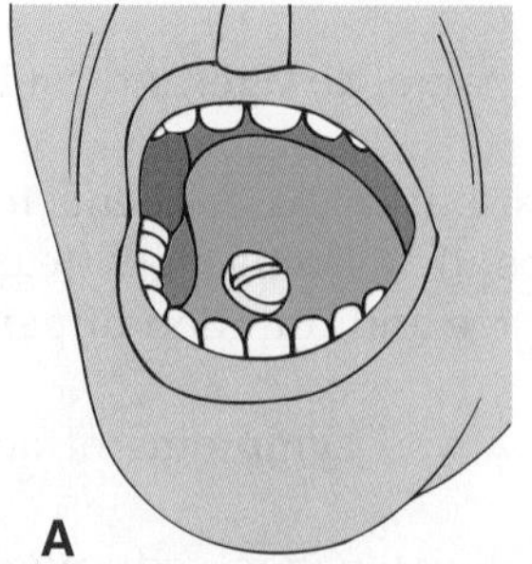

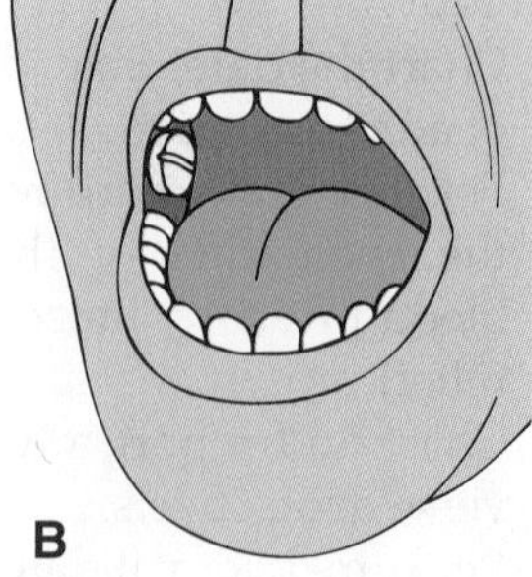

FIGURE **8-5** Placing medication in the mouth. **A,** Under the tongue (sublingual). **B,** In the buccal pouch.

RIGHT DOSE
RIGHT TIME OF ADMINISTRATION

3. Provide privacy for the patient and give a thorough explanation of the procedure.
4. Put on a glove and place the medication under the tongue (sublingual) (see Figure 8-5, *A*) or between the upper molar teeth and the cheek (buccal) (see Figure 8-5, *B*). The tablet is meant to dissolve in these locations. Do not administer with water. Encourage the patient to allow the drug to dissolve where placed and hold saliva in mouth until tablet is dissolved.
5. Remove glove and dispose of it according to policy.
6. Wash your hands thoroughly.

Patient Teaching

Explain the exact placement of the medication and the dosage and frequency of doses. The patient should be told what side effects to expect, what adverse effects to report, where to carry the medication, how to store the medication, and how to refill the prescription when needed.

Documentation

Provide the RIGHT DOCUMENTATION of the medication administration and responses to drug therapy.

1. Chart the date, time, drug name, dose, site, and route of administration.
2. Perform and record regular patient assessments for the evaluation of therapeutic effectiveness (e.g., blood pressure, pulse, degree and duration of pain relief, number of doses taken, etc.).
3. Chart and report any signs and symptoms of adverse drug effects.
4. Perform and validate essential patient education about the drug therapy and other essential aspects of intervention for the disease process affecting the individual.

   Note: When the patient is self-administering a medication, the nurse is still responsible for all aspects of the charting and monitoring parameters to document the drug therapy and response achieved.

Administration of Eye Drops, Ointment, and Disks

Dose Form

Medications for use in the eye are labeled **ophthalmic.** If not labeled as such, do not administer to the eye. Ocular solutions are sterile, easily administered, and usually do not interfere with vision when instilled. Allow eye medication to warm to room temperature before administration.

Ocular ointments do cause alterations in visual acuity. However, they have a longer duration of action than solutions. Always use a separate bottle or tube of eye medication for each patient.

Perform premedication assessments. See individual drug monographs.

Equipment

Gloves
Eye drops, ointment prescribed (check strength carefully), or disk
Dropper (use only the dropper supplied by the manufacturer)
Paper tissues and/or sterile cotton balls
Sterile eye dressing (pad), as appropriate
Normal saline solution, if needed for cleaning off exudates
MAR or medication profile

Site

Administer to the eye(s).

Technique

1. Wash your hands and assemble *ophthalmic* medication.
2. Use the five RIGHTS of medication preparation and administration throughout the procedure.

   RIGHT PATIENT
   RIGHT DRUG
   RIGHT ROUTE OF ADMINISTRATION
   RIGHT DOSE
   RIGHT TIME OF ADMINISTRATION
3. Provide privacy for the patient and give a thorough explanation of the procedure.
4. Position the patient so that the back of the head is firmly supported on a pillow and the face is directed toward the ceiling. With children, restraints may be necessary if the child is too young to cooperate voluntarily. Always ensure patient safety.
5. Check to be certain that you have the correct medication according to the five RIGHTS. Put on gloves. Inspect the affected eye to determine the current status. As appropriate, remove exudate from the eyelid and eyelashes using sterile saline solution. Always use a separate cotton ball for each wiping motion. A clean washcloth may also be used, using a separate part of the cloth for each eye. Start at the inner canthus and wipe outward.
6. Expose the lower conjunctival sac by applying gentle traction to the lower lid at the bony rim of the orbit.
7. Approach the eye from below with the medication dropper or tube of ointment. (Never touch the eye dropper or ointment tip against the eye or face.)
8. At the conclusion of either procedure, remove the gloves and dispose of them according to the policy of the practice setting.
9. Wash your hands thoroughly.

Drops (Figure 8-6)

- Have the patient look upward over your head.
- Drop the specified number of drops into the conjunctival sac. Never drop directly onto the eyeball.
- After instilling the drops, apply gentle pressure, using a cotton ball or clean tissue, to the inner corner

FIGURE **8-6** Administering ophthalmic drops. **A,** Have the patient look upward; apply gentle traction to lower lid to expose conjunctival sac. Instill drops into sac. **B,** Using a tissue, apply gentle pressure to the inner corner of eyelid on bone for 1 to 2 minutes.

of the eyelid on the bone for approximately 1 to 2 minutes. This prevents the medication from entering the canal, where it would be absorbed in the vascular mucosa of the nose and produce systemic effects. It also ensures an adequate concentration of medication in the eye.

- When more than one type of eye drop is ordered for the same eye, wait 1 to 5 minutes between instillation of the different medications. Use only the dropper provided by the manufacturer. Apply a sterile dressing as ordered.

Ointment

- Gently squeeze the ointment in a strip fashion into the conjunctival sac (Figure 8-7). Do not allow the tip to touch the patient.
- Tell the patient to close the eye(s) gently and move the eyes with the lid shut, as if looking around the room, to spread the medication. Apply a sterile dressing as ordered.

Disk

- Open package to reveal the disk and gently press your fingertip against the disk so the convex side adheres to the finger.
- Ask the patient to look up as you gently pull the lower lid away from the eye, exposing the conjunctival sac.
- Insert the disk into the conjunctival sac between the iris and lower eyelid.
- Pull the patient's lower eyelid out over the disk and allow the disk to float on the sclera.
- To remove disk:
  Wash your hands and don gloves.
  Ask the patient to look up as you gently pull the lower lid away from the eye, exposing the disk in the sac.
  Use your opposite hand and grasp the disk, using your forefinger and thumb to gently pinch the disk and lift it out.
- Remove gloves and dispose of supplies.

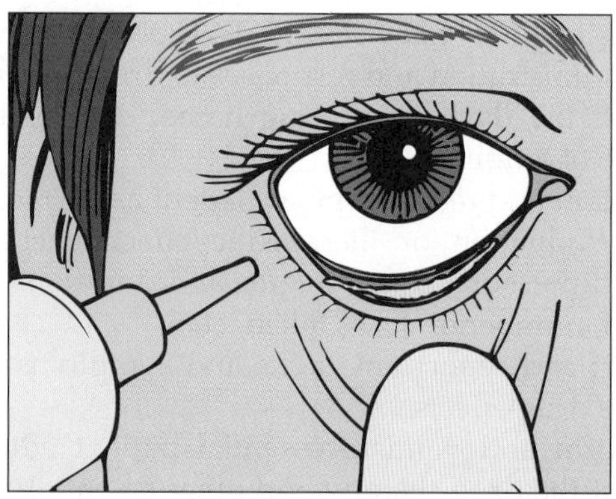

FIGURE **8-7** Administering ophthalmic ointment. To instill the ointment, gently pull the lower lid down as patient looks upward. Squeeze ophthalmic ointment into lower sac. Avoid touching tube to eyelid.

Patient Teaching

1. Guide the patient in learning how to apply his or her own ophthalmic medication.
2. Tell the patient to wipe the eye(s) gently from the nose outward to prevent contamination between the eyes and possible spread of infection, and to use a separate tissue to wipe each eye.
3. Have the patient wash hands often and avoid touching the eye or immediate areas surrounding it, espe-

cially when an infection is present. Dispose of tissues in a manner that prevents spread of an infection.
4. Stress punctuality in administration of eye medications, especially when used for treating infections or increased intraocular pressure.
5. Tell the patient to discard eye medications that have changed color, become cloudy, or contain particles. (If the patient's visual acuity is reduced, someone else should check clarity.)
6. The patient must not use OTC eyewashes without first consulting the health care provider who is managing the eye disorder.
7. Emphasize the need for careful follow-up of any eye disorder until the health care provider releases the patient from further care.

Documentation

Provide the RIGHT DOCUMENTATION of the medication administration and responses to drug therapy.

1. Chart the date, time, drug name, dosage, site, and route of administration.
2. Perform and record regular patient assessments for the evaluation of therapeutic effectiveness (e.g., redness, discomfort, visual acuity, changes in infection or inflammatory reaction, degree and duration of pain relief).
3. Chart and report any signs and symptoms of adverse drug effects.
4. Perform and validate essential patient education about the drug therapy and other essential aspects of intervention for the disease process affecting the individual.

Administration of Ear Drops

Dose Form

Ear drops are a solution containing a medication used for the treatment of localized infection or inflammation of the ear. Medications for use in the ear are labeled **otic.** If not labeled as such, they should not be administered to the ear. Ear drops should be warmed to room temperature before use, and separate bottles of ear drops should be used for each patient.

Perform premedication assessments. See individual drug monographs.

Equipment

Gloves
Otic solution prescribed
Dropper provided by the manufacturer
MAR or medication profile

Site

Administer to the ear(s).

Techniques

1. Review the policy of the practice setting and follow guidelines regarding whether gloves are to be worn during instillation of ear medications.
2. Wash your hands and assemble the equipment.
3. Use the five RIGHTS of medication preparation and administration throughout the procedure.
   RIGHT PATIENT
   RIGHT DRUG
   RIGHT ROUTE OF ADMINISTRATION
   RIGHT DOSE
   RIGHT TIME OF ADMINISTRATION
4. Provide privacy for the patient and give a thorough explanation of the procedure.
5. Position the patient so that the affected ear is directed upward; put on gloves (according to policy).
6. Assess the ear canal for wax accumulation. If wax is present, get an order to irrigate the canal before instilling the ear drops.
7. Allow the medication to warm to room temperature, shake well, and draw up into the dropper.
8. *Administration:* For children younger than 3 years of age, restrain the child, turn the head to the appropriate side, and gently pull the earlobe *downward* and *back* (Figure 8-8, *A*). Instill the prescribed number of drops into the canal. Do not allow the dropper tip to touch any part of the ear. For children older than 3 years and adults, enlist cooperation or restrain as necessary, turn the head to the appropriate side, and gently pull the earlobe *upward* and *back* (Figure 8-8, *B*) to straighten the external auditory canal. Instill the prescribed number of drops into the canal. Do not allow the dropper tip to touch any part of the ear.
9. Instruct the patient to remain on the side for a few minutes following instillation; insert a cotton plug *loosely* if ordered.
10. Repeat the procedure if ear drops are ordered for both ears.
11. Remove gloves and dispose of them according to policy.

Patient Teaching

1. Explain the importance of administering the medication as prescribed.
2. Teach self-administration or administration to another person as appropriate.

Documentation

Provide the RIGHT DOCUMENTATION of the medication administration and the responses to drug therapy.

1. Chart the date, time, drug name, dosage, site, and route of administration.
2. Perform and record regular patient assessments for the evaluation of therapeutic effectiveness (e.g., redness, pressure, degree and duration of pain relief, color and amount of drainage).
3. Chart and report any signs and symptoms of adverse drug effects.
4. Perform and validate essential patient education about the drug therapy and other essential aspects of intervention for the disease process affecting the individual.

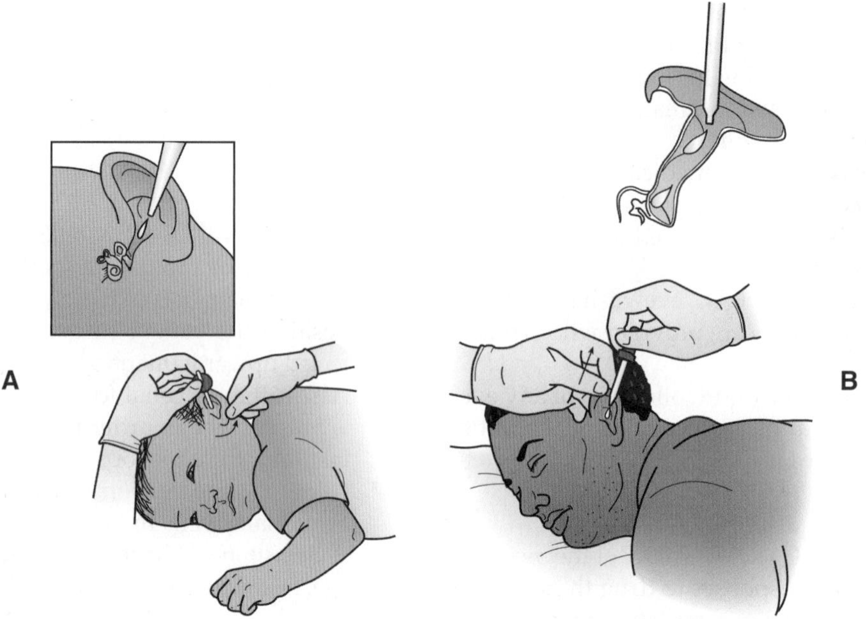

FIGURE **8-8** Administering ear drops. **A,** Pull earlobe downward and back in children younger than age 3 years. **B,** Pull earlobe upward and back in patients older than age 3.

Administration of Nose Drops

Nasal solutions are used to treat temporary disorders affecting the nasal mucous membranes. Always use the dropper provided by the manufacturer and give each patient a separate bottle of nose drops.

Perform premedication assessments. See individual drug monographs.

Equipment

Gloves
Nose drops prescribed
Dropper supplied by the manufacturer
Tissue to blow the nose
Penlight
MAR or medication profile

Site

Administer to the nostrils.

Technique

1. Review the practice setting policy and follow guidelines regarding whether gloves are to be used during the instillation of nose drops to prevent possible contact with body fluid secretions.
2. Wash your hands and assemble the equipment.
3. Use the five RIGHTS of medication preparation and administration throughout the procedure.
   RIGHT PATIENT
   RIGHT DRUG
   RIGHT ROUTE OF ADMINISTRATION
   RIGHT DOSE
   RIGHT TIME OF ADMINISTRATION
4. Provide privacy for the patient and give a thorough explanation of the procedure. Continue to explain the steps in the procedure to help the individual learn future self-administration.
5. Administration (Figure 8-9):
   For adults and older children:
   - Instruct the patient to blow the nose gently unless this is contraindicated (e.g., nosebleeds, risk of increased intracranial pressure). Use penlight to assess the nares.
   - Have the patient lie down and hang the head backward over the edge of the bed.
   - Draw the medication into the dropper. Hold the dropper just above the nostril and instill the medication.
   - After a brief time, have the patient turn the head to the other side and repeat the administration process in the second nostril, if needed.
   - Have the patient remain in this position for 2 to 3 minutes to allow the drops to remain in contact with the nasal mucosa.

   For infants and young children:
   - Position the infant or small child with the head over the edge of the bed or pillow, or use the "football" hold to immobilize the infant.
   - Administer nose drops in the same manner as for the adult.
   - For the child who is cooperative, offer praise. Provide appropriate comforting and personal contact for all children and infants.
6. Have paper tissues available for use if absolutely necessary to blow the nose.

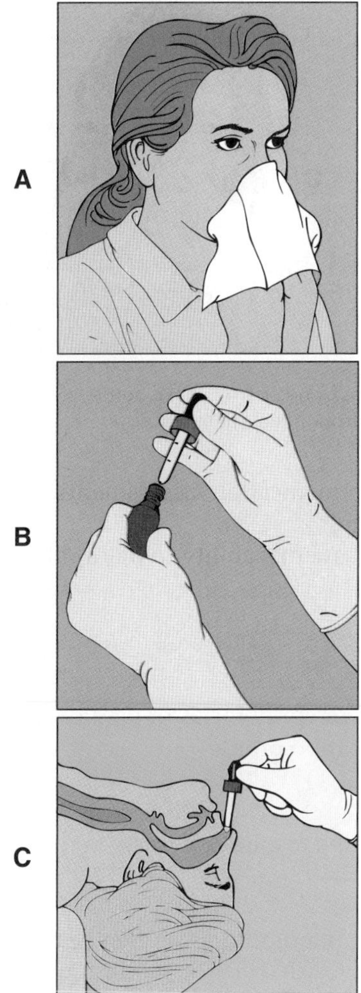

FIGURE 8-9 Administering nose drops. **A,** Gently blow nose. **B,** Open medication and draw up to calibration on dropper. **C,** Instill medication. Have patient remain in position for 2 to 3 minutes. Repeat on other side if necessary.

Patient Teaching

Guide the patient in learning self-administration of nose drops, if necessary. Tell the patient that overuse of nose drops can cause a "rebound effect," which causes the symptoms to become worse. If symptoms have not resolved after a week of nasal drop therapy, the health care provider should be consulted again.

Documentation

Provide the RIGHT DOCUMENTATION of the medication administration and responses to drug therapy.

1. Chart the date, time, drug name, dosage, site, and route of administration.
2. Perform and record regular patient assessments for the evaluation of the therapeutic effectiveness (e.g., nasal congestion, degree and duration of relief achieved, improvement in overall status), and reassess condition of nares periodically.
3. Chart and report any signs and symptoms of adverse drug effects.
4. Perform and validate essential patient education about the drug therapy and other essential aspects of intervention for the disease process affecting the individual.

Administration of Nasal Spray

The mucous membranes of the nose absorb aqueous solutions very well. When applied as a spray, the small droplets of solution containing medication coat the membranes and are rapidly absorbed. The advantage of spray over drops is less waste of medication because some of the drops often run down the back of the throat before absorption can take place. As with drops, each patient should have a personal container of spray.

Perform premedication assessments. See individual drug monographs.

Equipment

Gloves
Nasal spray prescribed
Paper tissues to blow the nose
Penlight
MAR or medication profile

Site

Administer to the nostrils.

Techniques

1. Review the policy of the practice setting and follow guidelines regarding whether gloves are to be used during the instillation of nasal sprays.
2. Wash your hands and assemble the equipment.
3. Use the five RIGHTS of medication preparation and administration throughout the procedure.
   RIGHT PATIENT
   RIGHT DRUG
   RIGHT ROUTE OF ADMINISTRATION
   RIGHT DOSE
   RIGHT TIME OF ADMINISTRATION
4. Don gloves.
5. Provide privacy for the patient and give a thorough explanation of the procedure.
6. Instruct the patient to gently blow the nose (Figure 8-10, *A*), unless this is contraindicated (e.g., nosebleeds, risk of increased intracranial pressure).
7. Have the patient assume the upright sitting position. Use penlight to inspect nares.
8. Block one nostril (see Figure 8-10, *B*).
9. Holding the spray bottle upright, shake the bottle.
10. Immediately after shaking, insert the tip into the nostril (Figure 8-10, *C*). Ask the patient to inhale through the open nostril and squeeze a puff of spray into the nostril at the same time.
11. Have paper tissues available for use if absolutely necessary to blow the nose.

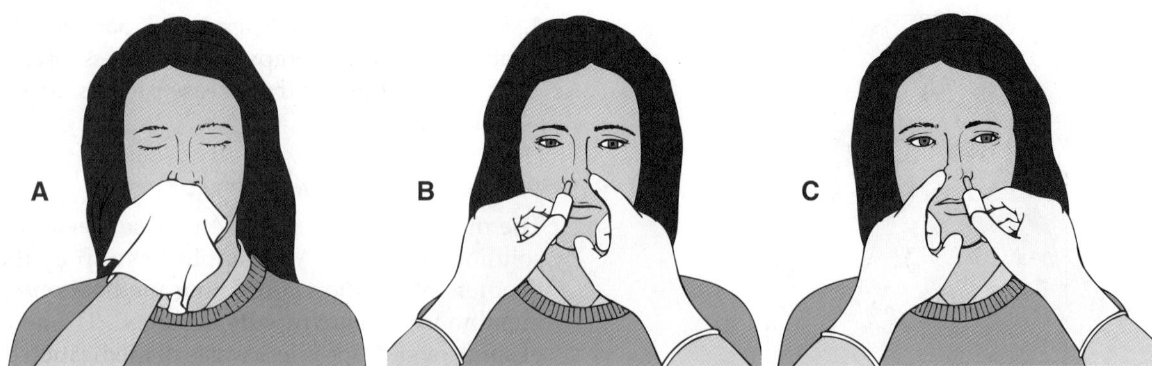

FIGURE **8-10** Administering nasal spray. **A,** Gently blow nose. **B,** Block one nostril; shake bottle. **C,** Insert tip into nostril, and squeeze a puff of spray while inhaling through the open nostril.

12. Remove gloves and dispose of them according to policy.
13. Wash your hands.

Patient Teaching

Guide the patient in learning self-administration of nasal spray, if necessary. Tell the patient that overuse of nasal spray can cause a "rebound effect," which causes the symptoms to become worse. If symptoms have not resolved after a week of nasal spray therapy, the health care provider should be consulted again.

Documentation

Provide the RIGHT DOCUMENTATION of the medication administration and responses to drug therapy.

1. Chart the date, time, drug name, dosage, site, and route of administration.
2. Perform and record regular patient assessments for the evaluation of therapeutic effectiveness (e.g., nasal congestion, degree and duration of relief achieved, improvement in overall status).
3. Chart and report any signs and symptoms of adverse drug effects.
4. Perform and validate essential patient education about the drug therapy and other essential aspects of intervention for the patient's disease process.

ADMINISTRATION OF MEDICATIONS BY INHALATION

The respiratory mucosa may be medicated by means of inhalation of sprays (nebulae [neb'-u-li') or aerosols. **Nebulae** are sprayed into the throat by a nebulizer. **Aerosols** use a flow of air or oxygen under pressure to disperse the drug throughout the respiratory tract. Oily preparations should not be applied to the respiratory mucosa, because the oil droplets may be carried to the lungs and cause lipid pneumonia. Although saliva as a body fluid has not been implicated in the transmission of the human immunodeficiency virus (HIV) at the time of this writing, the practice-setting policy manual should reflect current standards of universal precautions for all patients and health care personnel. Follow these procedures faithfully to prevent the transmission of this disease.

Perform premedication assessments. See specific drug monograph.

Assess the patient's ability to manipulate the nebulizer.

Equipment

Gloves
Liquid aerosol or spray forms of medications
MAR or medication profile

Site

Administer to the respiratory tract.

Techniques

1. Wash your hands and assemble the equipment.
2. Use the five RIGHTS of medication preparation and administration throughout the procedure.
   RIGHT PATIENT
   RIGHT DRUG
   RIGHT ROUTE OF ADMINISTRATION
   RIGHT DOSE
   RIGHT TIME OF ADMINISTRATION
3. Don gloves.
4. Provide privacy for the patient and give a thorough explanation of the procedure.
5. Have the patient assume a sitting position. This allows maximum lung expansion.
6. Prepare the medication according to the prescribed directions and fill the nebulizer with diluent. (This may be done before sitting the patient up if time is a factor to the patient's well-being.)
7. Direct the patient to exhale through pursed lips.
8. Put the nebulizer mouthpiece in the mouth: DO NOT seal the lips completely.
9. Activate the inhalation equipment while simultaneously having the patient inhale and breathe to full capacity.
10. Direct the patient to exhale *slowly* through pursed lips.
11. WAIT approximately 1 minute and repeat the sequence according to the health care provider's directions or until all of the medication in the nebulizer is used.

12. Clean the equipment according to the manufacturer's directions.
13. Assist the patient to a comfortable position.
14. Remove gloves and dispose of them; wash your hands.

Patient Teaching

1. As appropriate to the circumstances, teach the patient, family, or significant others to operate the nebulizer to be used at home.
2. Explain the operation and cleansing of the equipment.
3. Before being discharged, have the patient, family, or significant others administer the treatment using the equipment and medications prescribed for at-home use.
4. Stress the need to perform the procedure exactly as prescribed and to report any difficulties experienced after discharge for the health care provider's evaluation.

Documentation

Provide the RIGHT DOCUMENTATION of the medication administration and responses to drug therapy.

1. Chart the date, time, drug name, dosage, and route of administration.
2. Perform and record regular patient assessments for the evaluation of therapeutic effectiveness (e.g., blood pressure, pulse, improvement or quality of breathing, cough and productivity, degree and duration of pain relief, ability to operate the nebulizer, activity and exercise restrictions).
3. Chart and report any signs and symptoms of adverse drug effects.
4. Perform and validate essential patient education about the drug therapy and other essential aspects of intervention for the disease process affecting the individual.

ADMINISTRATION OF MEDICATIONS BY ORAL INHALATION

Dose Forms

Bronchodilators and corticosteroids may be administered by inhalation through the mouth using either an aerosolized, pressurized **metered-dose inhaler** (MDI) or a **dry powder inhaler** (DPI) (Figure 8-11). The primary advantage of the inhalers is that the medication is applied directly to the site of action, the bronchial smooth muscle. Smaller doses are used, with rapid absorption and onset of action. The valve of the pressurized container (MDI) or the dry powder packs of the DPI also helps ensure that the same dose of medication is administered with each inhalation.

Approximately 25% of patients do not use MDIs properly, and therefore do not receive the maximal benefit of the medication. Devices known as "extenders" or "spacers" (Figure 8-12) have been designed for patients who cannot coordinate the release of the medication with inhalation. The extender devices can be adapted to most pressurized canisters of the MDIs. These devices "trap" the aerosolized medication in a chamber through which the patient inhales within a few seconds after releasing the medication into the chamber.

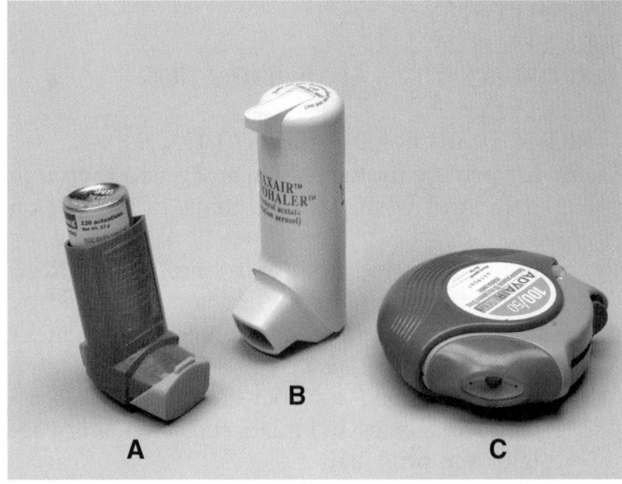

FIGURE 8-11 *A,* Metered-dose inhaler (MDI). *B,* Automated MDI. *C,* Dry powder inhaler (DPI).

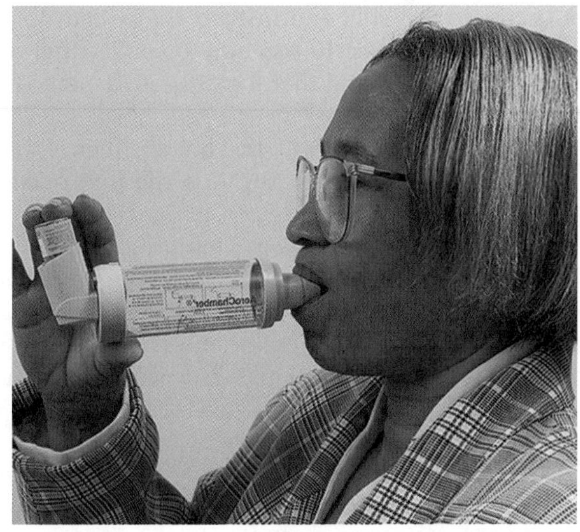

FIGURE 8-12 Metered-dose inhaler with an extender or spacer.

Perform premedication assessments. See individual drug monographs.

Equipment

Gloves
Prescribed medication packaged in an MDI or DPI
MAR or medication profile

Site

Administer to the respiratory tract.

Technique

Aerosolized Metered-Dose Inhaler

1. Wash your hands and assemble the equipment.
2. Use the five RIGHTS of medication preparation and administration throughout the procedure.

RIGHT PATIENT
RIGHT DRUG
RIGHT ROUTE OF ADMINISTRATION
RIGHT DOSE
RIGHT TIME OF ADMINISTRATION

3. Provide privacy for the patient and give a thorough explanation of what you are going to do; put on gloves.
4. The following principles apply to all MDIs. Read and adapt the technique to directions provided by the manufacturer for a specific inhaler and extender if needed.
   - If the medication is a suspension, shake the canister. This disperses and mixes the active bronchodilator and propellant.
   - Open the mouth and place the canister outlet 2 to 4 inches in front of the mouth, or use an extender. This space allows the propellant to evaporate and prevents large particles from settling in the mouth.
   - Activate the MDI and instruct the patient to inhale deeply over 10 seconds to ensure that airways are open and that the drug is dispersed as deeply as possible.
   - Have the patient hold the breath, then exhale slowly to permit the drug to settle into pulmonary tissue.
   - If prescribed, repeat in 2 to 3 minutes. Using small doses with two or three inhalations enhances deposition of the drug in the smaller, peripheral airways for longer therapeutic effect.
   - If the inhaled medication is a corticosteroid, rinse the mouth with water when administration is complete.
   - Cleanse the apparatus according to the manufacturer's recommendations; remove gloves and dispose of them according to hospital policy.

Dry Powder Inhaler

1. Wash your hands and assemble the equipment.
2. Use the five RIGHTS of medication preparation and administration throughout the procedure.
   RIGHT PATIENT
   RIGHT DRUG
   RIGHT ROUTE OF ADMINISTRATION
   RIGHT DOSE
   RIGHT TIME OF ADMINISTRATION
3. Provide privacy for the patient and give a thorough explanation of what you are going to do; put on gloves.
4. The following principles apply to all DPIs. Read and adapt the technique to directions provided by the manufacturer for a specific inhaler and extender if needed.
   - Remove the cover and check that the device and the mouthpiece are clean.
   - Make the medication available for inhalation by twisting the container, pulling the cartridge out and pushing in, or sliding the lever, depending on the model of inhaler. Keep the inhaler horizontal.
   - Have the patient breathe out away from the device.
   - Place the mouthpiece gently in the mouth and close the lips around it.
   - Have the patient breathe in quickly, forcefully, and deeply until a full breath has been taken.
   - Remove the inhaler from the mouth.
   - Hold the breath for about 10 seconds before breathing out.
   - Always check the number in the dose counter window to see how many doses remain.
   - If the patient drops the inhaler or breathes into it after the dose has been loaded, the dose may be lost. To ensure proper dosage, load another dose into the inhaler before using it.
   - Clean the device according to the manufacturer's instructions.

Patient Teaching

Explain the procedure and allow the patient to demonstrate the technique. Teaching aids of MDIs and DPIs without active ingredients are available from the pharmacy department to encourage patients to practice the technique before medication administration. In addition to technique, the patient should be told what side effects to expect, what adverse effects to report, how to carry the medication, how to store it, and how to have it refilled when needed.

Have the patient perform the self-administration of the prescribed amount of ordered medication. Have the patient demonstrate the ability to read the canister counter to determine the amount of medication remaining in the container.

Documentation

Provide the RIGHT DOCUMENTATION of the medication administration and responses to drug therapy.

1. Chart the date, time, drug name, dose, site, and route of administration.
2. Perform and record regular patient assessments for the evaluation of therapeutic effectiveness (blood

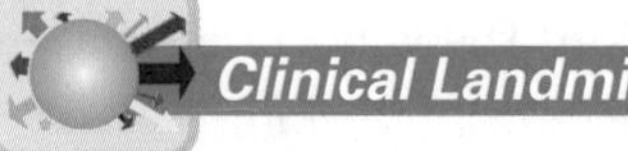

The patient should not wait until the canister is empty before having the prescription refilled. The last few doses in a canister are often subtherapeutic because of an imbalance in the remaining amounts of medication and propellant. Consult the manufacturer's information on how to determine if the canister is almost empty. The commonly used float test is inaccurate for many aerosolized metered-dose inhalers.

pressure, pulse, improvement of quality of breathing, cough and productivity, degree and duration of pain relief, ability to operate the MDI, activity and exercise restrictions, and so on).
3. Chart and report any signs and symptoms of adverse drug effects.
4. Perform and validate essential patient education about the drug therapy and other essential aspects of intervention for the disease process affecting the patient.

Administration of Vaginal Medications

Women with gynecologic disorders may require the administration of a medication intravaginally, usually for localized action. Vaginal medications may be creams, jellies, tablets, foams, suppositories, or irrigations (douches). The creams, jellies, tablets, and foams are inserted using special applicators provided by the manufacturer; suppositories are usually inserted with a gloved index finger. (See Administration of a Vaginal Douche, p. 128.)

Perform premedication assessment. See individual drug monograph.

Equipment

Prescribed medication
Vaginal applicator
Perineal pad
Water-soluble lubricant (for suppository)
Gloves
Paper towel
MAR or medication profile

Site

Administer to the vagina.

Techniques

1. Wash your hands and assemble the equipment.
2. Use the five RIGHTS of medication preparation and administration throughout the procedure.
   RIGHT PATIENT
   RIGHT DRUG
   RIGHT ROUTE OF ADMINISTRATION
   RIGHT DOSE
   RIGHT TIME OF ADMINISTRATION
3. Provide privacy for the patient and give a thorough explanation of the procedure. Have the patient void to ensure that the bladder is empty. Put on gloves.
4. Fill the applicator with the prescribed tablet, jelly, cream, or foam.
5. Place the patient in the lithotomy position and elevate the hips with a pillow. Drape the patient to prevent unnecessary exposure.
6. *Administration:* For *creams, foams,* and *jellies,* use the gloved nondominant hand to spread the labia and expose the vagina. Assess the status of presenting symptoms (e.g., color of discharge, volume, odor, level of discomfort). Gently insert the vaginal applicator as far as possible into the vagina and push the plunger to deposit the medication (Figure 8-13). Remove the applicator and wrap it in a paper towel for cleaning later. For *suppositories,* unwrap a vaginal suppository that has warmed to room temperature and lubricate it with a water-soluble lubricant. Lubricate the gloved dominant index finger. With the gloved nondominant hand, spread the labia to expose the vagina. Insert the suppository (rounded end first) as far into the vagina as possible with the dominant index finger.
7. Remove glove by turning inside out; place on paper towel for later disposal.
8. Apply a perineal pad to prevent drainage onto the patient's clothing or bed.
9. Instruct the patient to remain in a supine position with hips elevated for 5 to 10 minutes to allow melting and spreading of the medication.
10. Dispose of all waste and wash your hands.

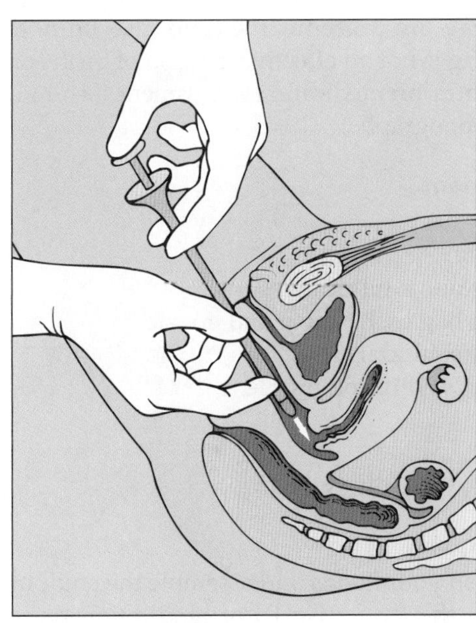

FIGURE 8-13 Applying vaginal medication. Gently insert the vaginal applicator as far as possible into the vagina and push plunger to deposit the medication.

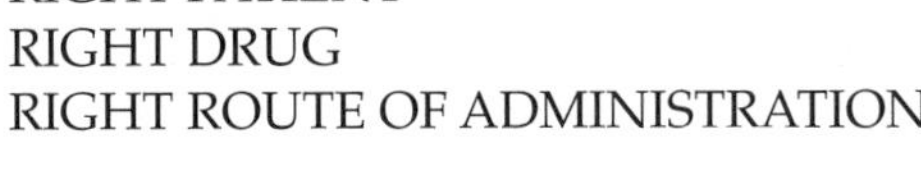

Medicines Administered by Inhalation

When muscle coordination is not fully developed (as in a younger child, or when dexterity has diminished in an older adult patient), it may be beneficial to use a spacer device (see Figure 8-12) for medicines administered by inhalation.

When administering medicines by aerosol therapy to an older adult, make sure the patient has the strength and dexterity to self-operate the equipment before discharge.

Patient Teaching

1. Guide the patient in learning how to administer the medication correctly.
2. The applicator should be washed in warm soapy water after *each* use.
3. Review personal hygiene measures such as wiping from the front to the back after voiding or defecating.
4. Tell the patient not to douche and to abstain from sexual intercourse after inserting the medication.
5. With most types of infection, both the male and female partners require treatment. To prevent reinfection, partners should abstain from sexual intercourse until both are cured.

Documentation

Provide the RIGHT DOCUMENTATION of the medication administration and responses to drug therapy.

1. Chart the date, time, drug name, dosage, and route of administration.
2. Perform and record regular patient assessments for the evaluation of the therapeutic effectiveness (e.g., type of discharge present, irritation of labia, discomfort, degree and duration of pain relief).
3. Chart and report any signs and symptoms of adverse drug effects.
4. Perform and validate essential patient education about the drug therapy and other essential aspects of intervention for the disease process affecting the individual.

Administration of a Vaginal Douche

Douches (irrigants) are used for washing the vagina. This procedure is not necessary for normal female hygiene but may be required if a vaginal infection and discharge are present. It should also be noted that douching is not an effective method of birth control.

Perform premedication assessment. See individual drug monograph.

Equipment

IV pole
Gloves
Water-soluble lubricant
Douche bag with tubing and nozzle
Douche solution
MAR or medication profile

Site

Administer to the vagina.

Techniques

1. Wash your hands and assemble the equipment.
2. Use the five RIGHTS of medication preparation and administration throughout the procedure.
   RIGHT PATIENT
   RIGHT DRUG
   RIGHT ROUTE OF ADMINISTRATION
   RIGHT DOSE
   RIGHT TIME OF ADMINISTRATION
3. Provide privacy for the patient and give a thorough explanation of the procedure.
4. Ask the patient to void before the procedure.
5. If teaching this procedure to a patient for home use, the patient would customarily recline in a bathtub. Depending on the patient's condition in the hospital, this too could occur. However, it may be necessary to place the patient on a bedpan and drape for privacy.
6. Hang the douche bag on an IV pole, about 12 inches above the vagina; put on gloves; apply water-soluble lubricant to plastic vaginal tip.
7. Cleanse the vulva by allowing a small amount of solution to flow over the vulva and between the labia.
8. Gently insert the nozzle, directing the tip backward and downward 2 to 3 inches.
9. Hold the labia together to facilitate filling the vagina with solution. Rotate nozzle periodically to help irrigate all parts of the vagina.
10. Intermittently release the labia allowing the solution to flow out.
11. When all the solution has been used, remove the nozzle. Have the patient sit up and lean forward to thoroughly empty the vagina.
12. Pat the external area dry.
13. Clean all equipment with warm soapy water after *every* use; rinse with clear water and allow to dry.
14. Thoroughly clean and disinfect the bathtub, if used. Remove gloves and dispose of according to hospital policy.
15. Wash your hands.

Patient Teaching

1. Guide the patient in learning how to correctly administer the douche.
2. Explain that the bag and tubing should be washed in warm soapy water after each use so as not to become a source of reinfection.
3. Review personal hygiene measures such as wiping from the front to the back after voiding or defecating.
4. Explain that douching is not recommended during pregnancy.
5. With most types of infection, both the male and female partners require treatment. To prevent reinfection, partners should abstain from sexual intercourse until both are cured.

Documentation

Provide the RIGHT DOCUMENTATION of the medication administration and responses to drug therapy.

1. Chart the date, time, drug name, dosage, and route of administration.
2. Perform and record regular patient assessments for the evaluation of therapeutic effectiveness (e.g., type

of discharge present, irritation of labia, discomfort, degree and duration of pain relief).
3. Chart and report any signs and symptoms of adverse drug effects.
4. Perform and validate essential patient education about the drug therapy and other essential aspects of intervention for the patient's disease process.

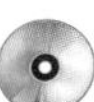

Go to your Companion CD-ROM for Appendices, an Audio Glossary, animations, Drug Dosage Calculators, customizable Patient Self-Assessment forms, and Review Questions for the NCLEX® Examination.

evolve Be sure to visit the companion Evolve site at http://evolve.elsevier.com/Clayton for WebLinks and additional online resources.

MEDICATION SAFETY REVIEW

CRITICAL THINKING QUESTIONS

1. Discuss the procedure used to remove and apply nitroglycerin ointment, including essential patient education.
2. Discuss proper application technique, frequency of changing patches, dosages of drugs available, and essential patient education for nitroglycerin, clonidine, estrogen, nicotine, scopolamine, Ortho Evra and fentanyl.
3. Explain premedication assessments that should be completed before administering the different types of percutaneous medications.

CONTENT REVIEW QUESTIONS

1. A drug-free period of ________ is usually recommended when nitroglycerin ointment is being prescribed.
   1. 3 to 4 hours off q24h
   2. 5 to 10 hours off q24h
   3. 10 to 12 hours off q24h
   4. 12 to 14 hours off q24h
2. Fentanyl patches do not usually achieve a sufficient blood level for pain control until _____ hours after initial application.
   1. 6
   2. 8
   3. 10
   4. 12
3. A client is to receive a medication via the buccal route. The nurse plans to implement the following action:
   1. place the medication inside the back of the cheek.
   2. crush the medication before administration.
   3. offer the client a glass of water or juice after administration.
   4. use sterile technique to administer the medication.
4. A client has a prescription for a medication that is administered via an inhaler. To determine whether the client requires a spacer for the inhaler, the nurse will determine the:
   1. dosage of medication required.
   2. coordination of the client.
   3. time of administration.
   4. use of a dry powder inhaler (DPI).
5. A client is ordered to have eye drops administered daily to both eyes. Eye drops should be instilled on the:
   1. sclera.
   2. outer canthus.
   3. lower conjunctival sac.
   4. opening of the lacrimal duct.

CHAPTER 9 Enteral Administration

evolve http://evolve.elsevier.com/Clayton

Chapter Content

The routes of drug administration can be classified into three categories: enteral, parenteral, and percutaneous. With the enteral route, drugs are administered directly into the gastrointestinal (GI) tract by oral, rectal, or nasogastric (NG) methods. The oral route is safe, most convenient, and relatively economical, and dose forms are readily available for most medications. In the event of a medication error or intentional drug overdose, much of the drug can be retrieved for a reasonable time after administration. The major disadvantage of the oral route is that it has the slowest and least dependable rate of absorption (and thus onset of action) of the commonly used routes of administration because of frequent changes in the GI environment produced by food, emotion, and physical activity. Another limitation of this route is that a few drugs, such as insulin and gentamicin, are destroyed by digestive fluids and must be given parenterally for therapeutic activity. This route should not be used if the drug may harm or discolor the teeth, or if the patient is vomiting, has gastric or intestinal suction, is likely to aspirate, or is unconscious and unable to swallow.

For patients who cannot swallow or who have had oral surgery, the NG method may be employed. The primary purpose of the NG method is to bypass the mouth and pharynx. Advantages and disadvantages are quite similar to those of the oral route. The irritation caused by the tube in the nasal passage and throat must be weighed against the relative immobility associated with continuous intravenous (IV) infusions, expense, and the pain and irritation of multiple injections.

Administration via the rectal route has the advantages of bypassing the digestive enzymes and avoiding irritation of the mouth, esophagus, and stomach. It may also be a good alternative when nausea or vomiting is present. Absorption via this route varies depending on the drug product, the ability of the patient to retain the suppository or enema, and the presence of fecal material.

ADMINISTRATION OF ORAL MEDICATIONS

Objectives

1. Correctly define and identify oral dose forms of medications.
2. Identify common receptacles used to administer oral medications.

Key Terms

capsules	unit dose packaging
lozenges	bar code
tablets	soufflé cup
elixirs	medicine cup
emulsions	medicine dropper
suspensions	oral syringe
syrups	

Dose Forms

Capsules

Capsules are small cylindrical gelatin containers that hold dry powder or liquid medicinal agents (Figure 9-1). They are available in a variety of sizes and are a convenient way of administering drugs that have an unpleasant odor or taste. They do not require coatings or additives to improve the taste. The color and shapes of capsules, as well as the manufacturer's symbols on the capsule surface, are means of identifying the product.

Timed Release Capsules. Timed release or sustained release capsules provide a gradual but continuous release

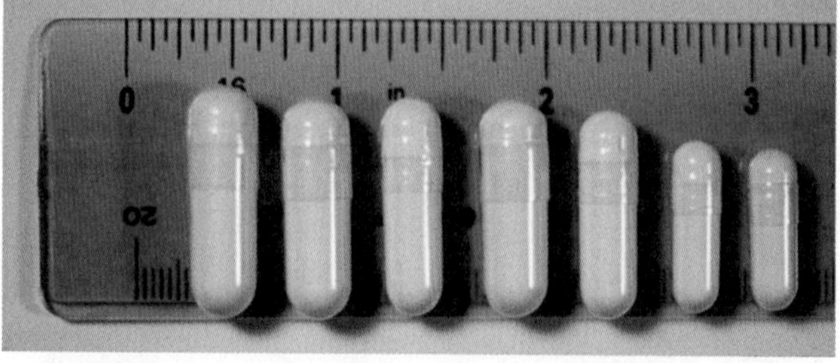

FIGURE 9-1 Various sizes and numbers of gelatin capsules, actual size.

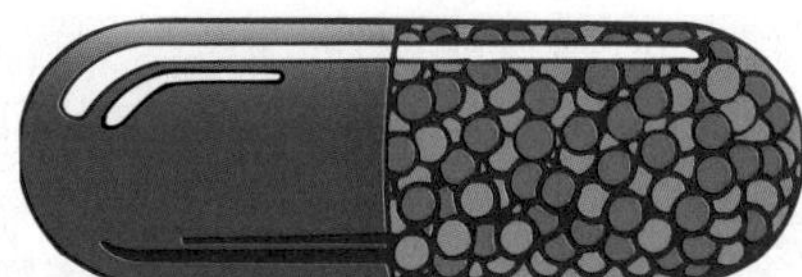

FIGURE 9-2 Timed release capsule.

The timed release capsules should NOT be crushed or chewed or the contents emptied into food or liquids because this may alter the absorption rate and could result in either drug overdose or subtherapeutic activity.

of a drug because the granules within the capsule dissolve at different rates (Figure 9-2). The advantage of this delivery system is that it reduces the number of doses administered per day. Trade names indicating that the drug is a timed release product are Spansules, Gyrocaps, and Plateau Caps.

Lozenges or Troches

Lozenges are flat disks containing a medicinal agent in a suitably flavored base. The base may be a hard sugar candy or the combination of sugar with sufficient mucilage to give it form. Lozenges are held in the mouth to dissolve slowly, thus releasing the therapeutic ingredients.

Pills

Pills are an obsolete dose form that is no longer manufactured as a result of the development of capsules and compressed tablets. However, the term is still used to refer to tablets and capsules.

Tablets

Tablets are dried, powdered drugs that have been compressed into small disks. In addition to the drug, tablets also contain one or more of the following ingredients: binders (adhesive substances that allow the tablet to hold together); disintegrators (substances that encourage dissolution in body fluids); lubricants (required for efficient manufacturing); and fillers (inert ingredients to make the tablet size convenient). Tablets are sometimes scored or grooved (Figure 9-3, *A*); the indentation may be used to divide the dose. When possible, it is best to request that the exact dose be prescribed rather than to attempt to divide even a scored tablet.

Tablets can be formed in layers (see Figure 9-3, *B*). This method allows otherwise incompatible medications to be administered at the same time.

An enteric-coated tablet has a special coating that resists dissolution in the acidic pH of the stomach but is dissolved in the alkaline pH of the intestines (see Figure 9-3, *C*). Enteric-coated tablets are often used for

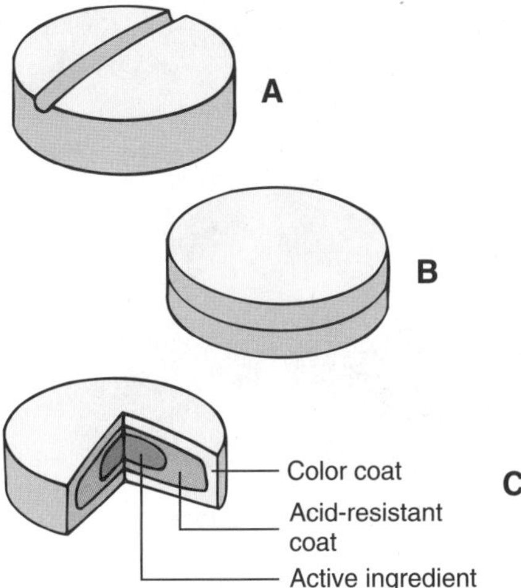

FIGURE 9-3 **A,** Scored tablet. **B,** Layered tablet. **C,** Enteric-coated tablet.

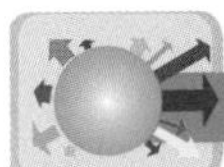

Enteric-coated tablets must NOT be crushed or chewed, or the active ingredients will be released prematurely and be destroyed in the stomach.

administering medications that are destroyed in an acid pH.

Elixirs

Elixirs are clear liquids made up of drugs dissolved in alcohol and water. Elixirs are used primarily when the drug will not dissolve in water alone. After the drug is dissolved in the elixir, flavoring agents are often added to improve taste. The alcohol content of elixirs is highly variable, depending on the solubility of the drug.

Emulsions

Emulsions are dispersions of small droplets of water in oil or oil in water. The dispersion is maintained by emulsifying agents such as sodium lauryl sulfate, gelatin, or acacia. Emulsions are used to mask bitter tastes or provide better solubility to certain drugs.

Suspensions

Suspensions are liquid dose forms that contain solid, insoluble drug particles dispersed in a liquid base. All suspensions should be shaken well before administration to ensure thorough mixing of the particles.

Syrups

Syrups contain medicinal agents dissolved in a concentrated solution of sugar, usually sucrose. Syrups are particularly effective for masking the bitter taste of a drug. Many preparations for pediatric patients are syrups because children tend to like the flavored base.

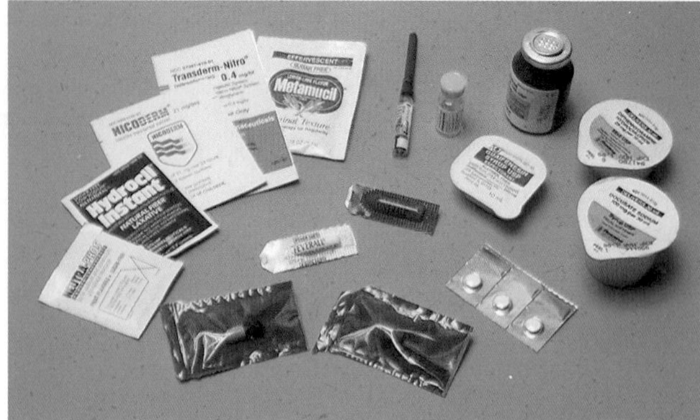

FIGURE **9-4** Unit dose packages.

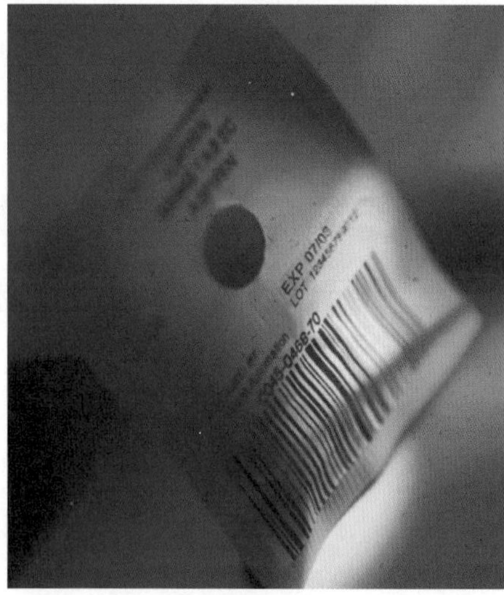

FIGURE **9-5** Most unit dose package labels include a bar code for electronic charting of medication administration and inventory control.

Equipment

Unit Dose or Single Dose

Unit dose packaging, or single-dose packaging, provides a single dose of medication in one package, ready for dispensing (Figure 9-4). The package is labeled with generic and brand names, manufacturer, lot number, and date of expiration. Depending on the distribution system, the patient's name may be added to the package by the pharmacy. Most unit dose package labels include a bar code for electronic charting of medication administration and inventory control (Figure 9-5).

Soufflé Cup

A soufflé cup is a small paper or plastic cup used to transport solid medication forms such as a capsule or tablet to the patient to prevent contamination by handling (Figure 9-6). A tablet that must be crushed can be placed between two soufflé cups and then crushed with a pestle. This powdered form of the tablet can then be administered in a solution if soluble, or it may be mixed with a small amount of food such as applesauce.

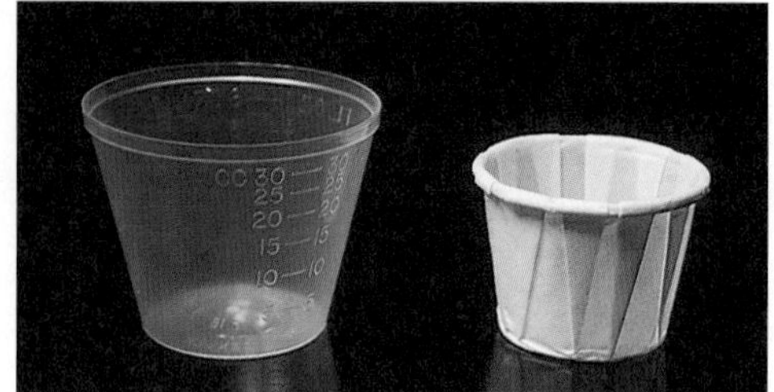

FIGURE **9-6** Soufflé cup.

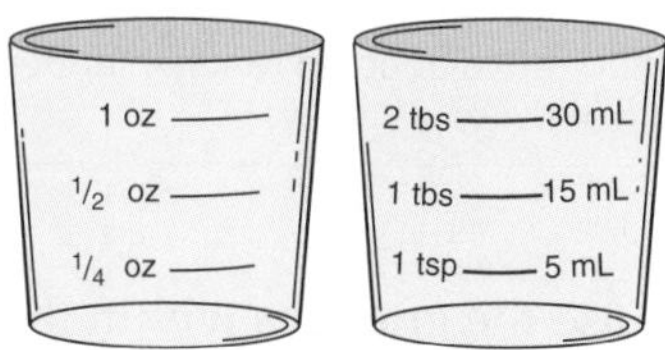

FIGURE **9-7** Medicine cup.

Table 9-1 ***Commonly Used Measurement Equivalents***

HOUSEHOLD MEASUREMENT	APOTHECARY MEASUREMENT	METRIC MEASUREMENT
2 tbs	1 oz	30 mL
1 tbs	1/2 oz	15 mL
2 tsp	1/3 oz	10 mL
1 tsp	1/6 oz	5 mL

Medicine Cup

The medicine cup is a glass or plastic container with three scales (apothecary, metric, and household) to measure liquid medications (Figure 9-7). Examine the medicine cup carefully before pouring any medication to ensure that the proper scale is being used for measurement (Table 9-1). The medicine cup is inaccurate for measuring doses smaller than 1 teaspoonful, although it is reasonably accurate for larger volumes. A syringe comparable to the volume to be measured should be used for smaller volumes. For volumes less than 1 mL, a tuberculin syringe should be used.

Medicine Dropper

The medicine dropper may be used to administer eye drops, ear drops, and occasionally, pediatric medications (Figure 9-8). There is a great variation in the size of the drop formed, so it is quite important to use only the dropper supplied by the manufacturer for a specific liquid medication. Before drawing medication into a dropper, it is necessary to become familiar with the calibrations on the barrel. Once the medication is drawn into the barrel, the dropper should not be tipped upside down. The medication will run into the bulb, causing some loss of the medication. Medications should not be drawn into the dropper and then transferred to another container for administration because part of the

2.0 mL
1.5 mL
1.0 mL
0.5 mL

FIGURE 9-8 Medicine dropper.

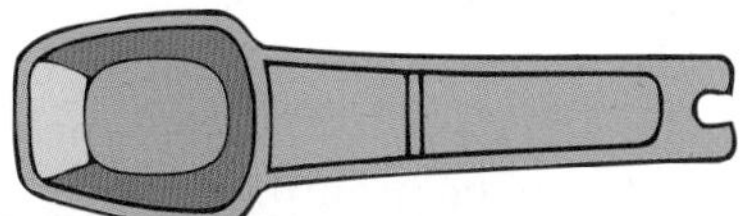

FIGURE 9-9 Measuring teaspoon.

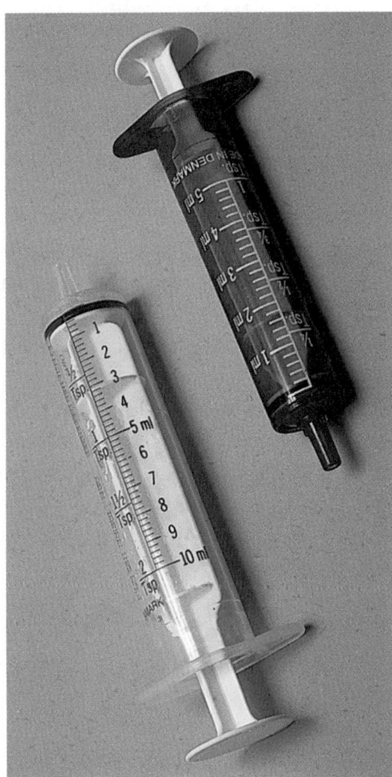

FIGURE 9-10 Plastic oral syringe.

medication will adhere to the second container, thus diminishing the dose delivered.

Teaspoon

Doses of most liquid medications are prescribed in terms using the teaspoon as the unit of measure (Figure 9-9).

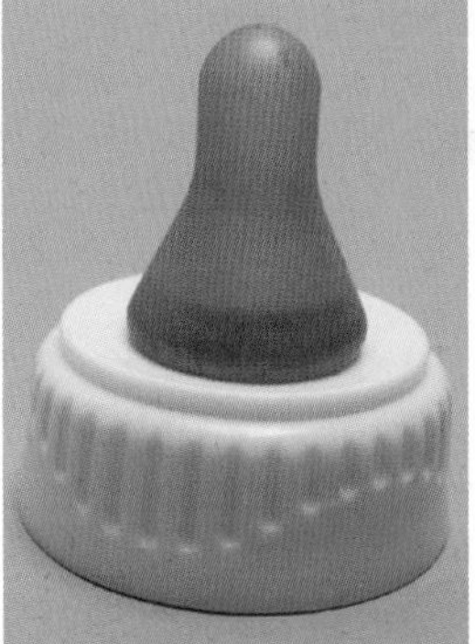

FIGURE 9-11 Nipple.

However, there is great variation between the volumes measured by various teaspoons within the household. Within the hospital, 1 teaspoonful is converted to 5 mL (see Table 9-1) and is read on the metric scale of the medicine cup. For home use, an oral syringe is recommended. If not available, a teaspoon used specifically for baking may be used as an accurate measuring device.

Oral Syringe

A plastic oral syringe may be used to measure liquid medications accurately (Figure 9-10). Various sizes are available to measure volumes from 0.1 mL to 15 mL. Note that a needle will not fit on the tip.

Nipple

An infant feeding nipple with additional holes may be used for administering oral medications to infants (Figure 9-11). (See General Principles of Liquid-Form Oral Medication Administration, For an Infant, p. 137.)

ADMINISTRATION OF SOLID-FORM ORAL MEDICATIONS

Objective

1. Describe general principles of administering solid forms of medications and the different techniques used with a medication card, and a computer-controlled and unit dose distribution system.

Medication Card System

Perform premedication assessment. See individual drug monographs for details.

Equipment

Medication tray
Soufflé cup or medicine cup
Medication cards

Technique

1. Wash your hands.
2. Gather medication cards and verify against Kardex and the health care provider's order for accuracy.

3. Gather remainder of equipment.
4. Read the entire medication card.
5. Obtain the prescribed medication from the cabinet.
6. COMPARE the label on the container against the medication card.
   RIGHT PATIENT
   RIGHT DRUG
   RIGHT ROUTE OF ADMINISTRATION
   RIGHT DOSE
   RIGHT TIME OF ADMINISTRATION
7. Open the lid of the bottle; pour the correct number of capsules or tablets into the lid; return any extras to the container using the lid. (DO NOT touch the medication with your hands!)
8. Transfer the correct number of tablets or capsules from the lid to a soufflé cup or medicine cup.
9. COMPARE the information on the medication card against the label on the stock bottle and the quantity of drug placed in the cup.
10. Replace the lid of the container.
11. RECHECK the FIVE RIGHTS of the medication order.
12. Return the medication container to the shelf in the cabinet.
13. Place the patient's medication cup on the medication tray with the medication card.
14. Proceed to the patient's bedside when all medications are assembled for administration.
    - Check the patient's identification bracelet and verify against the medication card. Have the patient state his or her name and birth date or other identifier.
    - Explain carefully to the patient what you are doing.
    - Check pertinent patient monitoring parameters (e.g., apical pulse, respiratory rate).
    - Hand the medication to the patient for placement into the mouth.

UNIT DOSE SYSTEM

Perform premedication assessment. See individual drug monographs for details.

Equipment

Medication cart
Medication profile

Technique

1. Wash your hands.
2. Read the patient medication profile for drugs and times of administration.
3. Obtain the prescribed medication from the drawer in the medication cart that is assigned to the patient.
4. Check the label on the unit dose package against the patient medication profile. Check the expiration date on all medication labels.
   RIGHT PATIENT
   RIGHT DRUG
   RIGHT ROUTE OF ADMINISTRATION
   RIGHT DOSE
   RIGHT TIME OF ADMINISTRATION
5. Check the number of doses remaining in the drawer. (If the number of doses remaining is not consistent, investigate!)
6. Check the FIVE RIGHTS of the medication order on the patient medication profile and unit dose package as it is removed from the drawer.
7. Proceed to the bedside:
   - Check the patient's identification bracelet and verify against the profile. Have the patient state his or her name and birth date or other identifiers.
   - Explain carefully to the patient what you are doing.
   - Check pertinent patient monitoring parameters (e.g., apical pulse, respiratory rate).
8. Hand the medication to the patient and allow him or her to read the package label.
9. Retrieve the unit dose package and open it, placing the contents in the patient's hand or medication cup for placement into the mouth.

ELECTRONIC CONTROL SYSTEM

Perform premedication assessment. See individual drug monographs for details.

Equipment

Computerized medication system
Medication profile

Technique

1. Wash your hands.
2. Obtain and read the medication profile or medication administration record (MAR) for drugs and time of administration.
3. Access the computerized medication system using the security access code and password.
4. Select the patient's name from the list of patients on the unit.
5. Review the on-screen profile and select the medications to be administered at this time.
6. Check all aspects of the on-screen order against the medication profile or MAR.
7. Check the label on the unit dose package against the patient medication profile. Check the expiration dates on all medication labels.
   RIGHT PATIENT
   RIGHT DRUG
   RIGHT ROUTE OF ADMINISTRATION
   RIGHT DOSE
   RIGHT TIME OF ADMINISTRATION
8. Check the FIVE RIGHTS of the medication order on the patient medication profile and unit dose package as it is removed from the drawer.
9. Proceed to the bedside:
   - Check the patient's identification bracelet and verify against the profile. Have the patient state his or her name and birth date, or two other identifiers.

- With a computerized scanner system, scan the patient identification, the bar code on the unit dose medication container, and the nurse's badge.
- Explain carefully to the patient what you are doing.
- Check pertinent patient monitoring parameters (e.g., apical pulse, respiratory rate).
- Hand the medication to the patient and allow him or her to read the package label.
- Retrieve the unit dose package and open it, placing the contents in the patient's hand for placement into the mouth.

General Principles of Solid-Form Medication Administration

1. Give the most important medication first.
2. Allow the patient to drink a small amount of water to moisten the mouth, so that swallowing the medication is easier.
3. Have the patient place the medication well back on the tongue. Offer appropriate assistance.
4. Give the patient liquid to swallow the medication. Encourage keeping the head forward while swallowing.
5. Drinking a full glass of fluid should be encouraged to ensure that the medication reaches the stomach and is diluted to decrease the potential for irritation.
6. Always remain with the patient while the medication is taken. DO NOT leave the medication at the bedside unless an order exists to do so (medication such as nitroglycerin may be ordered for the bedside).
7. Discard the medication container (such as a soufflé cup or unit dose package).
8. If the patient has difficulty swallowing and liquid medications are not an option, you may use a pill-crushing device. Ensure that the medication is not a capsule or enteric coated. Follow the guidelines for using the crushing device. Mix the crushed medication in a small amount of soft food such as applesauce, ice cream, custard, or jelly. This will help to counteract the bitter taste and consistency of the mixture (Figure 9-12).

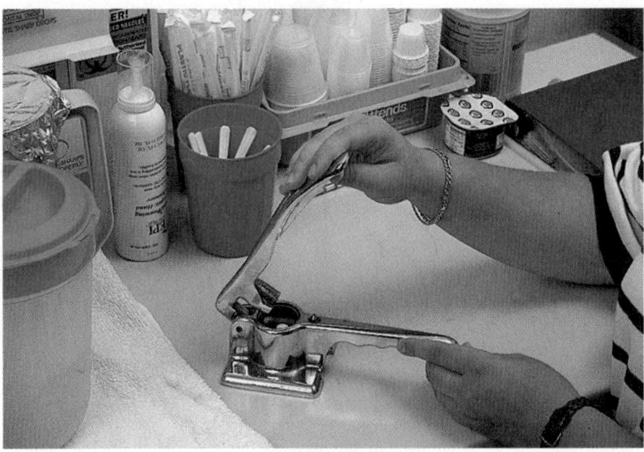

FIGURE 9-12 Tablet crusher.

Documentation

Provide the RIGHT DOCUMENTATION of medication administration and responses to drug therapy.

If using an electronic control system, the date, time, drug name, dose, and route of administration are automatically charted in the electronic MAR when the patient's identification badge, the bar-coded unit dose medication container, and the nurse's badge have been scanned.

1. Chart the date, time, drug name, dosage, and route of administration.
2. Perform and record regular patient assessments for the evaluation of the therapeutic effectiveness (e.g., blood pressure, pulse, intake and output, improvement or quality of cough and productivity, degree and duration of pain relief).
3. Chart and report any signs or symptoms of adverse drug effects.
4. Perform and validate essential patient education about the drug therapy and other essential aspects of intervention for the disease process affecting the individual.

ADMINISTRATION OF LIQUID-FORM ORAL MEDICATIONS

Objective

1. Compare techniques used to administer liquid forms of oral medication using medication card and unit dose systems of distribution.

Medication Card System

Perform premedication assessment. See individual drug monographs for details.

Equipment

Medication tray
Plastic syringe or medicine cup
Medication cards

Technique

1. Wash your hands.
2. Gather medication cards and verify against Kardex, the health care provider's order, or both, for accuracy.
3. Gather remainder of equipment.
4. Read the entire medication card.
5. Obtain the medication prescribed from the cabinet.
6. COMPARE the label on the container against the medication card.
   RIGHT PATIENT
   RIGHT DRUG
   RIGHT ROUTE OF ADMINISTRATION
   RIGHT DOSE
   RIGHT TIME OF ADMINISTRATION
7. Shake the medication, if required.
8. Remove the lid and place it upside down on a flat surface to prevent contamination.

9. Proceed with one of the following measuring techniques.

   Measuring with a medicine cup:
   - Hold the bottle of liquid so that the label is in the palm of the hand. This prevents the contents from smearing the label during pouring.
   - Examine the medicine cup and locate the exact place where the measured volume should be measured; place your fingernail at this level.
   - While holding the medicine cup straight at eye level, pour the prescribed volume.
   - Read the volume accurately at the level of the meniscus (Figure 9-13).
   - COMPARE the information on the medication card against the label on the stock bottle and the quantity of drug placed in the cup.
   - Replace the lid on the container.
   - RECHECK the FIVE RIGHTS of the medication order.
   - Return the medication container to the shelf of the cabinet.
   - Place the patient's medication cup on the medication tray with the medication card (Figure 9-14).
   - Proceed to the patient's bedside when all medications are assembled for administration.

   Measuring with an oral syringe:
   - See Chapter 10 for reading calibrations of a syringe.
   - Select a syringe in a size comparable to the volume to be measured.
   - *Method 1:* With a large-bore needle attached to the syringe, draw up the prescribed volume of medication. The needle is not necessary if the bottle opening is large enough to receive the syringe (Figure 9-15).
   - *Method 2:* Using the cup and method 1, pour the amount of medication needed into a medicine cup, then use a syringe to measure the prescribed volume (Figure 9-16).
10. COMPARE the information on the medication card against the label on the stock bottle and the quantity of drug placed in the syringe.
11. Replace the lid on the container.
12. RECHECK the FIVE RIGHTS of the medication order.
13. Return the medication container to the shelf of the cabinet.
14. Place the patient's medication syringe on the medication tray with the medication card directly under the syringe.
15. Proceed to the patient's bedside when all medications are assembled for administration.

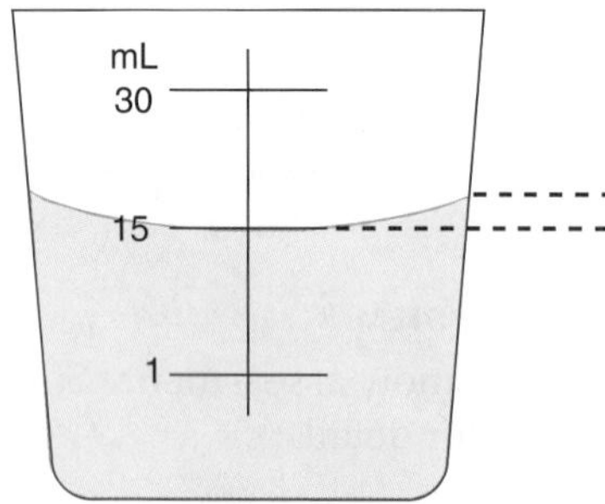

FIGURE **9-13** Reading meniscus. The meniscus is caused by the surface tension of the solution against the walls of the container. The surface tension causes the formation of a concave or hollowed curvature on the surface of the solution. Read the level at the lowest point of the concave curve.

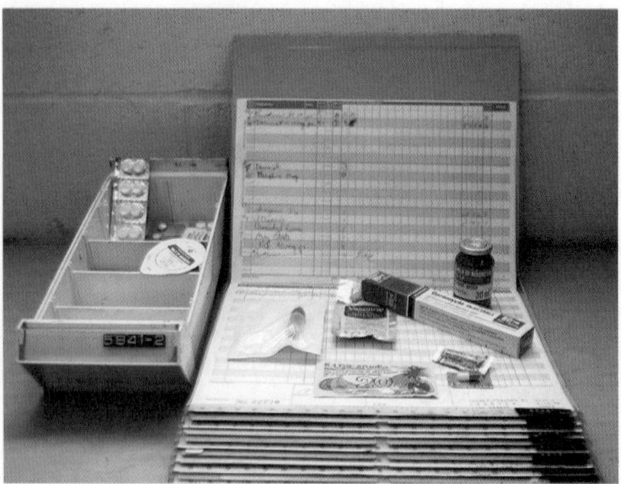

FIGURE **9-14** Tray for medication card system.

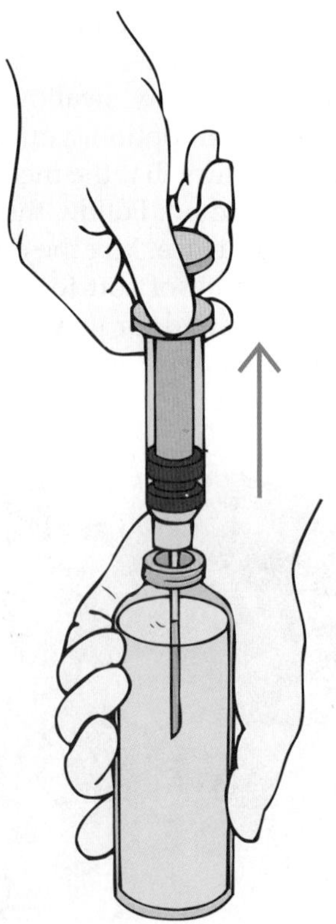

FIGURE **9-15** Removing medication directly from a bottle.

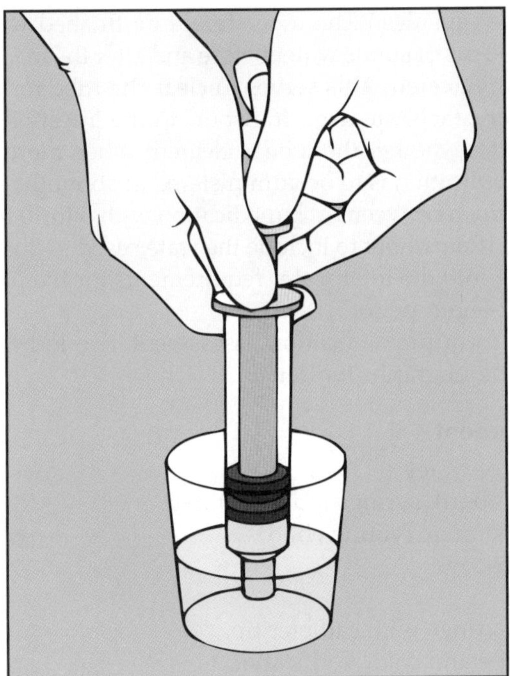

FIGURE **9-16** Filling a syringe directly from a medicine cup.

Now that the medication is ready to be administered, proceed as follows:

1. Check the patient's identification bracelet and verify against the medication card. Have the patient state his or her name and birth date, or two other identifiers.
2. Explain carefully to the patient what you are doing.
3. Check pertinent patient monitoring parameters (e.g., apical pulse, respiratory rate).
4. Hand the medication cup to the patient for placement of the contents into the mouth, or administer via the oral syringe.

Unit Dose System

Perform premedication assessment. See individual drug monographs for details.

Equipment

Medication cart
Medication profile

Technique

1. Wash your hands.
2. Read the patient medication profile for drugs and times of administration.
3. Obtain the prescribed medication from the drawer in the medication cart assigned to the patient.
4. Check the label on the unit dose package against the patient medication profile. Check the expiration dates on all medication labels.
   RIGHT PATIENT
   RIGHT DRUG
   RIGHT ROUTE OF ADMINISTRATION
   RIGHT DOSE
   RIGHT TIME OF ADMINISTRATION
5. Check the number of doses remaining in the drawer. (If the number of doses remaining is not consistent, investigate!)
6. Check the FIVE RIGHTS of the medication order on the patient medication profile and unit dose package as it is removed from the drawer.
7. Proceed to the bedside:
   - Check the patient's identification bracelet and verify against the profile. Have the patient state his or her name and birth date, or two other identifiers.
   - Explain carefully to the patient what you are doing.
   - Check pertinent patient monitoring parameters (e.g., apical pulse, respiratory rate).
8. Hand the unit dose medication to the patient and allow him or her to read the package label.
9. Retrieve the unit dose package and open it, placing the container in the patient's hand for placement of the contents into the patient's mouth.

General Principles of Liquid-Form Oral Medication Administration

For an Adult or Child

1. Give the most important medication first.
2. Never dilute a liquid medication unless specifically ordered to do so.
3. Always remain with the patient while the medication is taken. DO NOT leave the medication at the bedside unless an order exists to do so.

For an Infant

1. Check the infant's identification bracelet and verify against the medication card or profile.
2. Be certain that the infant is alert.
3. Position the infant so that the head is slightly elevated (Figure 9-17).
4. Administration:
   - *Oral syringe or dropper:* Place the syringe or dropper between the cheek and gums, halfway back into the mouth. This placement will reduce the chance that the infant will spit out the medication with tongue movements. Slowly inject, allowing the infant to swallow the medication. (Rapid administration may cause choking and aspiration!)
   - *Nipple:* When the infant is awake (and preferably hungry), place the nipple in the infant's mouth. When the baby starts to suck, place the medication in the back of the nipple with a syringe or dropper and allow the baby to suck it in (see Figure 9-17). (The size of the nipple holes may need to be enlarged for suspensions and syrups.) Follow with milk or formula, if necessary.

Documentation

Provide the RIGHT DOCUMENTATION of the medication administration and responses to drug therapy.

1. Chart the date, time, drug name, dosage, and route of administration.

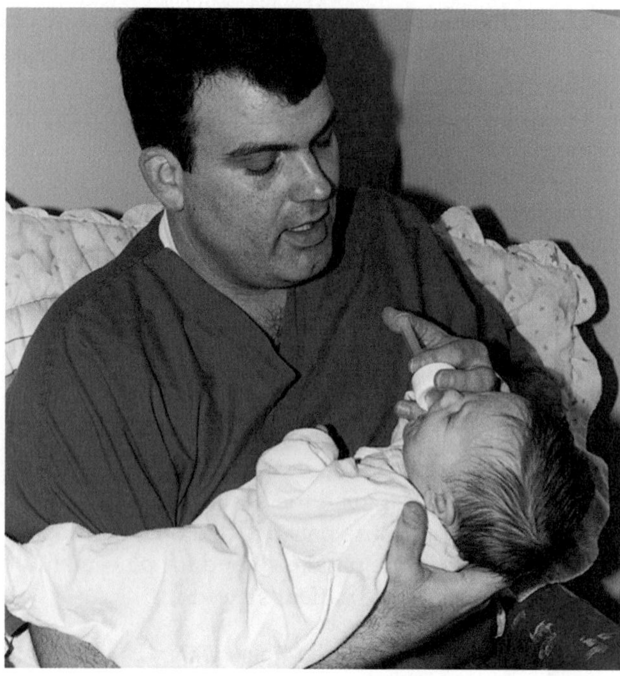

FIGURE 9-17 Position the infant in a "football hold" with the head slightly elevated. Place the nipple in the infant's mouth. When the baby starts to suck, place the medication in the back of the nipple and allow the baby to suck.

2. Perform and record regular patient assessments for the evaluation of therapeutic effectiveness (e.g., blood pressure, pulse, output, improvement or quality of cough and productivity, degree and duration of pain relief).
3. Chart and report any signs and symptoms of adverse drug effects.
4. Perform and validate essential patient education about the drug therapy and other essential aspects of intervention for the disease process affecting the individual.

ADMINISTRATION OF MEDICATIONS BY NASOGASTRIC TUBE

Objective

1. Cite the equipment needed, techniques used, and precautions necessary when administering medications via a nasogastric tube.

Key Term

nasogastric tube

Medications are administered via a **nasogastric** (NG) **tube** to patients who have impaired swallowing, are comatose, or have a disorder of the esophagus. Whenever possible, a liquid form of a drug should be used for NG administration. If it is necessary to use a tablet or capsule, the tablet should be crushed or the capsule pulled apart, and the powder sprinkled in approximately 30 mL of water. (DO NOT crush enteric-coated tablets or timed release capsules.) The tube should be flushed with at least 30 mL of sterile water before and after the medicine is administered. This serves to clear the tube for drug delivery, facilitate drug transport to the intestine, and indicates whether the tube is cleared. When more than one medication is to be administered at about the same time, flush between each medication with 5 to 10 mL of water. (Remember to include the water used to flush the tubing into the total water requirements for the patient for a 24-hour period.)

Perform premedication assessment. See individual drug monographs for details.

Equipment

Glass of water
20- to 30-mL syringe (adult patient)
1-mL syringe (young child)
Stethoscope
MAR
Bulb syringe with catheter tip
pH tape and color verification
Gloves

Technique

Refer to the sections on the administration of solid-form or liquid-form oral medications for preparation of doses.

1. Proceed to the patient's bedside when all medications are assembled for administration.
2. Check the patient's identification bracelet and verify against the medication card or drug profile. Have the patient state his or her name and birth date, or two other identifiers.
3. Put on disposable gloves.
4. Explain carefully to the patient what you are going to do.
5. Sit the patient upright and check the location of the NG tube before administering any liquid (Figure 9-18, *A*). (Note: x-ray confirmation of NG tube placement is performed when the tube is initially inserted. Thereafter, pH and color testing may be used to confirm placement.)

   Method 1: pH and color testing of gastric contents to check for tube placement
   - Put on gloves.
   - Flush the tube with 20 to 30 mL of air using a 30-mL or larger syringe. Aspirate part of the stomach contents using the bulb syringe. If unable to aspirate contents, reposition the patient on the left side and try aspirating again.
   - Check aspirated fluid color; color verification guidelines:
     Gastric fluid = green with sediment or off white
     Intestinal fluid = yellow (bile colored)
     Pleural fluid = clear to straw colored
     Tracheobronchial fluid = off white or tan
   - Check the pH of gastric contents. Stomach pH is <3, intestinal fluid pH is 6 to 7, respiratory fluid

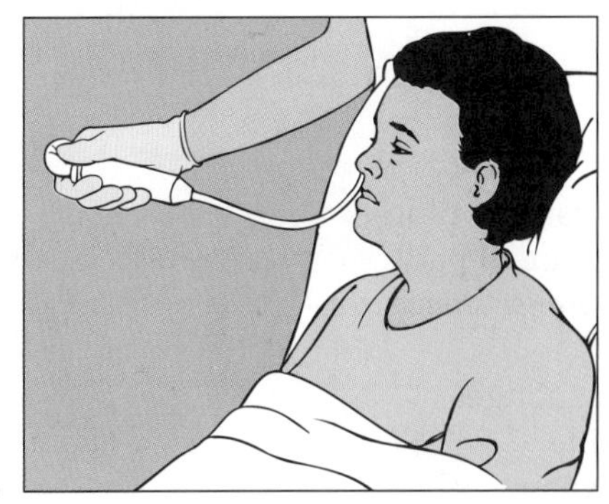

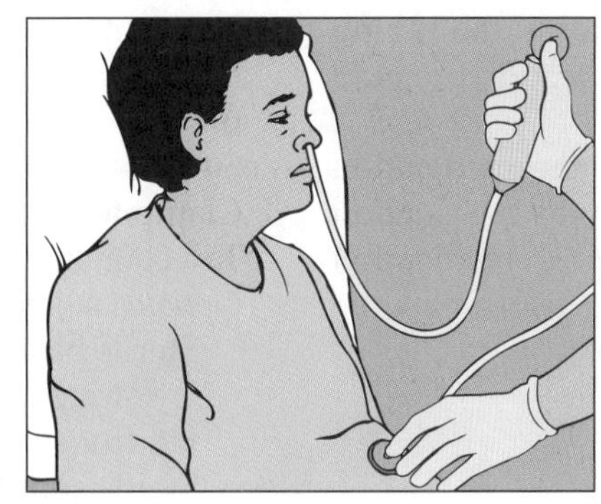

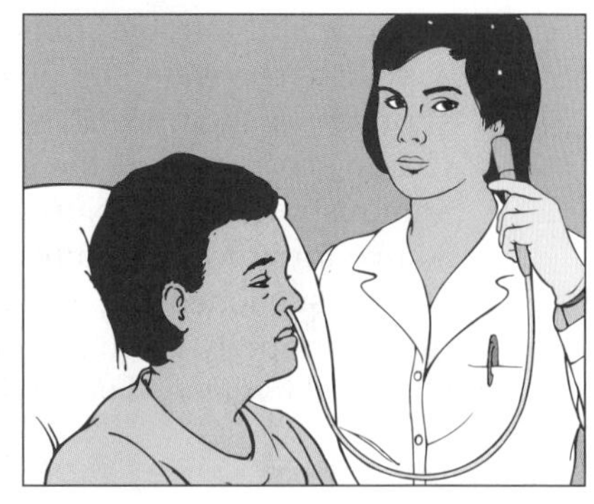

FIGURE **9-18** Checking the location of the nasogastric (NG) tube. **A,** Aspiration of stomach contents. **B,** Place a stethoscope over the stomach area; listen for a "gurgling" sound as air is inserted. **C,** Listen for "crackling" sounds indicating placement of the NG tube in the lung. Many clinical sites no longer use auscultation as a method to verify NG tube placement but have switched to pH testing and x-ray verification. It is no longer recommended to place the end of the NG tube in a glass of water. Although bubbling with respirations indicates placement of the tube in the lung, the patient may inadvertently inhale additional water from the glass into the lungs.

pH is >7. H_2 antagonists (ranitidine, cimetidine, famotidine, nizatidine) affect the aspirated fluid pH in the following ways:

People ***not*** receiving H_2 blockers
   Gastric = 1.0 to 4.0
   Intestinal = >6.0
People receiving H_2 blockers
   Gastric = 1.0 to 6.0
   Intestinal = >6.0
   Tracheobronchial/pleural aspirate = 7.0 or greater

- Return the stomach contents after confirmation of correct tube placement.

6. Once the placement of the NG tube in the stomach is confirmed, do the following:
   - Clamp the tubing and attach the bulb syringe; pour the medication into the syringe while the tubing is still clamped (Figure 9-19, *A*).
   - Unclamp the tubing and allow the medication to run in by gravity (see Figure 9-19, *B*); add the specified amount of water (at least 50 mL) (see Figure 9-19, *C*) to flush the medication through

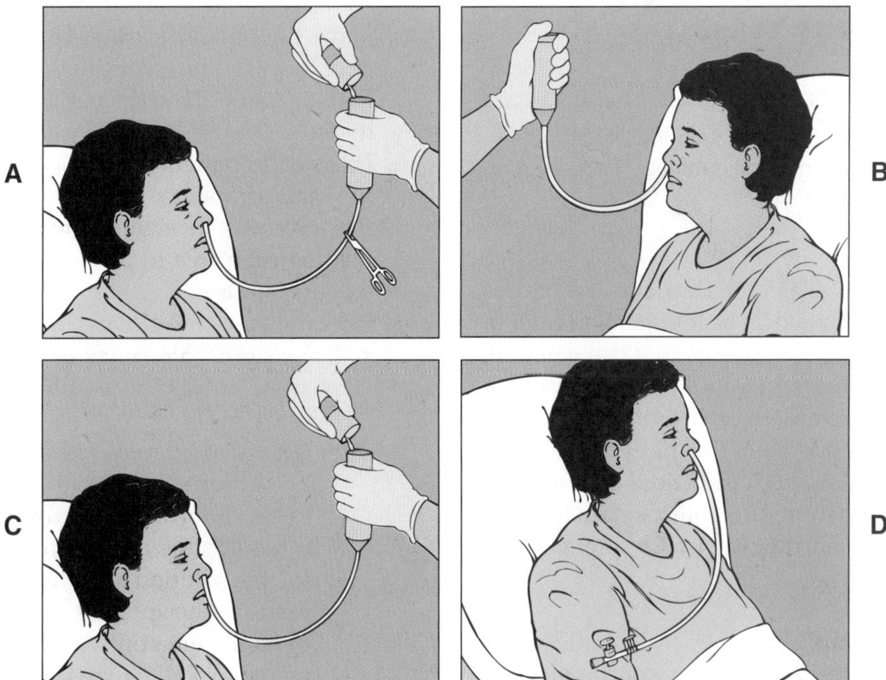

FIGURE **9-19** Administering medication via nasogastric (NG) tube. **A,** Clamp NG tube, attach a bulb syringe, and pour prescribed medication into syringe portion. **B,** Unclamp tubing and allow the medication to flow in by gravity. **C,** When medication is low in the syringe portion, pour in water to allow for thorough flushing of the medication from the tubing. **D,** Clamp tubing and secure end in place. Do not reattach to suction (if being used) for at least 30 minutes.

the tube and into the stomach; clamp the tubing as soon as the water has flowed through the bulb syringe (see Figure 9-19, *D*).

- Clamp the tubing at the end of the medication administration. DO NOT attach to the suction source for at least 30 minutes, or the medication will be suctioned out. Check to ensure that the tube is properly taped and secure.
- Give oral hygiene, if needed.

Documentation

Provide the RIGHT DOCUMENTATION of medication administration and responses to drug therapy.

1. Chart the verification of the NG tube placement.
2. Chart the date, time, drug name, dosage, and route of administration. Include all fluids (including fluid used to flush the tube) administered on the intake record.
3. Perform and record regular patient assessments for the evaluation of the therapeutic effectiveness (e.g., blood pressure, pulse, output, improvement or quality of cough and productivity, degree and duration of pain relief).
4. Chart and report any signs and symptoms of adverse drug effects.
5. Perform and validate essential patient education about the drug therapy and other essential aspects of intervention for the disease process affecting the individual.

ADMINISTRATION OF ENTERAL FEEDINGS VIA GASTROSTOMY OR JEJUNOSTOMY TUBE

Objective

1. Meet the person's basic metabolic requirements and provide adequate nutritional intake through the use of enteral nutrition support.

Dose Form

Enteral formulas are available in a variety of mixtures to meet the individual's needs. The four general categories are (1) intact nutrient (polymeric), (2) elemental, (3) disease or condition specific, and (4) modular nutrient. The type of formula ordered will be selected by the health care provider to meet the patient's energy requirements to maintain body functions and growth demands, and to repair tissue that is damaged or depleted by illness or injury. (See also Chapter 48.)

Equipment

Prescribed enteral formula
Disposable or ready-to-hang bag for continuous administration
Infusion pump specific for enteral formulas
Blood glucose testing materials (if blood glucose levels ordered)
Toomey syringe
50 mL of water
Measuring container/graduate
pH indicator tape
Stethoscope
Clamp (C-clamp or ostomy plug)
Towel or small incontinent pad
Optional supplies to cleanse stoma area:
Sterile basin
4 × 4-inch gauze sponges
Hydrogen peroxide
Sterile saline or water
Tape
Gloves

Technique

Place the patient in a semi-Fowler's position, 30 degrees head-of-bed (HOB) elevation for 30 minutes before starting feeding.

1. Wash your hands and assemble the necessary equipment and the prescribed formula.
2. Check date, time, and strength of solution and type of formula against the health care provider's order.
   RIGHT PATIENT
   RIGHT DRUG (FORMULA)
   RIGHT ROUTE OF ADMINISTRATION
   RIGHT DOSE (AMOUNT, DILUTION, STRENGTH)
   RIGHT TIME OF ADMINISTRATION
3. Proceed to the patient's bedside.
4. Check the patient's identification bracelet and verify against the medication card or drug profile. Have the patient state his or her name and birth date, or two other identifiers.
5. Explain carefully to the patient what you are going to do.
6. Provide for patient privacy; check patient positioning and drape to avoid unnecessary exposure. Place a towel or small incontinent pad under the feeding tube area to protect the area in case of accidental spills.
7. Put on disposable gloves.
   - If the stoma site needs cleansing, which should be done at least once daily or PRN, proceed as follows:
     - If crusted, place 4 × 4-inch gauze sponges in a solution of half-and-half hydrogen peroxide and normal saline or water. Place a saturated sponge around the stoma area, allowing the solution to soften the crusted exudate. Remove the sponges and wipe from the tube or stoma area outward. Rinse with saline- or water-soaked gauze sponges; pat dry.
8. Verify tube placement and initiate feeding:
   - *Gastrostomy tube:* Attach a Toomey syringe to the unclamped tube; release the clamp. Slowly withdraw the plunger to aspirate the residual. Observe the color and check the pH of aspirated

contents. (Use principles described in Administration of Medications by Nasogastric Tube to aspirate gastric contents.) Notify the health care provider if the residual is greater than 100 mL (or amount specified) since the last bolus feeding 4 hours earlier. Reintroduce the gastric contents aspirated.
- *Jejunostomy tube:* Aspirate the intestinal secretions using the same method as for a gastrostomy tube. Observe the color and check the pH.

9. Flush the tube with 30 mL of water.
10. Clamp the tube (gastrostomy or jejunostomy).
11. Proceed with one of the following feeding techniques.

Intermittent tube feeding:
- Remove a Toomey syringe from the container and remove the plunger. Reattach the Toomey syringe to the tubing while it is still clamped, pour the formula into the syringe, and unclamp the tubing and allow the contents to flow in by gravity. Continue filling the Toomey as it drains until the prescribed amount is instilled. Do not allow air to enter the stomach and cause distention.
- Flush the tubing with 50 mL of water. This removes the formula from the tubing, maintains the patency of the tube, and prevents the formula remaining in the tube from supporting bacterial growth.
- Clamp or plug the ostomy tube; remove the Toomey syringe.
- Tell the patient to remain in a sitting position or turn on the right side for 30 minutes to 1 hour to aid in normal digestion of feeding, and to prevent gastric reflux (with possible aspiration) or leakage.
- Wash all reusable equipment and dry and store in a clean area in the patient environment until the next feeding. Change the equipment according to institution policy, often every 72 hours.

Continuous tube feeding:
- Fill a disposable feeding container with enough of the prescribed formula for an 8-hour period. Store the remaining formula in the refrigerator. Label with the date and time initially used. The formula must be at room temperature at the time of initiation.
- Hang the container on an IV pole, clear air from the tubing, and thread the tubing through the pump in a manner prescribed by the pump's manufacturer.
- Connect the tube from the enteral feeding source to the end of the feeding tube. Release the clamp from the tube.
- Set the flow rate of the enteral formula at the prescribed rate to deliver the formula in the correct volume over the specified time span. When initiating tube feedings, the rate is started slowly and gradually advanced at specified intervals.

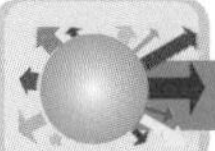

Clinical Landmine

Formula should be properly labeled with time, date, type of formula, and strength. Check date/time of preparation on formula mixed in the hospital pharmacy, discard unused portion every 24 hours. Commercially prepared vacuum-sealed formulas are generally stored at room temperature until used. Check the expiration date and return if outdated. If opened, discard in accordance with manufacturer's recommendations or institutional policy.

For patients receiving enteral nutrition via intermittent tube feedings (using facility guidelines).
- Check the residual volume before each feeding.
- Check to ensure the presence of bowel sounds. Absence of bowel sounds indicates the need to contact the health care provider for orders before proceeding.
- Check the position of the tube to ensure that it is still in the stomach.
- During initiation of enteral feedings by intermittent or continuous methods, blood glucose testing may be ordered.

- Wash all reusable equipment, dry and store in a clean area in the patient environment until the next feeding. Change the equipment every 24 hours.

12. Blood glucose assessment may be performed and recorded every 6 hours during the initiation of tube feedings. Assessments are continued until glucose levels are maintained within a specified range for a 24-hour period after the rate of enteral feeding has reached the prescribed maximum flow.
13. Inspect the nares at regular intervals to detect any pressure irritation created by the feeding tube.
14. Before the next scheduled feeding, a gastric residual volume should be checked using a bulb syringe for aspiration to ensure that the formula is leaving the stomach and passing into the intestine for absorption. If there is more than 100 mL residual volume, the physician should be notified.

Documentation

Provide the RIGHT DOCUMENTATION of the formula administered, cleansing of the stoma, and therapeutic response to the enteral feedings.

1. Chart date, time, and amount, color, and pH of residual aspirated, along with the amount, type, and strength of formula instilled, and amount of water used to rinse tubing.

ADMINISTRATION OF RECTAL SUPPOSITORIES

Objective

1. Cite the equipment needed and technique required to administer rectal suppositories.

Dose Form

Suppositories (Figure 9-20) are a solid form of medication designed for introduction into a body orifice. At body temperature, the substance dissolves and is

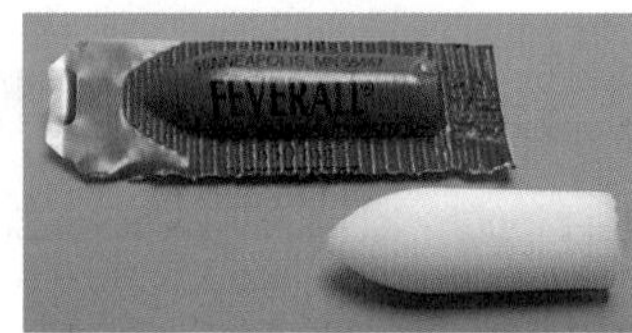

FIGURE **9-20** Rectal suppositories.

absorbed by the mucous membranes. Suppositories should be stored in a cool place to prevent softening. If a suppository becomes soft and the package has not yet been opened, hold the foil-wrapped suppository under cold running water, or place in ice water for a short time until it hardens. Rectal suppositories should generally not be used for patients who have had recent prostatic or rectal surgery, or recent rectal trauma.

Perform premedication assessment.

Equipment

Finger cot or disposable glove
Water-soluble lubricant
Prescribed suppository

Technique

1. Wash your hands and assemble the necessary equipment and the prescribed rectal suppository.
2. COMPARE the label on the container against the medication card or drug profile.
   RIGHT PATIENT
   RIGHT DRUG
   RIGHT ROUTE OF ADMINISTRATION
   RIGHT DOSE
   RIGHT TIME OF ADMINISTRATION
3. Proceed to the patient's bedside.
4. Check the patient's identification bracelet and verify against the medication card or drug profile. Have the patient state his or her name and birth date, or two other identifiers.
5. Explain carefully to the patient what you are going to do.
6. Check pertinent patient monitoring parameters (e.g., time of last defecation, severity of nausea or vomiting, respiratory rate) as appropriate to the medication to be administered.
7. Whenever possible, have the patient defecate before administering the suppository.
8. Provide for patient privacy; position and drape the patient to avoid unnecessary exposure (Figure 9-21, *A*). Generally, the patient is placed on the left side (Sims' position).
9. Put on a disposable glove or finger cot (index finger for an adult; fourth finger for infants).
10. Ask the patient to bend the uppermost leg toward the waist.
11. Unwrap the suppository and apply a small amount of water-soluble lubricant to the tip. (If lubricant is not available, use plain water to moisten; DO NOT use petroleum jelly or mineral oil as it may reduce absorption of the medicine) (Figure 9-21, *B* and *C*).
12. Place the tip of the suppository at the rectal entrance; ask the patient to take a deep breath and exhale through the mouth (many patients will have an involuntary rectal gripping when the suppository is pressed against the rectum). Gently insert the suppository about an inch beyond the orifice past the internal sphincter (Figure 9-21, *D*).
13. Ask the patient to remain lying on the side for 15 to 20 minutes to allow melting and absorption of the medication.
14. In children, it is necessary to gently but firmly compress the buttocks and hold in place for the same period to prevent expulsion.
15. Discard used materials and wash your hands thoroughly.

Documentation

Provide the RIGHT DOCUMENTATION of medication administration and responses to drug therapy.

1. Chart the date, time, drug name, dosage, and route of administration.
2. Perform and record regular patient assessments for the evaluation of therapeutic effectiveness (e.g., when given as a laxative, chart the color,

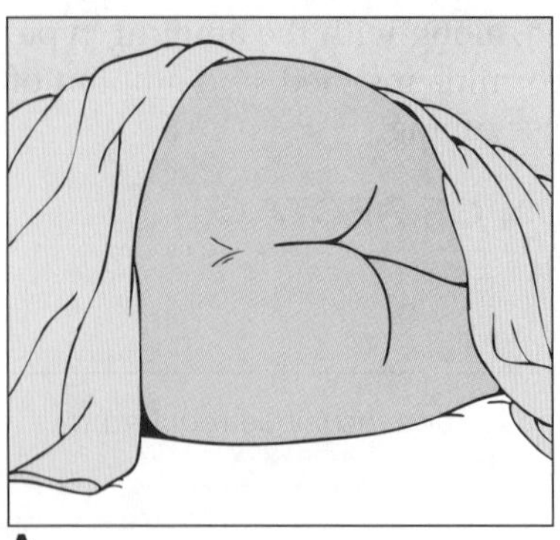
A

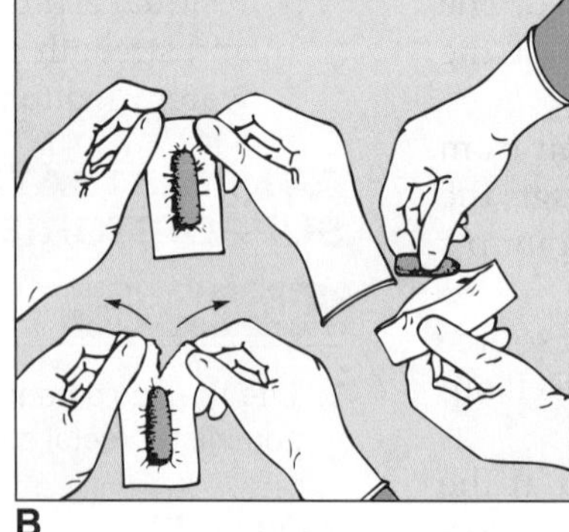
B

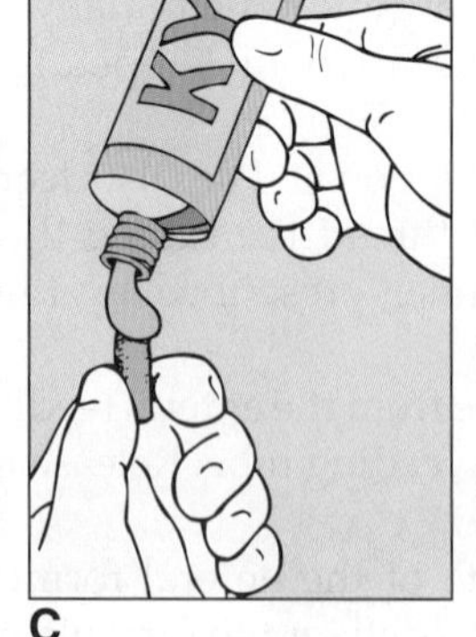

C

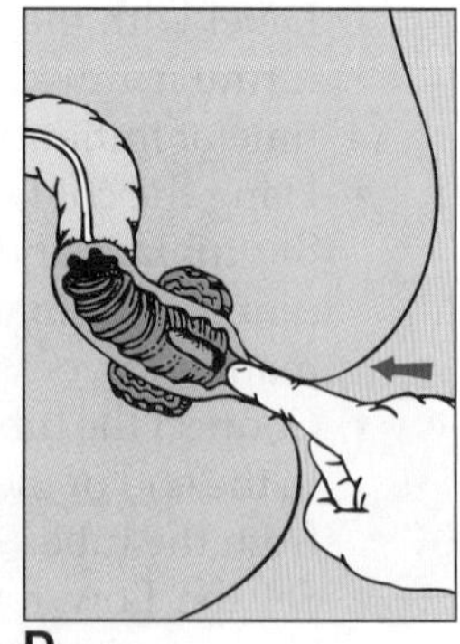
D

FIGURE **9-21** Administering a rectal suppository. **A,** Position patient on side and drape. **B,** Unwrap suppository and remove from package. **C,** Apply water-soluble lubricant. **D,** Gently insert suppository about 1 inch past the internal sphincter.

amount, and consistency of stool; if given for pain relief, chart the degree and duration of pain relief; if given as an antiemetic, the degree and duration of relief of nausea and vomiting).
3. Chart and report any signs and symptoms of adverse drug effects.
4. Perform and validate essential patient education about the drug therapy and other essential aspects of intervention for the disease process affecting the individual.

ADMINISTRATION OF A DISPOSABLE ENEMA

Objective

1. Cite the equipment needed and technique used to administer a disposable enema.

Dose Form

A prepackaged, disposable enema solution of the type prescribed by the health care provider.

Perform premedication assessment.

Equipment

Toilet tissue
Bedpan, if patient is not ambulatory
Water-soluble lubricant
Gloves
Prescribed disposable enema kit

Technique

1. Wash your hands and assemble the necessary equipment and prescribed rectal enema.
2. COMPARE the label on the container against the medication card or drug profile.
   RIGHT PATIENT
   RIGHT DRUG
   RIGHT ROUTE OF ADMINISTRATION
   RIGHT DOSE
   RIGHT TIME OF ADMINISTRATION
3. Proceed to the patient's bedside.
4. Check the patient's identification bracelet and verify against the medication card or drug profile. Have the patient state his or her name and birth date, or two other identifiers.
5. Explain carefully to the patient what you are going to do.
6. Check pertinent patient monitoring parameters (time of last defecation).
7. Provide for patient privacy; position the patient on the left side, and drape to avoid unnecessary exposure (Figure 9-22, *A*).
8. Put on gloves, remove protective covering from the rectal tube, and lubricate (Figure 9-22, *B*).

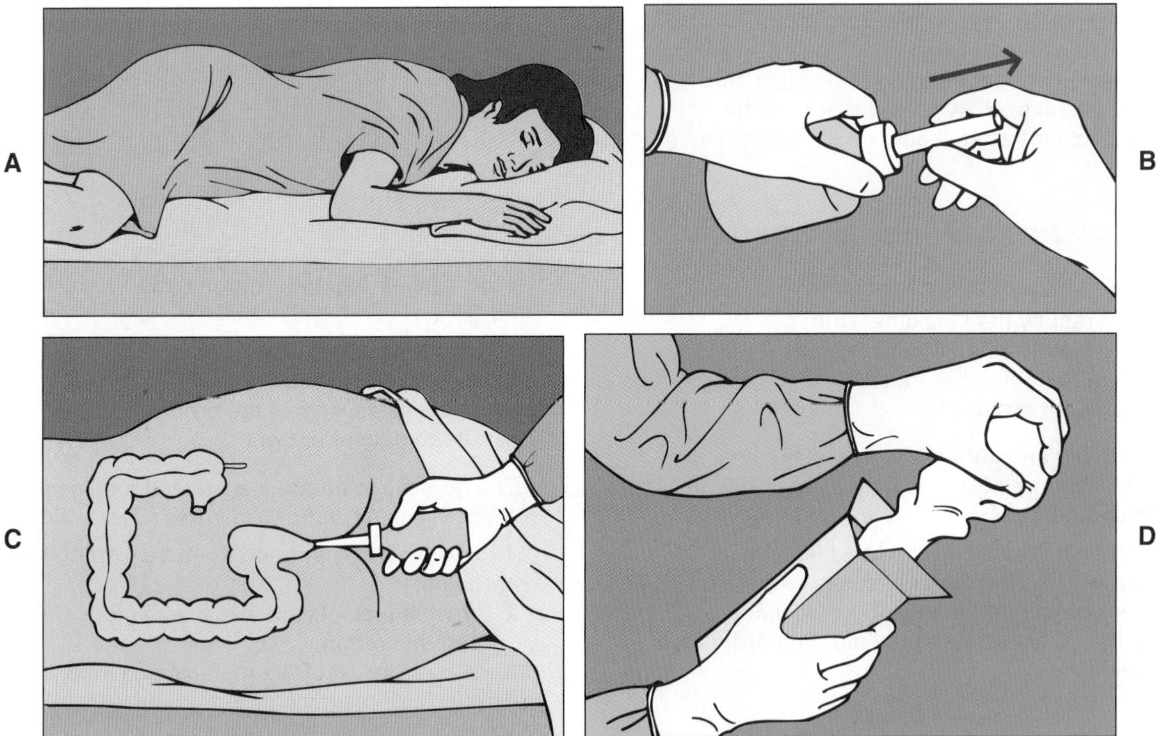

FIGURE **9-22** Administering a disposable enema (Fleet enema). **A,** Place patient in a left lateral position, unless knee-chest position has been specified. **B,** Remove protective covering from rectal tube, and lubricate tube. **C,** Insert lubricated rectal tube into rectum and dispense solution by compressing plastic container. **D,** Replace used container in original wrapping for disposal.

9. Insert the lubricated rectal tube into the rectum and insert the solution by compressing the plastic container (Figure 9- 22, *C*).
10. Replace the used container in its original package for disposal (Figure 9-22, *D*).
11. Encourage the patient to hold the solution for about 30 minutes before defecating.
12. Assist the patient to a sitting position on the bedpan or to the bathroom, as orders permit.
13. Tell the patient NOT to flush the toilet until you return and can see the results of the enema. Instruct the patient regarding the location of the call light in case assistance is needed.
14. Wash your hands thoroughly.

Documentation

Provide the RIGHT DOCUMENTATION of medication administration and responses to drug therapy.

1. Chart the date, time, drug name, dosage, and route of administration.
2. Perform and record regular patient assessments for the evaluation of the therapeutic effectiveness (e.g., color, amount, and consistency of stool).
3. Chart and report any signs and symptoms of adverse drug effects.
4. Perform and validate essential patient education about the drug therapy and other essential aspects of intervention for the disease process affecting the individual.

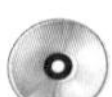

Go to your Companion CD-ROM for Appendices, an Audio Glossary, animations, Drug Dosage Calculators, customizable Patient Self-Assessment forms, and Review Questions for the NCLEX® Examination.

evolve Be sure to visit the companion Evolve site at http://evolve.elsevier.com/Clayton for WebLinks and additional online resources.

MEDICATION SAFETY REVIEW

CRITICAL THINKING QUESTIONS

1. Discuss problems that may be encountered when administering oral medications. What are some possible solutions?
2. Explain why many medications should not or cannot be given via the oral administration route.
3. Clinical problem: A new nasogastric tube has been placed in a patient. The pH of the gastric aspirate was checked and found to be 6. Where is the aspirated fluid from, what is the basis of the conclusion, and what should be done about it?
4. When and why should residual volumes be checked when patients are receiving enteral feedings?
5. Explain the rationale for checking blood glucose every 6 hours during initiation of tube feedings.
6. Describe the different forms of oral medications available and the procedural guidelines for administering each kind.

CONTENT REVIEW QUESTIONS

1. Medications given orally are absorbed:
   1. more rapidly than via other routes.
   2. more rapidly when food is present.
   3. slower than by other routes.
   4. rapidly but erratically.
2. When giving an intermittent enteral feeding, the residual aspirate obtained in an adult is 150 mL. The nurse should:
   1. administer the next scheduled feeding.
   2. stop feeding for 30 minutes and recheck residual.
   3. check procedural manual for guidelines.
   4. notify the health care provider if no orders are specified.
3. When giving oral medications, the nurse should FIRST:
   1. give the patient water to drink.
   2. identify the patient.
   3. check all aspects of the order.
   4. sit the patient upright.
4. The nurse is to administer several medications to the client via an NG tube. The nurse's first action is to:
   1. add the medication to the tube feeding being given.
   2. crush all tablets and capsules before administration.
   3. administer all of the medications mixed together.
   4. check for placement of the tube.

CHAPTER

10 Parenteral Administration: Safe Preparation of Parenteral Medications

evolve http://evolve.elsevier.com/Clayton

Chapter Content

The term *parenteral* means administration by any route other than the enteral, or gastrointestinal, tract. As ordinarily used, *parenteral route* refers to intradermal, subcutaneous (subcut), intramuscular (IM), or intravenous (IV) injections.

When drugs are given parenterally rather than orally, (1) the onset of drug action is generally more rapid but of shorter duration, (2) the dose is often smaller because drug potency tends not to be immediately altered by the stomach or liver, and (3) the cost of drug therapy is often greater. Drugs are administered by injection when all of the drug must be absorbed as rapidly and completely as possible or at a steady, controlled rate, or when a patient is unable to take a medication orally because of nausea and vomiting.

SAFE PREPARATION, ADMINISTRATION, AND DISPOSAL OF PARENTERAL MEDICATIONS AND SUPPLIES

Drug preparation and administration errors have been identified as contributing factors to the high incidence of adverse drug events (ADEs) discussed in Chapter 7. The actual rate of errors occurring during the preparation and administration of medicines is not known, but the potential is high. Thus the nurse must be diligent to prevent errors from occurring.

The role of the nurse in providing accurate drug administration necessitates attention to details in all facets of pharmacotherapy. It is essential that nurses preparing and administering medications focus on (1) the basic knowledge needed regarding the individual drugs being ordered, prepared, and administered; (2) symptoms for which the medication is prescribed, and collection of baseline data to be used for evaluation of the therapeutic outcomes desired for the prescribed medicine; and (3) the nursing assessments needed to detect, prevent, or ameliorate adverse events. Finally, the nurse must exercise clinical judgment about the scheduling of new drug orders, missed dosages, modified drug orders or substitution of therapeutically equivalent medicines by the pharmacy, or changes in the patient's condition that require consultation with the physician, health care provider, or pharmacist.

Injection of drugs requires skill and special care because of the trauma at the site of needle puncture, possibility of infection, and chance of allergic reaction, in addition to the fact that once it is injected, the drug is irretrievable. Therefore, medications must be prepared and administered carefully and accurately. The aseptic technique is used to avoid infection, and accurate drug dosing, along with the correct rate and site of injection, is followed to avoid injury such as abscess formation, necrosis, skin sloughing, nerve injuries, prolonged pain, or periostitis. Thus parenteral administration of medicines requires specialized knowledge and manual skill to ensure safety and therapeutic effectiveness for patients.

Health care professionals place the safety of their patients first and foremost, but the Occupational Safety and Health Administration (OSHA) reports that more than 5 million workers in the health care industry and related occupations are at risk of occupational exposure to blood-borne pathogens, including such devastating diseases as human immunodeficiency virus, hepatitis B virus, and hepatitis C virus. It is estimated that there are 600,000 to 800,000 needlestick and percutaneous injuries to health care workers annually. Studies indicate that nurses sustain the majority of these injuries and that as many as one third of all "sharps" injuries (i.e., from needles, lancets, scalpels) are related to the disposal process. The Centers for Disease Control and Prevention (CDC) estimate that 62% to 88% of sharps injuries can be prevented by using safer medical devices. (See pages 151 to 154 for further discussion of safety for health care professionals in the development of needleless access devices and proper disposal of sharps.)

Consequently, nurses have three primary safety concerns: that of the patient, themselves, and other health care workers. Paramount to the safe administration of medicines is the need for nurses to follow established policies and procedures while checking orders; transcribing orders; preparing, administering, recording, and monitoring therapeutic responses to drug therapy; and disposing of parenteral supplies and equipment.

EQUIPMENT USED IN PARENTERAL ADMINISTRATION

Objectives

1. Name the three parts of a syringe.
2. Read the calibrations of the minim and cubic centimeter or milliliter scale on different types of syringes.
3. Identify the sites where the volume of medication is read on a glass syringe and a plastic syringe.
4. Give examples of volumes of medications that can be measured in a tuberculin syringe rather than a larger volume syringe.
5. State the advantages and disadvantages of using prefilled syringes.
6. Explain the system of measurement used to define the inside diameter of a syringe.
7. Identify the parts of a needle.
8. Explain how the gauge of a needle is determined.
9. Compare the usual volume of medication that can be administered at one site when giving a medication by intradermal, subcutaneous, or IM routes.
10. State the criteria used for the selection of the correct needle gauge and length.
11. Identify examples of the safety-type syringes and needles.

Key Terms

barrel
plunger
tip
minim scale
milliliter scale
tuberculin syringe
insulin syringe
prefilled syringe
insulin pen
needle gauge
safety devices

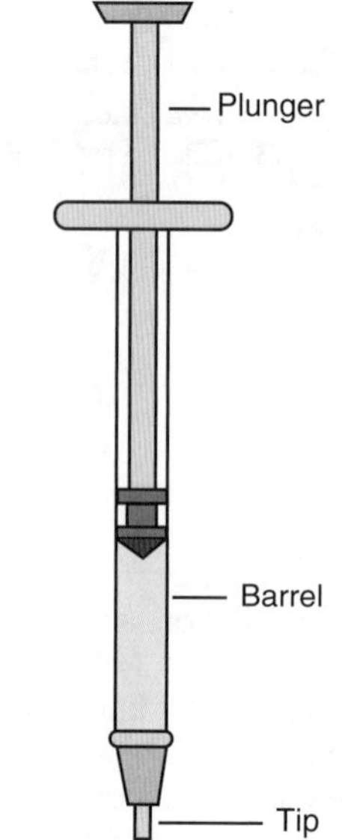

FIGURE **10-1** Parts of a syringe.

Syringes

The syringe has three parts (Figure 10-1). The **barrel** is the outer portion on which the calibrations for the measurement of the drug volume are located (Figure 10-1; Figure 10-2). The **plunger** is the inner cylindrical portion that fits snugly into the barrel. This portion is used to draw up and eject the solution from the syringe. The **tip** is the portion that holds the needle.

All syringes, regardless of the manufacturer, are available with either a luer slip or a luer lock tip. The luer system consists of two parts, the male tapered end (Figure 10-3, *A*), and the reverse tapered female connector with an outer flange (Figure 10-3, *B*).

The two types of syringe tips are the luer slip, a male tapered end (Figure 10-4, *A*), and the luer lock (see Figure 10-4, *B*), a threaded locking collar outside the male luer slip, that will lock the flange of the female connector securely, "locking" it in place.

When the female connector is placed on a male luer slip with a locking collar and given a half twist, it is securely locked in place. However, if a female adapter

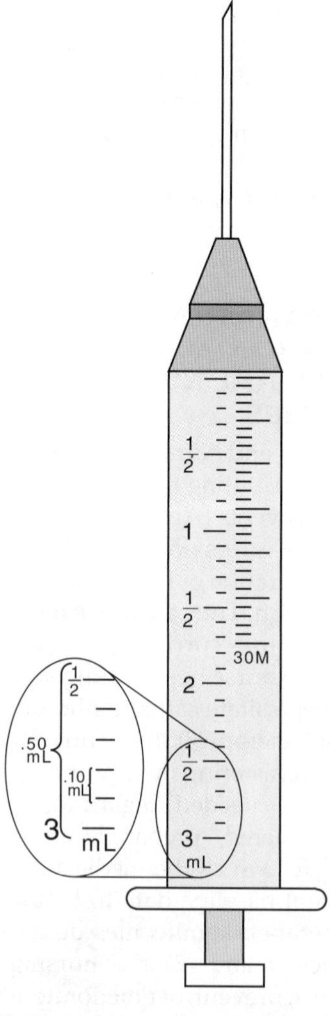

FIGURE **10-2** Reading the calibrations of a 3-mL syringe.

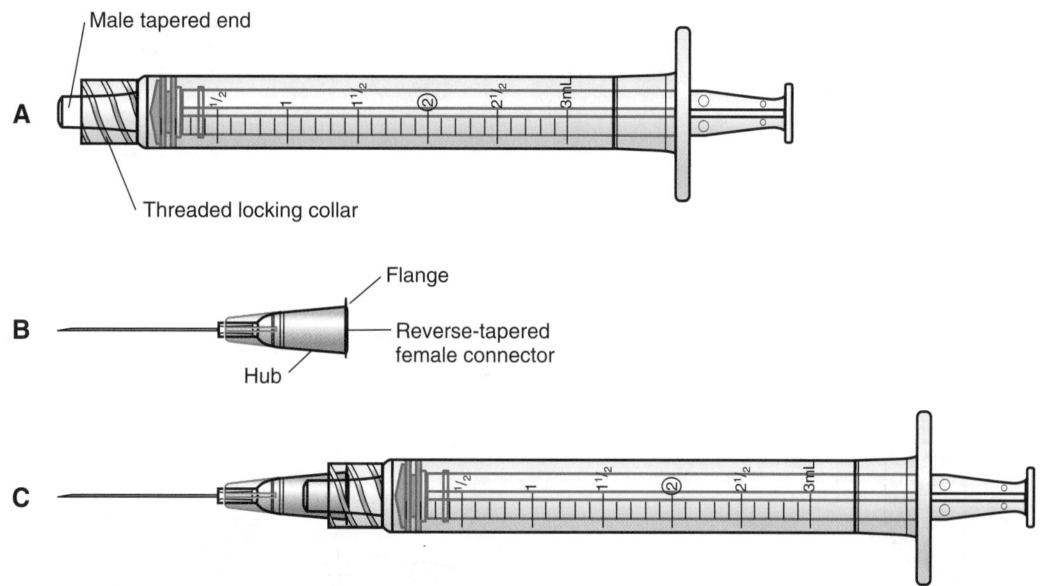

FIGURE **10-3** The Luer system consists of two parts, the male tapered end **(A)** and the reverse female tapered connector with an outer flange **(B)**. **C,** The two components joined together. The hub of the female connector slips over the male tapered end and is twisted so that the flange on the hub locks into the threads of the locking collar.

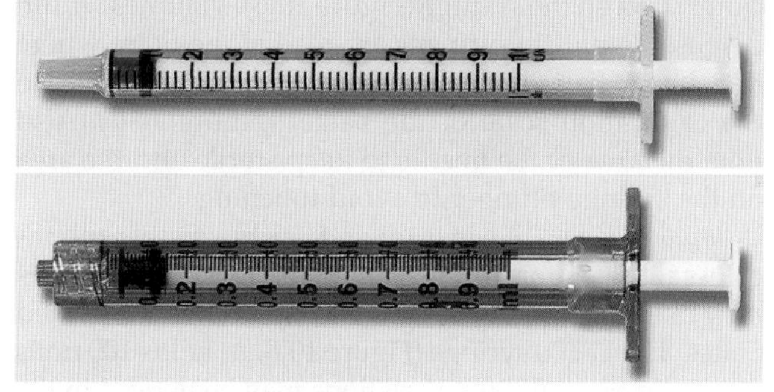

FIGURE **10-4** **A,** Male slip adapter tip (luer slip). **B,** Male slip adapter with outer locking collar (luer lock). (Courtesy of Baxter Healthcare Corp. All rights reserved.)

is placed on a male luer slip, there is no locking collar, so the connection is only relatively secure.

Syringes are made of glass or hard plastic. Each type has advantages and disadvantages.

Glass Syringe

Advantages of the glass syringe include economy, easy-to-read calibrations, and availability in a wide range of sizes. In addition, they can be cleaned, packaged, sterilized, and reused. Disadvantages of the glass syringe are that it is easily breakable; it is time-consuming to clean and sterilize again; and the plunger may become loose with extended use, which causes medication to "creep" between the plunger and the barrel. This results in an inaccurate dose administered to the patient. Glass syringes are seldom used today for routine subcutaneously (subcut) and IM injections.

Plastic Syringe

Advantages of the plastic syringe include availability in a wide range of sizes, prepackaging with and without needles in a wide variety of gauges and needle lengths, disposability, and convenience. Disadvantages of the plastic syringe include expense, one-time use, and, in some instances, unclear calibrations.

Syringe Calibration

The syringe is calibrated in *minims* (♏) and *milliliters* (mL) or *cubic centimeters* (cc) (see Figure 10-2). The most commonly used syringes are 1, 3, and 5 mL, but syringes of 10, 20, and 50 mL are also available.

Note: Technically, *milliliter* is a measure of volume, whereas *cubic centimeter* is a three-dimensional measure of space. Although it is technically inappropriate, many syringes are labeled with *cc* rather than *mL.*

Reading the Calibration of the Syringe

Minim Scale (♏). The use of the minim scale should be discouraged.

Milliliter Scale (mL). The milliliter scale is more accurate and represents the units by which medications are routinely ordered. For volumes of 1 mL or less, use a 1-mL or *tuberculin* syringe for more precise measurement of the drug. Milliliters (or cc) are read on the scale marked mL or cc (see Figures 10-2 and 10-6). The shorter lines represent 0.1 mL. The longer lines on this scale each represent 0.5 mL (1 mL = 1 cc).

Tuberculin Syringe. The tuberculin syringe, or 1-mL syringe, was originally designed to administer tuberculin inoculations (Figure 10-5). Today it is used to

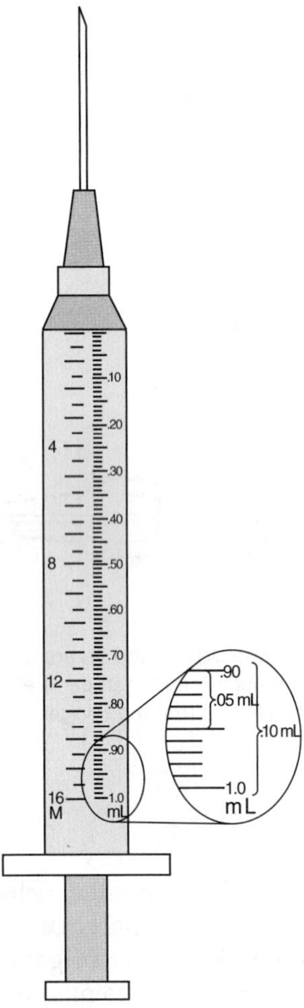

FIGURE **10-5** Tuberculin syringe calibration.

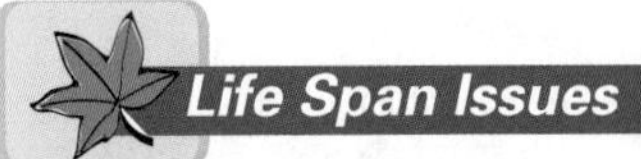

Tuberculin Syringe

The tuberculin syringe, using the metric system of measurement, will provide the most accurate measurement of doses for parenteral medications of 1 mL or less.

The practice of adding 0.2 mL of air bubbles to thoroughly empty all the medication contained in the needle of a syringe can significantly increase a drug dose, especially when small volumes of medicine are being administered to neonates or infants. Check the institutional policy on medication administration for the procedure to be used.

measure small volumes of medication accurately. The volume should be measured on the milliliters scale to achieve the greatest degree of accuracy. The syringe holds a total of 1 cc, or 16 minims. On the minim scale, the longer lines represent 1 minim, whereas the shorter lines measure 0.5 ($^5/_{10}$ or $^1/_2$) minim; however, the use of the minim scale should be discouraged. On the milliliter scale, each of the longest lines represents 0.1 ($^1/_{10}$) mL, the intermediate lines equal 0.05 ($^5/_{100}$) mL, and the shortest lines are 0.01 ($^1/_{100}$) mL.

The volumes within glass syringes are read at the point where the plunger is directly parallel with the

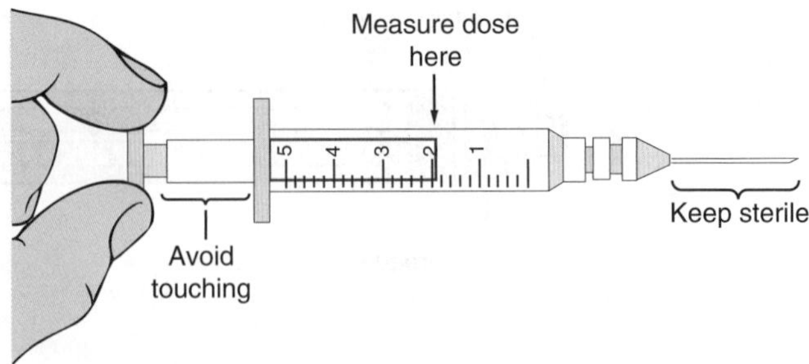

FIGURE **10-6** Reading measured amount of medication in a glass syringe.

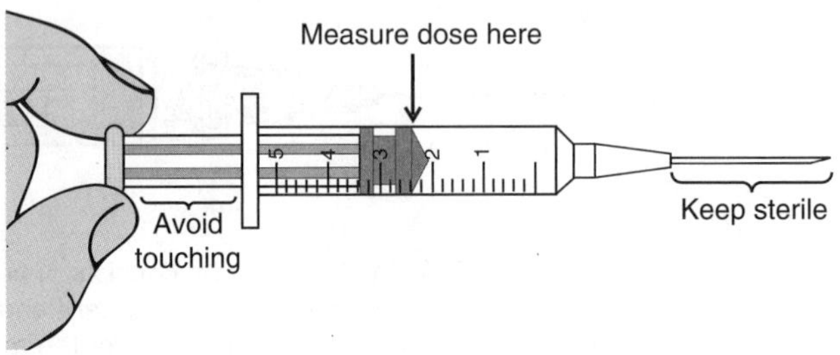

FIGURE **10-7** Reading measured amount of medication in a plastic syringe.

calibration on the syringe (Figure 10-6). Volumes within disposable plastic syringes are read at the point where the rubber flange of the syringe plunger is parallel to the calibration scale of the barrel (Figure 10-7). Also note the area of the needle to keep sterile and the area on the syringe plunger to avoid touching.

Insulin Syringe. The insulin syringe has a scale specifically calibrated for the measurement of insulin. Insulin is now manufactured in U-100 concentration in the United States. The U-100 syringe (Figure 10-8, *A*) holds 100 units of insulin per milliliter. Variations may be noticed in the way units are marked on the scale, but in general, the shorter lines represent 2 units measured, whereas the longer lines measure 10 units of insulin. Low-dose insulin syringes (see Figure 10-8, *B*) may be used for patients receiving 50 units or less of U-100 insulin. The shorter lines on the scale of the low-dose insulin syringe measure 1 unit, whereas the longer lines each represent 5 units. If traveling internationally, be aware that U-40 concentration insulin (40 units of insulin per mL) is commonly available. A specific insulin syringe calibrated for U-40 insulin should be used with the U-40 insulin.

Insulin delivery aids (e.g., nonvisual insulin measurement devices, syringe magnifiers, needle guides, and vial stabilizers) are available for people with visual impairments. Information about these products is available in the American Diabetes Association's annual diabetes resource guide published each January.

Prefilled Syringes

Several manufacturers supply a premeasured amount of medication in a disposable cartridge-needle unit, or prefilled syringe. These units are called by brand

FIGURE **10-8** Calibration of **A,** U-100 insulin syringe, and **B,** low-dose insulin syringe. Low-dose syringes are available in 25-, 30-, and 50-unit sizes to more accurately measure U-100 insulin.

names such as Tubex and Carpuject. The cartridge contains the amount of drug for one standard dose of medication. The drug name, concentration, and volume are clearly printed on the cartridge. Certain brands of prefilled cartridges require a holder that corresponds to the type of cartridge used (Figure 10-9). Advantages of the prefilled syringe include the time saved in preparing a standard amount of medication for one injection and the diminished chance of contamination between patient and hospital personnel (the cartridge is in a sealed unit, which is used once and discarded). Disadvantages include additional expense, the need for different holders for different cartridges, and the limitation of the volume of a second medication that may be added to the cartridge.

Many hospital pharmacies prefill syringes for specific doses of medication for some patients. The syringe is labeled with the drug name, dosage, patient's name, room number, and date of preparation and expiration.

Insulin is also available in a prefilled syringe known as an **insulin pen** (Figure 10-10). When capped, the pens look very much like an ink pen, allowing the person to carry insulin in a discreet manner. When needed, the cap is removed, a needle is attached, air bubbles are removed, the dose is dialed in, the needle is inserted in the subcutaneous tissue, and a "trigger" is pushed to inject the measured dose. When completed, the needle is removed and the cap replaced, again taking on the appearance of a pen. The pens are available in a variety of colors and styles including a prefilled, disposable model; a smaller, low-dose model; and a refillable model in which a new cartridge can be inserted when needed.

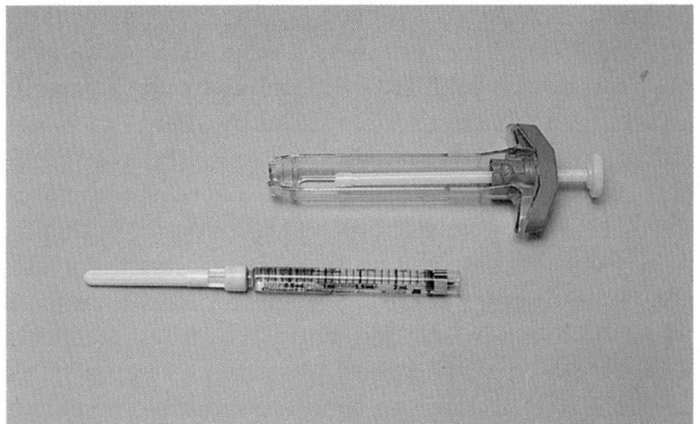

A

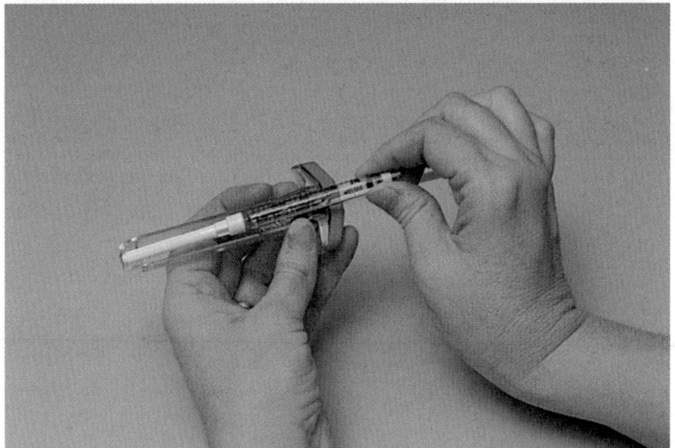

B

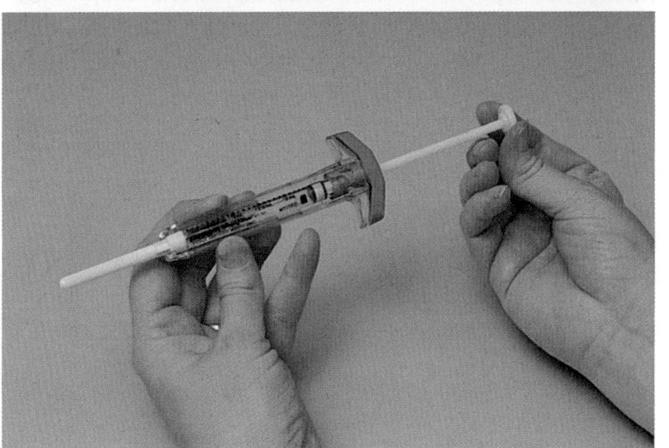

C

FIGURE **10-9** **A,** Carpuject syringe and prefilled sterile cartridge with needle. **B,** Assembling the Carpuject. **C,** Cartridge slides into syringe barrel, turns, and locks at needle end. Plunger then screws into cartridge end.

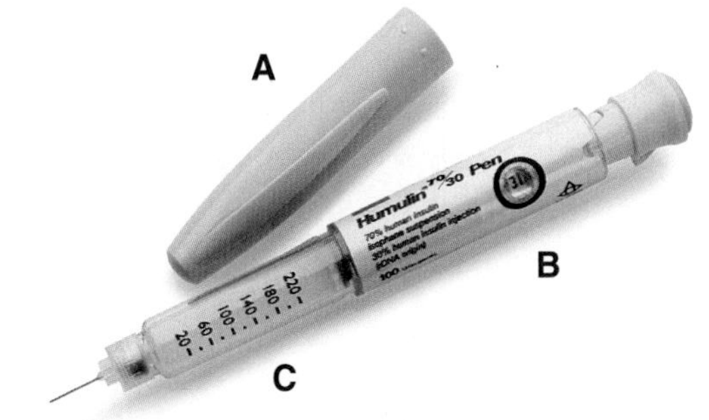

FIGURE **10-10** Elements of the insulin pen. *A,* Pen cap; *B,* measuring device; *C,* prefilled syringe and needle in protective cap.

Another type of prefilled syringe is the EpiPen (Figure 10-11). The syringe is a disposable automatic injection device prefilled with epinephrine for use in an emergency, such as that caused by allergy to insect stings or bites, foods, or drugs. When held perpendicular against the thigh and activated, a needle penetrates the skin into the muscle and a single dose of epinephrine is injected into the muscle. This product is available in adult and pediatric dosages for use at home or when traveling for people who have strong reactions when exposed to allergens. Once the epinephrine is administered, the person should go to the emergency department because additional treatment may be necessary.

The Needle

Parts of the Needle

The needle parts are the hub, shaft, and beveled tip (Figure 10-12). The angle of the bevel can vary; the longer the bevel, the easier the needle penetration.

Needle Gauge

The **needle gauge** is the diameter of the hole through the needle. The larger the gauge number, the smaller the hole. The gauge number is marked on the hub of the needle and on the outside of the disposable package. The proper needle gauge is usually selected based on the viscosity (thickness) of the solution to be injected. A thicker solution requires a larger diameter, so a smaller gauge number is chosen (Figure 10-13). Finer needles (e.g., 27, 29, and 31 gauge) are available for specialty use.

Selection of the Syringe and Needle

The size of the syringe used is determined by the volume of medication to be administered, the degree of accuracy needed in measurement of the dose, and the type of medication to be administered.

Needle selection should be based on the correct gauge for the viscosity of the solution and the correct needle length for delivery of the medication to the correct site (subcut, IM, or IV). Table 10-1 may be used as a guide to select the proper volume of syringe and length and gauge of needle for adult patients.

In small children and older infants, the usual maximum volume for IM injection at one site is 1 mL. In small infants the muscle mass may only be able to tolerate a volume of 0.5 mL using a ½-inch-long needle. For older children, the volume should be individualized; generally, the larger the muscle mass, the greater the similarity to the adult volume for one injection site. Pediatric IM injections routinely use a 25- to 27-gauge needle that is 1 to 1½ inches long, depending on assessment of the depth of the muscle mass in the child. Also available for pediatric use are 31-gauge, ½-inch needles.

Clinical Example: Selection of Needle Length

Assess the depth of the patient's tissue for administration (muscle tissue for IM administration, subcutaneous tissue for subcutaneous [subcut] injection) and choose a needle length to correspond with the findings.

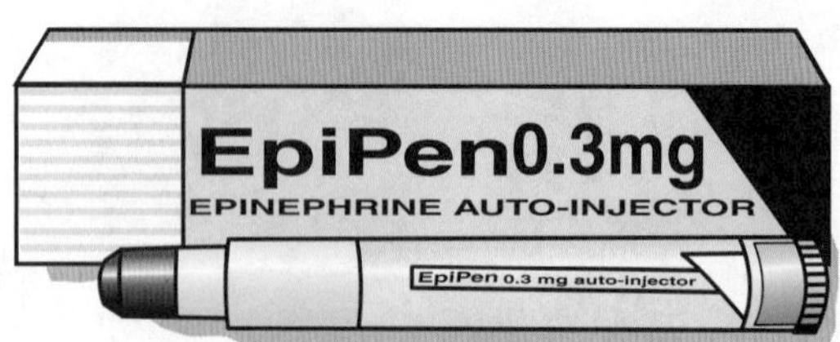

FIGURE **10-11** Prefilled syringe and needle containing epinephrine for use in emergencies.

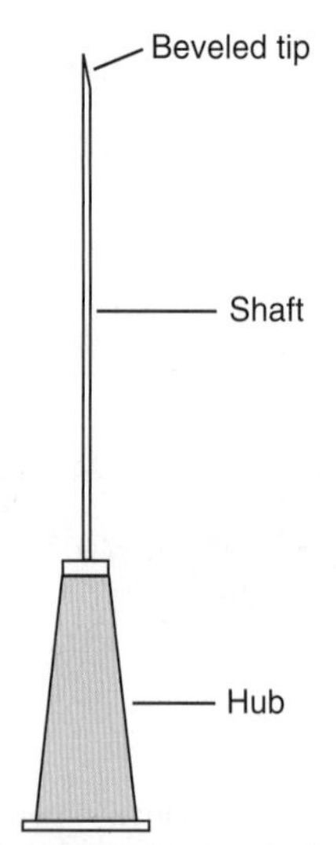

FIGURE **10-12** Parts of a needle.

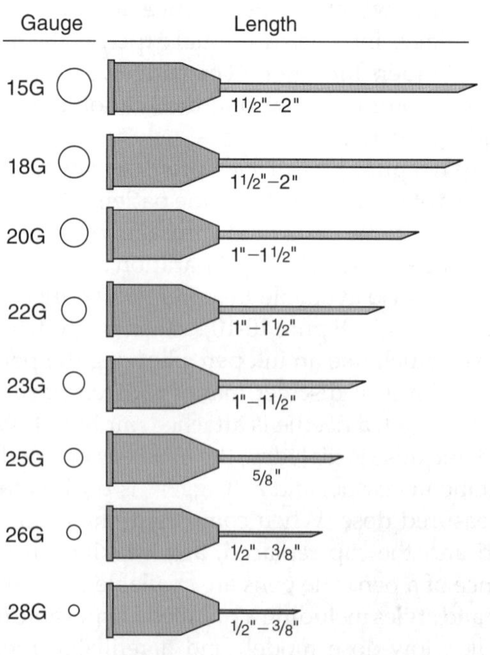

FIGURE **10-13** Needle length and gauge.

Table 10-1 Selection of Syringe and Needle

ROUTE	VOLUME	GAUGE	LENGTH*
Intradermal	0.01-0.1 mL	26-29 g	⅜-½ inch
Subcutaneous	0.5-2 mL	25-27 g	Individualize based on depth of appropriate tissue at site
Intramuscular	0.5-2 mL†	20-22 g	
Intravenous‡	1-2000 mL	20-22 g (solutions) 15-19 g (blood)	½-1¼ inches (butterfly) ½-2 inches (regular needles)

*When judging the needle length, allow an extra ¼ to ½ inch to remain above the skin surface when the injection is administered. In the rare event of a needle breaking, this allows a length of needle to protrude above the skin to grasp for removal.
†Divided doses are generally recommended for volumes that exceed 2 to 3 mL, particularly for medications that are irritating to the tissues.
‡See Chapter 12 for discussion of central access devices and ports.

EXAMPLE:
Compare the muscle depth of a 250-pound obese, sedentary woman with the muscle depth of a 105-pound debilitated adult patient. The obese individual may require a 3- to 5-inch needle, the frail person a 1- to 1½-inch needle. A child may require a 1-inch needle (Figure 10-14).

Packaging of Syringes and Needles

The sterility of the syringe and needle to be used should always be inspected and verified when preparing and administering a parenteral medication. Wrappers should be checked for holes, signs of moisture penetrating the wrapper, and the date of expiration. With prepackaged disposable items, continuity of the wrapper, loose lids or needle guards, and any penetration of the paper or plastic container by the needle should also be checked.

Safety Systems for Parenteral Preparation, Administration, and Disposal

The CDC estimate that 62% to 88% of sharps injuries can potentially be prevented by using medical devices. In response to this important public health concern, Congress passed the Needlestick Safety and Prevention Act in 2000. This act requires that OSHA revise its standards on blood-borne pathogens for closer monitoring and reporting of needlestick injuries, and to mandate development of new safety equipment in the health care industry. One of the major new developments is the broader use of "needleless systems." Needleless systems have been used for several years in the preparation of piggyback solutions such as the ADD-Vantage Needleless Drug Delivery System (see p. 195). But under new OSHA regulations, needleless systems are required for (1) the collection of body fluids or withdrawal of body fluids after initial venous or arterial access is established; (2) the administration of medication or fluids; or (3) any other procedure involving the potential for occupational exposure to blood-borne pathogens as a result of percutaneous injuries from contaminated sharps. Needleless systems provide an alternative to needles for routine procedures, thereby reducing the risk of percutaneous injury involving contaminated sharps. An example of a needleless system is the IV medication delivery system that administers medication or fluids through a catheter port or connector site using a blunt cannula or other nonneedle connection (see Chapter 12). Another new delivery system under development is a jet injection system that delivers subcutaneous injections of liquid medication (e.g., insulin, vaccine) through the skin without use of a needle.

Blunt Access Devices

The blunt access device (spike) is a safety innovation created to reduce the frequency of needle injuries. Note in Figure 10-15 that needleless access devices do not have a stainless steel needle suitable for injection. The spike is used when drawing liquid from a rubber diaphragm-covered vial. Another type of blunt access device, more commonly known as a filter needle, looks similar to other spikes, but contains an internal filter. This device is used to withdraw liquid from an ampule. The filter screens out glass particles that may have fallen into the ampule when the top is broken off. In addition to preventing needlestick injuries, these blunt access devices have the advantage of drawing larger fluid volumes more rapidly from the container. After the spike is used to draw up a medication, it is removed and the appropriate-size needle is attached to the syringe if the medication is intended for injection directly into the patient.

Safety devices have also been developed for syringes and needles. The BD Safety-Lok Syringe (Figure 10-16, *A* to *E*) provides a sleeve that is stored around the syringe barrel while the syringe is being filled through the needle. After administration, the sleeve is pulled forward fully, locking the shield permanently in place, covering the needle. Another type of safety device is the BD SafetyGlide shielding hypodermic needle (Figure 10-17, *A* to *D*). This is a device attached to the needle hub. After the medicine is injected, the health care provider pushes the hinged shield forward, covering the needle. The BD SafetyGlide Syringe Tiny Needle Technology is available for short needles (Figure 10-18, *A* to *D*). The newest technology available, the BD Integra Syringe System, is a spring-loaded syringe that retracts the needle into the syringe after

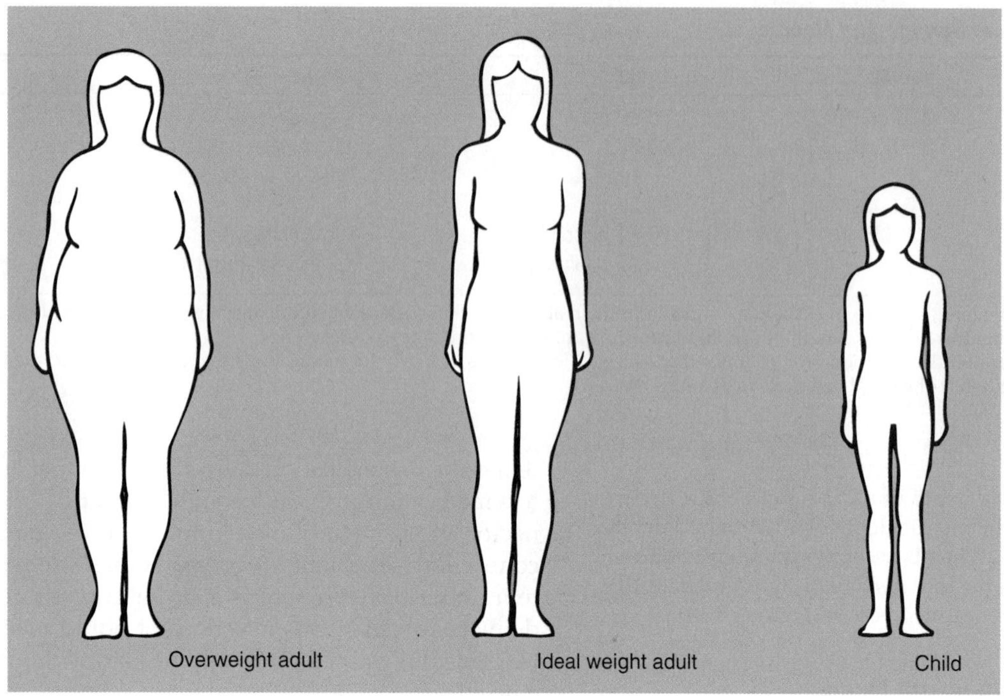

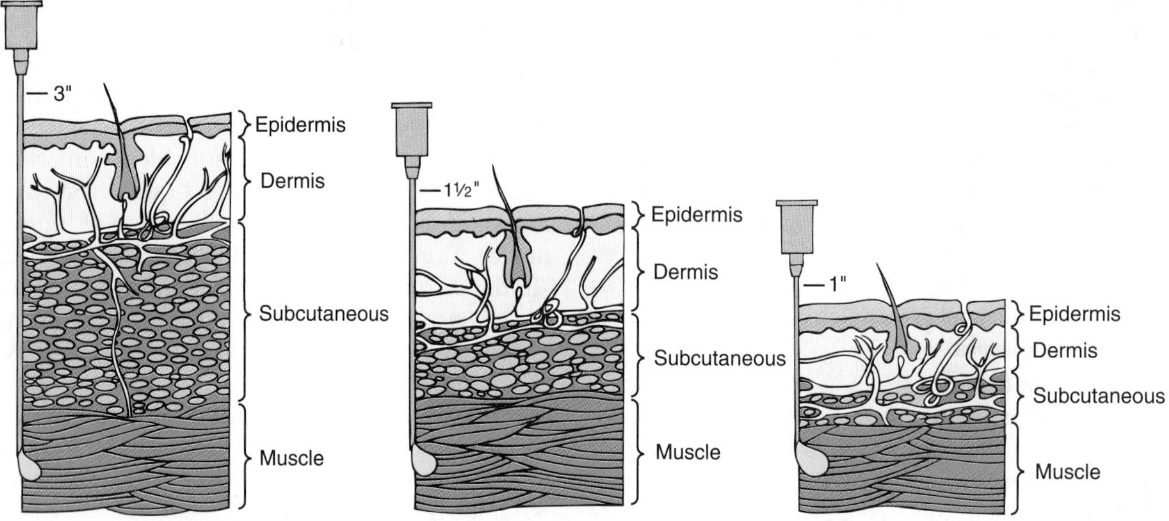

FIGURE **10-14** Clinical example: selection of needle length for intramuscular administration.

injection. The system also uses a new technology called Tru-lock Technology, an apparatus similar to luer-locking technology. It allows changing the needle between aspiration and administration, locks the syringe and needle together securely, and has a very low waste space in the hub. Like all safety-designed syringe/needles, it is necessary to read the accompanying literature for adjustments that need to be made when operating the devices.

Appropriate disposal of used syringes and needles, including those with needle protection devices, is crucial to preventing needle injury and transfer of blood-borne pathogens. To help minimize accidental needlesticks, a needle disposal container is commonly used for all sharps (Figure 10-19). Once full, the sharps container lid stays in place and the entire container is disposed of in a specific manner to comply with OSHA standards. Teach self-injecting patients how to protect themselves and others from accidental stick injury. Recent changes in regulations now encourage patients to purchase "Sharps by Mail Disposal Systems" at their pharmacy for disposal of syringes, needles, and lancets. Previously, individuals were taught to place used needles and syringes into a plastic container, such as a liquid detergent or bleach bottle, to provide protection from accidental sticks. Unfortunately, it has been found that trash compactors can rupture these containers, exposing sanitation workers

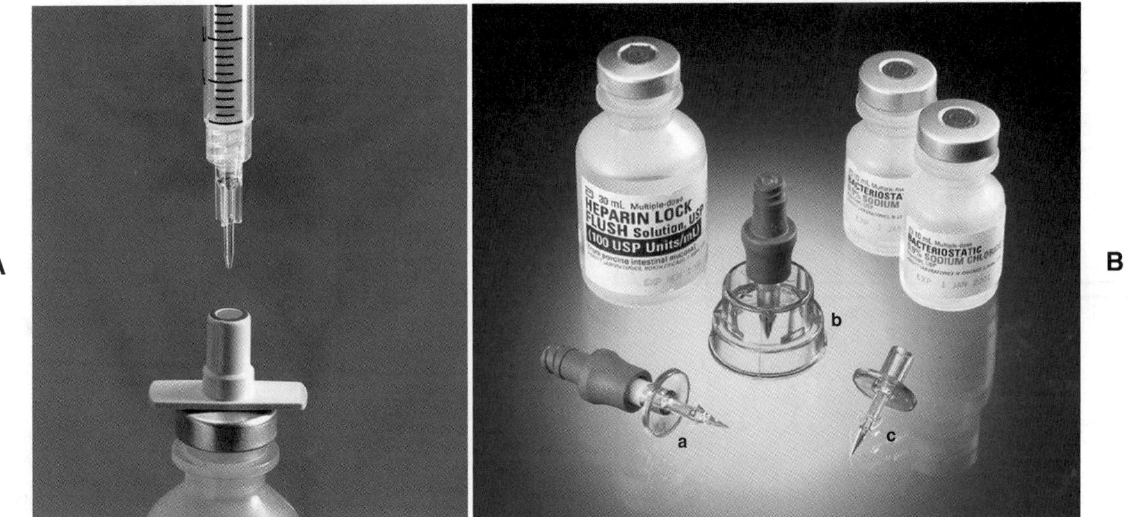

FIGURE **10-15** Needleless access devices. **A,** Interlink Vial Access Cannula entering a universal vial adapter. **B,** CLAVE Access System: *a,* needle-free multidose vial adapter; *b,* snaps onto the top of standard 20-mm medication vials; *c,* single-dose vial adapter. (**A,** Courtesy of Baxter Healthcare Corp. All rights reserved; **B,** courtesy of ICU Medical, Inc.)

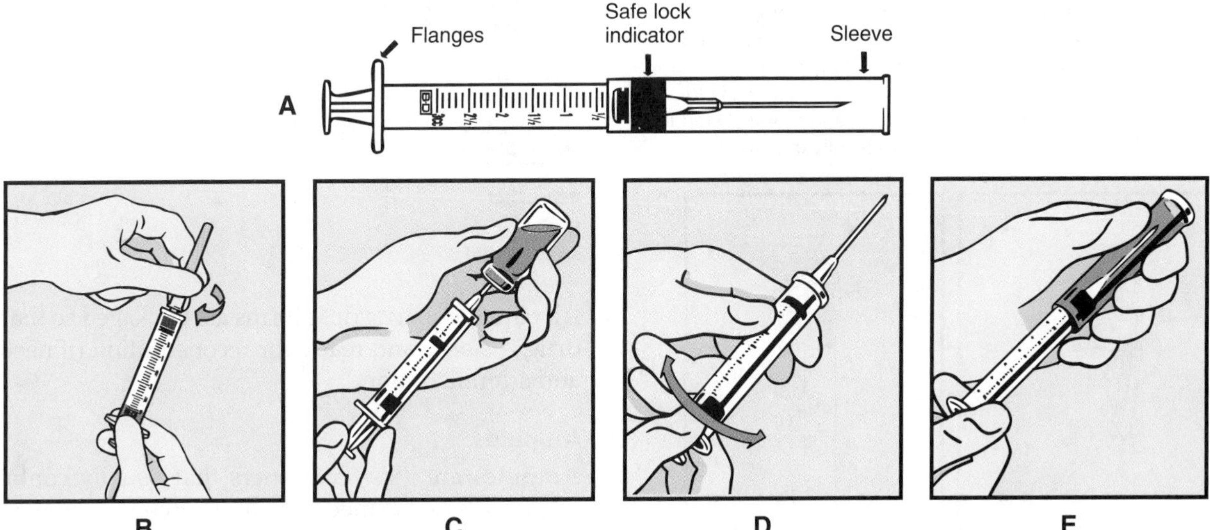

FIGURE **10-16** BD Safety-Lok Syringe. **A,** Syringe showing sleeve covering needle with safe lock indicator. **B,** Assemble by holding needle and syringe by flanges (wings) and twist needle until firmly seated. **C,** During aspiration, press index finger against flanges to prevent sleeve movement. (Note: If necessary to transport filled syringe to point of administration, use a safe, passive, one-handed recapping technique, per OSHA standards, to cover the needle before transport to point of use.) **D,** After injection, grasp sleeve firmly and twist flanges to loosen the sleeve. **E,** Fully retract the needle into sleeve until it locks in the protected position. When Safety-Lok Indicator green band fully covers the red band and an audible click is heard, the sleeve is locked into position.

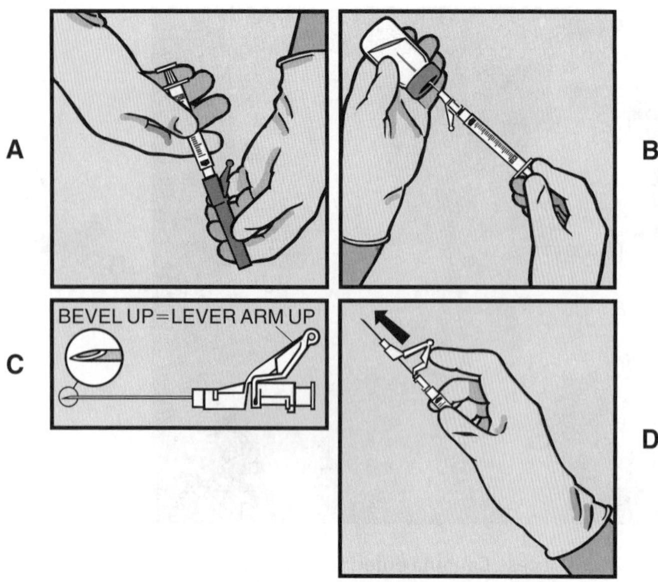

FIGURE **10-17** BD SafetyGlide Shielding Hypodermic Needle. **A,** Attach the BD SafetyGlide Shielding Hypodermic Needle to any standard luer-lock or luer-slip syringe; twist until firmly seated; pull shield straight off needle to avoid damaging needle point. **B,** Aspirate medication into syringe as per your usual technique. (Note: If necessary to transport filled syringe to point of administration, use a safe, passive, one-handed recapping technique, per OSHA standards, to cover the needle before transport to point of use.) **C,** Administer injection following established technique. **D,** After injection, immediately apply a single finger stroke to the activation-assist lever arm to activate the shielding mechanism. (Note: Activate away from self and others, listen for the click, and visually confirm needle tip is fully covered.)

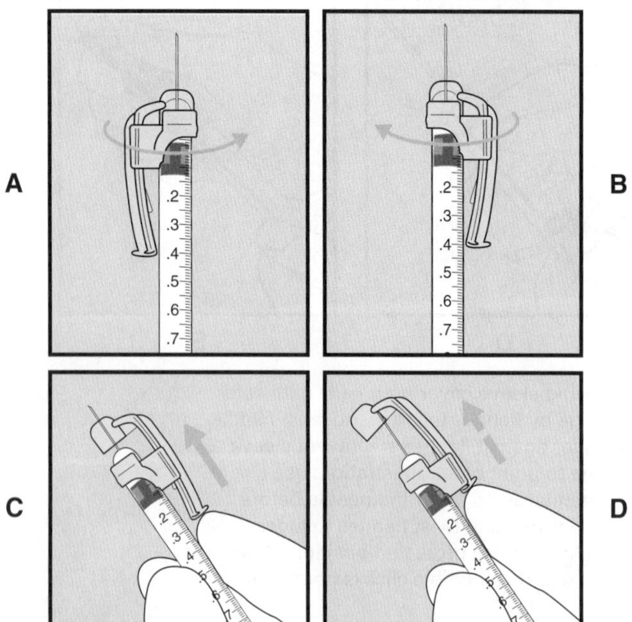

FIGURE **10-18** BD SafetyGlide Syringe Tiny Needle Technology. **A,** Aspirate medication into syringe as per your usual technique. Safety arm can be rotated for scale readability. **B,** Administer injection; to facilitate a low angle of injection, the safety arm can be rotated so it is oriented to the needle bevel. **C,** After injection apply a single finger stroke to activate the safety arm by moving it completely forward. **D,** Safety arm is locked and fully extended when you hear the click and the needle tip is covered.

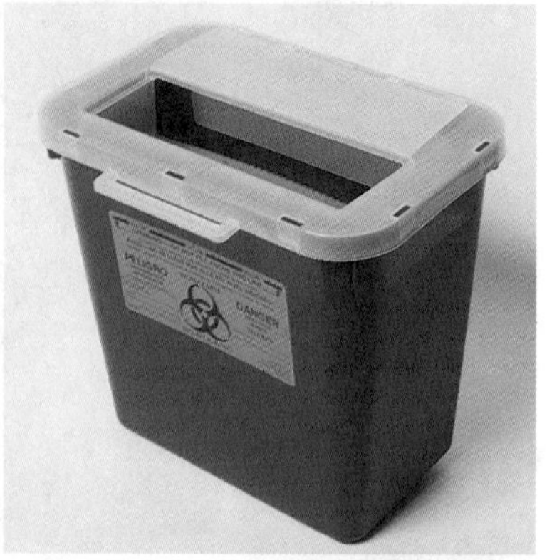

FIGURE **10-19** Needle disposal container.

to the sharp objects. The new mail system provides a sharps container, outer shipping box, and prepaid postage labels so that when the container is filled, it is mailed to an appropriate disposal center. If uncertain of the safest procedure for disposal of used syringes and needles, the individual should contact the local sanitation department.

PARENTERAL DOSE FORMS

Objective

1. Differentiate among ampules, vials, and Mix-O-Vials.

Key Terms

ampules
vials
Mix-O-Vials

All parenteral drug dose forms are packaged so that the drug is sterile and ready for reconstitution (if needed) and administration.

Ampules

Ampules are glass containers that usually contain a single dose of a medication. The container may be scored (Figure 10-20, *A*) or have a darkened ring around the neck (Figure 10-20, *B*). This marking is the location at which the ampule is broken open for withdrawing the medication.

Vials

Vials are glass containers that contain one or more doses of a sterile medication. The mouth of the vial is covered with a thick rubber diaphragm through which a needle is passed to remove the medication (Figure 10-21, *B*). Before use, the rubber diaphragm is sealed by a metal lid to ensure sterility (Figure 10-21, *A*). The medication in the vial may be in solution, or it may be a sterile powder to be reconstituted just before administration. The drug also can be withdrawn from the vial using a spike attached to the syringe (see Figure 10-15).

FIGURE 10-20 **A,** Scored and **B,** ringed ampules.

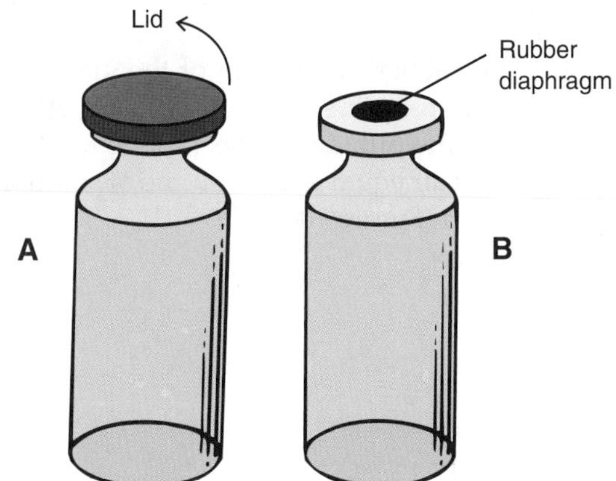

FIGURE 10-21 **A,** Metal lid and **B,** rubber diaphragm vials.

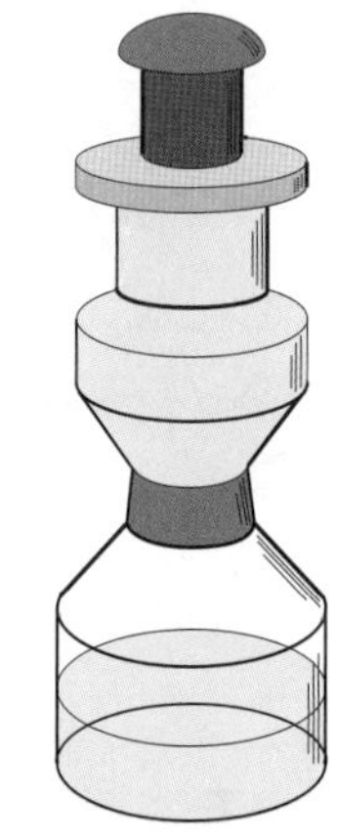

FIGURE 10-22 Mix-O-Vial.

Mix-O-Vials

Mix-O-Vials are glass containers with two compartments (Figure 10-22). The lower chamber contains the drug (solute), and the upper chamber contains a sterile diluent (solvent). Between the two areas is a rubber stopper. A single dose of medication is normally contained in the Mix-O-Vial. At the time of use, pressure is applied on the top rubber diaphragm plunger. This forces the solvent and the rubber stopper to fall into the bottom chamber, dissolving the drug.

PREPARATION OF PARENTERAL MEDICATION

Objectives

1. List the equipment needed for the preparation of parenteral medications.
2. Describe, practice, and perfect the preparation of medications using the various dose forms for parenteral administration.
3. Describe, practice, and perfect the technique of preparing two different drugs in one syringe, such as insulin or preoperative medications.

Perform premedication assessments. See individual drug monograph.

Equipment

Drug in sterile, sealed container
Syringe of the correct volume
Needles of the correct gauge and length
Needleless access device
Antiseptic swab
MAR or medication profile

Technique

The standard procedures for preparing all parenteral medications are as follows:

1. Wash your hands *before* preparing any medication or handling of sterile supplies. During the actual preparation of a parenteral medication, the primary rule is "sterile-to-sterile" and "unsterile-to-unsterile" when handling the syringe and needle.
2. Use the five RIGHTS of medication preparation and administration throughout the procedure:
   RIGHT PATIENT
   RIGHT DRUG
   RIGHT ROUTE OF ADMINISTRATION
   RIGHT DOSE (AMOUNT AND CONCENTRATION)
   RIGHT TIME OF ADMINISTRATION
3. Check the drug dose form ordered against the source you are holding.
4. Check compatibility charts or contact the pharmacist before mixing two medications or adding medication to an IV solution.
5. Check medication calculations. When in doubt about a dose, check it with another qualified nurse. (Most hospital policies require fractional doses of medications and doses of heparin and insulin to be checked by two qualified personnel before administration.)
6. Know the hospital policy regarding limitations on the types of medications to be administered by nursing personnel.
7. Prepare the drug in a clean, well-lighted area, using aseptic technique throughout the entire procedure.

8. Concentrate on this procedure; ensure accuracy in preparation.
9. Check the expiration date on the medication container.

Guidelines for Preparing Medications

Preparing a Medication from an Ampule

1. Move all of the solution to the bottom of the ampule, flicking the side of the glass container with the fingers to displace the medication from the top portion of the ampule (Figure 10-23, *A*).
2. Cover the ampule neck area with a sterile gauze pledget or antiseptic swab while breaking the top off (Figure 10-23, *B*). Discard the swab and top in a sharps container.
3. Using an aspiration (filter) needle (Figure 10-23, *C*), withdraw the medication from the ampule (Figure 10-23, *D* and *E*). Lower the needle as solution is withdrawn from the ampule.
4. Remove the aspiration needle from the ampule and point the needle vertically (Figure 10-23, *F*). Pull back on the plunger (this allows air to enter the syringe) (Figure 10-23, *G*) and replace the filter needle with a new sterile needle (Figure 10-23, *H* and *I*) of the appropriate gauge and length for administration.
5. Push the plunger slowly until the medication appears at the tip of the needle (Figure 10-23, *J*) or measure the amount of air to be included to allow total clearance of the medication from the needle when injected. (Never add air to a syringe that is to be used to administer an IV medication.)

Drugs in a *vial* may be in solution ready for administration or powdered form for reconstitution before administration.

Preparing a Medication from a Vial

Reconstitution of a Sterile Powder

1. Read the accompanying literature from the manufacturer and follow specific instructions for reconstituting the drug ordered. Add only the diluent specified by the manufacturer.
2. Cleanse the rubber diaphragm of the vial of diluent with an antiseptic swab (Figure 10-24, *A*).
3. Pull back on the plunger of the syringe to fill with an amount of air equal to the volume of solution to be withdrawn (Figure 10-24, *B*).

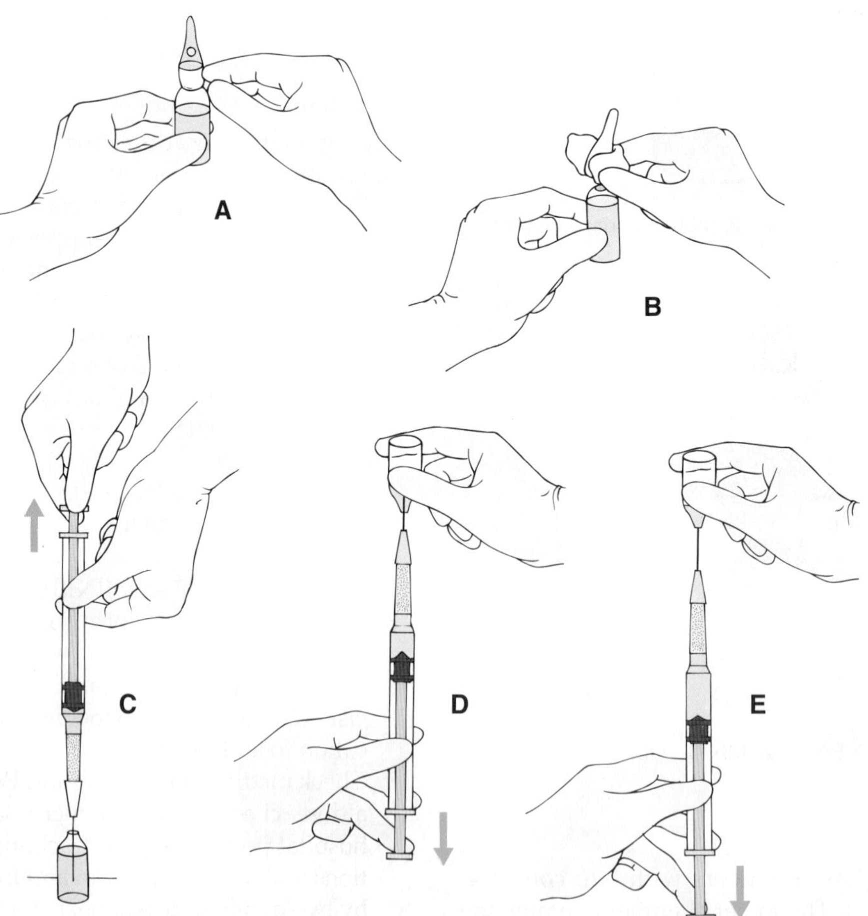

FIGURE **10-23** Withdrawing from an ampule and changing needle. **A,** Displace medication from top portion of ampule. **B,** Cover ampule neck area with gauze sponge while breaking top off. **C,** Filter needle. **D,** Withdraw medication from ampule. **E,** Note that needle must be lowered to withdraw all solution from ampule.

4. Insert the needle or needleless access device through the rubber diaphragm; inject air (Figure 10-24, *C*).
5. Withdraw the measured volume of diluent required to reconstitute the powdered drug (Figure 10-24, *D* and *E*). Remove the needle from the diaphragm of the diluent container.
6. Recheck the type and volume of diluent to be injected against the type and amount required.
7. Tap the vial containing the powdered drug to break up the caked powder (Figure 10-24, *F*). Wipe the rubber diaphragm of the vial of powdered drug with a new antiseptic swab (Figure 10-24, *G*).
8. Insert the needle or needleless access device in the diaphragm and inject the diluent into the powder (Figure 10-24, *H*).
9. Remove the syringe and needle from the rubber diaphragm.
10. MIX THOROUGHLY to ensure that the powder is entirely dissolved BEFORE withdrawing the dose (Figure 10-24, *I*).
11. Label the reconstituted medication including date and time of reconstitution, volume and type of dilu-

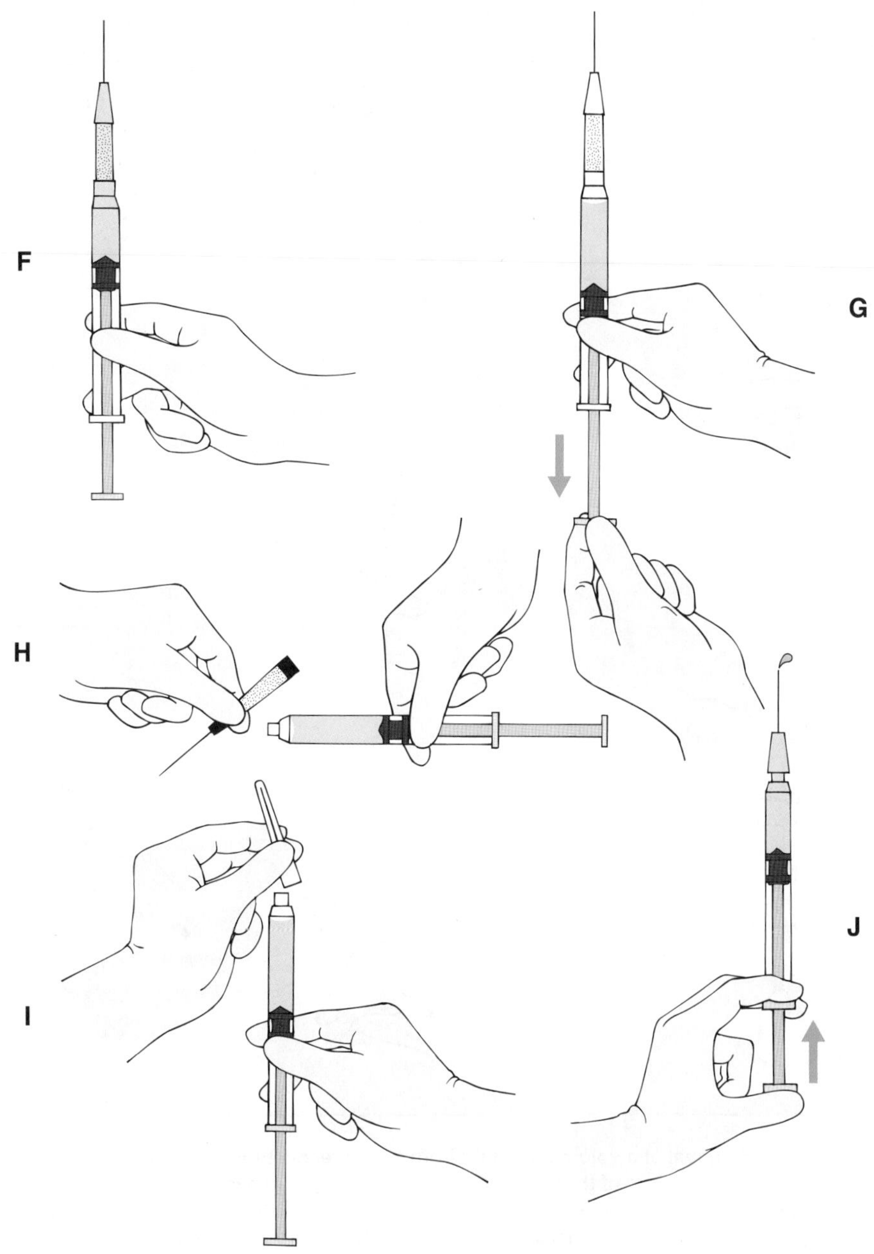

FIGURE **10-23, cont'd** **F,** Remove the filter needle from ampule and point needle vertically. **G,** Pull plunger downward to remove drug from needle. **H,** Remove filter needle. **I,** Replace filter needle with correct size needle for administering medication. **J,** Slowly push plunger until a drop of medication appears at needle tip. Recheck medication prepared against drug order.

ent added, name of reconstituted drug, concentration of reconstituted drug, expiration date and time, and name of person reconstituting drug. Store according to manufacturer's instructions.

12. Change the needle as described earlier (use principles illustrated in Figure 10-23, *H* to *J*) or remove the needleless access device. Attach a needle of the correct gauge and length to administer the medication to the patient.

Removal of a Volume of Liquid from a Vial (Figure 10-24, A to E)

1. Calculate the volume of medication required for the prescribed dose of medication to be administered.

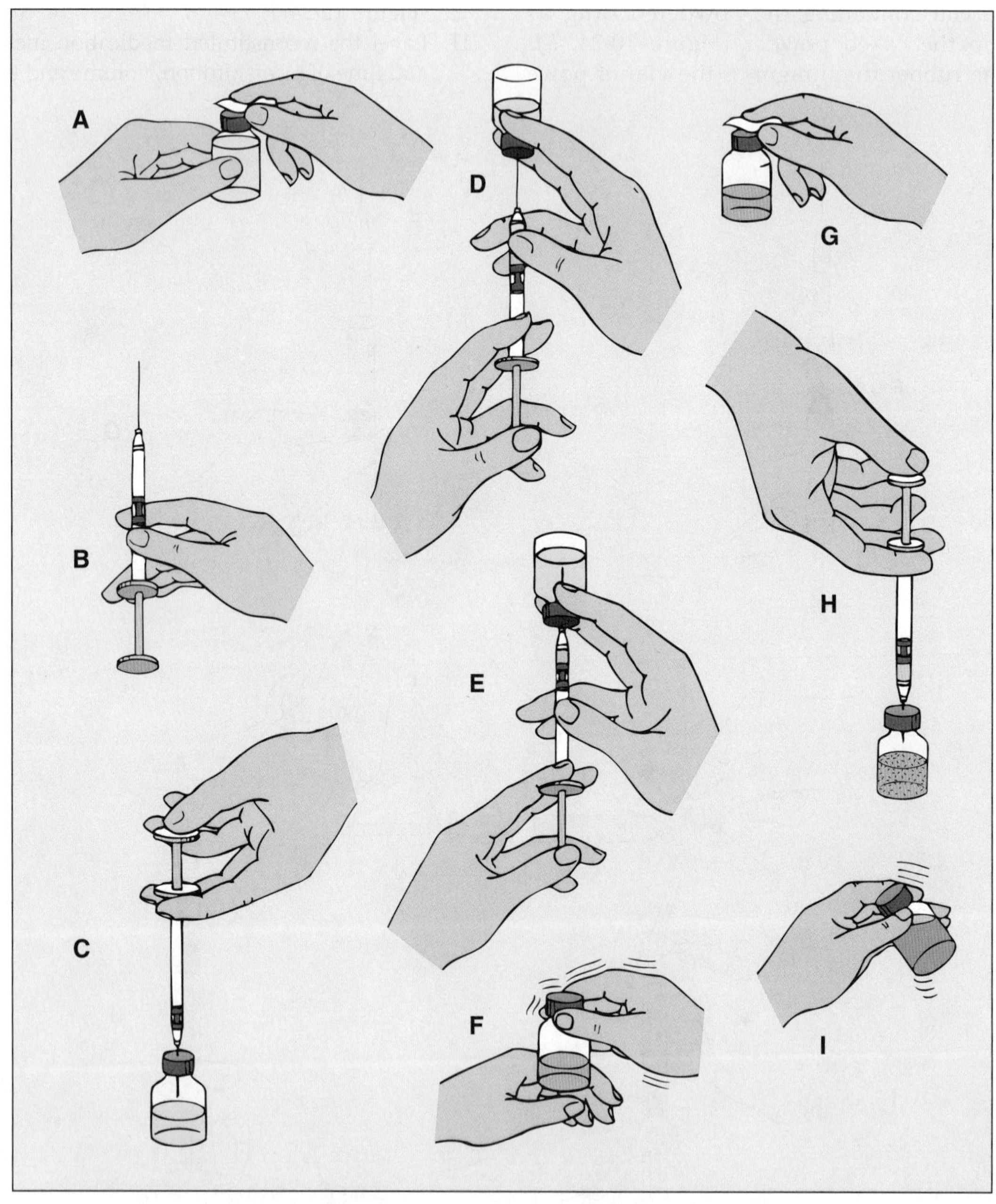

FIGURE **10-24** Removal of a volume of liquid from a vial; reconstitution of a powder. **A,** Cleanse rubber diaphragm of the vial. **B,** Pull back on plunger of syringe to fill with an amount of air equal to the volume of solution to be withdrawn. **C,** Insert the needle through the rubber diaphragm; inject air with vial sitting in downward position. **D,** Withdraw the volume of diluent required to reconstitute the drug. **E,** Move needle downward to facilitate removal of diluent. Change the needle as illustrated in Figure 10-23, *H* to *J*. **F,** Tap the container with the powdered drug to break up the "caked" powder. **G,** Wipe the rubber diaphragm of the vial of powdered drug with a new antiseptic swab. **H,** Insert the needle in the rubber diaphragm and inject the diluent into the powdered drug. **I,** Mix thoroughly to ensure the powdered drug is dissolved before withdrawing the prescribed dose.

2. Cleanse the rubber diaphragm of the vial of diluent with an antiseptic pledget.
3. Pull back on the plunger of the syringe to fill with an amount of air equal to the volume of solution to be withdrawn.
4. Insert the needle or needleless access device through the rubber diaphragm; inject air.
5. Withdraw the volume of drug required to administer the prescribed dose.
6. Recheck all aspects of the drug order.
7. Change the needle or remove the needleless access device and attach the needle, as described earlier (see Figure 10-23, *H* to *J*). Attach a needle of the correct gauge and length to administer the medication to the patient.

Preparing a Drug from a Mix-O-Vial

1. Check the drug order against the medication you have for administration.
2. To mix:
   - Tap the container in the hand a few times to break up the caked powder.
   - Remove the plastic lid protector (Figure 10-25, *A*).
   - Push firmly on the diaphragm-plunger. The downward pressure dislodges the divider between the two chambers (Figure 10-25, *B* and *C*).
   - Mix thoroughly to ensure that the powder is COMPLETELY DISSOLVED before drawing up the medication for administration.
   - Cleanse the rubber diaphragm and remove the drug in the same manner as described for removal of a volume of liquid from a vial (see Figure 10-24, *A* to *E*).

Preparing Two Medications in One Syringe

Occasionally two medications may be drawn into the same syringe for a single injection. This is most commonly done when preparing a preoperative medication or when two types of insulin are ordered to be administered at the same time. Mixing insulin is a routine procedure, so it will be used to illustrate the technique (Figure 10-26).

1. Check the compatibility of the two drugs to be mixed before starting to prepare the medications.
2. Check the labels of the medications against the medication order.
3. Check the following:
   Type: NPH, regular, lente, Humulin, other
   Concentration: U-100 (U-100 = 100 units/mL)
   Expiration date: Do NOT use if outdated
   Appearance: Clear, cloudy, precipitate present?
   Temperature: Should be at room temperature
4. The American Diabetes Association's 2003 guidelines state that "when mixing rapid- or short-acting insulin with intermediate or long-acting insulin, the clear rapid- or short-acting insulin should be drawn into the syringe first." When teaching a patient to mix insulin for self-administration, using a consistent method of preparing the mixture should be stressed so that the patient forms a habit. This can help prevent the patient from inadvertently reversing the dose of short- and long-acting insulin in the mixture.
5. Procedure
   - Check the expiration date on the vial of insulin.
   - To resuspend the insulin, roll the vial or pen between the palms of the hands to thoroughly mix the contents or shake gently.

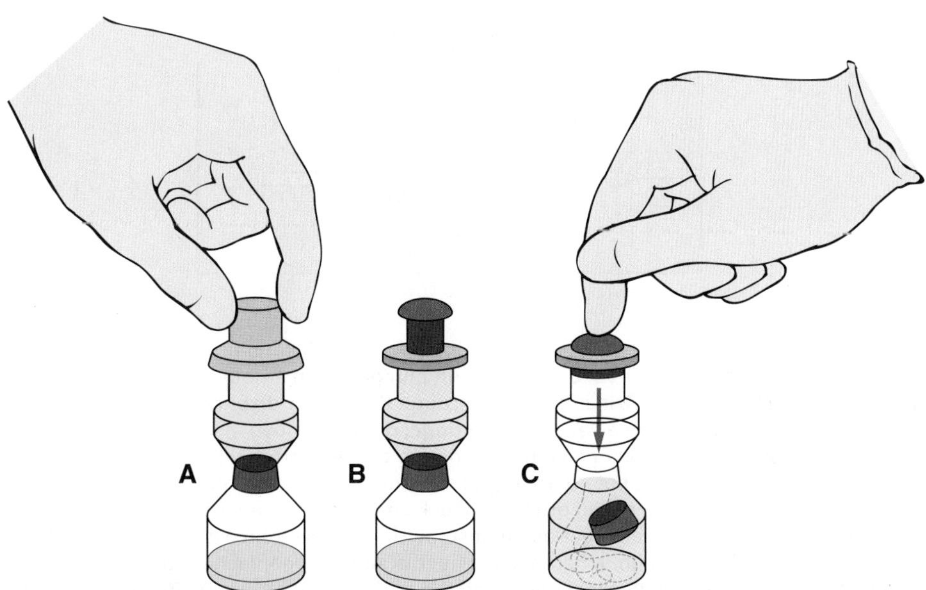

FIGURE **10-25** Mix-O-Vial. **A,** Remove plastic lid protector. **B,** Powdered drug is in lower half; diluent is in upper half. **C,** Push firmly on the diaphragm plunger. Downward pressure dislodges the divider between the two chambers.

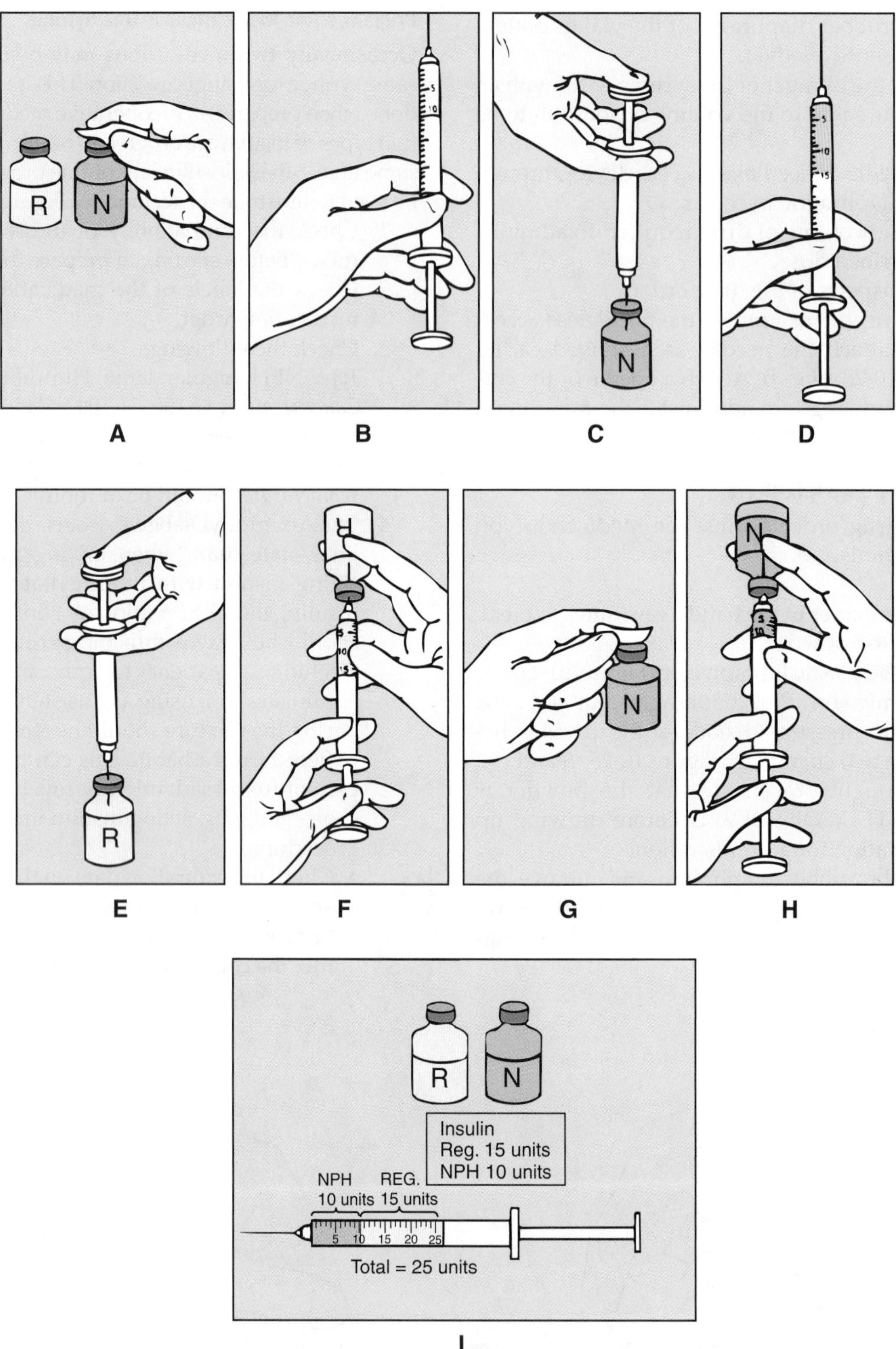

FIGURE **10-26** Preparing two drugs in one syringe. **A,** Check insulin order; cleanse top of both vials with an antiseptic swab. **B,** Pull back on plunger to an amount equal to the volume of longer-acting insulin. **C,** Insert needle through the rubber diaphragm of the longer-acting insulin; inject air. Remove needle and syringe; do not remove insulin. **D,** Pull back the plunger on the syringe to a point equal to the volume of the shorter-acting insulin ordered. **E,** Insert needle through the rubber diaphragm; inject air. **F,** Invert the bottle and withdraw the volume of shorter-acting insulin ordered. Check amount withdrawn against amount ordered. **G,** Rewipe the lid of the longer-acting insulin. **H,** Insert needle; withdraw the specified amount of longer-acting insulin. **I,** Remove the needle and syringe; recheck the drug order against the labels on the insulin containers and the amount in the syringe. Pull plunger back slightly and proceed to mix two insulins (tilt syringe back and forth gently); change needle.

- Check the insulin order and calculations of the preparation with another qualified nurse, in accordance with institution policy.
- Cleanse the top of BOTH vials with separate antiseptic swabs (Figure 10-26, *A*).
- Pull back the plunger on the syringe to an amount equal to the volume of the longer-acting insulin ordered (Figure 10-26, *B*).
- Insert the needle through the rubber seal of the longer-acting insulin bottle; inject air (Figure 10-26, *C*). Do not bubble air through the insulin solution because it may break up insulin particles.
- Remove the needle and syringe. Do not withdraw insulin at this time.
- Pull back the plunger on the syringe to an amount equal to the volume of the shorter-acting insulin ordered (Figure 10-26, *D*).
- Insert the needle through the rubber seal of the second bottle; inject air (Figure 10-26, *E*). Invert the bottle and withdraw the volume of shorter-acting insulin ordered (Figure 10-26, *F*).
- NOTE: Check for bubbles in the insulin in the syringe; flick the side of the syringe with the fingers to displace the bubbles, then recheck the amount in the syringe.
- Check the medication order against the label of the container and the amount in the syringe.
- Wipe the lid of the longer-acting insulin container again (Figure 10-26, *G*); recheck the drug order against this container; insert the needle of the syringe containing the shorter-acting insulin, and withdraw the specified amount of longer-acting insulin (Figure 10-26, *H*). Be careful NOT to inject any of the first type of insulin already in the syringe into the vial.
- Remove the needle and syringe; recheck the drug order against the label on the insulin container and the amount in the syringe (Figure 10-26, *I*).
- Withdraw a small amount of air into the syringe and mix the two medications. Remove air carefully so that part of the medication is not displaced.
- Administer subcutaneously.

Preparing Medications for Use in the Sterile Field during a Surgical Procedure

The following principles apply to drugs used in the operating room:

1. All medications used during an operative procedure must remain sterile.
2. All medication containers (e.g., ampules, vials, piggyback, blood bags) used during the surgical procedure should remain in the operating room until the entire procedure is completed. If a question arises, the container is then available.
3. Do not save an unused portion of medication for use in another surgical procedure. Discard at the end of the surgical procedure or send the patient's medication to the patient care unit with the patient, if appropriate (e.g., antibiotic ointment for a patient having ophthalmic surgery).
4. Adhere to hospital policies concerning handling and storage of medications in the operating room.
5. ALWAYS tell the surgeon the name and dosage or concentration of the medication or solution being handed to him or her.
6. ALWAYS repeat the entire medication order back to the surgeon at the time the request is made to verify all aspects of the order. If in doubt, repeat again until accuracy is certain.

The following technique is used to prepare medications for use in the sterile surgical field:

1. Prepare the drug prescribed according to the directions.
2. Always check the accuracy of the drug order against the medication being prepared at least three times during the preparation phase: (1) when first removed from the drug storage area, (2) immediately before removing the solution for use on the sterile field, (3) immediately after completing the transfer of the medication/solution to the sterile field. ALWAYS tell the surgeon the name and dose or concentration of the medication/solution when passing it to him or her for use.
3. The circulating (nonsterile) nurse retrieves the medication from storage, reconstitutes as needed, and turns the medication container so the scrubbed (sterile) person can read the label. It is best to read the label aloud to ensure that both individuals are verifying the contents against the verbal order from the surgeon.

The following two methods may be used:

Method 1

1. The circulating (nonsterile) nurse cleanses the top of the vial or breaks off the top of the ampule, as described earlier.
2. The scrubbed (sterile) person chooses a syringe of the correct volume for the medication to be withdrawn and attaches a large-bore needle to facilitate removal of the solution from the container.
3. The circulating (nonsterile) nurse holds the ampule or vial in such a way that the scrubbed (sterile) person can easily insert the sterile needle tip into the medication container (Figure 10-27, *A*).
4. The scrubbed person pulls back the plunger on the syringe until all the medication prescribed has been withdrawn from the container and from the needle used to withdraw the medication.
5. The needle is disconnected from the syringe and left in the vial or ampule (see Figure 10-27, *B*).
6. The medication container is again shown to the scrubbed person and read aloud to verify all components of the drug prepared against the medication/solution requested.

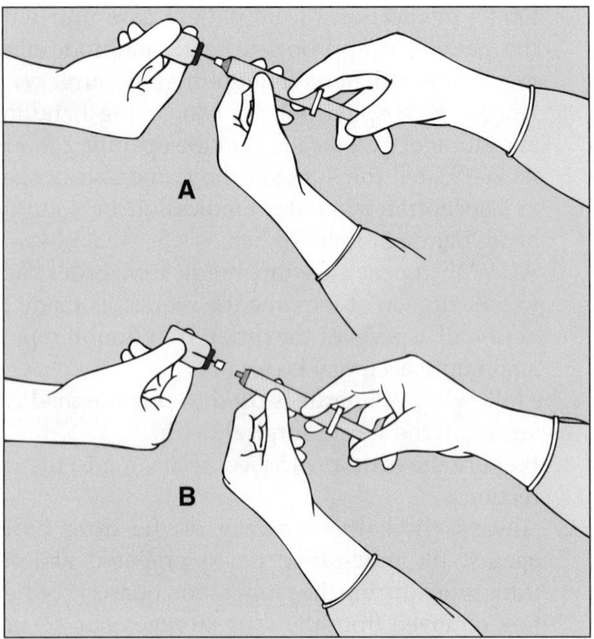

FIGURE **10-27** Preparing a medication in the operating room. **A,** Circulating (unsterile) nurse holds vial to facilitate the scrubbed (sterile) person to insert the sterile needle tip into the medication container. **B,** The needle is disconnected from the syringe and left in the vial.

Method 2

1. The circulating (nonsterile) nurse removes the entire lid of the vial with a bottle opener, cleanses the rim of the vial, and pours the medication directly into a sterile medicine cup held by the scrubbed nurse.
2. The scrubbed person continues drug preparation on the sterile field in accordance with the intended use (such as irrigation or injection).

Regardless of the method used to transfer the medication to the sterile field, both the sterile scrubbed person and the nonsterile circulating nurse should know the location and exact disposition of each medication on the sterile field.

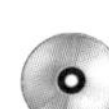

Go to your Companion CD-ROM for Appendices, an Audio Glossary, animations, Drug Dosage Calculators, customizable Patient Self-Assessment forms, and Review Questions for the NCLEX® Examination.

evolve Be sure to visit the companion Evolve site at http://evolve.elsevier.com/Clayton for WebLinks and additional online resources.

MEDICATION SAFETY REVIEW

CRITICAL THINKING QUESTIONS

1. Examine selected syringes such as tuberculin, insulin, and 3-mL syringes, and differentiate among the calibrations on the syringe.
2. Differentiate among procedures used in the preparation of parenteral medications from an ampule, a vial, and a Mix-O-Vial.
3. Discuss the policies on proper disposal of sharps in the clinical setting and in long-term care settings where assigned.

CONTENT REVIEW QUESTIONS

1. Proper disposal of sharps is controlled by:
   1. Joint Commission on Hospital Accreditation.
   2. Occupational Safety and Health Administration.
   3. Intravenous Nurses Society.
   4. American Medical Association.
2. When removing a parenteral medication from an ampule, the nurse must:
   1. inject air equal to the amount of medication to be removed.
   2. use a needleless spike for removing the medication.
   3. use a filter needle to ensure no glass is in the medication.
   4. depress the top rubber diaphragm to displace the stopper.
3. The nurse is teaching the client how to prepare 10 units of regular insulin and 5 units of NPH insulin for injection. The nurse instructs the client to:
   1. inject air into the regular insulin, then into the NPH.
   2. withdraw the regular insulin first.
   3. inject air into and withdraw the NPH immediately.
   4. inject air into both vials and withdraw the regular insulin first.

CHAPTER

11 Parenteral Administration: Intradermal, Subcutaneous, and Intramuscular Routes

evolve http://evolve.elsevier.com/Clayton

Chapter Content

ADMINISTRATION OF MEDICATION BY THE INTRADERMAL ROUTE

Objective

1. Describe the technique used to administer a medication via the intradermal route.

Key Terms

intradermal
erythema
anergic

Intradermal injections are made into the dermal layer of skin just below the epidermis (Figure 11-1). Small volumes, usually 0.1 mL, are injected. The absorption from intradermal sites is slow, making it the route of choice for allergy sensitivity tests, desensitization injections, local anesthetics, and vaccinations.

Perform premedication assessments. See individual drug monograph.

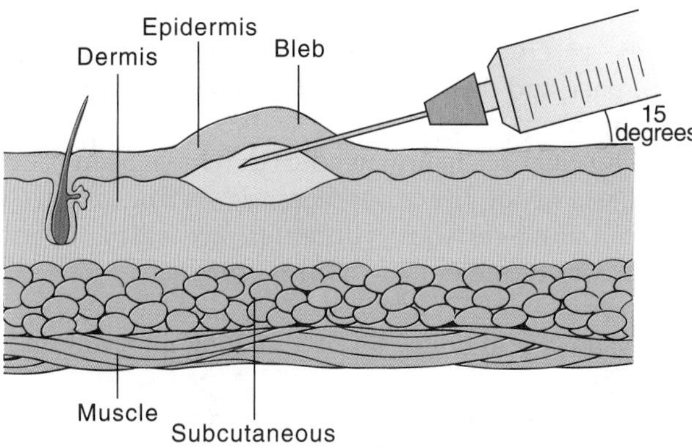

FIGURE **11-1** Intradermal injection technique.

Equipment

Medication to be injected (see medication administration record [MAR])
Tuberculin syringe with 26-gauge, ¼-, ⅜-, or ½-inch needle, *or* a special needle and syringe for allergens
Metric ruler, if skin-testing procedure
Gloves
Antiseptic pledget
Physician's order sheet

Sites

Intradermal injections may be made on any skin surface, but the site should be hairless and receive little friction from clothing. The upper chest, scapular areas of the back, and the inner aspect of the forearms are most commonly used (Figure 11-2, *A* and *B*).

Technique

This example of technique uses allergy sensitivity testing. Caution: Do not start any type of allergy testing unless emergency equipment is available in the immediate area in case of an anaphylactic response. Nurses should be familiar with the procedure to follow if an emergency does arise.

1. Check with the patient before starting the testing to ensure that he or she has not taken any antihistamines or antiinflammatory agents (e.g., aspirin, ibuprofen, corticosteroids) for 24 to 48 hours before the tests or is receiving immunosuppressant therapy. If the patient has taken antihistamines, certain sleep medications (e.g., doxylamine or diphenhydramine), or antiinflammatory agents, check with the health care provider before proceeding with the testing.
2. Cleanse the selected area thoroughly with an antiseptic pledget. Use circular motions starting at the planned site of injection, continuing outward in circular motions to the periphery. Allow the area to air dry.
3. Two methods can be used to administer allergy testing. One method requires the intradermal injection of the allergens; the other is completed by using the skin-prick method.
   Intradermal injection method:
   - Prepare the designated solutions for injection using aseptic technique. Usual volumes to be injected range between 0.01 and 0.05 mL. A pos-

A

1 2 3 4
9 10 11 12
17 18
21 22
5 6 7 8
13 14 15 16
19 20
23 24
25 26
27 28
29 30
31 32
33 34
35 36
37
38
39
40
41
42

B

43 44 45
46 47 48
49 50 51
52 53 54
55
56
57
58
59
60

Reading Chart for Intradermal Testing

Patient Name ______________________________
Identification Number ______________________
Physician Name ____________________________

C

DATE	TIME	AGENT	CONCENTRATION	DOSAGE	SITE NUMBER*	Reading Time in Hours or Minutes, e.g., 30 min or 24, 48, or 72 hr		

*Refer to diagram of sites in Figure 11-2, *A* and *B*.

- Follow directions for the "reading" of the skin testing performed
- Inspect sites in a good light
- Record reaction in upper half of box using the following guidelines, e.g., 2+
  - + (1+) No wheal, 3 mm flare
  - ++ (2+) 2 to 3 mm wheal with flare
  - +++ (3+) 3 to 5 mm wheal with flare
  - ++++ (4+) >5 mm wheal
- Record measurement of induration (process of hardening) in mm in lower half of box, e.g.,

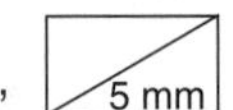

FIGURE **11-2** Intradermal sites. **A,** Posterior view. **B,** Anterior view. **C,** Reading chart for intradermal testing.

itive control solution using histamine and a negative control solution using saline or the diluent of the allergen are also administered. Wear gloves.

- Insert the needle at a 15-degree angle with the needle bevel upward. (NOTE: There is a controversy on whether the needle bevel should be upward or downward. Check the procedure manual for facility policy.) The solution being injected is deposited in the space immediately below the skin; remove the needle quickly. A small *bleb* will appear on the surface of the skin as the solution enters the intradermal area (Figure 11-1). Be careful not to inject into the subcutaneous space and do not wipe the site with alcohol after injection.
- DO NOT recap any needles that have been used. Dispose of used needles and syringes into a puncture-resistant container, according to the policy of the employing institution.

Skin-prick test (SPT) method:

- Make a grid on the test site at 2-cm intervals with a pen.
- Place a drop of each allergen in the grid on the site. A positive control solution using histamine and a negative control solution using saline or

the diluent of the allergen are also administered.
- Using a lancet with a 1-mm point, prick the skin through the allergen drop. Wipe the lancet with dry gauze between each prick to prevent carry-over of the allergen from the previous site.
- Gently blot the excess allergen off the site.
- The SPT can be read in 10 to 20 minutes after administration, depending on protocol.

4. Remove gloves and dispose of them according to agency policy. Thoroughly wash your hands.
5. Chart the times, agents, concentrations, and amounts administered (Figure 11-2, *C*). Make a diagram in the patient's chart, numbering each location. Record what agent and concentration was injected at each site. (Subsequent "readings" of each area are then performed and charted on this record.)
6. Follow directions for the time of the "reading" of the skin testing being performed. Inspection of the injection sites should be performed in good light. Generally, a positive reaction (development of a wheal) to a diluted strength of suspected allergen is considered clinically significant. Measure the diameter in millimeters of wheal and **erythema**, and palpate and measure the size of any induration. No reaction to the allergens, especially the positive control, is known as an **anergic** reaction. *Anergy* is associated with immunodeficiency disorders. Record this information in the patient's chart.

The injection technique can easily be modified for desensitization injections and vaccinations.

Patient Teaching

Tell the patient the time, date, and place to return to have the test sites read, if necessary. Tell the patient not to wash or scrub the area until the injections have been read.

If the patient develops an area of severe burning or itching, he or she should try not to scratch. Tell the patient to report immediately the development of any breathing difficulty, severe hives, or rashes and to go to the nearest emergency department if unable to reach the health care provider who prescribed the skin tests.

Documentation

Provide the RIGHT DOCUMENTATION of the medication administration and responses to drug therapy.

1. Chart the date, time, drug name (agent, concentration, amount), dosage, and site of administration (see Figure 11-2).
2. Perform a reading of each site after the application, as directed by the health care provider or the policy of the health care agency.
3. Chart and report any signs and symptoms of adverse drug effects.
4. Perform and validate essential patient education about the drug therapy and other essential aspects of intervention for the disease process affecting the individual.

The following is a list of commonly used readings of reactions and appropriate symbols:

+ (1+)	No wheal, 3-mm flare
++ (2+)	2- to 3-mm wheal with flare
+++ (3+)	3- to 5-mm wheal with flare
++++ (4+)	>5-mm wheal

Generally, a positive reaction to *delayed hypersensitivity* skin testing (to evaluate in vivo cell-mediated immunity) requires an *induration* of at least 5 mm in diameter.

ADMINISTRATION OF MEDICATION BY THE SUBCUTANEOUS ROUTE

Objective

1. Identify the equipment needed and describe the technique used to administer a medication via the subcutaneous route.

Key Term

subcutaneous

Subcutaneous (subcut) injections are made into the loose connective tissue between the dermis and muscle layer (Figure 11-3). Absorption is slower and drug action is generally longer with subcutaneous injections than with intramuscular (IM) or intravenous (IV) injections. If the circulation is adequate, the drug is completely absorbed from the tissue.

Many drugs cannot be administered by this route because no more than 2 mL can ordinarily be deposited at a subcutaneous site. The drugs must be quite soluble and potent enough to be effective in small volume, without causing significant tissue irritation. Drugs commonly injected into the subcutaneous tissue are heparin and insulin.

Perform premedication assessments. See individual drug monograph.

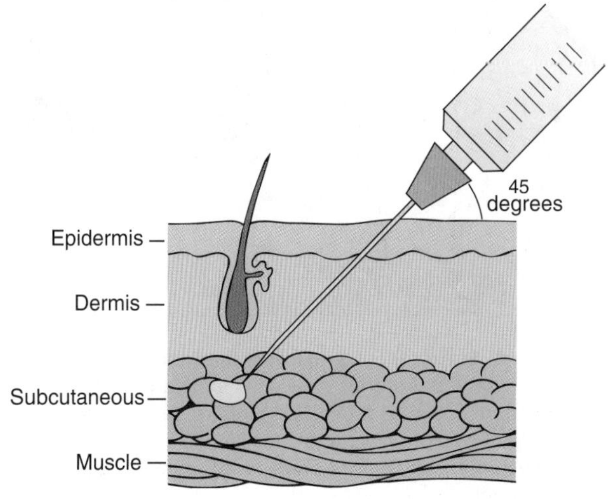

FIGURE 11-3 Subcutaneous injection technique.

Equipment

Medication to be injected (see MAR).

Syringe Size

Choose a syringe that corresponds to the volume of drug to be injected at one site. The usual amount injected subcutaneously at one site is 0.5 to 2 mL. Correlate syringe size with the size of the patient and the tissue mass.

Needle Length

Assess each patient so that the needle length selected will deposit the medication into the subcutaneous tissue, not muscle tissue. Needle lengths of 3/8, 1/2, and 5/8 inch are routinely used. It is prudent to leave an extra 1/4 inch of needle extending above the skin surface in case the needle breaks.

Needle Gauge

Commonly used gauges for subcutaneous injections are 25 to 29 gauge.

Sites

Common sites used for the subcutaneous administration of medications include upper arms, anterior thighs, and abdomen (Figure 11-4). Less common areas are the buttocks and upper back or scapular region.

A plan for rotating injection sites should be developed for all patients who require repeated injections (Figure 11-4). The anterior view (Figure 11-4, *B*) illustrates areas easily used for self-administration. The posterior view (Figure 11-4, *A*) illustrates less commonly used areas that may be used by other people injecting the medication.

When administering insulin subcutaneously, it is important to rotate the injection sites to prevent lipohypertrophy or lipoatrophy, which slows the absorption rate of the insulin. The American Diabetes Association Clinical Practice Recommendations state that insulin injection sites should be rotated systematically within one area before progressing to a new site for injection (see Figure 11-4). It is felt that this will decrease variations in insulin absorption. Absorption is known to be fastest when administered in the abdomen followed by the arms, thighs, and buttocks. Because exercise is also known to affect the rate of insulin absorption, site selection should take this factor into consideration.

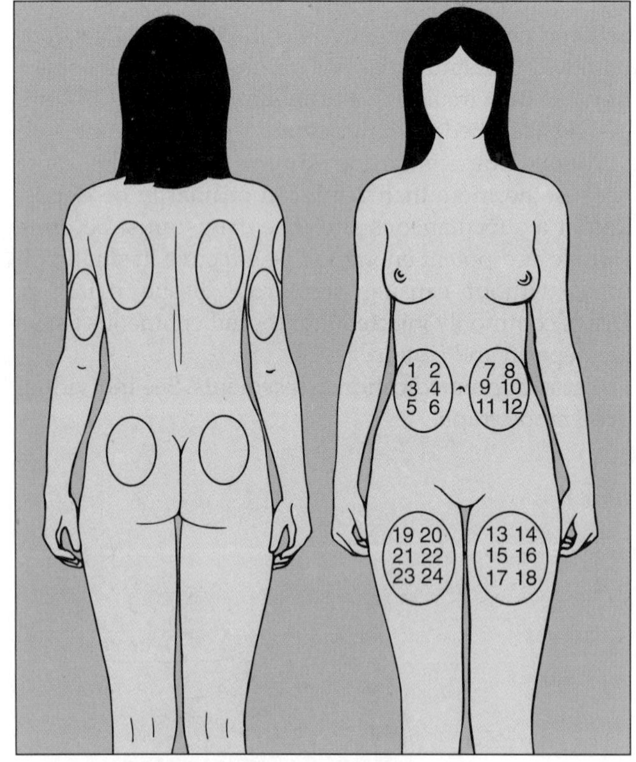

FIGURE **11-4** Subcutaneous injection sites and rotation plan. **A,** Posterior view. **B,** Anterior view. This illustrates commonly used subcutaneous sites for self-administration and provides an example of a rotation schedule for insulin injection using one site systematically before proceeding to the next site of administration.

Technique

1. Prepare the medication as described earlier.
2. Check the accuracy of the drug order against the medication being prepared at least three times during the preparation phase: (1) when first removing the drug from the storage area, (2) immediately after preparation, and (3) immediately before administration.
3. Check your hospital policy regarding whether 1 to 2 minims of air are added to the syringe AFTER accurately measuring the prescribed volume of drug for administration.

   NOTE: The rationale for adding the air is that it will result in the needle being completely cleared of all medication at the time of injection. Conversely, if the volume of medication is completely drawn into the syringe before changing the needle, the drug volume ordered will still be administered as long as the same size needle is used for drawing up and injecting the medication. Therefore the needle should not need to be completely cleared of medication by air during administration. This issue can be critical when small volumes of potent drugs are administered to neonates or infants.
4. Consult the master rotation schedule for the patient so that the drug is administered at the correct site.
5. Identify the patient before administration of the medication by checking the bracelet. Have the patient state his or her name and birth date, or two other identifiers.

6. Explain carefully to the patient what you are going to do.
7. Position the patient appropriately.
8. Expose the selected site and locate the landmarks. Put on gloves.
9. Cleanse the skin surface with an antiseptic pledget starting at the injection site and working outward in a circular motion toward the periphery.
10. Let the area air dry.
11. Consult the institution's policy regarding which of the following methods to use.

    Method 1
    - Grasp the skin area of the site selected and create a small roll or "bunch." Insert the needle quickly at a 90-degree angle, and slowly inject the medication.

    Method 2
    - Grasp the skin area of the site selected, spread, hold firmly, and insert the needle quickly at a 45-degree angle; and slowly inject the medication. American Diabetes Association Clinical Practice Recommendations state that "thin individuals or children may need to pinch the skin and inject at a 45-degree angle to avoid intramuscular injection, especially in the thigh area."
12. As the needle is withdrawn, apply gentle pressure to the site with an antiseptic pledget.
13. DO NOT recap any needles that have been used. Dispose of used needles and syringes into a puncture-resistant container according to the policy of the employing institution.
14. Remove gloves and dispose of them according to agency policy. Thoroughly wash your hands.
15. Provide emotional support for the patient.

Patient Teaching

Perform appropriate patient teaching as described in related drug monograph(s).

Documentation

Provide the RIGHT DOCUMENTATION of the medication administration and the patient's response to drug therapy.

1. Chart the date, time, drug name, dose, and route of administration.
2. Perform and record regular patient assessments for the evaluation of the therapeutic effectiveness (e.g., blood pressure, pulse, output, improvement or quality of cough and productivity, degree and duration of pain relief).
3. Chart and report any signs and symptoms of adverse drug effects.
4. Perform and validate essential patient education about the drug therapy and other essential aspects of intervention for the disease process affecting the individual.

ADMINISTRATION OF MEDICATION BY THE INTRAMUSCULAR ROUTE

Objectives

1. Describe the technique used to administer medications in the vastus lateralis muscle, rectus femoris muscle, ventrogluteal area, dorsogluteal area, or the deltoid muscle.
2. For each anatomic site studied, describe the landmarks used to identify the site before medication is administered.
3. Identify suitable sites for intramuscular administration of medication in an infant, a child, an adult, and an older adult.

Key Terms

intramuscular
vastus lateralis
rectus femoris
ventrogluteal area
dorsogluteal area
deltoid muscle
Z-track method

Intramuscular (IM) injections are made by penetrating a needle through the dermis and subcutaneous tissue into the muscle layer. The injection deposits the medication deep within the muscle mass (Figure 11-5). Absorption is more rapid than from subcutaneous injections because muscle tissue has a greater blood supply. Site selection is especially important with IM injections because incorrect placement of the needle may cause damage to nerves or blood vessels. A large, healthy muscle free of infection or wounds should be used.

Perform premedication assessments. See individual drug monograph.

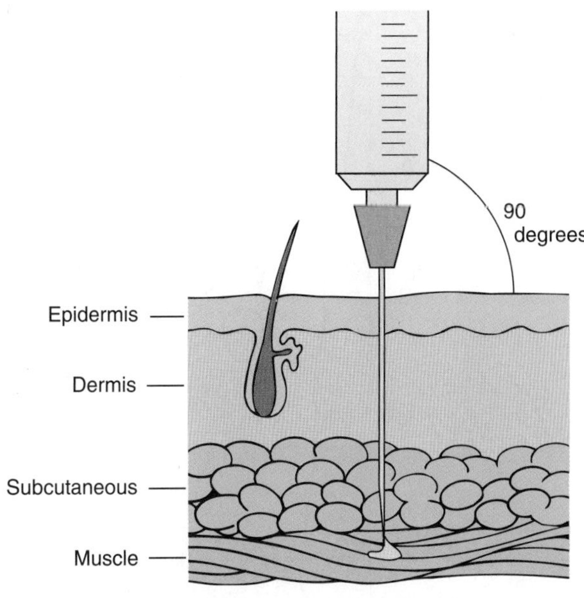

FIGURE 11-5 Intramuscular injection technique.

Equipment

Medication to be injected (see MAR)

Syringe Size

Choose a syringe that corresponds to the volume of drug to be injected at one site. The usual amount injected IM at one site is 0.5 to 2 mL. In infants and children, the amount should not range between 0.5 and 1 mL, not exceeding 1 mL. Correlate syringe size with the size of the patient and the tissue mass. In adults, divided doses are generally recommended for amounts in excess of 3 mL; 1 mL may be injected in the deltoid area. Other factors that influence syringe size include the type of medication and site of administration, thickness of subcutaneous fatty tissue, and the age of the individual.

Needle Length

Assess each patient so that the needle length selected will deposit the medication into the muscular tissue (Figure 11-6). There is a significant difference among needle lengths appropriate for an obese patient, an infant, or an emaciated or debilitated patient. Needles commonly used are 1 to 1½ inches long, although longer lengths may be required for an obese person. When estimating needle length, it is prudent to leave an extra ¼ inch of needle extending above the skin surface in case the needle breaks.

Needle Gauge

Commonly used gauges for IM injections are 20 to 22 gauge.

Sites

Common sites used for the IM administration of medication include the following:

Vastus Lateralis Muscle

This muscle is located on the anterior lateral thigh away from nerves and blood vessels. The midportion is one handbreadth below the greater trochanter and one

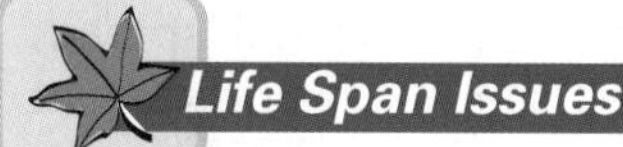

Injection Sites

The *vastus lateralis* injection site is preferred in infants. In the older, debilitated, or nonambulatory adult, carefully assess the sufficiency of the muscle mass before using this site for injection. The gluteal site must not be used in children younger than 3 years of age because the muscle is not well developed yet.

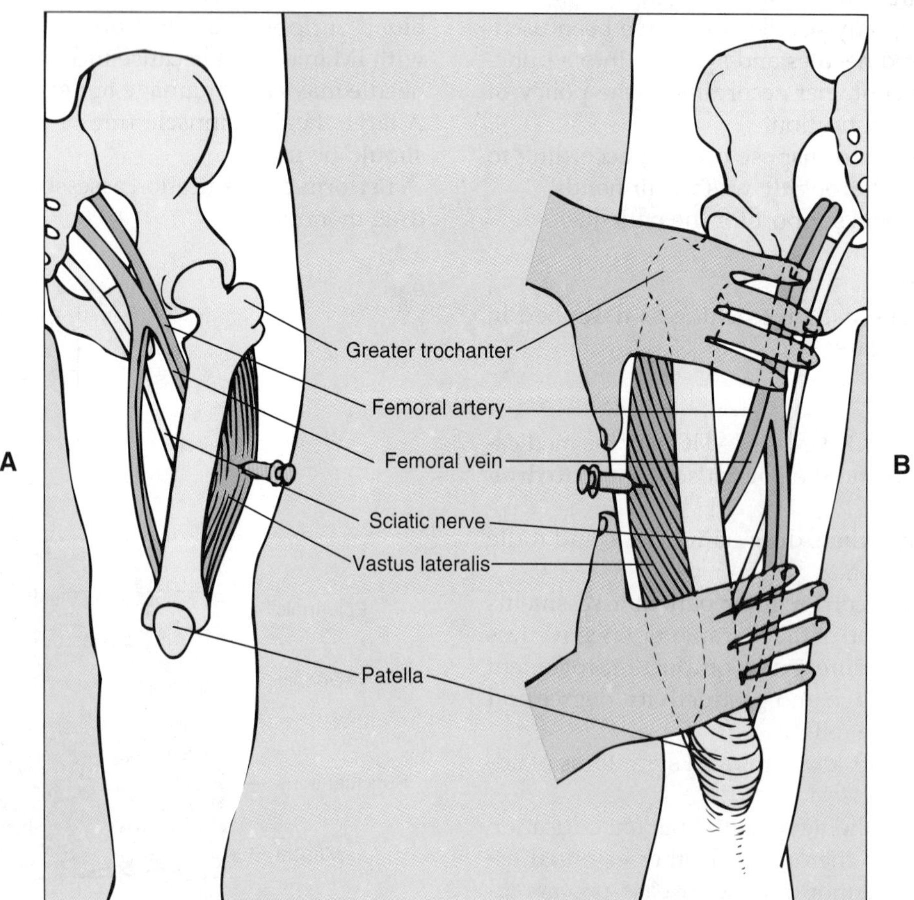

FIGURE 11-6 Vastus lateralis muscle. **A,** Child/infant. **B,** Adult.

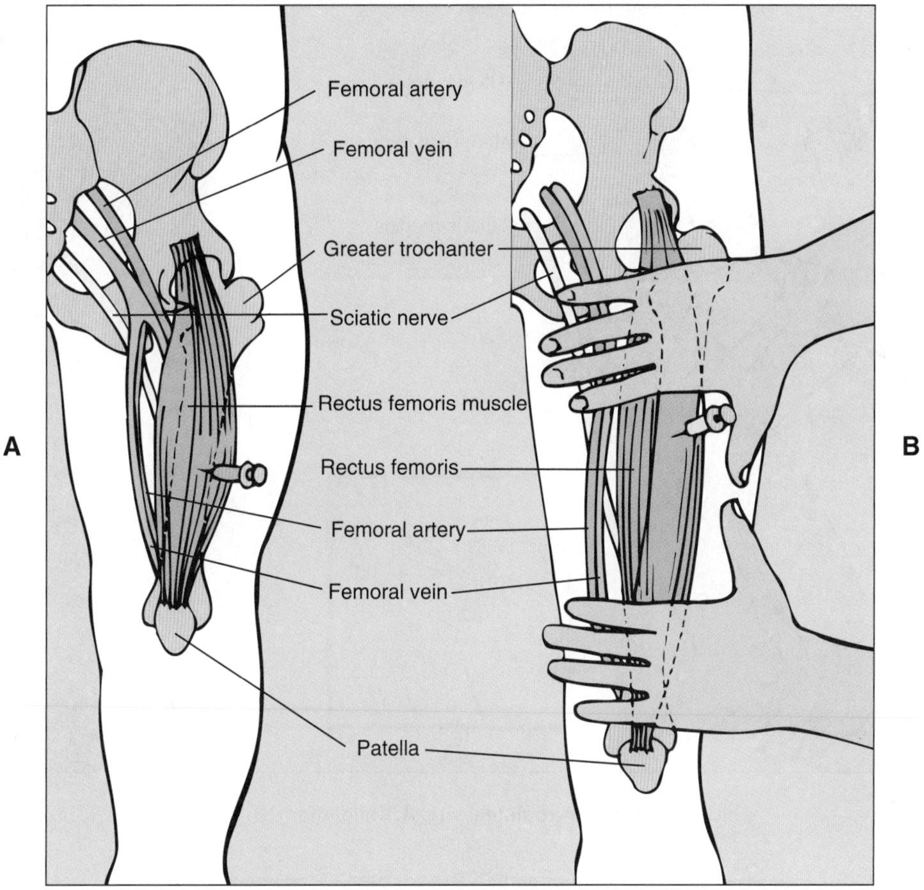

FIGURE 11-7 Rectus femoris muscle. **A,** Child/infant. **B,** Adult.

handbreadth above the knee (see Figure 11-6). It is generally the preferred site for IM injections in infants because it has the largest muscle mass for that age-group. The vastus lateralis muscle is also a good choice for an injection site in healthy, ambulatory adults (Figure 11-6, *B*). It accommodates a large volume of medication and permits good drug absorption. In the older adult, debilitated, or nonambulatory adult, the muscle should be carefully assessed before injection because significantly less muscle mass may be present. If muscle mass is insufficient, an alternative site should be selected.

Rectus Femoris Muscle

The rectus femoris muscle (Figure 11-7) lies just medial to the vastus lateralis muscle but does not cross the midline of the anterior thigh. The injection site is located in the same manner as the vastus lateralis muscle. It may be used in both children and adults when other sites are unavailable. A primary advantage to its use is that it may be used more easily by patients for self-administration. A disadvantage is that the medial border is quite close to the sciatic nerve and major blood vessels (see Figure 11-7). If the muscle is not well developed, injections in this site may also cause considerable discomfort.

Gluteal Area

The gluteal area is a commonly used site of injection because it is free of major nerves and blood vessels. *It must not be used in children younger than 3 years of age because the muscle is not yet well developed from walking.* The area may be divided into two distinct injection sites: (1) the ventrogluteal area and (2) the dorsogluteal area.

- Ventrogluteal area: This site is easily accessible when the patient is in a prone, supine, or side-lying position. It is located by placing the palm of the hand on the lateral portion of the greater trochanter, the index finger on the anterior superior iliac spine, and the middle finger extended to the iliac crest. The injection is made into the center of the V formed between the index and middle fingers, with the needle directed slightly upward toward the crest of the ilium (Figure 11-8). Pain on injection can be minimized if the muscle is relaxed. The patient can aid in relaxation by pointing the toes inward while lying in a prone position (Figure 11-9) or by flexing the upper leg if lying on the side (Figure 11-10).
- Dorsogluteal area: To use this injection site (Figure 11-11), the patient must be placed in a prone position on a flat table surface. The site is identified by drawing an imaginary line from the

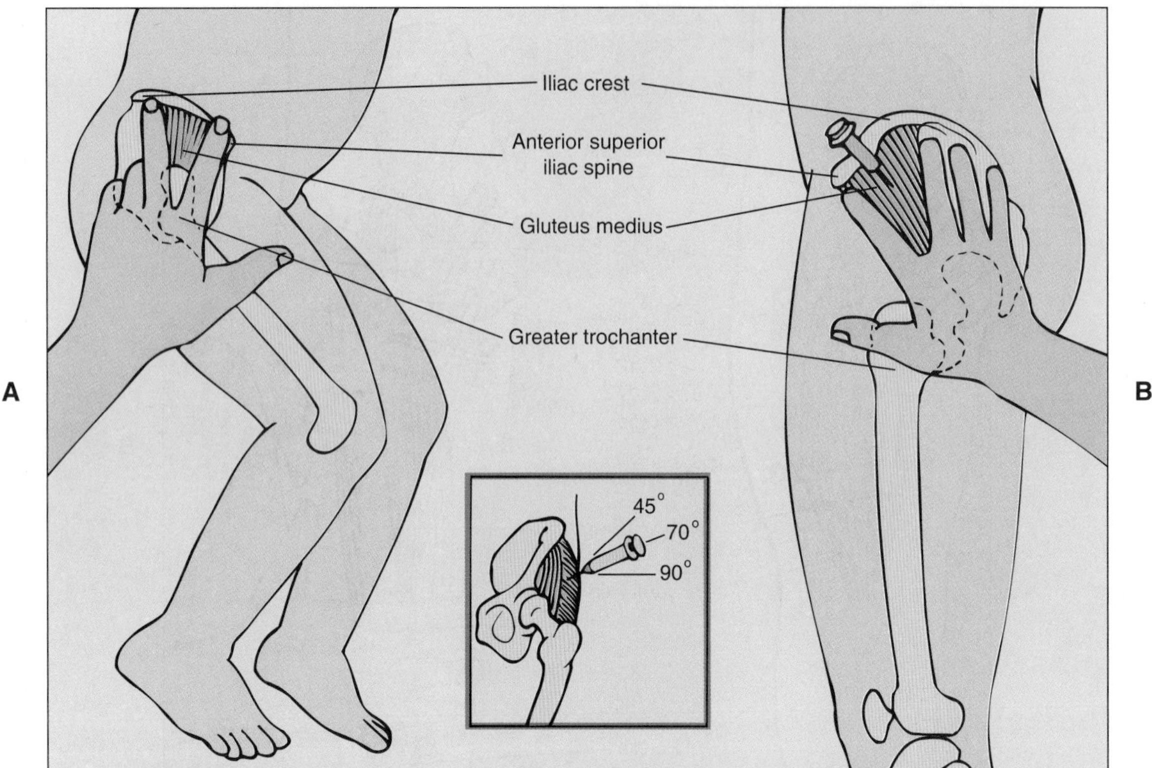

FIGURE **11-8** Ventrogluteal site. **A,** Child/infant. **B,** Adult.

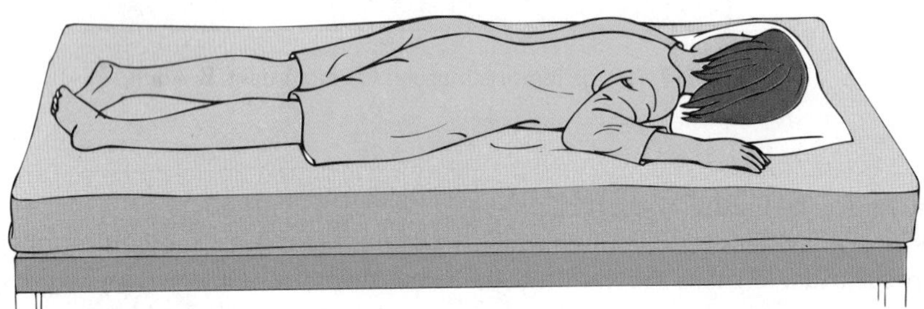

FIGURE **11-9** Prone position. Toes pointed to promote muscle relaxation.

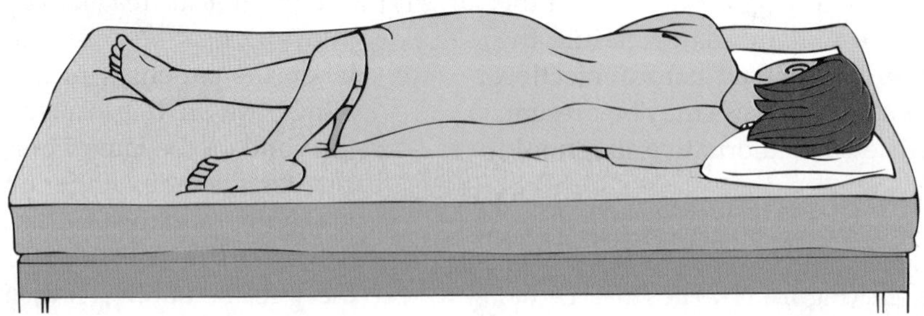

FIGURE **11-10** Patient lying on side. Flexing the upper leg promotes muscle relaxation.

posterior superior iliac spine to the greater trochanter of the femur. The injection should be given at any point between the imaginary straight line and below the curve of the iliac crest (hip bone). The syringe should be held perpendicular to the flat table surface with the needle directed on a straight back-to-front course. Pain on injection can be minimized if the muscle is relaxed. The patient can aid in relaxation by pointing the toes inward while lying in a prone position (see Figure 11-9).

Deltoid Muscle

The **deltoid muscle** is often used because of ease of access in the standing, sitting, or prone positions. However, it should be used in infants only when the

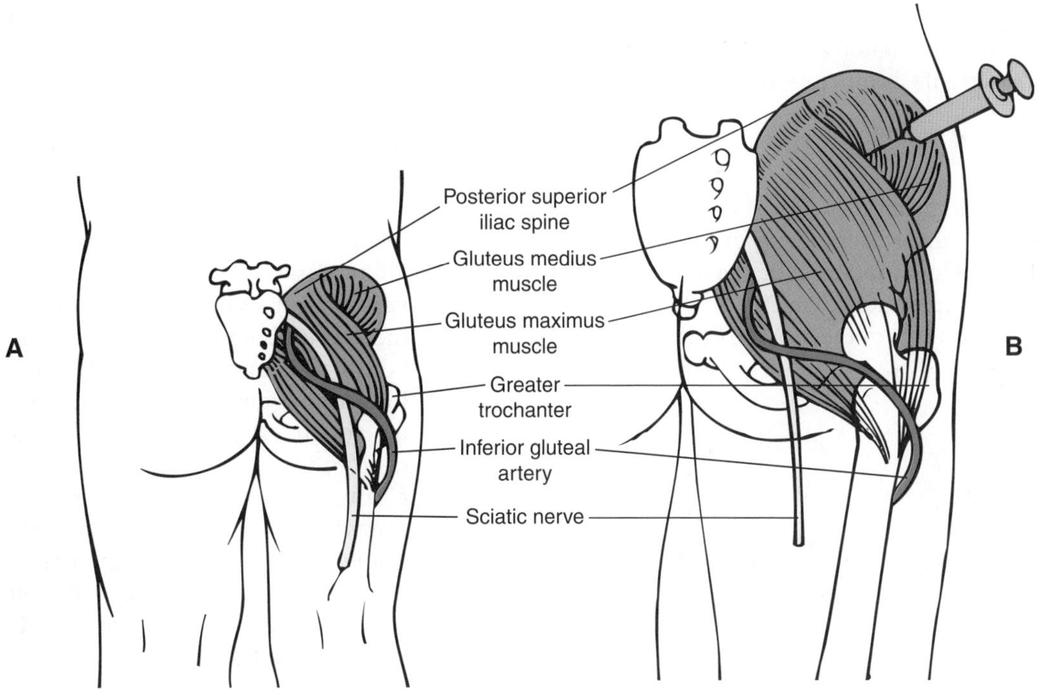

FIGURE **11-11** Dorsogluteal site. **A,** Child/infant. **B,** Adult.

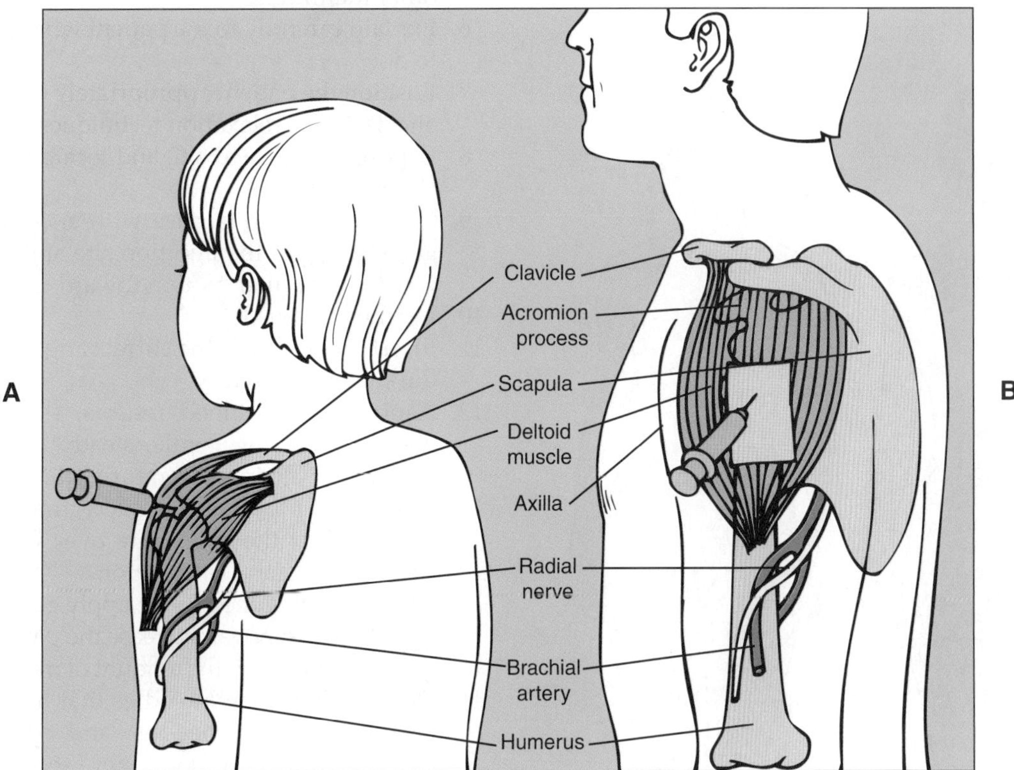

FIGURE **11-12** Deltoid muscle site. **A,** Child/infant. **B,** Adult.

volume to be injected is quite small, the drug is nonirritating, and the dose will be quickly absorbed. In adults, the volume should be limited to 2 mL or less and the substance must not cause irritation. Caution must also be exercised to avoid the clavicle, humerus, acromion, the brachial vein and artery, and the radial nerve.

The injection site (Figure 11-12) of the deltoid muscle is located by drawing an imaginary line across the armpit at the level of the axilla and the lower edge of the acromion. The lateral borders of the rectangle are vertical lines parallel to the area one third and two thirds of the way around the outer lateral aspect of the arm.

Site Rotation

A master plan for site rotation should be developed and used for all patients requiring repeated injections (Figure 11-13).

Technique

1. Prepare the medication as described earlier.
2. Check the accuracy of the drug order against the medication being prepared at least three times during the preparation phase: (1) when first removing the drug from the storage area; (2) immediately after preparation; and (3) immediately before administration.
3. Check your hospital policy regarding whether 0.1 or 0.2 mL of air should be added to the syringe AFTER accurately measuring the prescribed volume of drug for administration.
   Note: The rationale for adding the air is that it will result in the needle being completely cleared of all medication at the time of injection. Conversely, if the volume is completely drawn into the syringe before changing the needle, the drug volume ordered will still be administered as long as the same size needle is used for drawing up and injection. Thus the needle should not need to be completely cleared of medication by air during administration. This issue can be critical when small volumes of potent drugs are administered repeatedly to infants.
4. Consult the master rotation schedule for the patient so that the drug is administered at the correct site (see Figure 11-13).
5. Identify the patient before administration of the medication by checking the bracelet. Have the patient state his or her name and birth date, or two other identifiers.
6. Explain carefully to the patient what you are going to do.
7. Position the patient appropriately (see Figures 11-9 and 11-10 for relaxation techniques).
8. Expose the selected site and locate the landmarks. Wear gloves.
9. Cleanse the skin surface with an antiseptic pledget, starting at the injection site and working outward in a circular motion toward the periphery.
10. Let the area air-dry.
11. Insert the needle at the correct angle and depth for the site being used.
12. Aspirate. If no blood returns, slowly inject the medication using gentle, steady pressure on the plunger. If blood does return, place an antiseptic pledget over the injection site as the needle is withdrawn. Start the procedure over with a new syringe, needle, and medication.
13. After removing the needle, apply gentle pressure to the site. Massage can increase the pain if the muscle mass is stressed by the amount of medication given.
14. DO NOT recap any needles that have been used. Dispose of used needles and syringes into a puncture-resistant container according to the policy of the employing institution.
15. Remove gloves and dispose of them according to agency policy. Thoroughly wash your hands.
16. Apply a small bandage to the site.
17. Provide emotional support to the patient. Children should be comforted during and after the injection. Sometimes letting a child hold your hand or say "ouch" helps. Praise the patient for assistance and cooperation.

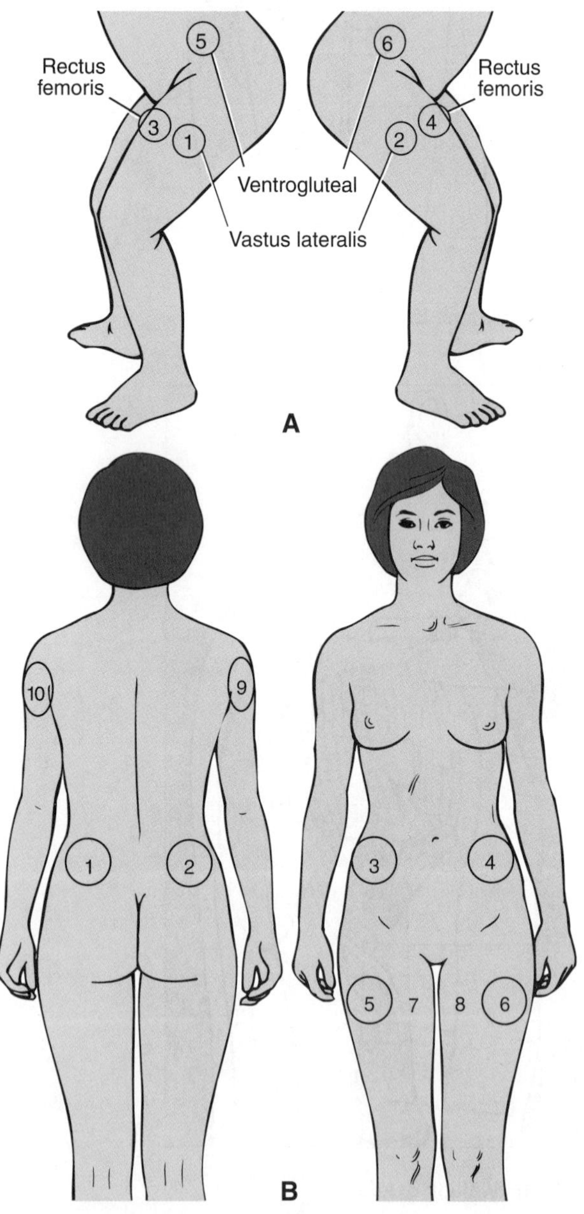

FIGURE **11-13** Intramuscular master rotation plan. **A,** Infant/child. Note that the deltoid site may also be used in an infant or child; however, the volume of medication must be quite small and the drug nonirritating. **B,** Adult. In an adult, avoid using the rectus femoris (numbers 7 and 8) unless other sites are not available, because of the pain produced when this site is used and the location of the sciatic nerve, femoral artery, and vein. If used, be certain to insert the needle lateral to the midline.

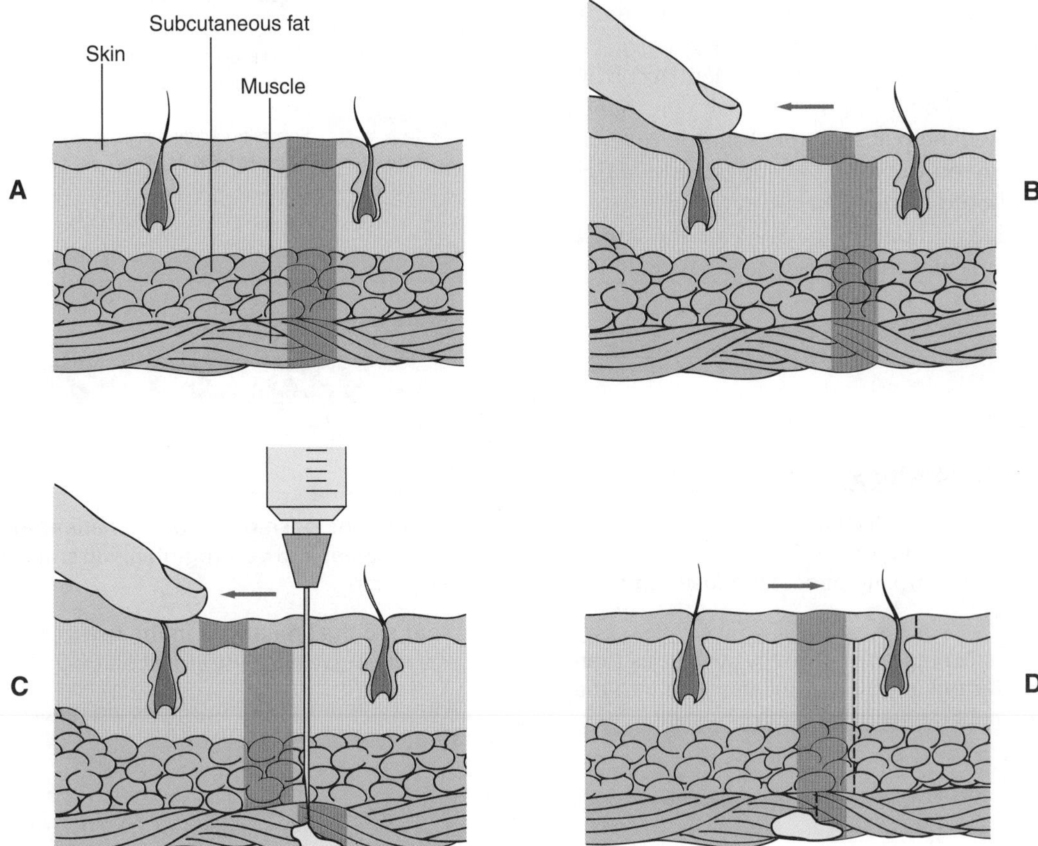

FIGURE **11-14** Z-track method of intramuscular injection. **A,** Before starting Z-tracking. **B,** Stretch skin slightly to one side, approximately 1 inch. **C,** Inject the medication; wait approximately 10 seconds. **D,** Remove needle and allow skin to return to normal position. Do not massage injection site.

Patient Teaching

Perform appropriate patient teaching as described in related drug monographs.

Documentation

Provide the RIGHT DOCUMENTATION of the medication administration and response to drug therapy.

1. Chart the date, time, drug name, dose, and route of administration.
2. Perform and record regular patient assessments for the evaluation of the therapeutic effectiveness (e.g., blood pressure, pulse, output, improvement or quality of cough and productivity).
3. Chart and report any signs and symptoms of adverse drug effects.
4. Perform and validate essential patient education about the drug therapy and other essential aspects of intervention for the disease process affecting the individual.

The Z-track Method

The use of a **Z-track method** (Figure 11-14) may be appropriate for medications that are particularly irritating or that stain the tissue. Check the hospital policy concerning which personnel may administer by this method.

1. Expose the dorsogluteal site (Figure 11-14, *A*). Calculate and prepare the medication, then add 0.5 mL of air to ensure that the drug will clear the needle. Position the patient and cleanse the area for injection as previously described. Never inject into the arm or other exposed site. Wear gloves.
2. Stretch the skin approximately 1 inch to one side (Figure 11-14, *B*).
3. Insert the needle. Choose a needle of sufficient length to ensure *deep* muscle penetration.
4. Aspirate and follow previous guidelines for use of the dorsogluteal site.
5. Gently inject the medication and wait approximately 10 seconds (Figure 11-14, *C*).
6. Remove the needle and allow the skin to return to the normal position (Figure 11-14, *D*).
7. DO NOT massage the injection site.
8. If further injections are to be made, alternate between dorsogluteal sites.
9. DO NOT recap any needles that have been used. Dispose of used needles and syringes into a

puncture-resistant container according to the policy of the employing institution.

10. Remove gloves and dispose of them according to agency policy. Thoroughly wash your hands.
11. Walking will help absorption. Vigorous exercise or pressure on the injection site (such as a tight girdle) should be temporarily avoided.

Documentation and patient teaching are the same as for other intramuscular injections.

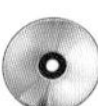
Go to your Companion CD-ROM for Appendices, an Audio Glossary, animations, Drug Dosage Calculators, customizable Patient Self-Assessment forms, and Review Questions for the NCLEX® Examination.

evolve Be sure to visit the companion Evolve site at http://evolve.elsevier.com/Clayton for WebLinks and additional online resources.

MEDICATION SAFETY REVIEW

CRITICAL THINKING QUESTIONS

1. Explain the details of selecting the injection site, the needle and the syringe for administration of medications intradermally, subcutaneously, and intramuscularly.
2. Use an anatomic diagram to identify structures that are targeted for the injection of medications into the intradermal, subcutaneous, and intramuscular sites.
3. Describe the positioning of the patient for dorsogluteal and ventrogluteal intramuscular injections.
4. What are the limitations in the use of the vastus lateralis muscle for intramuscular injections?
5. What type of rotation plan should be used for the administration of insulin?

CONTENT REVIEW QUESTIONS

1. The instructor requests that you gather the equipment needed to perform an intradermal injection. Which of the following would be appropriate?
   1. 3-mL syringe, 25-gauge 1-inch needle
   2. TB syringe, 26-gauge ⅜-inch needle
   3. 3-mL syringe, 21-gauge 1-inch needle
   4. TB syringe, 21-gauge ⅜-inch needle
2. When reading a reaction to an allergen you observe no wheal and a 3-mm flare. This would be recorded as a _____ reaction.
   1. 1+
   2. 2+
   3. 3+
   4. 4+
3. The American Diabetes Association (ADA) recommends insulin sites be rotated by rotating injections:
   1. within one area before going to the next site (arms, legs, abdomen, back).
   2. using a new site (the arm, leg, abdomen, or back) each time.
   3. using the arm in the morning and the legs in the evening.
   4. using the abdomen and legs.
4. The student nurse reads the order to give a 1-year-old patient an intramuscular injection. The appropriate and preferred muscle to select for a child is the:
   1. deltoid.
   2. dorsogluteal.
   3. ventrogluteal.
   4. vastus lateralis.
5. A nurse administers an intramuscular medication of iron by the Z-track method. The medication was administered by this method to:
   1. provide faster absorption of the medication.
   2. reduce discomfort from the needle.
   3. provide more even absorption of the drug.
   4. prevent the drug from irritating sensitive tissue.

CHAPTER

12 Parenteral Administration: Intravenous Route

evolve http://evolve.elsevier.com/Clayton

Chapter Content

INTRAVENOUS THERAPY

Objectives

1. Define intravenous (IV) therapy.
2. Describe the processes used to establish guidelines for nurses to perform infusion therapy.

Key Terms

intravenous
Infusion Nurses Society

Intravenous (IV) administration refers to the introduction of fluids directly into the venous bloodstream. Its advantages are that large volumes of fluids can be rapidly administered into the vein and there is usually less irritation. IV administration is the most rapid of all parenteral routes because it bypasses all barriers to drug absorption. Drugs may be given by direct injection with a needle in the vein, but more commonly they are administered intermittently or by continuous infusion through an established peripheral or central IV line.

IV drug administration is usually more comfortable for the patient, especially when several doses of medication must be administered daily. However, use of the IV route requires time and skill to establish and maintain an IV site, the patient tends to be less mobile, and there is a greater possibility for infection and for severe adverse reactions from the drug.

"IV nursing" is defined by the Infusion Nurses Society as the use of the nursing process as it relates to technology and clinical application, fluids and electrolytes, pharmacology, infection control, pediatrics, transfusion therapy, oncology, parenteral nutrition, and quality assurance. Before a nurse is eligible to perform IV therapy procedures, he or she must meet the institutional guidelines pertaining to infusion therapy. Some hospitals use infusion therapy teams, but many now assign the responsibility for infusion therapy to nurses with earned credentials. The nurse performing venipuncture and infusion therapy must be well versed in the techniques described in the above definition of IV nursing. All IV therapy requires a written order from a health care provider that is dated, specifies the type of solution or medication to be administered, the dosage, and the rate and frequency of administration.

Many institutions nationwide have acknowledged the value of the licensed practical/vocational nurse (LPN/LVN) as a member of the IV team. Most state laws recognize the role of the LPN/LVN in IV therapy, but delegate the scope of practice to be defined in policies and procedures of individual practice sites. The nurse should check with her particular state board of nursing to determine the current guidelines and education requirements. In general, LPN/LVN responsibilities do not include administration of IV medication, blood products, and antineoplastic agents.

Before any nurse administers IV therapy, he or she should ask the following questions:

- "Does law in this state delegate this function to the nurse?"
- "Does the written policy of the institution or agency through which I am employed, with the approval of the medical staff, permit a nurse with my level of education and experience to administer IV therapy?"
- "Does the institution or agency policy limit the types of fluids and medications that I may administer?"
- "Is the order written by a health care provider for a specific patient?"

Certification in infusion therapy is available for registered nurses by taking a written examination offered by the Infusion Nurses Certification Corporation (INCC). The nurse can use the initials "CRNI" in his or her title (certified registered nurse infusion) after passing the certification process for a period of 3 years. The nurse must meet the established criteria for recertification at 3-year intervals. Clinical sites and other local agencies also offer courses in infusion therapy at both an introductory and advanced level. The local state board governing nursing can provide information on the requirements for registered and licensed practical nurses to perform infusion therapy.

The Infusion Nurses Society (INS), a professional nursing organization, publishes the *Infusion Nursing Standards of Practice* and the Centers for Disease Control and Prevention (CDC) publish recommendations for infection control relating to infusion therapy. These are excellent sources to consult when reviewing standards for IV therapy.

EQUIPMENT USED FOR INTRAVENOUS THERAPY

Objectives

1. Describe equipment used to perform IV therapy (e.g., winged or butterfly needle, over-the-needle catheter, administration sets, and IV access devices).
2. Differentiate among peripheral, midline, central venous, and implantable access devices used for IV therapy.

Key Terms

- IV administration sets
- nonvolumetric IV controllers
- volumetric IV controllers
- syringe pumps
- peripheral devices
- midline catheters
- central devices
- implantable venous infusion ports
- winged, butterfly, or scalp needles
- over-the-needle catheters
- saline, heparin, or medlock
- in-the-needle catheters
- peripherally inserted central venous catheters (PICCs)
- tunneled central venous catheters
- implantable infusion ports

Intravenous Administration Sets

IV administration sets are the apparatus that connects a large volume of parenteral solution with the IV access device in the patient's vein. All sets (Figure 12-1) have

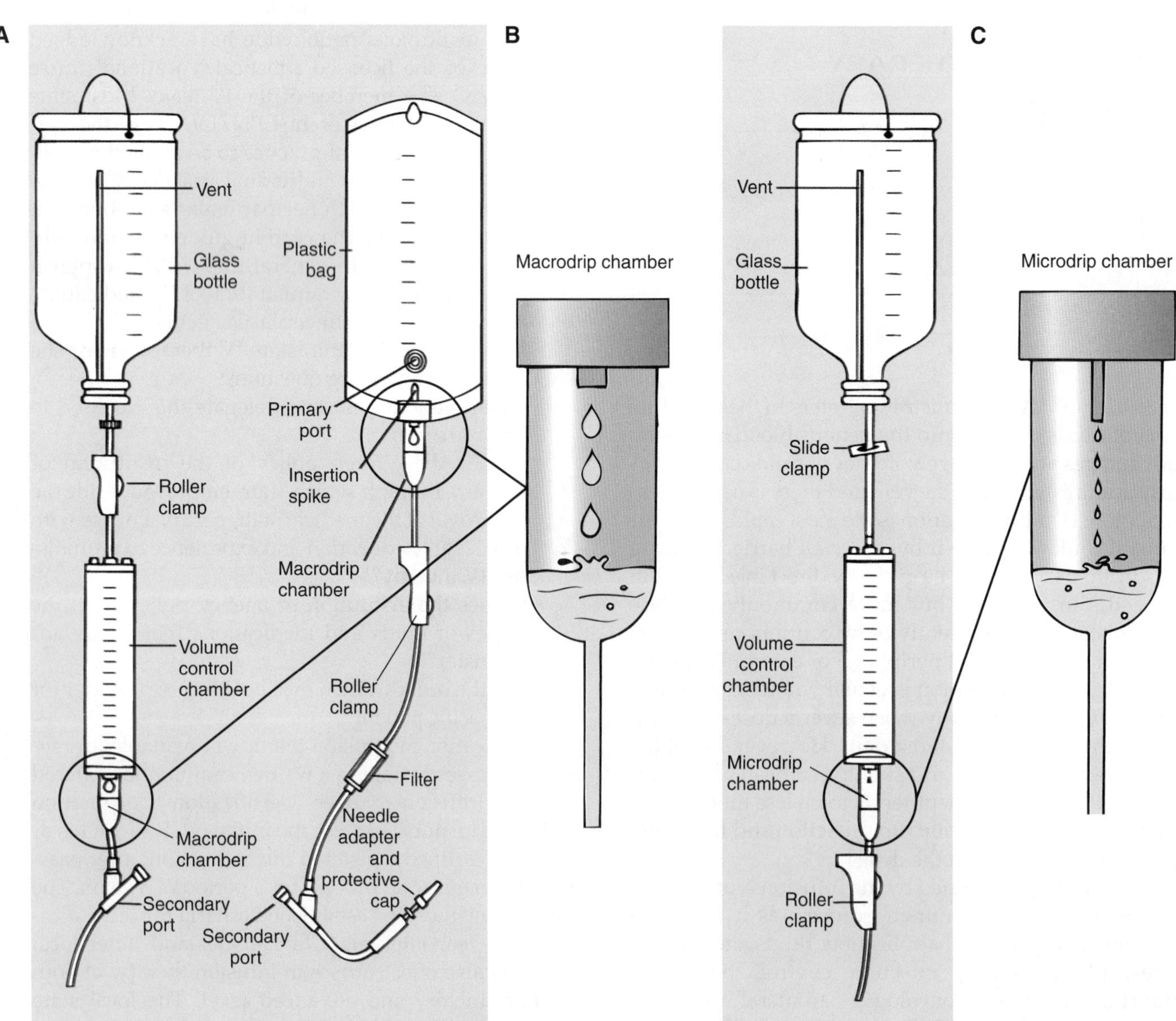

FIGURE **12-1** **A** and **B,** Different types of IV administration sets using a macrodrip chamber. **C,** An administration set using a microdrip chamber.

an insertion spike, a drip chamber, plastic tubing with a rate control clamp, a rubber injection portal, a needle adapter, and a protective cap over the needle adapter. Depending on the manufacturer, the sets are available with a variety of additional attachments (e.g., volume and size of drip chamber, "piggyback" portals, filters, style of control clamp [Figure 12-1]). The type of system used by a particular hospital is usually determined by the manufacturer of the IV solutions used by the institution. Each manufacturer makes adapters to fit a specific type of plastic or glass large-volume solution container. A crucial point to remember about administration sets is that the drops delivered by drip chambers vary among manufacturers. Macrodrip chambers (Figure 12-1, *A* and *B*) provide 10, 15, or 20 drops/mL, whereas microdrip chambers (Figure 12-1, *C*) deliver 60 drops/mL of solution (see p. 176). Microdrip administration sets are used when a small volume of fluid is being administered such as with a *to keep open* (TKO) order or for accurate volume administration for neonatal and pediatric patients. Volume-control chambers (Figure 12-1, *A* and *C*) are also used as a safety factor to limit the volume administered. In many clinical settings, microdrip sets are used for all volumes of IV fluid ordered that administer less than 100 mL per hour. It is essential to read the label on the box before opening it to ensure that you have the correct administration set. The nurse must know the number of drops per milliliter administered to calculate the flow rate for the IV solution.

Equipment Used in Conjunction with IV Therapy

A large variety of connector and access devices are available for various components of infusion therapy. The nurse must become familiar with the IV access systems and the terminology used at the clinical site to maintain sterility and safety.

Types of Infusion Control Devices

Devices have been developed to more safely and accurately control infusion rates of intravenous solutions, particularly those that must be administered at a very precise rate for therapeutic effect (e.g., continuous heparin infusion for anticoagulation) or prevention of toxicity (e.g., a specific rate for administration of aminoglycosides to prevent nephrotoxicity or ototoxicity). Infusion devices can be classified as controllers, pumps, and syringe pumps.

Controllers

The basic IV infusion through a peripheral IV access site (see Intravenous Access Devices, pp. 178 to 181) depends on gravity for administration. The IV container must be 24 to 36 inches above the IV site so that the pressure of the infusion solution in the tube is greater than the resistance (backpressure) from the vein, allowing the infusion to flow into the vein. If the height changes significantly because patient changes positions, or if the fluid volume remaining in the IV container is minimal, the IV infusion will slow down or stop. The simplest rate controllers are the roller and slide clamps (Figure 12-2, *A* and *B*) that accompany IV administration sets. These constricting devices regulate flow by being adjusted while the nurse counts the number of drops that pass through the drip chamber per minute. (Remember, the macrodrip chambers form 10 to 20 drops/mL, whereas the microdrip chambers form 60 drops/mL.)

Electronic control devices can be categorized as either nonvolumetric control devices or volumetric control devices. The **nonvolumetric IV controllers** monitor only the gravity infusion rate by counting the drops that drip through the chamber. They protect the patient by sounding an alarm if the clamp slips and results in

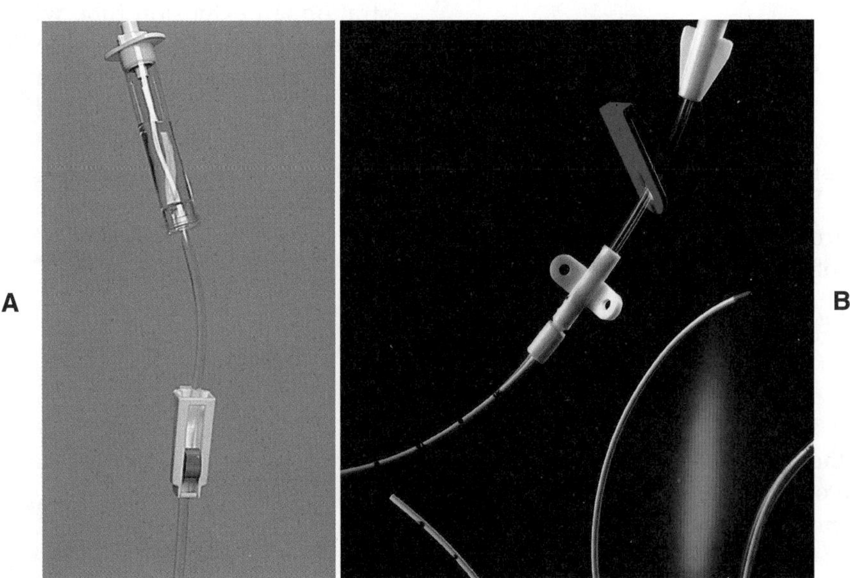

FIGURE 12-2 Control clamps for IV administration sets. **A,** Roller clamp. **B,** Slide clamp.

an inadvertent gravity free-flow, or if the number of drops per minute slow down or stop because of patient position changes, air in the tubing, or low solution volume. Nonvolumetric controllers have no moving parts, so maintenance costs are modest compared to pumps, but non-volumetric controllers are less accurate with viscous solutions such as blood products.

Pumps

The volumetric IV controllers are actually pumps that apply external pressure to the administration set tubing to squeeze the solution through the tubing at a specific rate (e.g., mL/minute or mL/hour). Volumetric control devices can be programmed for a specific volume over time and are much more accurate than the non-volumetric controllers. These pumps also have an alarm system that sounds if there is resistance in the IV line caused by a developing occlusion from thrombus formation or a kink in the administration set line because of patient movement. Disadvantages of pumps are cost of equipment and training of personnel, cost of maintenance, more equipment at the bedside, and the potential for more serious infiltration than from gravity-flow administration.

Syringe Pumps

Syringe pumps hold a prefilled syringe and apply positive pressure to the plunger, delivering a specific volume of medicine over a set time. Syringe pumps are more commonly used when small volumes need to be administered. Some models of syringe pumps can be operated by batteries or a spring, making them much more portable. Examples of small syringe pumps are those that continually infuse insulin into subcutaneous tissue of patients with diabetes mellitus, or the patient-controlled analgesia (PCA) pumps that allow patients receiving pain medications to administer continual infusions and intermittent boluses of the medicine for comfort.

Volumetric pumps and syringe pumps have become quite sophisticated and much safer (e.g., alarm systems, automatic stop capability, preprogrammed to prevent calculation errors, monitored from a distant site using a modem), allowing home infusions of medicines. It is important that the nurse become familiar with the specific devices used at the clinical setting for safety and efficiency of patient care.

Intravenous Access Devices

IV access devices are often subdivided into four groups based on the location of the terminal tip of the access device: (1) peripheral devices are for short-term use in peripheral veins in the hand or forearm; (2) midline catheters are for use over 2 to 4 weeks, inserted into intermediate-sized veins and advanced into larger vessels; (3) central devices are inserted into intermediate sized vessels and advanced into central veins for maximal mixing with large volumes of blood; and (4) the implantable venous infusion ports are placed into central veins for long-term therapy.

Peripheral Access Devices

All needles, if long enough, may be used to administer medications or fluids intravenously, but special equipment has been designed for this purpose. Winged needles, also known as butterfly or scalp needles, are short sharp-tipped needles (Figure 12-3) originally designed for venipuncture of small veins in infants and for geriatric use. These needles are available in sizes ranging from 17 to 29 gauge and are designed to minimize tissue injury during insertion. The winged area is pinched together to form a handle while the needle is being inserted, then laid flat against the skin to form a base for anchoring with tape. Two types are now available, one with a short length of plastic tubing and a permanently attached resealable injection port, and the other with a variable length of plastic tubing with a female luer adapter for attachment of a syringe or an administration set (Figure 12-3). The patency of the needle is maintained by use of either a heparin or saline flush routine as established by hospital policy.

Over-the-needle catheters, also known as short peripheral venous catheters, are recommended for routine peripheral infusion therapy. The needles are stainless steel and coated with a Teflon-like plastic catheter (Figure 12-4, *A*). After the needle penetrates the vein in the hand or forearm, the catheter is advanced into the vein, and the metal needle is removed, leaving the plastic catheter in place. An IV administration set is then attached to the catheter for continuous infusion. This unit is used when IV therapy is expected to continue for a few days. The rationale for use of the plastic catheter is that it does not have a sharp tip that may cause venous irritation and extravasation.

When a patient no longer needs IV fluid therapy but venous access is still needed for medicine administration, an extension tube with an injection port is attached to the catheter and the IV fluid discontinued. The intravenous access device is then referred to at

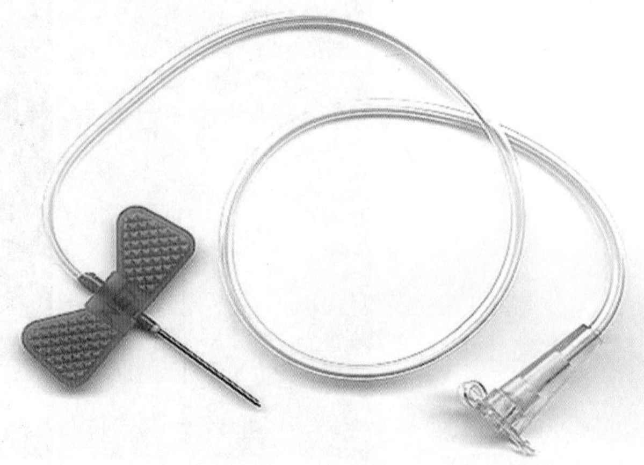

FIGURE 12-3 Winged needle with female luer adapter.

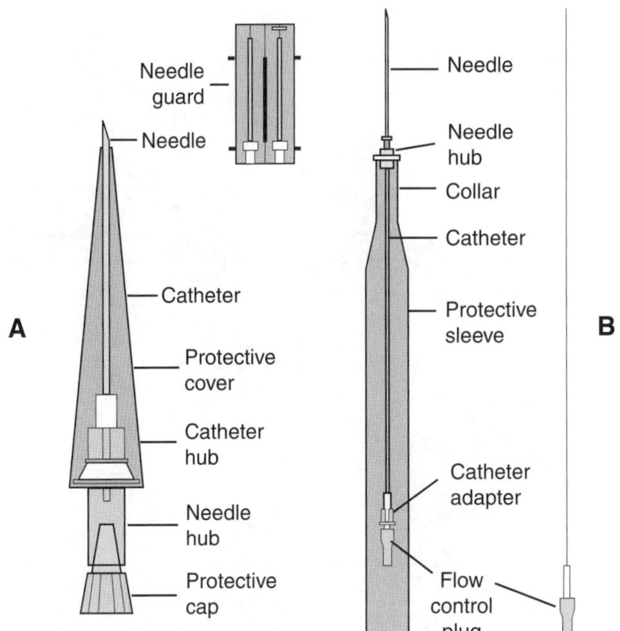

FIGURE **12-4** **A,** Over-the-needle catheter. This unit is the most commonly used type of catheter when IV therapy is expected to continue for several days. **B,** In-the-needle catheters use a large-bore needle for venipuncture, then a 4- to 6-inch sterile, small-gauge plastic catheter is advanced through the needle into the vein. The needle is withdrawn and the skin forms a seal around the plastic catheter. The intracatheter is infrequently used today.

different clinical sites as a saline, heparin, or medlock. The term "heparin lock" originated when both saline and heparin were used to flush the short peripheral venous catheter to prevent blockage by clot formation. Research indicates that normal saline flushing is sufficient to prevent clotting and maintain the peripheral catheter integrity, so a more appropriate term is a saline lock or medlock (for medication lock). Generally, peripheral catheters should be changed every 72 to 96 hours to prevent infection and phlebitis. Blood samples should not be drawn from peripheral catheters. If sites for venous access are limited and no evidence of infection is present, peripheral venous catheters can remain in place, although the patient and the insertion site should be monitored closely for signs and symptoms of phlebitis and infection. The CDC recommends that peripheral catheters not be changed for pediatric patients unless it is clinically indicated.

In-the-needle catheters use a large-bore needle for venipuncture (Figure 12-4, *B*). A 4- to 6-inch sterile, smaller-gauge plastic catheter is then advanced through the needle into the vein. The needle is withdrawn and the skin forms a seal around the plastic catheter. The IV administration set is attached directly to the plastic catheter. In-the-needle catheters are seldom used today for peripheral IVs because of the risk of shearing the through-the-needle catheter.

Midline access catheters are selected for use if it is anticipated that IV access will be needed for 7 days or more. They are often left in place for 2 to 4 weeks. Midline catheters are flexible, 3 to 8 inches long, and are inserted at the antecubital fossa into the cephalic or basilic vein and advanced to the distal subclavian vein. They do not enter the superior vena cava. Midline catheters appear to be associated with lower rates of phlebitis than short peripheral catheters, have a lower rate of infection, and cost less than central venous catheters. The CDC recommends replacement of the catheter and rotation of the injection site no more frequently than every 72 to 96 hours, but does not give recommendations regarding the maximum length of time it may remain in place. Many institutions require that the health care provider write an order indicating that the IV may be left in place for more than 72 hours. Midline catheters are used for continuous access, repeated access, or high flow rate IV solutions. This type of catheter needs to be flushed with saline and heparin solution after each use or at least once daily if not in use. Blood should not be drawn through this catheter.

Central Access Devices

Central IV access devices (also known as indwelling catheters) are used when the purpose of therapy dictates (e.g., large volumes, irritating medicine, or hypertonic solutions such as total parenteral nutrition are to be infused); when peripheral sites have been exhausted because of repeated use or the condition of veins for access is poor; when long-term or home therapy is required; and when emergency conditions mandate adequate vascular access.

The central venous sites most commonly used for central venous catheters are the subclavian and jugular veins. When upper body veins are not acceptable, the femoral veins may be accessed for short-term or emergency use. A physician can also elect to perform a venisection or "cutdown" to insert this type of catheter into the basilic or cephalic veins in the antecubital fossa. Three types of devices based on placement of the catheter's proximal tip are routinely used for central catheters: peripheral, tunneled, and implantable devices.

Peripherally inserted central venous catheters (PICCs) are inserted into the superior vena cava or just outside the right atrium by way of the cephalic or basilar veins of the antecubital space, providing an alternative to subclavian or jugular vein catheterization. PICCs are available in 14 to 28 gauge, with various lengths, thereby making them available for pediatric use. The catheter itself can have an open tip or valved (Groshong) tip and comes with either a single or a double lumen. The PICC line has the advantage of ease of insertion because the procedure can be performed at the bedside by a qualified nurse. Peripherally inserted central venous catheters are associated with fewer mechanical complications (e.g., thrombosis, hemothorax), cost less than other central venous catheters, are easier to maintain than short peripheral catheters because there is less frequent infiltration and phlebitis, and require less frequent site rotation. Because of the smaller lumen, in general, blood should not be drawn through PICC lines; neither should total parenteral nutrition fluids be administered. PICC lines routinely remain in place for 1 to 3 months, but can last for a year or more if cared for properly. When not in use, the IV is disconnected and the catheter is flushed and capped. The line should be flushed with a saline-heparin solution after every use or daily, if not used.

The **tunneled central venous catheters** are surgically placed in an outpatient procedure under local anesthesia. Through an incision the terminal tip of the catheter is inserted into the subclavian vein and advanced to the superior vena cava. The proximal end of the catheter is tunneled about 6 inches away under the skin on the chest, exiting near a nipple. A Dacron cuff is often placed around the catheter under the skin, which anchors the catheter and forms a seal around the catheter as the skin heals, helping keep the tunnel sterile.

Three types of catheters frequently used are the Hickman, Broviac, and the Groshong (Figure 12-5, *A* to *C*). The Broviac catheter is a single-lumen catheter with a larger external diameter and a standard end-hole. The Hickman catheter is larger in diameter than the Broviac catheter, but contains two or three lumens. It also has a standard end-hole. When not in use, both of these catheters are clamped to prevent contamination, clotting, and air embolism. These catheters must also be flushed with a saline-heparin solution after every medication administration or at least once daily if not in use. The Groshong catheter contains one to three lumens, each with a rounded, valved tip. The Groshong valve opens inward for blood sampling and outward for infusion, but remains closed when not in use. Because the valve remains closed when not in use, it seals the fluid inside the catheter and prevents it from coming into contact with the patient's blood. Thus, weekly flushing with saline solution is all that is required to keep the catheter patent. The valve also eliminates the need for routine clamping of the catheter, although it should remain capped when not being used.

The **implantable infusion ports** (e.g., Infus-A-Port, Port-A-Cath) are used when long-term therapy is required and intermittent accessing of the central vein is required for administering IV fluids, medications, total parenteral nutrition (TPN), and blood products. The implantable devices are similar in placement to the tunneled devices, except that the proximal end of the single- or double-lumen catheter is attached to a single- or double-lumen access port (Figure 12-6), implanted and sutured into a subcutaneous pocket in the chest area or upper arm. The double ports are designed to allow for administration of two IV solutions, two IV medications, or one of each simultaneously. One port can also be reserved for drawing blood samples. The ports contain a self-sealing silicone rubber septum specifically designed for repeated injections over an extended period. A special noncoring, 90-degree-angle Huber needle is used to penetrate the skin and the septum of the implanted device to minimize damage to the self-sealing septum. To prolong the life of the septum, only the smallest-gauge noncoring needles should be used. The chest port is estimated to withstand up to 2000 punctures, whereas the arm port has an estimated life of 1000 punctures.

A newer port model, the CathLink20 (Figure 12-7), is designed for placement in the upper arm or in the chest of a smaller patient. This port is designed for use

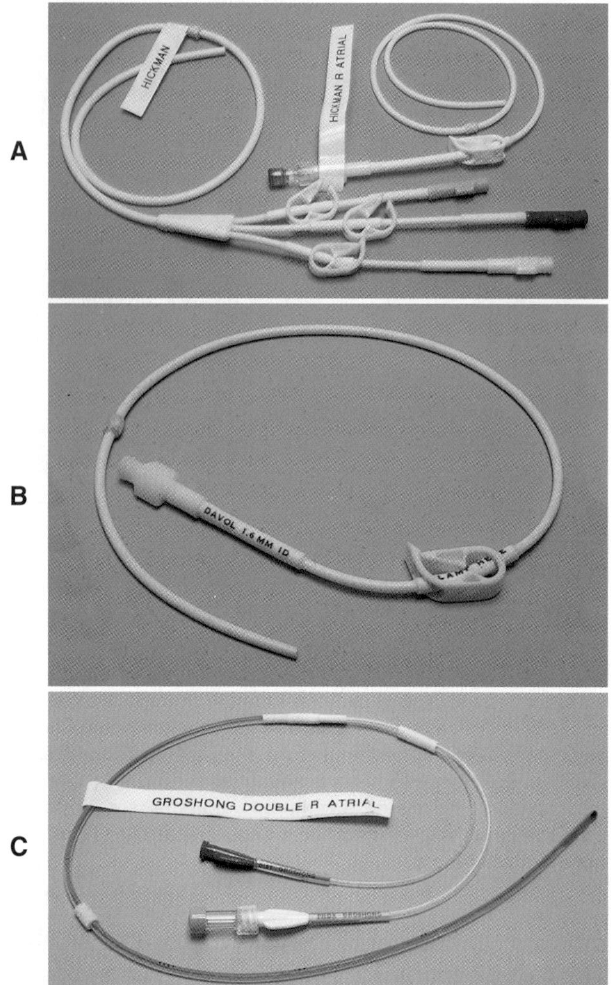

FIGURE **12-5** **A,** Hickman catheter. **B,** Broviac catheter. **C,** Groshong catheter.

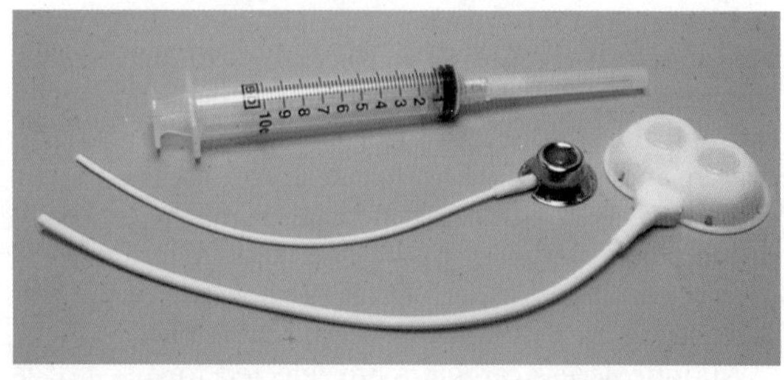

FIGURE **12-6** Silicone venous catheter with infusion ports.

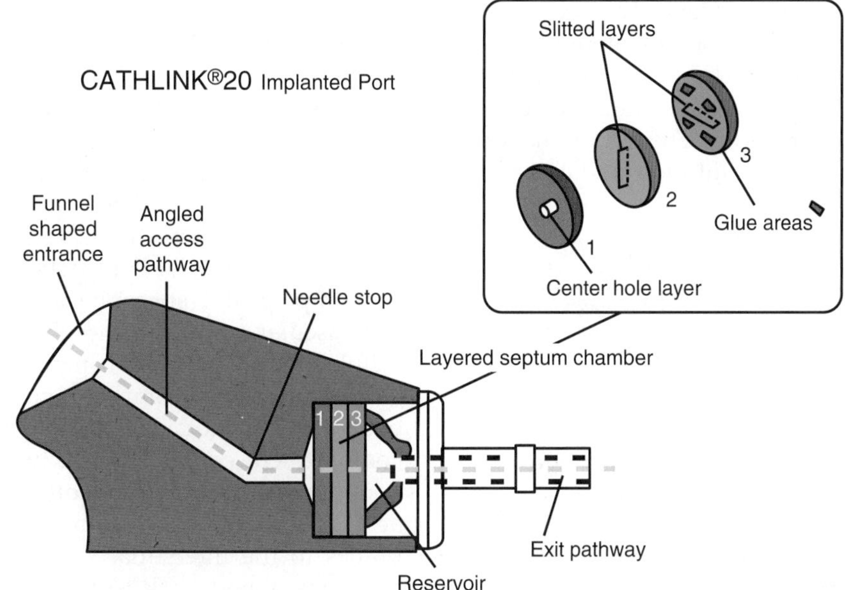

FIGURE 12-7 A newer port model, the CathLink20, is designed for placement in the upper arm or in the chest of smaller patients. This port is designed for use with a standard over-the needle IV catheter rather than 90-degree Huber noncoring needles.

with a standard over-the-needle IV catheter rather than 90-degree Huber noncoring needles. The funnel-shaped entrance to the port guides the over-the-needle catheter assembly into the angled access pathway to the needle stop. The needle cannot pass beyond the needle stop area, but once the needle is retracted, the flexible catheter tip is advanced farther through the layered septum. The septum helps maintain sterility of the catheter, and the angled access pathway and the septum stabilize and anchor the catheter.

An implanted central venous access catheter may remain in place for more than a year and requires only a saline-heparin solution flush after every access or once monthly. Because the entire port and catheter are under the skin, there is no daily maintenance, although the site should be viewed regularly to check for swelling, redness, or drainage. This type of central venous catheter gives the patient the greatest flexibility in terms of daily activities and exercise, including swimming, although contact sports should be avoided.

All central venous access devices require a postinsertion x-ray to verify the location of the device and to check for the presence of a pneumothorax with catheters tunneled on the chest. The CDC recommends that central venous catheters not be routinely replaced to prevent catheter-related infection.

INTRAVENOUS DOSE FORMS

Objectives

1. Differentiate among isotonic, hypotonic, and hypertonic intravenous solutions.
2. Explain the usual circumstances for administering isotonic, hypotonic, and hypertonic IV solutions.
3. Describe the three intravascular compartments and the distribution of body water among them.
4. Describe the different types of large-volume solution containers.

Key Terms

- intravenous (IV) solutions
- electrolytes
- intravascular compartment
- isotonic
- hypotonic
- hypertonic
- tandem setup, piggyback (IVPB), or IV rider

Review Chapter 10 for use of ampules, vials, and Mix-O-Vials. All parenteral drug dose forms are packaged so that the drug is sterile and ready for reconstitution (if needed) and administration.

Types of Intravenous Solutions

Under normal, healthy conditions, the body loses water and electrolytes (see definition following) daily through urine, perspiration, and feces; fluids are replenished by absorption of water in the gastrointestinal (GI) tract from the liquids and foods that are consumed. In many disease states (e.g., vomiting, diarrhea, GI suctioning, hemorrhage, drainage from a wound, decreased intake, nausea, anorexia, fever, excess loss from disease [e.g., uncontrolled diabetes mellitus, diabetes insipidus]), however, patients are unable to ingest sufficient quantities of fluid and electrolytes to offset losses. When this happens, intravenous infusion of solutions may be necessary for replacement. See a medical-surgical textbook for patient assessments for deficient fluid volume.

Intravenous (IV) solutions (Table 12-1) consist of water (the solvent) containing one or more types of dissolved particles (solutes). The solutes most commonly dissolved in IV solutions are sodium chloride, dextrose, and potassium chloride. The solutes that dissolve in water and dissociate into ion particles (e.g., Na^+ and Cl^-, K^+, and Cl^-) are called **electrolytes** because these ions give water the ability to conduct electricity. Total parenteral solutions contain all electrolytes, plus carbohydrates (usually dextrose), amino acids, and fatty acids to sustain life.

Table 12-1 *Types of Intravenous Solutions**

SOLUTION	INGREDIENTS	ABBREVIATION
Electrolyte solutions	5% Dextrose in water	D5W
	10% Dextrose in water	D10W
	0.45% Sodium Chloride	0.45 NS
	0.9% Sodium chloride (normal saline)	NS
	Lactated Ringer's solution	LR
	5% Dextrose in 0.2% sodium chloride	D5/0.2 NS
	5% Dextrose in 0.45% sodium chloride	D5/0.45 NS
	5% Dextrose in 0.9% sodium chloride	D5/0.9 NS
	5% Dextrose in lactated Ringer's solution	D5/LR
	5% Dextrose in 0.2% sodium chloride + 20 mEq potassium chloride	D5/0.2 NS + 20 KCl
Nutrient solutions		
• Carbohydrate	Dextrose 5%-25%	D5-25
• Amino acids	Novamine	
	Aminosyn	
	Travasol	
	ProcalAmine	
	NephrAmine	
	TrophAmine	
	BranchAmin	
	HepatAmine	
• Lipids	Intralipid	
	Liposyn	
Blood volume expanders	Hetastarch	
	Dextran	
	Albumin	
	Plasma	
Alkalinizing solutions	Sodium bicarbonate	
	Tromethamine	THAM
	Citrate citric acid solutions	
	Sodium lactate	
Acidifying solutions	Ammonium chloride	

*A representative listing, not intended to be inclusive.

From a physiologic standpoint, the water in the body is distributed among three compartments: the **intravascular compartment** (arteries, veins, capillaries), the intracellular compartment, and the interstitial compartment (spaces between the cells, outside of the vascular compartment) (Figure 12-8). The extracellular compartment is composed of the intravascular and interstitial compartments and contains about one third of the total body water, and the intracellular compartment contains about two thirds of the total body water. The spontaneous movement of water across the intravascular compartment capillary membranes to the interstitial spaces and across the cell membranes and back to the intravascular capillary space is called osmosis. The water moves from an area of high concentration of water (low electrolyte concentration) to an area of low water concentration (high electrolyte concentration). The electrolyte and protein content of each compartment is what draws water into the compartment until there is an equilibrium between compartments. The force caused by the electrolytes and proteins is called osmotic pressure. The concentration of the dissolved particles in each compartment is known as the osmolality. Normal blood serum osmolality is 295 to 310 milliosmoles/liter (mOsm/L). Because IV solutions also contain dissolved particles, they also have an osmolality. If the IV solution and the blood have approximately the same osmolality, the solution is said to be **isotonic.** Solutions that have fewer dissolved particles than the blood are known as being **hypotonic,** and those with a higher concentration of dissolved particles are considered to be **hypertonic** solutions. A 0.9% solution of sodium chloride, also known as normal saline or physiologic saline, is an isotonic solution with an osmolality of 308 mOsm/L. See Table 12-2 for commonly used IV solutions, their electrolyte concentrations,

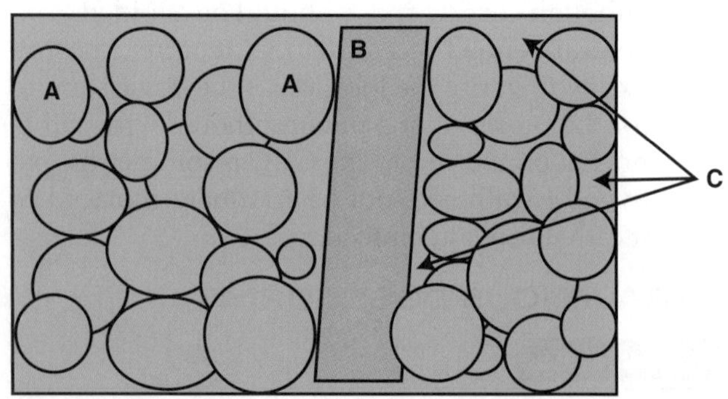

FIGURE 12-8 Fluid compartments of the body. *A*, Intracellular, *B*, vascular (within arteries, veins, capillaries), and *C*, interstitial spaces (spaces between cells). The body maintains a water and electrolyte balance between the compartments for homeostasis.

and osmolality. Those solutions with an osmolality between approximately 295 and 310 mOsm/L and less are considered hypotonic, and those above are hypertonic.

Isotonic solutions (e.g., 0.9% sodium chloride, lactated Ringer's [LR]) are ideal replacement fluids for the patient with an intravascular fluid deficit (e.g., acute blood loss from hemorrhage, GI bleeding, or from an accident). This type of fluid is used for hypovolemic, hypotensive patients to increase vascular volume to support blood pressure; however, patients must be monitored for fluid overload (potentially pulmonary edema), especially if the patient has congestive heart failure. Another isotonic solution, dextrose 5% with 0.2% sodium chloride (D5/0.2NS), is a standard solution for maintaining hydration and electrolytes (e.g., potassium chloride), administering continuous infusion IV medications, and to keep open (TKO) IV therapy for intermittent administration of medications. D5/0.2NS solutions are infused as isotonic solutions, but rapidly become hypotonic solutions as the dextrose is metabolized. Therefore D5/0.2NS solutions, even though initially isotonic, should not be used to maintain vascular volume in a patient who is hypovolemic and hypotensive.

Hypotonic solutions (e.g., 0.2% or 0.45% sodium chloride) have lower osmolality than the serum. This type of solution contains fewer electrolytes and more "free water," so the water is rapidly pulled from the vascular compartment into the interstitial and intracellular fluid compartments. Although these solutions are useful in conditions of cellular dehydration, administering them too rapidly might cause a sudden shift of fluids being drawn from the intravascular space into the other compartments.

Hypertonic *solutions* have an osmolality higher than the serum. Whereas hypotonic and isotonic solutions are used in particular situations because of their tonicity, hypertonic solutions are rarely used in this way, because hypertonic solutions have the potential to pull fluid from the intracellular and interstitial compartments into the intravascular compartment, causing cellular dehydration and vascular volume overload. Hypertonic solutions also have the disadvantage of causing phlebitis and spasm with infiltration and extravasation in peripheral veins. In general, solutions with osmolality greater than approximately 600 to 700 mOsm/L should not be administered in peripheral veins. Hypertonic solutions (e.g., parenteral nutrition solutions) must be administered though central infusion lines where the solution can be rapidly diluted by large volumes of rapidly flowing blood, such as that in the superior vena cava, near the entrance to the right atrium.

Large-Volume Solution Containers

IV solutions are available in both plastic and glass containers in a variety of types and concentrations (see Table 12-1; Table 12-2) and volumes ranging from 100 to 2000 mL. Both the glass and plastic containers are vacuum sealed. The glass bottles are sealed with a hard rubber stopper, then a metal disk, followed by a metal cap. Right before use, the metal cap and disk are removed, exposing the hard rubber stopper. The insertion spike of the IV administration set is pushed into a specifically marked area on the rubber stopper. Some brands also have another opening in the rubber stopper that serves as an air vent (see Figure 12-1, *A* and *C*). As the solution runs out of the container, it is replaced with air. Other brands use a flexible plastic container (see Figure 12-1, *B*). As the solution runs out of the bag, the flexible container collapses.

Plastic bags are somewhat different in that the entire bag and solution is sealed inside another plastic bag for removal just before administration. When the insertion spike is forced into the specially marked portal, an internal seal is broken, allowing the solution to flow into the tubing.

Small-Volume Solution Containers

Some medicines, such as antibiotics, are administered by intermittent infusion through an apparatus known as a **tandem setup, piggyback (IVPB),** or **IV rider** (Figure 12-9). These medicines are given by a setup that is hung in tandem and connected to the primary setup. The secondary setup may consist of a drug infusion from a small volume of fluid in a small bag or bottle (up to 250 mL) (see Figure 12-9) or a volume-control set (also known as a Volutrol or Buretrol) (see

Table 12-2 ***Intravenous Solutions, Electrolyte Concentrations, and Osmolality***

SOLUTION	Na^+ (mEq/L)	Cl^- (mEq/L)	GLUCOSE (g/L)	OSMOLALITY (mOsm/L)
0.2 NS	34	34	0	77
0.45 NS	77	77	0	154
0.9 NS	154	154	0	308
D5/0.2	34	34	50	320
D5/0.45	77	77	50	405
D5/0.9	154	154	50	560
Lactated Ringer's solution*	130	109	0	273

*K^+ = 4; lactate =28; Ca^{++} = 3.

Figure 12-1, *A* and *C*). A volume-control set is composed of a calibrated chamber hung under the primary IV solution container that can provide the necessary 50 to 250 mL of diluent per dose of drug. Most intermittent diluted-drug infusions are infused over 20 to 60 minutes.

ADMINISTRATION OF MEDICATIONS BY THE INTRAVENOUS ROUTE

Objectives

1. Identify the dose forms available, the types of sites of administration, and general principles of administering medications via the IV route.
2. List criteria used for the selection of an IV access site.
3. Describe the correct techniques for administering medications by means of an established peripheral or central IV line, a heparin lock, an IV bag, a bottle or volume-control device, or through a secondary piggyback set.
4. Describe the recommended guidelines and procedures for IV catheter care (including proper maintenance of patency of IV lines and implanted access devices), IV line dressing changes, and for peripheral and central venous IV needle or catheter changes.

Key Terms

SASH guideline

Dose Forms

Medications for IV administration are available in ampules, vials, prefilled syringes, and large-volume IV solution bags. Be certain that the label specifically states that the medication is "for IV use." IV fluid and electrolyte solutions come in a variety of volumes and concentrations in glass or plastic containers (see Table 12-1).

Equipment

Gloves
Tourniquet
Administration set with appropriate needle or needleless connector, drip chamber, and filter
Medication
Physiologic solution ordered
Sterile dressing materials
Antiseptic solution
Syringe and needle or needleless connector (if giving by bolus)

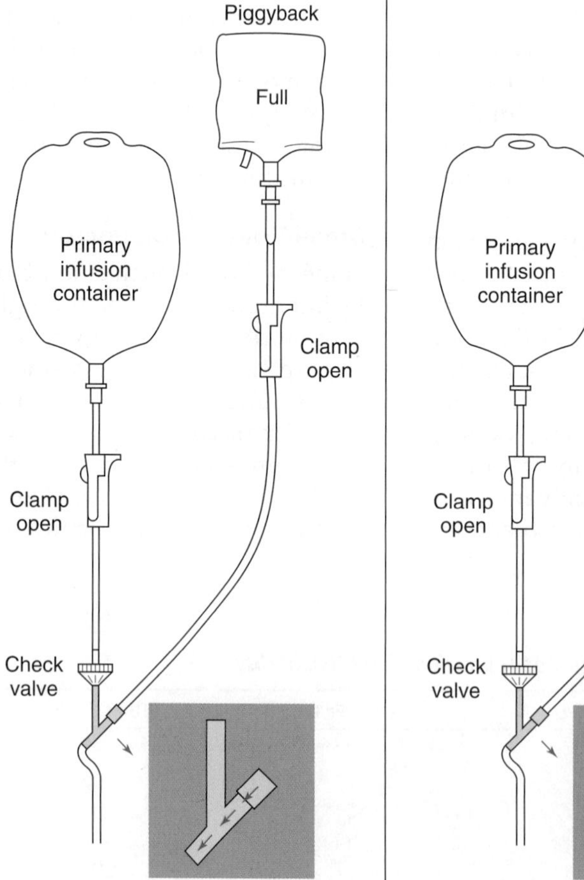

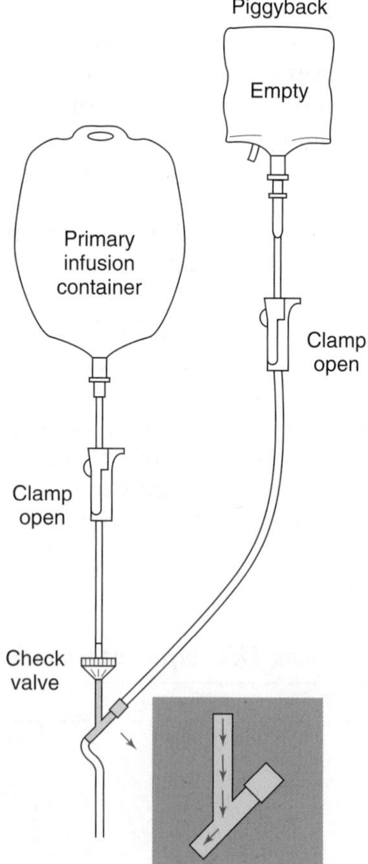

FIGURE 12-9 Tandem, secondary, or piggyback intermittent administration setup. A piggyback setup is shown. Note that the smaller bag is hung higher than the primary bag.

Heparin (saline) lock adapter
Armboard
Tape
Standard IV pole or rod
Heparin (saline) solution, piggyback, and additional solutions as appropriate

Additional supplies may be required to access, flush, change IV administration sets, inline filters or dressings, depending on the type of peripheral, central, or implantable device being used.

Sites

Peripheral IV Access

When selecting an IV site, consider the length of time the IV will be required; condition and location of veins; purpose of infusion, for example, rehydration, delivery of nutritional needs (TPN), chemotherapy, and antibiotics; and patient status, cooperation, and patient preference for and amount of self-care of the injection site (if appropriate).

Peripheral IV devices include wing-tipped needle (see Figure 12-3), over-the-needle catheter (see Figure 12-4, *A*), and inside-the-needle catheter (see Figure 12-4, *B*). The over-the-needle catheters are the most commonly used venous access system used to enter peripheral veins.

If a prolonged course of treatment is anticipated, start the first IV in the hand (Figure 12-10). The metacarpal veins, dorsal vein network, cephalic, and basilic vein are commonly used. To avoid irritation and leakage from a previous puncture site, the subsequent venipuncture sites should be made above the earlier site. See Figure 12-11 for the veins of the forearm area that could be used for additional venipuncture sites.

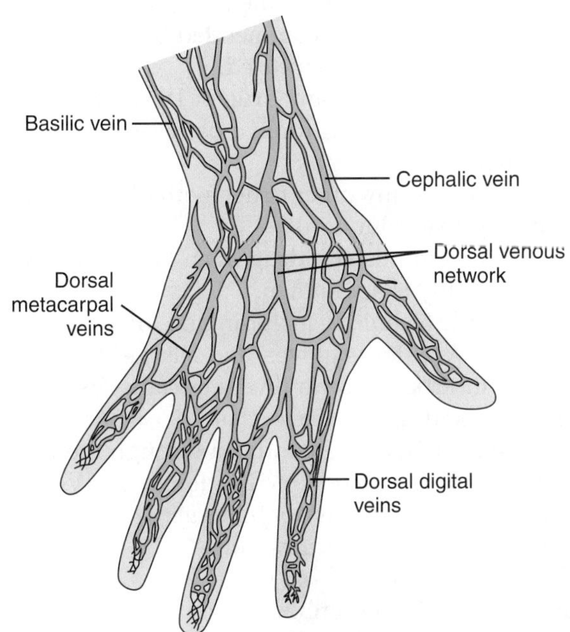

FIGURE **12-10** IV sites on the hand.

Central IV Access

Central IV access devices (see p. 179) are used when the purpose of therapy dictates (e.g., large volume, high concentration, or hypertonic solutions are to be infused); when peripheral sites have been exhausted because of repeated use or condition of veins for access is poor; when long-term or home therapy is required; and when emergency condition mandates adequate vascular access.

The central veins most commonly used for central venous catheters are the subclavian and jugular veins. When upper body veins are not acceptable, the femoral veins may be accessed for short-term or emergency use.

General Principles of Intravenous Medication Administration

- The nurse shall have passed a skill competency that demonstrates knowledge of the IV administration procedure.
- If it is institution policy to use a local anesthetic to anesthetize the IV site before insertion, the nurse must determine allergies to anesthetic agents.
- Use appropriate barrier precautions (universal blood and body fluid precautions) to prevent transmission of any infectious diseases, including human immunodeficiency virus (HIV), as recommended by the CDC.
- Gloves should be worn throughout the venipuncture procedure. Care should be taken to wash the skin surface if the area is contaminated with blood.
- When the procedure is complete, remove the gloves and dispose of them in accordance with the policies of the practice setting. Wash your hands thoroughly as soon as the gloves are removed. Care should be taken not to contaminate the IV tubing and rate regulator.
- Any used needles, syringes, venipuncture catheters, or vascular access devices should be placed in a puncture-resistant container in the immediate vicinity for disposal according to the policies of the practice setting.
- Never recap, bend, or break used needles because of the danger of inadvertently puncturing the skin.
- Whenever possible, use needle protector systems such as blunt needles/injection ports, needle sheaths, or needleless systems to prevent inadvertent needlesticks and risk of introducing pathogens into oneself.
- Be certain medications to be administered intravenously are thoroughly dissolved in the correct volume and type of solution. Always follow the manufacturer's recommendations.
- Most clinical practice sites now use transparent dressings over the IV insertion site that are changed in accordance with hospital policies, generally every 72 hours. Some clinical practice sites still use gauze dressings. When gauze is used, the four edges

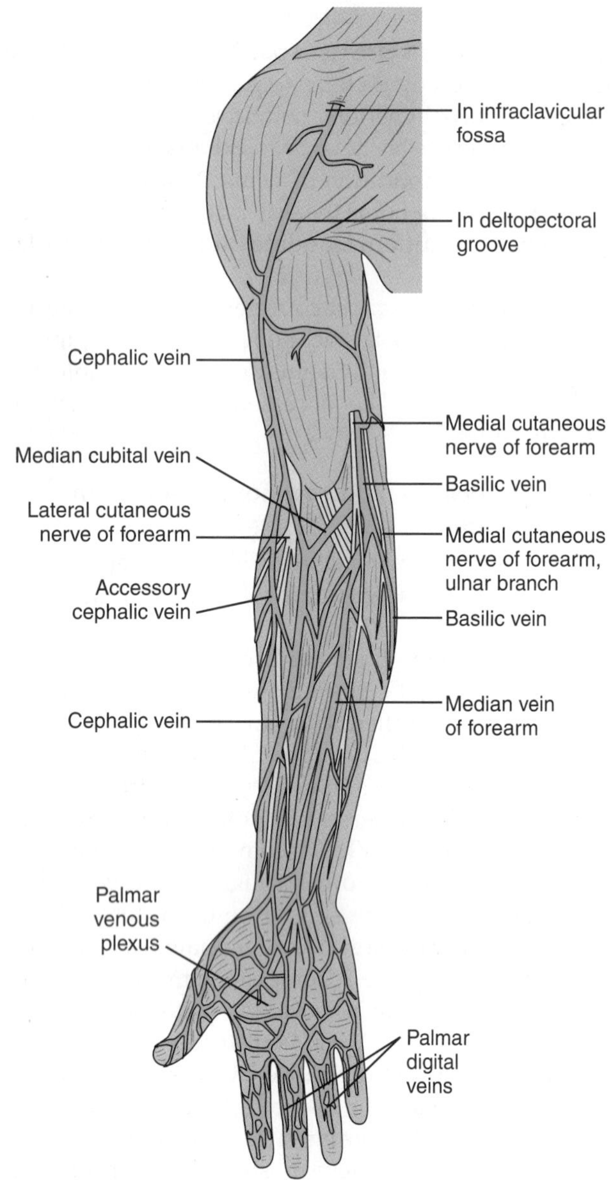

FIGURE **12-11** Veins in the forearm used as IV sites.

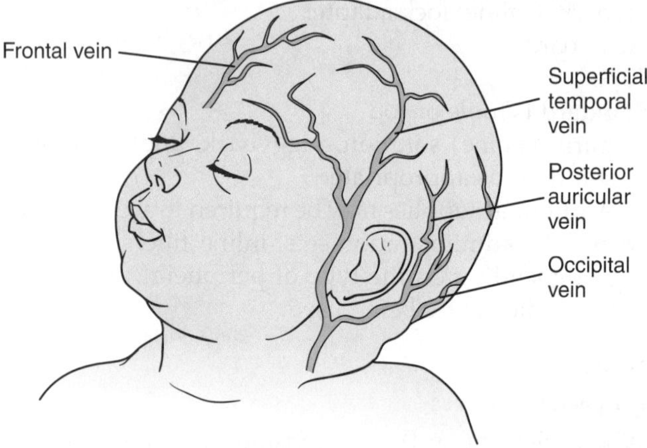

FIGURE **12-12** Veins in infants and children used as IV sites.

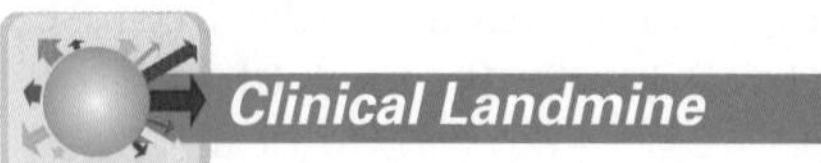

Clinical Landmine

- Note: Never start an IV in an artery!
- Whenever possible, initiate the IV in the nondominant arm.
- Do not initiate an IV in an arm with compromised lymphatic or venous flow such as mastectomy or axillary node dissection or in an extremity with a dialysis/pheresis catheter or shunt inserted.
- Avoid the use of blood vessels over bony prominences or joints unless absolutely necessary.
- In the older adult, using the veins in the hand area may be a poor choice because of the fragility of the skin and veins in this area.
- Veins commonly used in infants and children for IV administration are on the back of the hand, dorsum of the foot, or the temporal region of the scalp (Figure 12-12).
- When possible, avoid using the veins of the lower extremities because of the danger of developing thrombi and emboli.

of the dressing should be sealed with tape. To prevent skin irritation, place tincture of benzoin on the skin directly under the edge of the gauze and allow it to dry before applying the dressing tape. Always check the specific policies of the employing institution, as well as the health care provider's orders for frequency of dressing changes.

- Do not use topical antibiotic ointment or creams on insertion sites (except when using dialysis catheters) because of the potential to promote fungal infections and antimicrobial resistance.
- At the time of the dressing change on any type of IV site, the area should be thoroughly inspected for any drainage, redness, tenderness, irritation, or swelling. The presence of any of these symptoms should be reported to the health care provider immediately. (Also take the patient's vital signs and report these at the same time.)
- Use inline filters as recommended by the manufacturer of the drug to be infused.
- DO NOT administer any drug or IV solution that is hazy or cloudy or has foreign particles or a precipitate in it.
- DO NOT mix any other drugs with blood or blood products (e.g., albumin).
- DO NOT administer a drug in an IV solution if the compatibility is not known.
- Use aseptic technique including use of a cap, mask, sterile gown, sterile gloves, and a large sterile sheet for the insertion of central venous catheters (including PICCs) or guidewire exchange.
- Drugs must be entirely infused through the IV line before adding a second medication to the IV line.
- Drugs given by IV push or bolus generally are given following the **SASH guideline:**

  Saline flush first
  Administer the prescribed drug
  Saline flush following the drug
  Heparin flush line, depending on type of line, such as a Hickman catheter (check institution policy)

- Once mixed, know the length of time an agent remains stable; all unused IV solutions should be returned to the pharmacy if not used within 24 hours.
- Check the hospital policy for the definition of TKO. It is usually interpreted as *an infusion rate of 10 mL/hr* and should infuse less than 500 mL/24 hr.
- Shade IV solutions that contain drugs that should be protected from light (e.g., certain hyperalimentation solutions, amphotericin B, nitroprusside).
- All IV solution bag/bottles should be changed every 24 hours (check hospital policy) to minimize the development of new infections. Label all IV solutions with the date and time initiated and the nurse's initials. DO NOT use marking pens directly on plastic IV containers because the ink may penetrate the plastic into the IV solution.
- IV administration sets used to deliver blood or blood products should be changed after the unit is administered. Sets used to infuse lipids or TPN should be changed every 24 hours. Administration sets used only for physiologic IV fluids (e.g., D5/0.2NS) may be changed every 72 hours (check hospital policy). The sets/tubing must be labeled with the date and time initiated, the date to change the set, and the nurse's initials.
- Whenever a patient is receiving IV fluids, monitor intake and output accurately. Report declining hourly outputs and those of less than 30 to 40 mL/hr.
- Never "speed up" an IV flow rate to "catch up" when the volume to be infused has fallen behind. In certain cases this could be dangerous. The health care provider should be consulted, particularly with patients who have cardiac, renal, or circulatory impairment.

Preparing an Intravenous Solution for Infusion

Dose Form

Check the health care provider's order for the specific IV solution ordered and for any medication to be added to the container. If not already prepared by the pharmacy, check the accuracy of the drug order against the medication and/or solution being prepared at least three times during the preparation phase: (1) when first removing the drug/solution from the storage area, (2) immediately after preparation, and (3) immediately before administration. Check the expiration date on any additives and the primary solution. If an IV medication is to be added, ensure that the drug is approved for administration by nurses.

Perform preintravenous access assessments.

Equipment

Administration set with appropriate drip chamber (microdrip or macrodrip) (see Figure 12-2), needle, IV catheter, and inline filter (if used); the primary line administration set is usually labeled "universal" or "continuous flow"

IV start set/kit (antiseptic pads, nonsterile gloves, site labels, tape, transparent dressing materials, tourniquet)

Medications for IV delivery and label

Physiologic solution ordered

IV pole or IV pump

Sites

The most commonly used veins for IV administration in infants and children are in the temporal region of the scalp, back of hand, and dorsum of the foot.

Technique

1. Assemble equipment and thoroughly wash your hands.
2. Check the vein for the size and type of needle required to access the vein selected for venipuncture or for the type of needle required to access an implanted access device for the delivery of the IV solution or medication.
3. Check the health care provider's order against the physiologic solution chosen for administration.
4. Inspect the IV container for cloudiness, discoloration, or the presence of any precipitate. Verify the expiration date on the IV fluid container.
5. Remove the plastic cover from the IV container and inspect the plastic IV bag to be certain it is intact; squeeze gently to detect any punctures. Inspect a glass container of IV solution for any cracks.
6. Choose the administration set appropriate for the type of solution ordered, the rate of delivery requested (microdrip or macrodrip), and for the type of IV container being used. Plastic bag IV containers DO NOT require an air vent in the administration set. Glass containers for IV delivery must be vented or have an administration set with an air filter vent in it. Remove the administration set from its container and inspect for any faults or contamination.
7. Move the roller or slide clamp to the upper portion of the IV line 6 to 8 inches from the drip chamber; close the clamp.
8. *Plastic IV bags:* Remove the tab from the spike receiver port; remove the tab from the administration set spike; insert the spike firmly into the bag port. Maintain sterility of port and spike throughout the process.

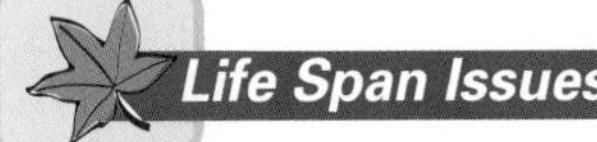

Intravenous Sites

The most commonly used veins for IV administration in infants and children are in the temporal region of the scalp, back of hand, and dorsum of the foot.

Glass IV bottle: Peel back the metal tab and lift the protective metal disk from the container; remove the latex-type covering (if present) from the top of the rubber stopper. As the latex diaphragm is removed, a sudden noise should be heard as the vacuum within the glass container is released. If the noise is not heard, the contents of the IV container may not be sterile and should be discarded. Remove the tab from the administration set spike; insert the spike firmly into the port in the rubber stopper. Maintain sterility of the port and spike throughout the process.

Note: When additive medications are ordered, they should be added to the large-volume container before tubing is attached to help ensure a uniform mixing of the medication and the physiologic solution. If medication is added to an existing IV solution, clamp the line before adding the medication to the container and make sure adequate mixing takes place before the infusion is started again. (See technique used for adding a medication to an IV solution, p. 195.)

9. Hang the solution on an IV pole; squeeze the drip chamber, and fill halfway; prime the IV line by removing the protective tab or cap from the distal end of the IV line; invert the back-check valve, open the roller or slide clamp and allow the solution to run until all the air is removed from the line. If using a pump, prime the tubing according to hospital policy. Cover the end of the IV tubing with a sterile cap. Inspect entire length of tubing to be certain all air is removed from line. Place an IV measuring device/tape strip on the plastic bag or glass IV container. Label the container with the patient's name, along with the date and time of preparation. If medication has been added, all details of the medication must be marked on the container's label: drug name, dose, rate of administration requested in health care provider's order, and the nurse's name who prepared IV. The IV tubing is labeled with the date and time it is opened and the date and time to be changed. The CDC recommends that IV tubing should be changed every 72 hours. Administration sets used to deliver blood or blood products may be changed after each unit is infused as defined by institution policy or within 24 hours of initiating the infusion. Lipid solutions have special tubing that should be changed every 24 hours if administered by continuous infusion or after every unit if administered intermittently. Follow institutional policies.

   Note: It may be necessary to add inline filters to the setup if recommended for the administration of the medication ordered. Purge air from the line before attaching the filter.

10. The IV solution can now be taken to the bedside for attachment after a venipuncture is performed or for addition to an existing IV system. For safety, all aspects of the IV order should be checked again immediately before attaching the IV for infusion.

    Note: Always identify the patient by checking the bracelet before initiating any procedure. Have the patient state his or her name and birth date or other identifiers.

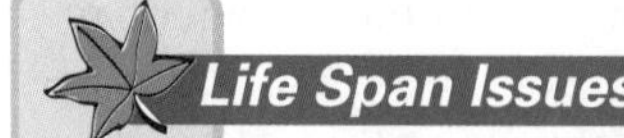

Intravenous Fluid Monitoring

The infusion of IV fluids necessitates careful monitoring for patients of all ages. The microdrip chamber, which delivers 60 drops (gtt)/mL is used whenever a small volume of IV solution is ordered to be infused over a specific time. Many clinical sites interpret a small volume as less than 100 mL/hr. In pediatric units, volume-control chamber devices, such as a Buretrol or SoluSet, and syringe pump controllers are commonly used to regulate the volume of fluid infused.

INTRAVENOUS FLUID MONITORING

The infusion of IV fluids necessitates careful monitoring for patients of all ages. The microdrip chamber, which delivers 60 drops (gtt)/mL, is used whenever a small volume of IV solution is ordered to be infused over a specific time. Many clinical sites interpret a small volume as less than 100 mL/hr. In pediatric units, controlled-volume chamber devices, such as a Buretrol or SoluSet, and syringe pump controllers are commonly used to regulate the volume infused.

BASIC GUIDELINES OF INTRAVENOUS ADMINISTRATION OF MEDICINES

Equipment

Medication administration record (MAR)
Drug in sterile, sealed container
Syringe of the correct volume
Needles of the correct gauge and length
Antiseptic swab
Special equipment based on the route of administration, such as a radiopaque, over-the-needle catheter for insertion, and IV administration set for starting IV infusion

Premedication Assessments

1. Know basic patient data, diagnosis, symptoms of disorder or disease process for which the medication is ordered, and the desired action of the drug for this specific individual.
2. Obtain baseline vital signs.
3. Check for any drug allergies or prior drug reactions.
4. Check the accuracy of the drug order against the medication or solution being prepared at least three times during the preparation phase: (1) when first removing the drug/solution from the storage area; (2) immediately after preparation; and (3) immediately before administration.
5. Check the expiration date on the solution.

6. Review the individual drug monograph to identify laboratory studies recommended before or intermittently during therapy, calculation of dose, side effects to expect and side effects to report, monitoring parameters recommended for the specific drug prescribed, and so on. (With certain light-sensitive medications [e.g., amphotericin B, nitroprusside], it is necessary to shield the IV bag with a dark plastic bag to prevent degradation of the drug.)
7. Know the type of IV access the patient has in place, the date and time of insertion, the type of IV fluid or medication running, and the rate of flow prescribed.

Technique

The standard procedures for preparing all parenteral medications are as follows:

1. Wash your hands *before* preparing any medication or handling sterile supplies. During the actual preparation of a parenteral medication, the primary rule is "sterile-to-sterile" and "unsterile-to-unsterile" when handling the syringe and needle.
2. Use the five RIGHTS of medication preparation and administration throughout the procedure:
   RIGHT PATIENT
   RIGHT DRUG
   RIGHT ROUTE OF ADMINISTRATION
   RIGHT DOSE (AMOUNT AND CONCENTRATION)
   RIGHT TIME OF ADMINISTRATION
3. Check the drug dose form ordered against the source you are holding to prepare.
4. Check compatibility charts or contact the pharmacist before mixing two medications or adding medication to an IV solution.
5. Check medication calculations. When in doubt about a dose, check it with another qualified nurse. (Most hospital policies require fractional doses of medications and doses of heparin and insulin to be checked by two qualified personnel before administration.)
6. Know the hospital policy regarding limitations on the types of medications to be administered by nursing personnel.
7. Prepare the drug in a clean, well-lighted area, using aseptic technique throughout the entire procedure.
8. Concentrate on this procedure; ensure accuracy in preparation.
9. Check expiration date on medication.
10. Before administering a drug IV, the nurse should check the list of drugs approved for administration by nurses in the clinical care setting.

Research the medication ordered as an IV additive (procedure also applies for direct push or bolus administration):

1. Name of drug
2. Usual dose (take into consideration patient's age, weight, and hydration state)
3. Compatibility of drug with existing IVs and drugs infusing
4. For IV push or bolus, does drug need to be diluted or can it be given undiluted (i.e., IV push)? If diluted, what types and amounts of diluent can be used? If being added to an existing IV, is the drug compatible with the primary solution?
5. Recommended rate of infusion

VENIPUNCTURE

Perform the following preintravenous assessments:

- Assess the patient's demeanor. Does the patient appear cooperative or will assistance be needed? (Always have sufficient assistance with pediatric patients.)
- Check for and avoid previously used IV sites, areas of impaired circulation, and any fistulas present in the extremities.
- Examine extremities for potential sites and estimate the size of the veins available for use.

Equipment

IV start set/kit
Antiseptic pads
One pair latex gloves
Site label
Tape
Transparent dressing materials
Two gauze sponges, 2 × 2 inches
One roll transparent tape
Latex tourniquet
One change label
Armboard
As appropriate, medications and/or physiologic solution ordered for IV delivery and IV equipment needed
For a saline/heparin/medlock, obtain correct extension tubing and injection cap, as appropriate; use saline/heparin flush solution in accordance with institution policy. (Use 10-mL syringes containing an appropriate volume of solution for flushing.)
IV pump, if required

Selection of the Catheter or Butterfly Needle

When selecting a catheter or butterfly needle for use, choose the smallest size feasible to administer the specific type of fluid ordered. Catheters are available in 27 gauge, ⅝ inch to 14 gauge, 2½ inches; and the butterfly needles are available in sizes 17 to 29 gauge. A more viscous fluid like blood requires a larger-diameter catheter. As with other needles, the lower the number of the gauge, the larger the diameter of the opening of the catheter. During the assessment process the nurse needs to note the size of the vein to be accessed.

For a pediatric patient, obtain a sheet or blanket for wrapping the child for the procedure.

Prepare the IV solution and/or medication (if ordered) (see pp. 187 to 188).

Technique

1. Assemble equipment and thoroughly wash your hands.
2. Check all aspects of the health care provider's orders.
3. Recheck the size and type of butterfly or catheter needed to access the vein selected, and any extension tubing or injection caps needed to prepare the site for future intermittent or continuous use for the prescribed IV therapy.
4. If ordered, the IV solution and medication should be prepared and taken to the bedside for attachment after a venipuncture is performed. For safety, all aspects of the IV therapy orders should be checked again immediately before initiating the venipuncture and attaching the IV for infusion.
   Note: Always identify the patient by checking the bracelet before initiating any procedure. Have the patient state his or her name and birth date or other identifiers.
5. Take equipment to the bedside.
6. Identify the patient and explain the procedure. Have the patient state his or her name and birth date, or two other identifiers.
7. Position the patient appropriately. Immobilize an infant or child for patient safety, if necessary. (Be sure the patient is wearing the type of hospital gown that has openings on the shoulder seams.)
8. Cut tape for stabilizing the IV catheter/butterfly before starting the procedure. Be careful not to contaminate the tape by placing it on a contaminated surface before use. Turn the ends of the tape back on themselves to form a tab that will not adhere to a glove when the tape is to be applied or removed. The nurse must consider his or her gloves to be contaminated when they come into contact with blood. If the gloves come into contact with the tape and dressing materials used at the venipuncture site, the outside of the dressings and tape are then potentially contaminated. Therefore during the procedure the nurse must focus on allowing contamination only of the dominant gloved hand; the nondominant hand must be maintained as uncontaminated to handle the taping and stabilization of the peripheral access device. Once the needle or catheter is stabilized, the gloves can be removed; wash your hands thoroughly and apply the gauze or occlusive type of dressing materials according to the practice-setting policies.
9. When an extension tubing is used with the catheter or the butterfly needle, fill the extension tubing with saline and purge of all air.
10. Apply the tourniquet using a slipknot 2 to 6 inches above the site chosen (shaded area in Figure 12-13, *A*). Inspect the area to identify a vein of sufficient size to accommodate the catheter and provide adequate anchorage.
11. Put on nonsterile gloves. As the vein dilates, palpate the vein to feel the depth and direction (see Figure 12-13, *B* and *C*). To dilate the vein, it may be necessary to place the extremity in a dependent position; massage the vein against the direction of blood flow; have the patient open and close the hand repeatedly; lightly thump the vein with your fingertips; or remove the tourniquet and apply a heating pad or warm, wet towels to the extremity for 15 to 20 minutes and then restart the process.
12. Cleanse the skin surface with the antiseptic, starting at the site of entry and working outward in a circular motion toward the periphery (see Figure 12-13, *D*). Do not retouch area where the puncture site will be made. (An alternative is to put a sterile glove on one hand so that the site can be touched again, or to prepare the fingertip with antiseptic.)
13. Let the area air dry.
14. Hold the butterfly or catheter to be inserted in the dominant hand and remove the protective cover while maintaining sterility of the catheter and/or butterfly needle. Approach the vein either directly from above or slightly to one side of the vein. Provide tension on the skin surface to stretch the skin and stabilize the vein.
    For peripheral over-the-needle catheter (see Figure 12-4, A):
    - Inspect the IV catheter and loosen the catheter needle by rotating the catheter. Hold the flash chamber with the thumb and forefinger and insert the catheter with needle at a 10- to 30-degree angle (bevel up) (see Figure 12-13, *E*) (check individual manufacturer's product directions for recommended angle of entry) and assess the depth of the vein—the deeper the vein the greater the angle of entry to puncture the skin and venous wall. Watch for blood in flashback chamber; once seen, advance the needle and catheter an additional $\frac{1}{16}$ to $\frac{1}{4}$ inch into the vein. Withdraw the needle from the catheter (see Figure 12-13, *F*), lower the angle of the catheter slightly, and advance the catheter into the vein. Hold the catheter hub in place while applying gentle pressure on the catheter tip to prevent excessive backflow of blood while the needle is removed from the catheter and the catheter and the IV is attached (see Figure 12-13, *G*).

    For butterfly insertion:
    - Prepare site as above. Hold the butterfly needle by the tabs and align the needle, bevel up, with the vein that has been selected. Puncture skin and vein surface as described above. Once the vein is entered, lower the angle and advance the needle into the vein until the tabbed area of the butterfly is adjacent to the puncture site.
15. Release the tourniquet and secure the connection of the IV tubing to the over-the-needle plastic needle hub (see Figure 12-13, *H*) or to the butterfly apparatus.

16. Cleanse the area to eliminate any blood that may have contacted the skin or IV tubing, remove gloves, and anchor the needle and tubing to the arm or hand with tape and dressing as prescribed in the practice setting policy. (Because it is difficult to handle tape with gloves on, it is helpful to have a second person anchor the needle and tubing, and adjust the flow rate.)
17. If no continuously flowing IV is attached, flush the catheter in accordance with institution policy.

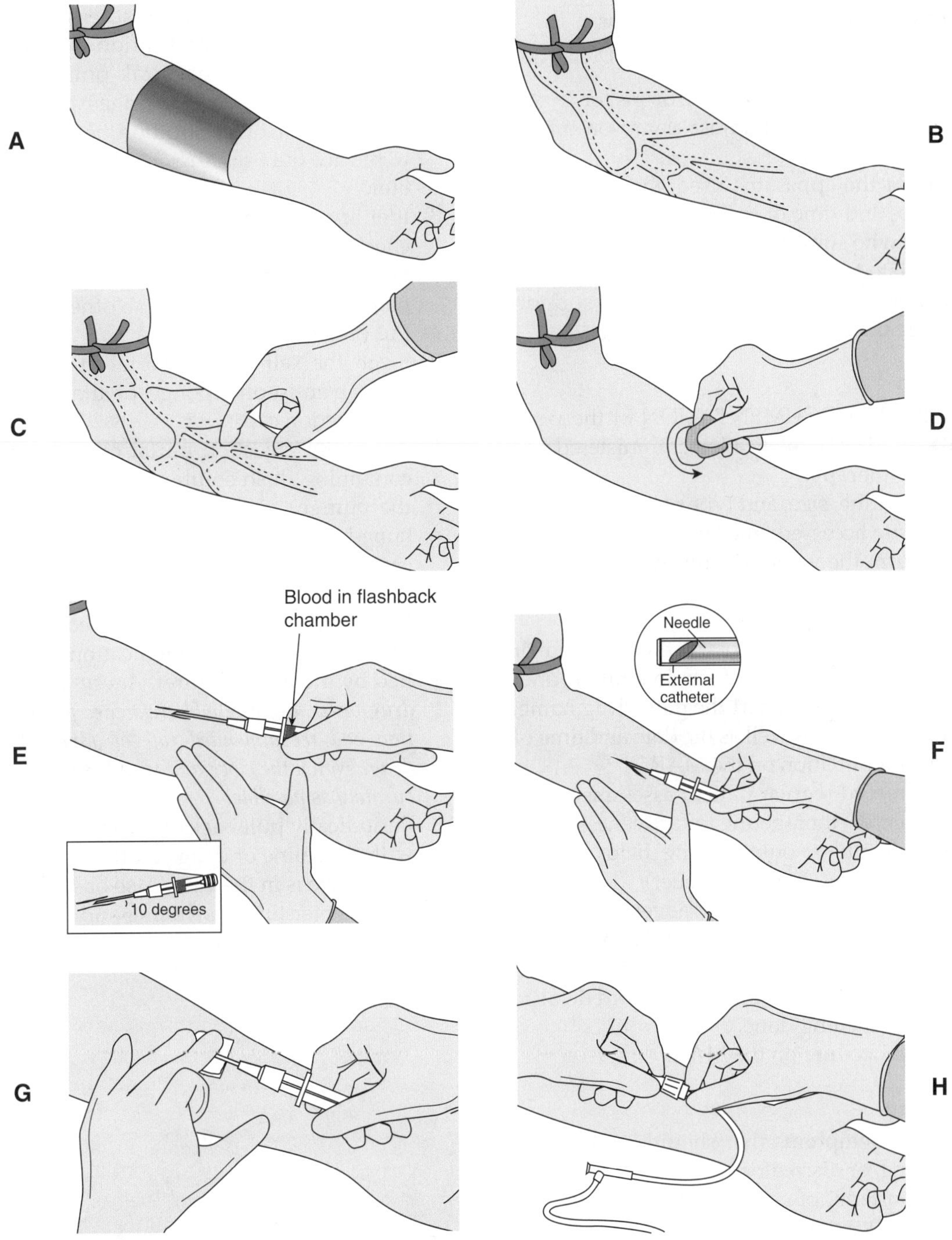

FIGURE **12-13** **A,** Apply tourniquet using a slipknot 2 to 6 inches above the chosen (shaded) area. **B,** Allow the veins to dilate. **C,** Palpate vein to feel depth and direction. **D,** Cleanse the skin surface with an antiseptic, starting at the anticipated site of entry and working outward in a circular motion to the periphery. **E,** For the over-the-needle catheter, hold the flash chamber with the thumb and forefinger and insert the catheter with the needle at a 10- to 30-degree angle (or at the angle as directed in specific manufacturer's directions) with the bevel up. **F,** Withdraw the needle from the catheter. **G,** Apply gentle pressure over the catheter tip to prevent excessive backflow of blood while the needle is removed and the IV is attached. **H,** Secure connection of IV tubing to hub of catheter.

18. The individual performing the venipuncture can dispose of all soiled dressings and contaminated supplies according to the practice setting's policy.
19. Remove gloves and wash your hands thoroughly.
20. Adjust the rate of flow solution or set the rate on the pump.

$$\frac{\text{mL of solution}}{\text{Hours of administration}} \times \frac{\text{Number of drops/mL}}{\text{60 minutes/hr}} = \text{Drops/min}$$

21. Regulate the flow by counting the drops for 15 seconds, multiply by 4, and adjust clamp on tubing for the appropriate rate.
22. Regardless of the apparatus used, mark the label with the date and time of insertion and the initials of the nurse who started it
23. As appropriate to age, site, and orientation of the individual, attach a padded armboard to support and stabilize the infusion site.

Documentation

Provide the RIGHT DOCUMENTATION of the venipuncture: IV started or IV medication administered and response to drug therapy:

1. Chart the date, time, size, and type of butterfly or IV catheter, the site accessed, and number of attempts made to perform the venipuncture. Make entries in appropriate IV site flow sheets used in the clinical site.
2. Chart the type and amount of IV fluid started or added to an existing line; rate of administration; and, if medication was added chart the date, drug name, amount added (dose), as well as the date and time of preparation and initiation on the MAR.
3. Perform and record regular patient assessments for the evaluation of therapeutic effectiveness (e.g., blood pressure, pulse, output, lung field sounds, and degree and duration of pain relief).
4. Chart any signs and symptoms of adverse effects to drugs given or problems encountered during the venipuncture procedure. If more than one attempt was required to perform the venipuncture, record details.
5. Record patient teaching done.
6. Record flush procedure on the MAR.

Patient Teaching

Teach the patient symptoms that should be reported (e.g., pain, swelling, or discomfort) at the insertion site.

1. Stress the importance of not trying to self-adjust the rate of an IV or IV medications being administered.
2. Explain the purposes of the dressing on the IV site and the need to leave it intact.

Administration of Medication by a Heparin/Saline/Medlock (Figure 12-14)

Perform premedication assessments. See individual drug monograph.

1. Select a syringe several milliliters larger than that required by the volume of the drug. This allows room for aspiration of blood to ensure proper placement of the needle or catheter in the vein and to allow blood to mix with the drug solution. Place a needleless access device on the syringe, or syringe is used in needleless system.
2. Research and prepare the medication as described earlier. Prepare saline and/or heparin in syringes with needleless access devices to flush before and after medication administration, in accordance with hospital policy. It is recommended that 10-mL syringes containing a few milliliters of flush solution be used for flushing to reduce the pressure exerted in the vein or catheter.
3. Identify the patient by checking the bracelet; recheck the medication order and explain what you are going to do. Have the patient state his or her name and birth date, or two other identifiers.
4. Put on gloves.
5. Swab the self-sealing portal of the injection site with an antiseptic sponge, or attach the syringe via the injection cap.
6. Access the injection portal or cap with a syringe containing flush solution and gently pull back on the plunger for blood return. If return is not obtained or resistance is felt, stop and evaluate the cause. Do not force insertion of the solution or a clot could be dislodged.
7. When blood return is established, inject saline for flush followed by the medication at the rate specified by the manufacturer. *Always carefully check the drug order and a reliable reference for the proper dilution and recommended rate of administration of the drug. Watch the clock and time the injection rate as accurately as possible!*
8. Periodically pull back on the plunger to mix blood with the saline or drug solution and to ensure that the needle is in the vein. Also observe the IV site at the catheter tip for swelling and monitor for complaints of discomfort.

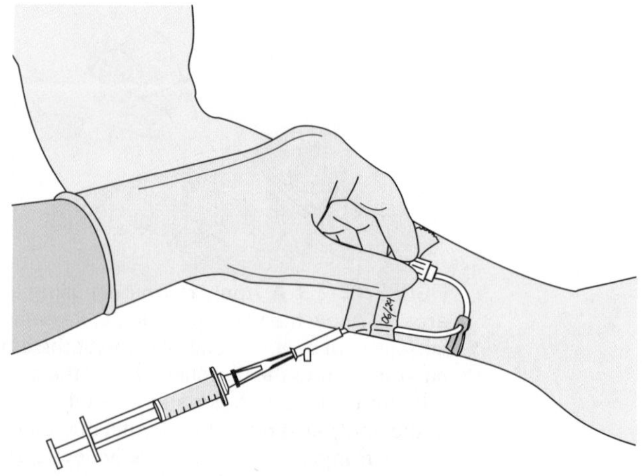

FIGURE 12-14 Heparin/saline/medlock with an extension tubing taped in place ready for access.

9. After administration, withdraw the needleless device from the diaphragm and dispose of it in a sharps safety container.
10. Access the injection cap, insert another syringe containing (usually) 1 to 2 mL of normal saline to flush the remaining drug from the catheter.
11. *Optional:* In accordance with hospital policy, flush the lock with 1 mL of heparin (10 to 100 Units/mL). Maintain constant pressure on the plunger of the syringe while simultaneously withdrawing the needle from the diaphragm to prevent backflow of blood. Always verify the heparin dose with another qualified nurse.
12. Cleanse the site of any blood or fluids. Remove gloves and dispose of properly. Wash your hands thoroughly. Dispose of equipment according to Occupational Safety and Health Administration (OSHA) standards.

The heparin/saline/medlock should be flushed when initially placed, after administering medications, after withdrawing blood samples, or every 8 hours if medications are not administered more frequently. Check the hospital policy to determine how long a lock may remain in place before changing it. Monitor the venipuncture site as you would any other venipuncture site.

Documentation

In the patient's MAR, document date, time, drug, dosage, rate of administration, and assessment data obtained such as how well the procedure was tolerated.

Patient Teaching

Explain to the patient the purpose of the medication administered and any side effects that should be reported.

Administration of Medications into an Established Intravenous Line (IV Bolus)

Perform premedication assessments. See individual drug monograph.

1. Research, then prepare the medication as described earlier. Ensure that the drug to be prepared is compatible with the IV solution currently being infused. Always carefully check the drug order and a reliable reference for the proper dilution and recommended rate of administration of the drug. Many medications ordered as IV push or bolus must be administered slowly over several minutes. An excessive rate of administration can result in shock and cardiac arrest.

Life Span Issues

Benzyl Alcohol Preservative

Do not use bacteriostatic water or saline containing the benzyl alcohol preservative to reconstitute or dilute medications or to flush IV catheters of newborns because the preservative is toxic to these patients.

2. Identify the patient by checking the bracelet, and explain what you are going to do. Have the patient state his or her name and birth date, or two other identifiers.
3. Recheck the medication order.
4. Put on gloves. It is helpful to keep one gloved hand uncontaminated.
5. Swab the self-sealing portal of the injection site with an antiseptic sponge; or attach a syringe via the injection cap.
6. Using a needleless device on the syringe, puncture the portal site (Figure 12-15); or for an injection cap (Figure 12-16), attach the syringe with medication directly.
7. Draw back the plunger of the syringe until blood flow is seen in the tubing to ensure that the line is open into the vein.

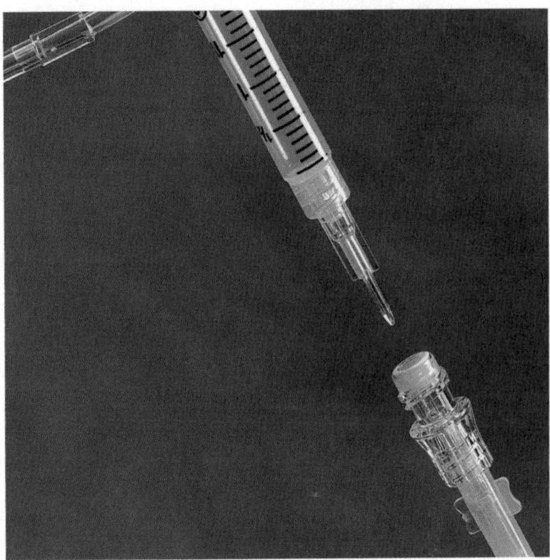

FIGURE **12-15** Syringe with blunt access cannula, attached by a luer-lock approaching as a portal on an IV administration set.

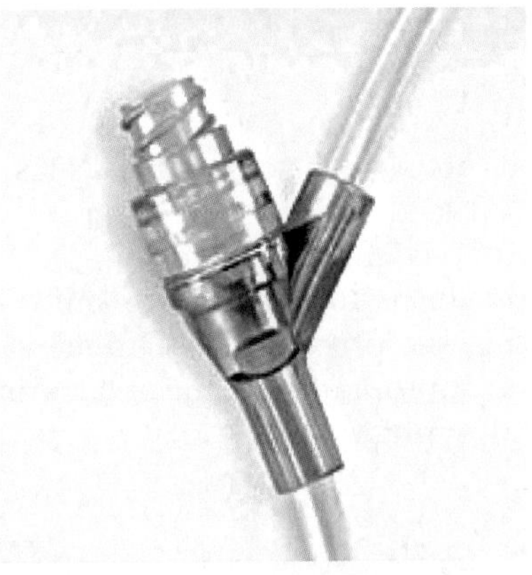

FIGURE **12-16** The Baxter Clearlink Access System allows a syringe with a luer-lock collar to be attached directly to an IV line. Clearlink's double seal design helps prevent back pressure and leakage since the seal tightens in relation to increased back pressure. The clear housing enables visualization of the fluid path to monitor for precipitates from incompatible drugs or blood clots resulting from inadequate flushing. (Courtesy of Baxter Healthcare Corp. All rights reserved.)

8. While pinching the IV tubing *above* the portal to stop flow (use the uncontaminated gloved hand), inject the prescribed medication into the IV line at a rate recommended by the manufacturer.
   If the medication and IV solution are not compatible:
   - Swab the injection port nearest the catheter with an alcohol pledget.
   - Insert a needleless device into the port; stop the primary infusion, and inject 2 mL of 0.9% normal saline (NS) (saline flush), in accordance with hospital policy, via IV push.
   - Swab the port with an alcohol pledget; insert the needleless device with medication, and administer at the prescribed rate.
   - Remove the medication syringe, swab the port again, and inject 2 mL of 0.9% NS (saline flush), in accordance with hospital policy, via IV push. If injecting into a central line, follow policy about the need to irrigate with saline and heparin solution.
9. When all the medication is administered, open the established IV line and readjust the flow rate to correspond with the health care provider's order, using the uncontaminated gloved hand. Remove gloves, and wash your hands thoroughly.

Documentation

In the patient's MAR, document date, time, drug, dosage, rate of administration, and assessment data obtained such as how well the procedure was tolerated and observations of the venipuncture site.

Patient Teaching

Explain to the patient the purpose of the medication administered and any side effects that should be reported.

Administration of Medication Through an Implanted Venous Access Device

Perform premedication assessments. See individual drug monograph.

Equipment

Dressing kits are used in some clinical sites.
Two pairs sterile gloves
2 to 10 mL 0.9% NS flush syringes
One heparin flush (10 to 100 Units/mL), amount as specified in site procedure; use 10-mL syringe containing an appropriate volume of heparin solution
Sterile 10-mL syringe

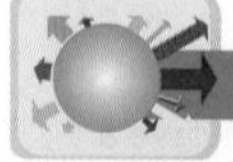

Clinical Landmine

Flushing the IV line by speeding the IV solution is not recommended because the medication still in the line would be administered too rapidly. This is contrary to the manufacturer's safety recommendation. Sudden boluses of certain medications may also cause severe hypotension or other signs of toxicity.

Needleless access device
18- to 22-gauge ⅝-inch needle
Povidone-iodine solution or swab sticks
Alcohol swabs
Huber needle
Extension tubing

Technique

1. Research and prepare the medication as described earlier.
2. Add medication to an IV piggyback bag.
3. Insert the administration set into the IV container, prime the IV line to remove all air, and cover the end of the IV line with a sterile cap.
   or Leave the prescribed medication in a sterile syringe.
4. Take all supplies and IV medication to the patient's bedside.
5. Identify the patient by checking the bracelet; recheck the drug order and explain what you are going to do. Have the patient state his or her name and birth date, or two other identifiers.
6. Recheck all aspects of the medication order.
7. Wash your hands.
8. If the implanted port is not already accessed, palpate the site to identify landmarks.
9. Open the dressing kit, set up and prepare the flushing supplies, and prime the infusion set, maintaining sterility of the Huber needle.
10. Put on sterile gloves.
11. Use the nondominant gloved hand to cleanse the skin over the implanted port with alcohol; cleanse from the intended site of insertion outward in widening circles. Repeat the cleansing process two more times. Allow the alcohol to dry, then repeat the cleansing process using povidone-iodine swab sticks.
12. Using the sterile gloved hand, grasp the Huber needle by the winged flanges, attach to the syringe containing saline, and insert the needle perpendicular to the patient's skin until the needle tip comes into contact with the bottom of the port. Support the Huber needle with folded 2 × 2-inch sponges.
13. Withdraw the plunger of the saline syringe slightly until blood returns; inject normal saline to flush the port of heparin; and attach the syringe with medication or IV piggyback container with medicine. (If administering from the syringe, use the bolus technique described on p. 193.) If administering as an infusion with the IV piggyback container (see Adding a Medication with a Piggyback Set, p. 195), attach the primed administration set to the Huber needle and adjust the rate of infusion. Provide support for the IV line. Apply transparent or gauze dressing and tape it in place. When medication administration is completed, flush with saline and heparin in accordance with institution policy. Maintain steady pressure on the plunger of

the syringe as the needle is withdrawn from the access device to prevent the backflow of blood.

14. Label the site with date of access, size/length of the Huber needle, and initial and date the dressing.
15. If the Huber needle is removed from a healed site at this time, cleanse the injection site with an antiseptic pledget and apply an adhesive bandage.
16. Dispose of used needles into a sharps safety container. Dispose of used extension tubing and other supplies according to institution policy.
17. Remove and dispose of gloves properly. Wash your hands thoroughly.

Documentation

In the patient's MAR, document date, time, drug, dosage, rate of administration, and assessment data obtained such as how well the procedure was tolerated and observations of the injection site.

Patient Teaching

1. Stress importance of preventing infection in the port and that the patient should avoid touching the site. If medication is being given intermittently using a pump, have the patient put the call light on when the machine alarm sounds.
2. Explain to the patient the purpose of the medication administered and any side effects that should be reported.

Adding a Medication to an Intravenous Bag, Bottle, or Volume Control

Perform premedication assessments. See individual drug monograph.

1. Prepare and research the medication as described earlier.
2. Identify the patient by checking the bracelet, and explain what you are going to do. Have the patient state his or her name and birth date, or two other identifiers.
3. Identify the injection port on the specific type of IV container or volume-control set being used; cleanse the portal with an antiseptic swab.
4. Clamp the IV tubing.
5. Insert the sterile access device into the port and slowly add the prescribed medication to the IV solution. Always check to be certain that the medication is being added to a compatible solution of sufficient volume to ensure proper dilution of the medication as specified by the manufacturer. Agitate the bag, bottle, or volume controller to thoroughly disperse the medication in the fluid.
6. For a volume-control apparatus, fill the volume chamber with the specified amount of IV solution (see Figure 12-1, *A* and C), and clamp the tubing between the IV bottle or bag and the volume-control chamber. Add the medication, as described before, via the cleansed injection port. Be sure medication is dispersed in the solution; adjust the rate of the flow solution.

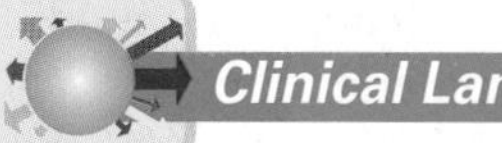

Clinical Landmine

When IV medications are administered by a volume-control apparatus, calculation of the rate of infusion to administer the drug over the proper time must include an allowance for the volume of the fluid in the IV tubing and the volume of medication.

7. Affix a label to the container. Indicate the medication name, dose, date and time prepared, rate of infusion, length of infusion time, and the nurse's signature.

Documentation

In the patient's MAR, document date, time, drug, dosage, rate of administration, and assessment data obtained such as how well the procedure was tolerated.

Patient Teaching

Explain to the patient the purpose of the medication administered and any side effects that should be reported.

Adding a Medication with a Piggyback Set

1. Research then prepare the medication as described earlier and add to an IV piggyback bag.
   a. If reconstituting a powder using a preassembled piggyback:
      (1) An example of a preassembled intravenous medication system is the ADD-Vantage System (Figure 12-17), a needleless system with two distinctly separate components, an ADD-Vantage diluent container (a plastic piggyback bag) containing 0.9% NS, D_5W (5% dextrose), or 0.45% sodium chloride and

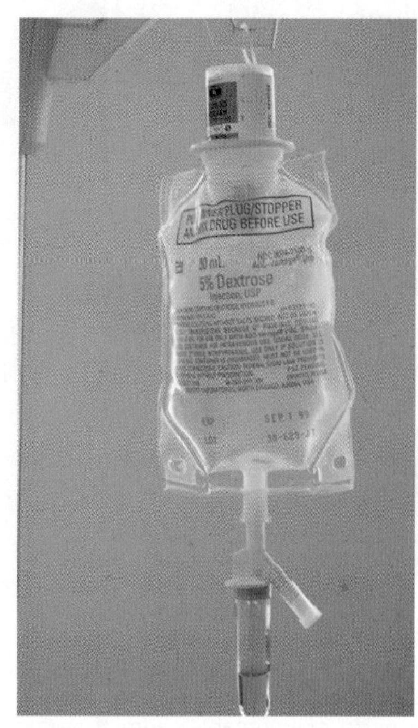

FIGURE **12-17** The ADD-Vantage drug delivery system.

an ADD-Vantage drug vial (containing medicines such as ampicillin powder).

b. Immediately before use, check all aspects of the drug order against the drug container.
   (1) Hold the ADD-Vantage vial and plastic container in a vertical position by the bottom of the attached drug vial (the vial is actually upside down), reach "through" the flexible container of diluent, grasp the inner stopper in the vial by the plastic ring that surrounds it, and pull straight down on the ring; the stopper disconnects and falls into the diluent solution. The drug powder also falls out and, with a few squeezes of the diluent bag, mixes with the diluent to reconstitute the drug.
   (2) The ADD-Vantage container is now ready for attachment of the secondary IV tubing when taken to the bedside.

2. Identify the patient by checking the bracelet, and explain what you are going to do. Have the patient state his or her name and birth date, or two other identifiers.
3. Insert the administration set into the piggyback container, attach a needleless device, fill the tubing purging the line of air, and clamp the tubing.
4. Connect to the primary IV tubing by arranging the piggyback container so that it is *elevated higher* than the primary container (see Figure 12-9). Cleanse the portal on the primary line with an antiseptic swab and insert the needleless device connector (Figure 12-18), attaching the piggyback tubing to the port of the tubing of the primary solution. Secure in place.
5. Check the specific orders for the infusion rate and sequence of solution or medication administration.

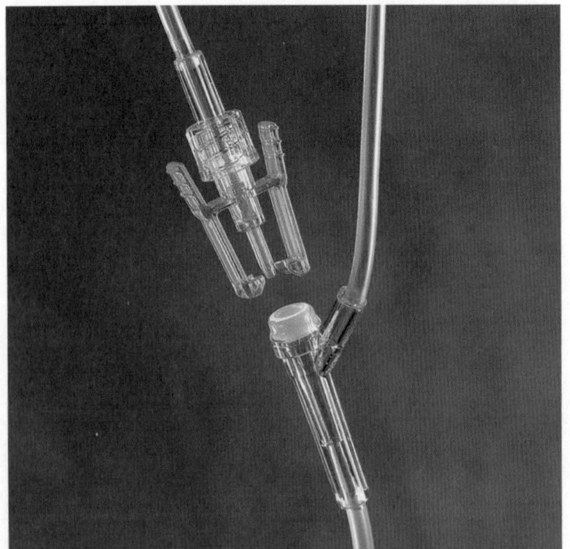

FIGURE **12-18** A male luer-lock with an Interlink Leverlock cannula attached. This illustrates how a (needleless) blunt plastic cannula-tipped adapter can be used to attach a piggyback container to a portal of a primary IV administration set.

6. Affix a label to the container. Indicate the medication name, dose, date and time prepared, rate of infusion, length of infusion time, and the nurse's signature.
7. When the piggyback empties, the check valve in the primary line releases and the primary infusion resumes. If a pump is used, the primary infusion will resume when the piggyback or secondary infusion is complete.

Documentation

In the patient's MAR, document date, time, drug, dosage, rate of administration, and assessment data obtained such as how well the procedure was tolerated.

Patient Teaching

Explain to the patient the purpose of the medication administered and any side effects that should be reported.

Changing to the Next Container of Intravenous Solution

1. Monitor the rate of infusion at least once per hour. When the container nears completion, notify the nurse responsible for adding the next container.
2. Slow the rate to keep the vein open if the level of solution in the container is low.
3. Check the IV site, dates on the IV lines, and compatibility of the IV solution running with the new container of IV solution to be added. (Medications may have been added to the IV solution per the health care provider's orders.)
4. Prepare the IV as previously described (see p. 187). Hang the new IV on the IV pole.
   If the same tubing is used, clamp the tubing on the primary IV line and, using aseptic technique, quickly exchange the new container for the empty one.
   If new tubing is used, attach the administration set to the solution container, fill the chamber on the IV line half full, prime the line to purge the air, and attach to the venous access device. Date and initial the new tubing with the label used in the clinical site. If a pump is used, prime the IV tubing, connect the tubing to the venous access device, and start the pump.
5. Unclamp the tubing and adjust the flow rate as previously described; inspect the venipuncture site.
6. Recheck all aspects of the IV order.

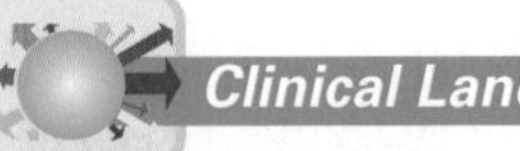

One of the most common mistakes in using preassembled IV medication containers (for safety and ease of reconstitution) is forgetting to activate the system and mix the drug powder with the diluent before hanging it for administration.

Documentation

1. In the patient's MAR, document date, time, IV solution, rate of administration, and assessment data collected.
2. Record amount of fluid infused on the intake and output sheet and any flow sheets maintained in the clinical site.

Patient Teaching

Explain to the patient the purpose of the IV solution.

Care of Peripheral Sites, Central Venous Catheters, and Implanted Ports

- Gauze or transparent semipermeable membranes are the two types of dressing materials used most frequently for IV dressings. When using gauze dressings, always seal all the edges with tape.
- Always label the dressing with the date, time of dressing change, gauge and length of the catheter, and name of the nurse inserting the catheter or changing the dressing.
- Always stabilize the catheter when changing a dressing to prevent movement of the catheter and irritation of the vein.

Flushing of Peripheral Catheters

See page 187 or SAS or SASH procedure and consult procedures used in the clinical site.

Peripheral Site Dressing Changes

The CDC recommends that venipuncture-site dressings are changed when they become damp, loose, or soiled, or whenever the venipuncture site is changed. Most clinical sites use this procedure for midline catheters as well.

Equipment

Dressing change kit
Sterile gloves

Technique

1. Gather supplies and check the health care provider order and/or clinical site guidelines.
2. Identify the patient by checking the bracelet, and explain what is to be done. Have the patient state his or her name and birth date, or two other identifiers.
3. Wash your hands.
4. Put on unsterile gloves to remove and discard the existing dressing (stabilize the catheter to minimize movement and irritation).
5. Assess the IV insertion site and surrounding tissue for redness, swelling, drainage, and warmth.
6. Cleanse the site with 70% alcohol swabs; start at the insertion site and continue outward in concentric circles until an area approximately 6 inches in diameter is covered; repeat three times. Allow to dry.
7. Repeat step 6 using povidone-iodine swabs or chlorhexidine; allow to dry.
8. Cover the site with transparent dressing or sterile gauze dressing in accordance with clinical site guidelines. Affix a label to the site as appropriate with the date, time, catheter gauge and length, and initials of the person doing the procedure.

Documentation

1. Document dressing change in the patient record and on any IV flow sheets maintained by the clinical site. State the date, time, and the name of the nurse performing the procedure. The nurse should also record observations of the peripheral site whenever the procedure is performed and at least once per shift daily.
2. If the IV access device was flushed, it should be documented on the flow sheet and on the MAR.

Patient Teaching

The patient and significant others should be taught the signs and symptoms of infection (e.g., temperature, redness, swelling, drainage). If the patient is immunocompromised or receiving analgesic-antipyretics (e.g., acetaminophen), the temperature may not be elevated or may only be minimally elevated.

Flushing of Central Venous Catheters

Equipment

Two 10-mL syringes with 0.9% NS, usually 5 to 10 mL; consult clinical policy manual for amount used in facility
One 10-mL syringe with heparin (10 units/mL), usually 2.5 to 5 mL; consult clinical policy manual for amount used in facility
Gloves
Alcohol or iodine wipes

Technique

1. Gather equipment needed and check the health care provider's order.
2. Identify the patient by checking the bracelet, and explain what is to be done. Have the patient state his or her name and birth date, or two other identifiers.
3. Wash your hands, prepare the equipment, and check the condition of the insertion site, dates on the insertion site, and all IV tubing in use; put on gloves.
4. Cleanse the injection cap with alcohol or povidone-iodine wipes and allow to dry.
5. Eliminate all air from the syringes immediately before performing the SAS or SASH (non-Groshong) procedure!
6. Insert the syringe into the center "bull's eye" of the injection cap; release the clamp; aspirate a small amount of blood, and inject the solution using a pause-push technique.
7. Continue with steps 4 through 6 until the SAS (for Groshong) or SASH procedure (see p. 187) of flushing is completed. Always close the clamp as the last

0.5 mL of solution is inserted to prevent backflow into non-Groshong catheters.
8. Check the injection cap; be certain it is securely in place and then resume IV therapy as prescribed. Check the rate of any infusing IV solutions before leaving the area.

Documentation

1. Document the condition of the insertion site and dressing in the patient record and record any IV tubing changes if done at this time on the IV flow sheets maintained by the clinical site.
2. Document the flushes used on the MAR.
3. Document any problems with catheter function in the record as well as measures taken to rectify the problem. Always record notification of the health care provider, additional orders obtained, and the patient's condition.

Patient Teaching

During the flushing procedure, explain to the patient what is being done and why; offer reassurance.

Dressing Changes for Central Lines

Check individual practice setting guidelines for frequency of dressing changes. In general, gauze dressings on central venous access sites are changed every 48 hours and semipermeable transparent dressings are changed every 3 to 7 days. However, it should be emphasized that whenever the site dressing is loose or sterility is compromised, the dressing should be changed.

Equipment

Mask
Sterile gloves
Nonsterile gloves
Dressing materials: transparent or gauze in accordance with site practice guidelines
Alcohol and iodine wipes

Technique

1. Gather supplies and check the health care provider order and/or clinical site guidelines.
2. Identify the patient and explain what is to be done. Have the patient state his or her name and birth date, or two other identifiers.
3. Wash your hands; put on mask.
   Note: Some clinical sites require that the patient also wear a mask during the central line dressing change.
4. Put on unsterile gloves to remove and discard the existing dressing (stabilize catheter to minimize movement).
5. Assess the IV insertion site and surrounding tissue for redness, swelling, drainage, and warmth.
6. Remove unsterile gloves and put on sterile gloves.
7. Cleanse the site with 70% alcohol swabs; start at the insertion site and continue outward in concentric circles until an area approximately 6 inches in diameter is covered; repeat three times. Allow to dry.
8. Repeat step 7 using povidone-iodine swabs or chlorhexidine; allow to dry.
9. Cover the site with transparent dressing or sterile gauze dressing in accordance with clinical site guidelines. Affix a label to the site as appropriate with the date, time, and initials of the person doing the procedure.

Documentation

1. Document the dressing change in the appropriate patient records. State the date, time, and the name of the nurse performing the procedure. The nurse should also record observations of the peripheral site whenever the procedure is performed and at least once per shift daily.
2. If the IV access device was flushed, it should be documented on the flow sheet and on the MAR.

Patient Teaching

The patient and significant others should be taught the signs and symptoms of infection (e.g., temperature, redness, swelling, drainage). If the patient is immunocompromised or receiving analgesic-antipyretics (e.g., acetaminophen), the temperature may not be elevated or may only be minimally elevated.

Care of Venous Ports

Generally, Huber infusion sets are changed every 7 days or when contaminated or not functioning. Check the IV flow sheet and labeling on the dressing for the date of insertion of the Huber needle.

Equipment

Appropriate dressing kit
Noncoring Huber needle infusion set (correct size and length)
   Note: For flushing an arm port, ½- or ¾-inch Huber needle of 20 gauge or smaller is preferred
SAS or SASH flushing equipment (depending on whether the catheter has a Groshong valve and institution policy); use a 10-mL or larger syringe for routine flushing and medication administration
2 × 2-inch gauze pads to support the Huber needle
Tape
Sharps safety container for used needle as well as a receptacle for the old dressing material that is removed
Face mask for nurse and patient
Sterile gloves

Technique

1. Gather equipment needed and check the health care provider's order.
2. Identify the patient and carefully explain what you plan to do. Have the patient state his or her name and birth date, or two other identifiers.

3. The nurse and the patient should put on sterile masks. (Explain to the patient that this is to keep microorganisms in the respiratory tract from depositing on the site.)
4. Wash your hands, put on sterile gloves, and palpate the port. Hold the port firmly in place with the thumb and middle finger to stabilize it as you remove the dressing, infusion set, and needle. Keep the needle in a straight line while pulling it upward; do not twist or bend from side to side to prevent inadvertently sticking yourself or the patient, or causing discomfort or a scratch to the patient as the needle is withdrawn.
5. Remove sterile gloves; wash your hands again.
6. Put on a new pair of sterile gloves.
7. Maintain aseptic technique throughout the procedure.
8. Open the sterile dressing kit and prepare the flushing supplies.
9. Use the gloved, dominant hand to handle sterile supplies. Use the nondominant gloved hand for nonsterile supplies.
10. Attach an access or injection cap to the extension tubing and prime the infusion set with 0.9% NS (leave saline syringe attached), maintaining sterility of the Huber infusion set.
11. Clean the injection site with 70% alcohol, starting at the center of the port working outward in concentric circular motions covering an area approximately 6 inches in diameter; allow to dry for 30 seconds; repeat three times. Repeat the procedure using povidone-iodine swabs or chlorhexidine gluconate; allow to dry.
12. Grasp the Huber needle firmly and support the edges of the port as the Huber needle is inserted in a straight line through the skin into the septum until the needle reaches the bottom of the port reservoir. Support the Huber needle with folded 2 × 2-inch gauze sponges.
13. Aspirate to view a small amount of blood return.
14. Flush the port with 10 mL 0.9% NS in a 10-mL syringe using the push-pause technique to create turbulence in the reservoir and thoroughly flush the port. If the port is not going to be used immediately, flush it with 5 mL heparin (100 units/mL) in a 10-mL syringe, or follow institutional policy. Anchor the Huber needle using sterile tape and 2 × 2-inch folded gauze pads to support the needle and keep it from shifting.
15. Apply transparent dressing.
16. Remove gloves and anchor the edges of the dressings with tape as well as tape the infusion set to anchor it in place.
17. Fill out the label with the date, time of access, size and length of the Huber needle, and the initials of the nurse performing the procedure.
18. Discard the used Huber needle in a sharps safety container and the dressing materials in the proper biohazard receptacle as established by clinical policy.
19. Wash your hands.

Documentation

1. Document the insertion and dressing change in the patient record and on any IV flow sheets maintained by the clinical site.
2. State the date, time of access, size and length of the Huber needle, and the initials of the nurse performing the procedure. The nurse should also record the observation of the port site whenever the procedure is performed and at least once per shift daily.
3. Document the flushes used on the MAR.
4. Document the dressing changes in the patient's record as well as the condition of the port site.

Patient Teaching

1. The patient and significant others should be taught the signs and symptoms of infection (e.g., temperature, redness, swelling, drainage at the port site), as well as the actual catheter care procedures. Explain throughout the procedure what is being done and why.
2. At the time of discharge, flush the port with saline and heparin. Have specific orders regarding when, where, and who will be performing future care of the port. Stress the importance of keeping appointments to maintain port function!

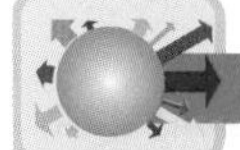

Clinical Landmine

- The flushing of central lines is an important aspect of maintaining the patency of the central venous access device. Two types of solutions are used to maintain patency of vascular access devices. Heparin is used to prevent clot formation and 0. 9% NS is used to clean the interior diameter of the device of blood or particles of medication. It is recommended that a 10-mL syringe be used for flushing lines and medication administration to prevent excessive pressure within the catheter that could result in rupture. Always follow institutional guidelines for the recommended procedures to maintain line patency.
- Preventing infection is a major concern with all IV devices. Appropriate procedures for cleansing the area and access device with the recommended antiseptics are mandatory.
- If unable to aspirate blood when performing a flush procedure, the catheter may be occluded. Never force the solution into the IV line! Start interventions by doing the simple things—check that the clamp is open and that the catheter and IV tubing are not kinked. Reposition the patient's upper body. Have the patient perform a Valsalva maneuver. (Check institutional policy for removal and replacement of the injection cap.) It may be necessary to remove the injection cap, attach a 20-mL syringe, and aspirate the blood clot. Immediately following aspiration of the blood clot; replace injection cap with a new sterile cap and institute 0. 9% NS and heparin (100 units/mL) flushing of the catheter in accordance with clinical guidelines. Report malfunctioning of the catheter to the health care provider. Radiographic evaluation as well as instillation of a thrombolytic agent (e.g., urokinase) may be necessary.

Discontinuing an Intravenous Infusion

Equipment

Tourniquet
Sterile sponges
Gloves
Dressing materials
Tape
Sharps safety container for needles, butterfly, or other types of IV catheter
If being converted to saline/heparin/medlock:
Extension tubing with cap
Saline flush in 10-mL syringe

Technique

If the IV site is being discontinued completely:

1. Check the health care provider's orders. Verify that all IV solutions and medications have been completed.
2. Check the patient's identity using the bracelet, and carefully explain what you are going to do. Have the patient state his or her name and birth date, or two other identifiers.
3. Wash your hands.
4. Adequately expose the IV site.
5. Clamp the IV tubing; turn off the electronic controller/pump.
6. Prepare a gauze sponge and tape for use on the venipuncture site.
7. Loosen the tape at the site while simultaneously stabilizing the needle to prevent venous damage. If the IV site is contaminated by blood or drainage, put on gloves before handling the tape.
8. Review hospital policy regarding the placement of a tourniquet. (Some health care agencies state that a tourniquet should be applied before removal of the needle or IV catheter in case the tip breaks during removal. Other agencies state that the tourniquet should be loosely attached to the limb, but not tightened unless necessary.)
9. Put on gloves.
10. Using a gauze pad, gently apply pressure with the nondominant hand to the venipuncture site. Withdraw the needle/catheter, pulling it out parallel to the skin surface. Inspect the tip of the needle or catheter to be sure it is intact. Release the tourniquet, if in place. Place the needle/catheter in the sharps safety container.
11. Cleanse the area if contaminated with any blood or fluid.
12. Continue to hold the IV site firmly until all bleeding ceases. If the venipuncture site was in the antecubital fossa, have the patient flex the elbow to hold the gauze in place.
13. Check for bleeding after 1 to 2 minutes. Remove the gauze and discard with other contaminated dressings. Cleanse the area as appropriate.
14. Remove and discard gloves according to policy and wash your hands thoroughly.
15. Apply a small dressing or adhesive bandage as stated by policy.
16. Provide patient comfort.

If the IV site is to be converted to a saline lock when the large volume solution is discontinued:

1. Perform steps 1 through 6 above.
2. Prepare a saline flush; attach the syringe to the extension tubing and purge air from tubing; clamp the extension tubing. Leave the syringe attached.
3. Clamp the tubing on the IV line; shut off the infusion equipment, if present.
4. Put on gloves; cleanse the connector site with antiseptic swab. Let dry.
5. Stabilize the catheter hub while disconnecting the IV primary tubing and quickly connect the extension tubing.
6. Unclamp the extension tubing and flush the catheter with saline in accordance with institution policy; clamp the tubing as the last 0.5 mL is injected.
7. Tape the site securely and label and date the extension tubing.

Documentation

Provide the RIGHT DOCUMENTATION of termination of IV therapy.

1. Chart the date and time of termination of the IV site or the conversion to a saline lock.
2. Perform and record regular patient assessments (e.g., site data, size of site, and color of skin at the venipuncture site).
3. Chart and report any signs of adverse effects (e.g., redness, warmth, swelling, or pain at the venipuncture site).
4. Record the total amount infused on intake and output record, and any flow sheets used in the clinical site.
5. Record the saline flush on the MAR.

MONITORING INTRAVENOUS THERAPY

Objectives

1. Discuss the proper baseline patient assessments needed to evaluate the IV therapy.
2. Explain the signs, symptoms, and treatment of complications associated with IV therapy (e.g., phlebitis, thrombophlebitis, localized infection, septicemia, infiltration, extravasation, air in tubing, pulmonary edema, catheter embolism, and "speed shock").

Key Terms

phlebitis	air embolism
thrombophlebitis	pulmonary edema
septicemia	pulmonary embolism
infiltration	"speed shock"
extravasation	
infiltration scale	

Before initiating therapy, perform baseline patient assessments to evaluate the patient's current status. Report at appropriate intervals throughout the course of treatment.

Immediately after receiving a report on your assigned patients, check the MAR or Kardex for IV medications and IV infusion orders for the patients assigned. Make rounds to perform a baseline assessment. Data that should be gathered and analyzed with reference to IV therapy include the following:

- Check that the ordered IV solution with or without medications is being administered to the correct patient at the correct rate of infusion.
- Check the total amount infused against the amount that should have infused. Is the volume of infused IV solution or IV medication "on target," "ahead," or "behind"? Inspect the volume-infused strips attached to the infusing solution bag or bottle.
- Calculate the drip rate. If the IV tubing is running by gravity, adjust it to the correct rate of infusion to deliver the milliliters per hour ordered. If a controller is being used, check to be certain the drop sensor is positioned superior to the fluid level in the drip chamber and inferior to the port from where the fluid drops. If an infusion pump is being used, ensure that the pump is set to deliver the prescribed volume (mL) per hour.
- Check for inline filters. If one is recommended for the medicine being infused, is it being used?
- Check the date and time the infusing IV solution or IV medication was hung. Identify when the infusing IV solution, administration set and tubing, IV site, IV catheters, and/or dressing is to be changed in accordance with policies of the practice setting. The CDC recommends that venipuncture-site dressings are changed when they become damp, loose, or soiled, or whenever the venipuncture site is changed.
- Check the date and time that procedures are ordered to maintain the patency of the established IV lines. (Follow the practice-setting policies.) The following are general guidelines:
  - Peripheral intermittent IV lines are usually flushed every 8 hours, using 1 to 2 mL of saline solution. Use positive pressure to prevent backflow of blood and possible occlusion.
  - Central venous IV lines are usually flushed with a minimum of 10 mL of normal saline solution whenever irrigated. Use a push-pause method to irrigate, rather than continuous pressure. To prevent excessive pressure within the line, always use at least a syringe of a 10-mL capacity to irrigate and maintain the patency of a central line. Follow institutional policy for the use of saline and heparin solutions.
  - Groshong catheters have a two-way valve that prevents backflow; therefore these catheters do not require heparin. Groshong catheters are flushed with 5 mL normal saline weekly or at an interval determined by institutional policy for lumens not in use. After medication administration or TPN infusion, flush with 10 mL of normal saline. After blood sample draws or blood product infusion, flush with 20 mL of sterile normal saline solution.
  - The amount of solution used to flush a Hickman, Broviac, or Groshong catheter varies and must be sufficient to equal two times the volume required to fill the catheter lumen plus the volume of any extension tubing being used.
  - Implantable vascular access ports (e.g., Port-A-Cath, Infus-A-Port) require that the port be filled with sterile heparinized solution, usually 100 units/mL, after each use. If not accessed regularly, flushes may only be performed once each month or at an interval cited by institutional policy.
  - Prevent damage to central venous catheters by clamping only the catheter with a padded hemostat or a smooth-edged clamp.
  - Change the injection caps for lumen hubs on central venous catheters every 72 hours or as stated in the institutional policy.
  - Check the IV tubing for any obstructions or air in the line. If running by gravity, ensure that the tubing is not hanging below the level of the insertion site.
  - The patient and the venipuncture site should be checked at least every hour for flow rate, infiltration (e.g., tenderness, redness, puffiness), and adverse effects. Report and take immediate action if the infusion is infiltrated, improperly infusing, or if signs of infection exist. If the flow rate is falling behind schedule:
    - Check for mechanical obstruction of the tubing (e.g., closed clamp, kinking) or filter and either irrigate or change the tubing.
    - Check the drip chamber. If less than half full, squeeze it to fill more completely. Do not overfill.
    - Check to make sure that the IV container is not empty. Also check to make sure the container is higher than 3 feet above the venipuncture site. The incorrect height may inadvertently occur if the patient is repositioned or the bed height is readjusted.
    - Check for tubing that has fallen below the venipuncture site. If a significant length has fallen, elevate and carefully coil the tubing near the site of venipuncture.
- Wear gloves to inspect the IV site. Check the transparent dressing for date the infusion device was started; palpate gently around the catheter or needle for edema, coolness, or pain, indicating infiltration. Check for any signs of redness or

heat, indicating an inflammatory process is occurring.

- Check to determine whether the bevel of the needle is pushing against the wall of the vein. Do this by CAUTIOUSLY raising or lowering the angle of the needle slightly to see if flow is restored. If so, reposition slightly using a gauze pad in the most appropriate location.
- Check the temperature of the solution being infused. Cold solutions can cause spasms in the vein.
- Check to ensure that a restraint or blood pressure cuff applied to the arm has not interfered with the flow.
- If it appears that the intravenous access device is clotted, DO NOT attempt to clear the needle by flushing with fluid. This will dislodge the clot and may cause a thromboembolus. Aspiration of the needle or catheter with a syringe to dislodge the clot is no longer recommended; rather the site should be discontinued and the IV restarted.
- Remain alert at all times for complications associated with IV therapy of any type (e.g., phlebitis, infection, air in the tubing, circulatory overload, pulmonary edema, pulmonary embolism, or drug reactions from the IV medications).
- Document all findings and procedures performed in association with IV therapy.

During your shift report, identify the exact volume of IV solution or medication that has been infused on the current shift and the volume remaining to be infused during the next shift. Also report any IV sites that are functioning poorly or that require frequent site changes.

Complications Associated with Intravenous Therapy

Complications that can occur with IV therapy include phlebitis, thrombophlebitis, localized infection, septicemia, infiltration, extravasation, air in tubing, pulmonary edema, catheter embolism, and "speed shock."

Phlebitis, Thrombophlebitis, and Local Infection

Phlebitis is the inflammation of a vein and **thrombophlebitis** is inflammation of the vein with the formation of a thrombus in the area of inflammation. Three primary causes of phlebitis are as follows:

1. Irritation of the vein by the catheter (e.g., catheter is too large for the vein; improper insertion; improper anchoring with excessive movement of the catheter)
2. Chemical irritation from medicines (e.g., solutions infused too rapidly or the volume was too large for vein; solution is irritating to the vein)
3. Infection caused by improper aseptic technique during accessing or care, or from long-term catheter placement

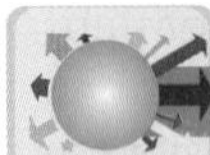

Clinical Landmine

Note: ONLY A HUBER NEEDLE IS USED TO ACCESS AN IMPLANTED PORT, except the new CathLink20 port.

If signs of redness (erythema), warmth, tenderness, swelling, and burning pain along the course of the vein are present, phlebitis or thrombophlebitis and infection may be developing (Figure 12-19). Confirm the presence of these signs with the supervising nurse. Treatment of phlebitis depends on the cause of venous irritation. If the IV line is a peripheral IV and there is evidence of infiltration (Figure 12-20), the IV is discontinued and a new IV using all new equipment is inserted at a different location. For people with any type of midline catheter (e.g., PICC), the health care provider should be notified. Not all midline catheters are removed when infection occurs; some may be treated with antibiotic therapy. Many hospitals also require that the infection control nurse be notified. If purulent drainage is present, a sample of the drainage is obtained for culture and sensitivity. If a fever and chills (signs of septicemia) accompany these symptoms, cultures of the patient's blood and the catheter tip may also be indicated. Check practice setting policies about whether a health care provider's order is necessary to do this or whether standing orders exist as part of the infection control procedures. Generally, follow-up treatment includes elevation and application of warm, moist compresses to the site. Document findings, treatment administered, and ongoing assessments.

Septicemia

When pathogens associated with a local infection invade the bloodstream and are carried to other parts of the body and trigger an inflammatory (fever, chills) response, the infection is no longer local, but is now systemic and called **septicemia.** People who already have an infection or who are immunocompromised are

Score	Descriptors
0	No clinical symptoms
1	Erythema at access site with or without pain
2	Pain at the access site with erythema and/or edema
3	Pain at the access site with erythema, streak formation, and/or palpable venous cord + or − 1 inch in length
4	Pain at the access site with erythema, streak formation, palpable venous cord >1 inch in length, and/or purulent drainage

FIGURE **12-19** Assessing the severity of phlebitis. An example of how signs and symptoms of phlebitis can be more uniformly described using a phlebitis score.

Grade	Clinical Criteria
0	No symptoms
1	Skin blanched Edema <1 inch in any direction
2	Cool to touch With or without pain Skin blanched Edema 1-6 inches in any direction
3	Cool to touch With or without pain Skin blanched, translucent Gross edema >6 inches in any direction
4	Cool to touch Mild–moderate pain Possible numbness Skin blanched, translucent Skin tight, leaking Skin discolored, bruised, swollen Gross edema >6 inches in any direction Deep pitting tissue edema Circulatory impairment Moderate–severe pain Infiltration of any amount of blood product, irritant or vesicant

FIGURE **12-20** Infiltration scale. An example of how signs and symptoms of infiltration can be more uniformly described using an infiltration scale.

at higher risk of developing septicemia. The importance of maintaining aseptic technique throughout all aspects of catheter insertion and maintenance care cannot be overemphasized. The potential for contamination exists during every aspect of intravenous therapy, starting at the time of manufacture and packaging of IV fluids and equipment, throughout the actual preparation and administration of the intravenous therapy. The risk of septicemia also increases with the frequency with which the catheter and site are manipulated and with the length of time an IV catheter remains in place. Perform catheter site inspection according to practice site policy. Suspect localized infection at the catheter site if redness, edema, or purulent drainage is present at the entry site or if the patient has an elevated temperature or elevated white blood count. Keep in mind that the immunocompromised patient, or those receiving an antipyretic (e.g., acetaminophen, ibuprofen) may not develop a fever.

Suspect septicemia if the patient develops sudden onset of flushing; fever; chills; general malaise; a weak, rapid pulse; headache; nausea; vomiting; hypotension; and shock. Take vital signs and notify the health care provider immediately of all findings. Obtain health care provider's orders, which will usually include blood cultures, discontinuation of the IV catheter, and antibiotic therapy once cultures are obtained. Return the unused portion of the IV solution to the pharmacy or laboratory for testing as specified by hospital policy.

Document findings, treatment administered, and ongoing assessments.

Infiltration and Extravasation

Infiltration is leakage of an intravenous solution into the tissue surrounding the vein. **Extravasation** is the leakage of an irritant chemical (e.g., the medicine being infused) into the tissue surrounding the vein. Infiltration/extravasation may be accompanied by redness and warmth, coolness and blanching of the skin, swelling, and a dull ache to a severe pain at the venipuncture site (Figure 12-20, *Infiltration Scale*). Infiltration or extravasation occurs most commonly when a needle tip punctures the vein and the IV solution leaks into the tissue surrounding the vein. Serious tissue damage may occur, particularly if the medicine in the solution is irritating to the tissue (e.g., calcium salts) or causes vasoconstriction (e.g., levarterenol) to the vasculature in the area.

The nurse should always do patient education regarding the signs and symptoms so that the patient can report early discomfort and early interventions can be initiated in the event infiltration does occur.

Inspect the IV site at regular intervals for infiltration. Whenever a change in the limb's color, size, or skin integrity is observed, compare with the opposite limb. If present, apply a tourniquet *proximal* to the infusion site to constrict the flow. Continued flow with the tourniquet in place confirms infiltration. DO NOT rely on blood backflow into the tubing when the container is lowered. The infusion could still be patent, but a laceration in the vessel may allow infiltration. Know the policies of your institution concerning the treatment of infiltration.

General guidelines are as follows:

- For an infiltration, stop the infusion. Elevate the affected limb. Assess for circulatory compromise–check capillary refill and pulses proximal and distal to the area of infiltration. If the infiltration is caused by an IV solution, remove the catheter as directed by policy, and as described on page 200. Whether cold or heat is applied to the site depends on the specific type of IV solution and the type of medication that has infiltrated. Consult institutional guidelines. Describe using the infiltration scale.
- For extravasation, the protocol will call for the IV infusion to be stopped, but the catheter is left in place. With authorization from the health care provider, attempts may be made to aspirate the medication, with orders that an antidote may be injected or infused to minimize tissue damage. Elevate the extremity. Apply ice (per site policy), not heat, for 24 hours except for vincristine or vinblastine, which require heat rather than cold. Document on the chart as 4+ infiltration and describe the visual appearance and measurements of the size of the site where extravasation has

occurred. Photographs of the site may be part of the protocol. Once the protocol for extravasation is complete, restart the IV solution at a new site proximal to the area of infiltration.
- Document findings, treatment administered, and ongoing assessments.

Air in Tubing/Air Embolus

If an air bubble is found in IV tubing, clamp the tubing immediately. Swab either the injection site in the rubber hub near the needle or the piggyback portal (whichever is closer to the air bubble) with an antiseptic sponge. Using sterile technique, insert a needleless access device on a syringe into the portal below the air bubble, and withdraw the air pocket.

Air embolism occurs as a result of an air bubble entering the cardiovascular system. Symptoms of an air embolism may include patient complaints of palpitations, chest pain, shortness of breath, cyanosis, hypotension, and a weak thready pulse. If air has actually entered the patient via the IV tubing, turn the patient onto the left side with the head in a dependent position. Administer oxygen and notify the health care provider immediately. Monitor vital signs. Be prepared for possible orders to draw arterial blood gases (ABGs) and for ventilatory support, if necessary. Air emboli can be prevented by clamping catheters when not in use, instructing the patient in the Valsalva maneuver during tubing and injection cap changes, using proper in-line filters, not allowing IV containers to run dry, and removing all air from tubing or syringes before connecting to an IV access device. Always purge the flush or medication syringe of air before attachment and injection.

Document findings, treatment administered, and ongoing assessments.

Circulatory Overload and Pulmonary Edema

Circulatory overload leading to **pulmonary edema** is caused by infusing fluid too rapidly or giving too much fluid, particularly to older adults, infants, or patients with cardiovascular disease. Signs of circulatory overload are engorged neck veins, dyspnea, reduced urine output, edema, bounding pulse, and shallow, rapid respirations. The signs of pulmonary edema are dyspnea, cough, anxiety, rales, rhonchi, possible cardiac dysrhythmias, thready pulse, elevation or drop in blood pressure depending on severity, and frothy sputum. When these symptoms develop, slow the IV immediately to keep an open (TKO) rate. Place the patient in a high Fowler's position, start oxygen, collect vital signs, and summon the health care provider immediately. In severe respiratory distress, the patient may require intubation and a mechanical ventilator to improve oxygen delivery. Anticipate health care provider orders for medications such as diuretics, vasodilators, and morphine sulfate.

Document findings, treatment administered, and ongoing assessments.

Pulmonary Embolism

A **pulmonary embolism** may occur from foreign materials injected into the vein or from a blood clot that breaks loose, traveling to the lungs, where it lodges in the arterioles. Symptoms include sudden onset of apprehension and dyspnea, pleuritic pain, sweating, tachycardia, cough, unexplained hemoptysis, low-grade fever, and cyanosis. When suspected, immediately place the patient in semi-Fowler's position, administer oxygen, take vital signs and notify the health care provider. Anticipate orders for drawing blood for ABGs, a lung scan to verify the presence of the pulmonary embolism, and baseline prothrombin time before initiating anticoagulant therapy.

Foreign-particle emboli can be prevented by using an inline filter, using proper diluents for reconstitution, ensuring complete dissolution of any medications added to a solution, and ensuring no visible signs of foreign matter in IV solutions. Thromboemboli can be avoided by not using the veins in the lower extremities in adults, and using a 10-mL syringe when flushing all central lines. A 10-mL syringe decreases the pressure exerted within the vascular system. (The smaller the syringe the greater the pressure exerted.) Whenever flushing catheters, never force the flush solution because this may dislodge a clot.

Document findings, treatment administered, and ongoing assessments.

"Speed Shock"

"Speed shock" occurs as a systemic reaction to a foreign substance given too rapidly into the bloodstream. This can occur when an IV drug is administered too rapidly into the circulation most commonly by IV push. The rapid delivery of the IV drug creates a concentrated plasma level in the patient that may result in shock, syncope, and cardiac arrest. Resources (e.g., *AHFS Drug Information, Physicians' Desk Reference*) and package inserts accompanying a medication state the recommended rate of injection or flow rate to prevent complications from rapid infusion rate. Nurses need to time the administration of an IV push medication by directly observing the infusion time on a clock or watch. The nurse also needs to check the flow rate of gravity IV infusions frequently; use infusion control devices for all central lines and potent drugs; and resist "speeding up" medications or IV rates when therapy is "behind schedule." Assess the patient before initiating an IV drug to obtain baseline data such as vital signs, and continue with monitoring during IV therapy for dizziness; flushing; tightness in the chest; rapid, irregular pulse; hypotension; and anaphylactic shock. Immediately upon suspecting speed shock, stop the infusion, maintain IV patency at a TKO rate, take vital signs, and notify the health care provider. Anticipate treatment of shock. Check institutional policy.

Documentation

Provide the RIGHT DOCUMENTATION of the medication administration, responses to drug therapy, and any complications or untoward reactions to the prescribed therapy.

1. Chart the date, time, drug name, dosage, and route of administration.
2. Perform and record regular patient assessments for the evaluation of therapeutic effectiveness (e.g., blood pressure, pulse, intake and output, lung-field sounds, respiratory rate, pain at infusion site).
3. Perform regular assessments of the patient and the IV access sites for complications associated with IV therapy or the administration of IV drug therapy.
4. Chart and report any signs and symptoms of adverse drug effects of therapy. Notify the health care provider of complications.
5. Chart dressing changes performed and cite any signs and symptoms of complications at the insertion site (e.g., redness, tenderness, swelling, drainage).
6. Chart any difficulty with irrigation of any venous access device and notify the health care provider as appropriate.
7. Chart the date and times that procedures are performed to maintain the patency of the IV site, needle, peripheral or midline catheter, central venous catheter, or port (e.g., heparinized flush or for Groshong catheter, the saline flush).
8. Perform and validate essential patient education about the drug therapy, and other essential aspects of intervention for the disease process affecting the individual.
9. Perform and validate essential patient education about the drug therapy, site or central venous catheter care, dressing care, or flushing of the IV system being used to administer medication. Always teach the patient (and significant others) signs and symptoms of complications that should be reported immediately to the health care provider. Depending on the type of IV delivery system used to administer the medication, instruct people being treated on an outpatient or home health setting when to return for the catheter to be changed and when to return for the next visit to the health care provider or clinic.

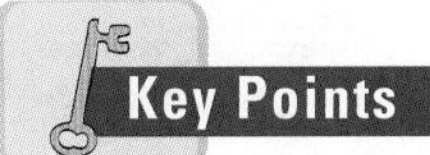

- IV nursing is defined by the Infusion Nurses Society as the use of the nursing process as it relates to technology and clinical application, fluids and electrolytes, pharmacology, infection control, pediatrics, transfusion therapy, oncology, parenteral nutrition, and quality assurance.
- As more medications have become available for IV use and as new IV access technologies have grown, the nurses' scope of practice has expanded to encompass more responsibilities for IV administration of very potent medications. It is necessary for nurses to be knowledgeable about the medications prescribed and IV procedures used, as well as to be familiar with current scope of practice statements, competencies, and educational requirements for the performance of IV therapy.
- Whenever IV medications are prescribed, the nurse needs to perform assessments to determine essential patient data before or during IV therapy.
- Patient assessments:
  - Review the chart to determine the medical and nursing diagnosis, patient history, allergies, and significant presenting symptoms.
  - Review baseline assessment data, current vital signs, laboratory/diagnostic data, and type and use of any IV access devices (e.g., peripheral IV site [catheter size, date of insertion], midline access devices, tunneled central venous access, implantable infusion ports).
  - Refer to a medical-surgical nursing text for further coverage of assessment of fluid and electrolyte therapy.
  - After the IV site is established, the IV solution or blood product is hung, or an IV medication is administered; an ongoing assessment is required to monitor the patient's condition, the IV site, and the patient's response to the IV therapy delivered.
- Nurses need to be familiar with all policies and procedures for infusion therapy used in the practice setting where providing care.
- Patient education needs to be implemented. All aspects of the patient's care needs must be explained to the patient and family. Additionally, community resources must be arranged to assist with the home infusion therapy.

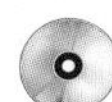

Go to your Companion CD-ROM for appendices, an Audio Glossary, animations, Drug Dosage Calculators, customizable Patient Self-Assessment forms, and Review Questions for the NCLEX® Examination.

evolve Be sure to visit the companion Evolve site at http://evolve.elsevier.com/Clayton for WebLinks and additional online resources.

MEDICATION SAFETY REVIEW

CRITICAL THINKING QUESTIONS

1. In a group setting with the instructor, discuss the ways in which common IV therapy problems may be resolved:
   a. IV fluid in a primary (gravity flow) line stops running.
   b. Obstruction is encountered when flushing a saline/medlock.
   c. The Huber needle in a port has come out while an IV medication is being infused.
   d. An air bubble is seen in the IV tubing.
   e. Two medications ordered for IV administration at the same time are not compatible.
   f. A saline/medlock has stopped functioning while a medicine is infusing.
2. The primary nurse tells you your patient's central line dressing needs to be changed. What steps would you take BEFORE seeking your instructor's assistance?
3. The instructor tells you to prepare to discontinue an IV infusion and to collect the supplies needed to convert the site to a saline lock. What equipment would you assemble and how is this procedure done?
4. Investigate the clinical guidelines in the practice setting where assigned for the "flushing" guidelines used for: peripheral sites, PICC lines, central access lines, and implanted venous ports.

CONTENT REVIEW QUESTIONS

1. If air is seen in the IV tubing, the nurse should:
   1. immediately close the clamp on the tubing.
   2. notify the primary nurse.
   3. get the instructor.
   4. disregard it if less than 2 mL.
2. A patient's skin at the site of a running IV in a peripheral IV access site appears swollen and feels cool and the patient complains of discomfort. The nurse should:
   1. apply a tourniquet and check patency.
   2. flush the site with saline.
   3. lower the IV bottle to check for blood return.
   4. notify the health care provider.
3. After changing a primary IV, it will not run. The nurse should first check for:
   1. type of IV solution hung.
   2. clamps not released.
   3. height of container.
   4. piggyback or rider set needed.
4. When initiating an IV access device for the first time in an extremity, it should be placed:
   1. near the antecubital space.
   2. in the biggest vein visible.
   3. in the dominant hand.
   4. in the metacarpal vein if large enough.
5. When planning to insert a Huber needle into a port, the nurse should:
   1. use aseptic technique throughout the procedure.
   2. use clean technique throughout the procedure.
   3. use latex examination gloves.
   4. put on mask and use sterile technique with gloves and supplies.
6. To minimize the risk of phlebitis, routine IV tubing should be changed at what frequency?
   1. 24 hours
   2. 36 hours
   3. 48 hours
   4. 72 hours
7. Which of the following is NOT a sign of infusion phlebitis?
   1. Redness
   2. Swelling
   3. Tenderness
   4. Blanched skin

13 Drugs Affecting the Autonomic Nervous System

evolve http://evolve.elsevier.com/Clayton

Chapter Content

Objectives

1. Differentiate between afferent and efferent nerve conduction within the central nervous system.
2. Explain the role of neurotransmitters at synaptic junctions.
3. Name the most common neurotransmitters known to affect central nervous system function.
4. Identify the two major neurotransmitters of the autonomic nervous system.
5. Cite the names of nerve endings that liberate acetylcholine and those that liberate norepinephrine.
6. Explain the action of drugs that inhibit the actions of the cholinergic and adrenergic fibers.
7. Identify two broad classes of drugs used to stimulate the adrenergic nervous system.
8. Name the neurotransmitters that are called catecholamines.
9. Review the actions of adrenergic agents to identify conditions that would be affected favorably and unfavorably by these medications.
10. Explain the rationale for use of adrenergic blocking agents for conditions that have vasoconstriction as part of the disease pathophysiology.
11. Describe the benefits of using beta-adrenergic blocking agents for hypertension, angina pectoris, cardiac arrhythmias, and hyperthyroidism.
12. Identify disease conditions that preclude the use of beta-adrenergic blocking agents.
13. List the neurotransmitters responsible for cholinergic activity.
14. List the predictable side effects of cholinergic agents.
15. List the predictable side effects of anticholinergic agents.
16. Describe the clinical uses of anticholinergic agents.

Key Terms

central nervous system
afferent nerves
efferent nerves
peripheral nervous system
motor nervous system
autonomic nervous system
neuron
synapse
neurotransmitters
norepinephrine
acetylcholine
cholinergic fibers
adrenergic fibers
cholinergic agents
adrenergic agents
anticholinergic agent
adrenergic blocking agent
catecholamine
alpha receptor
beta receptor
dopaminergic receptors

THE CENTRAL AND AUTONOMIC NERVOUS SYSTEMS

Control of the human body as a living organism comes primarily from two major systems: the nervous and endocrine systems. In general, the endocrine system controls the body's metabolism. The nervous system regulates the body's ongoing activities (e.g., heart and respiratory muscle contractions), rapid response to sudden changes in the environment, and the rates of secretions of some glands.

The brain and the spinal cord make up the **central nervous system** (CNS). The CNS receives signals from sensory receptors (e.g., vision, pressure, pain, cold, warmth, touch, smell) throughout the body that are transmitted to the spinal cord and brain by way of **afferent nerves.** The CNS processes these signals and controls body response by sending signals through **efferent nerves,** which leave the CNS to carry impulses to other parts of the body. The efferent and afferent nerves are known collectively as the **peripheral nervous system.** The efferent nerves transmit signals that control contractions of smooth and skeletal muscle and some glandular secretions.

The efferent system is subdivided into the **motor nervous system,** which controls skeletal muscle contractions, and the **autonomic nervous system.** The autonomic nervous system helps regulate such body functions as heart rate, blood pressure, thermal control, light regulation by the eyes, and many other activities.

Each nerve of the central and peripheral nervous systems is actually composed of a series of segments called **neurons.** The junction between one neuron and the next is called a **synapse.** The transmission of nerve signals or impulses occurs because of the activity of chemical substances called **neurotransmitters** (transmitters of nerve impulses). A neurotransmitter is released into the synapse at the end of one neuron, activating receptors on the next neuron in the chain or at the end of the nerve chain, stimulating the end organ (the heart, smooth muscle, or gland). Neurotransmitters can be either excitatory, stimulating the next neuron, or inhibitory, inhibiting the neuron. Because a single neuron releases only one type of neurotransmitter, the CNS is composed of different types of neurons that secrete separate neurotransmitters. Research indicates that there are more than 30 different types of neurotransmitters: the more common throughout the CNS are acetylcholine, norepinephrine, epinephrine, dopamine, glycine, gamma-aminobutyric acid (GABA), and glutamic acid. Substance P and the enkephalins and endorphins regulate the sensation of pain, and serotonin regulates mood. Other neurotransmitters include the prostaglandins, histamine, cyclic adenosine monophosphate (cAMP), and amino acids and peptides. Neurotransmitter regulation by pharmacologic agents (medicines) is a major mechanism by which we can control diseases that are caused by either an excess or deficiency of these neurotransmitters. Use of inhibitory and excitatory neurotransmitters to control illnesses is explained in the chapters in Unit Three.

AUTONOMIC NERVOUS SYSTEM

With the exception of skeletal muscle, the autonomic nervous system controls most tissue function. This nervous system helps control blood pressure, gastrointestinal (GI) secretion and motility, urinary bladder function, sweating, and body temperature. In general, it maintains a constant internal environment (homeostasis) and responds to emergency situations. The word autonomic means *self-governing* or *automatic;* thus the autonomic nervous system has also been called the involuntary nervous system because we have little or no control over it. We do, however, have control over much of the motor nervous system, which controls skeletal muscle. The two major neurotransmitters of the

Table 13-1 ***Actions of Autonomic Nerve Impulses on Specific Tissues***

TISSUE	RECEPTOR TYPE*	ADRENERGIC RECEPTORS (SYMPATHETIC)	CHOLINERGIC RECEPTORS (PARASYMPATHETIC)
BLOOD VESSELS			
Arterioles			
Coronary	α; β_2	Constriction; dilation	Dilation
Skin	α	Constriction	Dilation
Renal	α_1; β_1 and β_2	Constriction; dilation	—
Skeletal muscle	α; β_2	Constriction; dilation	Dilation
Veins (systemic)	α_1; β_2	Constriction; dilation	—
EYE			
Radial muscle, iris	α_1	Contraction (mydriasis)	—
Sphincter muscle, iris	—	—	Contraction (miosis)
Ciliary muscle	β	Relaxation for far vision	Contraction for near vision
GASTROINTESTINAL TRACT			
Smooth muscle	α; β_1 and β_2	Relaxation	Contraction
Sphincters	α	Contraction	Relaxation
HEART	β_1	Increased heart rate, force of contraction	Decreased heart rate
KIDNEY	Dopamine	Dilates renal vasculature, increasing renal perfusion	—
LUNG			
Bronchial muscle	β_2	Smooth muscle relaxation (opens airways)	Smooth muscle contraction (closes airways)
Bronchial glands	α_1; β_2	Decreased secretions; increased secretions	Stimulation
METABOLISM	β_2	Glycogenolysis (increases blood glucose)	—
URINARY BLADDER			
Fundus (detrusor)	β	Relaxation	Contraction
Trigone and sphincter	α	Contraction	Relaxation
UTERUS	α; β_2	Pregnancy: contraction (α); relaxation (β_2)	Variable

*α, α_1, Alpha receptors; β_1, beta-1 receptors; β_2, beta-2 receptors.

autonomic nervous system are norepinephrine (nohr ep′ in ef′ rin) and acetylcholine (ah see′ til koh′ leen). The nerve endings that liberate acetylcholine are called cholinergic (koh′ lin er′ gek) fibers; those that secrete norepinephrine are called adrenergic (ad′ rin er′ gek) fibers. Most organs are innervated by both adrenergic and cholinergic fibers, but they produce opposite responses such as in the heart, where adrenergic agents increase the heart rate and cholinergic agents slow the heart rate, and in the eyes, where adrenergic agents cause pupillary dilation and cholinergic agents cause pupillary constriction (Table 13-1).

Medications that cause effects in the body similar to those produced by acetylcholine are called cholinergic agents or parasympathomimetic agents because they mimic the action produced by stimulation of the parasympathetic division of the autonomic nervous system. Medications that cause effects similar to those produced by the adrenergic neurotransmitter are called adrenergic agents, or sympathomimetic agents. Agents that block or inhibit cholinergic activity are called anticholinergic agents, and those that inhibit the adrenergic system are referred to as adrenergic blocking agents. See Figure 13-1 for a diagram of the autonomic system and representative stimulants and inhibitors.

DRUG CLASS: Adrenergic Agents

Actions

The adrenergic nervous system may be stimulated by two broad classes of drugs: catecholamines (kat eh col′ ah meens) and noncatecholamines. The body's naturally occurring neurotransmitter catecholamines are norepinephrine, epinephrine, and dopamine. Norepinephrine is secreted primarily from nerve terminals, epinephrine primarily from the adrenal medulla, and dopamine at selected sites within the brain, kidneys, and GI tract. All three agents are also synthetically manufactured and may be administered to produce the same effects as those that are naturally secreted. Noncatecholamines have actions that are somewhat similar to those of the catecholamines but are more selective for certain types of receptors, are not quite as fast acting, and have a longer duration.

As illustrated in Figure 13-1, the autonomic nervous system can be subdivided into the alpha, beta, and dopaminergic (doh′ pah min er′ gek) receptors. When stimulated by chemicals of certain shapes, these receptors produce a specific action. In general, stimulation of the alpha-1 receptors causes vasoconstriction of blood vessels. The alpha-2 receptors appear to serve as mediators of negative feedback, preventing further release of norepinephrine. Stimulation of beta-1 receptors causes an increase in the heart rate, and stimulation of beta-2 receptors causes relaxation of smooth muscle in the bronchi (bronchodilation), uterus (relaxation), and peripheral arterial blood vessels (vasodilation). Stimulation of the dopaminergic receptors in the brain improves the symptoms associated with Parkinson's disease. Dopamine also increases urine output because of stimulation of specific receptors in the kidneys that results in better renal perfusion.

Uses

As noted in Table 13-2, many drugs act on more than one type of adrenergic receptor. Fortunately each agent can be used for a specific purpose without many adverse effects. If recommended doses are exceeded, however, certain receptors may be stimulated excessively, causing serious adverse effects. An example of this is terbutaline, which is primarily a beta stimulant. With normal doses, terbutaline is an effective bronchodilator. In addition to bronchodilation, higher doses of terbutaline cause central nervous system stimulation, resulting in insomnia and wakefulness. See Table 13-2 for clinical uses of the adrenergic agents.

NURSING PROCESS *for Adrenergic Agents*

See also nursing process for respiratory tract disease, bronchodilators, and decongestants (Chapters 30 and 31).

Premedication Assessment

1. Take baseline vital signs of heart rate and blood pressure.
2. See also premedication assessment for respiratory tract disease, bronchodilators, and decongestants (Chapters 30 and 31).

Planning

Availability

See Table 13-2.

Implementation

Dosage and Administration

See Table 13-2.

Evaluation

Side effects associated with adrenergic agents are usually dose related and resolve when the dosage is reduced or discontinued. Patients who are potentially more sensitive to adrenergic agents are those with impaired hepatic function, thyroid disease, hypertension, and heart disease. Patients with diabetes mellitus may also have increased frequency of episodes of hyperglycemia.

Side Effects to Expect

Palpitations, Tachycardia, Skin Flushing, Dizziness, Tremors

These side effects are usually mild and tend to resolve with continued therapy. Encourage the patient not to discontinue therapy without first consulting the physician.

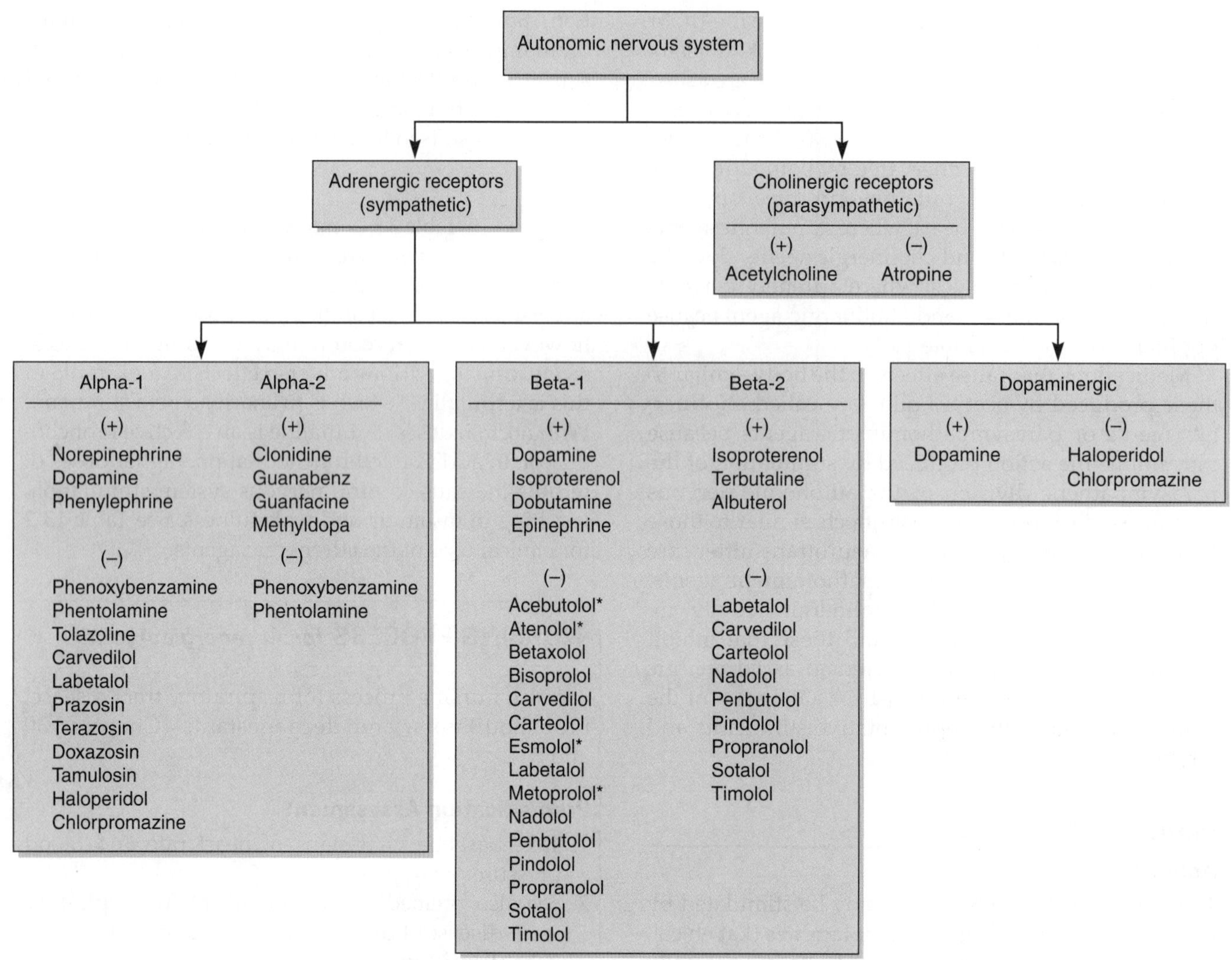

FIGURE **13-1** Receptors of the autonomic nervous system. (+) Stimulates receptors; (–) inhibits receptors; asterisks indicate representative examples of selective beta-1 antagonists only.

Orthostatic Hypotension

Although infrequent and generally mild, adrenergic agents may cause some degree of orthostatic hypotension manifested by dizziness and weakness, particularly when therapy is initiated. Monitor the blood pressure daily in both the supine and standing positions. Anticipate the development of postural hypotension and take measures to prevent an occurrence. Teach the patient to rise slowly from a supine or sitting position; encourage the patient to sit or lie down if feeling faint.

Side Effects to Report

Dysrhythmias, Chest Pain, Severe Hypotension, Hypertension, Anginal Pain, Nausea, Vomiting

Discontinue therapy immediately and notify the health care provider. Ask the patient if there has been a recent change in prescription, nonprescription, or herbal medicines in addition to those prescribed.

Drug Interactions

Agents That May Increase Therapeutic and Toxic Effects

Monoamine oxidase inhibitors (i.e., phenelzine, tranylcypromine); tricyclic antidepressants (i.e., amitriptyline, imipramine, others); guanethidine, atropine, and cyclopropane or halothane anesthesia. Many over-the-counter (OTC) medications such as cold remedies and appetite suppressants (diet pills) (pseudoephedrine, ephedrine, ma huang) contain adrenergic medicines that can have an additive effect when taken with a prescribed adrenergic agent. Monitor patients for tachycardia, serious dysrhythmias, hypotension, hypertension, and chest pain.

Agents That Inhibit Therapeutic Activity

Concurrent use of beta-adrenergic blocking agents (e.g., propranolol, nadolol, timolol, pindolol, atenolol, metoprolol), alpha-adrenergic blocking agents (e.g.,

Drug Table 13-2 ADRENERGIC AGENTS

GENERIC NAME	BRAND NAME	AVAILABILITY	ADRENERGIC RECEPTOR	ACTION	CLINICAL USE
albuterol*	Proventil, Ventolin	Aerosol: 90 mcg per puff Tablets: 2, 4 mg Syrup: 2 mg/5 mL Tablets: extended-release 4, 8 mg	Beta-2	Bronchodilator	Asthma, emphysema
dopamine		IV: 40, 80, 160 mg/mL in 5, 10, 20 mL ampules	Alpha, beta-1, dopaminergic	Vasopressor	Shock, hypotension, inotropic agent
dobutamine	Dobutrex	IV: 250 mg/20 mL vials	Beta-1	Cardiac stimulant	Inotropic agent
ephedrine*		Subcutaneous, IM, IV: 50 mg/mL in 1 mL ampules Capsules: 25 mg	Alpha, beta	Bronchodilator, vasoconstrictor	Nasal decongestant, hypotension
epinephrine*	Adrenalin	IV:1:1000 in 1 mL ampules; 1:10,000 in 10 mL prefilled syringes	Alpha, beta	Allergic reactions, vasoconstrictor, bronchodilator, cardiac stimulant	Anaphylaxis, cardiac arrest, topical vasoconstrictor
isoetharine*	—	Inhalation: 1% solutions	Beta-2	Bronchodilator	Inhalation therapy in bronchospasm, asthma
isoproterenol	Isuprel	Subcutaneous, IM, IV: 1:5000 solution, 1, 5 mL vials; 1:50,000 solution in 10 mL prefilled syringes	Beta	Bronchodilator, cardiac stimulant	Shock, digitalis toxicity, bronchospasm
metaproterenol	Alupent	Aerosol: 0.65 mg/puff Nebulization: 0.4, 0.6, 5% solution	Beta-2	Bronchodilator	Bronchospasm
metaraminol	Aramine	Subcutaneous, IM, IV: 10 mg/mL in 10 mL vials	Alpha-1	Vasoconstrictor	Shock, hypotension
norepinephrine (Levarterenol)	Levophed	IV: 1 mg/mL in 4 mL ampules	Alpha-1	Vasoconstrictor	Shock, hypotension
phenylephrine†	Neo-Synephrine	Subcutaneous, IM, IV: 1% in 1 mL ampules Ophthalmic drops: 0.12, 2.5, 10% Nasal solutions: 0.125, 0.25, 0.5, 1% Tablets: 10 mg	Alpha-1	Vasoconstrictor	Shock, hypotension, nasal decongestant, ophthalmic vasoconstrictor, mydriatic
terbutaline*	Brethine, ✤ Bricanyl	Tablets: 2.5, 5 mg Subcutaneous: 1 mg/mL in 1 mL ampules	Beta-2	Bronchodilator, uterine relaxant	Emphysema, asthma, premature labor

✤ Available in Canada.
*See also Bronchodilators.
†See also Decongestants.

phenoxybenzamine, phentolamine), guanethidine, reserpine, and bretylium tosylate with adrenergic agents is not recommended. ■

DRUG CLASS: Alpha- and Beta-Adrenergic Blocking Agents

Actions

The alpha- and beta-adrenergic blocking agents act by plugging the alpha or beta receptors, which prevents other agents, usually the naturally occurring catecholamines, from stimulating the specific receptors.

The beta blockers can be subdivided into nonselective and selective beta antagonists. The nonselective blocking agents have an equal affinity for beta-1 and beta-2 receptors and inhibit both. These agents are propranolol, nadolol, pindolol, penbutolol, carteolol, sotalol, and timolol. The selective beta-1 blocking agents exhibit action against the heart's beta-1 receptors (cardioselective) and do not readily affect the beta-2 receptors of the bronchi. Selective beta-1 antagonists are esmolol, metoprolol, acebutolol, betaxolol, bisoprolol, and atenolol. This selective action is beneficial in patients, such as those with asthma, in whom nonselective beta blockers may induce bronchospasm. It is important to note, however, that the selectivity of these agents is only relative. In larger doses, these agents will also inhibit the beta-2 receptors. There are no selective beta-2 blockers available. Labetalol and carvedilol exhibit both selective alpha-1 and nonselective beta-adrenergic blocking activity. Alpha and beta blockers are listed in Figure 13-1 and Table 13-2.

Uses

Because a primary action of the alpha-receptor stimulants is vasoconstriction, it would be expected that alpha blocking agents are indicated in patients with diseases associated with vasoconstriction. In fact, phenoxybenzamine and tolazoline are used as vasodilators in peripheral vascular diseases such as Raynaud's disease and Buerger's disease. (See Chapter 26 for the clinical use of these agents.) Phentolamine is used in the diagnosis and treatment of pheochromocytoma, a tumor that secretes epinephrine. Alpha blockers (e.g., prazosin, terazosin, doxazosin) are used to treat hypertension (see Chapter 23). Terazosin, doxazosin, and tamsulosin are used to relax the smooth muscle of the bladder and prostate, treating urinary obstruction caused by benign prostatic hyperplasia (see Chapter 41).

Beta-adrenergic blocking agents (beta blockers) are used extensively to treat hypertension, post-myocardial infarction, angina pectoris, cardiac dysrhythmias, symptoms of hyperthyroidism, and "stage fright." Beta blockers must be used with extreme caution in patients with respiratory conditions such as bronchitis, emphysema, asthma, or allergic rhinitis. A beta blockade produces severe bronchoconstriction and may aggravate wheezing, especially during the pollen season.

Beta blockers should be used with caution in patients with diabetes and those susceptible to hypoglycemia. Beta blockers further induce the hypoglycemic effects of insulin and reduce the release of insulin in response to hyperglycemia. All beta blockers mask most of the signs and symptoms of acute hypoglycemia.

Beta-adrenergic blocking agents should be used only in patients with controlled heart failure. Further hypotension, bradycardia, or heart failure may develop.

NURSING PROCESS *for Beta-Adrenergic Blocking Agents*

See also nursing process for patients with antidysrhythmic therapy (p. 393) and for patients with hypertension (p. 367).

Premedication Assessment

1. Take baseline vital signs of heart rate and blood pressure.
2. See also premedication assessment for patients with antidysrhythmic therapy (Chapter 24) and for patients with hypertension (Chapter 23).

Planning

Availability

See Table 13-3.

Implementation

Dosage and Administration

See Table 13-3.

Individualization of Dosage. Although the onset of activity is fairly rapid, it may often take several days to weeks for a patient to show optimal improvement and become stabilized on an adequate maintenance dosage. Patients must be periodically reevaluated to determine the lowest effective dosage necessary to control the disorder.

Sudden Discontinuation. Patients must be counseled against poor adherence or sudden discontinuation of therapy without a health care provider's advice. Sudden discontinuation has resulted in an exacerbation of anginal symptoms, followed in some cases by myocardial infarction. When discontinuing chronically administered beta blockers, the dosage should be gradually reduced over 1 to 2 weeks with careful patient monitoring. If anginal symptoms develop or become more frequent, beta blocker therapy should be restarted temporarily.

Evaluation

Most of the adverse effects associated with beta-adrenergic blocking agents are dosage related. Response by individual patients is highly variable. Many of these side effects may occur but may be transient. Strongly encourage patients to see their health care provider before discontinuing therapy. Minor dosage adjustment

Drug Table 13-3 BETA-ADRENERGIC BLOCKING AGENTS

GENERIC NAME	BRAND NAME	AVAILABILITY	CLINICAL USE	DOSAGE RANGE
acebutolol	Sectral ✱ Monitan	Capsules: 200, 400 mg	Hypertension, ventricular dysrhythmias	PO: Initial, 400 mg daily; maintenance, 800-1200 mg daily
atenolol	Tenormin ✱ Nu-Atenol	Tablets: 25, 50, 100 mg Inj: 0.5 mg/mL in 10 mL amps	Hypertension, angina pectoris, after myocardial infarction	PO: Initial, 50 mg daily; maintenance, up to 200 mg daily
betaxolol	Kerlone	Tablets: 10, 20 mg	Hypertension	PO: Initial, 10 mg daily; maintenance, 20 mg daily
bisoprolol	Zebeta	Tablets: 5, 10 mg	Hypertension	PO: Initial, 5 mg daily; maintenance, 10-20 mg daily
carteolol	Cartrol	Tablets: 2.5, 5 mg	Hypertension	PO: Initial, 2, 5 mg daily; maintenance, 2.5-10 mg daily
carvedilol	Coreg	Tablets: 3.125, 6.25, 12.5, 25 mg	Hypertension, heart failure, myocardial infarction	PO: Initial, 6.25 mg twice daily; maintenance, up to 50 mg daily
esmolol	Brevibloc	Inj: 10, 250 mg/mL in 10 mL amps	Supraventricular tachycardia, hypertension	IV: Initial, 500 mcg/kg/min for 1 min, followed by 50 mcg/kg/min for 4 min; then adjust to patient's needs
labetalol	Normodyne, Trandate	Tablets: 100, 200, 300 mg Inj: 5 mg/mL in 20, 40 mL vials	Hypertension	PO: Initial, 100 mg two times daily; maintenance, up to 2400 mg daily
metoprolol	Lopressor, Toprol XL ✱ Betaloc	Tablets: 50, 100 mg Tablets, extended release: 25, 50, 100, 200 mg Inj: 1 mg/mL in 5 mL amps	Hypertension, myocardial infarction, angina pectoris, heart failure	PO: Initial, 100 mg daily; maintenance, 100-450 mg daily
nadolol	Corgard ✱ Apo-Nadol	Tablets: 20, 40, 80, 120, 160 mg	Angina pectoris, hypertension	PO: Initial, 40 mg once daily; maintenance, 80-320 mg daily; maximum, 640 mg/day
penbutolol	Levatol	Tablets: 20 mg	Hypertension	PO: Initial, 20 mg daily; maintenance, 20 mg daily
pindolol	Visken ✱ Apo-Pindol	Tablets: 5, 10 mg	Hypertension	PO: Initial, 5 mg twice daily; maximum, 60 mg/day
propranolol	Inderal Inderal LA ✱ Detensol	Tablets: 10, 20, 40, 60, 80 mg Solution 4, 8, 80 mg/mL Sustained release capsules: 60, 80, 120, 160 mg IV: 1 mg/mL in 1 mL ampules	Dysrhythmias, hypertension, angina pectoris, myocardial infarction, migraine, tremor, hypertrophic subaortic stenosis	PO: Initial, 40 mg two times daily; maintenance, 120-640 mg daily IV: 1-3 mg under close ECG monitoring
sotalol	Betapace ✱ Sotacar	Tablets: 80, 120, 160, 240 mg	Dysrhythmias	PO: Initial, 80 mg two times daily; maintenance, up to 320 mg daily
timolol	Blocadren	Tablets: 5, 10, 20 mg	Hypertension, myocardial infarction, migraine, angina pectoris	PO: Initial, 10 mg twice daily; maintenance, up to 30 mg twice daily

✱ Available in Canada.

may be all that is required to eliminate most side effects.

Side Effects to Expect and Report

Bradycardia, Peripheral Vasoconstriction (Purple, Mottled Skin). Discontinue further doses until the patient is evaluated by a health care provider.

Bronchospasm, Wheezing. Withhold additional doses until the patient has been evaluated by a health care provider.

Diabetic Patients. Monitor for symptoms of hypoglycemia: headache, weakness, decreased coordination, general apprehension, diaphoresis, hunger, or blurred or double vision. Many of these symptoms may be masked by beta-adrenergic blocking agents. Notify the health care provider if you suspect that any of the symptoms described appear intermittently.

Heart Failure. Monitor patients for an increase in edema, dyspnea, crackles, bradycardia, and orthopnea. Notify the health care provider if these symptoms develop.

Drug Interactions

Antihypertensive Agents. All beta blocking agents have hypotensive properties that are additive with antihypertensive agents (e.g., guanethidine, methyldopa, hydralazine, clonidine, prazosin, minoxidil, captopril, reserpine). If it is decided to discontinue therapy in patients receiving beta blockers and clonidine concurrently, the beta blocker should be withdrawn gradually and discontinued several days before gradually withdrawing the clonidine.

Beta-Adrenergic Agents. Depending on the dosage, the beta stimulants (e.g., isoproterenol, metaproterenol, terbutaline, albuterol) may inhibit the action of beta blocking agents, and vice versa.

Lidocaine, Procainamide, Phenytoin, Disopyramide, Digoxin. When these drugs are occasionally used concurrently, the patient must be monitored carefully for additional arrhythmias, bradycardia, and signs of heart failure.

Enzyme-Inducing Agents. Enzyme-inducing agents (e.g., cimetidine, phenobarbital, nembutal, rifampin, phenytoin) enhance the metabolism of propranolol, metoprolol, pindolol, and timolol. This reaction probably does not occur with nadolol or atenolol because they are not metabolized but are excreted unchanged. The dosage of the beta blocker may have to be increased to provide therapeutic activity. If the enzyme-inducing agent is discontinued, the dosage of the beta blocker also will require reduction.

Nonsteroidal Antiinflammatory Agents. Indomethacin, salicylates, and possibly other prostaglandin inhibitors inhibit the antihypertensive activity of propranolol and pindolol. This results in loss of hypertensive control. The dose of the beta blocker may have to be increased to compensate for the antihypertensive inhibitory effect of indomethacin and perhaps other prostaglandin inhibitors. ■

DRUG CLASS: Cholinergic Agents

Actions

Cholinergic, also known as parasympathomimetic, agents produce effects similar to those of acetylcholine. Some cholinergic agents act by directly stimulating the parasympathetic nervous system, whereas others inhibit acetylcholinesterase, the enzyme that metabolizes acetylcholine once it is released by the nerve ending. These latter agents are known as indirect-acting cholinergic agents. Some of the cholinergic actions are slow heartbeat; increased GI motility and secretions; increased contractions of the urinary bladder, with relaxation of muscle sphincter; increased secretions and contractility of bronchial smooth muscle; sweating; miosis of the eyes, which reduces intraocular pressure; increased force of contraction of skeletal muscle; and sometimes decreased blood pressure.

Uses

See Table 13-4.

NURSING PROCESS *for Cholinergic Agents*

See also nursing process for patients with disorders of the eyes (Chapter 43), for patients with glaucoma (Chapter 43), for patients with urinary system disease (Chapter 42), and for patients with respiratory tract disease (Chapters 30 and 31).

Premedication Assessment

1. Take baseline vital signs of heart rate and blood pressure.
2. See also premedication assessment for patients with disorders of the eyes (Chapter 43), for patients with glaucoma (Chapter 43), for patients with urinary system disease (Chapter 42), and for patients with respiratory tract disease (Chapters 30 and 31).

Planning

Availability

See Table 13-4.

Evaluation

Because cholinergic fibers innervate the entire body, effects in most body systems can be expected. Fortunately, because all receptors do not respond to the same dosage, adverse effects are not always seen. The higher the dosage, however, the greater the likelihood for adverse effects.

Side Effects to Expect

Nausea, Vomiting, Diarrhea, Abdominal Cramping. These symptoms are extensions of the pharmacologic effects of the medication and are dosage related. Reducing the dosage may be effective in controlling adverse effects without eliminating the desired pharmacologic effect.

Drug Table 13-4 CHOLINERGIC AGENTS

GENERIC NAME	BRAND NAME	AVAILABILITY	CLINICAL USE
ambenonium	Mytelase	Tablets: 10 mg	Treatment of myasthenia gravis
bethanechol	Urecholine		See Chapter 42
edrophonium	Tensilon, Enlon, Reversol	Inj: 10 mg/mL in 1, 10, 15 mL vials	Diagnosis of myasthenia gravis Reverse nondepolarizing muscle relaxants such as tubocurarine
guanidine	Guanidine	Tablets: 125 mg	Treatment of myasthenia gravis
neostigmine	Prostigmin	Tablets: 15 mg Inj: 0.25, 0.5, 1 mg/mL	Treatment of myasthenia gravis Reverse nondepolarizing muscle relaxants such as tubocurarine
physostigmine	Antilirium	Inj: 1 mg/mL in 2 mL amp	Reverse toxicity of overdoses of anticholinergic agents (such as pesticides, insecticides)
pilocarpine	Isopto Carpine, Pilocar, Adsorbocarpine		See Chapter 43
pyridostigmine	Mestinon	Tablets: 60 mg Syrup: 60 mg/5 mL Sustained release tablets: 180 mg Inj: 5 mg/mL in 2 mL amp	Treatment of myasthenia gravis Reverse nondepolarizing muscle relaxants such as tubocurarine Reverse toxicity of overdoses of anticholinergic agents (such as pesticides, insecticides)

Dizziness, Hypotension

Monitor blood pressure and pulse. To minimize hypotensive episodes, instruct the patient to rise slowly from a supine or sitting position and perform exercises to prevent blood pooling while standing or sitting in one position for prolonged periods. Teach the patient to sit or lie down if feeling faint.

Side Effects to Report

Bronchospasm, Wheezing, Bradycardia. Withhold the next dose until the patient is evaluated by a health care provider.

Drug Interactions

Atropine, Antihistamines. Atropine, other anticholinergic agents, and most antihistamines antagonize the effects of cholinergic agents.

DRUG CLASS: Anticholinergic Agents

Actions

Anticholinergic agents, also known as cholinergic blocking agents or parasympatholytic agents, block the action of acetylcholine in the parasympathetic nervous system. These drugs act by occupying receptor sites at parasympathetic nerve endings, which prevents the action of acetylcholine. The parasympathetic response is reduced, depending on the amount of anticholinergic drug blocking the receptors. Inhibition of cholinergic activity (anticholinergic effects) includes mydriasis of the pupil with increased intraocular pressure in patients with glaucoma; dry, tenacious secretions of the mouth, nose, throat, and bronchi; decreased secretions and motility of the gastrointestinal tract; increased heart rate; and decreased sweating.

Uses

The anticholinergic agents are used clinically in the treatment of GI and ophthalmic disorders, bradycardia, Parkinson's disease, and genitourinary disorders; as a preoperative drying agent; and to prevent vagal stimulation from skeletal muscle relaxants or placement of an endotracheal tube (Table 13-5).

NURSING PROCESS *for Anticholinergic Agents*

See also nursing process for patients with Parkinson's disease (Chapter 15), for patients with disorders of the eyes (Chapter 43), and for antihistamines (Chapter 30).

Premedication Assessments

1. All patients should be screened for closed-angle glaucoma because anticholinergic agents may precipitate an acute attack. Patients with open-angle glaucoma can safely use anticholinergic agents in conjunction with miotic therapy.

Drug Table 13-5 ANTICHOLINERGIC AGENTS

GENERIC NAME	BRAND NAME	AVAILABILITY	CLINICAL USE
atropine	Atropine Sulfate	Inj: 0.05, 0.1, 0.3, 0.4, 0.5, 0.8, 1.0 mg/mL Tablets: 0.4 mg	Presurgery: reduce salivation and bronchial secretions; minimize bradycardia during intubation Treatment of pylorospasm and spastic conditions of the GI tract Treatment of urethral and biliary colic
belladonna	Belladonna Tincture	Tincture: 30 mg/100 mL	Indigestion, peptic ulcer Nocturnal enuresis Parkinsonism
dicyclomine	Bentyl, Antispas, Dibent, ✱ Bentylol	Tablets: 20 mg Capsules: 10 mg Syrup: 10 mg/5 mL Inj: 10 mg/mL	Irritable bowel syndrome Infant colic
glycopyrrolate	Robinul	Tablets: 1, 2 mg Inj: 0.2 mg/mL	Peptic ulcer disease Presurgery: reduce salivation and bronchial secretions; minimize bradycardia during intubation
mepenzolate	Cantil	Tablets: 25 mg	Peptic ulcer disease
propantheline	Pro-Banthine	Tablets: 7.5, 15 mg	Peptic ulcer disease

✱ Available in Canada.

2. Check for history of enlarged prostate. If present, anticholinergic agents may cause temporary inability to void.
3. Take baseline vital signs of heart rate and blood pressure. See also premedication assessment for patients with Parkinson's disease (Chapter 15), for patients with disorders of the eyes (Chapter 43), and for antihistamines (Chapter 30).

Planning

Availability

See Table 13-5.

Evaluation

Because cholinergic fibers innervate the entire body, effects from blocking this system occur throughout most systems. Fortunately, because all receptors do not respond to the same dose, all adverse effects are not seen to the same degree with all cholinergic blocking agents. The higher the dosage, however, the greater the likelihood for more adverse effects.

Side Effects to Expect

Blurred Vision, Constipation, Urinary Retention, Dryness of the Mucosa of the Mouth, Nose, and Throat. These symptoms are the anticholinergic effects produced by these agents. Patients taking these medications should be monitored for the development of these side effects.

Mucosa dryness may be alleviated by sucking hard candy or ice chips or by chewing gum.

If the patient develops urinary hesitancy, assess for bladder distention. Report to the health care provider for further evaluation. Give stool softeners as prescribed. Encourage adequate fluid intake and foods that provide sufficient bulk. Caution the patient that blurred vision may occur, and make appropriate suggestions for the patient's personal safety.

Side Effects to Report

Confusion, Depression, Nightmares, Hallucinations. Perform a baseline assessment of the patient's degree of alertness and orientation to name, place, and time before initiating therapy. Make regularly scheduled subsequent evaluations of mental status, and compare findings. Report development of alterations.

Provide for patient safety during these episodes. Reduction in the daily dosage may control these adverse effects.

Orthostatic Hypotension. Although this occurs infrequently and is generally mild, all anticholinergic agents may cause some degree of orthostatic hypotension manifested by dizziness and weakness, particularly when therapy is initiated.

Monitor the blood pressure daily in both the supine and standing positions. Anticipate the development of postural hypotension, and take measures to prevent it. Teach the patient to rise slowly from a supine or sitting position, and encourage the patient to sit or lie down if feeling faint.

Palpitations, Dysrhythmias. Report for further evaluation.

Glaucoma. All patients should be screened for closed-angle glaucoma before initiating therapy. Patients with open-angle glaucoma can safely use anticholinergic agents. Monitor intraocular pressures regularly.

Drug Interactions

Amantadine, Tricyclic Antidepressants, Phenothiazines. These agents may potentiate anticholinergic side effects. Confusion and hallucinations are characteristic of excessive anticholinergic activity.

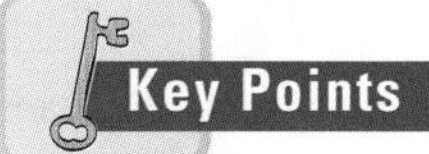

Key Points

- The nervous system is one of two primary regulators of body homeostasis and defense. The central nervous system is composed of the brain and spinal cord.
- The efferent nervous system is subdivided into the motor nervous system, which controls skeletal muscle, and the autonomic nervous system, which regulates smooth muscle and heart muscle and controls secretions from certain glands.
- Nerve impulses are passed between neurons and from neurons to end organs by neurotransmitters. The main neurotransmitters of the autonomic nervous system are acetylcholine and norepinephrine. Nerve endings that liberate acetylcholine are called cholinergic fibers; those that secrete norepinephrine are called adrenergic fibers.
- The CNS is composed of systems of different types of neurons that secrete separate neurotransmitters such as acetylcholine, norepinephrine, epinephrine, dopamine, serotonin, and GABA.
- Control of neurotransmitters is a primary way to alleviate symptoms associated with many diseases. As seen in Table 13-1, the administration of one type of autonomic nervous system drug can affect several organ systems, and adverse effects can be numerous. It thus requires monitoring of more than the symptoms for which the medicine was prescribed.

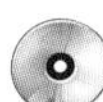

Go to your Companion CD-ROM for appendices, an Audio Glossary, animations, Drug Dosage Calculators, customizable Patient Self-Assessment forms, and Review Questions for the NCLEX® Examination.

evolve Be sure to visit the companion Evolve site at http://evolve.elsevier.com/Clayton for WebLinks and additional online resources.

MEDICATION SAFETY REVIEW

MATH REVIEW QUESTIONS

1. Order: Diphenhydramine (Benadryl) 40 mg PO tid

   Available: Benadryl 12.5 mg/5 mL

   Give __________.

2. Order: Propranolol (Inderal) 60 mg PO tid

   Available: Propranolol 40 mg tablets

   Give __________.

3. Order: Phenytoin (Dilantin) suspension 150 mg q8h

   Available: Dilantin suspension 125 mg/5 mL

   Give __________.

CRITICAL THINKING QUESTIONS

1. Based on a review of this chapter related to the actions, uses, and side effects of the primary drug classifications (adrenergic, adrenergic blocking agents, cholinergic, anticholinergic agents), develop a list of premedication assessments that should be made before using these drugs.
2. Summarize the actions of cholinergic and anticholinergic agents. Arrange the summaries in columns to compare the agents' actions.
3. Examine the drug actions listed for adrenergic blocking agents. Explain the mechanisms by which these drugs are beneficial in treating angina pectoris, cardiac arrhythmias, and hypertension.
4. Explain the effect of vasoconstriction and vasodilation of blood vessels on blood pressure.
5. What type of autonomic system drugs should generally not be used in patients with pulmonary disorders?

CONTENT REVIEW QUESTIONS

1. Which of the following components in the history and physical would cause the nurse to verify a preoperative medication order for atropine sulfate and morphine before administration?
   1. Episodes of hypertension
   2. Bradycardia
   3. Increased gastric motility
   4. Prostatic enlargement
2. Beta-adrenergic blocking drugs can cause:
   1. hypertension.
   2. angina pectoris.
   3. bronchoconstriction.
   4. cardiac dysrhythmias.

CHAPTER

14 Sedative-Hypnotics

evolve http://evolve.elsevier.com/Clayton

Chapter Content

Objectives

1. Differentiate among the terms sedative and hypnotic; initial, intermittent, and terminal insomnia; and rebound sleep and paradoxical excitement.
2. Identify alterations found in the sleep pattern when hypnotics are discontinued.
3. Cite nursing interventions that can be implemented as an alternative to administering a sedative-hypnotic.
4. Compare the effects of barbiturates and benzodiazepines on the central nervous system.
5. Explain the major benefits of administering benzodiazepines rather than barbiturates.
6. Identify laboratory tests that should be monitored when benzodiazepines or barbiturates are administered over an extended period.
7. Develop a plan for patient education for a patient receiving a hypnotic.

Key Terms

REM sleep
insomnia
hypnotic
sedative
rebound sleep

SLEEP AND SLEEP PATTERN DISTURBANCE

Sleep is a state of unconsciousness from which a patient can be aroused by appropriate stimulus. It is a naturally occurring phenomenon that occupies about one third of an adult's life. It is a different state of unconsciousness from that produced by deep anesthesia or coma.

Adequate sleep that progresses through the normal stages is important to maintain body function such as psychiatric equilibrium and strengthening of the immune system to ward off disease. Natural sleep is a rhythmic progression through phases that provide physical and mental rest. Based on brain wave activity, muscle activity, and eye movement, normal sleep can be divided into two phases—non–rapid eye movement (NREM) and rapid eye movement (REM). The NREM phase can be further divided into four stages. Each stage is characterized by a specific set of brain wave activities. Stage I is a transition phase between wakefulness and sleep and lasts only a few minutes. Some people experience it as wakefulness and others as drowsiness. Approximately 2% to 5% of sleep is stage I. Stage II comprises about 50% of normal sleep time. People often experience a drifting or floating sensation, and if awakened during this stage, will often deny being asleep, responding, "I was just resting my eyes." Stages I and II are light sleep periods from which a person is easily aroused. Stage III is a transition from the lighter to deeper sleep state of stage IV. Stage IV sleep is dreamless, very restful, and associated with a 10% to 30% decrease in blood pressure, respiratory rate, and basal metabolic rate. Stage IV is also referred to as delta sleep, based on the pattern of brain waves observed. Stage IV sleep comprises 10% to 15% of sleep time in young healthy adults. As we age, stage IV sleep diminishes, such that many people more than 75 years of age do not demonstrate any stage IV sleep patterns. Older adults also take longer to cycle through the relaxation stages of NREM sleep, with an increased frequency and duration of awakenings.

In a normal night of sleep, a person will rhythmically cycle from wakefulness through stages I, II, III, and IV, then back to stage III, stage II, and then to REM over about 90 minutes. The early episodes of **REM sleep** last only a few minutes, but as sleep progresses REM sleep increases, becoming longer and more intense around 5:00 AM. This type of sleep represents 20% to 25% of sleep time and is characterized by REM, dreaming, increased heart rate, irregular breathing, secretion of stomach acids, and some muscular activity. REM sleep appears to be an important time for our subconscious minds to release anxiety and tension and reestablish a psychiatric equilibrium.

Insomnia is the most common sleep disorder known: 95% of all adults experience insomnia at least once during their lives, and up to 35% of adults will have insomnia in a given year. **Insomnia** is defined as the inability to sleep. In general, insomnia is not a disease but a symptom of physical or mental stress. It is usually mild and lasts only a few nights. Common causes are changes in lifestyle or environment (e.g., hospitalization), pain, illness, excess consumption of products containing caffeine or alcohol, eating large or "rich" meals shortly before bedtime, or stress. *Initial* insomnia is the inability to fall asleep when desired, *intermittent* insomnia is the inability to stay asleep, and *terminal* insomnia is characterized by early awakening with the inability to fall asleep again. Insomnia is also classified according to its duration. A sleep disturbance lasting only a few nights is considered to be *transient* insomnia. A sleep disturbance lasting less than 3 weeks is referred to as *short-term insomnia* and is usually associated with travel across time zones, illness, or anxiety (e.g., job-related changes, financial stress, examinations, emotional relationships). *Chronic insomnia* requires at least 1 month of sleep disturbance to be diagnosed as a sleep disorder. About 10% of adults and up to 20% of elderly people report chronic insomnia. Women report suffering from insomnia twice as frequently as men. A higher incidence of insomnia is reported by the elderly, the unemployed, those of lower socioeconomic status, and the recently separated or widowed. As many as 40% of patients with chronic insomnia also suffer from psychiatric disorders (e.g., anxiety, depression, substance abuse). People with chronic insomnia often develop fatigue or drowsiness that interferes with daytime functioning and employment responsibilities. Recent studies also show that a reduced amount of sleep is associated with overweight and obesity, and the development of metabolic syndrome (see Chapter 21). Obesity itself is also detrimental to healthy sleep patterns, which can contribute to the development of sleep apnea.

SEDATIVE-HYPNOTIC THERAPY

Drugs used in conjunction with altered patterns of sleep are known as sedative-hypnotics. A **hypnotic** is a drug that produces sleep; a **sedative** quiets the patient and gives a feeling of relaxation and rest, not necessarily accompanied by sleep. A good hypnotic should provide the following action within a short period: restful natural sleep, duration of action that allows a patient to awaken at the usual time, natural awakening with no "hangover" effects, and no danger of habit formation. Unfortunately the ideal hypnotic is not available, although for short-term use, benzodiazepines and three benzodiazepine receptor agonists, zolpidem, zaleplon, and eszopiclone, are available. The most commonly used sedative-hypnotics increase total sleeping time, especially in stage II (light sleep); however, they also decrease the number of REM periods and the total time in REM sleep. REM sleep is needed to help maintain a mental balance during daytime activities. When REM sleep is decreased, there is a strong physiologic tendency to "make it up." Compensatory REM sleep, or **rebound sleep,** seems to occur even when hypnotics are used for only 3 or 4 days. After chronic administration of sedative-hypnotic agents, REM rebound may be severe, accompanied by restlessness and vivid nightmares. Depending on the frequency of hypnotic administration, normal sleep patterns may not be restored for weeks. The effects of REM rebound may enhance chronic use of and dependence on these agents to avoid the unpleasant consequences of rebound. Because of this, a vicious cycle occurs as the normal physiologic need for sleep is not met and the body attempts to compensate.

Recognizing that sedative-hypnotic agents have many side effects, especially with long-term use, medicines recognized for other primary uses are being used by health care providers for insomnia. Antidepressants such as amitriptyline, trazodone, and mirtazapine are prescribed in lower doses for their sedative effects to assist patients in getting to sleep (see Chapter 17). Anticonvulsants that are used in this way include gabapentin and topiramate (see Chapter 19). Antipsychotic agents such as quetiapine and olanzapine are prescribed for patients with psychoses who also have insomnia (see Chapter 18). It is important to note, however, that no extensive studies have been completed for using these antidepressants, antipsychotics, and anticonvulsants for insomnia, so long-term effects are not known and their use in treating chronic insomnia cannot be recommended.

Actions

Sedatives, used to produce relaxation and rest, and hypnotics, used to produce sleep, are not always different drugs. Their effects may depend on the dosage and condition of the patient. A small dose of a drug may act as a sedative, whereas a larger dose of the same drug may act as a hypnotic and produce sleep.

The sedative-hypnotics may be classified into three groups: barbiturates/benzodiazepines, and nonbarbiturate/nonbenzodiazepines, or miscellaneous sedative-hypnotic agents.

Uses

The primary uses for sedative-hypnotics are to improve sleep patterns for the temporary treatment of insomnia and to decrease the level of anxiety and increase relaxation and/or sleep prior to diagnostic or operative procedures.

NURSING PROCESS *for Sedative-Hypnotic Therapy*

Assessment

Central Nervous System Function. Because sedative-hypnotics depress overall central nervous system (CNS) function, identify the patient's level of alertness and orientation and ability to perform motor functions.

Vital Signs. Obtain current blood pressure, pulse, and respirations before initiating drug therapy.

Sleep Pattern. Assess the patient's usual pattern of sleep and obtain information on the pattern of sleep disruption (e.g., difficulty falling asleep, inability to sleep the entire night, or awakening in the early morning hours unable to return to a restful sleep).

Ask about the amount of sleep (hours) the patient considers normal and how insomnia is managed at home. Does the patient have a regular time to go to bed and wake up? If the patient is taking medications, determine the drug, dosage, and frequency of administration and whether this may be contributing to sleeplessness. (Medicines that may induce or aggravate insomnia include theophylline, caffeine, pseudoephedrine, ephedrine, nicotine, levodopa, corticosteroids, and selective serotonin reuptake inhibitor [SSRI] antidepressants.)

Patients with persistent insomnia should be carefully monitored for the number of naps taken during the day. Investigate the type of activities performed immediately before going to bed.

Anxiety Level. Assess the patient's exhibited degree of anxiety. Is it really a sedative-hypnotic the patient needs or is it someone to *listen?* Ask what stressors the patient has been experiencing in both personal and work environments.

Environmental Control. Obtain data relating to the possible disturbance present in the individual's sleeping environment that could potentially interfere with sleeping (e.g., room temperature, lights, noise, traffic, restlessness, or a snoring sleeping partner).

Nutritional Needs. Take a dietary history to identify sources of caffeinated products that may act as stimulants.

Alcohol Intake. Although alcohol causes sedation, it disrupts sleep patterns and may cause early-morning awaking.

Exercise. Obtain data relating to the patient's usual degree of physical activity and at what times during the day.

Respiratory Status. People with respiratory disorders and those who snore heavily may have low respiratory reserve and should not receive hypnotics because of the potential for causing respiratory depression.

Nursing Diagnosis

- Disturbed sleep pattern (indications)
- Risk for injury (side effects)
- Deficient knowledge related to medication regimen

Planning

Planning for patient care should be based on the assessment data, and interventions should be individualized to meet patient needs.

Central Nervous System Function. Schedule CNS assessments and monitoring of vital signs at least every 8 hours.

Sleep Pattern

Routine Orders. Many physicians order a sedative-hypnotic on an as-needed (PRN) basis. Do not offer it unless the patient is having difficulty sleeping and other measures to meet comfort and psychologic needs have failed to produce the desired effect.

- Never leave a medication at the bedside "in case" it is needed later.
- Reassess the underlying cause of sleeplessness. Is it really pain control that is needed? If so, repeating the order for a hypnotic will not meet the patient's needs because these medicines have no analgesic value and will often not work if the patient is suffering from pain.

Anxiety Level. Be aware of the possibility of a paradoxical response to sedative-hypnotic medicine, particularly in the elderly. If the patient is showing increasing signs of excitement, restlessness, euphoria, or confusion, it would be harmful to repeat the medication.

Environmental Control. Plan for the safety needs of the patient and protect from injury. Make sure that the call light is within reach and place the bed in the low position with side rails up. Leave a night-light on.

Organize nursing activities so that the patient is disturbed as infrequently as possible while maintaining safe patient care.

Nutritional Needs. Offer protein foods and dairy products at a specific time before sleep.

Exercise. Encourage adequate exercise during the day (not near bedtime) so the individual will be tired before trying to sleep.

Implementation

Vital Signs. Obtain vital signs periodically as the situation indicates.

Preoperative Medication. Give preoperative medications at the specified time.

Monitoring Effects

When a medication is administered, carefully assess the patient at regular intervals for therapeutic and adverse effects.

PRN. If giving PRN medications, assess the record for the effectiveness of previously administered therapy. It is sometimes necessary to repeat a medication if an order permits doing so. This is at the nurse's discretion based on the evaluation of a particular patient's needs.

Patient Education and Health Promotion

Bedtime. Encourage a standard time to go to bed to help the body establish a rhythm and routine.

Nutrition. Teach appropriate nutrition information concerning the food pyramid, adequate fluid intake, and vitamin use. Communicate the information at the educational level of the patient.

Avoid heavy meals late in the evening.

Alcohol and caffeine consumption should be reduced or discontinued, especially within several hours of bedtime. Introduce the patient to decaffeinated or herbal products that can be substituted for caffeinated foods. Help the patient avoid products containing caffeine, such as coffee, tea, soft drinks, and chocolate. Limit the total daily intake of these items and give warm milk and crackers as a bedtime snack. Protein foods and dairy products contain an amino acid that synthesizes serotonin, a neurotransmitter that is found to increase sleep time and decrease the time required to fall asleep.

PATIENT SELF-ASSESSMENT FORM Sleeping Medication

MEDICATIONS	COLOR	TO BE TAKEN

Patient ____________

Health Care Provider ____________

Health Care Provider's phone ____________

Next appt.* ____________

What I Should Monitor		Premedication Data	Date	Date	Date	Date	Date	Date	Comments
Time	Arising								
	Bedtime								
	Last cup of coffee								
Sleep pattern	Took _____ hr or min to get to sleep								
	Awaken during night; takes _____ hr or min to get back to sleep								
	Slept all night								
	Couldn't sleep								
	Went right to sleep								
Dreams	Dreamed all night								
	No. of dreams								
	Did not dream								
Feelings the next morning?	Very tired when I woke up								
	Awoke refreshed								
Exercise	No desire to exercise								
	Usual routine including work								
	Unable to work								
Stress level No time to relax — Time to relax 10 — 5 — 1									
Medication	Took _____ sleeping medication								
Other									

*Please bring this record with you to your next appointment.
Use the back of this sheet for additional information.

For insomnia, suggest warm milk about 30 minutes before the patient goes to bed.

Personal Comfort. Position the patient for maximum comfort, provide a backrub, encourage the patient to empty the bladder, and be certain that bedding is clean and dry. Take time to meet the patient's individual needs and calm fears. Foster a trusting relationship.

Environmental Control. Tell the patient to sleep in the proper environment such as a quiet, darkened room free from distractions and to avoid using the bedroom for watching television, preparing work for the following day, eating, and paying bills. Provide adequate ventilation, subdued lighting, correct room temperature, and control of traffic in and out of the patient's room.

For safety, instruct the patient to leave a night-light on and not smoke in bed after taking medication.

Activity and Exercise. Suggest the inclusion of exercise in daily activities so that the patient obtains sufficient exercise and is tired enough to sleep. For some individuals, plan a quiet "unwinding" time before retiring for the night. For children, try a bedtime story that is pleasant and soothing, not one that will cause anxiety or fear.

Stress Management. Explore personal and work stressors that may have a bearing on the insomnia. Some stressors may be within the work environment; therefore involvement of the occupational health nurse, along with a thorough exploration of work factors, may be appropriate. Stress produced within the dynamics of the family may require professional counseling.

Teach the patient relaxation techniques and personal comfort measures, such as a warm bath, to relieve stress. Playing soft music may also promote relaxation.

Make referrals for mastery of biofeedback, meditation, or other techniques to reduce stress levels.

Encourage the patient to express *feelings* openly regarding stress and insomnia. The adjustment to this situation involves working through great personal fears, frustrations, hostilities, and resentments.

Explore coping mechanisms the person uses in response to stress, and identify methods of channeling these toward positive realistic goals and alternatives to the use of medication.

Fostering Health Maintenance. Throughout the course of treatment, discuss medication information and how it will benefit the patient. Stress the importance of the nonpharmacologic interventions and the long-term effects that compliance with the treatment regimen can provide.

Provide the patient and/or significant others with important information contained in the specific drug monograph for the medicines prescribed. Additional health teaching and nursing interventions for the side effects to expect and report are described in the following drug monographs (e.g., barbiturates, benzodiazepines, and miscellaneous sedative-hypnotics).

Written Record. Enlist the patient's aid in developing and maintaining a written record of monitoring parameters (e.g., extent of insomnia, frequency) (see Patient Self-Assessment Form on p. 221). Complete the Premedication Data column for use as a baseline to track response to drug therapy. Ensure that the patient understands how to use the form and instruct the patient to bring the completed form to follow-up visits. During follow-up visits, focus on issues that will foster adherence with the therapeutic interventions prescribed.

DRUG THERAPY FOR SLEEP DISTURBANCE

DRUG CLASS: Barbiturates

The first barbiturate was placed on the market as a sedative-hypnotic in 1903. It became so successful that chemists identified some 2500 compounds, of which more than 50 were distributed commercially. Barbiturates became such a mainstay of therapy that fewer than a dozen other sedative-hypnotic agents were successfully marketed through 1960. The release of the first benzodiazepine (chlordiazepoxide) in 1961 started the decline in the use of barbiturates. However, several barbiturate compounds are still prescribed (Table 14-1).

Actions

Barbiturates can reversibly depress the activity of all excitable tissues. The CNS is particularly sensitive, but the degrees of depression (ranging from mild sedation to deep coma and death) depends on the dose, route of administration, tolerance from previous use, degree of excitability of the CNS at the time of administration, and condition of the patient. When used for hypnosis, barbiturates suppress REM and stage III and IV sleep patterns. Because barbiturates have long half-lives, residual daytime sedation is a common side effect.

Uses

Barbiturates are now rarely used for sedation-hypnosis, but when used, therapy should be limited to 2 weeks because tolerance to sedation and hypnosis develops during this time. The ultra–short-acting agents (methohexital, thiopental) may be administered intravenously as general anesthetics. The short-acting barbiturates (amobarbital, pentobarbital, secobarbital) are used for sedation before diagnostic procedures. The long-acting barbiturate, phenobarbital, is also used as an anticonvulsant.

Nursing Process for Barbiturate Therapy

Premedication Assessment

1. Seek information regarding prior use of sedative-hypnotic medications.
2. Obtain information relating to baseline neurologic function (e.g., degree of alertness).
3. Take vital signs (blood pressure, pulse, respirations, and pain rating).

Drug Table 14-1 **BARBITURATES**

GENERIC NAME	BRAND NAME	AVAILABILITY	ADULT ORAL DOSE	COMMENTS
amobarbital	Amytal	Inj: 250, 500 mg vials	Sedation: 30-50 mg IM two or three times daily Hypnosis: 100-200 mg IM 30 min before bedtime	Intermediate acting; Schedule II Used primarily as a sedative before anesthesia or during labor
butabarbital	Butisol	Tablets: 15, 30, 50, 100 mg Elixir: 30 mg/5 mL	Sedation: 15-30 mg three or four times daily Hypnosis: 50-100 mg at bedtime	Intermediate acting; Schedule III Elixir contains 7.5% alcohol Used primarily as a daytime sedative and bedtime hypnotic
mephobarbital	Mebaral	Tablets: 32, 50, 100 mg	Sedation: 32-100 mg three or four times daily Anticonvulsant: 400-600 mg daily	Long acting; Schedule IV Used primarily as an anticonvulsant; may also be used as a daytime sedative
pentobarbital	Nembutal	Capsules: 100 mg Elixir: 20 mg/5 mL Inj: 50 mg/mL	Sedation: 30 mg three or four times daily Hypnosis: 100 mg at bedtime	Short acting; Schedule II Used primarily as a daytime sedative and bedtime hypnotic; may also be used as a preanesthetic sedative Elixir contains 18% alcohol Also available for IM and IV use
phenobarbital	Luminal, Solfoton	Tablets: 15, 16, 30, 60, 100 mg Capsules: 16 mg Elixir: 15, 20 mg/5 mL Inj: 30, 60, 65, 130 mg/mL	Sedation: 8-30 mg two or three times daily Hypnosis: 100-320 mg Anticonvulsant: 60-100 mg two or three times daily	Long acting; Schedule IV Used most commonly now as an anticonvulsant; may also be used as a daytime sedative, preanesthetic, or hypnotic agent Also available for IM and IV use Elixir contains 13.5% alcohol
secobarbital	Seconal	Capsules: 100 mg	Hypnosis: 100-200 mg at bedtime	Short acting; Schedule II Used primarily as a daytime sedative or bedtime hypnotic Therapy is not recommended for longer than 14 days

Planning

Availability. See Table 14-1.

Implementation

Dosage and Administration. See Table 14-1.

Rapidly discontinuing barbiturates after long-term use of high dosages may result in symptoms similar to alcohol withdrawal. These may vary from weakness and anxiety to delirium and grand mal seizures. Treatment consists of cautious and gradual withdrawal over 2 to 4 weeks.

Evaluation

General adverse effects of barbiturates include drowsiness, lethargy, headache, muscle or joint pain, and mental depression.

Side Effects to Expect

Hangover, Sedation, Lethargy. Patients may complain of "morning hangover," blurred vision, and transient hypotension on arising. Hangover commonly occurs after administration of hypnotic doses of long-acting barbiturates. Patients may display a dulled affect, subtle distortion of mood, and impaired coordination. Explain to the patient the need to first rise to a sitting position, equilibrate, and then stand. Assistance with ambulation may be required.

If hangover becomes troublesome, there should be a reduction in the dosage, a change in the medication, or both.

People working around machinery, driving a car, pouring and giving medicines, or performing other duties in which they must remain mentally alert should not take these medications while working.

Side Effects to Report

Excessive Use or Abuse. Habitual use of barbiturates may result in physical dependence. Discuss the case with the physician and make plans to cooperatively approach gradual withdrawal of the medications being abused. Assist the patient to recognize the abuse problem. Identify underlying needs and plan for more appropriate management of those needs. Provide for emotional support of the individual; display an accepting attitude and be kind but firm.

Paradoxical Response. Elderly patients and those in severe pain may respond paradoxically to barbiturates with excitement, euphoria, restlessness, and confusion. Provide supportive physical care and safety during these responses. Assess the level of excitement and deal calmly with the individual. During periods of excitement, protect the patient from harm and provide for physical channeling of energy (e.g., walking). Seek change in the medication order.

Hypersensitivity. Reactions to barbiturates are infrequent, but may be serious. Report symptoms of hives, pruritus, rash, high fever, or inflammation of mucous membranes for evaluation by a health care provider. Withhold further barbiturate administration until the health care provider's approval has been granted.

Blood Dyscrasias. Blood dyscrasias are rare; however, laboratory studies (e.g., red blood cell [RBC], white blood cell [WBC], differential counts) should be scheduled when symptoms warrant. Stress the importance of the patient to return for this laboratory work. Monitor for the development of sore throat, fever, purpura, jaundice, or excessive and progressive weakness.

Drug Interactions

Drugs That Increase Toxic Effects. Drugs that increase toxic effects include antihistamines, alcohol, analgesics, anesthetics, tranquilizers, valproic acid, chloramphenicol, monoamine oxidase inhibitors, and other sedative-hypnotics. Monitor the patient for excessive sedation and reduce the dosage of the barbiturate if necessary.

Phenytoin. The effects of barbiturates on phenytoin are variable. Serum levels may be ordered, and a change in phenytoin dosage may be required. Observe patients for increased seizure activity and for signs of phenytoin toxicity: nystagmus, sedation, and lethargy.

Barbiturates reduce the effects of the following medicines:

- *Warfarin:* Monitor the prothrombin time and increase the dosage of warfarin if necessary.
- *Estrogens:* This drug interaction may be critical in patients receiving oral contraceptives containing estrogen. If patients develop spotting and breakthrough bleeding, a change in oral contraceptives and the use of alternative forms of contraception should be considered.
- *Corticosteroids, beta-adrenergic blockers, metronidazole, doxycycline, antidepressants, quinidine, and chlorpromazine:* The patient should be monitored for signs of increased activity of the illness for which the medication was prescribed. Dosage increases may be necessary or the barbiturate may have to be discontinued.

DRUG CLASS: Benzodiazepines

Benzodiazepines have been extremely successful products from a therapeutic and safety standpoint. A major advantage over the barbiturate and other nonbarbiturate sedative-hypnotics is the wide safety margin between therapeutic and lethal doses. Intentional and unintentional overdoses well above the normal therapeutic doses are well tolerated and not fatal.

More than 2000 benzodiazepine derivatives have been identified, and more than 100 have been tested for sedative-hypnotic or other activity. Although there are many similarities among the benzodiazepines, they are difficult to characterize as a class. This is because certain benzodiazepines are effective anticonvulsants, others serve as antianxiety and muscle relaxant agents, and others are used as sedative-hypnotics.

Actions

It is thought that the benzodiazepines have similar mechanisms of action as CNS depressants but that individual drugs within the benzodiazepine family act more selectively at specific sites, allowing for a variety of uses (e.g., sedative-hypnotic, muscle relaxant, antianxiety, and anticonvulsant). Those used as sedative-hypnotics bind to receptors that stimulate the release of gamma-aminobutyric acid (GABA), an inhibitory neurotransmitter in the CNS, initiating sleep and increasing total sleep time. They increase stage II sleep while decreasing stage III and IV sleep, and to a lesser extent, REM sleep.

Uses

Benzodiazepines are the most commonly used kind of sedative-hypnotic. Estazolam, flurazepam, quazepam, temazepam, and triazolam are the benzodiazepines marketed for hypnosis. Triazolam, a shorter-acting hypnotic, and estazolam and temazepam, intermediate-acting hypnotic agents, do not have active metabolites and therefore do not accumulate as readily after several days of dosing. Flurazepam and quazepam have long half-lives and active metabolites, making patients much more susceptible to next-day hangover.

When benzodiazepine therapy is started, patients feel a sense of deep or refreshing sleep. Benzodiazepine-induced sleep varies, however, from normal sleep in that there is less REM sleep. With chronic administration, the amount of REM sleep gradually increases as tolerance develops to the REM suppressant effects. When benzodiazepines are discontinued, a rebound increase in REM sleep may occur in spite of the tolerance. During the rebound period, the number of dreams stays about the same, but many of the dreams are reported to be bizarre. After long-term use of most benzodiazepines, there is also a rebound in insomnia. Consequently it is important to use these agents only for short courses (usually no more than 4 weeks) of therapy.

The short-acting benzodiazepines (e.g., midazolam) are used intramuscularly as a preoperative sedative and intravenously for conscious sedation before short diagnostic procedures or for induction of general anesthesia. Midazolam has a more rapid onset of action than diazepam and a much shorter duration. It also produces a greater degree of amnesia and shorter duration of action than diazepam, again making it beneficial for short diagnostic and operative procedures. Lorazepam is used as an antianxiety agent in general, but is particularly useful before diagnostic procedures when a longer duration of action is required, because a parenteral dosage form is available. It also has no active metabolites that may prolong sedation.

Therapeutic Outcomes

The primary therapeutic outcomes sought from benzodiazepine therapy are as follows:

- To produce mild sedation.
- For short-term use to produce sleep.
- Preoperative sedation with amnesia.

Nursing Process for Benzodiazepines

Premedication Assessment

1. Record baseline vital signs, particularly blood pressure, in sitting and lying positions.
2. Check for history of blood dyscrasias or hepatic disease or whether patient is in the first trimester of pregnancy.
3. Take vital signs (blood pressure, pulse, respirations, and pain rating).

Planning

Availability. See Table 14-2.

Pregnancy and Lactation. It is generally recommended that benzodiazepines not be administered during at least the first trimester of pregnancy. There may be an increased incidence of birth defects because these agents readily cross the placenta and enter fetal circulation.

Mothers who are breastfeeding should not receive benzodiazepines regularly. These agents readily cross into breast milk and exert a pharmacologic effect on the infant.

Implementation

Dosage and Administration. See Table 14-2.

The habitual use of benzodiazepines may result in physical and psychological dependence. Rapid discontinuance of benzodiazepines after long-term use may result in symptoms similar to alcohol withdrawal such as weakness, anxiety, delirium, and grand mal seizures. The symptoms may not appear for several days after discontinuation. Treatment consists of gradual withdrawal of benzodiazepines over 2 to 4 weeks.

Evaluation

Side Effects to Expect

Drowsiness, Hangover, Sedation, Lethargy. Patients may complain of "morning hangover," blurred vision, and transient hypotension on arising. Explain to the patient the need for arising first to a sitting position, equilibrating, and then standing. Assistance with ambulation may be required.

If hangover becomes troublesome, there should be a reduction in the dosage or a change in the medication, or both.

People who work around machinery, drive a car, pour and give medications, or perform other duties in which they must remain mentally alert should not take these medications while working.

Side Effects to Report

Confusion, Agitation, Hallucinations, Amnesia. All benzodiazepines have the potential to cause these symptoms, particularly in elderly patients who have been taking higher doses or for prolonged periods. Discuss the case with the physician and make plans to cooperatively approach gradual reduction of the medication to prevent withdrawal symptoms and rebound insomnia.

Excessive Use or Abuse. Habitual use of benzodiazepines may result in physical dependence. Discuss the case with the physician and make plans to cooperatively approach gradual withdrawal of the medications being abused. Assist the patient to recognize the abuse problem. Identify underlying needs and plan for more appropriate management of those needs. Provide for emotional support of the individual; display an accepting attitude. Be kind but firm.

Blood Dyscrasias. Routine laboratory studies (e.g., RBC and WBC counts, differential counts) should be scheduled. Stress the patient's returning for these tests. Monitor for the development of a sore throat, fever, purpura, jaundice, or excessive and progressive weakness.

Hepatotoxicity. The symptoms of hepatotoxicity are anorexia, nausea, vomiting, jaundice, hepatomegaly, splenomegaly, and abnormal liver function tests (e.g., elevated bilirubin, aspartate aminotransferase [AST], alanine aminotransferase [ALT], gamma glutamyl transferase [GGT], alkaline phosphatase, prothrombin time).

Drug Interactions

Drugs That Increase Toxic Effects. Antihistamines, alcohol, analgesics, anesthetics, tranquilizers, narcotics, cimetidine, disulfiram, isoniazid, rifampin, erythromycin, and other sedative-hypnotics increase toxic effects.

Smoking. Smoking enhances the metabolism of benzodiazepines. Larger doses may be necessary to maintain sedative effects in patients who smoke.

Drug Table 14-2 BENZODIAZEPINES USED FOR SEDATION-HYPNOSIS

GENERIC NAME	BRAND NAME	AVAILABILITY	ADULT ORAL DOSE	COMMENTS
estazolam	ProSom	Tablets: 1, 2 mg	Hypnosis: 1-2 mg at bedtime	Intermediate acting; Schedule IV Used to treat insomnia Tapering therapy recommended to reduce rebound insomnia Minimal morning hangover
flurazepam	Dalmane, ✱ Novo-Flupam	Capsules: 15, 30 mg	Hypnosis: 15-30 mg at bedtime	Long acting; Schedule IV Used for short-term treatment of insomnia, up to 4 wk Morning hangover may be significant Rebound insomnia and REM sleep occur less frequently
lorazepam	Ativan, ✱ Novo-Lorazepam	Tablets: 0.5, 1, 2 mg Oral solution: 2 mg/mL Inj: 2 mg and 4 mg/mL in 1, 10 mL vials ; 2, 4 mg/mL prefilled syringes	Hypnosis: 2-4 mg at bedtime	Used primarily to treat insomnia but may also be used for pre-operative anxiety IM, IV administration also available
midazolam	Versed ✱ Apo-Midazolam	Syrup: 2 mg/mL Inj: 1, 5 mg/mL in 1, 2, 5, 10 mL vials; 10 mg/2 mL prefilled syringes	Preop: IM, 0.07-0.08 mg/kg 1 hr before surgery Induction of anesthesia: IV, 0.2-0.3 mg/kg Endoscopy: IV, 0.1-0.15 mg/kg	Short acting; Schedule IV Onset: IM, 15 minutes; IV, 3-5 min Duration: IM, 30-60 min; IV, 2-6 hr Causes amnesia in most patients Lower dosage in patients over age 55
quazepam	Doral	Tablets: 7.5, 15 mg	Hypnosis: 7.5-15 mg at bedtime	Long acting; Schedule IV Used to treat insomnia Tapering therapy recommended to reduce rebound insomnia Morning hangover may be significant
temazepam	Restoril ✱ Nu-Temazepam	Capsules: 7.5, 15, 22.5, 30 mg	Hypnosis: 15-30 mg at bedtime	Intermediate acting; Schedule IV Used to treat insomnia Minimal if any morning hangover Rebound insomnia may occur
triazolam	Halcion ✱ Alti-Triazolam	Tablets: 0.125, 0.25 mg	Hypnosis: 0.125-0.5 mg at bedtime	Short acting; Schedule IV Used to treat insomnia but tends to lose effectiveness within 2 wk Tapering therapy is recommended to reduce rebound insomnia Rapid onset of action No morning hangover

✱ Available in Canada.

DRUG CLASS: Nonbarbiturate, Nonbenzodiazepine Sedative-Hypnotic Agents

Actions

The nonbarbiturate, nonbenzodiazepine sedative-hypnotics are listed in Table 14-3. They represent a variety of chemical classes, all of which cause CNS depression. These include the histamine-1 blockers (antihistamines), melatonin, a hormone secreted from the pineal gland (see Chapter 48), a melatonin receptor stimulant, and valerian, an herbal medicine (see Chapter 48). The newest class of agents are the benzodiazepine receptor agonists. All have somewhat variable effects on REM sleep, tolerance development, and rebound REM sleep and insomnia.

Uses

Antihistamines (particularly diphenhydramine and doxylamine) have sedative properties that may be used for short-term treatment of mild insomnia. They are common ingredients in over-the-counter (OTC) sleep aids. Tolerance develops after only a few nights of use; increasing the dose actually causes a more restless and irregular sleep pattern. Doxylamine has a longer half-life of approximately 10 hours, frequently causing morning hangover.

Melatonin is available OTC as a sleep aid. It appears to be particularly useful in patients who have been traveling through time zones and are suffering from "jet lag." Because this medicine is classified as a dietary supplement and is not regulated by the U.S. Food and Drug Administration (FDA), there may be inconsistencies in potency.

Ramelteon is a melatonin receptor stimulant, the first FDA-approved member of this class. It is used in patients with insomnia who have difficulty falling asleep.

Valerian, an herbal medicine, has been used for hundreds of years as a mild sedative. Its mechanism of action is unknown, but it may inhibit the enzyme that metabolizes GABA, prolonging the inhibitory neurotransmitter's duration of action. As with melatonin, valerian is classified as a dietary supplement and is not regulated by the FDA. There may be differences in strength and potency between distributors.

Because of the effect on sleep patterns and REM sleep, the use of benzodiazepines is diminishing in favor of the newer benzodiazepine receptor agonists, zaleplon, zolpidem, and eszopiclone, which bind to different GABA receptors in the CNS. In contrast to benzodiazepines and barbiturates, zaleplon, zolpidem, and eszopiclone have less effect on stage III, stage IV, and REM sleep. These agents are used as hypnotics to produce sleep. The recommended period of use for these benzodiazepine receptor agonists is 7 to 10 days, with reevaluation of the patient if use exceeds 2 to 3 weeks. Daytime drowsiness is generally

Drug Table 14-3 MISCELLANEOUS SEDATIVE-HYPNOTIC AGENTS

GENERIC NAME	BRAND NAME	AVAILABILITY	ADULT ORAL DOSE	COMMENTS
chloral hydrate	Aquachloral, ✤ PMS-Chloral Hydrate	Capsules: 500 mg Syrup: 250, 500 mg/5 mL Suppositories: 324, 648 mg	Sedation: 250 mg 3 times daily after meals Hypnosis: 500 mg to 1 g 15-30 min before bedtime	The original "Mickey Finn"; Schedule IV Used primarily as a bedtime hypnotic, but also is used as a preoperative sedative because it does not depress respirations or cough reflex May cause nausea; administer with full glass of water; do not chew capsules See Drug Interactions
dexmedetomidine	Precedex	Infusion: 100 mcg/mL in 9 mL vials	IV sedation: 1 mcg/kg over 10 min followed by infusion of 0.2-0.7 mcg/kg/hr using a controlled infusion device	For sedation of initially intubated and mechanically ventilated patients in an intensive care setting Infusion should not continue longer than 24 hours
diphenhydramine	Benadryl, ✤ Simply Sleep	Tablets: 12.5, 25, 50 mg Capsules: 25, 50 mg Liquid: 12.5 mg/5 ml	Sedation: 25-50 mg at bedtime	Over-the-counter availability Used for mild insomnia for up to 1 week. Tolerance develops, increased dosage causes more side effects with no more efficacy
doxylamine	Unisom	Tablets: 25 mg	Sedation: 25 mg at bedtime	Over-the-counter availability Morning hangover may be significant See diphenhydramine
eszopiclone	Lunesta	Tablets: 1, 2, 3 mg	Hypnosis: 2-3 mg	Onset within 45 min; duration 5-8 hr Older adult patients should start with 1 mg See Drug Interactions
melatonin				See Chapter 48, p. 841

✤ Available in Canada.

Continued

Drug Table 14-3 MISCELLANEOUS SEDATIVE-HYPNOTIC AGENTS—cont'd

GENERIC NAME	BRAND NAME	AVAILABILITY	ADULT ORAL DOSE	COMMENTS
paraldehyde	Paral	Liquid: 30 mL (for oral or rectal use)	Sedation: 4-8 mL	Schedule IV Bitter tasting, unpleasant odor; administer in milk or iced fruit juice to mask taste and odor Dispense only in a glass container; do not use a plastic spoon or container Used predominantly as a sedative in treating delirium tremens This agent imparts a strong, foul odor to the breath for up to 24 hr after administration; the patient is often unaware of the foul smell
ramelteon	Rozerem	Tablets: 8 mg	Hypnosis: 8 mg within 30 min of bedtime	Do not take with or immediately after a high-fat meal
valerian				See Chapter 48, p. 838
zaleplon	Sonata	Capsules: 5, 10 mg	Hypnosis: 10 mg at bedtime	Schedule IV Short acting; onset within 30 min; duration 2-4 hr Older adult or low-weight patients should start with 5 mg
zolpidem	Ambien Ambien CR	Tablets: 5, 10 mg Controlled release tablets: 6.25, 12.5 mg	Hypnosis: 10 mg at bedtime Hypnosis: 12.5 mg at bedtime	Schedule IV Short acting; onset within 30 min; duration 3-5 hr Older adult patients should start with 5 mg immediate release tablets or 6.25 controlled release tablets

not a problem with these agents because of their short half-lives, although it is more likely with eszopiclone. Rebound insomnia has been reported after their discontinuation. Zaleplon has a short onset of action and a duration of 2 to 4 hours. It is used clinically for people having difficulty getting to sleep and for those who wake in the middle of the night. Zolpidem has a similar onset of action, but a duration of 3 to 5 hours. It is more effective in helping patients get to sleep, and prolonging sleep duration without morning hangover. Eszopiclone is the newest agent. Its onset of action is somewhat slower than the other two agents, but its duration of action is 5 to 8 hours, making it more effective for patients with mid-night or early-morning awakening. It has been reported to cause morning hangover, especially in elderly patients and with higher doses.

Chloral hydrate is also used as a sedative for diagnostic procedures. Paraldehyde is occasionally used as a sedative in treating delirium tremens.

Therapeutic Outcomes

The primary therapeutic outcomes sought from miscellaneous sedative-hypnotic agents are as follows:

1. To produce mild sedation.
2. For short-term use to produce sleep.

Nursing Process for Miscellaneous Sedative-Hypnotic Agents

Premedication Assessment

1. Record baseline vital signs, particularly blood pressure, in sitting and lying positions.
2. Check for history of blood dyscrasias or hepatic disease.
3. Take vital signs (blood pressure, pulse, respirations, and pain rating).

Planning

Availability. See Table 14-3.

Implementation

Dosage and Administration. See Table 14-3.

The habitual use of sedative-hypnotic agents may result in physical dependence. Rapid discontinuance after long-term use may result in symptoms similar to alcohol withdrawal such as weakness, anxiety, delirium, and generalized seizures. Treatment consists of gradual withdrawal over 2 to 4 weeks.

Paraldehyde. Dilute oral form in milk or iced fruit juice to mask the taste and odor. Dispense only in a glass container; do not use a plastic spoon or container.

Zaleplon, zolpidem, and eszopiclone have a very rapid onset of action. These agents should be taken only immediately before going to bed or after the patient has gone to bed and has difficulty falling asleep.

Evaluation

General adverse effects include drowsiness, lethargy, headache, muscle or joint pain, and mental depression. Some people experience transient restlessness and anxiety before falling asleep. "Morning hangover" commonly occurs after administration of hypnotic doses of chloral hydrate, doxylamine, and the long-acting benzodiazepines, quazepam and flurazepam. It is also being reported with eszopiclone. Patients may display dulled affect, subtle distortion of mood, and impaired coordination.

Side Effects to Expect

Hangover, Sedation, Lethargy. Patients may complain of morning hangover, blurred vision, and transient hypotension on arising. Explain to the patient the need for first rising to a sitting position, equilibrating, and then standing. Assistance with ambulation may be required. If hangover becomes troublesome, the dosage should be reduced, medication should be changed, or both.

People who work around machinery, drive a car, pour and give medications, or perform other duties in which they must remain mentally alert should not take these medications while working.

Restlessness, Anxiety. These side effects are usually mild and do not warrant discontinuing the medication. Encourage the patient to try to relax and let the sedative effect take over.

Elderly patients and those in severe pain may respond paradoxically with excitement, euphoria, restlessness, and confusion.

Safety measures such as maintenance of bed rest, side rails, and observation should be used during this period.

Drug Interactions

Drugs that Increase Toxic Effects. Antihistamines, alcohol, analgesics, anesthetics, tranquilizers, narcotics, cimetidine, disulfiram, isoniazid, rifampin, erythromycin, ketoconazole, and other sedative-hypnotics increase toxic effects of all sedative hypnotic agents.

Fluvoxamine. Fluvoxamine specifically inhibits the metabolism of ramelteon, causing excessive sedation. Patients receiving fluvoxamine, a serotonin-reuptake inhibitor used as an antidepressant, should not take ramelteon.

Drugs that Decrease Therapeutic Effect. Rifampin significantly enhances the metabolism of eszopiclone and ramelteon, reducing therapeutic effect. Consider using zolpidem instead.

Warfarin. Chloral hydrate may enhance the anticoagulant effects of warfarin. Observe for petechiae, ecchymoses, nosebleeds, bleeding gums, dark tarry stools, and bright red or "coffee ground" emesis. Monitor the prothrombin time and reduce the dosage of warfarin if necessary.

Food. The presence of food, particularly food with high fat content, slows the absorption of zolpidem, zaleplon, eszopiclone, and ramelteon, slowing the onset of action. For faster onset of action, do not administer with or immediately after a meal.

Disulfiram. Disulfiram may prolong the activity of paraldehyde. Monitor the patient for excessive sedation.

Clinitest. Chloral hydrate may produce false-positive Clinitest results. Use Clinistix to measure urine glucose.

Key Points

- There are many types of sleep disorders, but by far the most common is insomnia.
- Most cases of insomnia are short lived and can be effectively treated by nonpharmacologic methods such as a backrub, eating a lighter meal in the evening, eliminating naps, and reducing the use of alcohol and stimulants such as caffeine and nicotine.
- People who have insomnia lasting longer than 1 month and who also suffer from daytime impairment in social and employment responsibilities should be referred to a physician for a good history and physical assessment. There may be other underlying conditions that must be treated before the patient resorts to the use of sedative-hypnotic agents.
- A variety of sedative-hypnotics are available for pharmacologic treatment; however, the drugs of choice are the newer nonbenzodiazepines (zaleplon, zolpidem, eszopiclone) because of their wide margin of safety.

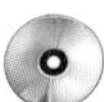

Go to your Companion CD-ROM for appendices, an Audio Glossary, animations, Drug Dosage Calculators, customizable Patient Self-Assessment forms, and Review Questions for the NCLEX® Examination.

evolve Be sure to visit the companion Evolve site at http://evolve.elsevier.com/Clayton for WebLinks and additional online resources.

MEDICATION SAFETY REVIEW

MATH REVIEW QUESTIONS

1. Order: Triazolam 0.5 mg at bedtime for 4 days only

   Available: Triazolam in 0.125- and 0.25-mg tablets

   Give ______.

2. Order: Chloral hydrate 400 mg 1 hour before patient undergoes a computed tomography scan

   Available: Chloral hydrate in 250- and 500-mg capsules and 250 and 500 mg/5 mL syrup

   Give: ______.

3. A patient is scheduled for an endoscopy at 9:00 AM tomorrow. He weighs 60 kg. A dose of midazolam 7.5 mg IV is scheduled to be administered a few minutes before the endoscopy. The normal midazolam dose is 0.1 to 0.15 mg/kg. Is the 7.5-mg dose reasonable for this patient?

CRITICAL THINKING QUESTIONS

1. Three hours after being given a hypnotic, a patient is still awake. She is having major surgery in the morning. Describe the actions you should initiate and the rationale for performing each.
2. Why should patients be cautioned against the use of alcohol when taking sedative-hypnotics?
3. Describe situations in which repeating a dose of a sedative-hypnotic would be appropriate.

CONTENT REVIEW QUESTIONS

1. As individuals age, their sleep becomes:
   1. more fragmented.
   2. more sound.
   3. characterized by fewer nocturnal awakenings.
   4. Both 2 and 3.
2. A patient receiving a benzodiazepine who also ingests alcohol may:
   1. experience erratic sleep and need less of the prescribed medication.
   2. experience additive effects of the alcohol and sedative-hypnotic agent.
   3. experience antagonist effects of the alcohol and sedative-hypnotic agent.
   4. require a higher dose of benzodiazepine and frequent assessments.
3. Long-term administration of benzodiazepines may result in:
   1. nephrotoxicity.
   2. withdrawal symptoms if withdrawn rapidly.
   3. a rush of morning energy with repeated usage.
   4. seizures during the time it is being administered.
4. A benefit of using zaleplon and zolpidem is:
   1. no rebound insomnia.
   2. their long half-life.
   3. they do not diminish stage III or IV or REM sleep as much as benzodiazepines.
   4. they can be used for only 2 weeks.

CHAPTER

15 Drugs Used for Parkinson's Disease

evolve http://evolve.elsevier.com/Clayton

Chapter Content

Objectives

1. Prepare a list of signs and symptoms of Parkinson's disease and accurately define the vocabulary used for the pharmacologic agents prescribed and the disease state.
2. Name the neurotransmitter that is found in excess and the neurotransmitter that is deficient in people with parkinsonism.
3. Describe reasonable expectations of medications prescribed for treatment of Parkinson's disease.
4. Identify the period necessary for a therapeutic response to be observable when drugs used to treat parkinsonism are initiated.
5. Name the action of bromocriptine, carbidopa, levodopa, entacapone, and apomorphine on neurotransmitters involved in Parkinson's disease.
6. List symptoms that can be attributed to the cholinergic activity of pharmacologic agents.
7. Cite the specific symptoms that should show improvement when anticholinergic agents are administered to the patient with Parkinson's disease.
8. Develop a health teaching plan for an individual being treated with levodopa.

Key Terms

Parkinson's disease
dopamine
neurotransmitter
acetylcholine
tremors
dyskinesia
propulsive, uncontrolled movement
akinesia
livedo reticularis
anticholinergic agents
levodopa

PARKINSON'S DISEASE

Parkinson's disease is a chronic progressive disorder of the central nervous system (CNS). It is the second most common neurodegenerative disease after Alzheimer's disease. An estimated 1% of the U.S. population older than age 50 and 2% older than age 60 have this disorder. Thirty percent of patients report onset of symptoms before age 50, 40% report the onset between ages 50 and 60, and the remainder, after age 60. The incidence is higher among men than women; all races and ethnic groups are affected. Characteristic symptoms include muscle tremors, slowness of movement in performing daily activities *(bradykinesia)*, muscle weakness with rigidity, and alterations in posture and equilibrium. The symptoms associated with parkinsonism are caused by a dopamine deficiency in the extrapyramidal system within the basal ganglia of the brain. The extrapyramidal system is responsible for maintaining posture and muscle tone and regulating voluntary smooth muscle activity. Normally a balance exists between **dopamine,** an inhibitory **neurotransmitter,** and **acetylcholine,** an excitatory neurotransmitter. With a deficiency of dopamine, a relative increase in acetylcholine activity occurs, causing the symptoms of parkinsonism. About 80% of the dopamine in the basal ganglia of the brain must be depleted for symptoms to develop.

There are two types of parkinsonism. Primary or idiopathic parkinsonism is caused by a reduction in dopamine-producing cells in the basal ganglia. The causes are not yet known, but there appear to be both genetic and environmental factors associated with its development. Approximately 10% to 15% of cases appear to be inherited. Secondary parkinsonism is caused by head trauma, intracranial infections, tumors, and drug exposure. Medicines that deplete dopamine, causing secondary parkinsonism, include dopamine antagonists such as phenothiazines, reserpine, methyldopa, and metoclopramide. In most cases of drug-induced parkinsonism, recovery is complete if the chemical is discontinued.

The symptoms of parkinsonism start insidiously and almost imperceptibly at first, with weakness and tremors, gradually progressing to involve movement disorders throughout the body (Figure 15-1). The symptoms usually begin on one side of the body such as a tremor of a finger or hand, and progress to become bilateral.

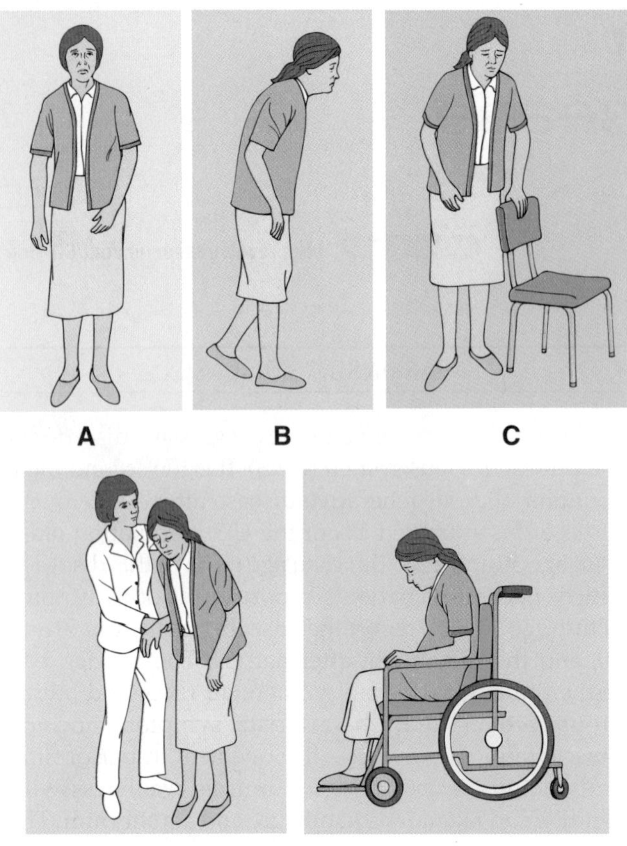

FIGURE **15-1** Stages of parkinsonism. **A,** Flexion of affected arm. Patient leans toward the unaffected side. **B,** Slow shuffling gait. **C,** Patient has increased difficulty walking and looks for sources of support to prevent falls. **D,** Further progression of weakness. Patient requires assistance from another person for ambulation. **E,** Profound disability. Patient may be confined to a wheelchair because of increasing weakness.

The upper part of the body is usually affected first. Eventually the individual has postural and gait alterations that result in the need for assistance with total care needs. Dementia, resembling Alzheimer's disease, occurs in a significant number of patients, but there is continuing debate as to whether it is part of the Parkinson's disease process or caused by concurrent drug therapy, Alzheimer's disease, or other factors. The diagnosis of Parkinson's disease is based on careful history taking and physical examination. There are no laboratory tests or imaging studies to confirm the diagnosis.

The patient and family should understand that Parkinson's disease often has a course over decades, the rate of progression varies greatly from one person to another, and many approaches are available to reduce symptoms. Patients should be counseled about exercise, including stretching, strengthening, cardiovascular fitness, and balance training. Patients and family often need assistance to learn the medical regimen used to control the symptoms and maintain the patient at an optimal level of participation in the activities of daily living (ADLs). Drug therapy presents the potential for many side effects that all involved parties must understand.

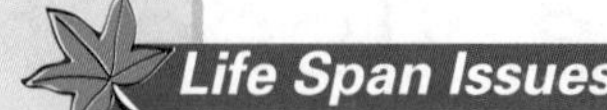

Parkinson's Disease

Parkinson's disease, which is most often seen in geriatric patients, causes a relative excess of acetylcholine because of a deficiency of dopamine. Drug therapy with dopaminergic agents increases dopamine availability, whereas anticholinergic medicines may be taken to counterbalance the availability of acetylcholine. Approximately 40% of patients with parkinsonism have some degree of clinical depression because of reduced availability of active metabolites of dopamine in the brain.

All drugs prescribed for Parkinson's disease produce a pharmacologic effect on the central nervous system. An assessment of the patient's mental status and physical functioning before initiation of therapy is essential to serve as a baseline so that comparisons can be made with subsequent evaluations.

Parkinson's disease is, at present, progressive and incurable. The goal of treatment is to moderate the symptoms and slow the progression of the disease. It is important to encourage the patient to take medications as scheduled and stay as active and involved in daily activities as possible.

Orthostatic hypotension is common with most of the medicines used to treat Parkinson's disease. In providing for patient safety, teach the patient to rise slowly from a supine or sitting position; encourage the patient to sit or lie down if feeling faint.

Constipation is a frequent problem with patients with Parkinson's disease. Instruct the patient to drink six to eight 8-ounce glasses of liquid daily and increase bulk in the diet to prevent constipation. Bulk-forming laxatives may also need to be added to the daily regimen.

Nurses can have a major influence in the positive use of coping mechanisms as the patient and family express varying degrees of anxiety, frustration, hostility, conflict, and fear. The primary goal of nursing intervention should be to keep the patient socially interactive and participatory in daily activities. This can be accomplished through physical therapy, adherence to the drug regimen, and management of the course of treatment.

DRUG THERAPY FOR PARKINSON'S DISEASE

Actions

The goal of treatment of parkinsonism is minimizing the symptoms, because there is no cure for the disease. Goals are to relieve symptoms and restore dopaminergic activity and neurotransmitter function as close to normal as possible. Treatment is usually started when symptoms progress to interfere with the patient's ability to perform at work or function in social situations. Drug therapy includes the use of selegiline to possibly slow the deterioration of dopaminergic nerve cells; bromocriptine, pergolide, ropinirole, pramipexole, amantadine, carbidopa-levodopa, or entacapone in various combinations to enhance dopaminergic activity; and anticholinergic agents to inhibit the relative excess in cholinergic activity. Therapy must be individualized, and realistic goals must be set for each patient. It is not possible to eliminate all symptoms of the disease because

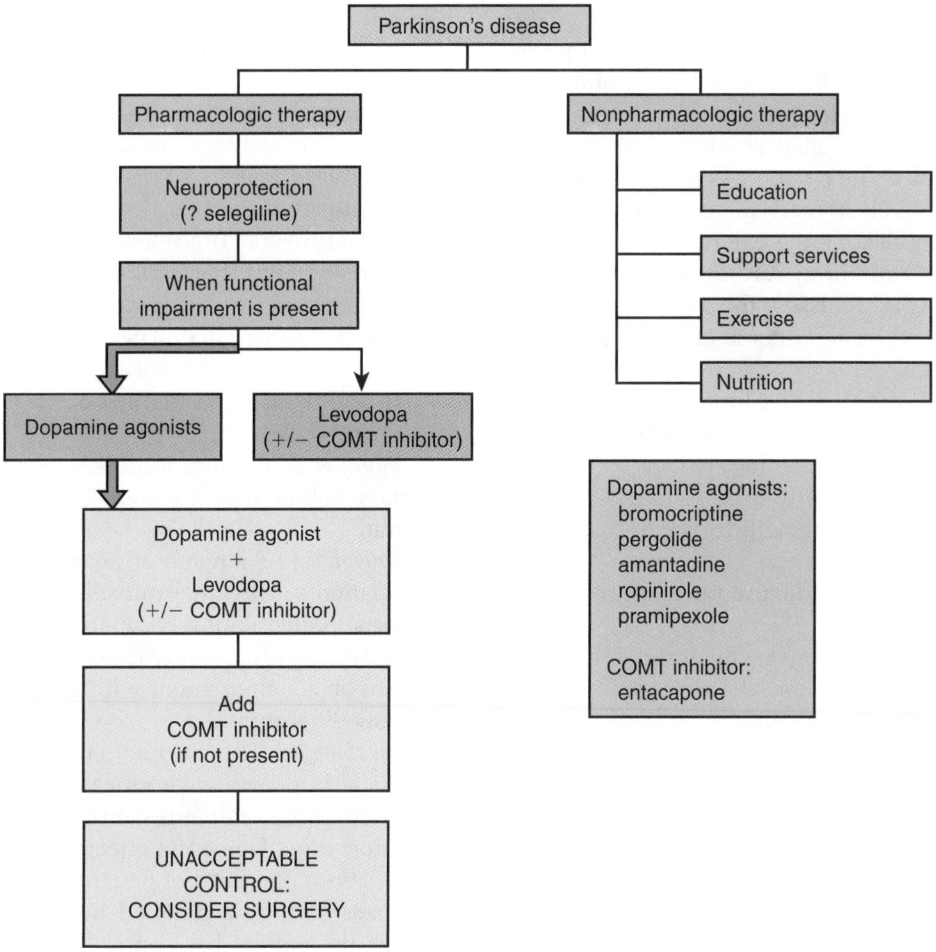

Parkinson's disease

Pharmacologic therapy

Neuroprotection (? selegiline)

When functional impairment is present

Dopamine agonists

Levodopa (+/− COMT inhibitor)

Dopamine agonist + Levodopa (+/− COMT inhibitor)

Add COMT inhibitor (if not present)

UNACCEPTABLE CONTROL: CONSIDER SURGERY

Nonpharmacologic therapy

Education

Support services

Exercise

Nutrition

Dopamine agonists: bromocriptine, pergolide, amantadine, ropinirole, pramipexole

COMT inhibitor: entacapone

FIGURE **15-2** Management of Parkinson's disease. Consider neuroprotective therapy as soon as diagnosis is made. When functional impairment starts, initiate a dopamine agonist; supplement with levodopa when dopamine agonist monotherapy no longer provides satisfactory clinical control. Consider introducing supplemental levodopa in combination with a COMT inhibitor to extend levodopa's duration of action. Consider surgical intervention when parkinsonism cannot be satisfactorily controlled with medical therapies.

the medications' side effects would not be tolerated. The trend is to use the lowest possible dose of medication so that as the disease progresses, dosages can be increased and other medicines added to get a combined effect.

Uses

Selegiline may be used to slow the course of Parkinson's disease by possibly slowing the progression of deterioration of dopaminergic nerve cells. A dopamine agonist such as bromocriptine, pergolide, amantadine, ropinirole, or pramipexole is initiated when the patient develops functional impairment. Carbidopa-levodopa continues to be the most effective drug to relieve symptoms, but after 3 to 5 years, the drug's effect gradually wears off and the patient suffers from "on-off" fluctuations in levodopa activity. A catechol-*O*-methyltransferase (COMT) inhibitor (entacapone) may be added to carbidopa-levodopa therapy to prolong the activity of the dopamine by slowing its rate of metabolism. Apomorphine may also be administered to treat "off" periods. Anticholinergic agents provide symptomatic relief from excessive acetylcholine. These agents are often used in combination to promote optimal levels of motor function (e.g., improve gait, posture, speech) and decrease disease symptoms (e.g., tremors, rigidity, drooling). See Figure 15-2 for an algorithm of treatment for Parkinson's disease.

NURSING PROCESS *for Parkinson's Disease Therapy*

Assessment

Unified Parkinson's Disease Rating Scale. The Unified Parkinson's Disease Rating Scale (UPDRS) is often used to identify the baseline of Parkinson's disease symptoms at the time of diagnosis and to monitor changes in symptoms that may require medicine dosage adjustment. The UPDRS evaluates (1) mentation, behavior, and mood; (2) ADLs; (3) motor examination; (4) complications of therapy; (5) modified Hoehn and Yahr staging; and (6) the Schwab and England ADL scale.

History of Parkinsonism. Obtain a history of exposure to known conditions associated with the development of parkinsonian symptoms such as head trauma, encephalitis, tumors, and drug exposure, including phenothiazines, reserpine, methyldopa, and metoclopramide. Also ask if the person has a history of being exposed to toxic levels of metals or carbon monoxide.

Obtain data to classify the extent of parkinsonism that the patient is exhibiting. A rating scale such as the UPDRS may be used to assess the severity of Parkinson's disease based on the degree of disability exhibited by the patient:

Stage 1: Involvement of one limb; slight tremor or minor change in speech, facial expression, posture or movement; mild disease

Stage 2: Involvement of two limbs; early postural changes, some social withdrawal, possible depression

Stage 3: Significant gait disturbances and moderate generalized disability

Stage 4: Akinesia (abnormal state of motor and psychic hypoactivity or muscle paralysis), rigidity, and severe disability; still able to walk or stand unassisted

Stage 5: Unable to stand or walk, perform all ADLs; wheelchair bound or bedridden unless aided

Motor Function. Patients with Parkinson's disease progress through the following symptoms.

Tremor. Tremors initially are so minor they are observed only by the patient. They occur primarily at rest, but are more noticeable during emotional turmoil or periods of increased concentration. The tremors are often observed in the hands and may involve the jaw, lips, and tongue. A "pill rolling" motion in the fingers and thumbs is characteristic. Tremors are usually reduced with voluntary movement. Emotional stress and fatigue may increase the frequency of tremors.

Assess the degree of tremor involvement and specific limitations in activities being affected by the tremors. Obtain a history of the progression of the symptoms from the patient.

Dyskinesia. Dyskinesia (dis kin eez' e ah) is the impairment of the individual's ability to perform voluntary movements. This symptom commonly starts in one arm or hand. It is usually most noticeable because the patient ceases to swing the arm on the affected side while walking.

As dyskinesia progresses, movement, especially in small muscle groups, becomes slow and jerky. This motion is often referred to as cogwheel rigidity. Muscle soreness, fatigue, and pain are associated with the prolonged muscle contractibility. The patient develops a shuffling gait, and may have difficulty in halting steps while walking (festination). When starting movement, there may be brief moments of immobility called *freezing*. Once-automatic movements such as getting out of a chair or walking require a concentrated effort.

Along with the shuffling gait, the head and spine flex forward and the shoulders become rounded and stooped.

As mobility deteriorates, steps quicken and become shorter. Propulsive, uncontrolled movement forward or backward is evident. Patient safety becomes a primary consideration.

Bradykinesia. Bradykinesia is the extremely slow body movement that may eventually progress to akinesia (a kin eez' e ah), or lack of movement.

Facial Appearance. The patient typically appears expressionless, as if wearing a mask; eyes are wide open and fixed in position. Some patients have almost total eyelid closure.

Nutrition. Complete an assessment of the person's dietary habits, recent weight loss, and difficulty with eating.

Salivation. As a result of excessive cholinergic activity, patients salivate profusely. As the disease progresses, patients may be unable to swallow all secretions and will frequently drool. If pharyngeal muscles are involved, the patient will have difficulty chewing and swallowing.

Psychologic. The chronic nature of the disease and physical impairment produce mood swings and serious depression. Patients commonly display a delayed reaction time. Dementia affects the intellectual capacity of about one third of patients.

Stress. Obtain a detailed history of the manner in which the patient has controlled physical and mental stress.

Safety/Self-Care. Assess the level of assistance needed for mobility and performance of ADLs and self-care.

Family Resources. Determine what family resources are available and the closeness of the family during daily as well as stress-producing events.

Nursing Diagnosis

- Risk for constipation (side effect)
- Deficient knowledge related to medication regimen
- Risk for injury (indications)
- Noncompliance related to drug side effects or lack of understanding of response time required for therapeutic response (side effects)
- Self-care deficits related to parkinsonian symptoms (indications)
- Imbalanced nutrition: less than body requirements related to dysphagia (indications)

Planning

History of Parkinsonism. Schedule a meeting to plan needed baseline assessments of the patient's functional abilities, including mental status, before initiating therapy and periodically throughout therapy to differentiate disease symptoms from drug-induced side effects.

Safety. Provide for patient safety. Obtain antislip pads for chair and/or other positioning devices.

Perform a safety check of the patient's environment to prevent accidents.

Care Needs. Coordinate care needs with other departments, for example, physical therapy and dietary and social services. Parkinson's disease is a progressive disorder, and it is important to plan for periodic evaluation of the patient's status.

Along with the patient and family, plan how the patient's daily care needs will be accomplished.

Make the patient/family/caretakers aware of the American Parkinson's Disease Association and the services and information available from this source. There are support groups for patients and families that can serve as a caring environment for people with similar experiences and concerns. Respite care may also be available, which provides temporary services to the dependent older adult either at home or in an institutional setting to provide the family with relief from the demands of daily patient care.

Medication Therapy. Schedule determination of vital signs on a routine basis, especially blood pressure monitoring. This is particularly important during initiation of therapy and when dose adjustments or medication changes are made.

Plan to stress that the effectiveness of medication therapy may take several weeks.

Schedule monitoring of behavioral changes on a consistent schedule established within the clinical practice setting.

Implementation

- Implement planned interventions consistent with assessment data and identify individual needs of the patient.
- Monitor and record vital signs, especially blood pressure, during the course of therapy. Report significant changes in blood pressure. These are most likely to occur during periods of dosage adjustment. Emphasize measures to prevent orthostatic hypotension.
- Monitor for degree of therapeutic response and side effects using forms provided by the clinical site to document changes in function.
- Monitor bowel function and implement measures to prevent constipation (e.g., adequate fluid intake, bulk in diet, exercise, use of stool softeners).
- Support the patient's efforts to remain mobile. Provide a safe environment by removing clutter and throw rugs; use correct equipment and supportive devices.
- Minimize deformities by encouraging erect posture. Maintain joint mobility through the use of active and passive exercises.
- Reinforce the principles taught for gait training.
- Nutritional needs must be carefully assessed because dietary modifications will be required as the disease progresses. Be vigilant for difficulty in swallowing and realize the patient may be prone to aspiration of food or water. Weigh the patient weekly; evaluate and report fluctuations in body weight to the dietitian or health care provider.
- Encourage self-maintenance and social involvement.
- Provide a restful environment and attempt to keep stressors at a minimum.
- Monitor mood and affect. Be alert for signs of depression. Mood alterations and depression are secondary to disease progression (for example, lack of ability to participate in sex, immobility, incontinence) and may be expected, but should not be ignored.
- Provide for patient safety during ambulation and delivery of care.

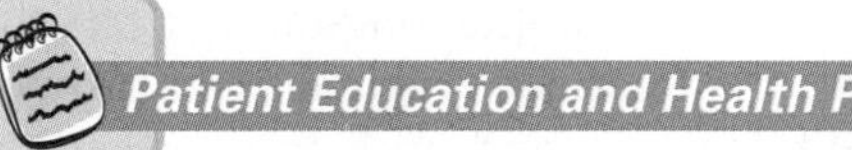

Patient Education and Health Promotion

Nutrition. Teach the patient to drink at least six to eight glasses of water or fluid per day to maintain adequate hydration. Because constipation is often a problem, instruct the patient to include bulk in the diet and use stool softeners as needed. As the disease progresses, the type and consistency of the foods eaten will need to be adjusted to meet the individual's needs. Because of fatigue and difficulty in eating, give assistance appropriate to the degree of impairment. Do not rush the individual when eating; cut foods into bite-size pieces. Teach swallowing techniques to prevent aspiration. Plan six smaller meals daily rather than three larger meals.

Instruct the patient to weigh weekly. Ask the patient to state the guidelines for weight loss or gain that should be reported to the health care provider.

Stress that vitamins should not be taken unless prescribed by the health care provider. Pyridoxine (B_6) will reduce the therapeutic effect of levodopa.

Stress Management. Explain to the patient and caregivers about the importance of maintaining an environment that is as stress-free as possible. Explain that symptoms such as tremors are enhanced by anxiety.

Self-Reliance. Encourage patients to perform as many ADLs as they can. Explain to caregivers that it is important not to "take over"; encourage self-maintenance, continued social involvement, and participation in activities such as hobbies. Use adaptive devices to aid in dressing, and purchase clothing with easy closures/fasteners such as Velcro. As mobility diminishes, use a bath chair and handheld shower nozzle.

Exercise. Instruct the patient and caregiver about the importance of maintaining correct body alignment, walking as erect as possible, and practicing the gait training taught by the physical therapy department. Gait training is essential if the patient is to delay the onset of shuffling and gait propulsion. Patients should wear sturdy, supportive shoes and use a cane, walker, or other assistive device to maintain mobility. Exercises to maintain the strength of facial muscles and the tongue help maintain speech clarity and the ability to swallow. Active and passive range-of-motion (ROM) exercises to all joints help minimize deformities. Explain that maintaining the exercise program can increase the patient's long-term well-being.

Mood Alterations. Explain to the patient and caregiver that depression and mood alterations are secondary to disease progression (e.g., inability to participate in sex, immobility, incontinence) and may be expected. Changes in mental outlook should be discussed with the health care provider.

Fostering Health Maintenance. Provide the patient and significant others with important information contained in the specific drug monograph for the medicines prescribed. Stress the importance of the nonpharmacologic interventions and the long-term effects that compliance with the treatment regimen can provide. Additional health teaching and nursing interventions for the side effects to expect and report are described in the drug monographs that follow.

Seek cooperation and understanding of the following points so that medication compliance is increased: name of medication, dosage, route, administration times, side effects to expect, and side effects to report.

Written Record. Enlist the patient's aid in developing and maintaining a written record of monitoring parameters (e.g., degree of tremor relief, stability, changes in mobility and rigidity, sedation, constipation, drowsiness, mental alertness, or deviations) (see Patient Self-Assessment Form on p. 237). Complete the Premedication Data column for use as a baseline to track response to drug therapy. Ensure that the patient understands how to use the form and instruct the patient to bring the completed form to follow-up visits. During follow-up visits, focus on issues that will foster adherence with the therapeutic interventions prescribed. ■

DRUG CLASS: Dopamine Agonists

amantadine hydrochloride (ah man′ ta deen)
▶ SYMMETREL (sim′ eh trel)

Amantadine is a compound developed originally to treat viral infections. It was administered to a patient with Asian influenza who also had parkinsonism. During the course of therapy for influenza, the patient showed definite improvement in the parkinsonian symptoms.

Actions

The exact mechanism of action is unknown but appears to be unrelated to the drug's antiviral activity. Amantadine seems to slow the destruction of dopamine, thus making the small amount present more effective. It may also aid in the release of dopamine from its storage sites. Unfortunately, about half the patients who benefit from amantadine therapy begin to notice a reduction in benefit after 2 or 3 months. A dosage increase or temporary discontinuation followed by a reinitiation of therapy several weeks later may restore the therapeutic benefits. When being discontinued, amantadine should be gradually withdrawn.

Uses

Amantadine is used for the relief of symptoms associated with Parkinson's disease and for the treatment of susceptible strains of viral influenza.

Therapeutic Outcomes

The primary therapeutic outcome sought from amantadine in treating parkinsonism is to establish a balance of dopamine and acetylcholine in the basal ganglia of the brain by enhancing delivery of dopamine to brain cells.

Nursing Process for Amantadine Therapy

Premedication Assessment

1. Perform a baseline assessment of parkinsonism using the UPDRS.
2. Amantadine should be used with caution in patients with a history of seizure activity, liver disease, uncontrolled psychosis, or congestive heart failure. Amantadine may cause an exacerbation of these disorders.
3. Take baseline blood pressures in supine and standing positions.

Planning

Availability. PO: 100 mg capsules, 50 mg/5 mL syrup.

Implementation

Dosage and Administration. *Adult:* PO: Initially 100 mg two times daily; maximum daily dose is 400 mg. Because of the possibility of insomnia, plan the last dose to be administered in the afternoon, not at bedtime.

Evaluation

Most of the adverse effects of amantadine therapy are dose related and reversible.

Side Effects to Expect

Confusion, Disorientation, Hallucinations, Mental Depression. Perform a baseline assessment of the patient's degree of alertness and orientation to name, place, and time before initiating therapy. Make regularly scheduled subsequent evaluations of mental status, and compare findings. Report alterations.

Dizziness, Lightheadedness, Anorexia, Nausea, Abdominal Discomfort. These side effects are usually mild and tend to resolve with continued therapy. Encourage the patient not to discontinue therapy without first consulting the health care provider. Provide patient safety during periods of dizziness or lightheadedness.

PATIENT SELF-ASSESSMENT FORM Antiparkinson Agents

MEDICATIONS	COLOR	TO BE TAKEN

Patient ______________________

Health Care Provider ______________________

Health Care Provider's phone ______________________

Next appt.* ______________________

What I Should Monitor		Premedication Data	Date	Date	Date	Date	Date	Date	Comments
Weight									
Blood pressure									
Pulse									
Tremor relief or pain relief Little relief (10) — Moderate relief (5) — Good relief (1)									
Mobility and rigidity: gait training, working or not No improvement (10) — 5 — Less rigidity (1)									
Control of secretions Worse (10) — 5 — No problem (1)									
Alertness and orientation to time, person, and place (TPP) Poor (10) — 5 — Good (1)									
Exercise: Note present level of activity: walking, getting out, performing range-of-motion (ROM) exercises									
Bowel and bladder	Check one: Constipated = C Normal = N	C ____ N ____	C ____ N ____	C ____ N ____	C ____ N ____	C ____ N ____	C ____ N ____	C ____ N ____	
	Difficulty urinating = D								
	Occasional problem urinating								
Dietary needs	No problem eating or drinking								
	Drinks (_____) glasses fluid per day								
	Needs frequent small meals								
	Needs a lot of time to eat								
Socialization Withdrawn (10) — 5 — Active involved (1)									
Other									

*Please bring this record with you to your next appointment.
Use the back of this sheet for additional information.

Livedo Reticularis (Skin Mottling). A dermatologic condition known as livedo reticularis is occasionally observed in conjunction with amantadine therapy. It is characterized by diffuse rose-colored mottling of the skin, often accompanied by ankle edema, predominantly in the extremities. It is more noticeable when the patient is standing or exposed to cold. It is reversible within 2 to 6 weeks after discontinuation of amantadine. However, discontinuing therapy is generally not necessary.

These side effects are usually mild and tend to resolve with continued therapy. Symptoms are enhanced by exposure to the cold or by prolonged standing. Encourage the patient not to discontinue therapy without first consulting the health care provider.

Side Effects to Report

Liver Disease. The symptoms of liver disease are anorexia, nausea, vomiting, jaundice, hepatomegaly, splenomegaly, and abnormal liver function tests (elevated bilirubin, aspartate aminotransferase [AST], alanine aminotransferase [ALT], gamma glutamyltransferase [GGT], alkaline phosphatase, prothrombin time).

Seizure Disorders, Psychosis. Provide patient safety during episodes of dizziness; report symptoms for further evaluation.

Dyspnea/Edema. If amantadine is used with patients who have a history of heart failure, assess lung sounds, additional edema, and weight gain on a regular basis.

Drug Interactions

Anticholinergic Agents (Trihexyphenidyl, Benztropine, Procyclidine, Diphenhydramine). Amantadine may exacerbate the side effects of anticholinergic agents that may also be used to control the symptoms of parkinsonism. Confusion and hallucinations may gradually develop. The dosage of amantadine or the anticholinergic agent should be reduced.

apomorphine (ah poh mor′ feen)
APOKYN (ah poh′ kin)

Action

Apomorphine is a nonergot dopamine agonist. It is thought to stimulate dopamine receptors in the brain, temporarily restoring motor function. It is chemically related to morphine, but does not have any opioid activity.

Use

As Parkinson's disease progresses, patients often experience episodes of lower responsiveness to levodopa, causing periods of hypomobility (e.g., inability to rise from a chair, speak, or walk). Apomorphine is used to treat hypomobility associated with the "wearing off" of dopamine agonists either near the end of a dosage cycle, or at unpredictable times ("on-off" phenomenon).

Therapeutic Outcomes

The primary therapeutic outcomes sought from apomorphine in treating parkinsonism are to improve motor and ADL scores, and to decrease "off" time.

Nursing Process for Apomorphine Therapy

Premedication Assessment

1. Perform a baseline assessment of parkinsonism using the UPDRS.
2. Obtain a history of cardiovascular symptoms, including baseline vital signs (e.g., blood pressure, heart rate).
3. Perform a baseline assessment of the patient's degree of mobility, alertness, and orientation to name, place, and time before initiating therapy. Ask specifically whether he or she may be taking other sedating medicines. Make regularly scheduled subsequent evaluations of blood pressure, pulse, mental status, and mobility, and compare findings.

Planning

Availability. Subcutaneously: 10 mg/mL in 2 mL glass ampules, and 3 mL cartridges.

Implementation

Dosage and Administration. NOTE: DO NOT ADMINISTER INTRAVENOUSLY. The apomorphine may crystallize in the vein and form a thrombus or embolism.

Apomorphine is administered most commonly using a manual, reusable, multidose injector pen that holds a 3-mL cartridge of medicine. To avoid potential confusion with the use of the pen and inadvertent overdose, it is recommended that the dose of the drug be identified in milliliters, not in milligrams. The pen is adjustable in 0.02-mL increments. A training pamphlet on the use of the injector pen is available for patient use.

Adult: Subcutaneously: Initially, a test dose of 0.2 mL (2 mg) should be administered in the stomach area, upper leg, or upper arm. Both supine and standing blood pressure should be determined before administering the dose and at 20, 40, and 60 minutes after administration. If significant orthostatic hypotension develops, therapy should be discontinued and the patient should receive no further doses of apomorphine.

If the patient tolerates the 0.2 mL dose and responds, the starting dose should be 0.2 mL used on a PRN basis to treat "off" events. If needed, the dose can be increased in 0.1 mL (1 mg) increments every few days on an outpatient basis. The maximum recommended dose is 0.6 mL (6 mg).

If a patient discontinues therapy for longer than 1 week and then wishes to go back to the use of apomorphine, therapy should be reinitiated at the starting dose of 0.2 mL, with gradual increases in dosage to optimal therapy.

Use of an Antiemetic. One of the pharmacologic actions of apomorphine is emesis. The antiemetic trimethobenzamide (Tigan) should be administered orally in a dosage of 300 mg three times a day for at least 3 days prior to the initial dose of apomorphine. It should be continued for at least the first 2 months of therapy. About 50% of patients are able to discontinue the antiemetic while continuing therapy with apomorphine. Do not use prochlorperazine (Compazine) or ondansetron (Zofran) as antiemetics. (See Drug Interactions.)

Evaluation

Most side effects observed with apomorphine agents are direct extensions of their pharmacologic properties.

Side Effects to Expect and Report

Nausea, Vomiting. These effects can be reduced by premedicating with trimethobenzamide and slowly increasing the dosage.

Orthostatic Hypotension. Apomorphine commonly causes orthostatic hypotension manifested by dizziness and weakness, particularly when therapy is being initiated. Patients with Parkinson's disease are at risk of falling due to the underlying postural instability associated with the disease, and apomorphine may increase the risk of falling by lowering blood pressure and altering mobility. Anticipate the development of postural hypotension and provide assistance when necessary. Monitor the blood pressure before and during apomorphine therapy in both the supine and standing positions.

Teach patients to rise slowly from a supine or sitting position; encourage them to sit or lie down if feeling faint.

Chewing Motions, Bobbing, Facial Grimacing, Rocking Movements. These involuntary movements (dyskinesias) occur in some patients, especially if they are also taking levodopa. A reduction in dosage of the levodopa or apomorphine may be beneficial.

Nightmares, Depression, Confusion, Hallucinations. Perform a baseline assessment of the patient's degree of alertness and orientation to name, place, and time before initiating therapy. Make regularly scheduled subsequent evaluations of mental status, and compare findings. Report alterations.

Provide for patient safety during these episodes. Reducing the daily dosage may control these adverse effects.

Tachycardia, Palpitations. Take the pulse at regularly scheduled intervals. Report for further evaluation.

Sudden Sleep Events. Sleep episodes have been reported with the dopamine agonists (e.g., apomorphine, bromocriptine, pergolide, pramipexole, ropinirole). These episodes are described as sleep attacks or sleep episodes including daytime sleep. Some sleep events have been reported as sudden and irresistible. Other sleep events have been preceded by sufficient warning to prevent accidents. Patients taking dopamine agonists should be informed about the possibility of daytime sleepiness and outright sleep attacks with these medicines and allowed to make their own decisions about driving based on past experiences with the medicines. Assessment of patients at risk of sleep attacks is possible with the Epworth Sleepiness Scale (ESS).

Penile Erection, Priapism. Apomorphine may cause penile erection, and rarely, priapism (prolonged painful erection). Apomorphine has been overused due to its ability to induce erection and increase libido. Indications of abuse include frequent erections, atypical sexual behavior, heightened libido, dyskinesias, agitation, confusion, and depression.

Drug Interactions

Ondansetron (Zofran), Dolasetron (Anzemet), Granisetron (Kytril), Palonosetron (Aloxi), Alosetron (Lotronex). The use of serotonin antagonists with apomorphine is contraindicated. Profound hypotension and loss of consciousness have been reported.

Phenothiazines, Including Prochlorperazine (Compazine), Butyrophenones (e.g., Haloperidol), Thioxanthines, Metoclopramide. These medicines are dopamine antagonists and will block the dopaminergic effect of apomorphine, aggravating parkinsonian symptoms.

Ethanol, Antihypertensive Agents, Vasodilators (e.g., Nitrates). Use of these agents concurrently with apomorphine significantly increases the frequency of orthostatic hypotension. Alcohol should be avoided when taking apomorphine. Dosage adjustment of the antihypertensive agent is often necessary because of excessive orthostatic hypotension.

bromocriptine mesylate (bro mo krip' teen)
▶ PARLODEL (par' lo del)

Actions

Bromocriptine is an ergot derivative that stimulates D_2 dopamine receptors in the basal ganglia of the brain.

Uses

Because parkinsonian patients are deficient of dopamine in the basal ganglia, there is marked improvement in the symptoms of the disease with bromocriptine therapy. Bromocriptine appears to be nearly as effective as levodopa in treating parkinsonism. It may be used alone in the treatment of mild symptoms or in combination with carbidopa-levodopa to reduce both the dose of carbidopa-levodopa and the parkinsonian symptoms.

Therapeutic Outcomes

The primary therapeutic outcome sought from bromocriptine in treating parkinsonism is to stimulate dopaminergic neurotransmission to relieve the rigidity, akinesia, and tremor associated with the dopamine deficiency of Parkinson's disease.

Nursing Process for Bromocriptine Therapy

Premedication Assessment

1. Perform a baseline assessment of parkinsonism using the UPDRS.
2. Take baseline blood pressures in supine and standing positions.

Planning

Availability. PO: 2.5 mg tablets, 5 mg capsules.

Implementation

Dosage and Administration. *Adult:* PO: Initially 1.25 mg two times daily with meals. Increase the dosage by 2.5 mg/day every 2 to 4 weeks. The dosage must be adjusted according to the patient's response and tolerance. Doses in the 50 to 100 mg daily range are not uncommon for maximal therapeutic benefit.

Side effects can be minimized by starting with small doses, then increasing the dosage gradually, and by administering medication with food in the evening. If severe side effects appear, they can be minimized by reducing the dosage for a few days, then increasing it more gradually.

Evaluation

Side Effects to Expect

Gastrointestinal Effects. Most of these effects may be minimized by temporary reduction in dosage, administration with food, and use of stool softeners for constipation.

Other Side Effects. Mouth dryness, double vision, nasal congestion, and metallic taste may also occur.

Side Effects to Report

Neurologic. Neurologic effects often occur with higher doses. Perform a baseline assessment of the patient's degree of alertness and orientation to name, place, and time before initiating therapy. Make regularly scheduled subsequent evaluations of mental status, and compare findings. Report alterations.

Provide patient safety, be emotionally supportive, and ensure the patient that these adverse effects dissipate within 2 to 3 weeks of discontinuing therapy.

Orthostatic Hypotension. Monitor the blood pressure daily in both the supine and standing positions.

Anticipate the development of postural hypotension and take measures to prevent an occurrence. Teach the patient to rise slowly from a supine or sitting position; encourage the patient to sit or lie down if feeling faint.

Hypertension. Although hypotension at the start of therapy is not uncommon, hypertension may begin in the first or second week of therapy. Monitor carefully and report if higher blood pressures develop. If the patient starts complaining of headaches and blood pressure is higher than normal, report to the health care provider immediately.

Sudden Sleep Events. Sleep episodes have been reported with the dopamine agonists (bromocriptine, pergolide, pramipexole, and ropinirole). These episodes are described as sleep attacks or sleep episodes, including daytime sleep. Some sleep events have been reported as sudden and irresistible and have caused accidents. Other sleep events have been preceded by sufficient warning to prevent accidents. Patients taking dopamine agonists should be informed about the possibility of daytime sleepiness and outright sleep attacks with these medicines and allowed to make their own decisions about driving based on past experiences with the medicines. Assessment of patients at risk of sleep attacks is possible with the ESS.

Drug Interactions

Levodopa. Bromocriptine and levodopa have additive neurologic effects. This interaction may be advantageous because it often allows a reduction in the dose of the levodopa.

Antihypertensive Agents. Dose adjustment of the antihypertensive agent is often necessary because of excessive orthostatic hypotension or development of hypertension.

carbidopa (kar bi doe' pa), **levodopa** (lee voe doe' pa)

▶ SINEMET (sin' eh met), PARCOPA (pahr-ko-pah)

Actions

Sinemet and Parcopa are combination products of carbidopa and levodopa used for treating the symptoms of Parkinson's disease. Carbidopa is an enzyme inhibitor that reduces the metabolism of levodopa, allowing a greater portion of the administered levodopa to reach the desired receptor sites in the basal ganglia. Carbidopa has no effect when used alone; it must be used in combination with levodopa.

Uses

Carbidopa is used to reduce the dose of levodopa required by approximately 75%. When administered with levodopa, carbidopa increases both plasma levels and the plasma half-life of levodopa. Parcopa is a formulation that dissolves in the mouth, reducing the incidence of choking secondary to attempting to swallow tablets.

Therapeutic Outcomes

The primary therapeutic outcome sought from Sinemet in treating parkinsonism is to establish a balance of dopamine and acetylcholine in the basal ganglia of the brain by enhancing delivery of dopamine to brain cells.

Nursing Process for Sinemet Therapy

Premedication Assessment

1. Perform a baseline assessment of parkinsonism using the UPDRS.
2. Review medicines prescribed that may need dose adjustments. Plan to perform focused assessments to detect responses to therapy that would need to be reported to the health care provider.
3. Review the symptoms manifested by the patient. Patients with irregular, "on-off" responses to levodopa do not benefit from Sinemet.

Planning

Availability. PO: Sinemet is a combination product containing both carbidopa and levodopa. The combination product is available in ratios of 10/100, 25/100, and 25/250 mg of carbidopa-levodopa. There are also sustained release products, Sinemet CR, which contains either 25 mg per 100 mg, or 50 mg per 200 mg of carbidopa-levodopa.

Parcopa is a combination product containing both carbidopa and levodopa. The combination product is available as orally disintegrating tablets in ratios of 10/100, 25/100, and 25/250 mg of carbidopa-levodopa.

Implementation

Dosage and Administration. *Adult:* PO: For patients not currently receiving levodopa, initially, Sinemet or Parcopa 10/100 or 25/100 three times daily, increasing by one tablet every other day until a dosage of six tablets daily is attained. As therapy progresses and patients show indications of needing more levodopa, substitute Sinemet 25/250, one tablet three or four times daily. Increase by one tablet every other day to a maximum of eight tablets daily. See the manufacturer's guidelines for switching a patient to the sustained release form of Sinemet.

Evaluation

Side Effects to Expect. Carbidopa has no effect when used alone; it must be used in combination with levodopa. The side effects seen with combined therapy are actually an enhancement of the effects of levodopa because the carbidopa is allowing more levodopa to reach the brain. See Levodopa below.

Drug Interactions. Sinemet may be used to treat parkinsonism in conjunction with dopamine agonists, COMT inhibitors, or anticholinergic agents. The dosages of all medications may need to be reduced because of combined therapy. See also Levodopa below.

levodopa (lee voe doe' pa)
▶ LARODOPA (lar oh doe' pah), DOPAR (do' par)

Actions

Dopamine, when administered orally, does not enter the brain. Levodopa does cross into the brain, is metabolized to dopamine, and replaces the dopamine deficiency in the basal ganglia. Dopamine stimulates D_1, D_2, and D_3 dopamine receptors.

Uses

About 75% of patients with parkinsonism respond favorably to levodopa therapy, but after a few years the response diminishes, becomes more uneven, and is accompanied by many more side effects. This loss of therapeutic effect reflects the progression of the underlying disease process.

Therapeutic Outcomes

The primary therapeutic outcome sought from levodopa in treating parkinsonism is to establish a balance of dopamine and acetylcholine in the basal ganglia of the brain by enhancing delivery of dopamine to brain cells.

Nursing Process for Levodopa Therapy

Premedication Assessment

1. Perform a baseline assessment of parkinsonism using the UPDRS.
2. Obtain a history of gastrointestinal (GI) and cardiovascular symptoms, including baseline vital signs (e.g., blood pressure, pulse).
3. Ask specifically about any symptoms of hallucinations or nightmares, dementia, or anxiety. Inquire about any urine testing being done.
4. All patients should be screened for the presence of angle-closure glaucoma before initiating therapy. Patients with open-angle glaucoma can safely use levodopa. Do not administer the medicine to people with a history of glaucoma unless specifically approved by the patient's health care provider.

Planning

Availability. PO: Dopar: 100, 250, and 500 mg capsules; Larodopa: 100, 500 mg tablets.

Implementation

Dosage and Administration. *Adult:* PO: Initially 0.5 to 1 g daily in divided doses and administered with food. Do not exceed 8 g per day. Administer medication with food or milk to reduce gastric irritation. Therapy for at least 6 months may be necessary to determine full therapeutic benefits.

Evaluation

Levodopa causes many side effects, but most are dose related and reversible. Side effects vary greatly, depending on the stage of the disease.

Side Effects to Expect

Nausea, Vomiting, Anorexia. These effects can be reduced by slowly increasing the dose, dividing the total daily dose into four to six doses, and administering the medication with food or antacids.

Orthostatic Hypotension. Although generally mild, levodopa may cause some degree of orthostatic hypotension manifested by dizziness and weakness, particularly when therapy is being initiated. Tolerance usually develops after a few weeks of therapy.

Monitor the blood pressure daily in both the supine and standing positions.

Anticipate the development of postural hypotension and take measures to prevent an occurrence. Teach patients to rise slowly from a supine or sitting position; encourage them to sit or lie down if feeling faint.

Side Effects to Report

Chewing Motions, Bobbing, Facial Grimacing, Rocking Movements. These involuntary movements occur in about half the patients taking levodopa more than 6 months. A reduction in dosage may be beneficial.

Nightmares, Depression, Confusion, Hallucinations. Perform a baseline assessment of the patient's degree of alertness and orientation to name, place, and time before initiating therapy. Make regularly scheduled subsequent evaluations of mental status, and compare findings. Report alterations.

Provide patient safety during these episodes.

Reducing the daily dosage may control these adverse effects.

Tachycardia, Palpitations. Take the pulse at regularly scheduled intervals. Report for further evaluation.

Drug Interactions

Phenelzine, Tranylcypromine. These monoamine oxidase inhibitor agents unpredictably exaggerate the effects of levodopa. They should be discontinued at least 14 days before the administration of levodopa.

Isoniazid. Use with caution in conjunction with levodopa. Discontinue isoniazid if patients taking levodopa develop hypertension, flushing, palpitations, and tremor.

Pyridoxine. Pyridoxine (vitamin B_6) in oral doses of 5 to 10 mg reverses the therapeutic and toxic effects of levodopa. Normal diets contain less than 1 mg of pyridoxine, so dietary restrictions are not necessary. However, the ingredients of multiple vitamins should be considered.

Diazepam, Chlordiazepoxide, Papaverine, Clonidine, Phenytoin. These agents appear to cause a deterioration in the therapeutic effects of levodopa. Use with caution in patients with parkinsonism and discontinue if the patient's clinical status deteriorates.

Phenothiazines, Reserpine, Haloperidol, Risperidone, Metoclopramide. A side effect associated with these agents is a parkinson-like syndrome. Because this will nullify the therapeutic effects of levodopa, do not use concurrently.

Ephedrine, Epinephrine, Isoproterenol, Amphetamines. Levodopa may increase the therapeutic and toxic effects of these agents. Monitor for tachycardia, dysrhythmias, and hypertension. Reduce the dosage of these agents if necessary.

Antihypertensive Agents. Dosage adjustment of the antihypertensive agent is frequently necessary because of excessive orthostatic hypotension.

Anticholinergic Agonists (Benztropine, Biperiden, Procyclidine, Diphenhydramine, Trihexyphenidyl). Even though these agents are used to treat parkinsonism, they increase gastric deactivation and decrease intestinal absorption of levodopa. Administration of doses of anticholinergic agents and levodopa should be separated by 2 hours or more.

Ketostix, Labstix, Acetest. Levodopa may produce false-positive urine ketone results with these products. Remind health care provider of this test interference.

Clinitest. Levodopa may produce a false-positive "trace" of urinary glucose.

Clinistix. Levodopa may produce false-negative urine glucose results with this product.

Bowl Cleaners. The metabolites of levodopa react with toilet-bowl cleaners to turn the urine red to black. This may also occur if the urine is exposed to air for long periods. Inform the patient that there is no cause for alarm.

pergolide mesylate (per' go lide)
PERMAX (per' maks)

Actions

Pergolide is an ergot derivative that is a potent D_1, D_2, and D_3 dopamine receptor stimulant. It is thought to exert its therapeutic effect in patients with Parkinson's disease by directly stimulating postsynaptic dopamine receptors in the nigrostriatal system of the brain.

Uses

Pergolide is used in combination with carbidopa-levodopa in the management of Parkinson's disease. In recent years there have been numerous reports of patients developing restrictive valvular heart disease while receiving pergolide. The risk of pergolide-induced cardiac valvular fibrosis may be related to cumulative dosage and duration of use. If pergolide must be used to treat parkinsonism, the lowest effective dosage should be used, and the patient should be evaluated periodically for development of restrictive valvular heart disease.

Therapeutic Outcomes

The primary therapeutic outcomes sought from pergolide in treating parkinsonism are as follows:

1. Improved motor and ADL scores.
2. Decreased "off" time.
3. Reduced dosage of levodopa.

Nursing Process for Pergolide Therapy

Premedication Assessment

1. Perform a baseline assessment of parkinsonism using the UPDRS.
2. Obtain a history of cardiovascular symptoms, including baseline vital signs (e.g., blood pressure, pulse).
3. Perform a baseline assessment of the patient's degree of alertness and orientation to name, place, and time before initiating therapy. Make regularly scheduled subsequent evaluations of mental status, and compare findings. Report alterations.

Planning

Availability. PO: 0.05, 0.25, and 1 mg tablets.

Implementation

Dosage and Administration. *Adult:* Dosage must be adjusted according to the patient's response and tolerance. Side effects can be minimized by starting with small doses, then increasing the dosage gradually. PO: Initiate with a daily dose of 0.05 mg for the first 2 days. Gradually increase the dosage by 0.1 or 0.15 mg/day every third day over the 12 days of therapy. The dosage may then be increased by 0.25 mg/day every third day until an optimal dosage is achieved. Pergolide is usually administered in divided doses three times daily. During dosage titration, the dose of concurrent carbidopa-levodopa should be cautiously decreased. The usual total daily dose of pergolide is 3 mg.

Evaluation

Side effects with pergolide are fairly common. About 25% of those patients receiving pergolide must discontinue therapy because of side effects.

Side Effects to Expect

GI Effects. GI effects include nausea, constipation, diarrhea, and upset stomach. Most of these effects may be minimized by temporary reduction in dosage, administration with food, and use of stool softeners for constipation.

Side Effects to Report

Neurologic. About 14% of patients develop hallucinations. Provide patient safety, be emotionally supportive, and assure the patient that these adverse effects usually dissipate as tolerance to the adverse effects develops over the next few weeks.

Orthostatic Hypotension. Monitor the blood pressure daily in both the supine and standing positions.

Anticipate the development of postural hypotension and take measures to prevent an occurrence. Teach the patient to rise slowly from a supine or sitting position; encourage the patient to sit or lie down if feeling faint.

Sudden Sleep Events. Sleep episodes have been reported with the dopamine agonists (bromocriptine, pergolide, pramipexole, and ropinirole). These episodes are described as sleep attacks or sleep episodes, including daytime sleep. Some sleep events have been reported as sudden and irresistible and have caused accidents. Other sleep events have been preceded by sufficient warning to prevent accidents. Patients taking dopamine agonists should be informed about the possibility of daytime sleepiness and outright sleep attacks with these medicines and allowed to make their own decisions about driving based on past experiences with the medicines. Assessment of patients at risk of sleep attacks is possible with the ESS.

Drug Interactions

Levodopa. Pergolide and levodopa have additive neurologic effects. This interaction may be beneficial because it often allows a reduction in dose of the levodopa.

Dopamine Antagonists. Dopamine antagonists include phenothiazines, butyrophenones, thioxanthenes, and metoclopramide. As dopamine antagonists, these agents will diminish the effectiveness of pergolide, a dopaminergic agonist.

Antihypertensive Agents. Dosage adjustment of the antihypertensive agent is often necessary because of excessive orthostatic hypotension.

pramipexole (pra mi pex' ole)
MIRAPEX (mihr ah' pex)

Action

Pramipexole is a nonergot dopamine agonist that stimulates D_2 and D_3 dopamine receptors.

Uses

Pramipexole may be used alone to manage early signs and symptoms of parkinsonism by improving ADLs, as well as motor manifestations such as tremor, rigidity, bradykinesia, and postural stability. It may also be used in combination with levodopa in advanced parkinsonism to manage similar signs and symptoms of the disease.

Therapeutic Outcomes

The primary therapeutic outcomes sought from pergolide in treating parkinsonism are as follows:

1. Improved motor and ADL scores.
2. Decreased "off" time.
3. Reduced dosage of levodopa.

Nursing Process for Pramipexole Therapy

Premedication Assessment

1. Perform a baseline assessment of parkinsonism using the UPDRS.
2. Obtain a history of GI and cardiovascular symptoms, including baseline vital signs (e.g., blood pressure, pulse).
3. Ask specifically about any symptoms of hallucinations, nightmares, dementia, or anxiety.

Planning

Availability. PO: 0.125, 0.25, 1.0, and 1.5 mg tablets.

Implementation

Dosage and Administration. *Adult:* PO: Initially 0.125 mg three times daily for 1 week. If tolerated, increase to 0.25 mg three times daily the second week. If tolerated, increase by increments of 0.25 mg three times daily through the seventh week. The usual maintenance dosage is 0.5 to 1.5 mg three times daily with or without levodopa therapy. When pramipexole is used with levodopa, consider reducing the levodopa.

Administer medication with food or milk to reduce gastric irritation.

If pramipexole is to be discontinued, the dosage should be gradually reduced over 1 week.

Evaluation

Pramipexole causes many side effects, but most are dose related and reversible. Side effects vary greatly, depending on the stage of the disease and the concurrent use of other medicines.

Side Effects to Expect

Nausea, Vomiting, Anorexia. These effects can be reduced by slowly increasing the dosage, dividing the total daily dose into three doses, and administering the medication with food.

Orthostatic Hypotension. Although generally mild, pramipexole may cause some degree of orthostatic hypotension manifested by dizziness and weakness, particularly when therapy is being initiated. Tolerance usually develops after a few weeks of therapy.

Monitor the blood pressure daily in both the supine and standing positions.

Anticipate the development of postural hypotension and take measures to prevent an occurrence. Teach patients to rise slowly from a supine or sitting position; encourage them to sit or lie down if feeling faint.

Side Effects to Report

Chewing Motions, Bobbing, Facial Grimacing, Rocking Movements. These involuntary movements occur in some patients, especially if they are also taking levodopa. A reduction in dosage of the levodopa may be beneficial.

Nightmares, Depression, Confusion, Hallucinations. Perform a baseline assessment of the patient's degree of alertness and orientation to name, place, and time before initiating therapy. Make regularly scheduled subsequent evaluations of mental status, and compare findings. Report alterations.

Provide for patient safety during these episodes. Reducing the daily dosage may control these adverse effects.

Tachycardia, Palpitations. Take the pulse at regularly scheduled intervals. Report for further evaluation.

Sudden Sleep Events. Sleep episodes have been reported with the dopamine agonists (e.g., bromocriptine, pergolide, pramipexole, and ropinirole). These episodes are described as sleep attacks or sleep episodes, including daytime sleep. Some sleep events have been reported as sudden and irresistible. Other sleep events have been preceded by sufficient warning to prevent accidents. Patients taking dopamine agonists should be informed about the possibility of daytime sleepiness and outright sleep attacks with these medicines and allowed to make their own decisions about driving based on past experiences with the medicines. Assessment of patients at risk of sleep attacks is possible with the ESS.

Drug Interactions

Cimetidine, Ranitidine, Diltiazem, Verapamil, Quinidine, Triamterene. These agents inhibit the urinary excretion of pramipexole. Dose reduction of pramipexole is often required to prevent toxic effects.

Dopamine Antagonists. Dopamine antagonists include phenothiazines, butyrophenones, thioxanthenes, and metoclopramide. As dopamine antagonists, these agents will diminish the effectiveness of pramipexole, a dopaminergic agonist.

Antihypertensive Agents. Dosage adjustment of the antihypertensive agent is often necessary because of excessive orthostatic hypotension.

ropinirole (roh pin' ihr ol)
REQUIP (re' kwip)

Action

Ropinirole is a nonergot dopamine agonist that stimulates D_2 and D_3 dopamine receptors.

Uses

Ropinirole may be used alone to manage early signs and symptoms of parkinsonism by improving ADLs, as well as motor manifestations such as tremor, rigidity, bradykinesia, and postural stability. It may also be used in combination with levodopa in advanced parkinsonism to manage similar signs and symptoms of the disease, and to reduce the degree of "on-off" symptoms often associated with long-term use of levodopa.

Therapeutic Outcomes

The primary therapeutic outcomes sought from ropinirole in treating parkinsonism are as follows:

1. Improved motor and ADL scores.
2. Decreased "off" time.
3. Reduced dosage of levodopa.

Nursing Process for Ropinirole Therapy

Premedication Assessment

1. Perform a baseline assessment of parkinsonism using the UPDRS.
2. Obtain a history of GI and cardiovascular symptoms, including baseline vital signs (e.g., blood pressure, pulse).
3. Ask specifically about any symptoms of hallucinations or nightmares, dementia, or anxiety.

Planning

Availability. PO: 0.25, 0.5, 1, 2, and 5 mg tablets.

Implementation

Dosage and Administration. *Adult:* PO: Initially 0.25 mg three times daily for 1 week. If tolerated, increase to 0.5 mg three times daily the second week. If tolerated, increase to 0.75 mg three times daily for the third week, and 1 mg three times daily through the fourth week. If necessary, the daily dosage may be increased by 1.5 mg/day on a weekly basis up to a daily dosage of 9 mg/day. Dosages may be further adjusted on weekly intervals up to a total dose of 24 mg/day.

Administer medication with food or milk to reduce gastric irritation.

When ropinirole is used with levodopa, consider reducing the levodopa. If ropinirole is to be discontinued, the dosage should be gradually reduced over 1 week.

Evaluation

Ropinirole causes many side effects, but most are dose related and reversible. Side effects vary greatly, depending on the stage of the disease and the concurrent use of other medicines.

Side Effects to Expect

Nausea, Vomiting, Anorexia. These effects can be reduced by slowly increasing the dosage, dividing the total daily dose into three doses, and administering the medication with food.

Orthostatic Hypotension. Although generally mild, ropinirole may cause some degree of orthostatic hypotension manifested by dizziness and weakness, particularly when therapy is being initiated. Tolerance usually develops after a few weeks of therapy.

Monitor the blood pressure daily in both the supine and standing positions.

Anticipate the development of postural hypotension and take measures to prevent an occurrence. Teach patients to rise slowly from a supine or sitting position; encourage them to sit or lie down if feeling faint.

Side Effects to Report

Chewing Motions, Bobbing, Facial Grimacing, Rocking Movements. These involuntary movements occur in some patients, especially if they are also taking levodopa. Reducing the dosage of levodopa may be beneficial.

Nightmares, Depression, Confusion, Hallucinations. Perform a baseline assessment of the patient's degree of alertness and orientation to name, place, and time before initiating therapy. Make regularly scheduled subsequent evaluations of mental status, and compare findings. Report alterations. Provide patient safety during these episodes. Reducing the daily dosage may control these adverse effects.

Tachycardia, Palpitations. Take the pulse at regularly scheduled intervals. Report for further evaluation.

Sudden Sleep Events. Sleep episodes have been reported with the dopamine agonists (e.g., bromocriptine, pergolide, pramipexole, and ropinirole). These episodes are described as sleep attacks or sleep episodes, including daytime sleep. Some sleep events have been reported as sudden and irresistible. Other sleep events have been preceded by sufficient warning to prevent accidents. Patients taking dopamine agonists should be informed about the possibility of daytime sleepiness and outright sleep attacks with these medicines and allowed to make their own decisions about driving based on past experiences with the medicines. Assessment of patients at risk of sleep attacks is possible with the ESS.

Drug Interactions

Ciprofloxacin. This antibiotic inhibits the metabolism of ropinirole. Dosage reduction of ropinirole is often required to prevent toxic effects.

Estrogens (Primarily Ethinyl Estradiol). Estrogen inhibits ropinirole excretion. If estrogen therapy is started or stopped during treatment with ropinirole, it may be necessary to adjust the dosage of ropinirole.

Dopamine Antagonists. Dopamine antagonists include phenothiazines, butyrophenones, thioxanthenes, and metoclopramide. As dopamine antagonists, these agents will diminish the effectiveness of ropinirole, a dopaminergic agonist.

Antihypertensive Agents. Dosage adjustment of the antihypertensive agent is often necessary because of excessive orthostatic hypotension.

DRUG CLASS: COMT Inhibitor

entacapone (en ta' ka pone)

▶ COMTAN (com' tan), STALEVO (stah lee' voh)

Actions

Entacapone is a potent COMT inhibitor that reduces the destruction of dopamine in the peripheral tissues, allowing significantly more dopamine to reach the brain to eliminate the symptoms of parkinsonism.

Uses

Carbidopa-levodopa are the current drugs of choice for the longer-term treatment of Parkinson's disease. Unfortunately, these agents lose effectiveness ("on-off" phenomenon) and develop more adverse effects (dyskinesias) over time. Adding entacapone inhibits the metabolism of dopamine, resulting in a more constant dopaminergic stimulation in the brain. This stimulation reduces motor fluctuations, increases on-time, reduces off-time, and often results in a reduction in the dosage of levodopa. Entacapone should always be administered with carbidopa-levodopa. Entacapone has no antiparkinsonian effect when used alone. Stalevo is a combination product containing levodopa, carbidopa, and entacapone.

Therapeutic Outcomes

The primary therapeutic outcomes sought from entacapone in treating parkinsonism are as follows:

1. Reduced motor fluctuations.
2. Increased "on" time, reduced "off" time.
3. Reduced total daily dosage of carbidopa-levodopa.

Nursing Process for Entacapone Therapy

Premedication Assessment

1. Perform a baseline assessment of parkinsonism using the UPDRS.
2. Obtain a history of bowel patterns and any ongoing GI symptoms.
3. Perform a baseline assessment of the patient's degree of alertness and orientation to name, place, and time before initiating therapy.
4. Check for any antihypertensive therapy currently prescribed. Monitor the blood pressure daily in both the supine and standing positions. If antihypertensive medications are being taken, report this to the health care provider for possible dosage adjustment.
5. Check hepatic function before initiation and periodically throughout the course of administration.

Planning

Availability. PO: Comtan: 200 mg tablets; Stalevo 50: 12.5 mg carbidopa, 50 mg levodopa, and 200 mg entacapone; Stalevo100: 25 mg carbidopa, 100 mg levodopa, and 200 mg entacapone; Stalevo 150: 37.5 mg carbidopa, 150 mg levodopa, and 200 mg entacapone.

Implementation

Dosage and Administration. Dosage must be adjusted according to the patient's response and tolerance. *Adult:* PO: Initially, one 200 mg tablet with each carbidopa-levodopa dose to a maximum of eight times daily (1600 mg entacapone). The dosage of carbidopa-levodopa will need to be reduced, particularly if the levodopa dose is higher than 600 mg/day if the patient has moderate or severe dyskinesias before the entacapone is started.

Evaluation

Entacapone may increase the adverse dopaminergic effects of levodopa such as chorea, confusion, or hallucinations, but these can be controlled by reducing the dosage of levodopa.

Side Effects to Expect

GI Effects. Diarrhea, usually of mild to moderate severity, may develop 1 to 12 weeks after initiation of therapy, especially when higher doses are used. These effects may be minimized by temporary reduction in dosage.

Sedative Effects. Patients may complain of drowsiness and lethargy, especially when initiating therapy. People should not drive or operate complex machinery or perform duties in which they must remain mentally alert until they have gained enough experience with entacapone to know whether it affects their mental and/or motor performance.

Urine Discoloration. Patients should be advised that entacapone may change the color of their urine to a brownish orange, but that it is harmless and there is no cause for alarm.

Side Effects to Report

Neurologic Effects. Entacapone may increase the adverse dopaminergic effects of levodopa, such as chorea, confusion, and hallucinations. Make regularly scheduled subsequent evaluations of mental status, and compare findings. Report alterations. Reduction of the carbidopa-levodopa dosage may be required to alleviate these effects.

Provide for patient safety, be emotionally supportive, and assure the patient that these effects usually dissipate as tolerance to them develops over the next few weeks.

Orthostatic Hypotension. Monitor the blood pressure daily in both the supine and standing positions.

Anticipate the development of postural hypotension and take measures to prevent an occurrence. Teach the patient to rise slowly from a supine or sitting position; encourage the patient to sit or lie down if feeling faint.

Drug Interactions

Levodopa. Entacapone and levodopa have additive neurologic effects. This interaction may be beneficial because it often allows a reduction in the dosage of the levodopa.

Antihypertensive Agents. Dosage adjustment of the antihypertensive agent is often necessary because of excessive orthostatic hypotension.

Apomorphine, Isoetharine, Bitolterol, Isoproterenol, Epinephrine, Levarterenol, Dopamine, Dobutamine, Methyldopa. These agents are metabolized by COMT. Concurrent administration of entacapone with these agents may prolong their duration of activity. Monitor blood pressure and heart rate.

DRUG CLASS: Anticholinergic Agents

Actions

Parkinsonism is induced by the imbalance of neurotransmitters in the basal ganglia of the brain. The primary imbalance appears to be a deficiency of dopamine, leaving a relative excess of the cholinergic neurotransmitter acetylcholine. Anticholinergic agents are thus used to reduce hyperstimulation caused by excessive acetylcholine.

Uses

The anticholinergic agents reduce the severity of the tremor and drooling associated with parkinsonism. Anticholinergic agents are more useful for patients with minimal symptoms and no cognitive impairment. Combination therapy with levodopa and anticholinergic agents is also successful in controlling symptoms of the disease more completely in about half the patients already stabilized on levodopa therapy. Anticholinergic agents have little effect on rigidity, bradykinesia, or postural abnormalities. If anticholinergic therapy is to be discontinued, it should be done so gradually to avoid withdrawal effects and acute exacerbation of parkinsonian symptoms, even in patients in whom there appears to have been no clinical response.

Therapeutic Outcomes

The primary therapeutic outcome sought from anticholinergic agents in treating parkinsonism is reduction in the severity of tremor and drooling that are caused by a relative excess of acetylcholine in the basal ganglia.

Nursing Process for Anticholinergic Agent Therapy

Premedication Assessment

1. Perform a baseline assessment of parkinsonism using the UPDRS.
2. Obtain baseline data relating to patterns of urinary and bowel elimination.
3. Perform a baseline assessment of the patient's degree of alertness and orientation to name, place, and time before initiating therapy.
4. Take blood pressure in both the supine and standing positions. Record pulse rate, rhythm, and regularity.
5. All patients should be screened for the presence of angle-closure glaucoma before initiation of therapy. Anticholinergic agents may precipitate an acute attack of angle-closure glaucoma. Patients with open-angle glaucoma can safely use anticholinergic agents. Monitor intraocular pressure regularly.

Planning

Availability. See Table 15-1.

Implementation

Dosage and Administration. *Adult:* PO: See Table 15-1. Administer medication with food or milk to reduce gastric irritation.

Evaluation

Most side effects observed with anticholinergic agents are direct extensions of their pharmacologic properties.

Side Effects to Expect

Blurred Vision; Constipation; Urinary Retention; Dryness of Mucosa of the Mouth, Throat, and Nose. These symptoms are the anticholinergic effects produced by these agents. Patients taking these medications should be monitored for the development of these side effects. Milder side effects, such as dry mouth and blurred vision, may subside with continued treatment. Provide for patient safety if blurred vision is present.

Dryness of the mucosa may be relieved by sucking hard candy or ice chips or by chewing gum.

If patients develop urinary hesitancy, assess for bladder distention. Report to the health care provider for further evaluation. Give stool softeners as prescribed. Encourage adequate fluid intake and foods to provide sufficient bulk and exercise as tolerated.

Drug Table 15-1 ANTICHOLINERGIC AGENTS

GENERIC NAME	BRAND NAME	AVAILABILITY	INITIAL DOSE (PO)	MAXIMUM DAILY DOSE (mg)
benztropine mesylate	Cogentin, ✱ Apo-Benztropine	Tablets: 0.5, 1, 2 mg Inj: 1 mg/mL in 2 mL amps	0.5-1 mg at bedtime	6
biperiden hydrochloride	Akineton	Tablets: 2 mg Inj: 5 mg/mL in 1 mL amps	2 mg three or four times daily	16
diphenhydramine hydrochloride	Benadryl, ✱ Allerdryl	Tablets: 12.5, 25, 50 mg Capsules: 25, 50 m g Elixir: 12.5 mg/5 mL Syrup: 12.5 mg/5 mL Inj: 50 mg/mL in 1, 10, 30 mL vials	25-50 mg three or four times daily	400
orphenadrine citrate	Banflex, Norflex	Tablets: 100 mg Sustained release tablets: 100 mg Inj: 30 mg/mL in 2, 10 mL vials	50 mg three times daily	150-250
procyclidine hydrochloride	Kemadrin	Tablets: 5 mg	2.5 mg three times daily	15-20
trihexyphenidyl hydrochloride	Artane, ✱ Trihexyphen	Tablets: 2, 5 mg Elixir: 2 mg/5 mL Sustained release capsules: 5 mg	1-2 mg daily	12-15

✱ Available in Canada.

Side Effects to Report

Nightmares, Depression, Confusion, Hallucinations. Make regularly scheduled subsequent evaluations of mental status, and compare findings. Report development of alterations.

Provide patient safety during these episodes.

Reducing the daily dosage may control these adverse effects.

Orthostatic Hypotension. Although the instance is infrequent and generally mild, all anticholinergic agents may cause some degree of orthostatic hypotension manifested by dizziness and weakness, particularly when therapy is being initiated.

Monitor the blood pressure daily in both the supine and standing positions.

Anticipate the development of postural hypotension and take measures to prevent an occurrence. Teach the patient to rise slowly from a supine or sitting position; encourage the patient to sit or lie down if feeling faint.

Palpitations, Dysrhythmias. Report for further evaluation.

Drug Interactions

Amantadine, Tricyclic Antidepressants, Phenothiazines. These agents may enhance the anticholinergic side effects. Confusion and hallucinations are characteristic of excessive anticholinergic activity. Dosage reduction may be required.

Levodopa. Large doses of anticholinergic agents may slow gastric emptying and inhibit absorption of levodopa. An increase in the dosage of levodopa may be required.

DRUG CLASS: Miscellaneous Antiparkinsonian Agents

selegiline (she ledge′ ah leen)

▶ ELDEPRYL (el′ deh pril), CARBEX (kar′ bex)

Actions

Selegiline is a potent monoamine oxidase-type B inhibitor that reduces the destruction of dopamine in the brain, allowing greater dopaminergic activity.

Uses

Carbidopa-levodopa are the current drugs of choice for the treatment of Parkinson's disease. Unfortunately these agents lose effectiveness (on-off phenomenon) and develop more adverse effects (dyskinesias) over time. It is often necessary to add other dopamine receptor agonists such as bromocriptine or pergolide or a COMT inhibitor (e.g., entacapone) to improve the patient response and tolerance. Selegiline has been found to have similar adjunctive activity to carbidopa-levodopa in the treatment of Parkinson's disease. The combination of selegiline and carbidopa-levodopa improves memory and motor speed and may increase life expectancy.

Selegiline may also have a "neuroprotective" effect by interfering with the ongoing degeneration of striated dopaminergic neurons. It is also used early in the treatment of Parkinson's disease to slow the progression of symptoms and delay the initiation of levodopa therapy. Selegiline was also recently approved to treat depression (see p. 268).

Therapeutic Outcomes

The primary therapeutic outcomes sought from selegiline in treating parkinsonism are as follows:

1. Slow the development of symptoms and progression of the disease.
2. Establish a balance of dopamine and acetylcholine in the basal ganglia of the brain by enhancing delivery of dopamine to brain cells.

Nursing Process for Selegiline Therapy

Premedication Assessment

1. Perform a baseline assessment of parkinsonism using the UPDRS.
2. Obtain a history of GI symptoms.
3. Perform a baseline assessment of the patient's degree of alertness and orientation to name, place, and time before initiating therapy.
4. Check for any antihypertensive therapy currently prescribed. Monitor the blood pressure daily in both the supine and standing positions. If antihypertensive medications are being taken, report this to the health care provider for possible dosage adjustment.
5. Check other medications prescribed and do not administer selegiline with meperidine.

Planning

Availability. PO: 5 mg tablets and capsules.

Implementation

Dosage and Administration. Dosage must be adjusted according to the patient's response and tolerance. *Adult:* PO: 5 mg at breakfast and lunch. Do not exceed 10 mg daily. After 2 to 3 days of treatment, the dosage of carbidopa-levodopa should start being titrated downward. Carbidopa-levodopa dosages may be able to be reduced by 10% to 30%.

Evaluation

Selegiline causes relatively few adverse effects. It may increase the adverse dopaminergic effects of levodopa such as chorea, confusion, or hallucinations, but these can be controlled by reducing the dosage of levodopa.

Side Effects to Expect

GI Effects. Most of these effects may be minimized by temporary reduction in dosage, administration with food, and use of stool softeners for constipation.

Side Effects to Report

Neurologic. Selegiline may increase the adverse dopaminergic effects of levodopa, such as chorea, confusion, and hallucinations. Make regularly scheduled subsequent evaluations of mental status, and compare findings. Report alterations.

Provide patient safety, be emotionally supportive, and assure the patient that these adverse effects usually dissipate as tolerance to them develops over the next few weeks.

Orthostatic Hypotension. Monitor the blood pressure daily in both the supine and standing positions.

Anticipate the development of postural hypotension and take measures to prevent an occurrence. Teach the patient to rise slowly from a supine or sitting position; encourage the patient to sit or lie down if feeling faint.

Drug Interactions

Levodopa. Selegiline and levodopa have additive neurologic effects. This interaction may be beneficial because it often allows a reduction in dose of the levodopa.

Meperidine. Fatal drug interactions have been reported between monoamine oxidase inhibitors and meperidine. Although this interaction has not been reported with selegiline, it is recommended that the two agents not be given concurrently.

Food. Patients should avoid food and beverages with a high tyramine content (e.g., Chianti wine, fava beans, cheeses), particularly if receiving selegiline in excess of 10 mg/day. Rare cases of hypertensive reactions have been reported.

Antihypertensive Agents. Dosage adjustment of the antihypertensive agent is often necessary because of excessive orthostatic hypotension.

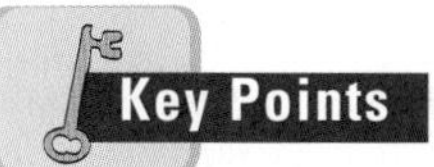

- Parkinson's disease is a progressive neurologic disorder caused by deterioration of dopamine-producing cells in the portion of the brain responsible for maintenance of posture and muscle tone and the regulation of voluntary smooth muscles.
- Normally a balance exists between dopamine, an inhibitory neurotransmitter, and acetylcholine, an excitatory neurotransmitter. The symptoms associated with Parkinson's disease develop because of a relative excess of acetylcholine in the brain.
- The goal of treatment is to restore dopamine neurotransmitter function as close to normal as possible and relieve symptoms caused by "excessive" acetylcholine.
- Therapy must be individualized, but selegiline therapy is often started first to slow the development of symptoms. As selegiline becomes less effective, levodopa is started, with or without selegiline.
- Dopamine agonists (amantadine, bromocriptine, pergolide, ropinirole, pramipexole) may be added to directly stimulate dopamine receptors.
- Entacapone may be added to levodopa therapy to reduce the metabolism of levodopa, prolonging its action.
- Anticholinergic agents may be added at any time to reduce the effects of the "excessive" acetylcholine.
- Nonpharmacologic treatment (e.g., diet, exercise, physical therapy) of Parkinson's disease is equally important in maintaining the long-term well-being of the patient.

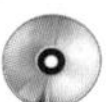

Go to your Companion CD-ROM for appendices, an Audio Glossary, animations, Drug Dosage Calculators, customizable Patient Self-Assessment forms, and Review Questions for the NCLEX® Examination.

evolve Be sure to visit the companion Evolve site at http://evolve.elsevier.com/Clayton for WebLinks and additional online resources.

MEDICATION SAFETY REVIEW

MATH REVIEW QUESTIONS

1. Order: Sinemet 25/100 at an initial dose of 1 tablet three times daily

   Available: Sinemet in 10/100, 25/100, 25/250, and 50/200 mg strengths

   Give: _____ strength and _____ tablets for each dose.

2. Order: Levodopa 0.25 g four times daily

   Available: Levodopa in 100, 250, and 500 mg strengths

   Give: _____ strength and _____ tablets for each dose.

3. Order: Bromocriptine at an initial dose of 1.25 mg two times daily with meals

   Available: Bromocriptine in 2.5 mg tablets and 5 mg capsules

   Give: ______.

CRITICAL THINKING QUESTIONS

1. What physiologic effect does stimulation of dopamine receptors have?
2. A patient's family asks you to explain the basic underlying problem that is causing the symptoms of Parkinson's disease in their mother. Give a simple explanation of the symptoms, appropriate for use with a layperson. Include an explanation of what a neurotransmitter is and the basic imbalances found with Parkinson's disease.
3. Discuss the normal course of progression of Parkinson's disease. Include the rationale for drug therapy to alleviate the symptoms.
4. Develop a teaching plan to be used with the patient and family of an individual being started on Sinemet for the treatment of Parkinson's disease.
5. Explain why baseline assessment of an individual's mental status and physical symptoms is important before and periodically throughout the course of treatment of Parkinson's disease.
6. A patient is being started on an anticholinergic drug as part of the treatment plan for Parkinson's disease. What symptoms can be expected to improve, and conversely, what problems could also arise from starting this medication?
7. Use the UPDRS to assess (1) a patient in the beginning stage of Parkinson's disease and (2) a patient with a more advanced stage of the disease. Document findings and modify the care plan appropriately to foster self-care and independence to the degree possible for the individual.

CONTENT REVIEW QUESTIONS

1. The use of selegilene (Eldepryl) in the early treatment of Parkinson's disease has the primary purpose of:
   1. reducing excessive acetylcholine stimulation.
   2. increasing dopamine in basal ganglia.
   3. slowing symptom progression; delaying initiation of levodopa therapy.
   4. reducing metabolism of levodopa, thereby making more available.
2. Which of the following may be used as initial treatment of early-stage Parkinson's symptoms?
   1. amitriptyline
   2. fluoxetine
   3. selegiline
   4. venlafaxine
3. Carbidopa in Parkinson's disease is to be used:
   1. as successful monotherapy
   2. in conjunction with levodopa to block peripheral conversion to dopamine
   3. to decrease the incidence of gastrointestinal side effects associated with levodopa
   4. 2 and 3
   5. 1, 2, and 3
4. Essential patient education for an individual receiving levodopa includes:
   1. the need to assess vitamins being taken daily.
   2. limiting daily intake of fluids.
   3. taking medication with food or milk.
   4. providing monthly gait training.

CHAPTER

16 Drugs Used for Anxiety Disorders

evolve http://evolve.elsevier.com/Clayton

Chapter Content

Objectives

1. Define key words associated with anxiety states.
2. Describe the essential components of a baseline assessment of a patient's mental status.
3. Cite the side effects of hydroxyzine therapy and identify those effects requiring close monitoring when used preoperatively.
4. Develop a teaching plan for patient education of people taking antianxiety medications.
5. Describe signs and symptoms the patient will display when a positive therapeutic outcome is being seen for the treatment of a high anxiety state.
6. Discuss psychological and physiologic drug dependence.

Key Terms

anxiety
generalized anxiety disorder
panic disorder
phobias
obsessive-compulsive disorder
compulsion
anxiolytics
tranquilizers

ANXIETY DISORDERS

Anxiety is a normal human emotion, similar to fear. It is an unpleasant feeling of apprehension or nervousness caused by the perception of potential or actual danger that threatens a person's security. *Mild anxiety* is a state of heightened awareness of the surroundings and is seen in response to day-to-day circumstances. This type of anxiety can be beneficial as a motivator for the individual to take action in a reasonable and adaptive manner. It is sometimes said that people "rise to the occasion." Patients are considered to have *anxiety disorder* when their responses to stressful situations are abnormal or irrational and impair normal daily functioning. The National Institute of Mental Health identifies anxiety disorders as the most commonly encountered mental disorder in clinical practice. Sixteen percent of the general population will experience an anxiety disorder during their lifetime. Anxiety disorders usually begin before the age of 30 and are more common in women than men. Patients often develop more than one anxiety disorder, major depression, or substance abuse. The most common disorders are generalized anxiety disorder, panic disorder, social phobia, simple phobia, and obsessive-compulsive disorder.

Generalized anxiety disorder is described as excessive and unrealistic worry about two or more life circumstances (e.g., finances, illness, misfortune) for 6 months or more. Symptoms are psychological (tension, fear, difficulty concentrating, apprehension) and physical (tachycardia, palpitations, tremor, sweating, and gastrointestinal [GI] upset). The disease has a gradual onset, usually in the 20- to 30-year age-group and is equally common in men and women. This illness usually follows a chronic fluctuating course of exacerbations and remissions triggered by stressful events in a person's life. Patients with generalized anxiety disorder often develop other psychiatric disorders such as panic disorder, obsessive-compulsive disorder, social anxiety disorder, and/or major depression at some time in their lives.

Panic disorder is recognized as a separate disease and not a more severe form of chronic generalized anxiety disorder. The average age of onset is in the late 20s; the disorder is often relapsing and may require lifetime treatment. Panic disorder is estimated to affect 1% to 2% of Americans at some time in their lives. Women are affected two to three times more frequently than men. Genetic factors appear to play a significant role in the disease because 15% to 20% of patients will have a close relative with a similar illness. Panic disorder begins as a series of acute or unprovoked anxiety (panic) attacks involving an intense, terrifying fear. The attacks do not occur on exposure to an anxiety-causing situation as phobias do. Initially the panic attacks are spontaneous, but later in the course of the illness, they may be associated with certain actions (e.g., driving a car, being in a crowded place). Symptoms include dyspnea, dizziness, palpitations, trembling, choking, sweating, numbness, and chest pain. There are usually feelings of impending doom or a fear of losing control. Patients with panic disorder often develop other psychiatric disorders such as generalized anxiety disorder, personality disorders, substance abuse, obsessive-compulsive disorder, social anxiety disorder, and/or major depression at some time in their lives.

Phobias are an irrational fear of a specific object, activity, or situation. Unlike other anxiety disorders, the object or activity that creates the feeling of fear is recognized by the patient, who also realizes that the fear is unreasonable. The fear persists, however, and the patient seeks to avoid the situation. *Social phobia* is described as a fear of certain social situations in which the person is exposed to scrutiny by others and fears doing something embarrassing. A social phobia toward public speaking is fairly common and is usually avoided. If the speaking is unavoidable, it is done with intense anxiety. Social phobias are rarely incapacitating but do cause some interference with social or occupational functioning. *Simple phobia* is an irrational fear of a specific object or situation such as heights (acrophobia), closed spaces (claustrophobia), air travel, or driving. Phobias to animals such as spiders, snakes, and mice are particularly common. If the person is exposed to the object, there is an immediate feeling of panic, sweating, and tachycardia. People are quite aware of the phobia and simply avoid the feared object.

Obsessive-compulsive disorder is the most disabling of the anxiety disorders, although it is responsive to treatment. The primary features of the illness are recurrent obsessions or compulsions that cause significant distress and interfere with normal occupational responsibilities, social activities, and relationships. The average age of onset for symptoms of obsessive-compulsive disorder is late adolescence to the early 20s. It occurs with equal frequency in men and women. There also appears to be a genetic component to the disease. An *obsession* is an unwanted thought, idea, image, or urge that the patient recognizes as time consuming and senseless but repeatedly intrudes into the consciousness, despite attempts to ignore, prevent, or counteract it. Examples of obsessions are recurrent thoughts of dirt or germ contamination, fear of losing things, need to know or remember, need to count or check, blasphemous thoughts, or concerns about something happening to self or others. An obsession produces a tremendous sense of anxiety in the person. A **compulsion** is a repetitive, intentional, purposeful behavior performed to decrease the anxiety associated with an obsession. The act is done to prevent a vague, dreaded event, but the person does not derive pleasure from the act. Common compulsions deal with cleanliness, grooming, and counting. When patients are prevented from performing a compulsion, there is a sense of mounting anxiety. In some individuals, the compulsion can become the person's lifetime activity. Obsessive-compulsive disorder is a complex condition that requires a highly individualized, integrated approach to treatment with pharmacologic, behavioral, and psychosocial components.

DRUG THERAPY FOR ANXIETY DISORDERS

Anxiety is a component of many medical illnesses involving the cardiovascular, pulmonary, digestive, and endocrine systems. It is also a primary symptom of many psychiatric disorders such as schizophrenia, mania, depression, dementia, and substance abuse. Therefore evaluation of the anxious patient requires a thorough history, as well as physical and psychiatric examination to determine whether the anxiety is a primary condition or secondary to another illness. Persistent irrational anxiety or episodic anxiety usually requires medical and psychiatric treatment. Treatment of anxiety disorders usually requires a combination of pharmacologic and nonpharmacologic therapies. When it is decided to treat the anxiety in addition to the other medical or psychiatric diagnoses, *antianxiety* medications, also known as **anxiolytics** or **tranquilizers,** are prescribed.

Actions

A great many medications have been used over the decades to treat anxiety. They range from the purely sedative effects of ethanol, bromides, chloral hydrate, and barbiturates to drugs with more specific antianxiety and less sedative activity, such as benzodiazepines, buspirone, extended release venlafaxine, meprobamate, and hydroxyzine. More recently, tricyclic antidepressants (e.g., imipramine), propranolol (a beta-adrenergic antagonist), serotonin agonists (selective serotonin reuptake inhibitors [SSRIs]), and serotonin antagonists (e.g., ondansetron) have been studied in treating anxiety disorders. See the individual monographs later in this chapter for mechanisms of action.

Uses

Generalized anxiety disorder is treated with psychotherapy and the short-term use of antianxiety agents. The U.S. Food and Drug Administration (FDA) has approved four classes of compounds or medications for treatment: specific benzodiazepines, paroxetine and escitalopram (SSRIs), extended release venlafaxine, and buspirone. To some extent, the beta-adrenergic blocking agents (see Chapter 13) are used. Barbiturates, meprobamate, and antihistamines such as hydroxyzine are infrequently prescribed. Panic disorders may be treated with a variety of agents in addition to behavioral therapy. Alprazolam and clonazepam (benzodiazepines), and sertraline, paroxetine, fluoxetine (SSRIs) are approved by the FDA for treatment of panic disorder. Other agents that show benefit are the tricyclic antidepressants desipramine and clomipramine, and mirtazapine and nefazodone (see Chapter 17). Phobias are treated by avoidance, behavior therapy and benzodiazepines or beta-adrenergic blockers such as propranolol or atenolol. Obsessive-compulsive disorder is treated with behavioral and psychosocial therapy in addition to paroxetine, sertraline, fluoxetine, or fluvoxamine.

NURSING PROCESS *for Antianxiety Therapy*

Assessment

History of Behavior. Obtain a history of the precipitating factors that may have triggered or contributed to the individual's current anxiety. Has the individual been using alcohol or drugs? Has the client had a recent loss such as job, relationship, death of loved one, or divorce? Has the individual witnessed or survived a traumatic event? Does the individual have any medical problems such as hyperthyroidism that could be attributed to these symptoms? Are there symptoms present that could be attributed to a panic attack, such as feeling of choking; palpitations; sweating; chest pain or discomfort; nausea; abdominal distress; or fear of losing control, going crazy, or fear of dying? Does the individual have symptoms of obsessions or compulsions? Does the individual have a history of agoraphobia (i.e., situations in which he or she feels trapped or unable to escape)? Did the attack occur in response to a social or performance situation? Is the client also depressed? What specific fears does the individual have?

Take a detailed history of all medications the individual is taking. Is there any use of central nervous system (CNS) stimulants such as cocaine, amphetamines, or CNS depressants such as alcohol or barbiturates?

Ask details regarding the length of time the individual has been exhibiting anxiety. Has the person been treated for anxiety previously? When did the symptoms start—during intoxication or withdrawal from a substance?

Basic Mental Status. Note general appearance and appropriateness of attire. Is the individual clean and neat? Is the posture stooped, erect, or slumped? Is the person oriented to date, time, place, and person?

What coping mechanisms has the individual been using to deal with the situation? Are they adaptive or maladaptive?

Assess the relationships that provide the individual with support. Identify support groups.

Mood/Affect. Is the individual tearful, excessively excited, angry, hostile, or apathetic? Is the facial expression tense, fearful, sad, angry, or blank? Ask the person to describe his or her feelings. Is there worry over real-life problems? Are the person's responses displayed as an intense fear, detachment, or an absence of emotions? If the patient is a child, are there episodes of tantrums or clinging?

Patients experiencing altered thinking, behavior, or feelings need careful evaluation of both verbal and nonverbal actions. Often the thoughts, feelings, and behaviors displayed are inconsistent with the so-called normal responses of individuals in similar circumstances.

Assess whether the mood being described is consistent with the circumstances being described. For example, is the person speaking of death, yet smiling?

Clarity of Thought. Evaluate the coherency, relevancy, and organization of thoughts. Ask specific questions regarding the individual's ability to make judgments and decisions. Is there any memory impairment?

Psychomotor Functions. Ask specific questions regarding the activity level the patient has maintained. Is the person able to work or go to school? Is the person able to fulfill responsibilities at work, socially, or within the family? How have the person's normal responses to daily activities been altered? Is the individual irritable, angry, easily startled, or hypervigilant? Observe for gestures, gait, hand tremors, voice quivering, and type of activity such as pacing or inability to sit still.

Obsessions or Compulsions. Does the individual have persistent thoughts, images, or ideas that are inappropriate and cause increased anxiety? Are there repetitive physical or mental behaviors such as handwashing, need to arrange things in perfect symmetric order, praying, silently repeating words? If obsessions or compulsions are present, how often do these occur? Do the obsessions or compulsions impair the person's social and/or occupational functioning?

Sleep Pattern. What is the person's normal sleep pattern, and how has it varied since the onset of the symptoms? Ask specifically whether insomnia is present. Ask the individual to describe the amount and quality of the sleep. What is the degree of fatigue present? Is the individual having recurrent, stressful dreams (after a traumatic event)? Is there difficulty falling or staying asleep?

Dietary History. Ask questions relating to appetite and note weight gains or losses not associated with intentional dieting.

Nursing Diagnoses

- Anxiety (indication)
- Ineffective coping (indication)
- Post-trauma syndrome (indication)
- Risk for injury (side effects)
- Noncompliance related to altered thought processes produced by anxiety state (indication)

Planning

History of Behavior

- Review data collected to identify an individual's ability to understand new information, follow directions, and provide self-care.
- Review medications being taken to specifically identify any that are CNS stimulants or depressants.

Basic Mental Status

- Plan to perform a baseline assessment of the individual's mental status at specific intervals throughout the course of treatment to identify the level of anxiety present and response to therapeutic interventions (including medication therapy).
- Identify events that trigger anxiety.
- Schedule specific times to discuss the patient's behavior and thoughts and foster understanding of it

with family members. Involve family or significant others in the discussion of the anxiety-producing events or circumstances and ways that they can be helpful to the patient in reducing the anxiety or coping more adaptively with stressors.

Mood/Affect. Review assessment data to plan strategies that will assist the individual to decrease the level of anxiety and identify management techniques to handle anxiety-producing situations effectively.

Clarity of Thought

- Identify areas in which the patient is capable of having input into setting goals and making decisions. (This will aid in overcoming a sense of powerlessness over life situations.) Provide an opportunity to plan for self-care. When the patient is unable to make decisions, plan to make them and set goals to involve the patient to the degree of his or her capability as abilities change with treatment.
- Identify signs of escalating anxiety; plan interventions to decrease escalation of anxiety.

Psychomotor Function

- Review activities offered within the clinical setting and plan for the individual to participate in those that will provide distraction and relaxation, as well as decrease the level of anxiety being exhibited.
- Provide a structured, safe environment for the individual to function.
- During severe or panic anxiety, provide a safe place for the release of energy.

Sleep Pattern. Plan for providing a nonstimulating environment (dim lighting, quiet area) that will encourage drowsiness and sleep.

Dietary Needs. Provide an opportunity for the individual to be involved in selecting foods appropriate to needs (to lose or gain weight).

Implementation

- Deal with problems as they occur; practice reality orientation.
- Provide a safe, structured environment; set limits on aggressive or destructive behaviors.
- Establish a trusting relationship with the patient by providing support and reassurance.
- Reduce stimulation by having interactions with the patient in a quiet, calm environment.
- Provide an opportunity for the individual to express feelings. Use active listening and therapeutic communication techniques. Be especially aware of cues that would indicate the patient may be considering self-harm. (If suspecting suicidal ideas, ask the patient directly if suicide is being considered and intervene to provide for safety.)

Allow patients to make decisions of which they are capable, make decisions when the client is not capable, and provide a reward for progress when decisions are initiated appropriately. Involve the patient in self-care activities. During periods of severe anxiety or during escalating anxiety, the individual may be unable to have insight and make decisions appropriately.

Encourage the individual to develop coping skills through the use of various techniques, for example, rehearsing or role-playing responses to threatening stressors. Have the individual practice problem solving; discuss possible consequences of the solutions offered by the patient.

Assist individuals with nonpharmacologic measures such as music therapy, relaxation techniques, or massage therapy.

Evaluation

Observe for therapeutic outcomes expected from drug therapy prescribed.

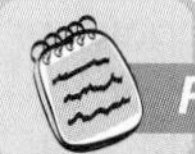

Patient Education and Health Promotion

- Orient the individual to the unit, explaining rules and the process of "privileges" and how they are obtained or lost. (The extent of the orientation and explanations given will depend on the individual's orientation to date, time, place, and abilities.)
- Explain the activity groups available and how and when the individual will participate. A variety of group process activities (e.g., social skills group, self-esteem groups, work-related groups, and physical exercise groups) exist within particular therapeutic settings. Meditation, biofeedback, and relaxation therapy may also be beneficial.
- Involve the patient and family in goal setting and integrate into the available group processes to develop positive experiences for the individual to enhance coping skills.
- Patient education should be individualized and based on assessment data to provide the individual with a structured environment in which to grow and enhance self-esteem. Initially the individual may not be capable of understanding lengthy explanations; therefore the approaches used should be based on the patient's capabilities.
- Explore coping mechanisms the person uses in response to stressors, and identify methods of channeling these toward positive realistic goals as an alternative to the use of medications.

Fostering Health Maintenance. Throughout the course of treatment, discuss medication information and how it will benefit the patient. Stress the importance of the nonpharmacologic interventions and the long-term effects that compliance with the treatment regimen can provide. Additional health teaching and nursing interventions for the side effects to expect and report are described in the drug monographs that follow. Seek cooperation and understanding of the following points so that medication compliance is increased: name of medication, dosage, route and times of administration, side effects to expect, and side effects to report. Instruct the patient not to suddenly discontinue medications prescribed after having been on long-term therapy. Withdrawal should be undertaken with health care provider

PATIENT SELF-ASSESSMENT FORM Antianxiety Medication

MEDICATIONS	COLOR	TO BE TAKEN

Patient ____________

Health Care Provider ____________

Health Care Provider's phone ____________

Next appt.* ____________

What I Should Monitor	Premedication Data	Date	Date	Date	Date	Date	Date	Comments
Weight								
Blood pressure AM PM								
Resting pulse rate								
I would like to be alone All the time (10) — Some of the time (5) — Not really (1)								
How I feel about my children Too much work (10) — 5 — Fun to be with (1)								
How I feel today Poor (10) — Fair (5) — Okay (1)								
Appetite Poor (10) — Fair (5) — Good (1) B								
L								
D								
S								
Has the family noted any problems? Judgment? Socialization?								
Does patient dress daily? (Yes/No)								
Does patient take pride in appearance? (Yes/No)								
Use of alcohol (Yes/No) Amount (e.g., one drink)								
General mood: tearful, excessively excited, angry, hostile, happy, or apathetic								
Sleep pattern: Amount of sleep per night: _______ hrs Degree of fatigue: rested, slightly fatigued, exhausted Insomnia (Yes/No)								
Other								

B, Breakfast; *L,* lunch; *D,* dinner; *S,* snack.

*Please bring this record with you to your next appointment.

Use the back of this sheet for additional information.

instructions and usually requires 4 weeks of gradual reduction in dosage and interval of administration.

Written Record. Enlist the patient's aid in developing and maintaining a written record of monitoring parameters (see Patient Self-Assessment Form on p. 255). Complete the Premedication Data column for use as a baseline to track response to drug therapy. Ensure that the patient understands how to use the form and instruct the patient to bring the completed form to follow-up visits. During follow-up visits, focus on issues that will foster adherence with the therapeutic interventions prescribed.

DRUG CLASS: Benzodiazepines

Benzodiazepines are most commonly used because they are more consistently effective, less likely to interact with other drugs, less likely to cause overdose, and have less potential for abuse than barbiturates and other antianxiety agents. They account for perhaps 75% of the 100 million prescriptions written annually for anxiety. Seven benzodiazepine derivatives are used as antianxiety agents (Table 16-1).

Actions

It is thought that the benzodiazepines have similar mechanisms of action as CNS depressants, but individual drugs within the benzodiazepine family act more selectively at specific sites, which allows for a variety of uses (e.g., sedative-hypnotic, muscle relaxant, antianxiety, and anticonvulsant). The benzodiazepines reduce anxiety by stimulating the action of an inhibitory neurotransmitter called *gamma-aminobutyric acid* (GABA) improving symptoms of sleep disturbance, tremor, and muscle tension.

In patients with reduced hepatic function or in older adults, alprazolam, lorazepam, or oxazepam may be most appropriate because they have a relatively short duration of action and no active metabolites. Oxazepam has been the most thoroughly investigated. The other benzodiazepines all have active metabolites that significantly prolong the duration of action and may accumulate to the point of excessive side effects with chronic administration. The primary active ingredient of both prazepam and clorazepate is desmethyldiazepam; therefore similar activity and patient response should be expected. Halazepam and diazepam are therapeutically active, but their major metabolite is also desmethyldiazepam; therefore a similar response should be expected with long-term administration.

Uses

Patients with anxiety reactions to recent events and those with a treatable medical illness that induces anxiety respond most readily to benzodiazepine therapy. In general, benzodiazepines are equally effective for treating anxiety. Patients generally respond to therapy within 1 week. Because all benzodiazepines have similar mechanisms of action, selection of the appropriate derivative depends on how the benzodiazepine is metabolized (see Actions). Oxazepam, lorazepam,

Drug Table 16-1 BENZODIAZEPINES USED TO TREAT ANXIETY

GENERIC NAME	BRAND NAME	AVAILABILITY	INITIAL DOSE (PO)	MAXIMUM DAILY DOSE (mg)
alprazolam	Xanax Nirvam	Tablets: 0.25, 0.5, 1, 2 mg Tablets, orally disintegrating: 0.25, 0.5, 1, 2 mg	0.25-0.5 mg three times daily	10
	Xanax XR	Tablets, extended release: 0.5, 1, 2, 3 mg Solution: 1 mg/mL	0.5-1 mg daily	6
chlordiazepoxide	Librium	Capsules: 5, 10, 25 mg Inj: 100 mg	5-10 mg three or four times daily	300
clorazepate	Tranxene Tranxene XR ✱ Novo-Clopate	Tablets: 3.75, 7.5, 11.25, 15, 22.5 mg Extended release tablets: 11.25 and 22.5 mg	10 mg one to three times daily	60
diazepam	Valium ✱ Apo-Diazepam	Tablets: 2, 5, 10 mg Liquid: 5 mg/5 mL Inj: 5 mg/mL in 2 mL prefilled syringe	2-10 mg two to four times daily	—
lorazepam	Ativan ✱ Nu-Loraz	Inj: 2, 4 mg/mL in 1, 10 mL vials Liquid: 2 mg/mL Tablets: 0.5, 1, 2 mg	2-3 mg two or three times daily	10
oxazepam	Serax ✱ Apo-Oxazepam	Tablets: 15 mg Capsules: 10, 15, 30 mg	10-15 mg three or four times daily	120

✱ Available in Canada.

chlordiazepoxide, diazepam, and clorazepate are approved for use in treating the anxiety associated with alcohol withdrawal. Oxazepam and lorazepam are the drugs of choice because they have no active metabolites. However, their use is somewhat limited in patients who cannot tolerate oral administration because of nausea and vomiting. Chlordiazepoxide, diazepam, or lorazepam may be administered intramuscularly in this case (see Chapter 49).

Therapeutic Outcomes

The primary therapeutic outcome expected from the benzodiazepine antianxiety agents is a decrease in the level of anxiety to a manageable level (e.g., coping is improved; physical signs of anxiety such as look of anxiety, tremor, and pacing are reduced).

Nursing Process for Benzodiazepines

Premedication Assessment

1. Record baseline data on level of anxiety present.
2. Record baseline vital signs, particularly blood pressure, in sitting and supine positions.
3. Check for history of blood dyscrasias or hepatic disease.
4. Determine whether the individual is pregnant or breastfeeding.

Planning

Availability. See Table 16-1.

Pregnancy and Lactation. It is recommended that benzodiazepines not be administered during at least the first trimester of pregnancy. There may be an increased incidence of birth defects because these agents readily cross the placenta and enter fetal circulation. If benzodiazepines are taken regularly during pregnancy, the infant should be monitored closely after delivery for signs of withdrawal, including sedation and hypotonia.

Mothers who are breastfeeding should not receive benzodiazepines regularly. The benzodiazepines readily cross into breast milk and exert a pharmacologic effect on the infant.

Implementation

Dosage and Administration. See Table 16-1.

The habitual use of benzodiazepines may result in physical and psychological dependence. Rapidly discontinuing benzodiazepines after long-term use may result in symptoms similar to alcohol withdrawal. Mild withdrawal symptoms have been reported in almost half of patients who received therapeutic doses for as few as 4 to 6 weeks. Common symptoms of withdrawal include restlessness, worsening of anxiety and insomnia, tremor, muscle tension, increased heart rate, and auditory hypersensitivity. More serious withdrawal symptoms include delirium and tonic-clonic seizures. The symptoms may not appear for several days after discontinuation. Prevention consists of gradual withdrawal of benzodiazepines over 4 weeks.

Evaluation

Side Effects to Expect

Drowsiness, Hangover, Sedation, Lethargy. Patients may complain of "morning hangover," blurred vision, and transient hypotension on arising. Explain to the patient the need for rising first to a sitting position, equilibrating, and then standing. Assist with ambulation if necessary.

If hangover becomes troublesome, the dosage should be reduced or the medication changed, or both.

People who work around machinery, drive a car, administer medication, or perform other duties in which they must remain mentally alert should not take these medications while working.

Side Effects to Report

Excessive Use or Abuse. Habitual benzodiazepine use may result in physical dependence. Discuss the case with the health care provider and make plans to cooperatively approach gradual withdrawal of the medications being abused. Assist the patient in recognizing the abuse problem. Identify underlying needs, and plan for more appropriate management of those needs. Provide emotional support of the individual, display an accepting attitude, and be kind but firm.

Blood Dyscrasias. Routine laboratory studies (e.g., red blood cell [RBC] and white blood cell [WBC] counts, differential counts) should be scheduled. Stress the patient's need to return for these tests. Monitor for a sore throat, fever, purpura, jaundice, or excessive and progressive weakness.

Hepatotoxicity. The symptoms of hepatotoxicity are anorexia, nausea, vomiting, jaundice, hepatomegaly, splenomegaly, and abnormal liver function tests (e.g., elevated bilirubin, aspartate aminotransferase [AST], alanine aminotransferase [ALT], gamma-glutamyltransferase [GGT], alkaline phosphatase, prothrombin time).

Drug Interactions

Drugs That Increase Toxic Effects. Antihistamines, alcohol, analgesics, anesthetics, probenecid, tranquilizers, narcotics, cimetidine, and other sedative-hypnotics may cause excessive sedation and impaired psychomotor function.

Oral Contraceptives, Cimetidine, Fluoxetine, Metoprolol, Propranolol, Isoniazid, Ketoconazole, Propoxyphene, Valproic Acid. These agents inhibit the metabolism of alprazolam, chlordiazepoxide, clorazepam, diazepam, and halazepam. Pharmacologic effects of the benzodiazepines may be increased and excessive sedation and impaired psychomotor function may result.

Smoking, Rifampin. Smoking and rifampin enhance the metabolism of benzodiazepines. Larger doses may be necessary to maintain anxiolytic effects in patients who smoke.

DRUG CLASS: Azaspirones

buspirone (byoo spy′ rone)
BuSpar (byoo sphar′)

Actions

Buspirone is an antianxiety agent that comes from the chemical class known as the *azaspirones,* which are chemically unrelated to the barbiturates, benzodiazepines, or other anxiolytic agents. The mechanism of action of buspirone is not fully understood. It is a partial serotonin and dopamine agonist and interacts in several ways with nerve systems in the midbrain; therefore it is sometimes called a *midbrain modulator.* It does not affect GABA receptors. Its advantage over other antianxiety agents is that it has lower sedative properties and does not alter psychomotor functioning. It requires 7 to 10 days of treatment before initial signs of improvement are evident, as well as 3 to 4 weeks of therapy for optimal effects.

Uses

It is approved for use in the treatment of anxiety disorders and for the short-term relief of the symptoms of anxiety. Buspirone has no antipsychotic activity and should not be used in place of appropriate psychiatric treatment. Because there is minimal potential for abuse with buspirone, it is not a controlled substance.

Therapeutic Outcomes

The primary therapeutic outcome expected from buspirone is a decrease in the level of anxiety to a manageable level (e.g., coping is improved, physical signs of anxiety such as look of anxiety, tremor, and pacing are reduced).

Nursing Process for Buspirone Therapy

Premedication Assessment

Record baseline data on the level of anxiety present.

Planning

Availability. PO: 5, 7.5, 10, 15, and 30 mg tablets. Schedule assessments periodically throughout therapy for development of slurred speech or dizziness, which are signs of excessive dosing.

Implementation

Dosage and Administration. *Adult:* PO: Initially, 5 mg three times daily. Doses may be increased by 5 mg every 2 to 3 days. Maintenance therapy often requires 30 mg daily in divided doses. Do not exceed 60 mg daily.

Evaluation

Side Effects to Expect

Sedation, Lethargy. The most common adverse effects of buspirone therapy are CNS disturbances (3.4%), which include dizziness, insomnia, nervousness, drowsiness, and lightheadedness.

People who work around machinery or perform other duties in which they must remain mentally alert should not take this medication while working.

Side Effects to Report

Slurred Speech, Dizziness. These are signs of excessive dosing. Report to the health care provider for further evaluation. Provide patient safety during these episodes.

Drug Interactions

Drugs That Increase Toxic Effects. The following drugs potentiate the toxicity of buspirone by inhibiting the metabolism of buspirone: itraconazole, erythromycin, nefazodone, clarithromycin, diltiazem, verapamil, fluvoxamine, grapefruit juice. If used together, the dose of buspirone should be reduced in half for a few weeks, then adjusted as needed.

Drugs That Reduce the Effects of Buspirone. The following drugs enhance the metabolism of buspirone: rifampin, phenytoin, phenobarbital, and carbamazepine. An increase in dose of buspirone may be needed.

Alcohol. Buspirone and alcohol generally do not have additive CNS depressant effects, but individual patients may be susceptible to impairment. Use with extreme caution.

DRUG CLASS: Selective Serotonin Reuptake Inhibitors

fluvoxamine (fluv ox′ ah meen)
Luvox (loo′ vox)

Actions

Fluvoxamine inhibits the reuptake of serotonin at nerve endings, thus prolonging serotonin activity.

Uses

Fluvoxamine is used in the treatment of obsessive-compulsive disorder when obsessions or compulsions cause marked distress, are time consuming, or interfere substantially with social or occupational responsibilities. Fluvoxamine reduces the symptoms of this disorder but does not prevent obsessions and compulsions. However, patients indicate that the obsessions are less intrusive and they have more control over them.

Therapeutic Outcomes

The primary therapeutic outcome expected from fluvoxamine is a decrease in the level of anxiety to a manageable level (e.g., coping with obsession is improved, frequency of compulsive activity is reduced).

Nursing Process for Fluvoxamine Therapy

See Chapter 17, Selective Serotonin Reuptake Inhibitors, p. 272.

DRUG CLASS: Miscellaneous Antianxiety Agents

hydroxyzine (hi drox′ ee zeen)
▶ VISTARIL (vis tar′ il), ATARAX (at′ a raks)

Actions

Defined strictly by chemical structure, hydroxyzine is an antihistamine. It acts within the CNS to produce sedation, antiemetic, anticholinergic, antihistaminic, antianxiety, and antispasmodic activity, making it a somewhat multipurpose agent.

Uses

Hydroxyzine is used as a mild tranquilizer in psychiatric conditions characterized by anxiety, tension, and agitation. It is also occasionally used as a preoperative or postoperative sedative to control vomiting, diminish anxiety, and reduce the amount of narcotics needed for analgesia. Hydroxyzine may also be used as an antipruritic agent to relieve the itching associated with allergic reactions.

Therapeutic Outcomes

The primary therapeutic outcomes expected from hydroxyzine are as follows:

1. A decrease in the level of anxiety to a manageable level (e.g., coping is improved; physical signs of anxiety such as look of anxiety, tremor, and pacing are reduced).
2. Sedation, relaxation, and reduction in analgesics before and after surgery.
3. Absence of vomiting when used as an antiemetic.
4. Itching controlled in allergic reactions.

Nursing Process for Hydroxyzine Therapy

Premedication Assessment

1. Perform baseline assessment of anxiety symptoms.
2. Determine level of anxiety present before and after surgical intervention; record and intervene appropriately.
3. For nausea and vomiting, administer when nausea first starts and determine effectiveness of control before giving subsequent doses.
4. For allergic reactions, perform baseline assessment of physical symptoms before administering dose; repeat before administration of subsequent doses to determine effectiveness.
5. Monitor for level of sedation present, slurred speech, or dizziness; report to health care provider if excessive before administering repeat doses.

Planning

Availability. PO: 10, 25, 50, and 100 mg tablets and capsules; 10 mg/5 mL syrup; 25 mg/5 mL suspension. IM: 25 and 50 mg/mL.

Implementation

Dosage and Administration

Adult

- Antianxiety: PO: 25 to 100 mg three or four times daily; IM: 50 to 100 mg every 4 to 6 hours.
- Pre- and postoperative: IM: 25 to 100 mg.
- Antiemetic: IM: 25 to 100 mg.

Evaluation

Side Effects to Expect

Blurred Vision; Constipation; Dryness of Mucosa of the Mouth, Throat, and Nose. These symptoms are the anticholinergic effects produced by hydroxyzine. Patients taking these medications should be monitored for the development of these side effects.

Mucosal dryness may be relieved by sucking hard candy or ice chips or by chewing gum.

The use of stool softeners such as docusate may be required for constipation. Caution the patient that blurred vision may occur and make appropriate suggestions for personal safety.

Sedation. People who work around machinery, drive a car, administer medication, or perform other duties in which they must remain mentally alert should not take these medications while working.

Side Effects to Report

Slurred Speech, Dizziness. These are signs of excessive dosing. Report to the health care provider for further evaluation. Provide patient safety during these episodes.

Drug Interactions

Drugs That Increase Toxic Effects. Antihistamines, alcohol, analgesics, anesthetics, tranquilizers, barbiturates, narcotics, and other sedative-hypnotics can increase toxic effects. Monitor the patient for excessive sedation and reduce the dosage of hydroxyzine if necessary.

meprobamate (mep roe ba′ mate)
▶ EQUANIL (ek′ wah nil), MILTOWN (mil′ towhn)

Actions

Meprobamate acts on multiple sites within the CNS to produce mild sedation, antianxiety, and muscle relaxation. The mechanism of action is unknown.

Uses

Meprobamate is used as an antianxiety agent and mild skeletal muscle relaxant for the short-term relief (less than 4 months) of anxiety and tension. It is of little use in the treatment of psychoses.

Therapeutic Outcomes

The primary therapeutic outcome expected from meprobamate is a decrease in the level of anxiety to a manageable level (e.g., coping is improved; physical signs of anxiety such as look of anxiety, tremor, and pacing are reduced).

Nursing Process for Meprobamate Therapy

Premedication Assessment

Record baseline data on the level of anxiety present.

Planning

Availability. PO: 200 and 400 mg tablets. Schedule assessments periodically throughout therapy for development of slurred speech or dizziness, which are signs of excessive dosing, use, or abuse.

Implementation

Dosage and Administration. Adult: PO: 400 mg three or four times daily. Smaller doses may work well in older adults and debilitated patients. Maximum daily doses should not exceed 2400 mg.

Evaluation

Side Effects to Expect

Sedation. People who work around machinery, drive a car, administer medication, or perform other duties in which they must remain mentally alert should not take these medications while working.

Side Effects to Report

Slurred Speech, Dizziness. These are signs of excessive dosing. Report to the health care provider for further evaluation. Provide patient safety during these episodes.

Excessive Use or Abuse. Psychological and physiologic dependence may occur in patients taking doses of 3.3 to 6.4 g per day for 40 or more days. Symptoms of chronic use and abuse of high doses include ataxia, slurred speech, and dizziness. Withdrawal reactions such as vomiting, tremors, confusion, hallucinations, and tonic-clonic seizures may develop within 12 to 48 hours after abrupt discontinuation. Symptoms usually decline within the next 12 to 48 hours. Withdrawal from high and prolonged doses should be completed gradually over 1 to 2 weeks.

Discuss the case with the health care provider and make plans to cooperatively approach gradual withdrawal of the medications being abused. Assist the patient in recognizing the abuse problem. Identify underlying needs and plan for more appropriate management of those needs. Provide emotional support of the individual, display an accepting attitude, and be kind but firm.

Orthostatic Hypotension (Dizziness, Weakness, Faintness). Although this effect is infrequent and generally mild, meprobamate may cause some degree of orthostatic hypotension manifested by dizziness and weakness, particularly when therapy is being initiated.

Anticipate the development of postural hypotension and take measures to prevent an occurrence. Teach the patient to rise slowly from a supine or sitting position; encourage the patient to sit or lie down if feeling faint. Monitor the blood pressure daily in both the supine and standing positions.

Paradoxical Excitement, Dysrhythmias. Withhold doses and report for further evaluation.

Hives, Pruritus, Rash. Report symptoms for further evaluation by the health care provider. Pruritus may be relieved by adding baking soda in the bathwater.

Drug Interactions

Drugs That Increase Toxic Effects. Antihistamines, alcohol, analgesics, tranquilizers, narcotics, and other sedative-hypnotics may increase toxic effects. Monitor the patient for excessive sedation and reduce the dosage of the meprobamate if necessary.

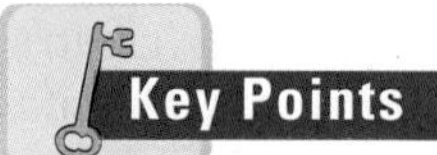

Key Points

- Anxiety is an unpleasant feeling of apprehension or nervousness caused by the perception of danger threatening the security of the person. In most cases, it is a normal human emotion.
- When a person's response to anxiety is irrational and impairs daily functioning, patients are said to have an anxiety disorder. Some 16% of the general population will experience an anxiety disorder during their lifetime.
- The most common types of anxiety disorders are generalized anxiety disorder, panic disorder, social phobia, simple phobia, and obsessive-compulsive disorder.
- Anxiety is a component of many medical illnesses involving the cardiovascular, pulmonary, digestive, and endocrine systems. It is also a primary symptom of many psychiatric disorders. Therefore evaluation of the anxious patient requires a thorough history, as well as a physical and psychiatric examination to determine whether the anxiety is a primary condition or is secondary to another illness. Persistent irrational anxiety or episodic anxiety usually requires medical and psychiatric treatment.
- Treatment of anxiety disorders usually requires a combination of pharmacologic and nonpharmacologic therapies.
- It is the responsibility of the nurse to educate patients about their therapy, monitoring for therapeutic benefit, side effects to expect, and side effects to report, intervening whenever possible to optimize therapeutic outcomes.

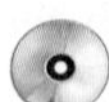

Go to your Companion CD-ROM for appendices, an Audio Glossary, animations, Drug Dosage Calculators, customizable Patient Self-Assessment forms, and Review Questions for the NCLEX® Examination.

evolve Be sure to visit the companion Evolve site at http://evolve.elsevier.com/Clayton for WebLinks and additional online resources.

MEDICATION SAFETY REVIEW

MATH REVIEW QUESTIONS

1. Order: hydroxyzine (Vistaril) 20 mg IM stat
   Available: hydroxyzine (Vistaril) 25 mg/mL
   Give: _____ mL.
2. Order: meprobamate (Equanil) 1600 mg PO daily in four divided doses
   How many milligrams per dose should be administered?
3. Order: lorazepam (Ativan) 2.5 mg IM stat
   Available: lorazepam (Ativan) 4 mg/mL
   Give: _____ mL.

CRITICAL THINKING QUESTIONS

A patient is admitted to the unit with symptoms of generalized anxiety disorder. During the admission interview the following information is obtained:

She is so fearful of losing her job that she discusses it several times a day as a possibility. This has been an increasing concern to her over the past 8 months. Her work performance was regarded as above average; however, over the past 2 months, she has had increasing difficulty concentrating and completing her responsibilities. Finally, last week her employer suggested she take a brief vacation to "get it together." Since then the symptoms have escalated significantly.

She is having difficulty falling asleep and frequently awakens with palpitations and clammy hands. When asked to describe her feelings she says, "I'm out of control; I'm going to lose my job. What am I ever going to do?"

1. What additional nursing assessments need to be made? Research a typical data intake assessment sheet used with anxiety disorders.
2. Her admission orders include giving alprazolam 0.25 mg three times daily. What schedule would be used to administer these doses?
3. Describe premedication assessment data needed and what additional assessments should be made after initiation of drug therapy using benzodiazepines.
4. How soon after initiation of drug therapy is it reasonable to expect a therapeutic response from an antianxiety medication?
5. Describe the behavior monitoring system and intervention flow records used in the clinical setting when assigned to detect the side effects of anxiolytic drugs.
6. What assessments and nursing interventions, including health teaching, need to be performed to deal with the possible physical dependence or tolerance known to occur with benzodiazepine therapy?

CONTENT REVIEW QUESTIONS

1. The benzodiazepine drug monograph states hepatotoxicity as a side effect to report. Laboratory tests to be reviewed to assess this include:
   1. bilirubin, alkaline phosphatase, gamma-glutamyltransferase (GGT), prothrombin time
   2. albumin, ferritin, prothrombin time
   3. aspartate aminotransferase (AST), GGT, ferritin
   4. creatinine, creatinine clearance, albumin
2. The following lab values should be monitored when a patient is receiving benzodiazepines:
   1. CBC with differential and liver function
   2. CBC and renal function
   3. WBC and biochemical profile
   4. Blood glucose
3. Patient teaching for antianxiety therapy should include:
   1. you may take this medication while operating machinery.
   2. when discontinuing the medication there is no need to gradually reduce the dose.
   3. notify doctor if hangover symptoms persist because the dose may need to be reduced or the medication changed.
   4. therapeutic effects of the drug take 4 to 6 weeks to occur.
4. Drugs that may increase the toxic effects of benzodiazepines are which of the following? *(Select all that apply.)*
   1. Antihistamines
   2. Alcohol
   3. Analgesics
   4. Beta blockers
5. For the case study listed above in the critical thinking section, which of the following would be an appropriate nursing diagnosis? *(Select all that apply.)*
   1. Anxiety
   2. Ineffective coping
   3. Deficient diversional activity
   4. Risk for injury

CHAPTER

17 Drugs Used for Mood Disorders

evolve http://evolve.elsevier.com/Clayton

Chapter Content

Objectives

1. Describe the essential components of a baseline assessment of a patient with depression or bipolar disorder.
2. Discuss the mood swings associated with bipolar disorder.
3. Compare drug therapy used during the treatment of the manic phase and depressive phase of bipolar disorder.
4. Cite monitoring parameters used for patients taking monoamine oxidase inhibitors (MAOIs), selective serotonin reuptake inhibitors (SSRIs), or tricyclic antidepressants.
5. Prepare a teaching plan for an individual receiving tricyclic antidepressants.
6. Differentiate between the physiologic and psychological therapeutic responses seen with antidepressant therapy.
7. Identify the premedication assessments necessary before administration of MAOIs, SSRIs, tricyclic antidepressants, and antimanic agents.
8. Compare the mechanism of action of SSRIs to that of other antidepressant agents.
9. Cite the advantages of SSRIs over other antidepressant agents.
10. Examine the drug monograph for SSRIs to identify significant drug interactions.

Key Terms

mood	mania
mood disorder	euphoria
neurotransmitters	labile mood
depression	grandiose delusions
cognitive symptoms	suicide
psychomotor symptoms	antidepressants
bipolar disorder	

MOOD DISORDERS

Mood is a sustained, emotional feeling perceived along a normal continuum of sad to happy. Mood is our perception of our surroundings. A **mood disorder** (affective disorder) is present when certain symptoms impair a person's ability to function for a time. Mood disorders are characterized by abnormal feelings of depression or euphoria. They involve prolonged, inappropriate expression of emotion that go beyond brief emotional upset from negative life experiences. In severe cases, other psychotic features may also be present. At least 10% of the U.S. population have a diagnosable mood disorder in their lifetime. Mood disorders are divided into depressive (unipolar) and bipolar disorders.

The first *Surgeon General's Report on Mental Health* (1999) recognized that the effect of mental illness on the health and productivity has been profoundly underestimated. Major depression currently ranks as the second leading cause of disease burden (years lived with the disability) in the United States (the leading cause is ischemic heart disease). Unfortunately the majority of people with depression receive no treatment. Undertreatment of mood disorders stems from many factors, including social stigma, financial barriers, underrecognition by health care providers, and underappreciation by the general public of the potential benefits to treatment. The symptoms of depression, such as feelings of worthlessness, excessive guilt, and lack of motivation, deter people from seeking treatment. Members of racial and ethnic minority groups often encounter additional barriers.

The underlying causes of mood disorders are still unknown. They are too complex to be completely explained by a single social, developmental, or biologic theory. A variety of factors appear to work together to cause depressive disorders. It is known that patients with depression have changes in the brain **neurotransmitters** norepinephrine, serotonin, dopamine, acetylcholine, and gamma-aminobutyric acid (GABA), but other unexpected negative life events (e.g., sudden death of a loved one, unemployment, medical illness, other stressful events) also play a major role. Endocrine abnormalities such as excessive secretion of cortisol and abnormal thyroid-stimulating hormone (TSH) have been found in 45% to 60% of patients with depression. Genetic factors also predispose patients to developing depression. Depressive disorders and suicide tend to cluster in families, and relatives of patients with depression are two to three times more likely to develop depression.

The onset of depressive disorder tends to be in the late 20s, although it can occur at any age. The lifetime frequency of depressive symptoms appears to be as high as 26% for women and 12% for men. Risk factors for depression include a personal or family history of depression; prior suicide attempts; female gender; lack of social support; stressful life events; substance abuse, especially alcohol and cocaine; and medical illness. The American Psychiatric Association classifies episodes of depression into mild, moderate, and severe. *Mild depression* causes only minor functional impairment. Patients with *severe depression* have several symptoms that exceed the minimum diagnostic criteria, and daily functioning is significantly impaired. Hospitalization may be required. *Moderate depression* is intermediate between mild and severe conditions for both symptomatology and functional impairment.

It is beyond the scope of this text to discuss mood disorders in detail, but general types of symptoms associated with mood disorders are described as follows. Patients experiencing **depression** display varying degrees of emotional, physical, cognitive, and psychomotor symptoms. *Emotionally,* the depression is characterized by a persistent, reduced ability to experience pleasure in life's usual activities such as hobbies, family, and work. Patients frequently appear sad, and a personality change is common. They may describe their mood as sad, hopeless, or blue. Patients often feel that they have let others down, although these feelings of guilt are unrealistic. Anxiety symptoms (see Chapter 16) are present in almost 90% of depressed patients. *Physical symptoms* often motivate the person to seek medical attention. Chronic fatigue, sleep disturbances such as frequent early morning awakening (terminal insomnia), appetite disturbances (weight loss or gain), and other symptoms such as stomach complaints or heart palpitations are common. **Cognitive symptoms,** such as the inability to concentrate, slowed thinking, confusion, and poor memory of recent events are particularly common in older patients with depression. **Psychomotor symptoms** of depression include slowed or retarded movements, thought processes, and speech, or conversely, agitation manifesting as purposeless, restless motion (e.g., pacing, hand wringing, and outbursts of shouting).

Bipolar disorder (formerly known as manic depression) is another of several mood disorders. It is characterized by distinct episodes of **mania** (main' e ah) (elation, euphoria) and depression, separated by intervals without mood disturbances. The patient displays extreme changes in mood, cognition, behavior, perception, and sensory experiences. At any one time, a patient with bipolar disorder may be manic or depressed, may exhibit symptoms of both mania and depression (mixed), or may be between episodes.

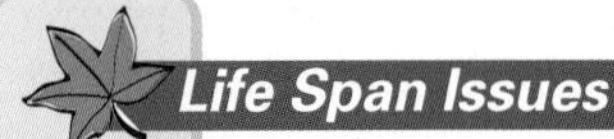

Depression

The patient and caregivers must understand the importance of continuing to take the prescribed antidepressant medication despite minimal initial response. The lag time of 1 to 4 weeks between initiation of therapy and therapeutic response must be emphasized. In most cases the symptoms of depression may improve within a few days (e.g., improved appetite, sleep, and psychomotor activity). The depression, however, still exists, and monitoring should be continued for negative thoughts, feelings, and behaviors. Suicide precautions should be maintained until assessment indicates that suicidal ideation is no longer present.

Suicide statistics are varied and not well documented. However, older adults with depression are more likely to commit suicide than are depressed people of other age-groups. It appears that the older adult is serious when attempting suicide because one of two attempts is successful.

Suicide is the third leading cause of death in adolescents; the incidence may be even higher because of underreporting. Suicide is a "call for help"; however, it is permanent when successfully completed. All comments of suicide or suicide gestures should be taken seriously.

The depressive state has been previously described. Symptoms of acute mania usually begin abruptly and escalate over several days. These symptoms are a heightened mood **(euphoria)** (u for' e ah), quicker thoughts (flight of ideas), more and faster speech (pressured speech), increased energy, increased physical and mental activities (psychomotor excitement), decreased need for sleep, irritability, heightened perceptual acuity, paranoia, increased sexual activity, and impulsivity. There is often a **labile mood,** with rapid shifts toward anger and irritability. The attention span is short, resulting in an inability to concentrate. Anything in the environment may change the topic of discussion, leading to flight of ideas. Social inhibitions are lost, and the patient may become interruptive and loud, departing suddenly from the social interaction and leaving everything in disarray. As the manic phase progresses, approximately two thirds of patients with bipolar disorder develop psychotic symptoms (see Chapter 18), primarily paranoid or **grandiose delusions,** if treatment interventions have not been initiated. Unfortunately, most manic patients do not recognize the symptoms of illness in themselves and may resist treatment.

Bipolar disorder occurs equally between men and women and has a prevalence rate of 0.4% to 1.6% of the adult population in the United States. The onset of bipolar disorder is usually in late adolescence or early 20s. It is rare in preadolescence and may occur as late as age 50. Approximately 60% to 80% of patients with bipolar disease will begin with a manic episode. Without treatment, episodes last 6 months to a year for depression and 4 months for mania.

Patients with mood disorders have a high incidence of attempting **suicide.** The frequency of successful suicide is 15%, 30 times higher than that in the general population. All patients with depressive symptoms should be assessed for suicidal thoughts. Factors that increase the risk of suicide include increasing age, being widowed, being unmarried, unemployment, living alone, substance abuse, previous psychiatric admission, and feelings of hopelessness. The presence of a detailed plan with intention and ability to carry it out indicates strong intent and a high risk of suicide. Other hints of potential suicidal intent include changes in personality, a sudden decision to make a will or give away possessions, and the recent purchase of a gun or hoarding a large supply of medication, including antidepressants, tranquilizers, or other toxic substances.

The prognosis for mood disorders is highly variable. Of patients with major depression, 20% to 30% recover fully and do not experience another bout of depression. Another 50% have recurring episodes, often with a year or more separating the events. The remaining 20% have a chronic course with persistent symptoms and social impairment. Most treated episodes of depression last approximately 3 months; untreated ones last 6 to 12 months. Patients with bipolar illness are more likely to have multiple subsequent episodes of symptoms.

TREATMENT OF MOOD DISORDERS

Treatment of mood disorders requires both nonpharmacologic and pharmacologic therapy. Cognitive-behavioral therapy, psychodynamic therapy, and interpersonal therapy and pharmacologic treatment have been more successful than any one treatment alone. Psychotherapy improves psychosocial function, interpersonal relationships, and day-to-day coping. Patients and family should be educated about recognizing the signs and symptoms of mania, as well as depression and the importance of treatment compliance to minimize recurrence of the illness. Patients should be encouraged to target symptoms to help them recognize mood changes and to seek treatment as soon as possible.

Most patients pass through three stages (i.e., acute, continuation, maintenance) prior to restoring full function. The acute stage is that period from diagnosis to initial treatment response. An "initial response" is defined as a significant reduction in symptoms such that the person no longer fits the criteria for the illness. The acute phase for medication typically takes 10 to 12 weeks, during which the patient is seen by the health care provider weekly or biweekly to monitor symptoms and side effects, make dosage adjustments, and give support. Psychotherapies are initiated at the same time. Treatment of the acute phase is often prolonged because about half of patients either become noncompliant with the medicine and psychotherapy or abandon the program. The goals of the continuation phase of therapy are to prevent relapse and to consolidate the initial response into a complete recovery (defined as being symptom-free for 6 months). The continuation phase is 4 to 9 months of combined pharmacotherapy and psychotherapy. Maintenance phase therapy is recommended for individuals with a history of three or more depressive episodes, chronic depression, or bipolar disorder. The goal of the maintenance phase therapy is to prevent recurrences of the mood disorder.

Another form of nonpharmacologic treatment for depression and bipolar illness is electroconvulsive therapy (ECT). Under guidelines provided by the American Psychiatric Association, ECT is safe and effective for all subtypes of major depression and bipolar disorders. It is more effective, more rapid in onset of effect, and safer in patients with cardiovascular disease than many drug therapies. A course of ECT usually consists of 6 to 12 treatments, but the number is individualized to the needs of the patient. Patients are now premedicated with anesthetics and neuromuscular blocking agents to prevent many of the adverse effects previously associated with ECT. Although it has been misused, ECT should be viewed as a treatment option that can be lifesaving for patients who otherwise would not recover from depressive illnesses. It is usually followed by drug therapy to minimize the rate of relapse.

DRUG THERAPY FOR MOOD DISORDERS

Actions

Pharmacologic treatment of depression is recommended for patients with symptoms of moderate to severe depression and should be considered for patients who do not respond well to psychotherapy. The treatment is accomplished with several classes of drugs collectively known as **antidepressants.** Antidepressants can be subdivided into the MAOIs, tricyclic antidepressants (TCAs), SSRIs, and a miscellaneous group of agents. All have varying degrees of effect on norepinephrine, dopamine, and serotonin by blocking reuptake and reducing destruction of these neurotransmitters, thereby prolonging their action. The development of a clinical antidepressant response requires at least 2 to 4 weeks of therapy at adequate dosages. In general, antidepressant therapy should be changed if there is no clear effect within 4 to 6 weeks. Although much is known about the pharmacologic actions of antidepressants, the exact mechanism of action of these agents in treating depression is still unknown. It is now understood, however, that depression is not simply a deficiency of neurotransmitters.

Uses

Two factors are important in selecting an antidepressant drug: the patient's history of response to previously prescribed antidepressants and the potential for adverse effects associated with different classes of antidepressants. Contrary to marketing claims, there are no differences among antidepressant drugs (with the exception of the MAOIs) in relative overall therapeutic efficacy and onset caused by full therapeutic dosages. There are, however, substantial differences in the adverse effects caused by different agents. It is not possible to predict which drug will be most effective in an individual patient, but patients do show a better response to a specific drug. About 30% of patients do not show much appreciable therapeutic benefit with the first agent used but may have a high degree of success with a change in medication. The history of previous treatment is helpful in selection of new treatment if illness returns. Approximately 65% to 70% of patients respond to antidepressant therapy; 30% to 40% achieve remission. Therapy is based on a patient's history of previous response, or the successful response of a first-degree relative who showed response to antidepressant therapy. Concurrent medical conditions such as obesity, seizure history, potential for dysrhythmias, presence of anxiety, and potential for drug interactions must also be considered in therapy selection. Certain types of mood disorders respond to medication more readily than others. Therapeutic success with tricyclic antidepressants can be improved by monitoring and maintaining therapeutic serum levels by adjusting dosages as needed. Serum levels of other classes of antidepressants generally do not correlate well with success in therapy, but may be helpful to determine whether the patient is adherent to the dosage regimen or is suffering from toxicities associated with higher serum levels.

Patients must be counseled on expected therapeutic benefits and adverse effects to be tolerated from antidepressant therapy. The physiologic manifestations of depression (e.g., sleep disturbance, change in appetite, loss of energy, fatigue, palpitations) begin to be alleviated within the first week of therapy. The psychological symptoms (e.g., depressed mood, lack of interest, social withdrawal) will improve after 2 to 4 weeks of therapy at an effective dose. Therefore it may take 4 to 6 weeks to adjust the dosage to optimize therapy and minimize side effects. Unfortunately, some adverse effects develop early in therapy, and patients who are already pessimistic because of their illness have a tendency to be noncompliant.

The pharmacologic treatment of bipolar disorder must be individualized because the clinical presentation, severity, and frequency of episodes vary widely among patients. Acute mania is initially treated with lithium, valproate, or an atypical antipsychotic agent (olanzapine, risperidone) as monotherapy. Once the patient is stabilized, most patients are placed on long-term lithium therapy to minimize future episodes. Therapy with carbamazepine, oxcarbazine, divalproex (valproic acid), lamotrigine, or gabapentin may be used for patients who do not adequately respond to lithium.

NURSING PROCESS *for Mood Disorder Therapy*

Assessment

History of Mood Disorder

- Obtain a history of the mood disorder. Is it depressive only, or are there both manic and depressive phases interspersed with periods of normalcy? What precipitating factors contribute to the changes in mood? Is it associated with a particular season? How often do the depressive, normal, and manic moods persist? Are there better or worse times of day? Has the patient been treated previously for a mood disorder? What is the patient's current status? Has the individual been using alcohol or drugs? Has there been a recent loss, for example, job, relationship, death of a loved one?
- Obtain a detailed history of all medications the individual is taking and those taken within the past 2 months to evaluate the patient's adherence to the treatment regimen. How compliant has the patient been with the treatment regimen?

Basic Mental Status

- Note general appearance and appropriateness of attire. Is the individual clean and neat? Is the posture erect, stooped, or slumped? Is the individual oriented to date, time, place, and person?
- What coping mechanisms has the individual been using to deal with the mood disorder? How adaptive are the coping mechanisms?

Interpersonal Relationships

- Assess the individual's interpersonal relationships. Identify people who are supportive.
- Identify whether interpersonal relationships have declined between the patient and people in the family, at work, or in social settings.

Mood/Affect

- Is the individual elated, overjoyed, angry, irritable, crying, tearful, or sad? Is the facial expression tense, worried, sad, angry, or blank? Ask the person to describe feelings. Be alert for expressions of loneliness, apathy, worthlessness, or hopelessness. Moods may change suddenly.
- Patients experiencing altered thinking, behavior, or feelings must be carefully evaluated for verbal and nonverbal actions. Many times, the thoughts, feelings, and behaviors displayed are inconsistent with the so-called normal responses of individuals in similar circumstances.
- Assess whether the mood being described is consistent with the circumstances being described. For example, is the person speaking of death, yet smiling?

Clarity of Thought. Evaluate the coherency, relevancy, and organization of thoughts; observe for flight of ideas, hallucinations, delusions, paranoia, or grandiose ideation. Ask specific questions regarding the individual's ability to make judgments and decisions. Is there evidence of memory impairment?

Thoughts of Death. If the individual is suspected of being suicidal, ask the patient if there have ever been thoughts about suicide. If the response is yes, get more details. Is a specific plan formulated? How often do these thoughts occur? Does the individual make direct or indirect statements regarding death, such as "things would be better" at death?

Psychomotor Function. Ask specific questions regarding the activity level the patient has maintained. Is the person able to work or go to school? Is the person able to fulfill responsibilities at work, socially, and within the family? How have the person's normal responses to daily activities been altered? Is the individual withdrawn and isolated or still involved in social interactions? Check gestures, gait, pacing, presence or absence of tremors, and ability to perform gross or fine motor movements. Is the patient hyperactive or impulsive? Note the speech pattern. Are there prolonged pauses before answers are given or altered levels of volume and inflection?

Sleep Pattern. What is the person's normal sleep pattern, and how does it vary with mood swings? Ask specifically whether insomnia is present and whether it is initial or terminal in nature. Ask the individual to describe the perception of the amount and quality of the sleep nightly. Are naps taken regularly?

Dietary History. Ask questions relating to appetite and note weight gains or losses not associated with intentional dieting. During the manic phase, the individual may become anorexic. Is the person able to sit down to eat a meal, or eat only small amounts while pacing?

Nonadherence. Nonadherence is usually expressed by denial of the severity of the disease. Monitor for denial of the severity of the depression; listen for excuses for not taking medicine (e.g., cannot afford medication, asymptomatic, "I don't like the way it changes me. I want to be myself!").

Nursing Diagnoses

- Risk for self-directed violence (indication)
- Hopelessness (indication)
- Dysfunctional grieving (indication)
- Ineffective coping (indication)
- Social isolation (indication)
- Disturbed sensory perception, visual or auditory (indication)

Planning

History of Mood Disorder

- Review data collected to identify individual's strengths and weaknesses.
- Review medications being taken to specifically identify any that are known to cause depression.

Basic Mental Status

- Plan to perform a baseline assessment of the individual's mental status at specific intervals throughout the course of treatment.
- Review coping mechanisms used. Plan to discuss those that are maladaptive. Plan to initiate changes by guiding the individual in the use of more adaptive coping strategies.
- Schedule specific times to discuss the patient's behavior and foster understanding of it with family members.

Mood/Affect

- Review assessment data to develop strategies to assist the individual to cope more effectively with exhibited behaviors. Reward positive accomplishments for progress made.
- It is difficult to plan activities with a patient in a manic phase because the patient's mood may be argumentative and aggressive and may tend toward self-injury. Be brief, direct, and to the point with these individuals. Setting limits will be necessary. Plan to approach the individual in a quiet, safe environment with other staff available in case the person is aggressive or threatens personal harm or harm to others.

Clarity of Thought. Identify areas in which the patient is capable of input to set goals and make decisions. (This will aid the individual to overcome a sense of powerlessness over life situations.) When the patient is unable to make decisions, plan to make them. Set goals to involve the patient as abilities change with treatment. Provide an opportunity to plan for self-care. Manic patients are often manipulative and argumentative, seek less vulnerable individuals with whom to pick fights, and project blame onto others. The nursing staff must plan collaboratively for these possible behaviors, and interventions must be consistent among all caregivers.

Thoughts of Death. Provide a safe environment for the individual. Search the surroundings for objects that could be used to inflict self-harm. Because the manic patient may also be harmful to others, a safe, structured environment must be maintained.

Psychomotor Function. Review activities offered within the clinical setting and plan for the individual to participate in those that will be beneficial and foster success, such as channeling for hyperactivity, yet being safe for the patient and others. During initiation of therapy the individual may not be capable of participating in group activities.

Sleep Pattern. For the patient with depression, provide specific parameters in which the patient can function that do not allow the individual to continually sleep. Design activities during the day that will stimulate the individual and promote sleep at night. Plan to use relaxation techniques. For patients in the manic phase, plan activities that will channel excessive energy. Recognize that sleep deprivation is a possibility with manic patients and can be life threatening. Select a quiet, nonstimulating environment in which to sleep. Plan to schedule specific rounds to evaluate the individual's sleep and safety.

Prescribed Antidepressant Therapy. Whenever sleep deprivation therapy, consisting of missing one night's sleep or more, or phototherapy, using exposure to bright artificial light, is prescribed, scheduling and intervention strategies need to be planned.

Dietary Needs. Provide an opportunity for the individual to be involved in selecting foods appropriate to needs (to lose or gain weight). Request a nutritional assessment by a dietitian to identify foods the person may eat (finger foods may work best). Supplemental feedings with nutritional preparations such as special high-calorie shakes may be needed. Obtain weights weekly or more frequently, and monitor intake and output.

Self-Care. During periods of severe depression, identify the level of assistance with the self-care the patient will require.

Adherence. When adherence is an issue, help the patient to identify alternative self-care approaches that are acceptable to the individual and the therapeutic regimen. Establish rewards for compliant behavior, and provide reinforcement when positive compliant behaviors are observed.

ECT. Review the health care provider's orders for the planned use of ECT as an approach to treatment of severe depression, and check for the health care provider's orders specific to the pre- and posttreatment of the patient receiving ECT.

Therapeutic Outcomes

Plan through the acute, continuation, and maintenance phases of care delivery to facilitate the patient to achieve the highest level of independent functioning.

Implementation

- Nursing interventions must be individualized and based on patient assessment data.
- Provide an environment of acceptance that focuses on the individual's strengths while minimizing the weaknesses. Sometimes it is necessary to provide a new environment for the patient during a period of depression. The individual may not be able to work, may need a new peer group, and may need to be away from family while restructuring and regrouping his or her resources, identifying strengths, and achieving a therapeutic drug level.
- Provide an opportunity for the individual to express feelings. Use active listening and therapeutic communication techniques. Provide an opportunity for the person to express feelings in nonverbal ways, for example, involvement in physical activities or occupational therapy. Recognize that patients are hyperactive and talkative during the manic phase; it may be necessary to interrupt talking and to give concise, simple directions.
- Remain calm, direct, and firm in providing care. Because patients in the manic phase tend to be argumentative, avoid getting involved in an argument. State the unit rules matter-of-factly and enforce them.
- Allow the patient to make decisions if capable; make those decisions the patient is not capable of making. Provide a reward for progress when decisions are initiated appropriately. Involve the patient in self-care activities.
- If suicidal, ask for details of the plan being formulated. Follow up on details obtained with appropriate family members or significant others, for example, have guns removed from home if this is part of the plan. Provide patient safety and supervision, and record observations at specified intervals consistent with severity of the suicide threat and policies of the practice site. This is the highest priority with severe mood disorders.
- Manic patients may be harmful to others; it may be necessary to limit interactions with other patients. Patients in the manic phase may require a quiet room.
- Stay with patients who are highly agitated.
- Administer PRN drugs ordered for hyperactivity. Make necessary observations for response to medications administered.
- Use physical restraints within the guidelines of the clinical setting as appropriate to the behaviors being exhibited. Use the least restrictive alternative possible for the circumstances. Have sufficient staff available to assist with violent behavior to demonstrate ability to control the situation while providing for the safety and well-being of the patient and fellow staff members.
- Provide for nutritional needs by having high-protein, high-calorie foods appropriate for the individual to eat while pacing or highly active. Have nutritious snacks the patient is known to like available on the unit, and offer them throughout the day. Administer vitamins and liquid supplemental feedings as ordered.
- Manipulative behavior must be handled in a consistent manner by all staff members. Use limit setting and consequences that are agreed to by all staff members. When the patient attempts to blame others, refocus on the patient's responsibilities. Give positive reinforcement for nonmanipulative behaviors when they occur.

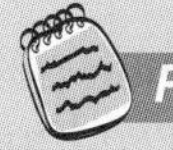

Patient Education and Health Promotion

Orient the individual to the unit, explaining rules and the process of privileges and how they are obtained or lost. (The extent of the orientation and explanations given will depend on the individual's orientation to date, time, place, and abilities.)

- Explain unit rules and therapeutic rules.
- Explain the activity groups available and how and when the individual will participate in these.
- A variety of group process activities (e.g., social skills group, self-esteem groups, and physical exercise groups) are available within particular therapeutic settings.
- The patient and family must be involved in goal setting and integrated into the appropriate group

processes to develop positive experiences for the patient to enhance coping skills.
- Patient education must be based on assessment data and individualized to provide the patient with a structured environment in which to grow and enhance self-esteem.
- Before discharge the patient and family must understand the desired treatment outcomes and the entire follow-up plan (e.g., frequency of therapy sessions, doctor visits, return-to-work goals).

Fostering Health Maintenance

- Throughout the course of treatment, discuss medication information and how it will benefit the patient. Drug therapy is not immediately effective in treating depression; therefore the patient and significant others must understand the importance of continuing to take the prescribed medications despite minimal initial response. The lag time of 2 to 4 weeks between initiation of drug therapy and therapeutic response must be stressed.
- Patients, families, and caregivers should be encouraged to be alert to the emergence of anxiety, agitation, panic attacks, insomnia, irritability, hostility, aggressiveness, impulsivity, akathisia (psychomotor restlessness), hypomania, mania, unusual changes in behavior, worsening of depression, and suicidality, especially early during antidepressant treatment and when the dose is adjusted up or down. Families and caregivers should be advised to observe for the emergence of such symptoms on a daily basis, because changes may be abrupt. Such symptoms should be reported to the patient's prescriber, especially if they are severe, abrupt in onset, or were not part of the patient's presenting symptoms. Symptoms such as these may be associated with an increased risk of suicidal thinking and behavior and indicate a need for very close monitoring and possible changes in the medicine.
- Emphasize the need for lithium blood levels to be taken at specified intervals. Give details of date, time, and place for these to be done.
- Stress the importance of adequate hydration (six to eight 8-ounce glasses of water per day) and sodium intake when receiving lithium therapy.
- Instruct the patient to weigh daily.
- Provide the patient or significant others with important information contained in the specific drug monograph for the medicines prescribed. The monographs also contain health teaching and nursing interventions for the side effects to expect and report.
- Seek cooperation and understanding of the following points so that medication adherence is increased: name of medication, dosage, route and time of administration, side effects to expect, and side effects to report. Encourage the patient not to discontinue or adjust drug dosage without consulting the health care provider.
- At the time of discharge, prescriptions should be written for the smallest quantity of tablets consistent with good patient management in order to reduce the risk of overdose.

Written Record. Enlist the patient's aid in developing and maintaining a written record of monitoring parameters (see Patient Self-Assessment Form on p. 269). Complete the Premedication Data column for use as a baseline to track response to drug therapy. Ensure that the patient understands how to use the form and instruct the patient to bring the completed form to follow-up visits. During follow-up visits, focus on issues that will foster adherence with the therapeutic interventions prescribed.

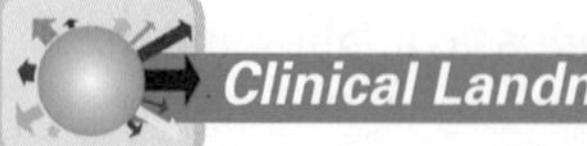

Clinical Landmine

Antidepressants may increase the risk of suicidal thinking and behavior (suicidality) in patients of all ages experiencing major depressive disorder. Patients who are started on antidepressants should be monitored by daily observation from families and caregivers for the emergence of agitation, irritability, unusual changes in behavior, as well as the emergence of suicidality, and report such symptoms immediately to health care providers.

DRUG THERAPY FOR DEPRESSION

DRUG CLASS: Monoamine Oxidase Inhibitors

In the early 1950s, isoniazid and iproniazid were released for the treatment of tuberculosis. It was soon reported that iproniazid had mood-elevating properties in tuberculosis patients. It was discovered in further investigation that iproniazid, in addition to its antitubercular properties, inhibited monoamine oxidase, whereas isoniazid did not. Other MAOIs were synthesized and used extensively to treat mental depression until the 1960s, when the tricyclic antidepressants became available.

Actions

MAOIs act by blocking the metabolic destruction of epinephrine, norepinephrine, dopamine, and serotonin neurotransmitters by the enzyme monoamine oxidase in the presynaptic neurons of the brain. They prevent the degradation of these central nervous system (CNS) neurotransmitters so that their concentration is increased. Although MAO inhibition starts within a few days of initiating therapy, the antidepressant effects require 2 to 4 weeks to become evident. Approximately 60% of the clinical improvement of symptoms of depression occurs in 2 weeks, and maximum improvement is usually attained within 4 weeks.

Uses

The MAOIs used today are phenelzine, tranylcypromine, isocarboxazid, and selegiline (Table 17-1). They are equally effective and have very similar side effects.

PATIENT SELF-ASSESSMENT FORM Antidepressants

MEDICATIONS	COLOR	TO BE TAKEN

Patient ______________________

Health Care Provider ______________________

Health Care Provider's phone ______________________

Next appt.* ______________________

What I Should Monitor	Premedication Data	Date	Date	Date	Date	Date	Date	Comments
Weight								
Blood pressure AM / PM								
Resting pulse rate								
I would like to be alone **All the time** (10) — **Some of the time** (5) — **Not really** (1)								
How I feel about my children **Too much work** (10) — 5 — **Fun to be with** (1)								
How I feel today **Poor** (10) — **Fair** (5) — **Okay** (1)								
Appetite **Poor** (10) — **Fair** (5) — **Good** (1) — B								
L								
D								
S								
Has the family noted any problems? Judgment? Socialization?								
Does patient dress daily? (Yes/No)								
Does patient take pride in appearance? (Yes/No)								
Use of alcohol? (Yes/No) Amount (e.g., one drink)								
General mood: Briefly describe whether tearful, excessively excited, happy, angry, hostile, depressed, sad, or having suicidal thoughts								
Anxiety level: Pacing, tremors, hyperactivity, or slow, retarded movements								
Other								

B, Breakfast; *L*, lunch; *D*, dinner; *S*, snack.

*Please bring this record with you to your next appointment.

Use the back of this sheet for additional information.

Drug Table 17-1 ANTIDEPRESSANTS

GENERIC NAME	BRAND NAME	AVAILABILITY	INITIAL DOSE (PO)	DAILY MAINTENANCE DOSE (mg)	MAXIMUM DAILY DOSE (mg)
MONOAMINE OXIDASE INHIBITORS (MAOIs)					
phenelzine	Nardil	Tablets: 15 mg	15 mg three times daily	15-60	90
tranylcypromine	Parnate	Tablets: 10 mg	10 mg twice daily	30	60
isocarboxazid	Marplan	Tablets: 10 mg	10 mg twice daily	40	60
selegiline	Emsam	Transdermal patch: 6, 9, 12 mg	6 mg patch daily	6	12
TRICYCLIC ANTIDEPRESSANTS					
amitriptyline		Tablets: 10, 25, 50, 75, 100, 150 mg IM: 10 mg/mL in 10 mL vials	25 mg three times daily	150-250	300
amoxapine		Tablets: 25, 50, 100, 150 mg	50 mg three times daily	200-300	400 (outpatients) 600 (inpatients)
clomipramine	Anafranil	Capsules: 25, 50, 75 mg	25 mg three times daily	100-150	250
desipramine	Norpramin	Tablets: 10, 25, 50, 75, 100, 150 mg	25 mg three times daily	75-200	300
doxepin	Sinequan, ✱ Apo-Doxepin	Capsules: 10, 25, 50, 75, 100, 150 mg Oral concentrate 10 mg/mL	25 mg three times daily	at least 150	300
imipramine	Tofranil, ✱ Apo-Imipramine	Tablets: 10, 25, 50 mg	30-75 mg daily at bedtime	150-250	300
nortriptyline	Aventyl, Pamelor	Capsules: 10, 25, 50, 75 mg Solution: 10 mg/5 mL	25 mg three or four times daily	50-75	100
protriptyline	Vivactil	Tablets: 5, 10 mg	5-10 mg three or four times daily	20-40	60
trimipramine	Surmontil	Capsules: 25, 50, 100 mg	25 mg three times daily	50-150	200 (outpatients) 300 (inpatients)

✱ Available in Canada.

They are most effective in atypical depression, panic disorder, obsessive-compulsive disorder, and some phobic disorders. They are also used when tricyclic antidepressant therapy is unsatisfactory and when ECT is inappropriate or refused. Selegiline is available as a transdermal patch that is to be changed once every 24 hours. Patients using the lowest strength available (6 mg) do not have dietary restrictions. Dietary restrictions are required for those using the 9- and 12-mg patches.

Therapeutic Outcomes

The primary therapeutic outcomes expected from MAOIs are elevated mood and reduction of symptoms of depression.

Nursing Process for MAOIs

Premedication Assessment

1. Obtain blood pressure and pulse rate before and at regular intervals after initiation of therapy.
2. If the patient is diabetic, monitor blood glucose to establish baseline values and to assess periodically during therapy. Because MAOIs cause hypoglycemia, a dosage adjustment in insulin or oral hyperglycemic therapy may be required. If the patient has a history of severe renal disease, liver disease, cerebrovascular disease, or congestive heart failure, do not give medication. Consult with prescribing health care provider.

Drug Table 17-1 ANTIDEPRESSANTS—cont'd

GENERIC NAME	BRAND NAME	AVAILABILITY	INITIAL DOSE (PO)	DAILY MAINTENANCE DOSE (mg)	MAXIMUM DAILY DOSE (mg)
SELECTIVE SEROTONIN REUPTAKE INHIBITORS (SSRIs)					
citalopram	Celexa	Tablets: 10, 20, 40 mg Liquid: 10 mg/5 mL	20 mg daily	20-40	60
duloxetine	Cymbalta	Sustained release capsules: 20, 30, 60 mg	40 mg daily	60	60
escitalopram	Lexapro	Tablets: 5, 10, 20 mg Liquid: 5 mg/5 mL	10 mg daily	10-20	20
fluoxetine	Prozac	Capsules: 10, 20, 40 mg Tablets: 10, 20 mg Solution: 20 mg/5 mL Weekly capsule: 90 mg	20 mg in morning	20-60	80
fluvoxamine	Luvox	Tablets: 25, 50, 100 mg	90 mg at bedtime	100-300	300
paroxetine	Paxil Paxil CR	Tablets: 10, 20, 30, 40 mg Suspension: 10 mg/5 mL Sustained release tablets: 12.5, 25, 37.5 mg	20 mg daily	20-50	50
sertraline	Zoloft	Tablets: 25, 50, 100 mg Oral concentrate: 20 mg/mL	50 mg daily	50-200	200

3. Complete a diet history to ensure that the patient has not ingested meals with a high tyramine content in the past few days.
4. Complete a medication history to ensure that the patient has not taken any of the following medicines in the past few days before therapy: dextromethorphan, ephedrine, phenylpropanolamine, amphetamine, methylphenidate, levodopa, or meperidine.

Planning

Availability. See Table 17-1.

Implementation

1. Instruct the patient on how to limit tyramine-containing foods that may cause a life-threatening hypertensive crisis if ingested concurrently with MAOIs.
2. The dosage should be taken in divided doses, with the last dose administered no later than 6:00 PM to prevent drug-induced insomnia. Caution the patient not to abruptly discontinue the medicine. If a dose is missed, take immediately and space the remainder of the daily dosage throughout the rest of the day.
3. Check to be certain the patient is not receiving meperidine.

Evaluation

Side Effects to Expect

Orthostatic Hypotension. The most common side effect of MAOIs is hypotension; it is more significant with phenelzine than tranylcypromine. Although generally mild, orthostatic hypotension manifested by dizziness and weakness is more common when therapy is started. Daily divided doses help minimize the hypotension. Tolerance usually develops after a few weeks of therapy.

Monitor the blood pressure daily in both the supine and standing positions.

Anticipate the development of postural hypotension, and take measures to prevent an occurrence. Teach patients to rise slowly from a supine or sitting position; encourage them to sit or lie down if feeling faint.

Drowsiness, Sedation. Phenelzine has mild to moderate sedating effects. These symptoms tend to disappear with continued therapy and possible readjustment of the dosage.

Inform the patient of possible sedative effects. The patient should use caution while driving or performing other tasks that require alertness. Consult with the health care provider to consider moving the daily dose to bedtime if sedation continues to be a problem.

Restlessness, Agitation, Insomnia. These effects are more common with tranylcypromine and are transient as the dosage is being adjusted. Take the last dose before 6:00 PM to minimize insomnia.

Blurred Vision; Constipation; Urinary Retention; Dryness of Mucosa of the Mouth, Throat, and Nose. These symptoms are the anticholinergic effects produced by these agents. Patients taking these medications should be monitored for these side effects.

Mucosa dryness may be relieved by sucking hard candy or ice chips or by chewing gum. If the patient develops urinary hesitancy, assess for bladder distention. Report to the health care provider for further evaluation.

Give stool softeners as prescribed. Encourage adequate fluid intake and foods to provide sufficient bulk. Caution the patient that blurred vision may occur, and make appropriate suggestions for personal safety of the individual.

Side Effects to Report

Hypertension. A major potential complication with MAOI therapy is that of hypertensive crisis, particularly with tranylcypromine. Because MAOIs block amine metabolism in tissues outside the brain, patients who consume foods or medications (see Drug Interactions) containing indirect sympathomimetic amines are at considerable risk for a hypertensive crisis. Foods containing significant quantities of tyramine include well-ripened cheeses (e.g., Camembert, Edam, Roquefort, Parmesan, mozzarella, cheddar); yeast extract; red wines; pickled herring; sauerkraut; overripe bananas, figs, or avocados; chicken livers; and beer. Foods containing other vasopressors include fava beans, chocolate, coffee, tea, and colas. Common prodromal symptoms of hypertensive crisis include severe occipital headache, stiff neck, sweating, nausea, vomiting, and sharply elevated blood pressure.

Drug Interactions

Drugs That Increase Toxic Effects. The following drugs potentiate the toxicity of MAOIs by raising neurotransmitter levels: dextromethorphan, carbamazepine, cyclobenzaprine, methylphenidate, tryptophan, sulfonamides, amphetamines, ephedrine, methyldopa, mazindol, phenylpropanolamine, levodopa, nefazodone, epinephrine, and norepinephrine.

Tricyclic Antidepressants. MAOIs and tricyclic antidepressants, especially imipramine and desipramine, should not be administered concurrently. It is recommended that at least 14 days lapse between the discontinuation of MAOIs and the initiation of another antidepressant.

SSRIs. Severe reactions including convulsions, hyperpyrexia, and death have been reported with concurrent use. It is recommended that at least 14 days lapse between discontinuing an MAOI and starting SSRI therapy. A 5-week interval is recommended between discontinuing fluoxetine and starting MAOIs.

General Anesthesia, Diuretics, Antihypertensive Agents. MAOIs may potentiate the hypotensive effects of general anesthesia, diuretics, and antihypertensive agents.

Insulin, Oral Hypoglycemic Agents. MAOIs have an additive hypoglycemic effect in combination with insulin and oral sulfonylureas. Monitor blood glucose; lower hypoglycemic doses if necessary.

Meperidine. When used concurrently, meperidine and MAOIs may cause hyperpyrexia, restlessness, hypertension, hypotension, convulsions, and coma. The effects of this interaction may occur for several weeks after discontinuing an MAOI. Use morphine instead of meperidine.

DRUG CLASS: Selective Serotonin Reuptake Inhibitors

Actions

SSRIs (see Table 17-1) are a newer class of antidepressant chemically unrelated to other antidepressants. They act by inhibiting the reuptake and destruction of serotonin from the synaptic cleft, thereby prolonging the action of the neurotransmitter. In addition to inhibiting serotonin, duloxetine also inhibits the reuptake of norepinephrine and to a lesser extent, dopamine.

Uses

SSRIs have become the most widely used class of antidepressants. They have been shown to be equally effective in treating depression as the tricyclic antidepressants. A particular advantage of the SSRIs is that they do not have the anticholinergic and cardiovascular side effects that often limit the use of the tricyclic antidepressants. As with other antidepressants, it takes 2 to 4 weeks of therapy to obtain the full therapeutic benefit in treating depression. Fluoxetine is the only SSRI that has been approved for use in treating depression in children and adolescents. The U.S. Food and Drug Administration (FDA) has recommended that paroxetine not be administered to patients younger than 18 years of age.

SSRIs are also being studied for the treatment of obsessive-compulsive disorder, obesity, eating disorders (anorexia nervosa, bulimia nervosa), bipolar disorder, panic disorder, autism, and several other disorders. Fluvoxamine, paroxetine, sertraline, and fluoxetine are approved for use in obsessive-compulsive disorder. Fluoxetine is marketed under the brand name of Sarafem for the treatment of premenstrual dysphoric disorder (PMDD). Duloxetine is also approved for treatment of diabetic peripheral neuropathic pain.

Therapeutic Outcomes

The primary therapeutic outcomes expected from the SSRIs are elevated mood and reduction of symptoms of depression.

Nursing Process for SSRI Therapy

Premedication Assessment

1. Obtain baseline blood pressures in supine, sitting, and standing positions; record and report significant lowering to health care provider before administering drug.
2. Obtain baseline weight; schedule weekly weights.
3. Note any GI symptoms present before the start of therapy.

4. Monitor CNS symptoms present, such as insomnia or nervousness.
5. Check hepatic studies before initiation and periodically throughout course of administration.

Planning

Availability. See Table 17-1.

Implementation

Dosage and Administration. See Table 17-1.

Observation. Symptoms of depression may improve within a few days (e.g., improved appetite, sleep, and psychomotor activity). The depression still exists, however, and it usually takes several weeks of therapeutic doses before improvement is noted. Suicide precautions should be maintained during this time.

Evaluation

Side Effects to Report

Restlessness, Agitation, Anxiety, Insomnia. This usually occurs early in therapy and may require short-term treatment with sedative-hypnotic agents. Avoiding bedtime doses may also help decrease the incidence of insomnia.

Sedative Effects. Tell the patient of possible sedative effects. The patient should use caution while driving or performing other tasks that require alertness. Consult with the health care provider to consider moving the daily dose to bedtime if sedation continues to be a problem.

Gastrointestinal Effects. Most of these effects may be minimized by temporary reduction in dosage and administration with food. Encourage the patient not to discontinue therapy without consulting the health care provider first.

Suicidal Actions. Monitor the patient for changes in thoughts, feelings, and behaviors during the initial stages of therapy.

Drug Interactions

Tricyclic Antidepressants. The interaction between SSRIs and tricyclic antidepressants is very complex. An increased toxicity results from tricyclic antidepressants. Observe patients for signs of toxicity, such as dysrhythmias, seizure activity, and CNS stimulation.

Lithium. Fluoxetine, citalopram, and fluvoxamine have been reported to reduce lithium levels and increase levels to induce lithium toxicity. Monitor for lithium toxicity manifested by nausea, anorexia, fine tremors, persistent vomiting, profuse diarrhea, hyperreflexia, lethargy, and weakness.

MAOIs. Severe reactions, including excitement, diaphoresis, rigidity, convulsions, hyperpyrexia, and death have been reported with concurrent use of MAOIs and SSRIs. It is recommended that at least 14 days lapse between discontinuing an MAOI and starting SSRI therapy. A 5-week stop interval is recommended between discontinuing fluoxetine and starting MAOIs.

Haloperidol. Fluoxetine and fluvoxamine increase haloperidol levels as well as the frequency of extrapyramidal symptoms (EPS). If used concurrently, the dosage of haloperidol may need to be decreased.

Phenytoin, Phenobarbital. Complex interactions occur when phenobarbital and phenytoin enhance the metabolism of paroxetine, requiring a dosage increase in paroxetine for therapeutic effect. In a similar fashion, paroxetine increases the metabolism of phenytoin and phenobarbital, thus requiring an increase in dosage of these two agents for maintaining therapeutic effect. Conversely, fluoxetine may diminish the metabolism of phenytoin, resulting in potential phenytoin toxicity.

Carbamazepine. Fluoxetine and fluvoxamine can increase carbamazepine concentrations, resulting in signs of toxicity, such as vertigo, tremor, headache, drowsiness, nausea, and vomiting. The dosage of carbamazepine may need to be reduced. Carbamazepine may enhance the excretion of citalopram, leading to decreased therapeutic effect. The dosage of citalopram may need to be increased.

Alprazolam. Fluoxetine, fluvoxamine, and sertraline prolong the activity of alprazolam, resulting in excessive sedation and impaired motor skills.

Propranolol, Metoprolol. Fluvoxamine and citalopram significantly inhibit the metabolism of these beta-adrenergic blocking agents. Monitor closely for bradycardia and hypotension. Reduce the dosage of the beta blocker as needed.

Cimetidine. Cimetidine inhibits the metabolism of paroxetine and sertraline. Patients should be closely monitored when cimetidine is added to paroxetine or sertraline therapy.

Warfarin. Fluoxetine, paroxetine, sertraline, citalopram, and fluvoxamine may enhance the anticoagulant effects of warfarin. Observe for petechiae, ecchymoses, nosebleeds, bleeding gums, dark tarry stools, and bright red or "coffee ground" emesis. Monitor the prothrombin time and INR; reduce the dosage of warfarin if necessary.

Smoking. Smoking enhances the metabolism of fluvoxamine. Dosages of fluvoxamine may need to be increased for full therapeutic response.

Amphetamines, Tryptophan, Dextromethorphan, Ephedrine, Phenylpropanolamine, Pseudoephedrine, Epinephrine. All these agents increase serotonin levels, potentially causing serotonin syndrome when taken by a person receiving SSRIs. These medicines should be used only under the supervision of a health care provider.

DRUG CLASS: Tricyclic Antidepressants

Actions

Until recently, tricyclic antidepressants (see Table 17-1) have been the most widely used medications in the treatment of depression. SSRIs now have that distinction, but long-term outcome is yet to be determined. The tricyclic antidepressants prolong the action of norepinephrine, dopamine, and serotonin to varying degrees by blocking the reuptake of these neurotransmitters in the synaptic cleft between neurons. The exact mechanism of action when used as antidepressants is unknown.

Uses

Tricyclic antidepressants produce antidepressant and mild tranquilizing effects. After 2 to 4 weeks of therapy, they elevate mood, improve the appetite, and increase alertness in approximately 80% of patients with endogenous depression. Combination therapy with phenothiazine derivatives may be beneficial in treating depression of schizophrenia or moderate to severe anxiety and depression observed with psychosis.

Tricyclic antidepressants are equally effective in treating depression, assuming that appropriate dosages are used for an adequate time. Consequently the selection of an antidepressant is based primarily on the characteristics of each agent. Sedation is more notable with amitriptyline, doxepin, and trimipramine. Protriptyline has no sedative properties and may actually produce mild stimulation in some patients. All tricyclic compounds display anticholinergic activity, with amitriptyline displaying the most and desipramine the least. This factor should be considered in patients with cardiac disease, prostatic hyperplasia, or glaucoma. Other factors to consider are that men tend to respond better to imipramine than do women, and older adults tend to respond better to amitriptyline than younger patients.

Doxapin is also approved for treating anxiety and imipramine is approved for treating enuresis in children ages 6 years and older. Clomipramine is not used to treat depression but is approved to treat obsessive-compulsive disorder.

Selected tricyclic antidepressants are also used to treat phantom limb pain, chronic pain, cancer pain, peripheral neuropathy with pain, postherpetic neuralgia, arthritic pain, eating disorders, premenstrual symptoms, and obstructive sleep apena.

Therapeutic Outcomes

The primary therapeutic outcomes expected from tricyclic antidepressants are elevated mood and reduction of symptoms of depression.

Nursing Process for Tricyclic Antidepressants

Premedication Assessment

1. Note consistency of bowel movements; constipation is common when taking tricyclic antidepressants.
2. Obtain baseline blood pressures in supine and standing positions; record and report significant hypotension to the health care provider before administering drug.
3. Check history for symptoms of dysrhythmias, tachycardia, or congestive heart failure; if present, consult the health care provider before starting therapy (may require electrocardiogram [ECG] before initiating therapy).
4. If patient has a history of seizures, check with the health care provider to see if a dosage needs to be adjusted in anticonvulsant therapy medications.

Planning

Availability. See Table 17-1.

Implementation

Dosage and Administration. *Adult:* PO: See Table 17-1. Dosage should be initiated at a low level and increased gradually, particularly in older or debilitated patients. Dosage increases should be made in the evening because increased sedation is often present.

Observation. Symptoms of depression may improve within a few days (e.g., improved appetite, sleep, and psychomotor activity). The depression still exists, however, and it usually takes several weeks of the therapeutic doses before improvement is noted. Suicide precautions should be maintained during this time.

Evaluation

Side Effects to Expect

Blurred Vision; Constipation; Urinary Retention; Dryness of Mucosa of the Mouth, Throat, and Nose. These symptoms are the anticholinergic effects produced by these agents. Patients taking these medications should be monitored for these side effects.

Mucosa dryness may be relieved by sucking hard candy or ice chips, or by chewing gum. The use of stool softeners such as docusate or the occasional use of a stimulant laxative such as bisacodyl may be required for constipation.

Caution the patient that blurred vision may occur, and make appropriate suggestions for personal safety of the individual.

Orthostatic Hypotension. All tricyclic antidepressants may cause some degree of orthostatic hypotension manifested by dizziness and weakness, particularly when therapy is being initiated.

Monitor blood pressure daily in both the supine and standing positions. Anticipate the development of postural hypotension, and take measures to prevent an occurrence. Teach the patient to rise slowly from a supine or sitting position; encourage the patient to sit or lie down if feeling faint.

Sedative Effects. Tell the patient of sedative effects, especially during the onset of therapy. Single doses at bedtime may diminish or relieve the sedative effects.

Side Effects to Report

Tremor. Approximately 10% of patients develop this adverse effect. The tremor can be controlled with small doses of propranolol.

Numbness, Tingling. Report for further evaluation.

Parkinsonian Symptoms. If these symptoms develop, the tricyclic antidepressant dosage must be reduced or discontinued. Antiparkinsonian medications will not control symptoms induced by tricyclic antidepressants.

Dysrhythmias, Tachycardia, Heart Failure. Report for further evaluation.

Seizure Activity. High doses of antidepressants lower the seizure threshold. Adjustment of anticonvulsant therapy may be required, especially in seizure-prone patients.

Suicidal Actions. Monitor the patient for changes in thoughts, feelings, and behaviors during the initial stages of therapy.

Drug Interactions

Enhanced Anticholinergic Activity. The following drugs enhance the anticholinergic activity associated with tricyclic antidepressant therapy: antihistamines, phenothiazines, trihexyphenidyl, benztropine, and meperidine. The side effects are usually not severe enough to warrant discontinuing therapy, but stool softeners may be required.

Enhanced Sedative Activity. The following drugs enhance the sedative activity associated with tricyclic antidepressant therapy: ethanol, barbiturates, narcotics, tranquilizers, antihistamines, anesthetics, and sedative-hypnotics. Concurrent therapy is not recommended.

Barbiturates. Barbiturates may stimulate the metabolism of tricyclic antidepressants. Dosage adjustments of the antidepressant may be necessary.

Bupropion. Bupropion may increase serum levels of tricyclic antidepressants. Dosages may need to be reduced.

Carbamazepine. Tricyclic antidepressants can increase carbamazepine concentrations, resulting in signs of toxicity, such as vertigo, tremor, headache, drowsiness, nausea, and vomiting. The dosage of carbamazepine may need to be reduced. Carbamazepine may also reduce serum levels of tricyclic antidepressants. Dosages of the antidepressant may need to be increased.

Valproic Acid, Methylphenidate, Thyroid Hormones. These agents may increase serum levels of the tricyclic antidepressants. This reaction has been advantageous in attempts to gain a faster onset of antidepressant activity, but an increased incidence of dysrhythmias also has been reported.

Guanethidine, Clonidine. Tricyclic antidepressants inhibit the antihypertensive effects of these agents. Concurrent therapy is not recommended.

MAOIs. Severe reactions, including convulsions, hyperpyrexia, and death, have been reported with concurrent use. It is recommended that 2 weeks lapse between discontinuing an MAOI and starting tricyclic antidepressants.

Phenothiazines. Concurrent therapy may increase serum levels of both drugs, causing an increase in anticholinergic and sedative activity. Dosages of both agents may be reduced.

SSRIs. The interaction between SSRIs and tricyclic antidepressants is complex. The net result is that there is an increased toxicity from tricyclic antidepressants. Observe patients for signs of toxicity, such as dysrhythmias, seizure activity, and CNS stimulation.

Amphetamines, Tryptophan, Dextromethorphan, Ephedrine, Phenylpropanolamine, Pseudoephedrine, Epinephrine. All these agents increase serotonin levels, potentially causing serotonin syndrome when taken by a person receiving tricyclic antidepressants. These medicines should be used only under the supervision of a health care provider.

Sparfloxacin. Sparfloxacin inhibits the metabolism of tricyclic antidepressants, potentially causing life-threatening cardiac dysrhythmias. Sparfloxacin therapy should be avoided in patients receiving tricyclic antidepressants.

Cimetidine. Cimetidine inhibits the metabolism of tricyclic antidepressants. Patients should be closely monitored for additional anticholinergic symptoms. In general, cimetidine therapy should be avoided in these patients. Ranitidine and famotidine may be used without drug interactions.

Smoking. Smoking enhances the metabolism of tricyclic antidepressants. Dosages of the antidepressant may need to be increased for full therapeutic response.

DRUG CLASS: Miscellaneous Agents

bupropion hydrochloride (byoo pro′ pee on)
WELLBUTRIN (wel byoo′ trihn)

Actions

Bupropion is a monocyclic antidepressant chemically related to phenylethylamine antidepressants. Its mechanism of action is unknown. Compared with tricyclic antidepressants, it is a weak inhibitor of the reuptake and inactivation of the neurotransmitters serotonin, norepinephrine, and dopamine.

Uses

It is approved for use in patients unresponsive to tricyclic antidepressants and who cannot tolerate the adverse effects of tricyclic antidepressants. Disadvantages include seizure activity and the requirement of multiple doses daily. It must not be used in patients with psychotic disorders because its dopamine agonist activity causes increased psychotic symptoms.

Therapeutic Outcomes

The primary therapeutic outcomes expected from bupropion therapy are elevated mood and reduction of symptoms of depression.

Nursing Process for Bupropion Therapy

Premedication Assessment

1. Obtain baseline weight.
2. Perform Dyskinesia Identification System: Condensed Use Scale (DISCUS) or Abnormal Involuntary Movement Scale (AIMS) (see Appendixes G and H) at specified intervals to detect and/or check on EPS; record and report according to policy.

Planning

Availability. PO: 75 and 100 mg tablets; 100, 150, 200, and 300 mg sustained release tablets.

Implementation

Dosage and Administration. Adult: PO: Initially 100 mg twice daily. This may be increased to 100 mg three times daily (at least every 6 hours) after several days of therapy. No single dose of bupropion should exceed 150 mg; do not exceed 450 mg daily. Avoid a dose shortly before bedtime.

Observation. Symptoms of depression may improve within a few days (e.g., improved appetite, sleep, and psychomotor activity). The depression still exists, however, and it usually takes several weeks of the therapeutic doses before improvement is noted. Suicide precautions should be maintained during this time.

Evaluation

Side Effects to Expect

Gastrointestinal Effects. Most of these effects (anorexia, constipation, diarrhea, nausea and vomiting) may be minimized by temporary reduction in dosage, administration with food, and use of stool softeners for constipation.

Restlessness, Agitation, Anxiety, Insomnia. This usually occurs early in therapy and may require short-term treatment with sedative-hypnotic agents. Avoiding bedtime doses may also help decrease the incidence of insomnia.

Side Effects to Report

Seizures. See Nursing Assessments for Patients with Seizure Disorders (p. 298).

Suicidal Actions. Monitor the patient for changes in thoughts, feelings, and behaviors during the initial stages of therapy.

Drug Interactions

Carbamazepine, Cimetidine, Phenobarbital, Phenytoin. Bupropion may be an inducer of hepatic enzymes that may metabolize these agents more quickly. The dosage of these medications may need to be increased if taken concurrently with bupropion.

Carbamazepine. Carbamazepine may decrease bupropion serum levels, leading to decreased pharmacologic effect.

Nicotine Replacement. Coadministration with bupropion may cause hypertension. Monitor blood pressure when products such as nicotine patches or nicotine gum are being used.

Ritonavir. Ritonavir may cause large increases in serum concentrations of bupropion. Monitor patients for tachycardia, headaches, dizziness, agitation, nausea and vomiting, and dry mouth.

Levodopa. Bupropion has some mild dopaminergic activity and may cause an increase in adverse effects from levodopa. If bupropion is to be added to levodopa therapy, it should be initiated in small doses with small increases in the dosage of bupropion.

maprotiline hydrochloride (ma proe' ti leen)

Actions

Maprotiline was the first of the tetracyclic antidepressants to be released for clinical use. The mechanism of action is unknown, but pharmacologic response is similar to that with tricyclic antidepressants. It acts by enhancing norepinephrine and serotonin at nerve endings. The frequency and severity of anticholinergic effects, cardiac dysrhythmias, and orthostatic hypotension are reported to be lower with maprotiline when compared with the tricyclic antidepressants. There is a threefold higher incidence of seizure activity and delirium associated with maprotiline therapy.

Uses

Maprotiline is used in the treatment of depression and the depressive phase of bipolar disorder and for the relief of anxiety associated with depression.

Therapeutic Outcomes

The primary therapeutic outcomes expected from maprotiline therapy are elevated mood and reduction of symptoms of depression.

Nursing Process for Maprotiline Therapy

Premedication Assessment

1. Obtain baseline blood pressures in supine, sitting, and standing positions; record and report significant hypotension to the health care provider before administering drug.
2. Obtain baseline weight; schedule weekly weights.
3. Check for history of seizures. If present, notify health care provider before starting therapy.
4. Check hepatic studies before initiation and periodically throughout course of administration.
5. Perform DISCUS or AIMS at specified intervals to detect and/or check on EPS; record and report according to policy.

Planning

Availability. PO: 25, 50, and 75 mg tablets.

Implementation

Dosage and Administration. Adult: PO: Initially 75 mg daily. Because of the long half-life of maprotiline, maintain the initial dosage for 2 weeks. It may then be increased gradually in 25 mg increments, as required and tolerated. The usual maintenance dose is 150 mg daily. The maximum dose is 225 mg daily. Therapeutic blood levels are 50 to 200 ng/mL. An increase in the dosage should be made in the evening because increased sedation is often present.

Observation. Symptoms of depression may improve (e.g., improved appetite, sleep, and psychomotor activity) within a few days. The depression still exists, however, and it usually takes several weeks of therapeutic doses before improvement in the depression is noted. Suicide precautions should be maintained during this time.

Evaluation

See Tricyclic Antidepressants (p. 273).

mirtazepine (mer taz′ ah peen)
REMERON (rem′ er on)

Actions

Mirtazepine is a tetracyclic antidepressant that is a serotonin antagonist. The mechanism of action is unknown, but pharmacologic response is similar to that of tricyclic antidepressants.

Uses

Mirtazepine is used to treat depression.

Therapeutic Outcomes

The primary therapeutic outcomes expected from mirtazepine therapy are elevated mood and reduction of symptoms of depression.

Nursing Process for Mirtazepine Therapy

Premedication Assessment

1. Obtain baseline blood pressures in supine, sitting, and standing positions; record and report significant hypotension to the health care provider before administering drug.
2. Obtain baseline weight; schedule weekly weights.
3. Check for history of seizures. If present, notify the health care provider before starting therapy.
4. Check hepatic studies before initiation and periodically throughout course of administration.
5. Perform DISCUS or AIMS at specified intervals to detect and/or check on EPS; record and report according to policy.
6. Obtain a baseline and periodic white blood cell count because agranulocytosis has been reported.

Planning

Availability. PO: 15, 30, and 45 mg tablets and orally disintegrating tablets (Soltabs).

Implementation

Dosage and Administration. Adult: PO: Initially 15 mg daily. Every 1 to 2 weeks, the dosage may be increased up to a maximum of 45 mg daily. Increases in dosage should be made in the evening because increased sedation is often present.

Observation. Symptoms of depression may improve (e.g., improved appetite, sleep, and psychomotor activity) within a few days. The depression still exists, however, and it usually takes several weeks of therapeutic doses before improvement in the depression is noted. Suicide precautions should be maintained during this time.

Evaluation

See Tricyclic Antidepressants (p. 273).

nefazodone (nehf as′ oh doan)
SERZONE (sur′ zone)

Actions

Nefazodone is an antidepressant similar in chemical structure to trazodone. It inhibits serotonin and norepinephrine reuptake from the neuronal cleft prolonging its action. It also blocks serotonin-2 receptors. Its mechanism of action as an antidepressant is unknown.

Uses

Nefazodone is used to treat depression. This agent appears to have less anticholinergic, hypotensive, and sedative activity relative to the tricyclic antidepressants. A major disadvantage of nefazodone is the potential for life-threatening liver failure.

Therapeutic Outcomes

The primary therapeutic outcomes expected from nefazodone therapy are elevated mood and reduction of symptoms of depression.

Nursing Process for Nefazodone Therapy

Premedication Assessment

1. Obtain blood pressures in the supine, sitting, and standing positions; report significant lowering to the health care provider before administering the medicine.
2. Obtain heart rate before and at regular intervals following initiation of therapy. An ECG may be required for baseline information before starting therapy. Report significant lowering in blood pressure

to the health care provider before administering the medicine.
3. Note any GI symptoms present before start of therapy.
4. Monitor CNS symptoms present (e.g., insomnia or nervousness).
5. Check hepatic studies before initiation and periodically throughout the course of administration.

Planning

Availability. PO: 50, 100, 150, 200, and 250 mg tablets.

Implementation

Dosage and Administration. Adult: PO: Initially 100 mg two times daily. At no less than weekly intervals, increase the dosage by 100 to 200 mg, again on a twice-daily schedule as tolerated. Several weeks of adjustment may be required for optimization of therapy. The normal dose range is 300 to 600 mg daily.

Observation. Symptoms of depression (e.g., improved appetite, sleep, and psychomotor activity) may improve within a few days. The depression still exists, however, and it usually takes several weeks of therapeutic doses before improvement is noted. Suicide precautions should be maintained during this time.

Evaluation

Side Effects to Expect

Drowsiness, Sedation. Nefazodone has mild to moderate sedating effects. These symptoms tend to disappear with continued therapy and possible readjustment of the dosage.

Inform the patient of possible sedative effects. The patient should use caution while driving or performing other tasks that require alertness. Consult with the health care provider to consider moving the daily dose to bedtime if sedation continues to be a problem.

Blurred Vision; Constipation; Urinary Retention; Dryness of Mucosa of the Mouth, Throat, and Nose. These symptoms are the anticholinergic effects produced by these agents. Patients taking these medications should be monitored for these side effects.

Dryness of the mucosa may be relieved by sucking hard candy or ice chips or by chewing gum.

The use of stool softeners such as docusate or the occasional use of a stimulant laxative such as bisacodyl may be required for constipation.

Caution the patient that blurred vision may occur, and make appropriate suggestions for personal safety of the individual.

Orthostatic Hypotension. Nefazodone may cause some degree of orthostatic hypotension manifested by dizziness and weakness, particularly when therapy is initiated. Monitor the blood pressure daily in both the supine and standing positions.

Anticipate the development of postural hypotension and take measures to prevent an occurrence. Teach the patient to rise slowly from a supine or sitting position; encourage the patient to sit or lie down if feeling faint.

Sedative Effects. Tell the patient of sedative effects, especially during the onset of therapy. Single doses at bedtime may diminish or relieve the sedative effects.

Side Effects to Report

Hepatotoxicity. The symptoms of hepatotoxicity are anorexia, nausea, vomiting, jaundice, hepatomegaly, splenomegaly, and abnormal liver function tests (e.g., elevated bilirubin, aspartate aminotransferase [AST], alanine aminotransferase [ALT], gamma-glutamyltransferase [GGT], alkaline phosphatase, prothrombin time).

Bradycardia. Monitor heart rate as therapy is initiated and dosing is adjusted. Bradycardias with a drop in 15 beats per minute and rates below 50 beats per minute have been reported. Notify the health care provider immediately. Withhold the next dose until specifically approved.

Suicidal Actions. Monitor the patient for changes in thoughts, feelings, and behaviors during the initial stages of therapy.

Drug Interactions

MAOIs. Severe reactions including excitement, diaphoresis, rigidity, convulsions, hyperpyrexia, and death have been reported with concurrent use of MAOIs and nefazodone. It is recommended that at least 14 days lapse between discontinuing an MAOI and starting nefazodone. It is further recommended that there be a 1-week drug-free interval between discontinuing nefazodone and starting MAOI therapy.

Haloperidol. Nefazodone inhibits the metabolism of haloperidol. It does not apparently increase the serum levels but does prolong the action of haloperidol. Doses may have to be given less often to prevent potential toxicity.

Carbamazepine. Nefazodone inhibits the metabolism of carbamazepine. Monitor for signs of toxicity: disorientation, ataxia, lethargy, headache, drowsiness, nausea, and vomiting.

Alprazolam, Triazolam. Nefazodone significantly increases serum levels of these benzodiazepines. Monitor closely for excessive sedation and impaired motor skills.

Digoxin. Nefazodone significantly increases serum levels of digoxin. Monitor serum levels and signs of toxicity (e.g., dysrhythmias, bradycardia).

St. John's Wort. Increased sedative-hypnotic effects may occur.

Sibutramine, Trazodone. When sibutramine or trazodone is used in conjunction with nefazodone, a serotonin syndrome may develop, with symptoms of irritability, increased muscle tone, shivering, myoclonus, and reduced consciousness.

Cisapride. Nefazodone may significantly increase the serum concentrations of cisapride, causing potentially fatal cardiac toxicities.

Herbal Interactions

St. John's Wort

St. John's wort may increase toxic effects of antidepressant medicines. Use of St. John's wort with other antidepressants should be done only with close supervision of a health care provider.

trazodone hydrochloride (tray′ zoh doan)
DESYREL (dez′ er el)

Actions

Trazodone was the first of the triazolopyridine antidepressants to be released for clinical use. The triazolopyridines are chemically unrelated to the other classes of antidepressants. The exact mechanisms of action of trazodone are unknown. The actions are complex and in some ways resemble those of the tricyclic antidepressants, benzodiazepines, and phenothiazines; however, the overall activity of trazodone is different from that of each of these classes of drugs.

Uses

Trazodone has been shown to be as effective in treating depression; depression associated with schizophrenia; and depression, tremor, and anxiety associated with alcohol dependence. Compared with other antidepressants, it has a low incidence of anticholinergic side effects, which makes trazodone particularly useful in patients whose antidepressant doses are limited by anticholinergic side effects and in patients with severe angle-closure glaucoma, prostatic hyperplasia, organic mental disorders, and cardiac dysrhythmias. Trazodone is commonly used to treat insomnia in patients with substance abuse because it is very sedating, improves sleep continuity, and the potential for tolerance and addiction is very minimal.

Therapeutic Outcomes

The primary therapeutic outcome expected from trazodone therapy is elevated mood and reduction of symptoms of depression.

Nursing Process for Trazodone Therapy

Premedication Assessment

1. Obtain baseline blood pressures in supine, sitting, and standing positions.
2. Record and report significant hypotension to health care provider before administering drug.

Planning

Availability. PO: 50, 100, 150, and 300 mg tablets.

Implementation

Dosage and Administration. *Adult:* PO: Initially 150 mg in three divided doses. Increase in increments of 50 mg daily every 3 to 4 days while monitoring clinical response. Do not exceed 400 mg daily in outpatients or 600 mg daily in hospitalized patients.

Dosage should be initiated at a low level and increased gradually, particularly in older adult, or debilitated patients. Dosage increases should be made in the evening because increased sedation is often present. Administer medication shortly after a meal or with a light snack to reduce adverse effects.

Observation. Symptoms of depression may improve (e.g., improved appetite, sleep, and psychomotor activity) within a few days. The depression still exists, however, and it usually requires several weeks of therapeutic doses before improvement is noted. Suicide precautions should be maintained during this time.

Evaluation

Side Effects to Expect and Report

Confusion. Perform a baseline assessment of the patient's degree of alertness and orientation to name, place, and time before starting therapy. Make regularly scheduled subsequent evaluations of mental status, and compare findings. Report alterations.

Dizziness, Lightheadedness. Provide patient safety during episodes of dizziness; report for further evaluation.

Drowsiness. People who work with machinery, drive a car, administer medicines, or perform other duties in which they must remain mentally alert should not take these medications while working.

Orthostatic Hypotension. Although episodes are infrequent and generally mild, trazodone may cause some degree of orthostatic hypotension manifested by dizziness and weakness, particularly when therapy is initiated. Monitor blood pressure daily in both the supine and standing positions.

Anticipate the development of postural hypotension and take measures to prevent an occurrence. Teach the patient to rise slowly from a supine or sitting position; encourage the patient to sit or lie down if feeling faint.

Dysrhythmias, Tachycardia. Report for further evaluation.

Drug Interactions

Enhanced Sedative Activity. The following drugs enhance the sedative effects associated with trazodone therapy: ethanol, barbiturates, narcotics, tranquilizers, antihistamines, anesthetics, phenothiazines, and sedative-hypnotics. Concurrent therapy is not recommended.

Nefazodone, Venlafaxine, MAOIs, SSRIs. When trazodone is used in conjunction with any of these agents, a serotonin syndrome may develop, with symptoms of irritability, increased muscle tone, shivering, myoclonus, and reduced consciousness. Use cautiously, initiating therapy at lower doses, with close monitoring for adverse effects listed.

venlafaxine (vehn lah fax′ een)

EFFEXOR (eef ex′ ohr)

Actions

Venlafaxine is a phenethylamine derivative antidepressant structurally related to bupropion. Although its antidepressant action is unknown, it is a potent inhibitor of reuptake of serotonin and norepinephrine and a weak inhibitor of dopamine reuptake in the neuronal cleft.

Uses

Venlafaxine is approved for use in patients for the treatment of depression and generalized anxiety disorder. The FDA has recommended that venlafaxine not be administered to patients younger than 18 years of age.

Therapeutic Outcomes

The primary therapeutic outcome expected from venlafaxine therapy is elevated mood and reduction of symptoms of depression and anxiety.

Nursing Process for Venlafaxine Therapy

Premedication Assessment

1. Obtain baseline weight and blood pressure.
2. Note any GI symptoms before starting therapy.
3. Monitor CNS symptoms, such as insomnia or nervousness.
4. Report any history of hypertension, substance abuse, or renal or hepatic disease to the health care provider.

Planning

Availability. PO: 25, 37.5, 50, 75, and 100 mg tablets; 37.5, 75, and 150 mg sustained release capsules.

Implementation

Dosage and Administration. *Adult:* PO: 75 mg daily, taken with food in two or three doses. Dosages may be increased by 75 mg daily at intervals greater than every 4 days. The maximum recommended dose is 375 mg daily, generally in three divided doses.

Discontinuation of Therapy. If the patient has taken the medicine for more than 1 week, the dosage should be tapered over the next few days. If venlafaxine has been taken for longer than 6 weeks, the dosage should gradually be tapered over the next 2 weeks.

Observation. Symptoms of depression may improve within a few days (e.g., improved appetite, sleep, and psychomotor activity). The depression still exists, however, and it usually requires several weeks of therapeutic doses before improvement is noted. Suicide precautions should be maintained during this time.

Evaluation

Side Effects to Expect

Dizziness, Drowsiness. People should be warned not to work with machinery, drive a car, administer medication, or perform other duties in which mental alertness is required until they are sure that these side effects do not impair judgment.

Nausea, Anorexia. Most of these effects may be minimized by temporary reduction in dosage and administration with food.

Restlessness, Agitation, Anxiety, Insomnia. This usually occurs early in therapy, and the patient may require short-term treatment with sedative-hypnotic agents. Avoiding bedtime doses may help decrease the incidence of insomnia.

Side Effects to Report

Suicidal Actions. Monitor the patient for changes in thoughts, feelings, and behaviors during the initial stages of therapy.

Drug Interactions

MAOIs. Severe reactions including excitement, diaphoresis, rigidity, convulsions, hyperpyrexia, and death have been reported with concurrent use of MAOIs and venlafaxine. It is recommended that at least 14 days lapse between discontinuing an MAOI and starting venlafaxine therapy, and vice versa.

Cimetidine. Cimetidine inhibits the metabolism of venlafaxine. Patients should be closely monitored for excessive effects of venlafaxine when cimetidine is added to the therapeutic regimen.

Trazodone. When trazodone is used in conjunction with venlafaxine, a "serotonin syndrome" may develop, with symptoms of irritability, increased muscle tone, shivering, myoclonus, and reduced consciousness.

Haloperidol. Venlafaxine increases haloperidol levels and increases the frequency of EPS. If used concurrently, the dosage of haloperidol may need to be decreased.

DRUG CLASS: Antimanic Agents

lithium carbonate (lith′ ee um)

ESKALITH (esk′ ah lith), LITHANE (lith′ ane)

Actions

Lithium is a monovalent cation that competes with other monovalent and divalent cations (i.e., potassium, sodium, calcium, magnesium) at cellular binding sites that are sensitive to changes in cation concentration. Lithium replaces intracellular and intraneuronal sodium, stabilizing the neuronal membrane. It also reduces the release of norepinephrine and increases the uptake of tryptophan, the precursor to serotonin. It also interacts with second-messenger cellular processes to inhibit intracellular concentrations of cyclic adenosine monophosphate. Because of the complexity of the CNS, the exact mechanisms of action of lithium in treating mood disorders are unknown. It has no sedative, depressant, or euphoric properties, differentiating it from all other psychotropic agents.

Uses

Lithium is used to treat acute mania and for the prophylaxis of recurrent manic and depressive episodes in bipolar disorder. In patients with bipolar disorder it is more effective in preventing signs and symptoms of mania than those of depression. It is also effective in some patients in reducing the recurrence of depressive episodes in unipolar disorder.

Therapeutic Outcome

The primary therapeutic outcome expected from lithium therapy is maintaining the individual at an optimal level of functioning with minimal exacerbations of mood swings.

Nursing Process for Lithium Therapy

Premedication Assessment

1. Before initiating lithium therapy, the following laboratory tests should be completed for baseline information: electrolytes, fasting blood glucose, blood urea nitrogen (BUN), serum creatinine, creatinine clearance, urinalysis, and thyroid function tests.
2. Obtain baseline blood pressures in supine, sitting, and standing positions; record and report significant hypotension to the health care provider before administering drug.
3. Weigh daily; check hydration of patient (e.g., moistness of mucous membranes, skin turgor, and firmness of eyeball); monitor urine specific gravity.
4. Lithium may enhance sodium depletion, which enhances lithium toxicity. Assess for early signs of lithium toxicity before giving medication, including nausea, vomiting, abdominal pain, diarrhea, lethargy, speech difficulty, mild dizziness, muscle twitching, and tremor.

Planning

Availability. PO: 150, 300, and 600 mg capsules and tablets; 300 and 450 mg slow-release tablets; and 300 mg/ 5 mL syrup.

Serum Lithium Levels. Levels are monitored once or twice weekly during initiation of therapy and monthly while on a maintenance dosage. Blood should be drawn approximately 12 hours after the last dose was administered. The normal serum level is 0.4 to 1.5 mEq/L. Report serum levels greater than these values to the health care provider promptly.

Good Nutrition. Lithium may enhance sodium depletion, which enhances lithium toxicity. It is important that patients maintain a normal dietary intake of sodium with adequate maintenance fluids (10 to 12, 8-ounce glasses of water daily), especially when initiating therapy, to prevent toxicity.

Implementation

Dosage and Administration. *Adult:* PO: 300 to 600 mg three or four times daily. Administer with food or milk. Adequate diet is important to maintain normal serum sodium levels and prevent toxicity. Onset of the acute antimanic effect of lithium usually occurs within 5 to 7 days; full therapeutic effect often requires 10 to 21 days.

Evaluation

Side Effects to Expect

Nausea, Vomiting, Anorexia, Abdominal Cramps. These side effects are usually mild and tend to resolve with continued therapy. Encourage the patient not to discontinue therapy without first consulting the health care provider.

If gastric irritation occurs, administer medication with food or milk. If symptoms persist or increase in severity, report for health care provider evaluation. These may also be early signs of toxicity.

Excessive Thirst and Urination, Fine Hand Tremor. These side effects are usually mild and tend to resolve within a week with continued therapy. Encourage the patient not to discontinue therapy without first consulting the health care provider. If these symptoms persist or become severe, the patient should consult the health care provider.

Side Effects to Report

Persistent Vomiting, Profuse Diarrhea, Hyperreflexia, Lethargy, Weakness. These are all signs of impending serious toxicity. Report immediately, and do not administer the next dose until reconfirmed by the health care provider.

Progressive Fatigue, Weight Gain. These may be early signs of hypothyroidism. Report for further evaluation.

Pruritus, Ankle Edema, Metallic Taste, Hyperglycemia. These are all rare side effects from lithium therapy. Report for further evaluation.

Nephrotoxicity. Monitor urinalysis and kidney function tests for abnormal results. Report an increasing BUN and creatinine, increasing or decreasing urine output or decreasing specific gravity (despite amount of fluid intake), and casts or protein in the urine.

Drug Interactions

Reduced Serum Sodium Levels. Therapeutic activity and toxicity of lithium are highly dependent on sodium concentrations. Decreased sodium levels significantly enhance the toxicity of lithium and high sodium levels result in low lithium levels.

Patients who are to begin diuretic therapy, a low-sodium diet, or activities that produce excessive and prolonged sweating should be observed particularly closely.

Methyldopa. Monitor patients on concurrent, long-term therapy for signs (nausea, vomiting, abdominal pain, diarrhea, lethargy, speech difficulty, mild dizziness, and tremor) of the development of lithium toxicity.

Indomethacin, Piroxicam. Indomethacin and piroxicam reduce the renal excretion of lithium, allowing it to accumulate to potentially toxic levels.

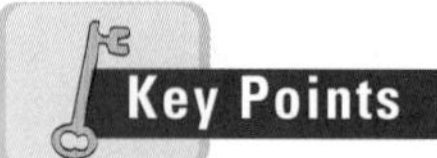

Key Points

- Mood disorders (affective disorders) are present when certain symptoms impair the person's ability to function for a period. At least 10% of people in the United States will suffer from a diagnosable mood disorder in their lifetime.
- Mood disorders are divided into depressive (unipolar) and bipolar disorders.
- Treatment of mood disorders requires both nonpharmacologic and pharmacologic therapy. Simultaneous psychotherapy and pharmacologic treatment has been shown to be more successful than either treatment alone.
- Antidepressant medications act on a variety of receptors both in the CNS and in the peripheral tissues and are associated with many side effects and drug interactions. It is a responsibility of the nurse to educate patients about therapy and monitoring for therapeutic benefit and side effects to expect and report, as well as intervene whenever possible to optimize therapeutic outcomes.

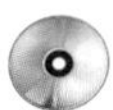

Go to your Companion CD-ROM for appendices, an Audio Glossary, animations, Drug Dosage Calculators, customizable Patient Self-Assessment forms, and Review Questions for the NCLEX® Examination.

evolve Be sure to visit the companion Evolve site at http://evolve.elsevier.com/Clayton for WebLinks and additional online resources.

MEDICATION SAFETY REVIEW

MATH REVIEW QUESTIONS

1. Order: Lithium carbonate 300 mg PO, twice daily
   Available: Lithium carbonate 150 mg tablets
   Give: ____ tablets
2. Order: Maprotiline 100 mg this AM
   Available: None found in medication container; consult drug monograph for dosage availability.
   What strength tablets would most likely be dispensed, and how would you administer the dose?

CRITICAL THINKING QUESTIONS

1. During her clinic visit, a patient complains to the nurse that since she started taking amitriptyline (Elavil) for depression, she has had a "terrible dry mouth," and she feels "sleepy all the time." What additional information would you elicit? What interventions to alleviate these symptoms could be suggested?
2. The next patient at the clinic is taking fluoxetine (Prozac). He is 5′ 6″ tall, weighs 120 lb, and has been receiving the medication for 6 weeks. He reports that he feels like a "cloud has been lifted from my mind." What additional data would be appropriate to collect during this visit?
3. When a patient is starting therapy with an MAOI, what health teaching is important?
4. When looking at the drug monograph for MAOI therapy, it states that one major potential complication of this therapy is a hypertensive crisis. Discuss what this is, how to recognize it, and the interventions that should be anticipated if it occurs.
5. Discuss the behavioral monitoring sheets used in clinical settings to assess for the development of EPS. How often are the assessments made, how are they recorded, and when is the health care provider notified of changes in the patient's behavior?
6. Review drug monographs to identify medications that are affected by smoking.
7. Access a website listed at end of chapter to research a topic related to mood disorders.
8. Cite four reasons given for depression to be undertreated or not treated.
9. Why should dosage increases of maprotiline be initiated in the evening hours?

Clinical Case: A 34-year-old patient is being treated for bipolar disorder with lithium 300 mg PO four times daily. She is being seen today in the clinic. During the intake interview she tells the nurse that her medicine "never works." Further exploration reveals that she has not taken the medication for the past 4 days.

CRITICAL THINKING QUESTIONS—cont'd

10. As the nurse in this situation, how would you proceed?

11. When reviewing the patient's history, the nurse reads that her lithium level taken the month before was 2 mEq/L. What symptoms might be seen with this lithium level?

12. The history also notes that the importance of adequate intake of water and sodium was discussed with the patient. How does the sodium level within the body influence the metabolism of lithium?

CONTENT REVIEW QUESTIONS

1. Fluoxetine (Sarafem), an SSRI used for mood disorders, is also approved for treatment of:
   1. hallucinations associated with psychosis.
   2. EPS.
   3. premenstrual dysphoric disorder (PMDD).
   4. neuroleptic malignant syndrome.

2. A patient taking an MAOI needs to be monitored for:
   1. blood dyscrasias.
   2. hyperglycemia.
   3. hypertension.
   4. hyperactivity.

3. Bupropion hydrochloride (Wellbutrin) may cause hypertension when combined with:
   1. nicotine.
   2. levodopa.
   3. anticholinergics.
   4. lithium carbonate.

4. A severe reaction can occur between SSRIs and which of the following?
   1. MAOIs
   2. Birth control pills
   3. Beta blockers
   4. Antihistamines

5. Patients who are being treated for depression should continually be monitored for thoughts of suicide. Which of the following behaviors would indicate suicidal behavior?
   1. Excessive appetite
   2. Poor hygiene
   3. Comments such as "things would be better at death"
   4. Sleeping throughout the day

CHAPTER

18 Drugs Used for Psychoses

evolve http://evolve.elsevier.com/Clayton

Chapter Content

Objectives

1. Identify signs and symptoms of psychotic behavior.
2. Describe major indications for the use of antipsychotic agents.
3. Identify common adverse effects observed with antipsychotic medications.
4. Develop a teaching plan for a patient taking haloperidol and one receiving clozapine.

Key Terms

psychosis
delusion
hallucinations
disorganized thinking
loosening of associations
disorganized behavior
changes in affect
target symptoms
typical (first generation) antipsychotic agents
atypical (second generation) antipsychotic agents
equipotent doses
extrapyramidal symptoms (EPS)
dystonia
pseudoparkinsonian symptoms
akathisia
tardive dyskinesia
abnormal involuntary movement scale
dyskinesia identification system: condensed user scale
neuroleptic malignant syndrome
depot antipsychotic medicine

PSYCHOSIS

Psychosis (si ko′ sis) does not have a single definition but is a clinical descriptor that means being out of touch with reality. Psychotic symptoms can be associated with many illnesses including dementias and delirium that may have metabolic, infectious, or endocrinologic causes. Psychotic symptoms are also common in mood disorders such as major depression and bipolar disorder. Psychosis can also be caused by many drugs (e.g., phencyclidine, opiates, amphetamines, cocaine, hallucinogens, anticholinergic agents, and alcohol). Psychotic disorders are characterized by loss of reality, perceptual deficits such as hallucinations and delusions, and deterioration in social functioning. Of the several psychotic disorders defined by the American Psychiatric Association in the *Diagnostic and Statistical Manual of Mental Disorders, 4th Edition, Text Revised (DSM-IVR)*, schizophrenia is the most common.

Psychotic disorders are extremely complex illnesses that are influenced by biologic, psychosocial, and environmental circumstances. Some of the disorders require several months of observation and testing before a final diagnosis can be determined. It is beyond the scope of this text to discuss psychotic disorders in detail, but general types of symptoms associated with psychotic disorders are described as follows.

A **delusion** (del ooh′ shun) is a false or irrational belief that is firmly held despite obvious evidence to the contrary. Delusions may be persecutory, grandiose, religious, sexual, or hypochondriac. Delusions of reference, in which the patient attributes a special, irrational, and usually negative significance to other people, objects, or events such as song lyrics or newspaper articles in relation to self are common. Delusions may be defined as "bizarre" if they are clearly irrational and do not derive from ordinary life experiences. A common bizarre delusion is the patient's belief that the thinking process, parts of the body, or actions or impulses are controlled or dictated by some external force.

Hallucinations (hal ooh sin a′ shuns) are false sensory perceptions that are experienced without an external stimulus but that nevertheless seem real to the patient. Auditory hallucinations, experienced as "voices" characteristically heard that are commenting negatively about the patient in the third person, are prominent in schizophrenia. Hallucinations of touch, sight, taste, smell, and bodily sensation also occur.

Disorganized thinking is commonly associated with psychoses. The thought disorders may consist of a **loosening of associations** so that the speaker jumps from one idea or topic to another unrelated one (derailment) in an illogic, inappropriate, or disorganized way. Answers to questions may be obliquely related or completely unrelated (tangentiality). At its most serious, this incoherence of thought extends into pronunciation itself, and the speaker's words become garbled or unrecognizable. Speech may also be overly concrete (loss of ability to think in abstract terms) and inexpressive; it may be repetitive, or although vociferous, it may convey little or no real information.

Disorganized behavior is another common characteristic of psychosis. Problems may be noted in any form of goal-directed behavior, leading to difficulties in performing activities of daily living (ADLs) such as organizing meals or maintaining hygiene. The patient may appear markedly disheveled, may dress in an unusual manner (e.g., wearing several layers of clothing, scarves, and gloves on a hot day), or may display clearly inappropriate sexual behavior (e.g., public masturbation) or unpredictable, nontriggered agitation (e.g., shouting or swearing). Disorganized behavior must be distinguished from behavior that is merely aimless or generally not purposeful and from organized behavior that is motivated by delusional beliefs.

Changes in affect may also be a symptom of psychosis. Emotional expressiveness is diminished; there is poor eye contact and reduced spontaneous movement. Patients appear to be withdrawn from others; the face appears immobile and unresponsive. Speech is often minimal with only brief, slow, monotone replies to questions. There is a withdrawal from areas of functioning in interpersonal relationships, work, education, and self-care.

TREATMENT OF PSYCHOSIS

The importance of initial assessment for accurate diagnosis cannot be underestimated in a patient with acute psychosis. A thorough physical and neurologic examination, mental status examination, complete family and social history, and laboratory workup must be performed to exclude other causes of psychoses, such as substance abuse. Both drug and nondrug therapies are critical to the treatment of most psychoses. Long-term outcome is improved in patients with an integrated drug and nondrug treatment regimen. Nonpharmacologic interventions such as individual psychotherapy to improve insight into the illness and assist the patient in coping with stress, group therapy to enhance socialization skills, behavioral or cognitive therapy, and vocational training are beneficial to patients.

Before initiation of therapy, the treatment goals and baseline level of functioning must be established and documented. Target symptoms must also be identified and documented. Target symptoms are critical monitoring parameters that are used to assess change in clinical status and response to medications. Examples of target symptoms include frequency and type of agitation, degree of suspiciousness, delusions, hallucinations, loose associations, grooming habits and hygiene, sleep patterns, speech patterns, social skills, and judgment. The ultimate goal is to restore behavioral, cognitive, and psychosocial processes and skills to as close to baseline levels as possible so that the patient is reintegrated into the community. Realistically, unless the psychosis is part of another medical diagnosis such as substance abuse, most patients will have recurring symptoms of the mental disorder most of their lives. Treatment is therefore focused at decreased severity of the target symptoms that most interfere with functioning. A variety of scales have been developed over recent years to assist in objective measurement of change in target symptoms due to psychotherapy and pharmacotherapy. These include the Brief Psychiatric Rating Scale (BPRS), the Positive and Negative Syndrome Scale for Schizophrenia (PANSS), the Clinical Global Impression (CGI) scale, and the Rating of Aggression Against People and/or Property (RAAPP) scale.

DRUG THERAPY FOR PSYCHOSIS

Pharmacologic treatment of psychosis is accomplished with several classes of drugs. The most specific are the first- and second-generation antipsychotic agents, but benzodiazepines (see p. 224) are often used for control of acute psychotic symptoms. The beta adrenergic–blocking agents (propranolol) (see p. 212), lithium (see p. 280), anticonvulsants (valproic acid, carbamazepine) (see p. 305), antiparkinsonian agents (see p. 232), and anticholinergic agents (see p. 215) occasionally play a role in controlling adverse effects of antipsychotic therapy.

Antipsychotic, also known as neuroleptic, agents can be classified in several ways. Traditionally they have been divided into phenothiazines and nonphenothiazines. Antipsychotic agents can also be classified as low-potency or high-potency drugs. *Low* and *high potency* refers only to the milligram doses used for these medicines and does not suggest any difference in effectiveness (e.g., 100 mg of chlorpromazine, a low-potency agent, is equivalent in antipsychotic activity to 2 mg of haloperidol, a high-potency agent). Chlorpromazine and thioridazine are low-potency agents, whereas trifluoperazine, fluphenazine, thiothixene, haloperidol, loxapine, and molindone are high-potency agents. Since 1990, antipsychotic agents have also been classified as typical, **or first-generation** or atypical, **or second-generation** antipsychotic agents, based on mechanism of action (Table 18-1). The atypical antipsychotic agents are aripiprazole, clozapine, olanzapine, quetiapine, risperidone, and ziprasidone. All of the remaining antipsychotic agents in Table 18-1 are typical antipsychotic agents.

Actions

The typical antipsychotic agents antagonize the neurotransmitter dopamine in the central nervous system (CNS). The atypical antipsychotic agents inhibit dopamine receptors, but also inhibit serotonin receptors to varying degrees. However, the exact mechanism by which these actions prevent psychotic symptoms is unknown. There is substantially more to the development of psychotic symptoms than elevated dopamine levels. There are at least five known types of dopamine receptors and several more types of serotonin receptors in various areas of the CNS. Antipsychotic agents also stimulate or block cholinergic, histaminic, nicotinic, and alpha and beta adrenergic neurotransmitter receptors to varying degrees, accounting for many of the adverse effects of therapy.

Uses

All antipsychotic agents are equal in efficacy when used in equipotent doses. There is some unpredictable variation between patients, however, and individual patients sometimes show a better response to particular drugs. In general, selection of medication should be based on the need to avoid certain side effects in concurrent medical or psychiatric disorders. Despite practice trends, no proof exists that agitation responds best to sedating drugs or that withdrawn patients respond best to nonsedating drugs. Medication history should be a major factor in drug selection. The final important factors in drug selection are the clinically important differences in frequency of adverse effects. No single drug is least likely to cause all adverse effects; thus individual response should be the best determinant of which drug is to be used. The atypical antipsychotic agents tend to be more effective in relieving negative and cognitive symptoms associated with schizophrenia, are more effective in refractory schizophrenia, and have a much lower incidence of extrapyramidal symptoms and hyperprolactinemia.

The initial goal of antipsychotic therapy is both to calm the agitated patient who may be a physical threat to self or others and to begin treatment of the psychosis and thought disorder. Combined therapy with

Drug Table 18-1 ANTIPSYCHOTIC AGENTS

GENERIC NAME	BRAND NAME	AVAILABILITY	ADULT DOSAGE RANGE (mg)	MAJOR SIDE EFFECTS			
				SEDATION	EPS*	HYPOTENSION	ACE†
TYPICAL (FIRST-GENERATION) ANTIPSYCHOTIC AGENTS							
Phenothiazines							
chlorpromazine	Thorazine, ✱ Largactil	Tablets: 10, 25, 50, 100, 200 mg Syrup: 100 mg/mL Injection: 25 mg/mL Suppository: 100 mg	30-1000	+++	++	+++	++
fluphenazine	Prolixin, ✱ Moditen	Tablets: 1, 2.5, 5, 10 mg Elixir: 2.5 mg/5 mL Injection: 2.5, 25 mg/mL	0.5-20	+	+++	+	+
perphenazine		Tablets: 2, 4, 8, 16 mg Concentrate: 16 mg/5 mL	12-64	+	+++	+	++
prochlorperazine	Compazine, ✱ Stemetil	Tablets: 5, 10, 25 mg Sustained release capsules: 30 mg Syrup: 5 mg/mL Injection: 5 mg/mL Suppository: 2.5, 5, 25 mg	15-150	+	+++	+	+
thioridazine		Tablets: 10, 15, 25, 50, 100, 150, 200 mg	150-800	+++	+	++	++
trifluoperazine		Tablets: 1, 2, 5, 10 mg	2-40	+	+++	+	+
Thioxanthenes							
thiothixene	Navane	Capsules: 1, 2, 5, 10, 20 mg	6-60	+	+++	+	+
Nonphenothiazines							
haloperidol	Haldol, ✱ Novo-Peridol	Tablets: 0.5, 1, 2, 5, 10, 20 mg Concentrate: 2 mg/mL	1-15	+	+++	+	+
loxapine	Loxitane, ✱ Loxapac	Capsules: 5, 10, 25, 50 mg	20-250	++	+++	++	+
molindone	Moban	Tablets: 5, 10, 25, 50 mg	15-225	++	++	++	+

+, low; ++, moderate; +++, high; ACE, anticholinergic effects; EPS, extrapyramidal symptoms.
✱ Available in Canada.

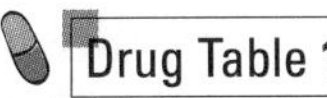

Drug Table 18-1 **ANTIPSYCHOTIC AGENTS—cont'd**

GENERIC NAME	BRAND NAME	AVAILABILITY	ADULT DOSAGE RANGE (mg)	MAJOR SIDE EFFECTS			
				SEDATION	EPS*	HYPOTENSION	ACE†
ATYPICAL (SECOND-GENERATION) ANTIPSYCHOTIC AGENTS							
aripiprazole	Abilify	Tablets: 5, 10, 15, 20, 30 mg	10-15	+	+	+	0
clozapine	Clozaril	Tablets: 12.5, 25, 100 mg Tablets, orally disintegrating: 25, 100 mg	300-900	+++	+	+++	++
olanzapine	Zyprexa	Tablets: 2.5, 5, 7.5, 10, 15, 20 mg Tablets, orally disintegrating: 5, 10, 15, 20, mg Injection: 10 mg	10-15	+++	+	++	+++
quetiapine	Seroquel	Tablets: 25, 100, 200, 300 mg	50-800	++	+	++	0
risperidone	Risperdal	Tablets: 0.25, 0.5, 1, 2, 3, 4 mg Tablets, orally disintegrating: 0.5, 1, 2, mg Solution: 1 mg/mL Injection: 25, 37.5, 50 mg	4-16	+	+	+	0
ziprasidone	Geodon	Capsules: 20, 40, 60 mg Injection: 20 mg	100-160	+	++	+	0

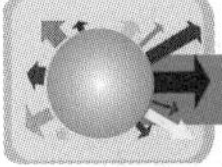

Clinical Landmine

During episodes of acute psychosis, the patient is out of touch with reality and often does not understand the need to take medicines that will help to stabilize the condition. The nurse must ensure that the patient has actually swallowed the medication when administered and not just "mouthed" or "cheeked" it. Outpatients often require supervision of medication administration to ensure adherence to the medication regimen. In some instances it is necessary to use injection of long-acting medicines to overcome the nonadherence problem in selected patients with psychotic symptoms.

benzodiazepines (often lorazepam) and antipsychotic agents allows lower doses of the antipsychotic agent to be used, reducing the risk of serious adverse effects more commonly seen with higher-dose therapy. Some therapeutic effects, such as reduced psychomotor agitation and insomnia, are observed within 1 week of therapy, but reductions in hallucinations, delusions, and thought disorder often require 6 to 8 weeks for full therapeutic effect. Rapid increases in the dosing of antipsychotic medicines will not reduce the antipsychotic response time. Patients, families, and the health care team must be educated to give antipsychotic agents an adequate chance to work before unnecessarily escalating the dosing and increasing the risk of adverse effects.

After an acute psychotic episode has resolved and the patient is free from overt psychotic symptoms, a decision must be made as to whether maintenance therapy is necessary. This will depend on the diagnosed psychotic disorder and the patient's tolerance of the adverse effects of the medicine. However, most psychotic disorders are treated with lower maintenance doses to minimize the risk of recurrence of the disorder (Box 18-1).

Box 18-1 ***Antipsychotic Medicines***

Patients beginning antipsychotic drug therapy can expect some therapeutic effect such as reduced psychomotor agitation and insomnia within 1 week of starting, but reduction in hallucinations, delusions, and thought disorders often requires 6 to 8 weeks for a full therapeutic response to be achieved. Rapid increases in dosages of antipsychotic medication will not reduce the antipsychotic response time but will increase the frequency of adverse effects.

Antipsychotic medicines may produce extrapyramidal effects. Tardive dyskinesia may be reversible in the early stages, but it becomes irreversible with continued use of the antipsychotic medication. Regular assessment for tardive dyskinesia should be completed for all patients receiving antipsychotic agents. Older adult patients should be observed for hypotension and tardive dyskinesia.

ADVERSE EFFECTS OF ANTIPSYCHOTIC DRUG THERAPY

Extrapyramidal Effects

Many of the serious adverse effects of antipsychotic agents can be attributed to the pharmacologic effect of blocking dopaminergic, cholinergic, histaminic, serotonergic, and adrenergic neurotransmitter receptors. Whereas these agents block D_2 receptors in the mesolimbic area of the brain to stop psychotic symptoms, blockade of the D_2 receptors in other areas of the brain explains the occurrence of extrapyramidal effects.

Extrapyramidal effects are the most troublesome side effects and the most common cause of nonadherence associated with antipsychotic therapy. There are four categories of **extrapyramidal symptoms (EPS):** dystonic reactions, pseudoparkinsonism, akathisia, and tardive dyskinesia.

Acute dystonia has the earliest onset of all the EPS. **Dystonias** are spasmodic movements (prolonged tonic contractions) of muscle groups such as tongue protrusion, rolling back of the eyes (oculogyric crisis), jaw spasm (trismus), or neck torsion (torticollis). These symptoms are often frightening and painful for the patient. Approximately 90% of all dystonic reactions occur in the first 72 hours of therapy. Dystonic reactions are most frequent in males, younger patients, and patients receiving high-potency medicines such as haloperidol. Dystonic reactions are generally brief and are the most responsive of the EPS to treatment. Acute dystonic reactions may be controlled by intramuscular injections of diphenhydramine, benztropine, diazepam, or lorazepam. The following rating scales assess patients with different forms of dystonias: the Toronto Western Spasmodic Torticollis Rating Scale (TWSTRS), Global Dystonia Scale (GDS), Unified Dystonia Rating Scale (UDRS), and the Fahn-Marsden Scale. See Related Websites for scales to assess and document dystonia.

Pseudoparkinsonian symptoms of tremor, muscular rigidity, masklike expression, shuffling gait, and loss or weakness of motor function typically begin after 2 to 3 weeks of antipsychotic drug therapy but may occur up to 3 months after starting therapy. They are more commonly seen in older adults. The cause of these symptoms is a relative deficiency of dopamine with cholinergic excess caused by antipsychotic agents. These symptoms are well controlled by anticholinergic antiparkinsonian agents (e.g., benztropine, diphenhydramine, trihexyphenidyl).

Akathisia is a syndrome consisting of subjective feelings of anxiety and restlessness and objective signs of pacing, rocking, and inability to sit or stand in one place for extended periods. Akathisia can increase aggression and is a frequent cause of noncompliance. It occurs more commonly when high-potency antipsychotic agents are used. The mechanism of action is not known. Reducing the dose of the antipsychotic agent or switching to a low-potency agent should be considered. Treatment with anticholinergic agents, benzodiazepines (e.g., diazepam, lorazepam), beta adrenergic–blocking agents (e.g., propranolol), and clonidine have shown varying degrees of success.

Tardive dyskinesia is a syndrome of persistent and involuntary hyperkinetic abnormal movements. It develops in about 20% to 25% of patients receiving typical antipsychotic agents on a long-term (e.g., months to years) basis. There appears to be a lower incidence in patients receiving atypical antipsychotic agents, but these agents are newer and it sometimes takes years for tardive dyskinesia to develop. This drug-induced, late-appearing neurologic disorder is noted for such symptoms as buccolingual masticatory (BLM) syndrome or orofacial movements. The BLM movements begin with mild forward, backward, or lateral tongue movement. As the disorder progresses, more obvious movements appear, including tongue thrusting, rolling, or fly-catching movement, as well as chewing or lateral jaw movements that produce smacking noises. Symptoms may interfere with the patient's ability to chew, speak, or swallow. Facial movements include frequent blinking, brow arching, grimacing, and upward deviation of the eyes. The severity of symptoms of tardive dyskinesia can fluctuate daily, and symptoms often will remit during sleep. The clinical manifestations of tardive dyskinesia are similar to those of EPS, but there are some significant differences. Tardive dyskinesia typically appears after antipsychotic dosage reduction or discontinuation, improves when the antipsychotic dosage is increased, worsens with administration of anticholinergic agents, and may persist for months or years after antipsychotic medicines are discontinued. The exact cause of tardive dyskinesia is unknown. Early signs of tardive dyskinesia may be reversible but over time may become irreversible, even with discontinuation of the antipsychotic medicine.

The best treatment approach to tardive dyskinesia is prevention. Patients who receive maintenance antipsychotic drug therapy should be assessed for early signs of tardive dyskinesia at least semiannually and preferably quarterly. Findings should be documented in patient records to ensure continuity of care and medicolegal protection. Because of the variability in severity and presentation, rating scales have been developed to standardize assessments and diagnoses. The **abnormal involuntary movement scale** (AIMS) rates dyskinetic movements but is not exclusively diagnostic for tardive dyskinesia (see Appendix H). The **dyskinesia identification system: condensed user scale** (DISCUS) rates the presence and severity of abnormal movements and considers other variables when formulating a conclusion. The DISCUS evaluation specifically describes the type of tardive dyskinesia and allows diagnoses to change over time (see Appendix G).

Treatment of tardive dyskinesia is not particularly successful. The most beneficial treatments are anticholinergic withdrawal, adrenergic blocking agents (e.g., beta blockers, clonidine), and benzodiazepines. Antipsychotic dosages may be increased but may only mask symptoms, and eventually will worsen tardive dyskinesia. Patients receiving typical antipsychotic therapy with severe symptoms of tardive dyskinesia who must be maintained on antipsychotic therapy may be candidates for atypical antipsychotic therapy.

Neuroleptic malignant syndrome (NMS) is a potentially fatal adverse effect of antipsychotic therapy in which the patient displays extrapyramidal manifestations as part of the symptoms of the disorder. It occurs in 0.5% to 1.4% of patients receiving antipsychotic therapy. It has been reported most often with high-potency antipsychotic agents given intramuscularly. It typically occurs after 3 to 9 days of treatment with antipsychotic agents and is not related to dosage or previous drug exposure. Once NMS begins, symptoms rapidly progress over 24 to 72 hours. Symptoms usually last 5 to 10 days after discontinuing oral medications and 13 to 30 days with depot antipsychotic medicine (*depot:* injectable, slow-release dose form). Most cases of NMS occur in patients younger than age 40, and it occurs twice as often in males. The syndrome is characterized by fever, severe EPS such as lead-pipe rigidity, trismus, choreiform movements, and opisthotonos; autonomic instability such as tachycardia, labile hypertension, diaphoresis, and incontinence; and alterations in consciousness such as stupor, mutism, and coma. Mortality rates have been as high as 30%, but prompt recognition of the symptoms has reduced the mortality rate to 4% in recent years. It is hypothesized that the cause of the symptoms is excessive dopamine depletion. Treatment includes bromocriptine or amantadine as dopamine agonists and dantrolene as a muscle relaxant. Fever is treated by using cooling blankets, adequate hydration, and antipyretics. Once the patient's condition is stabilized, a thorough evaluation of the medications being prescribed must be made. Resumption of the antipsychotic agent may result in a recurrence of NMS; therefore the lowest dose possible of an antipsychotic agent is prescribed, and close observation of the patient's response is required.

Seizures

Antipsychotic agents may lower the seizure threshold in patients with seizure disorders and in those with no previous history of seizures. The low-potency typical agents and clozapine, an atypical agent, have a higher incidence of inducing seizures.

Weight Gain

Antipsychotic drug therapy often causes substantial weight gain. There is a higher prevalence of obesity associated with schizophrenia, and the weight gain often contributes to nonadherence of therapy. Obesity leads to an increased risk of type 2 diabetes mellitus, dyslipidemia, hypertension, coronary heart disease, and stroke. The frequency and amount of weight gain generally are greater with atypical agents than with typical agents, although individual atypical agents vary in the extent to which they cause weight gain. Of the atypical agents, clozapine and olanzapine cause the most weight gain, moderate weight gain is reported with risperidone and quetiapine, and aripiprazole and ziprasidone cause the least weight gain.

Hyperglycemia

A relatively new adverse effect being reported particularly with atypical antipsychotic agents is hyperglycemia and the development of diabetes mellitus. The mechanism by which this occurs is unknown, and research in this area is more difficult because patients with schizophrenia also have a two- to threefold higher incidence of diabetes mellitus than the general population. Hyperglycemia occurs more frequently with clozapine, olanzapine, and quetiapine, but development of hyperglycemia by the other atypical agents cannot yet be ruled out because these agents are so new.

Dyslipidemia

Clozapine, olanzapine, and quietiapine appear to increase serum triglyceride levels. They do not increase cholesterol levels, although they may appear to because serum triglycerides are a component of total serum cholesterol values. The increase in serum triglycerides may occur without change in weight, although increased body weight will contribute to the hypertriglyceridemia.

Dysrhythmias

Thioridazine, ziparasidone, haloperidol, quetiapine, olanzapine and risperidone have rarely been associated with torsades de pointes (a ventricular dysrhythmia associated with prolongation of the QTc interval on the electrocardiogram), syncope, and sudden death. Bradycardia, electrolyte imbalance (hypokalemia, hypomagnesemia), the presence of congenital prolongation of the QTc interval, and the concomitant use of other medicines that may significantly prolong the QTc interval (e.g., quinidine, sotalol, moxifloxacin, sparfloxacin, dofetilide), can increase the risk of torsades de pointes and sudden death in patients receiving antipsychotic agents.

OTHER ADVERSE EFFECTS

Other adverse effects of antipsychotic therapy can also be predicted based on the receptor-blocking activity of the agents:

- Blocking the *cholinergic (acetylcholine) receptors* explains the anticholinergic effects (e.g., dry mouth, constipation, sinus tachycardia, blurred vision, inhibition or impairment of ejaculation, urinary retention) associated with antipsychotic agents.
- Blocking *histamine-1 receptors* causes sedation, drowsiness, and appetite stimulation, and contributes to the hypotensive effects and potentiation of CNS depressant drugs. Molindone has no histamine-1–blocking effect; therefore it causes no weight gain, compared with other antipsychotic agents.
- Antipsychotic agents also block *alpha-1* and *alpha-2 adrenergic receptors*, causing postural hypotension, sexual dysfunction, reflex tachycardia, and potentiation of antihypertensive agents. The most potent alpha-1 blockers are chlorpromazine, and

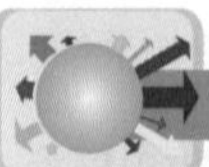

Clinical Landmine

Antipsychotic medicines may have side effects such as seizure activity, parkinsonian symptoms, tardive dyskinesia, and hepatotoxicity that require management by the prescribing health care provider. It is essential that the patient and those providing supervision understand the importance of communicating any of these symptoms promptly for appropriate interventions.

thioridazine, whereas molindone and haloperidol have virtually no effect on alpha-1 receptors.

Antipsychotic agents may produce many side effects other than those already listed. These include hepatotoxicity, blood dyscrasias, allergic reactions, endocrine disorders, skin pigmentation, and reversible effects in the eyes. Patients receiving clozapine are particularly susceptible to developing agranulocytosis. Regularly scheduled white blood cell (WBC) counts are mandatory.

NURSING PROCESS *for Antipsychotic Therapy*

Assessment

History of Behavior

- Gather information from the patient and other historians relating to the onset, duration, and progression of the patient's symptoms. Has the patient previously been treated for this or other mental disorders? Does the patient have any coexisting health conditions?
- Take a detailed history of all medications the individual is taking or has taken in the past 3 months.
- Inquire about the use of substances.

Basic Mental Status

- Note general appearance and appropriateness of attire. Is the individual clean and neat? Is the posture erect, stooped, or slumped? Is the patient oriented to date, time, place, and person?
- What coping mechanisms has the individual been using to deal with the situation? How adaptive are the coping mechanisms?
- Has the patient been able to carry out self-care activities and social and work obligations?
- Are symptoms of depression present? Symptoms may not be evident during the acute phase of schizophrenia.

Interpersonal Relationships. Assess the quality of relationships in which the individual is involved. Identify people who are supportive. Ask the family and significant others to describe the relationship they have with the patient. Has there been deterioration in their closeness and ability to interrelate effectively?

Mood/Affect. Patients experiencing altered thinking, behavior, or feelings require careful evaluation of both verbal and nonverbal actions. Often the thoughts, feelings, and behaviors displayed are inconsistent with the so-called normal responses of individuals in similar circumstances.

- Is the facial expression worried, sad, angry, or blank?
- Is the individual displaying behaviors that are inappropriate, blunted, or have a flat affect?
- Is the patient apathetic to normal situations?
- Is there consistency when expressing feelings verbally and nonverbally?
- Does the patient overreact to situations at times?

Clarity of Thoughts/Perception

- Does the patient suffer from delusions, disorganized speech pattern, flight of ideas, autism, grandiose ideas, or mutism? Ask about the presence of hallucinations (i.e., auditory, visual, tactile).
- Does the patient talk about unrelated topics (loose association) as though they are connected and related?
- Is the patient self-absorbed and not in contact with reality?
- Does the patient display interruption of thoughts?
- Does the patient display paranoid behavior?

Thoughts of Death. If the individual is suspected of being suicidal, ask if there have ever been thoughts about suicide. If the response is yes, get more details. Is a specific plan formulated? How often do these thoughts occur? Does the individual make direct or indirect statements regarding death, for example, things would be better at death?

Psychomotor Function. What is the patient's activity level? Is the individual unable to sit still, pacing continually? Is the patient catatonic, that is, immobile because of psychological functioning?

Sleep Pattern. What is the person's normal sleep pattern, and how has it varied since the onset of the psychotic symptoms? Ask specifically whether insomnia is present. Ask the individual to describe the perception of the amount and quality of sleep nightly. What is the level of fatigue? Are naps taken regularly?

Dietary History. Ask questions relating to appetite and note weight gains or losses not associated with intentional dieting.

Nursing Diagnoses

- Impaired adjustment (indication)
- Impaired verbal communication (indication)
- Ineffective coping (indication)
- Ineffective role performance (indication)
- Disturbed thought processes (indication)
- Risk for injury (side effects)

Planning

History of Psychotic Behavior

- Review data collected to identify individual's strengths and weaknesses.
- Review medications being taken to identify any that are known to cause any of the symptoms exhibited.

Basic Mental Status

- Plan to perform a baseline assessment of the individual's mental status at specific intervals throughout the course of treatment.
- Review coping mechanisms used. Plan to discuss those that are maladaptive. Plan to initiate changes by guiding the individual in the use of more adaptive coping strategies.
- Schedule specific times to discuss the patient's behavior with family members to foster understanding of it.

Mood/Affect. Review assessment data to develop strategies to assist the individual to cope more effectively with his or her exhibited behaviors. Reward positive accomplishments for progress made.

Clarity of Thought/Perception. Plan to monitor the patient carefully for altered thoughts and perceptions. Develop approaches that could be tried when the individual is having delusions or hallucinations. Decrease the stimuli within the patient's immediate environment. Identify areas in which the patient is capable of input to set goals and make decisions. When the patient is unable to make decisions, plan to make them. Set goals to involve the patient as abilities change with treatment. Provide an opportunity to plan for self-care.

Thoughts of Death. Provide for a safe environment for the individual. Search the surroundings for objects that could be used to inflict self-harm.

Psychomotor Function. Review activities offered within the clinical setting and plan for the individual to participate in those that will be beneficial and nonthreatening.

Sleep Pattern. Provide specific parameters in which the patient can function that meet the individual's need for sleep.

Dietary Needs. Provide an opportunity for the individual to be involved in selecting foods appropriate to needs (to lose or gain weight). If the person is paranoid and suspects being poisoned, allow the individual to self-serve food, open canned food, and perform other activities, as appropriate within the setting.

Implementation

- Nursing interventions must be individualized and based on patient assessment data.
- Provide the individual with a structured environment that is safe and decreases external stimuli.
- Provide an environment of acceptance that focuses on the individual's strengths while minimizing weaknesses.
- Provide an opportunity for the individual to express feelings. Use active listening and therapeutic communication techniques. Allow the person to express feelings in nonverbal ways (e.g., involve in physical activities or occupational therapy).
- Allow the patient to make decisions if capable; make those the client is not capable of making. Provide a reward for progress when decisions are initiated appropriately.
- Involve the patient in self-care activities. Assist with personal grooming, as needed. Ensure that the patient is dressed appropriately to prevent embarrassment.
- Set limits and enforce them in a kind, firm manner to handle inappropriate behaviors.
- Once the content is known, do not reinforce hallucinations or delusions.
- When the person has altered perceptions, provide diversionary activities and minimize interactions such as viewing television programs that may reinforce the distorted perceptions.
- Be open and direct in handling patients who are highly suspicious. Speak distinctly to be heard; do not whisper or laugh in circumstances the patient could misconstrue.
- If the patient is suicidal, ask for details of the plan being formulated. Follow up on details obtained with appropriate family members or significant others. For example, have guns removed from home if this is part of the plan. Provide patient safety and supervision and record observations at specified intervals consistent with severity of the suicide threat and policies of the practice site.
- Use physical restraints within the guidelines of the clinical setting as appropriate to the behaviors being exhibited. Use the least restrictive alternative possible for the circumstances. Have sufficient staff available to assist with violent behavior to demonstrate ability to control the situation while providing for the safety and well-being of the patient and fellow staff members.
- Provide for nutritional needs by having high-protein, high-calorie foods appropriate for the individual to eat while pacing or highly active. Have nutritious snacks the patient is known to like available on the unit. Offer these at specific intervals throughout the day. Administer vitamins and liquid supplemental feedings as ordered.
- Manipulative behavior must be handled in a consistent manner by all staff members. Use limit setting and consequences that are agreed to in advance by all staff members. When the patient attempts to blame others, refocus on the patient's responsibilities. Give positive reinforcement for nonmanipulative behaviors when they occur.

Patient Education and Health Promotion

- Orient the individual to the unit, explaining rules and the process of privileges, as well as how they are obtained or lost. (The extent of the orientation and explanations given depend on the individual's orientation to date, time, and place, as well as his or her abilities.)

- Explain unit rules and therapeutic rules. Keep explanations clear and concise.
- Patient education must be based on assessment data and individualized to provide the patient with a structured environment in which to grow and enhance self-esteem.
- Explain the activity groups available and how and when the individual will participate in these. A variety of group process activities (e.g., social skills group, self-esteem groups, and physical exercise groups) are available within particular therapeutic settings.
- The patient and family must be involved in establishing outcomes and integrating these into the appropriate group processes to develop positive experiences to enhance coping skills. Those patients who are disruptive or withdrawn, or who have impaired communication, need individualized approaches to improve patient education.
- Before discharge, the patient and family must understand the goals of treatment and the entire follow-up plan, such as frequency of therapy sessions, health care provider visits, and return to work goals.

Fostering Health Maintenance. Throughout the course of treatment, discuss medication information and how it will benefit the patient's symptoms and circumstances. Drug therapy is a major portion of antipsychotic therapy. Although symptoms may improve, they may not be totally eliminated. The onset of the drug's effectiveness varies widely, depending on the drug administered and the route of administration. Nonadherence is a major problem in this group of patients; therefore, tracking of the medications being taken needs careful scrutiny. On an outpatient basis, many of these patients require administration of their medication by another responsible individual. (The patient may find this stressful.) Nonadherence is thought to be a major cause of repeat hospitalization in this group of patients. Long-acting injections may be used on some patients in an attempt to overcome this problem. On an inpatient basis the nurse must always check to be sure the patient is actually swallowing the medication because there is a high incidence of "cheeking" it. Perform baseline clinical evaluation rating scales (e.g., BPRS, CGI, PANSS) and adverse effect scales (e.g., GDS, TWSTRS for dystonias, DISCUS or AIMS for extrapyramidal symptoms) at specified intervals; record and report according to agency policy.

Provide the patient and significant others with important information contained in the specific drug monograph for the medicines prescribed. Additional health teaching and nursing interventions for the side effects to expect and report are described in the drug monographs that follow.

Seek cooperation and understanding of the following points so that medication compliance is increased: name of medication, dosage, route and times of administration, side effects to expect, and side effects to report.

Written Record. Enlist the patient's aid in developing and maintaining a written record of monitoring parameters. Complete the Premedication Data column for use as a baseline to track response to drug therapy. Ensure that the patient understands how to use the form and instruct the patient to bring the completed form to follow-up visits. Because there are a number of debilitating side effects and others that are life-threatening if not acted on correctly, it is important that open communication with the health care provider, nurses, therapist, and pharmacist be encouraged throughout the course of therapy.

DRUG CLASS: Antipsychotic Agents

phenothiazines, thioxanthenes, haloperidol, molindone, loxapine, clozapine, olanzepine, aripiprazole, quetiapine, risperidone, ziprasidone

Actions

Although the antipsychotic agents are from distinctly different chemical classes, all are similar in that they act by blocking the action of dopamine in the brain. The atypical antipsychotic agents block serotonin receptors in addition to dopamine receptors. Because all of the antipsychotic agents work at different sites within the brain, the side effects are observed on different systems throughout the body. Atypical antipsychotic agents tend to be more effective and have fewer side effects than typical agents.

Uses

Antipsychotic agents are used to treat psychoses associated with mental illnesses such as schizophrenia, mania, psychotic depression, and psychotic organic brain syndrome. Medications used to treat these disorders are grouped into two broad categories: first-generation antipsychotic agents (also known as typical antipsychotic agents including the phenothiazines and nonphenothiazines—thioxanthenes, haloperidol, molindone, loxapine) and the second-generation antipsychotic agents (also known as atypical antipsychotic agents—aripiprazole, clozapine, olanzapine, quetiapine, risperidone, ziprasidone). Aripiprazole, olanzapine, quetiapine, rispridone, and ziprasidone are now considered to be first-line second-generation antipsychotic agents that provide significant relief of active psychotic symptoms such as hallucinations, delusion, and thought disorganization for approximately 70% of patients with schizophrenia. Clozapine is reserved for more resistant cases that do not respond adequately to the other atypical agents. All of these antipsychotic agents also significantly reduce the risk of recurrence.

As clinical experience is being gained with the relatively new second-generation antipsychotic agents, dramatic weight gain, diabetes mellitus, electrocardiographic changes (i.e., QT interval prolongation) and dyslipidemia have been reported. The risk of these potentially serious adverse effects is not the same with all agents, but the U.S. Food and Drug Administration (FDA) has issued precautionary statements that body weight, blood glucose, and serum lipids should be closely monitored in all patients receiving these antipsychotic agents.

Therapeutic Outcomes

The primary therapeutic outcome from antipsychotic therapy is maintaining the individual at an optimal level of functioning, with minimal exacerbations of psychotic symptoms and minimal adverse effects from medicines.

Nursing Process for Therapy with Antipsychotic Agents

Premedication Assessment

1. Obtain baseline blood pressures in supine, sitting, and standing positions; record and report significant lowering to the health care provider before administering the medicine.
2. Check electrolytes, body weight, height, blood glucose, lipid profile, hepatic function, cardiac function, and thyroid function before initiation and periodically throughout the course of administration.
3. Perform baseline clinical evaluation rating scales (e.g., BPRS, CGI, PANSS) and adverse effect scales, (e.g., GDS, TWSTRS for dystonias, DISCUS or AIMS for extrapyramidal symptoms) at specified intervals; record and report according to agency policy.
4. Use of clozapine requires a baseline and weekly WBC counts for the first 6 months of treatment because of the high incidence of agranulocytosis. Thereafter, if WBC counts are acceptable (greater than or equal to 3500/mm^3), and the absolute neutrophil count is greater than 2000/mm^3, WBC counts can be monitored every other week. WBC counts must be monitored weekly for at least 4 weeks after the discontinuation of clozapine.

Planning

Availability. See Table 18-1.

Implementation

Dosage and Administration. See Table 18-1. The dosage must be individualized according to the degree of mental and emotional disturbance. It will often take several weeks for a patient to show optimal improvement and become stabilized on an adequate maintenance dosage. As a result of the cumulative effects of antipsychotic agents, patients must be reevaluated periodically to determine the lowest effective dosage necessary to control psychiatric symptoms.

Evaluation

Side Effects to Expect

Chronic Fatigue, Drowsiness. Chronic fatigue and drowsiness are common problems associated with medicines used to treat psychoses. Sedative effects associated with antipsychotic therapy can be minimized by giving the dose of medication at bedtime. People who work around machinery, drive a car, administer medication, or perform other duties in which they must remain mentally alert should not take these medications while working.

Orthostatic Hypotension. All antipsychotic agents may cause some degree of orthostatic hypotension manifested by dizziness and weakness, particularly when therapy is being initiated. Monitor the blood pressure daily in the supine, sitting, and standing positions.

Anticipate the development of postural hypotension and take measures to prevent an occurrence. Teach the patient to rise slowly from a supine or sitting position; encourage the patient to sit or lie down if feeling faint.

Blurred Vision; Constipation; Urinary Retention; Dryness of Mucosa of the Mouth, Throat, and Nose. These symptoms are the anticholinergic effects produced by these agents. Patients should be monitored for the development of these side effects. Caution the patient that blurred vision may occur, and make appropriate suggestions for the individual's personal safety.

Mucosal dryness may be relieved by sucking hard candy or ice chips or by chewing gum.

A high-fiber diet, stool softeners such as docusate, or the occasional use of a stimulant laxative such as bisacodyl may be required for constipation.

Side Effects to Report

Seizure Activity. Provide patient safety during episodes of seizures; report for further evaluation. Adjustment of anticonvulsant therapy may be required, especially in seizure-prone patients.

Parkinsonian Symptoms. Report the development of drooling, cogwheel rigidity, shuffling gait, masklike expression, or tremors. Anticholinergic agents may be used to help control these symptoms.

Tardive Dyskinesia. Report the development of fine tremors of the tongue, "fly catching" tongue movements, and lip smacking. This is particularly important in patients who have been receiving antipsychotic agents and anticholinergic agents for several years.

Hepatotoxicity. The symptoms of hepatotoxicity are anorexia, nausea, vomiting, jaundice, hepatomegaly, splenomegaly, and abnormal liver function tests (e.g., elevated bilirubin, aspartate aminotransferase [AST], alanine aminotransferase [ALT], gamma-glutamyltransferase [GGT], alkaline phosphatase, prothrombin time).

Blood Dyscrasias. Routine laboratory studies (e.g., red blood cell [RBC], WBC, and differential counts) should be scheduled. This is particularly important for patients receiving clozapine. Monitor for sore throat, fever, purpura, jaundice, or excessive and progressive weakness.

Hives, Pruritus, Rash. Report symptoms for further evaluation by the health care provider.

Photosensitivity. The patient should be cautioned to avoid prolonged exposure to sunlight and ultraviolet light. Suggest wearing long-sleeved clothing, a hat, and sunglasses when exposed to sunlight. Advise against using artificial tanning lamps.

Drug Interactions

Drugs That Increase Toxic Effects. Antihistamines, alcohol, analgesics, anesthetics, tranquilizers, barbiturates, narcotics, St. John's wort, and sedative-hypnotics increase the toxic effects of antipsychotic drugs. Monitor the patient for excessive sedation and reduce the dosage of the above-mentioned agents if necessary.

Drugs That Decrease Therapeutic Effects. Dopamine agonists (levodopa, bromocriptine, pergolide, amantadine, ropinirole, pramipexole) will block the dopamine antagonist effects of the antipsychotic agents. Avoid concurrent use.

Carbamazepine. Carbamazepine stimulates the metabolism of haloperidol, clozapine, aripiprazole, olanzepine, risperidone, and ziprasidone. Dosage adjustment of the antipsychotic medicine may be required.

Erythromycin, Clarithromycin, Fluoxetine, Grapefruit Juice, Ketoconazole, Nefazodone. These substances inhibit the metabolism of aripiprazole, clozapine, quetiapine, and ziprasidone, causing an increase in serum levels and potential toxicity from the antipsychotic agent. Dosages of the antipsychotic may need to be reduced by up to 50% to avoid toxicities.

Cimetidine. Cimetidine inhibits the metabolism of quetiapine. The dosage of quetiapine may need to be reduced to prevent adverse effects.

Phenytoin. Phenytoin increases the metabolism of quetiapine, thioridazine, and haloperidol. Increases in dosage of the antipsychotic medicine may be necessary.

Guanethidine. Antipsychotic agents may inhibit the antihypertensive effect of guanethidine. Concurrent therapy is not recommended.

Beta-Adrenergic Blockers. Beta-adrenergic blocking agents (e.g., propranolol, timolol, nadolol, pindolol) significantly enhance the hypotensive effects of antipsychotic agents. Concurrent therapy is not recommended unless used to treat adverse effects of antipsychotic agents.

Barbiturates. Barbiturates may stimulate the rate of metabolism of phenothiazines. Dosage adjustments of the antipsychotic agent may be necessary.

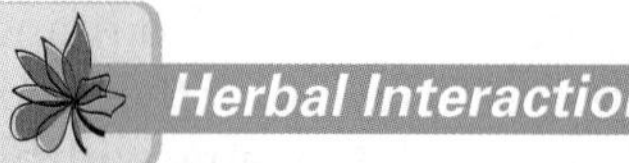

St. John's Wort

St. John's wort increases toxic effects of antipsychotic agents.

Insulin, Oral Hypoglycemic Agents. Diabetic or prediabetic patients must be monitored for the development of hyperglycemia, particularly during the early weeks of therapy. Assess regularly for glycosuria and report if it occurs with any frequency. Patients receiving oral hypoglycemic agents or insulin may require a dosage adjustment.

Venlafaxine. Venlafaxine significantly inhibits the metabolism of haloperidol. Doses of haloperidol may have to be given less often to prevent potential toxicity.

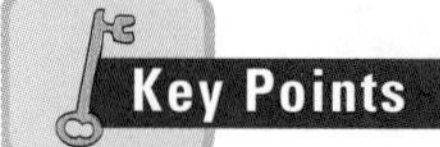

- Psychoses are symptoms of psychotic disorders, that is, illnesses in which the patient has lost touch with reality. The underlying illness must be treated, not just the psychosis.
- A combination of nonpharmacologic and pharmacologic therapies provides the most successful outcomes to therapy.
- The emphasis on community treatment has ensured that virtually all health care settings treat patients with psychotic symptoms. Community hospitals and health maintenance organizations now provide care to many psychiatric patients, and nurses increasingly serve residential care facilities. Many patients require years of antipsychotic drug treatment to prevent exacerbations of illness.
- Although antipsychotic agents cause many adverse effects, most can be minimized by patient education, manipulation of dosage and administration, and sometimes adjunctive drug treatments. These patients require careful monitoring of target symptoms to maximize response and minimize adverse effects.

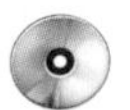

Go to your Companion CD-ROM for appendices, an Audio Glossary, animations, Drug Dosage Calculators, customizable Patient Self-Assessment forms, and Review Questions for the NCLEX® Examination.

evolve Be sure to visit the companion Evolve site at http://evolve.elsevier.com/Clayton for WebLinks and additional online resources.

MEDICATION SAFETY REVIEW

MATH REVIEW QUESTIONS

1. Order: chlorpromazine (Thorazine) 125 mg PO
   Available: chlorpromazine 100 mg/5 mL
   Give: _____ mL.
2. Order: benztropine mesylate (Cogentin) 1 mg PO at bedtime daily
   Available: benztropine mesylate 0.5-mg tablets
   Give: _____ tablets.
3. Order: trifluoperazine (Stelazine) 12 mg IM
   Available: trifluoperazine 10 mg/mL and 20 mg/mL
   Give: which concentration _____, what volume _____.

CRITICAL THINKING QUESTIONS

1. A patient is taking a high-potency antipsychotic medication.
   - **a.** What is meant by the term *high-potency antipsychotic,* and what drugs are included in this category?
   - **b.** What is meant by *extrapyramidal symptoms?*
   - **c.** How often should the patient be monitored for these symptoms?
   - **d.** When found, what nursing actions are appropriate?
2. It is decided that the patient should receive clozapine.
   - **a.** What are the side effects to expect and those to report with this medication?
   - **b.** Discuss monitoring for agranulocytosis.
3. Why is an anticholinergic agent often given in addition to haloperidol? What is its action?

CONTENT REVIEW QUESTIONS

1. Four major side effects of antipsychotic medications are:
   1. nausea, vomiting, diarrhea, sedation.
   2. orthostatic hypotension, blood dyscrasias, hepatotoxicity, sedation.
   3. EPS, hypertension, mucosa dryness, sedation.
   4. sedation, EPS, hypotension, anticholinergic effects.
2. Premedication assessments for antipsychotic agents should include checking for:
   1. history of cardiovascular disorders.
   2. daily weights.
   3. positional blood pressure reading.
   4. history of diabetes mellitus.

CHAPTER

19 Drugs Used for Seizure Disorders

evolve http://evolve.elsevier.com/Clayton

Chapter Content

Objectives

1. Prepare a chart to be used as a study guide that includes the following information:
   - Name of seizure type
   - Description of seizure
   - Medications used to treat each type of seizure
   - Nursing interventions and monitoring parameters for seizures
2. Describe the effects of the hydantoins on patients with diabetes and on people receiving oral contraceptives, theophylline, folic acid, or antacids.
3. Cite precautions needed when administering phenytoin or diazepam intravenously.
4. Explain the rationale for proper dental care for people receiving hydantoin therapy.
5. Develop a teaching plan for patient education for people diagnosed with a seizure disorder.
6. Cite the desired therapeutic outcomes for seizure disorders.
7. Identify the mechanisms of action thought to control seizure activity when anticonvulsants are administered.
8. Discuss the basic classification systems used for epilepsy.

Key Terms

seizures
epilepsy
generalized seizures
partial seizures
anticonvulsants
antiepileptic drug (AED)
tonic phase
clonic phase
postictal state
status epilepticus
atonic seizure
myoclonic seizures
absence (petit mal) epilepsy
seizure threshold
gamma-aminobutyric acid (GABA)
gingival hyperplasia
nystagmus
urticaria

SEIZURE DISORDERS

Seizures are symptoms of an abnormality in the nerve centers of the brain. They are brief periods of abnormal electrical activity in these nerve centers. Seizures may be convulsive (i.e., accompanied by violent, involuntary muscle contractions) or nonconvulsive. During seizure activity there is often a change in the person's consciousness, sensory and motor systems, subjective well-being, and objective behavior. Seizures may result from fever, head injury, brain tumor, meningitis, hypoglycemia, a drug overdose or withdrawal, or poisoning. It is estimated that 8% to 10% of all people will have a seizure during their lifetime. If the seizures are chronic and recurrent, the patient is diagnosed as having **epilepsy.** Epilepsy is the most common of all neurologic disorders. It is not a single disease but several different disorders that have one common characteristic: a sudden discharge of excessive electrical energy from nerve cells in the brain. An estimated 2.3 million Americans have these disorders, and approximately 125,000 new cases are diagnosed annually. The cause of epilepsy may be unknown (idiopathic), or it may be the result of a head injury, a brain tumor, meningitis, or a stroke.

Epilepsy has been classified in several ways. Traditionally the most important subdivisions have been *grand mal, petit mal, psychomotor,* and *jacksonian* types. They also can be grouped based on type of seizure, etiology, location of the brain involved, causal factors, age at onset, severity, frequency, and prognosis. An international commission has reclassified epilepsies into two broad categories based on clinical and electroencephalographic (EEG) patterns: generalized and partial (localized). **Generalized seizures** refer to those that affect both hemispheres of the brain, are accompanied by loss of consciousness, and may be subdivided into convulsive and nonconvulsive types. **Partial seizures** may be subdivided into simple and complex symptom types; a change in consciousness occurs with complex seizures. **Partial seizures** begin in a localized area in one hemisphere of the brain. Both simple and complex partial seizures can evolve into generalized seizures, a process referred to as *secondary generalization.* Epilepsy is treated almost exclusively with medications known as **anticonvulsants.** Another term gaining more widespread use is **antiepileptic drug (AED).**

DESCRIPTIONS OF SEIZURES

Generalized Convulsive Seizures

The most common generalized convulsive seizures are the tonic-clonic, atonic, and myoclonic seizures.

Tonic-Clonic (Grand Mal) Seizures

Tonic-clonic (grand mal) seizures are the most common type of seizure. In the tonic phase, patients suddenly develop intense muscular contractions that cause them to fall to the ground, lose consciousness, and lie rigid. The back may arch, arms may flex, legs extend, and the teeth clench. Air is forced up the larynx, extruding saliva as foam and producing an audible sound like a cry. Respirations stop and the patient may become cyanotic. The tonic phase usually lasts 20 to 60 seconds before diffuse trembling sets in. The clonic phase, manifested by bilaterally symmetric jerks alternating with relaxation of extremities, then begins. The clonic phase starts slightly and then gradually becomes more violent, involving the whole body. Patients often bite their tongues and become incontinent of urine or feces. Usually within 60 seconds this phase proceeds to a resting, recovery phase of flaccid paralysis and sleep, lasting 2 to 3 hours (postictal [post ik′ tal] state). The patient has no recollection of the attack on awakening. The severity, frequency, and duration of attacks are highly variable. They may last from 1 to 30 minutes and occur as frequently as daily or as infrequently as every few years. Status epilepticus is a rapidly recurring generalized seizure that does not allow the individual to regain normal function between seizures. It is a medical emergency that requires prompt treatment to minimize permanent nerve damage and death.

Atonic or Akinetic Seizures

A sudden loss of muscle tone is known as an atonic (a tah′ nik) seizure, or drop attack. This may be described as a head drop, the dropping of a limb, or slumping to the ground. A sudden loss of consciousness and muscle tone results in a dramatic fall. Seated patients may slump forward violently. The attacks are short, but frequent injury occurs from the uncontrolled falls. These patients often wear protective headgear to minimize the trauma.

Myoclonic Seizures

Myoclonic (my oh klon′ ik) seizures involve lightning-like repetitive contractions of the voluntary muscles of the face, trunk, and extremities. The jerks may be isolated events or rapidly repetitive. It is not uncommon for patients to lose their balance and fall to the floor. These attacks occur most often at night as the patient enters sleep.

Generalized Nonconvulsive Seizures

By far the most common generalized nonconvulsive seizure disorder is absence (petit mal) epilepsy. These seizures occur primarily in children and usually disappear at puberty, although the patient may develop a second type of seizure activity. Attacks consist of paroxysmal episodes of altered consciousness lasting for 5 to 20 seconds. There are no prodromal or postictal phases. Patients appear to be staring into space and may exhibit a few rhythmic movements of the eyes or head, lip smacking, mumbling, chewing, or swallowing movements. Falling does not occur, patients do not convulse, and they will have no memory of events occurring during the seizures.

Partial (Localized) Seizures

Partial seizures are subdivided into partial simple motor seizures and partial complex seizures. *Partial simple motor (jacksonian) seizures* involve localized convulsions of voluntary muscles. A single body part, such as a finger or extremity, may start jerking. The muscle spasm may end spontaneously or spread over the whole body. The patient does not lose consciousness unless the seizure develops into a generalized convulsion. *Partial seizures with complex symptoms (psychomotor seizures)* are manifested by a vast array of possible symptoms. The patient's outward appearance may be normal or there may be aimless wandering, unusual and repeated chewing, lip smacking, or swallowing movements. The person is conscious but may be in a confused, dreamlike state. The attacks, which may occur several times daily and last several minutes, commonly end in sleep or with a clouded sensorium, with no recollection of the events of the attack.

ANTICONVULSANT THERAPY

Identification of the cause of seizure activity is important in determining the type of therapy required. Contributing factors (e.g., head injury, fever, hypoglycemia, drug overdose) must be specifically treated to correct the underlying cause before chronic anticonvulsant therapy is started. Once the underlying cause is treated, it is rare that chronic antiepileptic therapy is needed. When seizure activity continues, drug therapy is the primary form of treatment. The goals of therapy are to reduce the frequency of seizure activity and minimize the adverse effects of the medicine. Therapeutic outcomes must be individualized for each patient. The selection of the medicine depends on the type of seizure, the age and gender of the patient, other medical conditions present, and the potential adverse effects of the individual medicines.

In general, anticonvulsant therapy should start with the use of a single agent selected from a group of first-line agents based on type of seizure (see Table 19-1 for antiepileptic drugs of choice for primary seizure disorders). The agents classified as first-line therapy are fairly similar in their potential to prevent seizures, but vary in side effects. Thus, the agent chosen is selected first on its ability to control a certain form of epilepsy, then on its adverse effect profile and likelihood for side effects in a particular patient. In general, if treatment is

Table 19-1 *Antiepileptic Drugs of Choice Based on Type of Seizure*

	GENERALIZED SEIZURES			
	GENERALIZED TONIC-CLONIC	ABSENCE	ATONIC, MYOCLONIC	PARTIAL SEIZURES
Drugs of choice	valproate, lamotrigine	valproate, ethosuximide, lamotrigine	valproate, lamotrigine	carbamazepine, phenytoin, oxcarbazepine, lamotrigine, valproate
Alternatives	topiramate, zonisamide, phenytoin, levetiracetam, phenobarbital	zonisamide, clonazepam, levetiracetam	clonazepam, topiramate, zonisamide, levetiracetam	levetiracetam, zonisamide, gabapentin, tiagabine, phenobarbital

Compiled from Karceski S, Morrell M, Carpenter D: The expert consensus guideline series, treatment of epilepsy, *Epilepsy Behav* 2:A1-A50, 2001.

not successful with the first agent chosen, it is discontinued and another first-line agent is started. If treatment fails with the second agent, the health care provider may decide to discontinue the second agent and start a third first-line agent, or may start combination therapy by adding an alternative medicine to one of the first-line therapies. Occasionally some patients will require multiple-drug therapy with a combination of agents and will still not be completely seizure-free.

Actions

Unfortunately the mechanisms of seizure activity are extremely complex and not well understood. In general, anticonvulsants increase the **seizure threshold** and regulate neuronal firing by either inhibiting excitatory processes or enhancing inhibitory processes. The medicines can also prevent the seizure from spreading to adjacent neurons. Phenytoin, carbamazepine, lamotrigine, zonisamide, and valproic acid act on sodium and calcium channels to stabilize the neuronal membrane and may decrease the release of excitatory neurotransmitters. Barbiturates, benzodiazepines, tiagabine, and gabapentin enhance the inhibitory effect of **gamma-aminobutyric acid (GABA)**, an inhibitory neurotransmitter that counterbalances the effect of excitatory neurotransmitters.

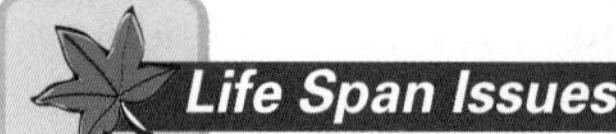

Anticonvulsant Therapy

In children, anticonvulsant therapy may cause a change in personality and possible indifference to school activities and family activities. Behavioral differences must be discussed with the health care provider, family, and teachers. The school nurse must be informed of medications prescribed.

Liquid dosage forms of anticonvulsants must be measured accurately to help maintain seizure control. It is extremely important to shake the liquid first to disperse the medicine uniformly in the suspension. The dosage should then be measured with an oral syringe to ensure accuracy before administration.

Medicines should be taken at the same time daily to maintain a constant blood level. Dosages should not be self-adjusted, and drugs should not be discontinued suddenly.

Monitoring response to anticonvulsant therapy is essential. Dosages may need to be adjusted weekly, especially during initiation of therapy.

Uses

Anticonvulsants are used to reduce the frequency of seizures.

NURSING PROCESS *for Anticonvulsant Therapy*

Nurses may play an important role in the correct diagnosis of seizure disorders. Accurate seizure diagnosis is crucial to the selection of the most appropriate medications for each patient. Because health care providers are not always able to observe patient seizures directly, nurses should learn to observe and record these events objectively.

Assessment

History of Seizure Activity

- What activities was the individual engaging in immediately before the last seizure?
- Has the individual noticed any particular activity that usually precedes attacks?
- When was the last seizure before the current one?
- Did the individual experience any changes in behavior before the onset of the seizure (e.g., increasing anxiety or depression)?
- Is the individual aware of a pre-seizure "aura" (a particular feeling or odor that occurs before a seizure onset)?
- Was there an "epileptic cry"?

Seizure Description

- Record the exact time of seizure onset and duration of each phase, a description of the specific body parts involved, and any progression of the affected body parts.
- Did the patient lose consciousness?
- Was stiffening and jerking present?
- Describe autonomic responses usually seen during the clonic phase: altered, jerky respirations or

frothy salivation, dilated pupils, or any eye movements, cyanosis, diaphoresis, or incontinence.

Postictal Behavior

- Record the level of consciousness: orientation to time, place, and person.
- Assess the degree of alertness, fatigue, or headache present.
- Evaluate the degree of weakness, alterations in speech, and memory loss.
- Patients often experience muscle soreness and extreme need for sleep. Record the duration of sleep.
- Evaluate any bodily harm that occurred during the seizure, such as bruises, cuts, or lacerations.

Nursing Diagnoses

- Injury, risk for (indication)
- Body image, disturbed (indication, side effects)
- Gas exchange, impaired (indication)
- Sensory perception, disturbed visual, tactile (indication)

Planning

Seizure Activity

- Identify the need for seizure precautions on a Kardex, care plan, or enter into computer record.
- Have equipment and supplies needed to care for a patient during seizure available in immediate area.
- Order periodic laboratory studies to detect adverse effects (e.g., blood dyscrasias, electrolytes, nephrotoxicity, hepatotoxicity, and anticonvulsant serum levels) at intervals specified by the health care provider.

Psychosocial Assessment

- Plan specific times to discuss the concerns of the patient, family, or significant others with regard to the seizure disorder. Set specific goals for health teaching needed.
- Arrange for a social worker to intervene with care needs in the school or work setting.

Emergency Equipment

- Know the location of equipment for suctioning and/or ventilating a patient.
- Have drugs available to treat status epilepticus or know the procedure for obtaining them stat.

Implementation

Management of Seizure Activity. Assist the patient during a seizure by doing the following:

- Protect the patient from further injury. Place padding around or under the head; do not try to restrain; loosen tight clothing. If in a standing position initially, lower the patient to a horizontal position.
- Once the patient enters the relaxation stage, turn slightly onto the side to allow secretions to drain out of the mouth.
- Remain calm and quiet and give reassurance to the patient when the seizure is over.
- Suction the patient as needed and initiate ventilatory assistance if breathing does not return spontaneously.
- Provide a place for the patient to rest immediately after a seizure. Summon appropriate assistance so that the individual can get home.
- Initiate nursing interventions appropriate to the underlying cause of the seizures (e.g., high fever, metabolic disorder, head trauma, drug/alcohol withdrawal).
- If the patient has another seizure, or if a seizure lasts longer than 4 minutes, immediately summon assistance; the patient may be going into status epilepticus.
- Observe all aspects of the seizure for detailed recording: aura (if present), time started/ended, body parts affected, order of progression of seizure action, autonomic signs (e.g., altered breathing, diaphoresis, incontinence, salivation, flushing, pupil dilation), postictal period observations (e.g., vital signs, level of consciousness, speech pattern/disorder, muscle soreness, weakness, or paralysis) and note time each phase lasted.

Psychological Implications

Lifestyle. Encourage maintenance of a normal lifestyle. Provide for appropriate limitations (e.g., limits on operating power equipment, a motor vehicle, or swimming) to ensure patient safety. Make the patient aware of the Rehabilitation Act of 1973 that was initiated to ensure that individuals with handicaps do not experience discrimination in employment. Contact the Epilepsy Foundation of America and state vocational rehabilitation agencies for information about vocational rehabilitation and employment.

Expressing Feelings. Allow patient to ventilate feelings. Seizures may occur in public and may be accompanied by incontinence. Patients are usually embarrassed about having a seizure in front of others. Provide for ventilation of any discrimination the patient feels at the workplace. Encourage open discussion of self-concept issues relating to the disease and its impact on daily activities, work, and the responsiveness of other individuals toward them.

School-Age Children. Acceptance by peers can present a problem to the patient. The school nurse can help teachers and other children understand seizures.

Denial. Be alert for signs of denial of the disease, indicated by increased seizure activity in a previously well-controlled patient. Question compliance with the drug regimen.

Adherence. Determine the patient's current medication schedule: name of medication, dosage, and time of last dose. Have any doses been skipped? If so, how many? If adherence appears to be a problem, try to determine the reasons for patient nonadherence so that appropriate interventions can be implemented.

Status Epilepticus

1. Provide patient protection and summon assistance for transportation of the patient to an emergency facility.
2. Administer oxygen; have suction and resuscitation equipment available.
3. Establish an intravenous (IV) line and have available drugs for treatment (e.g., lorazepam, diazepam, phenytoin, phenobarbital). When administering IV drugs, monitor for bradycardia, hypotension, and respiratory depression.
4. Monitor vital signs and neurologic status.
5. Insert a nasogastric tube if patient is vomiting.

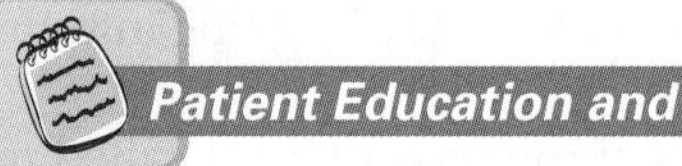

Patient Education and Health Promotion

Exercise and Activity. Encourage maintenance of a regular lifestyle with moderate activity. Avoid excessive exercise that would lead to excessive fatigue.

Nutrition. Avoid excessive use of stimulants (e.g., caffeine-containing products). Seizures are also known to follow the significant intake of alcoholic beverages; therefore ingestion should be avoided or limited. Ask the health care provider whether vitamin supplements are needed, because some anticonvulsants interfere with vitamin and mineral absorption.

Safety. Teach the patient to avoid operating power equipment or machinery. Driving may be minimized or prohibited. Check state laws regarding how or if an individual with a history of seizure activity may qualify for a driver's license. In the elderly, be especially alert to signs of confusion and impaired coordination. Provide safety.

Stress. Reduction of tension and stress within the individual's environment may reduce seizure activity in some patients.

Oral Hygiene. Encourage daily oral hygiene practices and scheduling regular dental examinations. **Gingival hyperplasia,** gum overgrowth associated with hydantoins (e.g., phenytoin, ethotoin), can be reduced by good oral hygiene, frequent gum massage, regular brushing, and proper dental care.

Medication Considerations

- If pregnancy is suspected, consult an obstetrician as soon as possible. Inform the health care provider of seizure medications. Do not discontinue medications unless told to do so by the health care provider.
- The patient should carry an identification card or bracelet.

Expectations of Therapy. Discuss the expectations of therapy (e.g., level of seizure control, degree of lethargy, sedation, frequency of use of therapy, relief of symptoms, sexual activity, maintenance of mobility, ability to maintain activities of daily living (ADLs) or work, limitations in operating power equipment or a motor vehicle). Assess changes in expectations as therapy progresses and the patient gains understanding and skill in the management of the diagnosis.

Fostering Health Maintenance. Throughout the course of treatment, discuss medication information and how it will benefit the patient. Recognize that nonadherence may be a means of denial. Explore underlying problems in acceptance of disease and the need for strict compliance for maximum seizure control. Provide the patient and significant others with important information contained in the specific drug monograph for the medicines prescribed. Additional health teaching and nursing interventions for the side effects to expect and report are described in the drug monographs that follow. Seek cooperation and understanding of the following points so that medication compliance is increased: name of medication, dosage, route and times of administration, side effects to expect, and side effects to report.

Written Record. Enlist the patient's aid in developing and maintaining a written record of monitoring parameters (e.g., degree of lethargy; sedation; oral hygiene for gum disorders; degree of seizure relief; nausea, vomiting, or anorexia present) (see Patient Self-Assessment Form on p. 301). Complete the Premedication Data column for use as a baseline to track response to drug therapy. Ensure that the patient and significant others understand how to use the form. Have others record the date, time, duration, and frequency of any seizure episodes. Also record the behavior immediately before and after seizures. Emphasize taking medications at the same time daily to help maintain a consistent therapeutic drug level. Consult with a pharmacist before taking over-the-counter (OTC) medications to prevent drug interactions. Have the patient bring the completed form to follow-up visits.

Difficulty in Comprehension. If it is evident that the patient or family does not understand all aspects of continuing prescribed therapy (e.g., administering and monitoring medications, managing seizure activity when present, diets, follow-up appointments, the need for lifelong management), consider using social services or visiting nurse agencies. ■

DRUG THERAPY FOR SEIZURE DISORDERS

DRUG CLASS: Benzodiazepines

Actions

The mechanism of action for benzodiazepines is not fully understood, but it is thought that benzodiazepines inhibit neurotransmission by enhancing the effects of GABA in postsynaptic clefts between nerve cells.

Uses

The three benzodiazepines approved for use as anticonvulsants are diazepam, clonazepam, and clorazepate. Clonazepam is useful in the oral treatment of absence, akinetic, and myoclonic seizures in children. Diazepam

PATIENT SELF-ASSESSMENT FORM Anticonvulsants

MEDICATIONS	COLOR	TO BE TAKEN

Patient ______

Health Care Provider ______

Health Care Provider's phone ______

Next appt.* ______

What I Should Monitor		Premedication Data	Date	Date	Date	Date	Date	Date	Comments
Previous seizure activity	Number/day								
	Lasted how long								
	Type, describe								
Present seizure activity	Number/day								
	Lasted how long								
	Type, describe								
	Slept after (Yes/No)								
Compliance	I take my medication as ordered								
	Sometimes I forget								
	I don't like to take my medication								
Drowsiness **Feel like sleeping all day** — **Feel like being active** **10** — **5** — **1**									
Disease acceptance **I don't want people to know I have epilepsy** — **I have epilepsy and take medication** **10** — **5** — **1**									
Oral hygiene: Brushing and flossing teeth	3 times a day								
	2 times a day								
	1 time a day								
	I forgot								
Condition of gums	No bleeding								
	Some bleeding (____) Times/day								
	Bleeding every time I brush								
Nausea and vomiting	All day								
	Sometimes (when)								
Other									

*Please bring this record with you to your next appointment.
Use the back of this sheet for additional information.

must be administered intravenously to control seizures and is the drug of choice for treatment of status epilepticus. Clorazepate is used with other antiepileptic agents to control partial seizures.

Therapeutic Outcomes

The primary therapeutic outcomes expected from the benzodiazepines are as follows:

1. Reduced frequency of seizures and reduced injury from seizure activity.
2. Minimal adverse effects from therapy.

Nursing Process for Benzodiazepines

Premedication Assessment

1. Review routine blood studies to detect blood dyscrasias and hepatotoxicity.
2. Perform a baseline assessment of the patient's speech patterns; degree of alertness; and orientation to name, place, and time before initiating therapy. Monitor behavioral responses to therapy.
3. Review the medical record to document frequency of seizure activity.

Planning

Availability. See Table 19-2.

Implementation

Dosage and Administration. See Table 19-2. NOTE: Rapidly discontinuing benzodiazepines after long-term use may result in symptoms similar to those of alcohol withdrawal. These may vary from weakness and anxiety to delirium and generalized tonic-clonic seizures. The symptoms may not appear for several days after discontinuation. Treatment consists of gradual withdrawal of benzodiazepines over 2 to 4 weeks.

Intravenous Administration. Do not mix parenteral diazepam in the same syringe with other medications; do not add to other IV solutions because of

Drug Table 19-2 ANTICONVULSANTS

GENERIC NAME	BRAND NAME	AVAILABILITY	ADULT DOSAGE RANGE	USE IN SEIZURES
BENZODIAZEPINES				
clonazepam	Klonopin, ✱ Rivotril	Tablets: 0.5, 1, 2 mg Tablets, orally disintegrating: 0.125, 0.25, 0.5, 1, 2 mg	Up to 20 mg/day	Absence, myoclonic seizures
clorazepate	Tranxene, ✱ Novoclopate	Tablets: 3.75, 7.5, 11.25, 15, 22 mg	Up to 90 mg/day	Focal seizures
diazepam	Valium, ✱ Apo-Diazepam	Tablets: 2, 5, 10 mg IV: 5 mg/mL Liquid: 1, 5 mg/mL Gel, rectal: 2.5, 5, 10, 15, 20 mg	Initially 5-10 mg, up to 30 mg	All forms of epilepsy; used in conjunction with other agents
lorazepam	Ativan, ✱ Novolorazepam	Tablets: 0.5, 1, 2 mg Oral solution: 2 mg/mL IM, IV: 2, 4 mg/mL	IV: 4-8 mg repeated at 10- to 15-minute intervals if seizing	Status epilepticus
HYDANTOINS				
ethotoin	Peganone	Tablets: 250 mg	2-3 g/day	Generalized tonic-clonic seizures; psychomotor seizures
fosphenytoin	Cerebyx	IV: 75 mg/mL in 2- and 10-mL vials	As for phenytoin	
phenytoin	Dilantin	Tablets: 50 mg Capsules: 30, 100 mg Suspension: 125 mg/5 mL Inj: 50 mg/mL in 2- and 5-mL ampules	300-600 mg/day	Generalized tonic-clonic seizures; psychomotor seizures
SUCCINIMIDES				
ethosuximide	Zarontin	Capsules: 250 mg Syrup: 250 mg/5 mL	1000-1250 mg/day	Absence seizures
methsuximide	Celontin	Capsules: 150, 300 mg	900-1200 mg/day	Absence seizures

✱ Available in Canada.

precipitate formation. Administer slowly at a rate of no more than 5 mg per minute. If at all possible, give under electrocardiogram (ECG) monitoring and observe closely for bradycardia. Stop boluses until the heart rate returns to normal.

Evaluation

Side Effects to Expect

Sedation, Drowsiness, Dizziness, Blurred Vision, Fatigue, Lethargy. The more common side effects of benzodiazepines are extensions of their pharmacologic properties. These symptoms tend to disappear with continued therapy and possible dosage readjustment. Encourage the patient not to discontinue therapy without first consulting the health care provider.

People who work around machinery, operate a motor vehicle, or perform other duties in which they must remain mentally alert should be particularly cautious. Provide patient safety during episodes of dizziness and ataxia; report for further evaluation.

Caution the patient that blurred vision may occur, and make appropriate suggestions for personal safety of the individual.

Side Effects to Report

Behavioral Disturbances. Behavioral disturbances such as aggressiveness and agitation have been reported, especially in patients who are mentally retarded or have psychiatric disturbances. Provide supportive physical care and safety during these responses.

Assess the level of excitement and deal calmly with the individual. During periods of excitement, protect people from harm and provide for physical channeling of energy (e.g., walk with them). Seek change in the medication order.

Blood Dyscrasias. Routine laboratory studies (red blood cell count [RBC], white blood cell count [WBC], and differential counts) should be scheduled. Monitor for sore throat, fever, purpura, jaundice, or excessive and progressive weakness.

Hepatotoxicity. The symptoms of hepatotoxicity are anorexia, nausea, vomiting, jaundice, hepatomegaly, splenomegaly, and abnormal liver function tests (e.g., elevated bilirubin, aspartate aminotransferase [AST], alanine aminotransferase [ALT], gamma-glutamyltransferase [GGT], alkaline phosphatase, prothrombin time [PT]).

Drug Interactions

Drugs That Increase Toxic Effects. Antihistamines, alcohol, analgesics, anesthetics, tranquilizers, narcotics, cimetidine, sedative-hypnotics, and other anticonvulsants. Monitor the patient for excessive sedation, and eliminate the nonanticonvulsants if possible.

Smoking. Smoking enhances the metabolism of benzodiazepines. Larger doses may be necessary to maintain effects in patients who smoke.

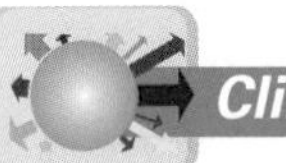

Clinical Landmine

Do not mix parenteral diazepam or phenytoin with other medications in the same syringe, and do not add either medication to other IV solutions because of precipitate formation. Always check for IV incompatibility before administering either medicine through an established IV line and use the SAS (saline flush, administer drug, saline flush) technique! Administer **diazepam slowly at a rate of 5 mg per minute.** Administer **phenytoin slowly at a rate of 25 to 50 mg per minute.** During administration of either medication it is recommended that an electrocardiograph monitor be used to closely observe for bradycardia. Should bradycardia occur, stop the bolus infusion until the heart rate returns to normal. Observe the patient during administration for respiratory depression and hypotension.

DRUG CLASS: Hydantoins

Actions

The mechanism of action of the hydantoins is unknown.

Uses

Hydantoins (phenytoin, ethotoin, and fosphenytoin) are anticonvulsants used to control partial (psychomotor) seizures and generalized tonic-clonic seizures. Phenytoin is by far the most commonly used anticonvulsant of the hydantoins. Fosphenytoin is a prodrug that is converted to phenytoin after administration.

Therapeutic Outcomes

The primary therapeutic outcomes expected from the hydantoins are as follows:

1. Reduced frequency of seizures and reduced injury from seizure activity.
2. Minimal adverse effects from therapy.

Nursing Process for Phenytoin

Premedication Assessment

1. Review routine blood studies to detect blood dyscrasias and hepatotoxicity.
2. Obtain baseline blood sugar levels in patients with diabetes, and monitor periodically at specified intervals because hyperglycemia may be caused by hydantoin therapy.
3. Perform a baseline assessment of the patient's speech patterns; degree of alertness; and orientation to name, place, and time before initiating therapy. Monitor behavioral responses to therapy.
4. Review the medical record to document frequency of seizure activity.

Planning

Availability. See Table 19-2.

Implementation

Dosage and Administration. See Table 19-2. Administer medication with food or milk to reduce gastric irritation. If an oral suspension is used, shake well first. Encourage the use of an oral syringe for accurate measurement. Intramuscular (IM): If at all possible, avoid IM administration. Absorption is slow and painful. IV: Do not mix parenteral phenytoin in the same syringe with other medications; because of precipitate formation, do not add to other IV solutions.

Administer slowly at a rate of 25 to 50 mg per minute. If at all possible, give under electrocardiogram (ECG) monitoring and observe closely for bradycardia. Stop boluses until the heart rate returns to normal. Therapeutic blood levels for phenytoin are 10 to 20 mg/L.

Evaluation

Side Effects to Expect

Nausea, Vomiting, Indigestion. These effects are common during initiation of therapy. Gradual increases in dosage and administration with food or milk will reduce gastric irritation.

Sedation, Drowsiness, Dizziness, Blurred Vision, Fatigue, Lethargy. These symptoms tend to disappear with continued therapy and possible dosage adjustment. Encourage the patient not to discontinue therapy without first consulting the health care provider.

People who work around machinery, drive a car, or perform other duties in which they must remain mentally alert should be particularly cautious. Provide patient safety during episodes of dizziness; report for further evaluation. Caution the patient that blurred vision may occur, and make appropriate suggestions for personal safety of the individual.

Confusion. Perform a baseline assessment of the patient's degree of alertness and orientation to name, place, and time before initiating therapy. Make regularly scheduled subsequent evaluations of mental status and compare findings. Report alterations.

Gingival Hyperplasia. The frequency of gum overgrowth may be reduced by good oral hygiene, including gum massage, frequent brushing, and proper dental care.

Side Effects to Report

Hyperglycemia. Hydantoins may elevate blood glucose levels, especially if higher doses are used; patients with diabetes mellitus are more susceptible to hyperglycemia. Particularly during the early weeks of therapy, diabetic or prediabetic patients must be monitored for the development of hyperglycemia.

Assess regularly for glycosuria and report if it occurs with any frequency. Patients receiving oral hypoglycemic agents or insulin may require a dosage adjustment.

Blood Dyscrasias. Routine laboratory studies (RBC, WBC, and differential counts) should be scheduled. Monitor for sore throat, fever, purpura, jaundice, or excessive and progressive weakness.

Hepatotoxicity. The symptoms of hepatotoxicity are anorexia, nausea, vomiting, jaundice, hepatomegaly, splenomegaly, and abnormal liver function tests (e.g., elevated bilirubin, AST, ALT, GGT, alkaline phosphatase, prothrombin time).

Dermatologic Reactions. Report a rash or pruritus immediately and withhold additional doses pending approval by the health care provider.

Drug Interactions

Drugs That Enhance Therapeutic and Toxic Effects. Warfarin, carbamazepine, oxcarbazepine (>1200 mg/day), topiramide, metronidazole, miconazole, omeprazole, phenothiazines, disulfiram, amiodarone, isoniazid, chloramphenicol, cimetidine, and sulfonamides enhance therapeutic as well as toxic effects. Monitor patients with concurrent therapy for signs of phenytoin toxicity: **nystagmus** (involuntary rhythmic, uncontrollable movements of one or both eyes), sedation, or lethargy. Serum levels may be ordered, and a reduced dosage of phenytoin may be required.

Drugs That Decrease Therapeutic Effects. Barbiturates, loxapine, nitrofurantoin, theophylline, ethanol (chronic ingestion), rifampin, sucralfate, folic acid, and antacids decrease therapeutic effects. Monitor patients with concurrent therapy for increased seizure activity. Monitoring changes in serum levels should help warn of possible increased seizure activity.

Disopyramide, Quinidine, Mexiletine. Phenytoin decreases serum levels of these agents. Monitor patients for redevelopment of dysrhythmias.

Prednisolone, Dexamethasone. Phenytoin decreases serum levels of these agents. Monitor patients for reduced antiinflammatory activity.

Oral Contraceptives. Spotting or bleeding may be an indication of reduced contraceptive activity. Using alternative forms of birth control is recommended.

Theophylline. Phenytoin decreases serum levels of theophylline derivatives. Monitor patients for a greater frequency of respiratory difficulty. The theophylline dosage may need to be increased 50% to 100% to maintain the same therapeutic response.

Valproic Acid. This agent may increase or decrease the activity of phenytoin. Monitor for increased frequency of seizure activity. Monitoring changes in serum levels should help warn of possible increased seizure activity. Monitor patients with concurrent therapy for signs of phenytoin toxicity: nystagmus, sedation, lethargy. Serum levels may be ordered, and a reduced dosage of phenytoin may be required.

Ketoconazole. Concurrent administration with ketoconazole may alter the metabolism of one or both drugs. Monitoring for both is recommended.

Cyclosporine. Phenytoin enhances the metabolism of cyclosporine. Increased dosages of cyclosporine may be necessary in patients receiving concomitant therapy.

DRUG CLASS: Succinimides

Actions

The mechanism of action of the succinimides is unknown.

Uses

Succinimides (e.g., ethosuximide, methsuximide) are used to control absence (petit mal) seizures.

Therapeutic Outcomes

The primary therapeutic outcomes expected from the succinimides are as follows:

1. Reduced frequency of seizures and reduced injury from seizure activity.
2. Minimal adverse effects from therapy.

Nursing Process for Succinimides

Premedication Assessment

1. Review routine blood studies to detect blood dyscrasias and hepatotoxicity.
2. Perform a baseline assessment of the patient's speech patterns; degree of alertness; and orientation to name, place, and time before initiating therapy. Monitor behavioral responses to therapy.
3. Review the medical record to document frequency of seizure activity.

Planning

Availability. See Table 19-2.

Implementation

Dosage and Administration. See Table 19-2.

Evaluation

Side Effects to Expect

Nausea, Vomiting, Indigestion. These effects are common during initiation of therapy. Gradual increases in dosage and administration with food or milk will reduce gastric irritation.

Sedation, Drowsiness, Dizziness, Fatigue, Lethargy. These symptoms tend to disappear with continued therapy and possible dosage adjustment. Encourage the patient not to discontinue therapy without first consulting the physician.

People who work around machinery, operate a motor vehicle, or perform other duties in which they must remain mentally alert should be particularly cautious. Provide patient safety during episodes of dizziness; report for further evaluation.

Drug Interactions

Drugs That Enhance Toxic Effects. Antihistamines, alcohol, analgesics, anesthetics, tranquilizers, other anticonvulsants, and sedative-hypnotics.

DRUG CLASS: Miscellaneous Anticonvulsants

carbamazepine (kar bah maz' e peen)
▶ TEGRETOL (teg' reh tol)

Actions

Carbamazepine blocks the reuptake of norepinephrine and decreases the release of norepinephrine and the rate of dopamine and GABA turnover. Despite knowing these pharmacologic effects, the mechanisms of action as an anticonvulsant, selective analgesic, and antimanic agent are unknown. Carbamazepine is structurally related to the tricyclic antidepressants.

Uses

Carbamazepine is an anticonvulsant often used in combination with other anticonvulsants to control generalized tonic-clonic and partial seizures. It is not effective in controlling myoclonic or absence seizures. Carbamazepine has also been used successfully to treat the pain associated with trigeminal neuralgia (tic douloureux). It may also be used to treat manic-depressive disorders when lithium therapy has not been optimal.

Therapeutic Outcomes

The primary therapeutic outcomes expected from carbamazepine are as follows:

1. Reduced frequency of seizures and reduced injury from seizure activity.
2. Minimal adverse effects from therapy.

Nursing Process for Carbamazepine

Premedication Assessment

1. As a result of serious adverse reactions, the manufacturer recommends that the following baseline studies be repeated at regular intervals: complete blood count (CBC), liver function tests, urinalysis, blood urea nitrogen (BUN), serum creatinine, and ophthalmologic examination.
2. Perform a baseline assessment of the patient's speech patterns; degree of alertness; and orientation to name, place, and time before initiating therapy. Monitor behavioral responses to therapy.
3. Review the medical record to document frequency of seizure activity.

Planning

Availability. PO: 100 and 200 mg tablets; 100, 200, and 400 mg extended release tablets; 200 and 300 mg extended release capsules; 100 mg/5 mL suspension.

Implementation

Dosage and Administration. *Adult:* PO: Initial dose is 200 mg two times daily in the first day. Increase gradually by 200 mg per day in divided doses at 6- to 8-hour intervals. Do not exceed 1600 mg daily. Therapeutic plasma levels for carbamazepine are 4 to 10 mg/L.

Evaluation

Side Effects to Expect

Nausea, Vomiting, Drowsiness, Dizziness. These effects can be reduced by slowly increasing the dose. They are usually mild and tend to resolve with continued therapy. Encourage the patient not to discontinue therapy without first consulting the health care provider.

Provide patient safety during episodes of drowsiness or dizziness. Patients must be warned about not working around machinery, operating a motor vehicle, or performing other duties in which they must remain mentally alert until it is known how they are affected by this medication.

Side Effects to Report

Orthostatic Hypotension, Hypertension. Monitor the blood pressure daily in both the supine and standing positions. Anticipate the development of postural hypotension and take measures to prevent an occurrence. Teach the patient to rise slowly from a supine or sitting position; encourage the patient to sit or lie down if feeling faint.

Dyspnea, Edema. If carbamazepine is used in patients with a history of heart failure, monitor daily weights, lung sounds, and accumulation of edema.

Neurologic Assessment. Perform a baseline assessment of the patient's speech patterns; degree of alertness; and orientation to name, place, and time before initiating therapy. Make regularly scheduled subsequent evaluations of mental status, and compare findings. Report alterations.

Nephrotoxicity. Monitor urinalysis and kidney function tests for abnormal results. Report an increasing BUN and creatinine; decreasing urine output or specific gravity despite amount of fluid intake; casts or protein in the urine; frank blood or smoky-colored urine; or RBC in excess of 0 to 3 on the urinalysis report.

Hepatotoxicity. The symptoms of hepatotoxicity are anorexia, nausea, vomiting, jaundice, hepatomegaly, splenomegaly, and abnormal liver function tests (elevated bilirubin, AST, ALT, GGT, alkaline phosphatase, and prothrombin time).

Blood Dyscrasias. Routine laboratory studies (RBC, WBC, and differential counts) should be scheduled. Monitor for sore throat, fever, purpura, jaundice, or excessive and progressive weakness.

Dermatologic Reactions. Report a rash or pruritus immediately and withhold additional doses pending approval by the health care provider.

Drug Interactions

Drugs That Enhance Therapeutic and Toxic Effects. Isoniazid, cimetidine, fluoxetine, fluvoxamine, ketoconazole, and macrolide antibiotics (erythromycin, clarithromycin) inhibit the metabolism of carbamazepine. Monitor for signs of toxicity, such as disorientation, ataxia, lethargy, headache, drowsiness, nausea, and vomiting. Dosage reductions in carbamazepine may be necessary.

Propoxyphene, Verapamil, Diltiazem, Danazol, Lamotrigine, Nefazodone. These drugs increase serum levels of carbamazepine. Monitor for signs of toxicity (e.g., disorientation, ataxia, lethargy, headache, drowsiness, nausea, vomiting). A 40% to 50% decrease in the carbamazepine dosage may be necessary.

Warfarin. Carbamazepine may diminish the anticoagulant effects of warfarin. Monitor the prothrombin time and increase the dosage of warfarin if necessary.

Phenobarbital, Phenytoin, Valproic Acid. Carbamazepine enhances the metabolism of these agents. Monitor for increased frequency of seizure activity. Monitoring changes in serum levels should help warn of possible increased seizure activity.

Doxycycline. Carbamazepine enhances the metabolism of this antibiotic. Monitor patients for signs of continued infection.

Oral Contraceptives. Carbamazepine enhances the metabolism of estrogens. Spotting or bleeding may be an indication of reduced contraceptive activity. Use of other forms of birth control is recommended.

gabapentin (gah bah pen′ tin)
▶ NEURONTIN (nuhr on′ tin)

Actions

The mechanism of action of gabapentin is unknown. It does not appear to enhance GABA.

Uses

Gabapentin is an anticonvulsant usually used in combination with other anticonvulsants to control partial seizures.

Therapeutic Outcomes

The primary therapeutic outcomes expected from gabapentin are as follows:

1. Reduced frequency of seizures and reduced injury from seizure activity
2. Minimal adverse effects from therapy

Nursing Process for Gabapentin

Premedication Assessment

1. Perform a baseline assessment of the patient's speech patterns; degree of alertness; and orientation to name, place, and time before initiating therapy. Monitor behavioral responses to therapy.
2. Review the medical record to document frequency of seizure activity.

Planning

Availability. PO: 100, 300, and 400 mg capsules; 100, 300, 400, 600, and 800 mg tablets; 250 mg/5 mL oral suspension.

Implementation

Dosage and Administration. *Adult:* PO: 900 to 1800 mg daily. Initially administer 300 mg at bedtime on day 1, 300 mg two times on day 2, then 300 mg three times on day 3. Adjust the dosage upward to a maximum of 1800 mg daily in three divided doses using a combination of 300 and 400 mg capsules. The maximum time between doses in the three-times-daily schedule should not exceed 12 hours.

If the patient also uses antacids, administer gabapentin at least 2 hours after the last dose of antacid. Antacids reduce the absorption of gabapentin.

Evaluation

Side Effects to Expect

Sedation, Drowsiness, Dizziness, Blurred Vision. These symptoms tend to disappear with continued therapy and possible dosage adjustment. Encourage the patient not to discontinue therapy without first consulting the health care provider.

Provide patient safety during episodes of drowsiness or dizziness. Patients must be warned about not working around machinery, operating a motor vehicle, or performing other duties in which they must remain mentally alert until it is known how they are affected by this medication.

Caution the patient that blurred vision may occur, and make appropriate suggestions for personal safety of the individual.

Side Effects to Report

Neurologic Assessment. Perform a baseline assessment of the patient's speech patterns; degree of alertness; and orientation to name, place, and time before initiating therapy. Make regularly scheduled subsequent evaluations of mental status and compare findings. Report alterations.

Drug Interactions

Enhanced Sedation. Central nervous system (CNS) depressants, including sleep aids, analgesics, tranquilizers, and alcohol enhance the sedative effects of gabapentin. Patients must be warned about not working around machinery, operating a motor vehicle, or performing other duties in which they must remain mentally alert until it is known how they are affected by this medication. Provide patient safety during episodes of drowsiness or dizziness.

Urine Protein. False-positive readings for protein in the urine have been reported by patients taking gabapentin when using the Ames N-Multistix SG dipstick test. The manufacturer recommends that the more specific sulfosalicylic acid precipitation procedure be used to determine the presence of urine protein.

lamotrigine (lah mot' rah geen)
LAMICTAL (lah mik' tahl)

Actions

Lamotrigine is a new anticonvulsant of the phenyltriazine class, unrelated to other antiepileptic medicines currently available. It is thought to act by blocking voltage-sensitive sodium and calcium channels in neuronal membranes. This stabilizes the neuronal membranes and inhibits the release of excitatory neurotransmitters such as glutamate that may induce seizure activity.

Uses

Lamotrigine is used in combination with other anticonvulsants to treat partial onset seizures and the generalized seizures of Lennox-Gastaut syndrome in pediatric and adult patients.

Therapeutic Outcomes

The primary therapeutic outcomes expected from lamotrigine are as follows:

1. Reduced frequency of seizures and injury from seizure activity
2. Minimal adverse effects from therapy

Nursing Process for Lamotrigine

Premedication Assessment

1. Perform a baseline assessment of the patient's speech patterns; degree of alertness; and orientation to name, place, and time before initiating therapy. Monitor behavioral responses to therapy.
2. Review the medication history to determine whether the patient is already taking valproic acid for seizure control.
3. Review the medical record to document frequency of seizure activity.

Planning

Availability. PO: 25, 100, 150, and 200 mg tablets; 2, 5, and 25 mg chewable tablets.

Implementation

Dosage and Administration. *Adult:* PO: If not already taking valproic acid for seizure control, initiate lamotrigine therapy at 50 mg once a day for 2 weeks, followed by 100 mg per day given in two divided doses for 2 weeks. Thereafter the usual maintenance dose is 300 to 500 mg per day in two divided doses. If the patient is already receiving valproic acid for seizure control, the dosing of lamotrigine is less than half these doses. See manufacturer's recommendations.

Evaluation

Side Effects to Expect

Nausea, Vomiting, Indigestion. These effects are common during initiation of therapy. Gradual increases in dosage and administration with food or milk will reduce gastric irritation.

Sedation, Drowsiness, Dizziness, Blurred Vision. These symptoms tend to disappear with continued therapy and possible dosage adjustment. Encourage the patient not to discontinue therapy without first consulting the health care provider.

Provide patient safety during episodes of drowsiness or dizziness. Patients must be warned not to work around machinery, operate a motor vehicle, or perform other duties in which they must remain mentally alert until it is known how they are affected by this medication.

Caution the patient that blurred vision may occur, and make appropriate suggestions for the individual's safety.

Side Effects to Report

Skin Rash. Approximately 10% of patients receiving lamotrigine develop a skin rash and urticaria in the first 4 to 6 weeks of therapy. Slower increases in each dosage adjustment are thought to decrease the incidence of rash. In most cases, the rash resolves with continued therapy; however, the health care provider should be promptly informed because the rash could also be an early indicator of a more serious condition. Combination therapy with valproic acid appears to be more likely to precipitate a serious rash.

Encourage the patient not to discontinue the lamotrigine until alternative anticonvulsant therapy can be considered to prevent renewed seizure activity.

Drug Interactions

Drugs That Enhance Therapeutic and Toxic Effects. Valproic acid reduces the metabolism of lamotrigine by as much as 50%. Significant lamotrigine dosage reductions may be required.

Drugs That Decrease Therapeutic Effects. Phenobarbital, phenytoin, primadone, carbamazepine, oxcarbazepine, ethosuximide, rifampin, acetaminophen, and progestin oral contraceptives enhance the metabolism of lamotrigine. Monitor for increased frequency of seizure activity. Monitoring changes in serum levels should help warn of possible increased seizure activity. Twice daily administration of lamotrigine may be necessary.

Enhanced Sedation. CNS depressants, including sleep aids, analgesics, tranquilizers, and alcohol enhance the sedative effects of lamotrigine. Patients must be warned about not working around machinery, operating a motor vehicle, or performing other duties in which they must remain mentally alert until it is known how they are affected by this medication. Provide patient safety during episodes of drowsiness or dizziness.

levetiracetam (lehv et tihr ah see' tahm)
KEPPRA (kep' rah)

Actions

Levetiracetam is classified as a pyrrolidine derivative chemically unrelated to other antiepileptic drugs available. Its mechanism of action is unknown. It does not appear to act on sodium, potassium, or calcium ion pathways, or stimulate GABA as other anticonvulsants do.

Uses

Levetiracetam is approved for use in combination with other anticonvulsants in the treatment of adult partial seizures.

Therapeutic Outcomes

The primary therapeutic outcomes sought from levetiracetam are as follows:

1. Reduced frequency of seizures and reduced injury from seizure activity.
2. Minimal adverse effects from therapy.

Nursing Process for Levetiracetam

Premedication Assessment

1. Review the medical record to document frequency of seizure activity.
2. Perform a baseline assessment of the patient's speech patterns; degree of alertness; and orientation to name, place, and time before initiating therapy.
3. Review the medical record to document frequency of seizure activity.
4. Review laboratory reports; report abnormal renal function (BUN, creatinine, creatinine clearance).

Planning

Availability. PO: 250, 500, and 750 mg tablets; 100 mg/mL oral solution.

Implementation

Dosage and Administration. *Adult:* PO: Initial dose is 500 mg two times daily. Dosage may be increased every 2 weeks by 500 mg two times daily until attaining a maximum dose of 3000 mg daily. NOTE: Dosage adjustment is necessary in patients whose creatinine clearance is less than 80 mL per minute. See the package insert for additional directions.

Evaluation

Side Effects to Expect

Weakness, Drowsiness, Dizziness. These effects can be reduced by slowly increasing the dosage. These effects are usually mild and tend to resolve with continued therapy. Encourage the patient not to discontinue therapy without first consulting the health care provider.

Provide patient safety during episodes of weakness and dizziness. Patients must be warned about not working around machinery, operating a motor vehicle, or performing other duties in which they must remain mentally alert until it is known how they are affected by this medication.

Side Effects to Report

Neurologic Assessment. Perform a baseline assessment of the patient's speech patterns; degree of alertness; and orientation to name, place, and time before initiating therapy. Make regularly scheduled subsequent evaluations of mental status and compare findings. Report alterations.

Drug Interactions

Enhanced Sedation. CNS depressants, including sleep aids, analgesics, tranquilizers, and alcohol enhance the sedative effects of levetiracetam. Patients must be warned about not working around machinery, operating a motor vehicle, or performing other duties in which they must remain mentally alert until it is known how they are affected by this medication.

oxcarbazepine (ox karb az′ e peen)

▶ TRILEPTAL (tri lehp′ tahl)

Actions

Oxcarbazepine is a prodrug that metabolizes into some of the active metabolites of carbamazepine. Oxcarbazepine interacts with sodium, potassium, and calcium ion channels, stabilizing the neurons, and preventing repetitive firing and propagation of electrical impulses thought to induce seizures.

Uses

Oxcarbazepine is used as monotherapy or combination therapy in treating partial seizures in adults and as combination therapy in treating partial seizures in children 4 to 16 years of age.

Therapeutic Outcomes

The primary therapeutic outcomes expected from oxcarbazepine are as follows:

1. Reduced frequency of seizures and injury from seizure activity.
2. Minimal adverse effects from therapy.

Nursing Process for Oxcarbazepine

Premedication Assessment

1. As a result of serious adverse reactions, the manufacturer recommends that serum electrolyte baseline studies be collected and then repeated periodically while the patient is receiving oxcarbazepine therapy.
2. Review the patient's medication history to ensure that the patient does not have an allergy to carbamazepine. If there is an allergy, inform the charge nurse and the health care provider immediately. Do not administer the medication without specific approval.
3. Perform a baseline assessment of the patient's speech patterns; degree of alertness; and orientation to name, place, and time before initiating therapy. Monitor behavioral responses to therapy.
4. Review the medical record to document frequency of seizure activity.

Planning

Availability. PO: 150, 300, and 600 mg tablets; 300 mg/5 mL suspension.

Implementation

Dosage and Administration. *Adult:* PO: Initial dosage is 300 mg two times daily for the first 3 days. The dosage may be increased by 300 mg per day every 3 days to a dosage of 1200 mg per day. Dosages of 2400 mg per day have been found to be effective in patients converted from other anticonvulsant therapy to monotherapy with oxcarbazepine.

Pediatric (ages 4 to 16): PO: Initial dosage is 4 to 5 mg/kg two times daily, not to exceed 600 mg per day. The dosage should be gradually increased over the next 2 weeks to a maintenance level based on body weight:

20-29 kg	900 mg/day
29.1-39 kg	1200 mg/day
>39 kg	1800 mg/day

Evaluation

Side Effects to Expect

Confusion, Poor Coordination, Drowsiness, Dizziness. These effects can be reduced by slowly increasing the dosage. They are usually mild and tend to resolve with continued therapy. Encourage the patient not to discontinue therapy without first consulting the health care provider.

Perform a baseline assessment of the patient's speech patterns; degree of alertness; and orientation to name, place, and time before initiating therapy. Make regularly scheduled subsequent evaluations of mental status, and compare findings. Report alterations.

Provide patient safety during episodes of drowsiness, confusion, or dizziness. Patients must be warned about not working around machinery, operating a motor vehicle, or performing other duties in which they must remain mentally alert until it is known how they are affected by this medication.

Side Effects to Report

Nausea, Headache, Lethargy, Confusion, Obtundation, Malaise. These are symptoms of hyponatremia. It is extremely important to notify the health care provider. Withhold additional doses of medicine until specifically told to administer the medication.

Drug Interactions

Drugs That Decrease Therapeutic Effects. Phenobarbital, primidone, phenytoin, valproic acid, carbamazepine, and verapamil may enhance the metabolism of oxcarbazepine. Monitor for increased frequency of seizure activity. Dosages of oxcarbazepine may need to be increased.

Oral Contraceptives. Oxcarbazepine enhances the metabolism of estrogens and progestins. Spotting or bleeding may be an indication of reduced contraceptive activity. Recommend using other forms of birth control.

phenobarbital (fee no barb′ it al)
LUMINAL (loom′ in al)

Actions

Phenobarbital, a long-acting barbiturate, elevates the seizure threshold and prevents the spread of electrical seizure activity by enhancing the inhibitory effect of GABA. The exact mechanism is unknown.

Uses

Phenobarbital is an effective anticonvulsant. Because of its sedative effects, however, it is now used primarily as an alternative when single, nonsedating anticonvulsants are unsuccessful in controlling seizures. Phenobarbital is most useful in treating partial and generalized tonic-clonic seizures and generalized myoclonic seizures, usually in combination with other anticonvulsants. Barbiturates are discussed in greater detail in Chapter 14.

Therapeutic Outcomes

The primary therapeutic outcomes expected from phenobarbital are as follows:

1. Reduced frequency of seizures and reduced injury due to seizure activity.
2. Minimal adverse effects from therapy.

primidone (prih′ mih doan)
MYSOLINE (my′ so leen)

Actions

Primidone is structurally related to the barbiturates. It is metabolized into phenobarbital and phenylethylmalonamide (PEMA), both of which are active anticonvulsants. The exact mechanism of anticonvulsant action is unknown.

Uses

Primidone is used in combination with other anticonvulsants to treat partial onset seizures and generalized tonic-clonic seizures.

Therapeutic Outcomes

The primary therapeutic outcomes expected from primidone are as follows:

1. Reduced frequency of seizures and reduced injury from seizure activity
2. Minimal adverse effects from therapy

Nursing Process for Primidone

Premedication Assessment

1. Review routine blood studies to detect blood dyscrasias.
2. Perform a baseline assessment of the patient's speech patterns; degree of alertness; and orientation to name, place, and time before initiating therapy. Monitor behavioral responses to therapy. In children, assess degree of excitability present.
3. Review the medical record to document frequency of seizure activity.

Planning

Availability. PO: 50 and 250 mg tablets

Implementation

Dosage and Administration. *Adult:* PO: Initially 100 to 125 mg daily at bedtime for 3 days. On days 4 through 6, increase the dosage to 100 to 125 mg two times daily. On days 7 through 9, increase the dosage to 100 to 125 mg three times daily. Increase by 100 to 125 mg daily every 3 or 4 days until therapeutic response or intolerance develops. The typical dosage is 750 to 1500 mg daily. Do not exceed 2000 mg daily.

Evaluation

Side Effects to Expect

Sedation, Drowsiness, Dizziness, Blurred Vision. These symptoms tend to disappear with continued therapy and possible dosage adjustment. Encourage the patient not to discontinue therapy without first consulting the health care provider.

People working around machinery, operating a motor vehicle, or performing other duties in which they must remain mentally alert should be particularly cautious until they know how this medication will affect them. Provide patient safety during episodes of dizziness; report for further evaluation. Caution the patient that blurred vision may occur.

Side Effects to Report

Blood Dyscrasias. Blood dyscrasias have rarely been reported with the use of primidone. Routine laboratory studies (e.g., RBC, WBC, differential counts) should be scheduled. Monitor for sore throat, fever, purpura, jaundice, or excessive and progressive weakness.

Paradoxical Excitability. Primidone may cause paradoxical excitability in children. During a period of excitement, protect people from harm and provide for physical channeling of energy (e.g., walk with them). Notify the health care provider for a possible change in medication.

Drug Interactions

Oral Contraceptives. Spotting or bleeding may be an indication of reduced contraceptive activity. Recommend alternate forms of birth control.

Phenytoin. Phenytoin may increase the phenobarbital serum levels when taken concurrently with primidone. Monitor patients for increased sedation.

tiagabine (tee ag′ ah bean)

▶ Gabatril (gab′ ah tril)

Actions

The mechanism of action of tiagabine is unknown. It does appear to prevent the reuptake of GABA into presynaptic neurons, permitting more GABA to be available to act as an inhibitory neurotransmitter.

Uses

Tiagabine is an anticonvulsant usually used in combination with other anticonvulsants to control partial seizures.

Therapeutic Outcomes

The primary therapeutic outcomes expected from tiagabine are as follows:

1. Reduced frequency of seizures and injury from seizure activity.
2. Minimal adverse effects from therapy.

Nursing Process for Tiagabine

Premedication Assessment

1. Perform a baseline assessment of the patient's speech patterns; degree of alertness; and orientation to name, place, and time before initiating therapy. Monitor behavioral responses to therapy.
2. Review the medical record to document frequency of seizure activity.

Planning

Availability. PO: 2, 4, 12, and 16 mg tablets.

Implementation

Dosage and Administration. Adult: PO: Initially 4 mg once daily. Increase the daily dosage by 4 to 8 mg at weekly intervals until clinical response is achieved or a total daily dosage of 56 mg has been achieved. A total daily dosage of 32 to 56 mg may be taken in two to four divided doses.

Evaluation

Side Effects to Expect

Sedation, Drowsiness, Dizziness. These symptoms tend to disappear with continued therapy and possible dosage adjustment. Encourage the patient not to discontinue therapy without first consulting the health care provider.

People working around machinery, operating a motor vehicle, or performing other duties in which they must remain mentally alert should be particularly cautious until they know how this medication will affect them. Provide patient safety during episodes of dizziness; report for further evaluation.

Side Effects to Report

Neurologic Assessment, Memory Loss. Perform a baseline assessment of the patient's speech patterns and degree of alertness, as well as orientation to name, place, and time before initiating therapy. Make regularly scheduled subsequent evaluations of mental status, and compare findings. Report alterations.

Drug Interactions

Drugs That Decrease Therapeutic Effects. Phenobarbital, primidone, phenytoin, carbamazepine may enhance the metabolism of tiagabine. Monitor for increased frequency of seizure activity. Monitoring changes in serum levels should help warn of the potential for increased seizure activity.

Enhanced Sedation. CNS depressants, including sleep aids, analgesics, tranquilizers, and alcohol enhance the sedative effects of tiagabine. Patients must be warned about not working around machinery, operating a motor vehicle, or performing other duties in which they must remain mentally alert until they know how they will be affected by this medication. Provide patient safety during episodes of drowsiness or dizziness.

topiramate (toh peer′ ah mate)

▶ Topamax (toh′ pah max)

Actions

The mechanism of action of topiramate as an anticonvulsant is unknown. Three potential mechanisms may support the anticonvulsant activity: (1) prolonged blockade of sodium channels in the neuronal membrane, (2) potentiation of the activity of the inhibitory neurotransmitter GABA, and (3) antagonism of certain receptors for the excitatory neurotransmitter.

Uses

Topiramate is an anticonvulsant used in combination with other anticonvulsants to control partial and generalized tonic-clonic seizures. It is also used in patients

2 years of age and older with seizures associated with Lennox-Gastaut syndrome.

Topiramate has also been approved for adults in the prevention (but not treatment) of migraine headaches.

Therapeutic Outcomes

The primary therapeutic outcomes expected from topiramate are as follows:

1. Reduced frequency of seizures and reduced injury from seizure activity.
2. Minimal adverse effects from therapy.

Nursing Process for Topiramate

Premedication Assessment

1. Perform a baseline assessment of the patient's speech patterns and degree of alertness, as well as orientation to name, place, and time before initiating therapy. Monitor behavioral responses to therapy.
2. Obtain a baseline weight for future reference. Weight loss may be a side effect of topiramate therapy.
3. Assess the baseline state of hydration. Rare cases of oligohydrosis (decreased sweating) and hyperthermia have been reported, particularly in children and those patients taking other medicines with anticholinergic activity. Proper hydration before and during activities such as exercise or exposure to warm temperatures is recommended.
4. Review the medical record to document frequency of seizure activity.
5. If used for migraine prevention, review the medical record to document frequency of migraine headaches.

Planning

Availability. PO: 25, 50, 100, and 200 mg tablets and 15 and 25 mg sprinkle capsules.

Implementation

Dosage and Administration

Anticonvulsant. *Adult:* PO: Initially 25 mg twice daily. Increase the daily dosage by 50 mg at weekly intervals until clinical response is achieved. The usual recommended daily dosage is 400 mg in two divided doses. Topiramate may be taken with or without food. The tablets should not be broken because they taste bitter. The sprinkle capsules may be swallowed whole or administered by carefully opening the capsule and sprinkling the entire contents on a small amount (teaspoon) of soft food. Swallow this drug/food mixture immediately; do not chew.

Migraine Prevention. *Adult*: PO: Use either the tablets or sprinkle capsules. Initially, week 1: 25 mg daily in the evening. Week 2: 25 mg morning and evening. Week 3: 25 mg in the morning, and 50 mg in the evening. Week 4 and thereafter: 50 mg in the morning and 50 mg in the evening. Do not use topiramate to treat migraine headaches.

Evaluation

Side Effects to Expect

Sedation, Drowsiness, Dizziness. These symptoms tend to disappear with continued therapy and possible dosage adjustment. Encourage the patient not to discontinue therapy without first consulting the health care provider.

People working around machinery, operating a motor vehicle, or performing other duties in which they must remain mentally alert should be particularly cautious while working until they know how the medication affects them. Provide patient safety during episodes of dizziness; report for further evaluation.

Side Effects to Report

Neurologic Assessment. Perform a baseline assessment of the patient's speech patterns and degree of alertness, as well as orientation to name, place, and time before initiating therapy. Make regularly scheduled subsequent evaluations of mental status, and compare findings. Report alterations.

Hydration Status. Decreased sweating and overheating have been reported with the use of topiramate, primarily in children. Most cases occurred in association with exposure to elevated environmental temperatures and/or vigorous activity. Proper hydration before and during activities such as exercise or exposure to warm temperatures is recommended.

Drug Interactions

Drugs That Decrease Therapeutic Effects. Phenobarbital, primidone, phenytoin, valproic acid, and carbamazepine may enhance the metabolism of topiramate. Monitor for increased frequency of seizure activity.

Enhanced Sedation. CNS depressants, including sleep aids, analgesics, tranquilizers, and alcohol enhance the sedative effects of topiramate. Patients must be warned about not working around machinery, operating a motor vehicle, or performing other duties in which they must remain mentally alert until it is known how they are affected by this medication. Provide patient safety during episodes of drowsiness or dizziness.

Oral Contraceptives. Spotting or bleeding may be an indication of reduced contraceptive activity. Recommend using alternative forms of birth control.

valproic acid (val proe′ ik ah′ sid)
DEPAKENE (dep′ ah keen)

Actions

Valproic acid is an anticonvulsant structurally unrelated to any other agent used to treat seizure disorders. Its mechanism of action is unknown; however, it appears to support GABA activity as an inhibitory neurotransmitter.

Uses

Valproic acid has broad activity against both partial seizures and generalized tonic-clonic seizures. It is the only available agent that can be used as single-drug therapy for treating patients with a combination of generalized tonic-clonic, absence, or myoclonic seizures. Valproic acid is also being tested to be used either alone or in combination with lithium or carbamazepine for treating acute mania of bipolar disorder in patients who do not respond to lithium therapy alone.

Therapeutic Outcomes

The primary therapeutic outcomes expected from valproic acid are as follows:

1. Reduced frequency of seizures and reduced injury from seizure activity.
2. Minimal adverse effects from therapy.

Nursing Process for Valproic Acid

Premedication Assessment

1. The manufacturer recommends that the following baseline studies be completed before therapy is initiated and at regular intervals thereafter: liver function tests, bleeding time determination, and platelet count.
2. *Patients with diabetes:* One of the metabolites of valproic acid is a ketone. It is excreted in the urine and may produce a false-positive test (Ketostix, Acetest) for urine ketones.
3. Review routine blood studies to detect blood dyscrasias and hepatotoxicity.
4. Perform a baseline assessment of the patient's speech patterns; degree of alertness; and orientation to name, place, and time before initiating therapy. Monitor behavioral responses to therapy.

Planning

Availability. PO: 250 mg capsules; 125 mg capsules containing coated particles; 125, 250, and 500 mg sustained release tablets; 250 mg/5 mL syrup; injection: 100 mg/mL in 5 mL vials.

Implementation

Dosage and Administration. *Adult:* PO: 5 mg/kg every 8 hours. Administer medication with food or milk to reduce gastric irritation. Increase by 5 to 10 mg/kg/day at weekly intervals. The maximum daily dosage is 30 mg/kg. Therapeutic blood levels are 50 to 100 mg/L. A capsule containing enteric-coated particles is available for patients who have persistent nausea and vomiting.

Evaluation

Side Effects to Expect

Nausea, Vomiting, Indigestion. These effects are common during initiation of therapy. Gradual increases in dosage and administration with food or milk reduce gastric irritation.

Sedation, Drowsiness, Dizziness, Blurred Vision. These symptoms tend to disappear with continued therapy and possible dosage adjustment. Encourage the patient not to discontinue therapy without first consulting the health care provider.

People working around machinery, operating a motor vehicle, or performing other duties in which they must remain mentally alert should not take these medications while working. Provide patient safety during episodes of dizziness; report for further evaluation. Caution the patient that blurred vision may occur, and make appropriate suggestions for the individuals' safety.

Side Effects to Report

Blood Dyscrasias. Routine laboratory studies (e.g., RBC, WBC, differential counts) should be scheduled. Monitor for sore throat, fever, purpura, jaundice, or excessive and progressive weakness.

Hepatotoxicity. The symptoms of hepatotoxicity are anorexia, nausea, vomiting, jaundice, hepatomegaly, splenomegaly, and abnormal liver function tests (e.g., elevated bilirubin, AST, ALT, GGT, alkaline phosphatase, prothrombin time).

Pancreatitis. The symptoms of pancreatitis are abdominal pain, nausea, vomiting, and/or anorexia. Report symptoms to the health care provider because of the potential for life-threatening complications.

Drug Interactions

Drugs That Decrease Therapeutic Effects. Phenobarbital, primidone, phenytoin, lamotrigine, and carbamazepine may enhance the metabolism of valproic acid. Monitor for increased frequency of seizure activity. Monitoring changes in serum levels should help warn of the potential for increased seizure activity.

Enhanced Sedation. CNS depressants, including sleep aids, analgesics, tranquilizers, and alcohol enhance the sedative effects of valproic acid. Patients must be warned about not working around machinery, operating a motor vehicle, or performing other duties in which they must remain mentally alert until it is known how they are affected by this medication. Provide patient safety during episodes of drowsiness or dizziness.

zonisamide (zoh nis′ am eyd)

▶ ZONEGRAN (zoh′ negh grahn)

Actions

Zonisamide is classified as a sulfonamide and is chemically unrelated to other anticonvulsants. Its mechanism of action is unknown, but it acts by blocking sodium and calcium channels to stabilize the neuronal membranes.

Uses

Zonisamide is approved for use in conjunction with other anticonvulsants in the treatment of adult partial seizures.

Therapeutic Outcomes

The primary therapeutic outcomes sought from zonisamide are as follows:

1. Reduced frequency of seizures and reduced injury from seizure activity.
2. Minimal adverse effects from therapy.

Nursing Process for Zonisamide

Premedication Assessment

1. Review the patient's medication history to ensure that the patient does not have an allergy to sulfonamide medicines (e.g., Bactrim, Septra). If the patient does, inform the charge nurse and the health care provider immediately. Do not administer the medication without specific approval.
2. Review the patient's medical record for a history of skin rashes. If the patient develops a rash, inform the charge nurse and the health care provider immediately. Do not administer the medication without specific approval.
3. Review the medical record to document frequency of seizure activity.
4. As a result of serious adverse reactions, the following baseline studies should be repeated at regular intervals: CBC, liver function tests, BUN, and serum creatinine.
5. Perform a baseline assessment of the patient's speech patterns; degree of alertness; and orientation to name, place, and time before initiating therapy.
6. Obtain baseline vital signs.

Planning

Availability. PO: 25, 50, and 100 mg capsules.

Implementation

Dosage and Administration. *Adult:* PO: Initial dose is 100 mg daily, taken with or without food. Due to sedative effects, it may be taken at bedtime. After 2 weeks, the dosage may be increased to 200 mg per day for at least 2 weeks. Both capsules may be taken at the same time. The dosage can be increased up to 600 mg per day, with at least 2 weeks between dosage changes to assess the therapeutic effects of therapy and monitor for adverse effects. Encourage the patient to drink six to eight 8-ounce glasses of water per day while taking this medicine.

Evaluation

Side Effects to Expect

Drowsiness, Dizziness. These effects can be reduced by slowly increasing the dosage. These effects are usually mild and tend to resolve with continued therapy. Encourage the patient not to discontinue therapy without first consulting the health care provider.

Provide patient safety during episodes of dizziness. Patients must be warned about not working around machinery, operating a motor vehicle, or performing other duties in which they must remain mentally alert until it is known how they are affected by this medication.

Side Effects to Report

Neurologic Assessment. Perform a baseline assessment of the patient's speech patterns; degree of alertness; and orientation to name, place, and time before initiating therapy. Make regularly scheduled subsequent evaluations of mental status, and compare findings. Report alterations.

Nephrotoxicity. Monitor kidney function tests for abnormal results. Report an increasing BUN and creatinine; frank blood or smoky-colored urine; or RBC in excess of 0 to 3 on the urinalysis report or back pain, abdominal pain, or pain on urination.

Blood Dyscrasias. Routine laboratory studies (e.g., RBC, WBC, differential counts) should be scheduled. Monitor for sore throat, fever, purpura, jaundice, or excessive and progressive weakness.

Dermatologic Reactions. Report a rash or pruritus with or without fever immediately and withhold additional doses until approved by the health care provider.

Drug Interactions

Enhanced Sedation. CNS depressants, including sleep aids, analgesics, tranquilizers, and alcohol enhance the sedative effects of zonisamide. Patients must be warned about not working around machinery, operating a motor vehicle, or performing other duties in which they must remain mentally alert until it is known how they are affected by this medication. Provide patient safety during episodes of drowsiness or dizziness.

Drugs That Decrease Therapeutic Effects. Phenobarbital, primidone, phenytoin, carbamazepine, and valproic acid may enhance the metabolism of zonisamide. Monitor for increased frequency of seizure activity. The dosage of zonisamide may have to be increased to prevent the return of seizures.

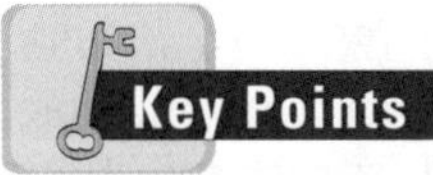

Key Points

- Seizures are the result of the sudden, excessive firing of a small number of neurons and the spread of electrical activity to adjacent neurons.
- There are several types and many causes of seizures. If the seizures are chronic and recurrent, the patient is diagnosed as having epilepsy.
- Epilepsy is treated almost exclusively with anticonvulsant medications.
- The effective treatment of epilepsy requires the cooperation of the patient and the health care provider.
- The desired therapeutic outcome of seizure treatment is to reduce the frequency of seizures while minimizing adverse effects of drug therapy. To attain this,

therapy must be individualized to consider the type of seizure activity and the age, gender, and concurrent medical condition of the patient.
- Patients as well as their families require education and support regarding their responsibilities in managing epilepsy.

Go to your Companion CD-ROM for appendices, an Audio Glossary, animations, Drug Dosage Calculators, customizable Patient Self-Assessment forms, and Review Questions for the NCLEX® Examination.

evolve Be sure to visit the companion Evolve site at http://evolve.elsevier.com/Clayton for WebLinks and additional online resources.

MEDICATION SAFETY REVIEW

MATH REVIEW QUESTIONS

1. Order: Dilantin 100 mg PO tid and at bedtime. What is your interpretation of the order, and how will you administer it to the patient?
2. A 10-year-old patient is to start on Tegretol suspension 50 mg PO qid. The suspension is 100 mg/5 mL. How will you administer this dose?
3. A 12-year-old, 110-pound newly diagnosed epileptic patient is to start on Depakene syrup, 5 mL PO tid. The normal starting dosage is 15 mg/kg daily. Is the order reasonable, and if so, how would you administer it?

CRITICAL THINKING QUESTIONS

1. Both diazepam and phenytoin have specific administration precautions when these agents are administered intravenously. What are these precautions?
2. A person suddenly had a tonic-clonic seizure while attending a class at college. When his family is notified of this and his need for transportation home, his wife tells you he has not been taking his medications regularly. Describe how you as a nurse would address this situation.
3. While working in the emergency department (ED), the rescue squad notifies the ED desk that a patient who is in status epilepticus is being transported. What medicines and equipment would you have ready for the patient's arrival?
4. What health teaching should be done for individuals recently diagnosed with epilepsy?

CONTENT REVIEW QUESTIONS

1. While administering intravenous phenytoin, the nurse should watch the patient for symptoms of which of the following adverse responses?
   1. Bradycardia
   2. Increased seizure activity
   3. Confusion
   4. Sedation
2. An infant is brought to the emergency department with observable twitching of the extremities and a temperature of 104.2° F reported by the parents. The priority action is to:
   1. take vital signs.
   2. call a health care provider.
   3. check the airway.
   4. take a history.
3. When caring for a patient with epilepsy who was hospitalized and successfully treated for status epilepticus, a precaution that the nurse institutes includes:
   1. placing oxygen and suction equipment at the bedside.
   2. assigning an assistant to stay with the patient at all times.
   3. keeping a tongue blade available to insert in case of a seizure.
   4. instructing the patient to stay in bed and call for assistance to go to the bathroom.
4. A nurse witnesses a patient with a seizure disorder as he suddenly jerks his arms and legs, falls to the floor, and regains consciousness immediately. The type of seizure demonstrated by this patient and that the nurse documents is:
   1. an atonic seizure.
   2. a myoclonic seizure.
   3. a complex partial seizure with automatisms.
   4. a simple partial seizure with motor symptoms.
5. Following recovery from a stroke, a 68-year-old patient developed complex partial seizures with motor symptoms beginning in the right arm with progression to unconsciousness. The physician prescribes phenytoin (Dilantin) for control of the seizures. A statement by the patient that indicates understanding of the self-care related to this drug includes:
   1. "I should use soft swabs rather than a toothbrush to clean my mouth."
   2. "If I have a seizure, I should call an ambulance to take me to the hospital."
   3. "I will take the medication at the beginning of the seizure before I lose consciousness."
   4. "As I start this drug, I will need to have my blood taken frequently to check the level of the drug."

CHAPTER

20 Drugs Used for Pain Management

evolve http://evolve.elsevier.com/Clayton

Chapter Content

Objectives

1. Differentiate among opiate agonists, opiate partial agonists, and opiate antagonists.
2. Describe monitoring parameters necessary for patients receiving opiate agonists.
3. Cite the side effects to expect when opiate agonists are administered.
4. Compare the analgesic effectiveness of opiate partial agonists when administered before or after opiate agonists.
5. Explain when naloxone can be used effectively to treat respiratory depression.
6. State the three pharmacologic effects of salicylates.
7. Prepare a list of side effects to expect, side effects to report, and drug interactions that are associated with salicylates.
8. Explain why synthetic nonopiate analgesics are not used for inflammatory disorders.
9. Prepare a patient education plan for a person being discharged with a continuing prescription for an analgesic.
10. Examine Table 20-5 and identify the active ingredients in commonly prescribed analgesic combination products. Identify products containing aspirin and compare the analgesic properties of agents available in different strengths.

Key Terms

pain experience
pain perception
pain threshold
pain tolerance
nociception
acute pain
chronic pain
nociceptive pain
somatic pain
visceral pain
neuropathic pain
idiopathic pain
analgesics
opiate agonists
opiate partial agonists
opiate antagonists
salicylates
nonsteroidal antiinflammatory agents
opiate receptors
nociceptors
addiction
drug tolerance
ceiling effect

PAIN

The International Association for the Study of Pain defines pain as "an unpleasant sensory and emotional experience associated with actual or potential tissue damage or described in terms of such damage." An unpleasant sensation that is part of a larger situation is called **pain experience.** The pain experience is highly subjective and influenced by behavioral, physiological, sensory, emotional (e.g., attention, anxiety, fatigue, suggestion, prior conditioning), and cultural factors for a particular person under a certain set of circumstances. This accounts for the wide variation in individual responses to the sensation of pain.

The three terms used in relationship to the pain experience are **pain perception, pain threshold,** and **pain tolerance.** *Pain perception* (also known as **nociception**) is an individual's awareness of the feeling or sensation of pain. *Pain threshold* is the point at which an individual first acknowledges or interprets a sensation as being painful. *Pain tolerance* is the individual's ability to endure pain.

Pain has physical and emotional components. Factors that decrease an individual's tolerance to pain include prolonged pain that is insufficiently relieved, fatigue accompanied by the inability to sleep, an increase in anxiety or fear, unresolved anger, depression, and isolation. Patients with severe, intractable pain fear that the pain cannot be relieved, and patients with cancer fear that new or increasing pain means the cancer is spreading or recurring.

Pain is usually described as acute or short term and as chronic or long term. **Acute pain** arises from sudden injury to the structures of the body (e.g., skin, muscles, viscera). The intensity of pain is usually proportional to the extent of tissue damage. The sympathetic nervous system is activated, resulting in an increase in the heart rate, pulse, respirations, and blood pressure. This also causes nausea, diaphoresis, dilated pupils, and elevated glucose. Continuing or persistent pain results from ongoing tissue damage or from chemicals released by the surrounding cells during the initial

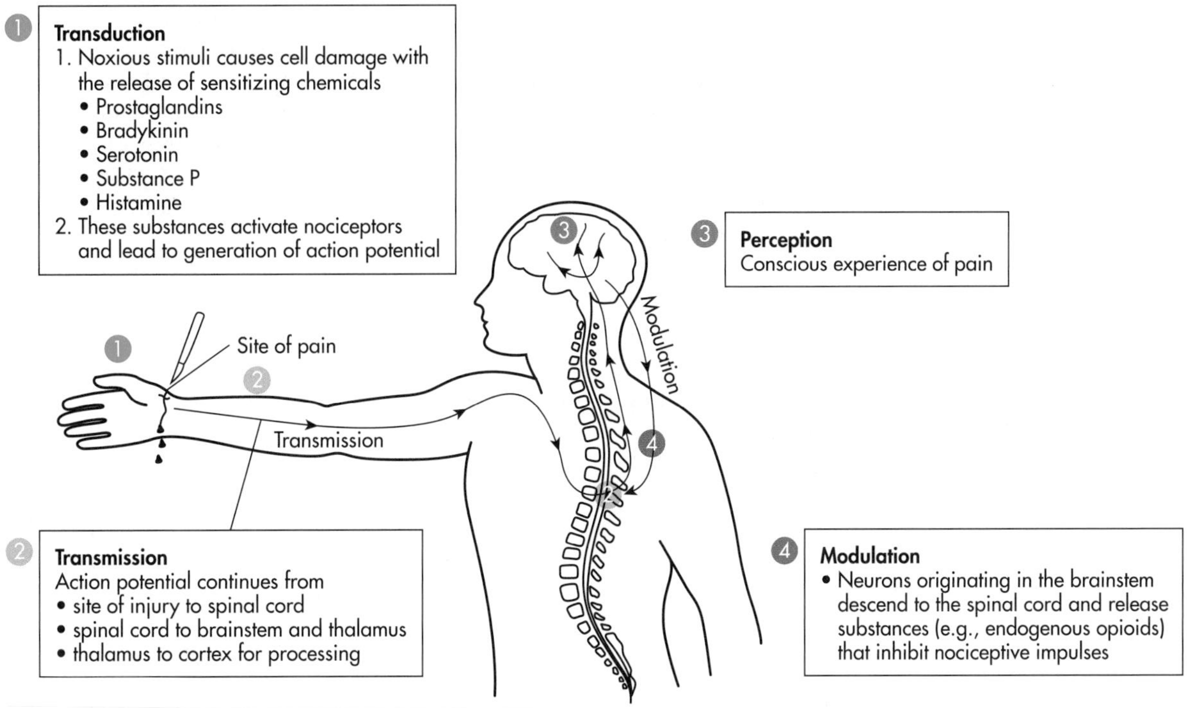

1 Transduction
1. Noxious stimuli causes cell damage with the release of sensitizing chemicals
   - Prostaglandins
   - Bradykinin
   - Serotonin
   - Substance P
   - Histamine
2. These substances activate nociceptors and lead to generation of action potential

3 Perception
Conscious experience of pain

1 Site of pain 2

Transmission

Modulation

2 Transmission
Action potential continues from
- site of injury to spinal cord
- spinal cord to brainstem and thalamus
- thalamus to cortex for processing

4 Modulation
- Neurons originating in the brainstem descend to the spinal cord and release substances (e.g., endogenous opioids) that inhibit nociceptive impulses

FIGURE **20-1** Nociceptive pain originates when the tissue is injured. *1,* Transduction occurs when there is release of chemical mediators. *2,* Transmission involves the conduct of the action potential from the periphery (injury site) to the spinal cord and then to the brain stem, thalamus, and cerebral cortex. *3,* Perception is the conscious awareness of pain. *4,* Modulation involves signals from the brain going back down the spinal cord to modify incoming impulses.

trauma (e.g., a crushing injury). The intensity diminishes as the stimulus is removed or tissue repair and healing take place. Acute pain serves an important protective physiologic purpose that warns of potential or actual tissue damage. **Chronic pain** has slower onset and lasts longer than 3 months beyond the healing process. Chronic pain does not relate to an injury or provide physiologic value. Depending upon the underlying etiology, it is often subdivided into malignant (cancer) or nonmalignant (causes other than cancer) pain. It may arise from visceral organs, muscular and connective tissue, or neurologic causes such as diabetic neuropathy, trigeminal neuralgia, or amputation. As chronic pain progresses, especially poorly treated pain, other physical and emotional factors come into play affecting almost every aspect of a patient's life—physical, mental, social, financial, and spiritual—causing additional stress, anger, chronic fatigue, and depression. Whereas pain has always been viewed as a symptom of a disease or a condition, chronic pain and its harmful physiologic effects are being looked upon as a disease itself.

Pain may also be classified by pathophysiology. **Nociceptive** (no se sep' tiv) **pain** is the result of a stimulus (e.g., chemical, thermal, mechanical) to pain receptors. Nociceptive pain is usually described by patients as dull and aching. It is called **somatic pain** if it originates from the skin, bones, joints, muscles, or connective tissue (e.g., arthritis pain) and **visceral pain** if it originates from the abdominal and thoracic organs. Nociception is the process by which a person becomes aware of the presence of pain. There are four steps in nociception: (1) transduction, (2) transmission, (3) perception, and (4) modulation (Figure 20-1).

Neuropathic pain results from injury to the peripheral or central nervous system (CNS) (e.g., trigeminal neuralgia). Patients describe neuropathic pain as stabbing and burning. Phantom limb pain is a neuropathic pain experienced by amputees in a body part that is no longer there. **Idiopathic pain** is a nonspecific pain of unknown origin. Anxiety, depression, and stress are often associated with this type of pain. Common areas associated with idiopathic pain are the pelvis, neck, shoulders, abdomen, and head.

PAIN MANAGEMENT

Analgesics are drugs that relieve pain without producing loss of consciousness or reflex activity. The search for an ideal analgesic continues, but it is difficult to find one that meets this definition. It should be potent so that it will afford maximum relief of pain; it should not cause dependence; it should exhibit a minimum of side effects such as constipation, hallucinations, respiratory depression, nausea, and vomiting; it should not cause tolerance; it should act promptly and over a long period with a minimum amount of sedation so that the patient is able to remain conscious and responsive; and it should be relatively inexpensive.

At present no completely satisfactory classification of analgesics is available. Historically they have been categorized based on potency (mild, moderate, and strong), origin (opium, semisynthetic, synthetic, coal-tar derivative), or addictive properties (narcotic and nonnarcotic).

Research into the control of pain over the past decade has given new insight into pathways of pain within the nervous system and a better understanding of precise mechanisms of action of analgesic agents. The current nomenclature for analgesics stems from these recent discoveries. In this section the medications have been divided into opiate agonists, opiate partial agonists, opiate antagonists, salicylates, nonsteroidal antiinflammatory agents (or drugs) (NSAIDs), and miscellaneous analgesic agents.

Actions

The pathways to pain transmission from the site of injury to the brain for processing and reflexive action have not been fully identified. The first step leading to the sensation of pain is the stimulation of receptors known as nociceptors (see Figure 20-1). These nerve endings are found in skin, blood vessels, joints, subcutaneous tissues, periosteum, viscera, and other tissues. These nociceptors are classified as thermal, chemical, and mechanical-thermal, based on the types of sensations that they transmit. The exact mechanism that causes stimulation of nociceptors is not understood; however, bradykinins, prostaglandins, leukotrienes, histamine, and serotonin sensitize these receptors. Receptor activation leads to action potentials that are transmitted along afferent nerve fibers to the spinal cord. A series of neurotransmitters (somatostatin, cholecystokinin, substance P) play roles in the transmission of nerve impulses from the site of damage to the spinal cord. Within the CNS, there may be at least four pain-transmitting pathways up the spinal cord to various areas of the brain for response.

Within the CNS is a series of receptors that control pain. These are known as opiate receptors because stimulation of these receptors by the opiates blocks the pain sensation. These receptors are subdivided into four types: the mu (μ), delta (δ), kappa κ), and epsilon (ϵ) receptors. Sigma (σ) is another receptor type that reacts to opioid agonists and partial agonists. The receptors are located in different areas of the CNS: κ-receptors are found in greatest concentration in the cerebral cortex and in the substantia gelatinosa of the dorsal horn of the spinal cord. They are responsible for analgesia at the levels of the spinal cord and brain. Stimulation of κ-receptors also produces sedation and dysphoria. μ-Receptors are located in the pain-modulating centers of the CNS and induce central analgesia, euphoria, physical dependence, miosis, and respiratory depression. δ-Receptors are located in the limbic area of the brain and in the spinal cord and may play a role in the euphoria that selected opiates produce. σ-Receptors are thought to produce the autonomic stimulation and psychotomimetic (e.g., hallucinations) and dysphoric effects of some opiate agonists and partial agonists. The functions of the ϵ receptors are under investigation. Research is focusing on building synthetic chemicals that are selective for specific receptors to maximize analgesia but minimize the potential for adverse effects such as addiction.

As described, other chemicals—histamine, prostaglandins, serotonin, leukotrienes, substance P, and bradykinins—released during trauma also contribute to pain. Developing pharmaceuticals that block these chemicals is another effective way of stopping pain. Antihistamines (e.g., diphenhydramine), prostaglandin inhibitors (e.g., NSAIDs), substance P antagonists (e.g., capsaicin), and antidepressants that prolong norepinephrine and serotonin activity (e.g., tricyclic antidepressants, selective serotonin reuptake inhibitors [SSRIs]) have analgesic properties.

Other pharmacologic agents can be used as adjuncts to pain suppression by a variety of mechanisms. Adrenergic agents such as norepinephrine and clonidine and gamma-aminobutyric acid (GABA) receptor stimulants (e.g., baclofen, gabapentin) produce significant analgesia by blocking nociceptor activity. Valproic acid, phenytoin, gabapentin, and carbamazepine act as analgesics by suppressing spontaneous neuronal firing, as occurs in trigeminal neuralgia. Tricyclic antidepressants inhibit the reuptake of serotonin and norepinephrine, causing the onset of analgesia to be more rapid, as well as improving the outlook of the person who is suffering from chronic pain and depression. Some antidepressants (e.g., amitriptyline) also block pain by antihistaminic and anticholinergic activity. The bisphosphonates (e.g., pamidronate) may be effective in treating pain associated with bony metastases.

Uses

The World Health Organization recommends a stepwise approach to pain management (Figure 20-2). Mild, acute pain is effectively treated with analgesics such as aspirin, NSAIDs, or acetaminophen. Pain associated with inflammation responds well to NSAIDs. Unrelieved or moderate pain is generally treated with a moderate potency opiate such as codeine or oxycodone, which are often used in combination with acetaminophen or aspirin (e.g., Empirin #3, Tylenol with Codeine No. 3, Percodan). Severe, acute pain is treated with opiate agonists (e.g., morphine, hydromorphone, levorphanol). Morphine sulfate is usually the drug of choice for the treatment of severe, chronic pain. Other agents may be used as adjunctive therapy with analgesics such as antidepressants or anticonvulsants, depending on the pain's etiology.

Unfortunately the health care delivery system in the United States has a long-standing history of inadequate pain management. The Joint Commission on Accreditation of Healthcare Organizations (JCAHO)

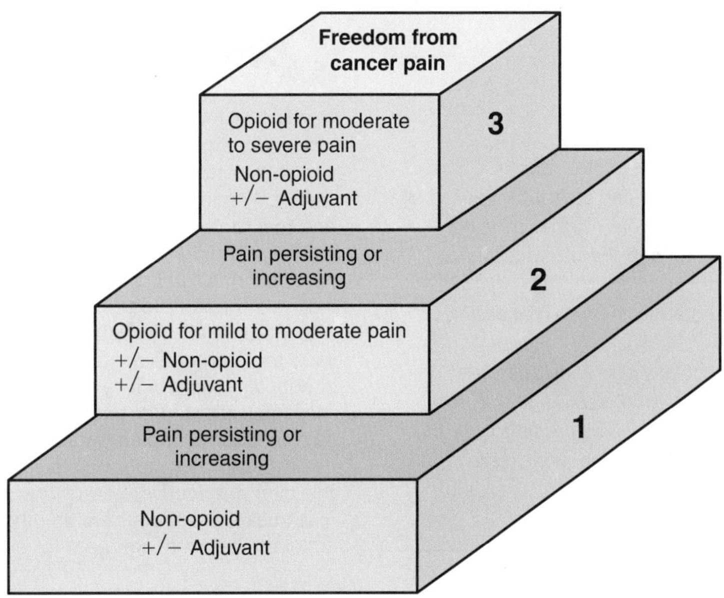

FIGURE **20-2** WHO's Pain Relief Ladder.

has developed new standards for assessing and relieving pain by health care providers.

The primary therapeutic outcomes from appropriate pain management therapy are as follows:

1. Relief of pain intensity and duration of pain complaint
2. Prevention of the conversion of persistent pain to chronic pain
3. Prevention of suffering and disability associated with pain
4. Prevention of psychological and socioeconomic consequences associated with inadequate pain management
5. Control of side effects associated with pain management
6. Optimization of the ability to perform activities of daily living (ADLs)

Although considered acceptable at one time, placebo therapy should never be used with pain management. One premise of pain management is that the patient should be believed when describing the presence of pain. The use of placebos implies a lack of belief in the patient's description, and can seriously damage the patient-provider relationship. The American Pain Society has declared that the use of placebos is unethical and should be avoided.

NURSING PROCESS *for Pain Management*

The management of all types of pain has clearly been a major health care concern for some time. The rating of pain as the fifth vital sign means that pain should be assessed every time vital signs are taken and recorded. Vital signs records have been revised to include this; pain flow sheets have also been developed (see Figure 7-6). Taking the pain rating only when doing vital signs, however, is not sufficient. The nurse should also evaluate the pain level immediately before and after pain medications are given, at 1-, 2-, and 3-hour intervals for oral medications and at 15- to 30-minute intervals after parenteral administration. Most assessment data sheets have a section on pain management containing the following elements: rating before and after medication, nonpharmacologic measures initiated, patient teaching performed, and breakthrough pain measures implemented. The pain flow sheet provides the health team members with a quick visual reference to evaluate the overall effectiveness of the pain management prescribed.

The American Pain Society publishes *Quality Improvement Guidelines for the Treatment of Acute Pain and Cancer Pain*. The American Pain Foundation has also developed the Pain Care Bill of Rights, which explains to the patient exactly what to expect and/or demand in the way of pain management (Table 20-1).

Nurses must assist the patient in managing pain. The first vital step in this process is to believe the patient's description of the pain being experienced. Pain brings with it a variety of feelings, such as anxiety, anger, loneliness, frustration, and depression. Part of the patient's response is tied to past experiences, sociocultural factors, current emotional state, and beliefs regarding pain.

Psychological, physical, and environmental factors all must be considered in managing pain. Never overlook the value of general comfort measures such as a backrub, repositioning, and the use of hot or cold applications. A variety of relaxation techniques, as well as diversional activities, may prove psychologically beneficial. Measures to decrease environmental stimuli and thereby provide successful periods of rest are essential.

Table 20-1 Pain Care Bill of Rights

As a Person with Pain, You Have the Right to:
Have your report of pain taken seriously and to be treated with dignity and respect by doctors, nurses, pharmacists, and other health care professionals.
Have your pain thoroughly assessed and promptly treated.
Be informed by your doctor about what may be causing your pain, possible treatments, and the benefits, risks, and costs of each.
Participate actively in decisions about how to manage your pain.
Have your pain reassessed regularly and your treatment adjusted if your pain has not been eased.
Be referred to a pain specialist if your pain persists.
Get clear and prompt answers to your questions, take time to make decisions, and refuse a particular type of treatment if you choose.

American Pain Foundation, available at www.painfoundation.org.

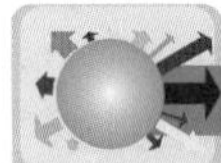

Clinical Landmine

All patients have a right to adequate management of pain. To help ensure appropriate analgesia, the rating of pain has been designated "the fifth vital sign." From a nursing standpoint, this means that pain should be assessed every time the vital signs are taken and recorded on the vital signs record and the pain flow sheet. Nurses should also evaluate the pain level immediately before administering a pain medication and afterward at 1-, 2-, and 3-hour intervals for oral medications and at a 15- to 30-minute intervals after parenteral administration. Although pain assessment forms vary, the elements contained in each collect similar information about pain: rating before and after medication, nonpharmacologic measures initiated, patient teaching performed, and breakthrough pain measures implemented. The pain flow sheet provides the health team members with a quick visual reference to evaluate the overall effectiveness of the pain management prescribed. Health care providers have an ethical duty to intercede to ensure adequate pain management for every patient.

It is important to evaluate the pain being experienced in a consistent manner. Therefore several assessment tools have been developed to gain some degree of uniformity in interpreting and recording the patient's description of pain.

There are a wide variety of pain assessment tools available such as the Riley Infant Pain Assessment Tool; the Face, Legs, Activity, Cry, Consolability (FLACC) Scale for use in nonverbal patients; the Pain Observation Scale for Young Children (POCIS) intended for children 1 to 4 years of age; the Modified Objective Pain Score (MOPS) intended for children 1 to 4 years of age after ear, nose, and throat surgery; Toddler-Preschooler Postoperative Pain Scale (TPPPS) for use in evaluating pain in smaller children during and following medical or surgical procedures; the Postoperative Pain Score (POPS) for infants having surgical procedures; and the Neonatal Infant Pain Scale (NIPS) for pain in preterm and full-term neonates used to monitor pain before, during, and after a painful procedure. The list of tools available is extensive and the preceding is only a partial listing. For further information on pain scales and the details of each, one need only log on to the Internet to find the data needed.

The Wong-Baker scale (Figure 20-3) has widespread use in people 3 years of age and older and is particularly useful in adults who have language barriers or who do not read, because they can select the face that best describes their pain. This rating scale is recommended for people ages 3 years and older.

Other pain assessment tools such as the McGill-Melzack Pain Questionnaire may be used to assist the patient in describing subjective pain experience (Figure 20-4). This tool uses descriptive words or phrases to identify the pain. It is especially useful for individuals who have chronic pain. When possible, chart the description in the patient's exact words. It may be necessary to seek additional data from significant others.

Scales such as that shown in Figure 20-5 are often used to assess acute pain. The most common scale used

Translations of Wong-Baker FACES Pain Rating Scale

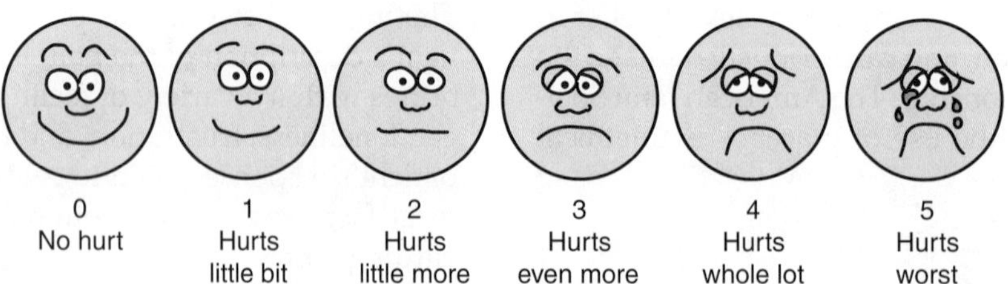

Original instructions:

Explain to the person that each face is for a person who feels happy because he has no pain (hurt) or sad because he has some or a lot of pain. **Face 0** is very happy because he doesn't hurt at all. **Face 1** hurts just a little bit. **Face 2** hurts a little more. **Face 3** hurts even more. **Face 4** hurts a whole lot. **Face 5** hurts as much as you can imagine, although you don't have to be crying to feel this bad. Ask the person to choose the face that best describes how he is feeling.

Rating scale is recommended for persons age 3 years and older.

FIGURE 20-3 Wong-Baker pain rating scale.

McGill-Melzack
Pain Questionnaire

Patient's name________________ Age____________
File No.________________ Date____________
Clinical category (e.g., cardiac, neurologic)
Diagnosis: ____________

Analgesic (if already administered):

1. Type____________
2. Dosage____________
3. Time given in relation to this test____________

Patient's intelligence: circle number that represents best estimate.

1 (low) 2 3 4 5 (high)

This questionnaire has been designed to tell us more about your pain. Four major questions we ask are:

1. Where is your pain?
2. What does it feel like?
3. How does it change with time?
4. How strong is it?

It is important that you tell us how your pain feels now. Please follow the instructions at the beginning of each part.

Part 1. Where Is Your Pain?

Please mark on the drawing below the areas where you feel pain. Put E if external, or I if internal, near the areas you mark. Put EI if both external and internal.

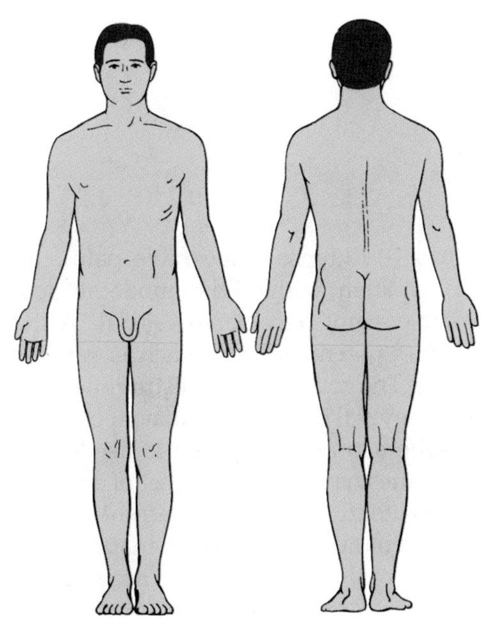

Part 2. What Does Your Pain Feel Like?

Some of the words below describe your present pain. Circle *ONLY* those words that best describe it. Leave out any category that is not suitable. Use only a single word in each appropriate category—the one that best applies.

1
Flickering
Quivering
Pulsing
Throbbing
Beating
Pounding

2
Jumping
Flashing
Shooting

3
Pricking
Boring
Drilling
Stabbing
Lancinating

4
Sharp
Cutting
Lacerating

5
Pinching
Pressing
Gnawing
Cramping
Crushing

6
Tugging
Pulling
Wrenching

7
Hot
Burning
Scalding
Searing

8
Tingling
Itchy
Smarting
Stinging

9
Dull
Sore
Hurting
Aching
Heavy

10
Tender
Taut
Rasping
Splitting

11
Tiring
Exhausting

12
Sickening
Suffocating

13
Fearful
Frightful
Terrifying

14
Punishing
Grueling
Cruel
Vicious
Killing

15
Wretched
Blinding

16
Annoying
Troublesome
Miserable
Intense
Unbearable

17
Spreading
Radiating
Penetrating
Piercing

18
Tight
Numb
Drawing
Squeezing
Tearing

19
Cool
Cold
Freezing

20
Nagging
Nauseating
Agonizing
Dreadful
Torturing

Part 3. How Does Your Pain Change with Time?

1. Which word or words would you use to describe the *pattern* of your pain?

1	2	3
Continuous	Rhythmic	Brief
Steady	Periodic	Momentary
Constant	Intermittent	Transient

2. What kind of things *relieve* your pain?

3. What kind of things *increase* your pain?

Part 4. How Strong Is Your Pain?

People agree that the following 5 words represent pain of increasing intensity. They are:

1	2	3	4	5
Mild	Discomforting	Distressing	Horrible	Excruciating

To answer each question below, write the number of the most appropriate word in the space beside the question.

1. Which word describes your pain right now? ______
2. Which word describes it at its worst? ______
3. Which word describes it when it is least? ______
4. Which word describes the worst toothache you ever had? ______
5. Which word describes the worst headache you ever had? ______
6. Which word describes the worst stomachache you ever had? ______

FIGURE **20-4** The McGill-Melzack Pain Questionnaire.

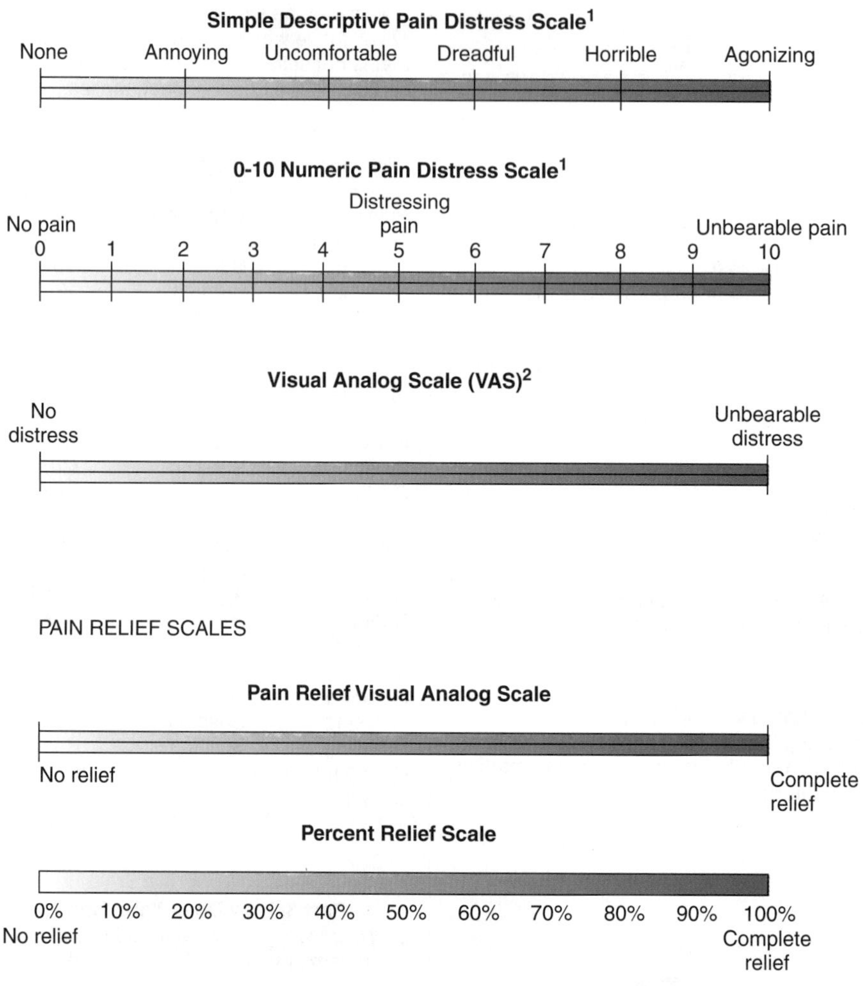

FIGURE **20-5** Pain-rating scales.

asks the patient to rate the pain being experienced on a scale of 0 (no pain) to 10 (intense or excruciating). The degree of relief for the pain after an analgesic is given is again rated using the same 0 to 10 scale. When different potencies of analgesic agents are ordered for the same patient, the nurse can use this numeric rating data in combination with the other data gathered to determine whether a more or less potent analgesic agent should be administered. Other scales sometimes used include faces depicting facial grimacing, smiles, and so forth. This approach is useful with children or people with a language barrier. The color scale is similar to a slide rule. The patient selects the hue or depth of color that corresponds with the pain being experienced. The nurse turns the slide rule scale over and a numeric value is identified that can be used to consistently record the patient's response.

Effective pain control must depend on the degree of pain experienced. The previously described scale of 0 (no pain) to 10 (intense/unbearable pain) can prove useful. For a patient with mild to moderate acute pain, a nonnarcotic agent may be successful. With severe, chronic pain, a potent analgesic such as morphine may be necessary. The route of administration chosen must be based on several factors. One major consideration is how soon the action of the drug is needed. The oral and rectal routes have a longer onset of action than the parenteral route. It is sometimes erroneously felt that the oral route of administration is inadequate to treat pain. In truth, oral medications can provide very good pain relief if appropriate doses are provided. Generally the oral route is used initially to treat pain if no nausea and vomiting are present. Patients may initially be treated effectively with administration via the oral route; however, the rectal, transdermal, subcutaneous, intramuscular, intraspinal, epidural, and intravenous (IV) routes may be required, depending on the patient and the course of the underlying disease.

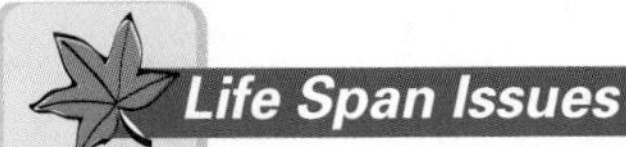

Life Span Issues

Analgesics

It is important to maintain a relatively steady blood level of analgesic to gain the best control of pain. However, drug absorption, metabolism, and excretion are affected by age. Dosages and frequency of administration of analgesics may have to be increased in children, especially teenagers, because many medicines are more rapidly metabolized and excreted in this age-group. Conversely, an older adult may need a somewhat smaller dose of an analgesic less frequently because of slower metabolism and excretion. In either situation, it is imperative that the nurse make regular assessments of the patient's pain level and contact the health care provider for adjustments in dosages and frequency based on the response to the analgesic.

Before initiating a pain assessment, assess the patient for hearing and visual impairment. Data collected may be invalidated by the person's inability to hear the questions or see the visual aids used to assess pain.

Nurses must evaluate and document in the patient's chart the effectiveness of the pain medications given. This requires careful assessments at intervals after the administration of the analgesics to validate the duration and degree of pain relief attained from the analgesic. Recording the patient's rating of the degree of pain relief at 1-, 2-, and 3-hour intervals after administration of oral medicines and 15 to 30 minutes after parenteral agents will provide useful information for evaluating future analgesic needs for the individual. Record and report all complaints of pain for analysis by the health care provider. The pattern of pain, particularly an increase in frequency or severity, may indicate new causes of pain. Major reasons for increased frequency or intensity of pain are pain from long-term immobility; pain from the treatment modalities used: surgery, chemotherapy, or radiation therapy; pain from direct extension of a tumor or metastasis into bone, nerve, or viscera; and pain unrelated to the original cause or the therapeutic modalities used.

Assessment

History of Pain Experience

- *Medication history:* What medications are being prescribed and how effective have they been? What dosage has been required to achieve adequate comfort? Is the patient experiencing side effects to the medications? If yes, get details of side effects and measures taken for management. What is the patient's attitude toward the use of pain medications (opioids, anxiolytics, and others)? What are the family or significant others' attitudes toward the use of medications to control the pain? Is there any history of substance abuse?
- *Patient's perception of pain:* Identify the causes of the patient's pain by having the patient describe the perception of the pain experienced. What does the patient feel is the cause of the pain? In the older adult, multiple chronic as well as acute pain problems may be present, making it difficult to determine which one of the problems is the most urgent or causing the most pain. Multiple pain complaints combined with hearing impairments, memory, and cognitive factors must be taken into consideration during the pain assessment.
- Listen to the patient and *believe the pain experience* being described regardless of whether the physical data substantiate the degree of discomfort described. *DO NOT* let personal biases or values interfere with establishing interventions that provide maximum pain relief for the individual. The myth that pain decreases with aging and that pain is expected with aging is INCORRECT!
- *Onset:* When was the pain first noticed? When was the most recent attack? Is the onset slow or abrupt? Is there any particular activity that starts the pain? Does the pain occur in response to eating certain foods?
- *Location:* What is the exact location of the pain? Having the patient shade in a human figure with the areas where the pain is felt may be helpful, especially with pediatric patients who can be given crayons as a means of identifying different intensities in addition to the location. With acute pain, the site of the pain can be more easily identified; however, with chronic pain, this may be more difficult because the normal physiologic responses of the sympathetic nervous system are no longer present.
- *Depth:* What is the depth of the pain? Does it radiate, having the sensation of spreading out or diffusing over an area, or is it localized in a specific site? It is important to recognize that the lack of physical symptoms comparable with the pain described *does not* mean that the patient's complaints should be ignored.
- *Quality:* What is the actual sensation felt when the pain is present—stabbing, dull, cramping, sore, burning, or other? Is the pain always in the same place and of the same intensity?
- *Duration:* Is the pain continuous or intermittent? How often does it occur, and once felt, how long does it persist? Is there a cyclic pattern to the pain?
- *Severity:* Have the patient rate the pain using the pain scale methodology that is standard for the clinical setting. Self-reporting pain assessment tools are used for most children 3 years and older. After age 8, children understand numerical values, so one of the visual analog scales or word-graphic scales can be used. There are numerous scoring systems available for neonates through adults. If these tools are not being used for consistency in pain assessment, it is not for lack of tools but the failure of the health care team to adequately assess the pain.

Nonverbal Observations. Note the patient's general body position during an episode of pain. Be particularly observant about subtle clues such as facial grimaces, immobility of a particular part, and holding or resisting movement of an extremity. With pediatric patients, facial expressions, squinting, grimacing, and crying may also be used as indicators of pain level and pain relief.

Developmental differences influence the pain experience and the way different age groups express pain. Realize that just because infants cannot speak does not mean they do not have pain. Infants may express pain through continual inconsolable crying; irritability, poor oral intake, and alterations in sleep pattern. Preschool children may verbalize pain; exhibit lack of cooperation; be "clingy" to parents, nurses, or significant others; and not want the site of the pain touched—they may actually push you away as you approach the area. Older children may deny pain in the presence of peers and display regressive behaviors in presence of support personnel. In the older adult it is useful to perform the Katz Activities of Daily Living Measurement and the "get up and go" test to determine the individual's functional status.

Pain Relief. What specific measures relieve the pain? What has already been tried for pain relief, and what if anything has been beneficial?

Physical Data. In the presence of pain, always examine the affected part for any alterations in appearance, change in sensation, or limitation in mobility or range of motion. In older adults it is particularly important to evaluate the musculoskeletal and neurologic systems during the physical examination.

Behavioral Responses. What coping mechanisms does the patient use to handle the pain experience—crying, anger, withdrawal, depression, anxiety, fear, or hopelessness? Is the individual introspective and self-focusing? Does the individual continue to perform activities of daily living (ADLs) despite the pain? Does the individual alter lifestyle patterns appropriately to enhance pain relief measures prescribed? Is the individual able to continue to work? Is the individual socially withdrawn? Is the person seeing more than one health care provider in hope of obtaining an answer to the origin of the pain?

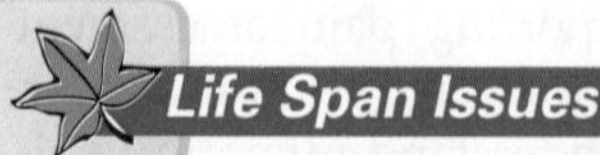

Life Span Issues

Pain in the Older Adult Patient

Pain assessment in the older adult patient must include more than a simple rating of pain using a pain scale. Because many older adults suffer from more than one chronic illness, a nursing history and a physical and functional assessment must be performed to understand the effect of pain on the patient's ability to meet self-care needs.

Nursing Diagnoses

- Pain, acute or chronic (indication)
- Constipation, risk for (side effect)
- Gas exchange, impaired, risk for (indication)
- Urinary retention (high risk for) (side effect)

Planning

History of Pain Experience

- Evaluate the pain according to location, depth, quality, duration, or severity.
- Perform baseline vital signs at least every shift or more often as dictated by patient's condition and type of medications administered. Pain assessment needs to take into consideration the therapeutic interventions used, and assessments should specifically target evaluation of the effectiveness of the interventions in place.

Pain Relief

- Goals of treatment should be established when initiating a treatment regimen. Prevention, reduction, or elimination of pain is an important therapeutic goal. The patient and caregivers should be involved in the establishment of these goals so that outcomes important to the patient are incorporated into the treatment goals, and the patient and caregiver have realistic expectations. Pain, especially chronic pain, may not be completely eliminated, but must be managed. Additional important goals include improving the patient's quality of life, functional capacity, and ability to retain independence. Specific therapeutic goals established may include:
  - Pain at rest <3 on pain scale
  - Pain with movement <5 on pain scale
  - Able to have at least 6 hours of sleep uninterrupted by pain
  - Able to work at a hobby (e.g., crafts, play cards, gardening) for 1 hour
- Update the Kardex and care plan with details of nursing interventions that are successful in reducing pain. This will allow all staff to intervene more knowledgeably.
- Plan to implement nonpharmacologic (physical, psychological, complementary) and pharmacologic measures for the control of pain.
- During the first 24 hours of pain treatment, reassessments should be done more frequently not only to evaluate the degree of pain relief but also to provide reassurance to the patient that the staff is serious about providing relief for discomfort. With children, the parents should be actively involved in the plan.

Environmental Control

- Provide a quiet environment with as little distraction as possible during periods of rest. Modify hospital schedules such as routine testing of vital signs and specimen collection so that the individual is not disturbed once asleep. Establish a

schedule that provides sufficient rest. (Fatigue and anxiety may increase the perception of pain.)
- Schedule diversional activities through the appropriate use of television, visitors, card games, and other patients to take the patient's mind off the pain.

Psychological Interventions

- During the planning process, it is important to stress to support people that they can be involved in a positive way by expressing understanding, providing diversional activities, and encouraging frequent rest periods, especially after the administration of analgesics, antidepressants, and antianxiety medications.

Medication Administration

- Plan to check often on the degree of pain relief being achieved and to administer medications as scheduled around the clock to achieve a steady blood level and consistently control the pain. Have orders available to deal with breakthrough pain on an as-needed (PRN) basis.
- Keep an adequate supply of pain medication available for immediate use on the unit so that the patient is not kept waiting because the drug has not been dispensed from the pharmacy.

Implementation

Comfort Measures

- Provide for the patient's basic hygiene and comfort. Use such techniques as backrubs, massage, hot and cold applications, or warm baths as ordered.
- Ask the patient what measures have been successful in the past in providing pain relief.
- Relieve pain by doing any or all of the following, as appropriate: (1) support an affected part during movement, provide appropriate assistance during movement or activities, or apply binders or splint an incisional area before initiating activities such as deep breathing and coughing; (2) give analgesics in advance of undertaking painful activities and plan for the activity to take place during the peak action of the medication given or use hot or cold applications, massage, warm baths, pressure, and vibration as interventions for pain relief.

Exercise and Activity. Unless contraindicated, moderate exercise should be encouraged. Many times, pain causes the individual not to move the affected part or to position it in a manner that provides relief. Stress the need to prevent complications by using a passive range of motion.

Regularly scheduled exercise is important to prevent further deterioration of the musculoskeletal system, especially in elderly patients who may also have a diminished capacity.

Nonpharmacologic Approaches. Use nonpharmacologic strategies to enhance the effects of the medication therapy such as relaxation techniques, visualization, meditation, biofeedback, and transcutaneous electrical nerve stimulation (TENS) units. (The patient will require education for use of each of these prescribed techniques.) Assist with referral to a pain clinic for management of pain, especially chronic pain.

Medication. Even though pain medicine administration may be scheduled, encourage the patient to request pain medication before the pain escalates and becomes severe. Encourage open communication between the patient and health care team regarding the effectiveness of the medications used. Although the smallest dose possible to control the pain is the goal of therapy, it is also important that the dose be sufficient to provide adequate relief. Therefore the patient must understand the importance of expressing the degree of relief being obtained so that appropriate dosage adjustments can be made.

The medication administration record (MAR) may list more than one analgesic order for the same patient. This requires the nurse to use judgment in choosing the correct medication for the patient based on pain assessment data collected.

The nurse must identify when the last dose of pain medication was administered by checking both the patient's MAR and the narcotic control record. It is common practice for analgesics to be ordered intermittently on a PRN basis every 3 to 4 hours. However, in the case of chronic pain or intractable pain, it has been found that giving analgesics to people on a scheduled basis every 3 to 4 hours will maintain a more constant plasma level of the drug, providing more effective analgesia. This approach can result in better control of the pain while using less of the analgesic ordered.

Patient-controlled analgesia (PCA) has gained acceptance in both the inpatient and ambulatory setting. Pumps are available for inpatient use and in ambulatory units for home or nursing home settings. The PCA method of administration allows the patient to control a small syringe pump containing an opiate agonist, usually morphine, which is connected to an indwelling IV catheter. When initiating the PCA pump procedure, a loading dose is often given to gain rapid blood levels necessary for analgesia. The patient then receives a slow, continuous infusion from the syringe pump. Depending on the activity level and the level of analgesia needed, the patient may push a button, self-administering a small bolus of analgesic to meet the immediate need. A timing device on the pump limits the amount and frequency of the dose that can be self-administered per hour. Additional adjustments of the dosing and frequency may be required as therapy continues. This approach allows the patient to have some control over the pain relief and eliminates the need for the patient to wait for a nurse to answer the call light, check the last dose of analgesics given, and prepare and administer the medication. After discharge from the hospital, this method of administration also allows significantly more freedom of movement for the patient and caregiver.

When PCA is used, the nurse should explain the use of the PCA pump to the patient and observe the patient using it to validate understanding. (It also should be explained to the family and significant others.) Record the amount used every shift and the amount remaining in the syringe at the end of the shift, and notify the pharmacy well in advance of the need for more medication so that it's available when needed. The degree of pain relief achieved should always be recorded. When pain relief is inadequate, assess for other causes, and contact the physician to discuss a modification of the regimen.

PCA pumps are also used for chronic pain; however, the dosage can be delivered intravenously or subcutaneously. For chronic pain treatment the largest dose of the medication is given continuously with demand. Continuous subcutaneous opioid analgesia uses either a butterfly-type needle (25 to 27 gauge) or a special needle device placed subcutaneously into the subclavicular tissue under the clavicle or in the abdomen. The needle should be inserted on the body's trunk, usually the abdomen, because of diminished circulation in the extremities.

Epidural analgesia has been used for a long time in obstetrics but is now recognized as an effective means controlling acute pain for a variety of postoperative procedures. Epidural analgesia most commonly delivers morphine or fentanyl (sometimes combined with bupivacaine) into the subarachnoid space. It can be administered continuously with an infusion pump, intermittently by bolus administration, or via an implanted port. Nursing responsibilities during epidural analgesia involve:

- Checking institutional policies for qualifications needed to administer and monitor the epidural analgesia.
- Use of assessment tools to assess pain medication administered and degree of pain relief, respiratory function, neurologic function, degree of sedation, and catheter status.
- Observing for narcotic-related side effects (respiratory depression, nausea and vomiting, pruritus, headaches) and catheter-related complications. Always have drugs and supplies in the immediate area to reverse a drug overdose.

Transdermal opioid analgesia uses fentanyl (Duragesic) for relief of chronic pain. It takes approximately 12 to 24 hours for the initial patch of medication to reach a steady blood level, so other analgesics must be used during this time. Once placed the patch provides relief for up to 72 hours. Intermittent "rescue" dosing may still be needed during the patch use. When terminated, the patient still needs to be monitored for an additional 24 hours because the drug may still be present.

Pain Control. Some patients will not ask for pain medication; therefore, it is important to intervene and anticipate their needs. It is important not to make the patient wait unnecessarily for pain medication.

Nutritional Aspects. The patient should eat a well-balanced diet high in B-complex vitamins; limit or eliminate sugar, nicotine, caffeine, and alcoholic intake; and drink 8 to 10, 8-ounce glasses of water per day to maintain normal elimination patterns. To minimize or avoid the constipating effects of opiates, increase intake of fiber and fluids. If long-term use of opiates is planned, stool softeners may be necessary.

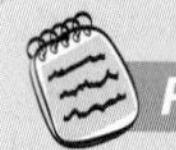

Patient Education and Health Promotion

Orient the patient, family, and significant others to the benefits of adequate pain control. Work with the patient, family, and significant others to determine their perception of pain management and the use of drug therapy, and nonpharmacologic approaches to pain management. If the patient is hesitant about these approaches, determine why. Stress that addiction is not a major factor with short-term use of analgesics and that during long-term use, such as with cancer, it is not the primary concern.

With long-term use of analgesics the major issues are obtaining sufficient pain control to ensure comfort, ensuring that the patient has ample rest, and enhancing the quality of life.

Teach the patient what medications are available for pain control and when and how to request them. Discuss the patient's expectations of pain management and how to rate the severity of pain honestly so that the expectations can be met. Ask what level of exercise is attainable without severe pain. Is the pain control adequate for the individual to maintain ADLs or work?

Assess changes in expectations as therapy progresses and the patient gains understanding and skill in the management of the diagnosis. In terminal illnesses, increasing pain necessitates careful management. The duration and intensity of the pain should be constantly reported to the health care provider for appropriate modifications of the medication regimen.

Assist the patient to learn to cope effectively with the pain. Discuss changes in lifestyle needed to support adequate pain control. Include family members in discussion of pain management. Give praise when techniques are tried regardless of whether success is achieved.

Teach the patient how to self-administer the analgesics ordered on an outpatient basis. This will include transdermal, transmucosal, oral, and rectal routes of administration and care of infusion ports and central lines. (Be sure to validate and record the degree of understanding of the prescribed pain regimen.)

Include social services in the patient education process, especially to connect with community resources available for the patient and family. Not everyone has the financial resources to obtain the medicine prescribed. The degree of professional support needed to implement the planned pain control regimen at home must be carefully evaluated.

PATIENT SELF-ASSESSMENT FORM Analgesics

MEDICATIONS	COLOR	TO BE TAKEN

Patient ____________

Health Care Provider ____________

Health Care Provider's phone ____________

Next appt.* ____________

What I Should Monitor			Premedication Data	Date	Date	Date	Date	Date	Date	Comments
Pain	Onset	Example 8 AM / 3 PM; 9 AM / 3 PM								
	Duration	Before taking medication								
	Relief	Example 6 hrs / 3 hrs								
Describe pain		Location								
		Check one: C = Constant I = Intermittent	C ___ I ___	C ___ I ___	C ___ I ___	C ___ I ___	C ___ I ___	C ___ I ___	C ___ I ___	
		Record: Sharp, dull, throbbing								
Pain *before* medication (Intense 10 — Moderate 5 — Low 1)		Time: e.g., 8 AM = 9								
Pain *after* medication (Intense 10 — Moderate 5 — Low 1 — None 0)		Time: e.g., 9 AM = 5								
		9 PM = 8								
		2 AM = 1								
Sleep (No 10 — Somewhat 5 — Yes 1)										
Appetite (Poor 10 — Decreased 5 — Normal 1)										
I enjoy life? (No 10 — Somewhat 5 — Yes 1)										
Activities of daily living (check one): Perform without difficulty										
Perform with difficulty										
Unable to function adequately										
Other										

*Please bring this record with you to your next appointment.
Use the back of this sheet for additional information.

Make sure the patient and family understand how to obtain assistance with pain medication administration and patient care needs (e.g., visiting nurse, hospice).

Fostering Health Maintenance. Throughout the course of treatment, discuss medication information and how it will benefit the patient. Drug therapy for the management of pain should be coupled with comfort measures, relaxation techniques, meditation, stress management, and meeting the total care needs of the individual to ensure maintenance of ADLs. Provide the patient and significant others with important information contained in the specific drug monograph for the medicines prescribed. Additional health teaching and nursing interventions for the side effects to expect and report are described in the drug monographs that follow.

Seek cooperation and understanding of the following points so that medication adherence is increased: name of medications, dosage, route and times of administration, side effects to expect, and side effects to report.

Written Record. Enlist the patient's aid in developing and maintaining a written record of monitoring parameters (e.g., frequency of pain attacks, activity performed when pain occurs, techniques used to control pain, degree of pain relief, exercise tolerance) (see Patient Self-Assessment Form on p. 327). Complete the Premedication Data column for use as a baseline to track response to drug therapy. Ensure that the patient understands how to use the form and instruct the patient to bring the completed form to follow-up visits. During follow-up visits, focus on issues that will foster adherence with the therapeutic interventions prescribed.

DRUG CLASS: Opiate Agonists

The term *opiate* was once used to refer to drugs derived from opium, such as heroin and morphine. It has been found that many other analgesics not related to morphine act at the same sites within the brain. It is now understood that opiate agonists or opiate antagonists are drugs that act at the same site as morphine either to stimulate analgesic effects (opiate agonists) or block the effects of opiate agonists (opiate antagonists).

Another outdated term is *narcotic.* Originally it referred to medications that induced a stupor or sleep. Over the past 80 years it has gradually come to refer to addictive, morphine-like analgesics. The Harrison Narcotic Act of 1914, which placed morphine-like products under governmental control, helped foster this association. With the development in recent years of analgesics that are as potent as morphine but do not have its sedative or addictive properties, the word *narcotic* should be abandoned in exchange for *opiate agonists* and *opiate partial agonists.*

Actions

Opiate agonists are a group of naturally occurring semisynthetic and synthetic drugs that have the capability to relieve severe pain without the loss of consciousness. The opiate agonists act by stimulation of the opiate receptors in the CNS. Most of these agents also have the ability to produce physical dependence and are thus considered controlled substances under the Federal Controlled Substances Act of 1970.

These agents can be subdivided into four groups: morphine-like derivatives, meperidine-like derivatives, methadone-like derivatives, and an "other" category (Table 20-2). Administration of these agents causes primary effects on the CNS (e.g., analgesia, suppression of the cough reflex, respiratory depression, drowsiness, sedation, mental clouding, euphoria, nausea and vomiting); there are also significant effects on the cardiovascular, gastrointestinal (GI), and urinary tracts.

With continued, prolonged use opiate agonists may produce tolerance or psychological and physical dependence **(addiction). Drug tolerance** occurs when a patient requires increases in dosing to receive the same analgesic relief. Development of tolerance seems to depend on the extent and duration of CNS depression. Patients who have prolonged depression by the continued use of opiate agonists have a higher incidence of developing tolerance. Patients who have developed tolerance to one opiate agonist usually require increased dosages of all opiate agonists.

Patients who are physically dependent on opiate agonists remain asymptomatic as long as they are able to maintain their daily opiate agonist requirement. Addiction may develop after 3 to 6 weeks of continual use of the opiate agonists if used for recreational purposes. Addiction following the use of opiates for acute pain management is infrequent. Early signs of withdrawal are restlessness, perspiration, gooseflesh, lacrimation, runny nose, and mydriasis. Over the next 24 hours, these symptoms intensify, and the patient develops muscular spasms; severe aches in the back, abdomen, and legs; abdominal and muscle cramps; hot and cold flashes; insomnia; nausea, vomiting, and diarrhea; severe sneezing; and increases in body temperature, blood pressure, and respiratory and heart rate. These symptoms reach a peak at 36 to 72 hours after discontinuation of the medication and disappear over the next 5 to 14 days.

Uses

The opiate agonists are used to relieve acute or chronic moderate to severe pain such as that associated with acute injury, postoperative pain, renal or biliary colic, myocardial infarction (MI), or cancer. These agents may be used to provide preoperative sedation and supplement anesthesia. In patients with acute pulmonary edema, small doses of the opiate agonists are used to reduce anxiety and produce positive cardiovascular hemodynamic effects to control edema.

Tramadol is a new synthetic opiate agonist that acts as an analgesic by selectively binding to the μ-receptors and inhibiting the reuptake of norepinephrine and serotonin.

Therapeutic Outcomes

The primary therapeutic outcomes from appropriate opiate agonist therapy are as follows:

1. Relief of pain intensity and duration of pain complaint
2. Prevention of the conversion of persistent pain to chronic pain
3. Prevention of suffering and disability associated with pain
4. Prevention of psychological and socioeconomic consequences associated with inadequate pain management
5. Control of side effects associated with pain management
6. Optimization of the ability to perform ADLs

Nursing Process for Opiate Agonists

Premedication Assessment

1. Perform baseline neurologic assessment, for example, orientation to date, time, and place; mental alertness; bilateral handgrip; and motor functioning.

Drug Table 20-2 OPIATE AGONISTS

GENERIC NAME	BRAND NAME	AVAILABILITY	INITIAL ADULT DOSE	DURATION (HOURS)	DOSE EQUAL TO MORPHINE (10 mg)	
					IM (mg)	ORAL (mg)
MORPHINE AND MORPHINE-LIKE DERIVATIVES						
codeine	Codeine Sulfate Codeine Phosphate	Tablets: 15, 30, 60 mg Inj: 30, 60 mg Oral solution: 15 mg/5 mL	PO, Subcut, IM, IV Analgesic: 15-60 mg q4-6h Antitussive: 10-20 mg q4-6h	4-6	130	200
hydromorphone	Dilaudid, Dilaudid-HP	Tablets: 2, 4, 8 mg Capsules, extended release: 12, 16, 24, 32 mg Liquid: 1 mg/mL Suppositories: 3 mg Inj: 1, 2, 4, 10 mg/mL	PO: 2 mg q4-6h Subcut, IM 2 mg q4-6h Rectal: 3 mg q6-8h	4-5	1.5	7.5
levorphanol	Levo-Dromoran	Tablets: 2 mg	PO: 2 mg	4-8	2	4
morphine	Roxanol, Morphine Sulfate, MSIR, Duramorph, MS Contin, Kadian	Tablets: 15, 30 mg Capsules: 15, 30 mg Sustained release tablets: 15, 30, 60, 100, 200 mg Solution: 10, 20, 100 mg/5 mL; 20 mg/mL Suppositories: 5, 10, 20, 30 mg Inj: 0.5, 1, 2, 4, 5, 8, 10 15, 25, 50 mg/mL	PO: 10-30 mg q4h Subcut, IM: 10 mg/70 kg IV: 4-10 mg slowly Rectal: 10-20 mg q4h	up to 7	10	60
oxycodone	Roxicodone Oxycontin	Tablets: 5 mg Tablets, controlled release: 10, 20, 40, 80, 160 mg Oral solution: 5 mg/5 mL; 20 mg/mL	PO: 5 mg q6h	4-5	15	30
oxycodone	Percodan (with aspirin)	Tablets: 5 mg	PO: 5 mg q6h	4-5	15	30
oxymorphone	Numorphan	Inj: 1, 1.5 mg/mL Suppositories: 5 mg	IV: 0.5 mg Subcut, IM: 1-1.5 mg q4-6h Rectal: 5 mg q4-6h	3-6	1	6

Continued

Drug Table 20-2 OPIATE AGONISTS—cont'd

GENERIC NAME	BRAND NAME	AVAILABILITY	INITIAL ADULT DOSE	DURATION (HOURS)	DOSE EQUAL TO MORPHINE (10 mg) IM (mg)	ORAL (mg)
MEPERIDINE-LIKE DERIVATIVES						
alfentanil	Alfenta	Inj: 500 mcg/mL in 2, 5, 10, 20 mL ampules	IV: variable	>45 min	—	—
fentanyl	Sublimaze	Inj: 0.05 mg/mL Lozenges: 100, 200, 300, 400 mcg	IM: 0.05-0.1 mg	1-2	0.1	—
	Actiq	Oral transmucosal lollipop: 200, 400, 600, 800, 1200, 1600 mcg	Buccal: 200 mcg	1-2	0.1	
	Duragesic	Transdermal patch: 2.5, 5, 7.5, 10 mg	Upper torso: 1 patch q48-72h	72		
meperidine	Demerol	Tablets: 50, 100 mg Syrup: 50 mg/5 mL Inj: 25, 50, 75, 100 mg/1 mL	PO, Subcut, IM: 50-150 mg q3-4h IV: 25-100 mg very slowly	2-4	75	300
sufentanil	Sufenta	Inj: 50 mcg/mL in 1, 2, 5 mL ampules	IV: variable	2-3	—	—
METHADONE-LIKE DERIVATIVES						
methadone	Methadone, Dolophine	Tablets: 5, 10, 40 mg Solution: 5, 10 mg/5 mL Inj: 10 mg/mL Oral concentrate: 10 mg/mL	Analgesia: PO, Subcut, IM: 2.5-10 mg q3-4h Maintenance: PO: 20-40 mg; up to 120 mg daily	4-6	10	20
OTHER OPIATE AGONISTS						
tramadol	Ultram	Tablets: 50 mg	PO: 50-100 mg	4-6	—	100

2. Take vital signs; hold medication if respirations are below 12 per minute and consult with health care provider. Check bowel sounds and note consistency of stools. Review the voiding pattern and urine output.
3. Check prior use of analgesics.
4. Perform pain assessment before administration of an opiate agonist and at appropriate intervals during therapy. Report poor pain control promptly and obtain modification in orders.

Planning

Availability. See Table 20-2.

Antidotes. Nalmefene, naloxone, naltrexone.

Implementation

Dosage and Administration. See Table 20-2.

Evaluation

Side Effects to Expect

Lightheadedness, Dizziness, Sedation, Nausea, Vomiting, Sweating. These effects tend to occur most often with the initial dose. Symptoms can be reduced by keeping the patient supine. Provide for patient safety, reassurance, and comfort.

Confusion, Disorientation. Perform a baseline assessment of the patient's degree of alertness and orientation to name, place, and time before initiating therapy. Make regularly scheduled subsequent evaluations of mental status, and report alterations from baseline. Provide for patient safety during these episodes.

Orthostatic Hypotension. Orthostatic hypotension, manifested by dizziness and weakness, occurs particularly when therapy is being initiated in a patient not in a supine position. Monitor blood pressure closely, especially if the patient complains of dizziness or faintness. Do not allow the patient to sit up.

Constipation. Continued use may cause constipation. Maintain the patient's state of hydration and obtain an order for stool softeners or bulk-forming laxatives if necessary. Encourage the inclusion of sufficient roughage, fresh fruits, vegetables, and whole-grain products in the diet.

Side Effects to Report

Respiratory Depression. Opiate agonists make the respiratory centers less sensitive to carbon dioxide, causing respiratory depression. This may occur before either the reduction in respiratory rate or tidal volume is noticeable. Check the respiratory rate and depth often. Have equipment for respiratory assistance available.

Urinary Retention. Opiate agonists may produce spasms of the ureters and bladder, causing urinary retention. Patients may also have difficulty in starting the stream for urination. If the patient develops urinary hesitancy, assess for bladder distention. Report to the health care provider for further evaluation. Try to stimulate urination by running water or placing the patient's hands in water; if permitted, have male patients stand to void; female patients should sit on a bedpan or toilet with receptacle.

Excessive Use or Abuse. Evaluate the *patient's* response to the analgesic. Identify underlying needs and plan for more appropriate management of those needs. Discuss the case with the health care provider and make plans to cooperatively approach gradual withdrawal of the medications being abused. Suggest a change to a milder analgesic when indicated.

Patients do not have to undergo the symptoms of withdrawal to be treated for addiction. Patients may be treated by gradual reduction of daily opiate agonist doses. If withdrawal symptoms become severe, the patient may receive methadone. Temporary administration of tranquilizers and sedatives may aid in reducing patient anxiety and craving for the opiate agonist.

Assist the patient in recognizing the abuse problem. Provide emotional support for the individual; display an accepting attitude—be kind but firm.

Drug Interactions

CNS Depressants. The following drugs may enhance the depressant effects of the opiate agonists: general anesthetics, phenothiazines, tranquilizers, sedative-hypnotics, tricyclic antidepressants, antihistamines, and alcohol.

Respiratory depression, hypotension, and profound sedation or coma may result from this interaction unless the dosage of the opiate agonist has been reduced appropriately (usually by one third to one half the normal dose).

Phenobarbital, Phenytoin, Rifampin, Chlorpromazine. These enzyme-inducing agents may enhance the metabolism of meperidine to normeperidine. Patients receiving long-term large oral doses of meperidine, those with renal impairment, and those with a highly acidic urine are predisposed to accumulating normeperidine. Evidence of toxic levels of normeperidine are excitation, tremors, and seizures.

Carbamazepine. Carbamazepine may enhance the metabolism of tramadol, reducing analgesic effect. If used concurrently, the dose of tramadol may need to be increased.

Selective Serotonin Reuptake Inhibitors, Monoamine Oxidase Inhibitors. All of these agents increase serotonin levels, potentially causing serotonin syndrome when taken by a person receiving tramadol. These medicines should be used only under the supervision of a health care provider.

Warfarin. The oral anticoagulant effect of warfarin may be increased by tramadol. Carefully monitor coagulation values and adjust the dose as needed when tramadol is initiated or discontinued.

DRUG CLASS: Opiate Partial Agonists

Actions

Opiate partial agonists (e.g., buprenorphine, butorphanol, nalbuphine, pentazocine) are an interesting class of drugs in that their pharmacologic actions depend on whether an opiate agonist has been administered previously and the extent to which physical dependence has developed to that opiate agonist. When used without prior administration of opiate agonists, the opiate partial agonists are effective analgesics. Their potency with the first few weeks of therapy is similar to that of morphine; however, after prolonged use, tolerance may develop. Increasing the dosage does not significantly increase the analgesia but definitely increases the incidence of side effects. This is called a ceiling effect in that, contrary to the action of the opiate agonists, a larger dose does not produce a significantly higher analgesic effect.

If an opiate partial agonist is administered to a patient addicted to an opiate agonist such as morphine or meperidine, the opiate partial agonist will induce withdrawal symptoms from the opiate agonist. If the patient is not addicted to the opiate agonist, there is no interaction and the patient will be relieved of pain.

Uses

Opiate partial agonists may be used for the short-term relief (up to 3 weeks) of moderate to severe pain associated with cancer, burns, renal colic, preoperative analgesia, and obstetric and surgical analgesia. Nalbuphine has minimal addiction liability and is not a controlled substance. Because nalbuphine has a ceiling effect for analgesia and respiratory depression, it is often used as an analgesic for obstetrics.

Therapeutic Outcomes

The primary therapeutic outcomes from opiate partial agonist therapy are as follows:

1. Relief of pain intensity and duration of pain complaint
2. Prevention of the conversion of persistent pain to chronic pain
3. Prevention of suffering and disability associated with pain
4. Prevention of psychological and socioeconomic consequences associated with inadequate pain management.

5. Control of side effects associated with pain management
6. Optimization of the ability to perform ADLs

Nursing Process for Opiate Partial Agonists

Premedication Assessment

1. Perform baseline neurologic assessment, for example, orientation to date, time, and place; mental alertness; bilateral handgrip; and motor functioning.
2. Take vital signs; hold medication if respirations are below 12 and consult with health care provider.
3. Check bowel sounds and note consistency of stools. Review voiding pattern and urine output.
4. Check for prior use of opiate agonists.
5. Perform pain assessment before administration of the opiate agonist and at appropriate intervals during therapy. Report poor pain control promptly and obtain modification in orders.

Planning

Availability. See Table 20-3.

Antidotes. Nalmefene, naloxone, naltrexone.

Implementation

Dosage and Administration. See Table 20-3.

Evaluation

Side Effects to Expect

Clamminess, Dizziness, Sedation, Nausea, Vomiting, Dry Mouth, Sweating. These effects tend to occur most often with the initial dose. Symptoms can be reduced by keeping the patient supine. Provide patient safety, assurance, and comfort.

Constipation. Continued use may cause constipation. Maintain the patient's state of hydration and obtain an order for stool softeners or bulk-forming laxatives if necessary. Encourage the inclusion of sufficient roughage, fresh fruits, vegetables, and whole-grain products in the diet.

Side Effects to Report

Confusion, Disorientation, Hallucinations. Butorphanol and pentazocine, and to a lesser degree, nalbuphine, may produce hallucinations. Patients may complain of seeing multicolored flashing patterns or animals, with and without sound, or may have very vivid dreams. These adverse effects have been reported after only one or two doses of medication and may occur in as many as one third of patients taking butorphanol or pentazocine.

Perform a baseline assessment of the patient's degree of alertness and orientation to name, place, and time before initiating therapy. Make regularly scheduled subsequent evaluations of mental status, and report alterations from baseline. Provide patient safety during these episodes. If recurring, seek a change in the medication order.

Respiratory Depression. Opiate partial agonists make the respiratory centers less sensitive to carbon dioxide, causing respiratory depression. This may occur before either the reduction in respiratory rate or tidal volume is noticeable. Check the respiratory rate and depth often.

Excessive Use or Abuse. Repeated use may lead to tolerance, dependence, and addiction. Evaluate the

Drug Table 20-3 OPIATE PARTIAL AGONISTS

GENERIC NAME	BRAND NAME	AVAILABILITY	ADULT DOSE	DURATION (HOURS)	DOSE EQUAL TO MORPHINE (10 mg)
buprenorphine	Buprenex, Subutex	Tablets: 2, 8 mg Inj: 0.3 mg/mL in 1 mL ampules	0.3-0.6 mg repeated in 5-6h	6	0.3 mg
butorphanol	Stadol	Inj: 1, 2 mg in 1, 2, 10 mL vials	IM: 2 mg, repeated in 3-4h; do not exceed single doses of 4 mg IV: 1 mg, repeated in 3-4h	(IM) 3-4	(IM) 2-3 mg
	Stadol NS	Nasal spray: 10 mg/mL	Nasal: 1 spray in each nostril repeated in 3-4h		
nalbuphine	Nubain	Inj: 10, 20 mg/mL in 1, 10 mL vials	Subcut, IM, IV: 10 mg/70 kg, repeat q3-6h; do not exceed 160 mg daily	3-6	10 mg
pentazocine	Talwin, Talwin NX*	Inj: 30 mg/mL in 1, 1.5, 2, 10 mL vials Tablets: (with naloxone) 50 mg	PO: 50-100 mg q3-4h; do not exceed 600 mg daily Subcut, IM, IV: 30 mg q3-4h; do not exceed 360 mg daily	2-3	30-60 mg

*Tablets contain naloxone to prevent abuse.

patient's response to the analgesic. Identify underlying needs and plan for more appropriate management of those needs. Discuss the case with the physician and make plans to cooperatively approach gradual withdrawal of the medications being abused. Suggest a change to a milder analgesic when indicated.

Patients do not have to experience the symptoms of withdrawal to be treated for addiction. Patients may be treated by gradual reduction of daily opiate agonist doses. If withdrawal symptoms become severe, the patient may receive methadone. Temporary administration of tranquilizers and sedatives may aid in reducing patient anxiety and craving for the opiate agonist.

Assist the patient in recognizing the abuse problem. Provide for emotional support of the individual; display an accepting attitude—be kind but firm.

Drug Interactions

CNS Depressants. The following drugs may enhance the depressant effects of the opiate partial agonists: general anesthetics, phenothiazines, tranquilizers, sedative-hypnotics, tricyclic antidepressants, antihistamines, and alcohol.

Respiratory depression, hypotension, and profound sedation or coma may result from this interaction unless the dosage of the opiate partial agonist has been reduced appropriately (usually by one third to one half the normal dose).

Opiate Agonists. Opiate partial agonists have weak antagonist activity. When administered to patients who have been receiving opiate agonists such as morphine or meperidine on a regular basis, it may precipitate withdrawal symptoms.

DRUG CLASS: Opiate Antagonists

nalmefene (nal' meh feen)
▶ REVEX (rev' ex)

Actions

Nalmefene is a pure opiate antagonist related to naltrexone. It has no effect of its own other than its ability to reverse the respiratory depression, sedation, and hypotension associated with opiate agonists and opiate partial agonists. Nalmefene has a longer duration of action than naloxone when reversing opiate effects. When administered to patients who have not recently received opiates, there is no respiratory depression, psychomimetic effect, circulatory changes, or other pharmacologic activity. If administered to a person addicted to the opiate agonists or the opiate partial agonists, withdrawal symptoms may be precipitated. Nalmefene is not effective in CNS depression induced by tranquilizers or sedative-hypnotics. Nalmefene may not completely reverse the effects of buprenorphine-induced respiratory depression possibly due to strong affinity and slow release of buprenorphine from receptor sites.

Uses

Nalmefene is a drug of choice for treatment of respiratory depression when excessive doses of opiate agonists or opiate partial agonists have been administered, or when the causative agent is unknown.

Therapeutic Outcomes

The primary therapeutic outcome expected from nalmefene is reversal of respiratory depression. When used for postoperative patients, the primary therapeutic outcome is to achieve reversal of excessive opioid effects without inducing a complete reversal and acute pain.

Nursing Process for Nalmefene

Premedication Assessment

1. Perform baseline neurologic assessment, for example, orientation to date, time, and place; mental alertness; bilateral handgrip; and motor functioning.
2. Take vital signs; blood pressure, pulse, and respirations should be taken at frequent intervals until resolution of CNS depression. Then schedule vital signs to be taken at appropriate intervals because the duration of action of nalmefene may be shorter than the duration of action of the opiate agonist.
3. Check prior use or dependence on opiate agonists or opiate partial agonists. Diagnostic testing for narcotic dependence may be performed in accordance with policies of the clinical site. Inform patient of risks involved.
4. Have supportive equipment available in immediate area to maintain respirations.
5. Check bowel sounds. Review voiding pattern and urine output.

Planning

Availability. Injection: 100 mcg/mL in 1 mL ampules for postoperative opiate depression and 1 mg/mL in 2 mL ampules for opiate overdose.

Implementation

Dosage and Administration

Postoperative Opiate Depression. *Adult:* Intravenous (IV): The goal of treatment in the postoperative setting is to achieve reversal of excessive opioid effects without inducing a complete reversal and acute pain. Initial dose: 0.25 mcg/kg followed by 0.25 mcg/kg incremental doses at 2- to 5-minute intervals, stopping as soon as the desired degree of opioid reversal is obtained.

Opiate Overdose. *Adult*: IV: Initially 0.5 mg/70 kg. A second dose of 1 mg/70 kg may be administered 2 to 5 minutes later. If a total dose of 1.5 mg/70 kg has been administered without clinical response, additional nalmefene is unlikely to have an effect; the depressive condition may be caused by a drug or disease process not responsive to nalmefene.

Evaluation

Side Effects to Expect

Mental Depression, Apathy, Nausea, Vomiting. Nalmefene rarely manifests any side effects. The following adverse effects have been reported very rarely when extremely high doses have been used: nausea, vomiting, chills, myalgia, dysphoria, abdominal cramps, and joint pain. These symptoms suggest blockade of naturally occurring opioids in the body.

Nalmefene should be given with caution to patients known or suspected to be physically dependent on opiates, including neonates born to women who are opiate dependent, because the drug may precipitate severe withdrawal symptoms. The severity of the symptoms depends on the dose of the nalmefene and the degree of dependence.

Drug Interactions. There are no drug interactions other than that of the antagonist activity toward opiate agonists and opiate partial agonists.

naloxone (nal oks' own)
NARCAN (nar' can)

Actions

Naloxone is a so-called pure opiate antagonist because it has no effect of its own other than its ability to reverse the CNS depressant effects of opiate agonists, opiate partial agonists, and propoxyphene. When administered to patients who have not recently received opiates, there is no respiratory depression, psychomimetic effect, circulatory changes, or other pharmacologic activity. If administered to a person addicted to opiate agonists or opiate partial agonists, withdrawal symptoms may be precipitated. Naloxone is not effective in CNS depression induced by tranquilizers or sedative-hypnotics.

Uses

Naloxone is a drug of choice for treatment of respiratory depression when excessive doses of opiate agonists, opiate partial agonists, or propoxyphene have been administered, or when the causative agent is unknown.

Therapeutic Outcomes

The primary therapeutic outcome expected from naloxone is reversal of respiratory depression.

Nursing Process for Naloxone

Premedication Assessment

1. Perform baseline neurologic assessment, for example, orientation to date, time, and place; mental alertness; bilateral handgrip; and motor functioning.
2. Monitor vital signs; blood pressure, pulse, and respirations should be taken at frequent intervals until resolution of CNS depression. Then schedule vital signs to be taken at appropriate intervals because the duration of action of naloxone is short.
3. Check prior use or dependence on opiate agonists or opiate partial agonists. Diagnostic testing for narcotic dependence may be performed in accordance with policies of the clinical site. Inform patient of risks involved.
4. Have supportive equipment available in immediate area to maintain respirations.
5. Check bowel sounds. Review voiding pattern and urine output.

Planning

Availability. Injection: 0.02 mg/mL in 2 mL vials (for neonatal use) and 0.4 mg/mL in 1 mL ampules, 1 mL syringes, and 1, 2, and 10 mL vials.

Implementation

Dosage and Administration. *Adult:* IV: Postoperative opiate depression—0.1 to 0.2 mg every 2 to 3 minutes until the desired response is achieved. Opiate overdose: 0.4 to 2 mg every 2 to 3 minutes. If no response is seen after 10 minutes, the depressive condition may be caused by a drug or disease process not responsive to naloxone.

Evaluation

Side Effects to Expect

Mental Depression, Apathy, Nausea, Vomiting. Naloxone rarely manifests any side effects. The following adverse effects have been reported very rarely when extremely high doses have been used: mental depression, apathy, inability to concentrate, sleepiness, irritability, anorexia, nausea, and vomiting. These adverse effects usually occurred in the first few days of treatment and dissipated rapidly with continued therapy.

Naloxone should be used with caution following the use of opiates during surgery because it may result in excitement, an increase in blood pressure, and a clinically important reversal of analgesia. The early reversal of opiate effects may induce nausea, vomiting, sweating, and tachycardia.

Naloxone should be given with caution to patients known or suspected to be physically dependent on opiates, including neonates born to women who are opiate dependent, because the drug may precipitate severe withdrawal symptoms. The severity of the symptoms depends on the dose of the naloxone and the degree of dependence.

Drug Interactions. There are no drug interactions other than that of the antagonist activity toward opiate agonists, opiate partial agonists, and propoxyphene.

naltrexone (nal trex' own)
REVIA (rhe vee' ah)

Actions

Naltrexone is a pure opioid antagonist that is closely related to naloxone. It differs, however, in that it is active after oral administration and has a considerably longer duration of action. Naltrexone blocks the effects of opioids by competitive binding at opioid receptors. The mechanism of action of naltrexone in alcoholism is not known.

Uses

Naltrexone is used clinically to block the pharmacologic effects of exogenously administered opiates in patients who are enrolled in drug abuse treatment programs. The rationale for using naltrexone as an adjunct in treatment is that naltrexone may diminish or eliminate opiate-seeking behavior by blocking the euphoric reinforcement produced by self-administration of opiates and by preventing the conditioned abstinence syndrome (i.e., opiate craving) that occurs after opiate withdrawal. Naltrexone has been added to pentazocine formulations (Talwin NX) to reduce its abuse, by blocking the euphoric high associated with pentazocine.

Naltrexone also has been approved as an adjunct in the treatment of alcoholism to support abstinence and reduce relapse rates, and alcohol consumption. It must be used with other treatment modalities; the expected effect of the drug treatment is a modest improvement in the outcome of conventional treatment.

Therapeutic Outcomes

The primary therapeutic outcomes expected from naltrexone are as follows:

1. Improved adherence with a substance abuse program because of reduced craving of opioids.
2. Improved adherence with an alcohol treatment program by diminishing craving for alcohol.

Nursing Process for Naltrexone

Premedication Assessment

1. Perform baseline neurologic assessment, for example, orientation to date, time, and place; mental alertness; bilateral handgrip; and motor functioning.
2. Monitor vital signs: temperature, blood pressure, pulse, and respirations.
3. Check laboratory values for hepatotoxicity; urine screen for opiate use.
4. Monitor for GI symptoms before and during therapy.
5. The manufacturer recommends that baseline determinations of liver function should be performed in all patients before initiation of therapy and repeated monthly for the next 6 months.
6. The manufacturer recommends a minimum of 7 to 10 days of abstinence from all opiates, a urinalysis to confirm the absence of opiates, and the use of a naloxone challenge test to ensure that the patient will not develop withdrawal symptoms.

Planning

Availability. PO: 50 mg tablets.

Implementation

Dosage and Administration

Behavior Modification. Naltrexone therapy in combination with behavioral therapy has been shown to be more effective than naltrexone or behavioral therapy alone in prolonging opiate or alcohol cessation in patients formerly physically dependent on opiates or alcohol.

Treatment of Narcotic Dependence. PO: Induction regimen of 25 mg. Observe for development of withdrawal symptoms. If none occur, administer 50 mg the next day. The maintenance regimen is 50 mg daily. Alternative regimens of 100 mg every other day or 150 mg every third day have been used to improve adherence during a behavior modification program (see Chapter 49).

Withdrawal Symptoms. Naltrexone may precipitate acute and severe withdrawal symptoms in patients who are physically dependent on opioids. Addicts must be completely detoxified and opioid-free before taking naltrexone. The manufacturer recommends a minimum of 7 to 10 days of abstinence from all opiates, a urinalysis to confirm the absence of opiates, and the use of a naloxone challenge test to ensure that the patient will not develop withdrawal symptoms.

Patients undergoing naltrexone therapy must be carefully instructed about the expectations of behavioral modification associated with therapy. They should also be advised that self-administration of small doses of opiates (e.g., heroin) during naltrexone therapy will not result in any pharmacologic effect and that large doses may result in serious pharmacologic effects, including coma and death. Patients should also be given identification to notify medical personnel that they are taking a long-acting opiate antagonist.

Treatment of Alcoholism. PO: 50 mg once daily. (See also Chapter 49.)

Evaluation

Many adverse effects have been associated with naltrexone therapy, but it is difficult to know exactly which adverse effects are secondary to naltrexone alone because some patients may experience mild opiate withdrawal symptoms as well. The adverse effects of drug and alcohol abuse and poor nutritional states may contribute to the patient's discomfort.

Side Effects to Expect

Nausea, Vomiting, Headache, Anorexia. Side effects are usually mild and tend to resolve with continued therapy. Encourage the patient not to discontinue therapy without first consulting the physician and treatment program.

Side Effects to Report

Hepatotoxicity. A major adverse effect is hepatotoxicity after doses of 300 mg daily for 3 to 8 weeks. The symptoms of hepatotoxicity are jaundice, nausea, vomiting, anorexia, hepatomegaly, splenomegaly, and abnormal liver function tests (e.g., elevated bilirubin, aspartate aminotransferase [AST], alanine aminotransferase [ALT], alkaline phosphatase, prothrombin time). Because many of these patients do not develop clinical symptoms but do develop abnormal liver function tests, strongly encourage patients to report for blood tests as scheduled. Report abnormal values to the appropriate health care provider.

Drug Interactions

Opiate-Containing Products. Patients taking naltrexone will probably not benefit from opioid-containing medicines such as analgesics, cough and cold preparations, and antidiarrheal preparations. These products should be avoided during naltrexone therapy when nonopiate therapy is available.

Clonidine. Clonidine may be administered in patients to reduce the severity of withdrawal symptoms precipitated or exacerbated by naltrexone.

DRUG CLASS: Salicylates

salicylates (sahl ih sil′ ates)

Actions

The **salicylates** are the most common analgesics used for the relief of slight to moderate pain. Salicylates were introduced into medicine in the late 19th century because of their three primary pharmacologic effects as analgesic, antipyretic, and antiinflammatory agents. Although the mechanisms of action are not fully known, most of the activity of the salicylates comes from inhibition of prostaglandin synthesis. Salicylates inhibit the formation of prostaglandins that sensitize pain receptors to stimulation causing pain (analgesia); they inhibit the prostaglandins that produce the signs and symptoms of inflammation (e.g., redness, swelling, warmth); and they inhibit the synthesis and release of prostaglandins in the brain that cause the elevation of body temperature (antipyresis). A major benefit of salicylates is that they do not dull the consciousness level and do not cause mental sluggishness, memory disturbances, hallucinations, euphoria, or sedation.

A unique property of aspirin, compared with other salicylates, is inhibition of platelet aggregation and enhancement of bleeding time. The platelet loses its ability to aggregate and form clots for the duration of its lifetime (7 to 10 days). The mechanism of action is inhibition of the synthesis of thromboxane A_2, a potent vasoconstrictor and inducer of platelet aggregation.

Uses

The combination of pharmacologic effects makes salicylates the drugs of choice for symptomatic relief of discomfort, pain, inflammation, or fever associated with bacterial and viral infections, headache, muscle aches, and rheumatoid arthritis. Salicylates can be taken to relieve pain on a long-term basis without causing drug dependence.

Because of its antiplatelet activity, aspirin is also indicated for reducing the risk of recurrent transient ischemic attacks (TIAs) or stroke in men. Aspirin is also used to reduce the risk of myocardial infarction (MI) in patients with previous MI or unstable angina pectoris.

Therapeutic Outcomes

The primary therapeutic outcomes expected from salicylates are reduced pain, reduced inflammation, and elimination of fever. The primary therapeutic outcomes expected from aspirin when used for antiplatelet therapy are reduced frequency of TIA, stroke, or MI.

Nursing Process for Salicylates

Premedication Assessment

1. Perform baseline neurologic assessment, for example, orientation to date, time, and place; mental alertness; bilateral handgrip; motor functioning; balance; and hearing.
2. Monitor vital signs: temperature, blood pressure, pulse, and respirations.
3. Check laboratory values for hepatotoxicity and renal impairment; clotting time.
4. Monitor for GI symptoms before and during therapy; conduct stool guaiac if suspecting GI tract bleeding.
5. Check for concurrent use of anticoagulant agents.
6. If on oral hypoglycemics, review baseline serum glucose level.
7. When used as analgesic, perform pain assessment before administering salicylate and at appropriate intervals during therapy. Report poor pain control promptly and obtain modification in orders.

Planning

Availability. See Tables 20-4 and 20-5.

Implementation

Dosage and Administration

Treatment of Pain. See Tables 20-4 and 20-5.

Prevention of Blood Clots. PO: 80 to 1300 mg daily. Dosing depends on whether the patient has a previous history of clot formation and other medications the patient may be receiving. The larger doses are usually subdivided into 325 mg two to four times daily.

Evaluation

As beneficial as the salicylates are, they are not without adverse effects. In normal therapeutic doses, they may produce GI irritation, occasional nausea, and gastric hemorrhage. Extreme caution should be used with administration to those patients with a history of peptic ulcer, liver disease, or coagulation disorders.

Side Effects to Expect

Gastric Irritation. If gastric irritation occurs, administer medication with food, milk, or antacids (1 hour later), or with large amounts of water. If symptoms

Drug Table 20-4 NONSTEROIDAL AND ANTIINFLAMMATORY AGENTS

GENERIC NAME	BRAND NAME	AVAILABILITY	USES AND DOSAGES	MAXIMUM DAILY DOSE (mg)
SALICYLATES				
aspirin	Zorprin, A.S.A., Empirin	Tablets: 81, 165, 325, 500, 650 mg Suppositories: 120, 200, 300, 600 mg	Minor aches and pains: 325-600 mg q4h Arthritis: 2.6-5.2 g/day in divided doses Acute rheumatic fever: 7.8 g/day Myocardial infarction prophylaxis: 325 mg daily	—
choline salicylate	Arthropan	Liquid: 870 mg/5 mL	Mild pain: 870 mg q3-4h (fewer GI side effects)	7000
diflunisal	Dolobid	Tablets: 250, 500 mg	Mild to moderate pain: Initially, 1000 mg, then 500 mg q8h Osteoarthritis and rheumatoid arthritis: 250-500 mg twice daily	1500
magnesium salicylate	Magan, Mobidin	Tablets: 467, 500, 545, 580, 600 mg	Mild aches and pains: 500-650 mg three or four times daily	9600
salsalate	Salsitab Artha-G	Tablets: 500, 750 mg	Mild pain: 500-700 mg four to six times daily	3000
sodium salicylate	Sodium Salicylate	Enteric-coated tablets: 325, 650 mg	Mild analgesia: 325-650 mg q4-8h (less effective than equal doses of aspirin)	3900
sodium thiosalicylate	Rexolate	Inj: 50 mg/mL in 2- and 30-mL vials	Acute gout: IM: 100 mg q3-4h for 2 days, then 100 mg/day Rheumatic fever: IM: 100-150 mg q4-6h for 3 days, then 100 mg twice daily	—
NONSTEROIDAL ANTIINFLAMMATORY AGENTS				
Cyclooxygenase-1 (COX-1) Inhibitors				
diclofenac	Cataflam, Voltaren, ✱ Novo-Difenac	Tablets: 50 mg Tablets, delayed release: 25, 50, 75, 100 mg	Rheumatoid and osteoarthritis, ankylosing spondylitis: 25-75 mg two or three times daily Primary dysmenorrhea: 50 mg three times daily	200
etodolac	Lodine, Lodine XL	Capsules: 200, 300 mg Tablets: 400, 500 mg Tablets, extended release: 400, 500, 600 mg	Osteoarthritis, pain: 300-400 mg three or four times daily	1200
fenoprofen	Nalfon	Capsules: 200, 300 mg Tablets: 600 mg	Rheumatoid and osteoarthritis: 300-600 mg three or four times daily Mild to moderate pain: 200 mg q4-6h	3200
flurbiprofen	Ansaid	Tablets: 50, 100 mg	Rheumatoid and osteoarthritis: 50-100 mg two or three times daily	300

✱ Available in Canada.

Continued

Drug Table 20-4 NONSTEROIDAL AND ANTIINFLAMMATORY AGENTS—cont'd

GENERIC NAME	BRAND NAME	AVAILABILITY	USES AND DOSAGES	MAXIMUM DAILY DOSE (mg)
NONSTEROIDAL ANTIINFLAMMATORY AGENTS—cont'd				
Cyclooxygenase-1 (COX-1) Inhibitors—cont'd				
ibuprofen	Motrin, Advil, ✱ Novoprofen	Tablets: 50, 100, 200, 400, 600, 800 mg Capsules: 200 Suspension: 100 mg/2.5 mL, 100 mg/5 mL Oral drops: 40 mg/mL	Rheumatoid and osteoarthritis: 300-600 mg three or four times daily Mild to moderate pain: 400 mg q4-6h Primary dysmenorrhea: 400 mg q4h Fever: Peds: 5-10 mg/kg three or four times daily	2400 40 mg/kg/24 hr
indomethacin	Indocin, ✱ Indocid	Capsules: 25, 50 mg Sustained release capsules: 75 mg Oral suspension: 25 mg/5 mL Suppository: 50 mg	Rheumatoid and osteoarthritis, ankylosing spondylitis: 25-50 mg three or four times daily Acute painful shoulder: 25-50 mg two or three times daily Acute gouty arthritis: 50 mg three times daily Closure of patent ductus arteriosus: IV—one to three doses at 12-24 h intervals	—
ketoprofen	Orudis ✱ Apo-Keto	Tablets: 12.5 mg Capsules: 50, 75 mg Extended release capsules: 100, 150, 200 mg	Rheumatoid and osteoarthritis: Initially 75 mg three times daily or 50 mg four times daily; reduce initial dose by ½ to ⅓ in elderly patients or those with impaired renal function Mild pain, primary dysmenorrhea: 25-50 mg three or four times daily	300
ketorolac	Toradol, Acular, ✱ Novo-Ketorolac	Tablets: 10 mg Injection: 15, 30 mg/mL in 1, 2 mL prefilled syringes	Injectable analgesic, antiinflammatory, antipyretic used for acute, short-term pain management; 30-60 mg IM, initially, 15-30 mg q6h PRN pain; then PO ≤40 mg/24 h; do not exceed 5 days of therapy	120-150
meclofenamate		Capsules: 50, 100 mg	Rheumatoid and osteoarthritis: 200-400 mg daily in three or four equal doses Mild to moderate pain: 50-100 mg three or four times daily Primary dysmenorrhea: 100 mg three times daily	400
mefenamic acid	Ponstel, ✱ Ponstan	Capsules: 250 mg	Moderate pain or primary dysmenorrhea: Initially 500 mg, then 250 mg q6h; do not exceed 7 days of therapy	1000
meloxicam	Mobic	Tablets: 7.5, 15 mg Liquid: 7.5 mg/5 mL	Osteoarthritis: 7.5-15 mg daily	15
nabumetone	Relafen	Tablets: 500, 750 mg	Rheumatoid and osteoarthritis: 1000-1500 mg daily in one or two doses	2000

Drug Table 20-4 **NONSTEROIDAL AND ANTIINFLAMMATORY AGENTS—cont'd**

GENERIC NAME	BRAND NAME	AVAILABILITY	USES AND DOSAGES	MAXIMUM DAILY DOSE (mg)
NONSTEROIDAL ANTIINFLAMMATORY AGENTS—cont'd				
Cyclooxygenase-1 (COX-1) Inhibitors—cont'd				
naproxen	Naprosyn, Aleve	Tablets: 200, 250, 375, 500 mg Extended release tablets: 375, 500 mg Oral suspension: 125 mg/5 mL	Rheumatoid and osteoarthritis, ankylosing spondylitis: 250-375 mg twice daily	1000
naproxen sodium	Anaprox, Anaprox DS	Tablets: 275 mg Tablets: 550 mg Tablets, extended release: 412, 550 mg	Acute gout: 750-825 mg initially, followed by 250-275 mg q8h Moderate pain, primary dysmenorrhea, acute tendonitis, bursitis: 500-550 mg followed by 250-275 mg	1100
oxaprozin	Daypro	Caplets: 600 mg	Rheumatoid arthritis, osteoarthritis: 1200 mg once daily	1800
piroxicam	Feldene, ✱ Nu-pirox	Capsules: 10, 20 mg	Rheumatoid and osteoarthritis: 20 mg once daily	200
sulindac	Clinoril, ✱ Apo-Sulin	Tablets: 150, 200 mg	Rheumatoid and osteoarthritis, ankylosing spondylitis: 150 mg twice daily Acute painful shoulder: 200 mg twice daily	400
tolmetin	Tolectin	Tablets: 200, 600 mg Capsules: 400 mg	Rheumatoid and osteoarthritis: 400-600 mg three times daily	2000
Cyclooxygenase-2 (COX-2) Inhibitors				
celecoxib	Celebrex	Capsules: 100, 200, 400 mg	Rheumatoid and osteoarthritis: 100-200 mg twice daily Ankylosing spondylitis: 200-400 mg daily Acute pain and primary dysmenorrhea: 400 mg initially, followed by 200 mg on the first day, then 200 mg twice daily Familial adenomatous polyposis (FAP): 400 mg twice daily taken with food	400

persist or increase in severity, report for health care provider evaluation. Aspirin is available in enteric-coated form to reduce gastric irritation.

Side Effects to Report

Gastrointestinal Bleeding. Dark tarry stools and bright red or "coffee ground" emesis. Test any suspicious stools or emesis for presence of occult blood.

Salicylism. Patients receiving higher doses on a continuing basis are susceptible to developing salicylate intoxication (salicylism). Symptoms include tinnitus (ringing in the ears), impaired hearing, dimming of vision, sweating, fever, lethargy, dizziness, mental confusion, nausea, and vomiting. This condition is reversible on dosage reduction. Massive overdoses may lead to respiratory depression and coma. There is no antidote; primary treatment is discontinuing the drug, gastric lavage, forcing IV fluids, and alkalizing the urine with IV sodium bicarbonate.

Patients who develop signs of salicylate toxicity should be reevaluated for other underlying disease and the possibility that other medications would be more effective.

Drug Interactions

NSAIDs. There is a controversy in the literature about the possibility that COX-1 inhibitors can reduce the platelet-inhibiting effects of aspirin when administered about the same time. The NSAID may be blocking the receptor on platelets that aspirin would

Drug Table 20-5 **INGREDIENTS OF SELECTED ANALGESIC COMBINATION PRODUCTS**

	NONCONTROLLED SUBSTANCE			CONTROLLED SUBSTANCE	
PRODUCT	**ASPIRIN (mg)**	**ACETAMINOPHEN (mg)**	**OTHER (mg)**	**CODEINE (mg)**	**OTHER (mg)**
Anacin Tablets	400		Caffeine 32		
Anacin Maximum Strength	500		Caffeine 32		
BC Powder	650		Caffeine 33 Salacylamide 195		
Darvocet-N 50		325			Propoxyphene napsylate 50
Darvocet-N 100		650			Propoxyphene napsylate 100
Darvon Compound-65	389		Caffeine 32		Propoxyphene HCl 65
Empirin					
Codeine #3	325			30	
Codeine #4	325			60	
Excedrin Extra-strength	250	250	Caffeine 65		
Fioricet		325	Caffeine 40		Butalbital 50
Fiorinal	325		Caffeine 40		Butalbital 50
Fiorinal w/Codeine	325		Caffeine 40	30	Butalbital 50
Lortab 10/500		500			Hydrocodone 10 mg
Percocet 7.5		500			Oxycodone 7.5
Percodan	325				Oxycodone 4.5
Percogesic		325	Phenyltolox-amine 30		
Talwin Compound Caplets	325				Pentazocine 12.5
Tylenol		325			
Tylenol					
Codeine #2		300		15	
Codeine #3		300		30	
Codeine #4		300		60	
Vicodin		500			Hydrocodone 5 mg

normally bind to, preventing the platelet inhibition caused by aspirin. One approach to avoid this interaction is to take aspirin several hours before the COX-1 NSAID. This might not be possible for the person with severe rheumatoid arthritis who needs the analgesic effects around the clock.

Sulfinpyrazone, Probenecid. Salicylates inhibit the excretion of uric acid by these agents. Although an occasional aspirin will not be sufficient to interfere with their effectiveness, regular use of salicylates or products containing salicylate should be discouraged. If analgesia is required, suggest acetaminophen.

Warfarin. Salicylates may enhance the anticoagulant effects of warfarin. Observe for petechiae, ecchymoses, nosebleeds, bleeding gums, dark tarry stools, and bright red or coffee-ground emesis. Monitor prothrombin time and reduce the dosage of warfarin if necessary.

Phenytoin. Monitor patients with concurrent therapy for signs of phenytoin toxicity, such as nystagmus, sedation, or lethargy. Serum levels may be ordered, and a reduced dosage of phenytoin may be required.

Oral Hypoglycemic Agents. Salicylates may enhance the hypoglycemic effects of these agents. Monitor for hypoglycemia, headache, weakness, decreased coordination, general apprehension, diaphoresis, hunger, or blurred or double vision. The dosage of the hypoglycemic agent may need to be reduced. Notify the health care provider if any of the above symptoms appear.

Methotrexate. Monitor for signs of methotrexate toxicity: bone marrow suppression, decreased white blood cell (WBC) count, red blood cell (RBC) count, sore throat, fever, or lethargy.

Corticosteroids. Although often used together, salicylates and corticosteroids may produce GI ulceration. Monitor for signs of GI bleeding: observe for the development of dark tarry stools and bright red or "coffee ground" emesis.

Ethanol. Patients should avoid aspirin within 8 to 10 hours of heavy alcohol use. Small amounts of GI bleeding often occur. If aspirin therapy is absolutely necessary, an enteric-coated product should be used.

Clinitest. Ingestion of 8 to 18, 325-mg tablets of aspirin daily may result in false-positive Clinitest urine glucose determinations. Blood glucose measurements may be required for an accurate reading.

DRUG CLASS: Nonsteroidal Antiinflammatory Agents

Actions

Nonsteroidal antiinflammatory agents/drugs (NSAIDs) are also known as "aspirin-like" drugs. They are chemically unrelated to the salicylates but are prostaglandin inhibitors and share many of the same therapeutic actions and side effects. NSAIDs act by blocking cyclooxygenase (COX-1 and COX-2). They all have varying degrees of analgesic, antipyretic, and antiinflammatory activity. Celecoxib, is a COX-2 selective inhibitor, whereas all other NSAIDs are nonselective COX-1 and COX-2 inhibitors.

Uses

In clinical studies, all of these agents (see Table 20-4) are superior to placebos and approach aspirin in effectiveness, but none is superior to aspirin. Depending on the agent used, the dosage, and the patient, the side effects of therapy tend to be somewhat less than those associated with salicylate therapy. Thus these agents are most effectively used as alternates for patients who do not tolerate aspirin. There is little difference between them in effectiveness or tolerance. Longer-acting NSAIDs may be useful for patients who have difficulty remembering to take frequent doses. The cost of therapy with NSAIDs is considerably higher than with aspirin treatment. There is also substantial cost difference between NSAIDs, so it makes sense to try the lower-cost agents before moving to the more expensive agents because they are similarly effective.

These agents are used to relieve the pain and inflammation of rheumatoid arthritis, osteoarthritis, ankylosing spondylitis, and gout. Certain agents (e.g., ibuprofen, ketoprofen, naproxen, diclofenac, celecoxib) are also approved for use to control the discomfort of primary dysmenorrhea. Ibuprofen, naproxen, and ketoprofen are available over the counter (OTC) to be used for the temporary relief of minor aches and pains associated with the common cold, headache, toothache, muscle aches, backaches, arthritis, and menstrual cramps, as well as to reduce fever. The COX-2 inhibitor appears to have the advantage of causing fewer GI side effects such as upper GI bleeding. This is quite significant because 7% to 8% of patients experience GI bleeding after using NSAIDs, and it is a primary cause of hospitalizations caused by adverse effects of medicines.

In April 2005, the U.S. Food and Drug Administration (FDA) issued a new warning about an increased risk of potentially fatal cardiovascular adverse effects (heart attack, stroke) that may be a class effect of NSAIDs. The FDA also reiterated the well-described risk of serious and potentially life-threatening GI bleeding associated with NSAIDs. If a decision is made to prescribe an NSAID for chronic use, the lowest effective dose for the shortest duration should be used. NSAIDS should not be used in patients who are immediately postoperative from coronary artery bypass graft (CABG) surgery.

Therapeutic Outcomes

The primary therapeutic outcomes expected from NSAIDs are reduced pain, reduced inflammation, and elimination of fever.

Nursing Process for NSAIDs

Premedication Assessment

1. Perform baseline neurologic assessment, for example, orientation to date, time, and place; mental alertness; bilateral handgrip; motor functioning; peripheral sensations; and vision and hearing.
2. Monitor vital signs: temperature, blood pressure, pulse, and respirations.
3. Check laboratory values for hepatotoxicity, nephrotoxicity, bleeding time, and blood dyscrasias.
4. Monitor for GI symptoms before and during therapy; conduct stool guaiac if suspecting GI tract bleeding.
5. Check bowel sounds and note stool consistency. Review voiding pattern and urine output.
6. Check for concurrent use of anticoagulant agents.
7. When used as an analgesic, perform pain assessment before administering NSAIDs and at appropriate intervals during therapy. Report poor pain control promptly and obtain modification in orders.

Planning

Availability. See Table 20-4.

Implementation

Dosage and Administration. See Table 20-4. NOTE: Do not administer to patients who are allergic to aspirin.

Evaluation

Side Effects to Expect

Gastric Irritation. If gastric irritation occurs, administer medication with food, milk, antacids, or large amounts of water. If symptoms persist or increase in severity, report for health care provider evaluation.

Constipation. The use of stool softeners or bulk-forming laxatives may be necessary. Maintain the patient's state of hydration. Encourage the inclusion of sufficient roughage, fresh fruits, vegetables, and whole-grain products in the diet.

Dizziness. Provide patient safety during episodes of dizziness.

Drowsiness. People who work around machinery, operate a motor vehicle, or perform other duties in which they must remain mentally alert should not take these medications while working.

Side Effects to Report

Gastrointestinal Bleeding. Observe for the development of dark tarry stools and bright red or "coffee ground" emesis.

Confusion. Perform a baseline assessment of the patient's degree of alertness and orientation to name, place, and time before initiating therapy. Make regularly scheduled subsequent evaluations of mental status, and report alterations from baseline.

Hives, Pruritus, Rash. Report symptoms for further evaluation by the health care provider.

Nephrotoxicity. Monitor urinalysis and kidney function tests for abnormal results. Report an increasing blood urea nitrogen (BUN) and creatinine, decreasing urine output or urine specific gravity despite amount of fluid intake, casts or protein in the urine, frank blood- or smoky-colored urine, or RBCs in excess of 0 to 3 on the urinalysis report.

Hepatotoxicity. The symptoms of hepatotoxicity are anorexia, nausea, vomiting, jaundice, hepatomegaly, splenomegaly, and abnormal liver function tests (e.g., elevated bilirubin, AST, ALT, alkaline phosphatase, prothrombin time).

Blood Dyscrasias. Routine laboratory studies (e.g., RBC, WBC, differential counts) should be scheduled. Monitor for sore throat, fever, purpura, jaundice, or excessive and progressive weakness.

Drug Interactions

Warfarin. NSAIDs may enhance the anticoagulant effects of warfarin. Observe for petechiae, ecchymoses, nosebleeds, bleeding gums, dark tarry stools, and bright red or "coffee ground" emesis. Monitor the prothrombin time (International Normalized Ratio [INR]) and reduce the dosage of warfarin if necessary.

Phenytoin. Monitor patients with concurrent therapy for signs of phenytoin toxicity, such as nystagmus, sedation, or lethargy. Serum levels may be ordered, and a reduced dosage of phenytoin may be required.

Valproic Acid. Aspirin inhibits valproic acid metabolism, increasing valproic acid blood levels. Monitor for valproic acid toxicity: sedation, drowsiness, dizziness, or blurred vision. Serum levels may be ordered, and a reduced dosage of valproic acid may be required.

Oral Hypoglycemic Agents. Monitor for hypoglycemia: headache, weakness, decreased coordination, general apprehension, diaphoresis, hunger, or blurred or double vision. The dosing of the hypoglycemic agent may need to be reduced. Notify the health care provider if any of the above-mentioned symptoms appear.

Furosemide, Thiazide Diuretics. NSAIDs inhibit the diuretic activity of these agents. The dosage of the diuretic agents may need to be increased or NSAIDs discontinued. Maintain accurate intake and output and blood pressure records, and monitor for a decrease in diuretic and antihypertensive activity.

Probenecid. Probenecid inhibits the excretion of NSAIDs. Monitor patients for signs of toxicity: headache, drowsiness, and mental confusion.

Lithium. NSAIDs (except possibly sulindac and aspirin) may induce lithium toxicity. Monitor patients for lithium toxicity manifested by nausea, anorexia, fine tremors, persistent vomiting, profuse diarrhea, hyperreflexia, lethargy, and weakness.

Aspirin. There is controversy in the literature about the possibility that COX-1 inhibitors can reduce the platelet-inhibiting effects of aspirin when administered about the same time. An NSAID may be blocking the receptor on platelets that aspirin would normally bind to, preventing the platelet inhibition caused by aspirin. One approach to avoid this interaction is to take the aspirin several hours before the COX-1 NSAID. This might not be possible for the person with severe rheumatoid arthritis who needs the analgesic effects around the clock.

Cholestyramine. Cholestyramine resins bind to NSAIDs in the gut, inhibiting absorption. Separate dosage administration by 2 hours. The NSAID dosage may need to be increased.

DRUG CLASS: Miscellaneous Analgesics

acetaminophen (a seat a min' o fen)

▶ TYLENOL (ty' le nol), DATRIL (day' tril), TEMPRA (tem' prah)

Actions

Acetaminophen is a synthetic nonopiate analgesic. The site and mechanism of action are unknown. Its antipyretic effectiveness and analgesic potency are similar to those of aspirin in equal doses.

Uses

Acetaminophen is an effective analgesic-antipyretic for fever and discomfort associated with bacterial and viral infections, headache, and conditions involving musculoskeletal pain. It is a good substitute for patients who cannot take products containing aspirin because of allergic reactions, hypersensitivities, anticoagulant therapy, or possible bleeding problems from gastric or duodenal ulcers, gastritis, and hiatus hernia. This drug has no antiinflammatory activity and is therefore ineffective (other than as an analgesic) in the relief of symptoms of rheumatoid arthritis or other inflammation.

Therapeutic Outcomes

The primary therapeutic outcomes expected from acetaminophen are reduced pain and fever.

Nursing Process for Acetaminophen

Premedication Assessment

1. Take vital signs: temperature, blood pressure, pulse, and respirations
2. Check laboratory values for hepatotoxicity or nephrotoxicity.
3. Monitor for GI symptoms before and during therapy.
4. Check bowel sounds and review voiding pattern and urine output.
5. When used as an analgesic, perform pain assessment before administering acetaminophen and at appropriate intervals during therapy. Report poor pain control promptly and obtain modification in orders.
6. When used as an antipyretic, take baseline temperature and continue monitoring temperature at appropriate intervals (e.g., every 2 to 4 hours, depending on severity of temperature elevation).

Planning

Availability. PO: 160, 325, 500, and 650 mg tablets; 80 and 160 mg chewable tablets; 325 and 500 mg capsules; 80- and 160-mg sprinkle capsules; 80 mg/0.8 mL drops; 80 mg/2.5 mL elixir; 80 mg/5 mL, 120 mg/5 mL, 160 mg/5 mL elixir; 160 mg/5 mL, 500 mg/15 mL liquid; 80 mg/1.66 mL, 100 mg/mL solution. Rectal: 80, 120, 125, 300, 325, or 650 mg suppositories.

Implementation

Dosage and Administration

- *Adult:* PO: 325 to 650 mg every 4 to 6 hours. Doses up to 1000 mg may be given four times daily for short-term therapy. Do not exceed 4 g daily.
- *Pediatric:* PO: 0 to 3 months, 40 mg; 4 to 11 months, 80 mg; 12 to 24 months, 120 mg; 2 to 3 years, 160 mg; 4 to 5 years, 240 mg; 6 to 8 years, 320 mg; 9 to 10 years, 400 mg; 11 to 12 years, 480 mg; older than 14 years, 650 mg. Rectal: Same as with oral doses.
- *Antidote:* Acetylcysteine

Evaluation

When used as directed, acetaminophen is essentially free of side effects.

Side Effects to Expect

Gastric Irritation. If gastric irritation occurs, administer medication with food, milk, antacids, or large amounts of water. If symptoms persist or increase in severity, report for health care provider evaluation.

Side Effects to Report

Overdose, Hepatotoxicity. Overdose due to acute and chronic ingestion has risen dramatically in the past few years. Severe life-threatening hepatotoxicity has been reported in patients who either ingest 5 to 8 g daily for several weeks or attempt suicide by consuming large quantities at one time.

Early indications of toxicity include anorexia, nausea, vomiting, low blood pressure, drowsiness, confusion, and abdominal pain—symptoms often attributed to other causes. Within 2 to 4 days, symptoms of hepatotoxicity develop (jaundice and a rise in the AST and ALT levels and prothrombin time). If acetaminophen toxicity is suspected, consult the manufacturer, a university drug information center, or a poison control center for the most current recommendations for therapy.

Drug Interactions

Barbiturates, Carbamazepine, Phenytoin, Rifampin, Sulfinpyrazone. If acetaminophen is taken in large doses or over the long term, these agents may enhance hepatotoxicity.

Alcohol. Chronic, excessive ingestion may increase the potential for hepatotoxicity of larger therapeutic doses or overdoses of acetaminophen.

propoxyphene (proe pox′ eh feen)
DARVON (dar′ von)

Actions

Propoxyphene is an effective, well-tolerated synthetic opiate agonist analgesic structurally related to methadone. It is one third to one half as potent as codeine. It is similar to aspirin in potency and duration of analgesic effect.

Uses

Propoxyphene is used for the relief of mild to moderate pain associated with muscular spasms, premenstrual cramps, bursitis, minor surgery and trauma, headache, and labor and delivery. Greater pain relief may be attained when used in combination with aspirin or acetaminophen.

Therapeutic Outcomes

The primary therapeutic outcome expected from propoxyphene is reduced pain.

Nursing Process for Propoxyphene

Premedication Assessment

1. Perform baseline neurologic assessment, for example, orientation to date, time, and place; mental alertness; and balance.
2. Take vital signs: temperature, blood pressure, pulse, and respirations.
3. Monitor urine pattern and amount.
4. Monitor for GI symptoms before and during therapy; monitor stools for consistency and number.
5. Perform pain assessments before administration of propoxyphene and at appropriate intervals during therapy. Report poor pain control promptly and obtain modification in orders.

Planning

Availability. PO: 65 mg capsules, 100 mg tablets. (The 65 mg capsules and the 100 mg tablets are equal in analgesic potency.) Propoxyphene is also available in combination: Darvocet (propoxyphene, acetaminophen), Darvon Compound (propoxyphene, aspirin, caffeine).

Implementation

Dosage and Administration

- *Adult:* PO: 65 mg (capsules) or 100 mg (tablets) every 4 hours as needed. Do not exceed 390 mg (capsules) or 600 mg (tablets) daily. If gastric irritation occurs, administer medication with food or milk.
- *Antidote:* Naloxone, naltrexone. Symptoms of acute overdose are coma, respiratory depression, pulmonary edema, and seizures. Symptoms of propoxyphene overdose may be complicated by salicylism, which may also develop as a result of an overdose of combination products containing both propoxyphene and aspirin.

Evaluation

Side Effects to Expect

Gastric Irritation. If gastric irritation occurs, administer medication with food or milk. If symptoms persist or increase in severity, report for health care provider evaluation.

Sedation. This side effect is usually mild and tends to resolve with continued therapy.

Dizziness. Provide patient safety during episodes of dizziness.

Side Effects to Report

Excessive Use or Abuse. Habitual use of propoxyphene may result in physical dependence. Discuss the case with the health care provider and make plans to cooperatively approach gradual withdrawal of the medications being abused. Assist the patient in recognizing the abuse problem. Identify underlying needs and plan for appropriate management. Provide emotional support for the individual; display an accepting attitude—be kind but firm.

Skin Rashes. Report for further evaluation.

Drug Interactions

Orphenadrine. Combined use with propoxyphene is not recommended. Cases of mental confusion, anxiety, and tremors have been reported.

Carbamazepine. Propoxyphene inhibits the metabolism of carbamazepine. Monitor patients for signs of carbamazepine toxicity: dizziness, nausea, drowsiness, or headache. Carbamazepine dosages usually need to be reduced.

Ritonavir, Lopinavir. These two antiviral agents inhibit the metabolism of propoxyphene, leading to potential toxicity. Concurrent use with propoxyphene is contraindicated.

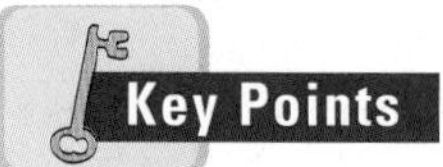

- Pain management has made significant progress over the past 15 years, primarily because of better understanding of the pain experience; however, there is still a great deal to do in educating patients, family, and some health care providers about appropriate pain management.
- Nurses can play an important role in providing counseling and guidance to these groups in understanding pain and how to maintain an appropriate balance between daily activities and timing of analgesics to optimize quality of life.

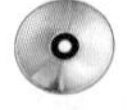

Go to your Companion CD-ROM for appendices, an Audio Glossary, animations, Drug Dosage Calculators, customizable Patient Self-Assessment forms, and Review Questions for the NCLEX® Examination.

evolve Be sure to visit the companion Evolve site at http://evolve.elsevier.com/Clayton for WebLinks and additional online resources.

MEDICATION SAFETY REVIEW

MATH REVIEW QUESTIONS

1. Order: Aspirin 650 mg PO qid

   Available: Aspirin 325 mg tablets

   Give _____ tablets for each dose.

2. The pediatrician orders a 75 mg PO dose of ibuprofen suspension for a child.

   Available: 100 mg/5 mL

   Give _____ mL.

3. Morphine, 15 mg IV q6h, has been ordered.

   Available: concentrations of 3, 4, 5, 8, 10, and 15 mg/mL

   Give _____ concentration, _____ volume.

4. Order: codeine 30 mg qid after wisdom tooth extraction. What is your interpretation of the order, and how will you administer it?

CRITICAL THINKING QUESTIONS

1. A terminal cancer patient returns to the unit with a morphine patient-controlled analgesia (PCA). His daughter comes to you alarmed that her father may "overuse" the morphine and become addicted. How would you, as the nurse, respond to her? (Support your answer with rationale.)
2. What is the difference between an order for morphine sulfate immediate release (MSIR) and an order for MS Contin?
3. An 86-year-old woman is taking enteric-coated aspirin for arthritis. She reports to the nurse that she thinks she saw a "whole tablet" in her stools. What follow-up would you do? The patient has been on continuous aspirin therapy for 2 years. Explain appropriate assessments that need to be made.
4. The head nurse sends the student nurse to evaluate a patient's postoperative pain. After entering the patient's room, the student observes the patient conversing and joking with her friends. The student decides not to further investigate the question of postoperative pain. Evaluate the correctness of the student's decision, and give underlying rationale for the views expressed.
5. Research the medications needed to treat respiratory depression during the administration of an epidural analgesic. Obtain a copy of the monitoring guidelines used in the clinical site where assigned and discuss the importance of collecting these data on a regularly scheduled basis throughout epidural analgesic use.

CONTENT REVIEW QUESTIONS

1. The length of time required for a transdermal fentanyl (Duragesic) to reach a steady blood level is _____ hours.
   1. 4
   2. 4 to 7
   3. 8 to 11
   4. 12 to 24
2. The management of respiratory depression (below 8 breaths/min) in a patient receiving an epidural analgesic should include the administration of:
   1. propoxyphene (Darvon).
   2. naloxone (Narcan).
   3. naltrexone (ReVia).
   4. bupivacaine (Marcaine).
3. Drug tolerance occurs when the patient requires:
   1. increased doses of the same analgesic to obtain the same relief.
   2. increased doses of a different analgesic to obtain the same relief.
   3. monitoring for respiratory depression.
   4. vital signs assessment at least q4h.
4. Opiate partial agonists such as butorphanol (Stadol) and nalbuphine (Nubain) are effective analgesics when:
   1. prior opiate antagonists have not been administered.
   2. dosages are increased following the use of prior opiate antagonists.
   3. prior NSAIDs have been administered.
   4. dosages are decreased following the use of prior opiate antagonists.
5. Which of the following medications contain codeine?
   1. Percogesic
   2. Tylenol #2, #3, #4
   3. Fioricet
   4. Darvon-N

Continued

CONTENT REVIEW QUESTIONS—cont'd

6. The nurse must frequently assess a client experiencing pain. When assessing the intensity of the pain, the nurse should:
   1. ask about what causes the pain.
   2. question the client about the location of the pain.
   3. offer the client a pain scale to objectify the information.
   4. use open-ended questions to find out about the pain.

7. A client will be going home on medication administered through a PCA (patient-controlled analgesia) system. To assist the family members with an understanding of how this therapy works, the nurse explains that the client:
   1. has control over the frequency of the IV analgesia.
   2. can choose the dosage of the drug received.
   3. may request the type of medication received.
   4. controls the route for administering the medication.

8. Nurses working with clients in pain need to recognize and avoid common misconceptions about pain. In regards to the pain experience, which of the following is correct?
   1. The client is the best authority on the pain experience.
   2. Chronic pain is mostly psychological in nature.
   3. Regular use of analgesics leads to drug addiction.
   4. The amount of tissue damage does not affect the perception of pain.

CHAPTER 21 Introduction to Cardiovascular Disease and Metabolic Syndrome

evolve http://evolve.elsevier.com/Clayton

Chapter Content

Objectives

1. Define metabolic syndrome.
2. List the major risk factors of metabolic syndrome.
3. List the diagnostic criteria for metabolic syndrome for men and women using the National Cholesterol Education Program guidelines.
4. State the importance of lifestyle modification in the treatment of metabolic syndrome.
5. List the treatment goals for type 2 diabetes management, lipid management, and hypertension management.
6. State why long-term control and adherence to medications are important in managing metabolic syndrome.

Key Terms

cardiovascular disease
coronary artery disease (CAD)
angina pectoris
myocardial infarction (MI)
stroke
hypertension
dysrhythmias
peripheral vascular disease
peripheral arterial disease
heart failure
insulin resistance syndrome
metabolic syndrome
body mass index (BMI)

CARDIOVASCULAR DISEASES

Cardiovascular disease is a collective term used to refer to disorders of the circulatory system (e.g., heart, arteries, veins) of the body. Cardiovascular disease affects approximately 65 million Americans at an annual cost of about $368 billion. Medical history has subdivided these diseases into the areas or organs of the body in which the pathology is most obvious, such as **coronary artery disease (CAD)** (see Chapter 22) pertaining to narrowing or obstruction of the arteries of the heart leading to **angina pectoris** (see Chapter 25) and **myocardial infarction (MI)**. **Stroke** (see Chapter 27) refers to either an obstruction or rupture of blood vessels in the brain. An increase in the pressure with which blood circulates through the arteries and veins is referred to as **hypertension** (see Chapter 23). **Dysrhythmias** (see Chapter 24) refer to abnormalities in the electrical conduction pathways of the heart that lead to inefficient pumping of blood through the circulatory system. **Peripheral vascular disease** refers to disorders of the blood vessels of the arms and legs. Peripheral vascular disease can be subdivided into two types based on arterial or venous origin: **peripheral arterial disease** (see Chapter 26) such as obstructive arterial disease, and venous disorders, such as acute deep vein thrombosis (see Chapter 27). The long-term pathology of any one or a combination of these diseases affecting the circulatory system leads to **heart failure** (see Chapter 28) and eventual death.

METABOLIC SYNDROME

There are many causes that lead to cardiovascular disorders (Box 21-1). Lifestyle is recognized as possibly the greatest contributor to a variety of diseases that reduce the quality of life and end lives prematurely. These diseases also cost the American economy billions upon billions of dollars that could be used in many more positive ways to benefit mankind. Although investigators have hypothesized about various factors that lead to cardiovascular disease since the 1920s, 1960s research indicated that persons with hypertension, diabetes mellitus, dyslipidemia, and obesity, alone or in combination, were found to be at greater risk for progressive cardiovascular disease. In

Box 21-1 ***Cardiovascular Disorders***

- Coronary artery disease
  - Angina pectoris
  - Acute myocardial infarction
- Congenital heart disease
  - Pulmonary stenosis
  - Coarctation of the aorta
  - Atrial septal defect
  - Ventricular septal defect
- Valvular heart disease
  - Mitral stenosis and regurgitation
  - Aortic stenosis and regurgitation
  - Tricuspid stenosis and regurgitation
- Disorders of heart rate and rhythm (dysrhythmias)
- Cardiomyopathies
- Pericarditis
- Rheumatic heart disease
- Cancers of the heart
- Heart failure

Table 21-1 Definitions and Characteristics of Metabolic Syndrome*

	NATIONAL CHOLESTEROL EDUCATION PROGRAM (NCEP)† (USA)		INTERNATIONAL DIABETES FEDERATION (IDF)‡ (INTERNATIONAL)	
RISK FACTOR DEFINING LIMIT	MEN	WOMEN	MEN	WOMEN
Waist circumference§ (inches)	>40	>36	>37	>31.5
HDL cholesterol† (mg/dL)	<40	<50	<40	<50
Triglycerides‡ (mg/dL)	>150	>150	>150	>150
Blood pressure¶ (mm Hg)	>130/85	>130/85	>130/85	>130/85
Fasting glucose (mg/dL)‖	>110	>110	>100	>100

*People with central obesity and at least two of the remaining four factors are considered to have metabolic syndrome.
†From Expert Panel on Detection, Evaluation, and Treatment of High Blood Cholesterol in Adults: *Third Report of the National Cholesterol Education Program (NCEP),* NIH Publication No. 02-5 215, September, 2002, National Heart, Lung, and Blood Institute/National Institutes of Health.
‡From International Diabetes Federation: The IDF Consensus Worldwide Definition of the Metabolic Syndrome.
§Specific circumferences for different ethnicities.
¶Or specific treatment for this abnormality.
‖Or previously diagnosed type 2 diabetes.

1988, a unifying pathway of insulin resistance was described and called Syndrome X. In 1998, the World Health Organization provided a working definition for this syndrome and named it "metabolic syndrome." Insulin resistance leads to type 2 diabetes and induces atherosclerosis, which leads to coronary artery disease. Over the past 20 years, the hypothesis of insulin resistance has been studied in great depth, and the syndrome has been renamed to be more descriptive of the underlying causes. Other terms include diabesity, and most recently, **insulin resistance syndrome. Metabolic syndrome** is still the most commonly used term worldwide. The key characteristics of metabolic syndrome are the presence of type 2 diabetes mellitus, abdominal obesity, hypertriglyceridemia, low high-density lipoproteins (HDLs), and hypertension. Although metabolic syndrome is a worldwide disease, an estimated 47 million adults (1 in 5) in the United States have metabolic syndrome. More than 4% of adolescents ages 12 through 19 also have metabolic syndrome. Within ethnic groups, African American males have the lowest rate at 14%, whereas Mexican-American women have the highest rate at 27%. Table 21-1 shows a comparison of criteria from the United States–based National Cholesterol Education Program (NCEP) and the International Diabetes Federation (IDF). People with central obesity and two of the four other criteria are defined as having metabolic syndrome.

Risk factors for the development of metabolic syndrome include poor diet, sedentary lifestyle (lack of exercise), and genetic predisposition. As a society "on the go," our dietary habits have changed significantly over the past 20 years, causing a dramatic increase in weight gain in the United States. Simply put, weight gain occurs when energy intake (food calories) exceeds energy expenditure (burning calories). The 1998 National Heart, Lung, and Blood Institute (NHLBI) expert report titled "Clinical Guidelines on the Identification, Evaluation and Treatment of Overweight and Obesity in Adults" describes weight in proportion to height as **body mass index (BMI).** It is measured by:

$$\frac{\text{weight in kilograms}}{(\text{height in meters})^2}$$

OR,

$$\frac{\text{weight in pounds} \times 703}{(\text{height in inches})^2}$$

The NHLBI guidelines also describe overweight and obesity in terms of the BMI. See Table 21-2 for the definitions of healthy weight, overweight, and obesity. In 1991, four states had obesity prevalence rates of 15% to 19% and no states had rates at or above 20%. In 2003, 15 states had prevalence rates of 15% to 19%; 31 states had rates of 20% to 24%; and 4 states had rates more than 25% (Figure 21-1) (CDC, 2004).

A sedentary lifestyle also contributes to overweight and obesity. New technologies ranging from labor-saving devices to remote control devices to the availability of entertainment though television and computers have significantly reduced daily caloric expenditure. Today, despite common knowledge that regular exercise is healthy, more than 60% of Americans are not regularly physically active, and 25% are not active at all. Increased working hours that lead to less time to prepare food at home and larger portions of commercially prepared food aggravate the problem. Ease and convenience of food preparation (e.g., fast-food restaurants, drive-throughs;

Table 21-2 Relationship between Body Mass Index and Categories of Obesity

BODY MASS INDEX (BMI) (kg/m²)	RELATIONSHIP WITH WEIGHT
<18.5	Underweight
18.5-24.9	Normal weight
25-29.9	Overweight
30-34.9	Obesity, class I
35-39.9	Obesity, class II
>40	Obesity, class III (extreme obesity)

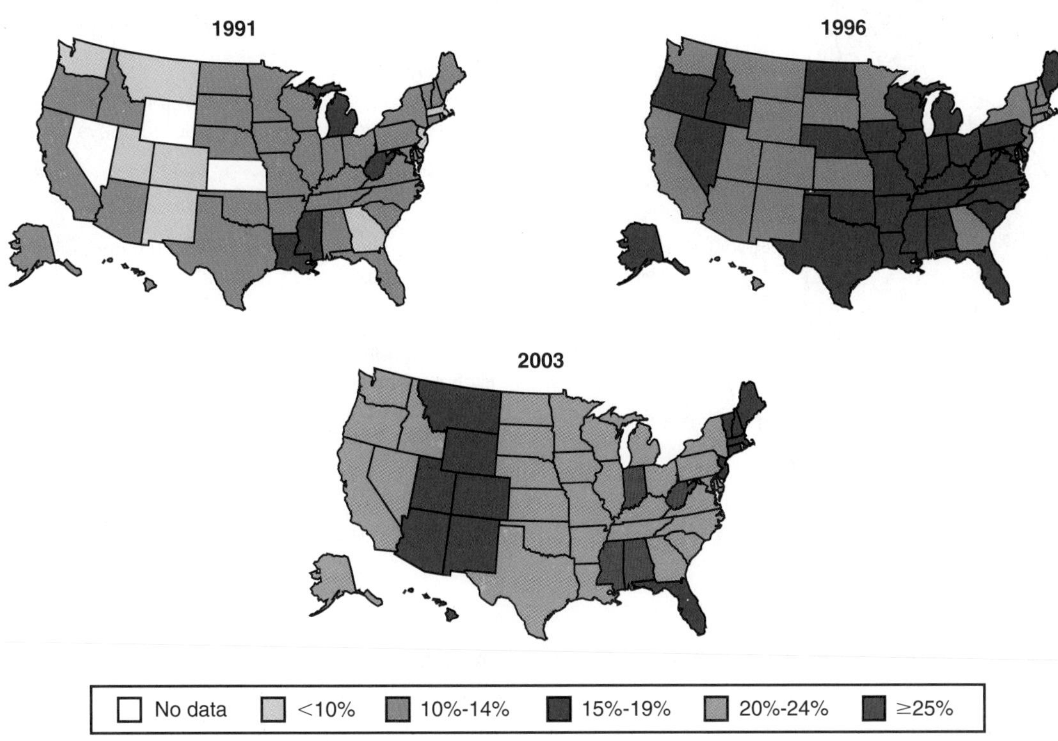

*BMI ≥30, or about 30 lbs overweight for 5'4" person

FIGURE **21-1** Growth in overweight and obesity in the United States, 1991-2003.

use of a microwave versus a convection oven), and increases in portion sizes ("supersize it, please!") have placed too many easily consumed calories on the table of the American public. Consequently, reduced physical activity and increased caloric intake have resulted in a national epidemic of obesity. Other negative lifestyle choices such as excessive consumption of alcohol and smoking aggravate metabolic syndrome. Excessive alcohol consumption causes fat accumulation in the liver, which is also associated with metabolic syndrome. Smoking is a major contributor to both pulmonary disease (see Chapter 31) and hypertension (see Chapter 23).

Genetic factors influence each component of the syndrome as well as the syndrome itself. A family history of first-degree relatives (e.g., parents, siblings) that includes type 2 diabetes, hypertension, and early heart disease (e.g., angina, "heart attack") greatly increases the likelihood that an individual will develop metabolic syndrome (Figure 21-2).

In addition to type 2 diabetes and heart disease, other consequences associated with metabolic syndrome include renal disease, obstructive sleep apnea, polycystic ovary syndrome, cognitive decline in the elderly, and dementia in the elderly.

Treatment of Metabolic Syndrome

The variety of factors associated with the presence of metabolic syndrome requires that an individualized approach to treatment is necessary based on a person's specific risk factors and diseases present. Lifestyle management is critical in preventing and treating the comorbidities that make up the metabolic syndrome. Research indicates that lifestyle changes alone may delay the onset of type 2 diabetes mellitus by more than 50%. The overall treatment goals for metabolic syndrome are listed in Box 21-2.

Weight loss and increased physical activity are usually the first steps to treatment. Reducing the number of calories consumed, while at the same time burning more calories, can have very positive effects in reducing metabolic syndrome. Even a 10- to 15-pound weight loss can improve hypertension and hyperglycemia. Initial therapeutics goals are a 7% to 10% weight reduction in the first year of treatment, with an ongoing goal of a body index of less than 25 kg/m^2. Several dietary approaches can be used to lose weight. Adopting the Dietary Approaches to Stop Hypertension (DASH) diet may be helpful for patients who also have hypertension (see Chapter 23). The Mediterranean diet, one that is rich in "good" fats (e.g., olive oil) and contains a reasonable amount of carbohydrates and proteins from fish and chicken is frequently recommended. Diet should reduce intake of saturated fat (<7% of total calories), *trans* fat, cholesterol levels (<200 mg/day), and total fat (25% to 35% of total calories). Most dietary fat should be unsaturated, and simple sugars should be reduced. Nonpharmacologic therapy must include elimination of smoking, restriction of alcohol intake, stress reduction, and sodium control (see Chapter 23).

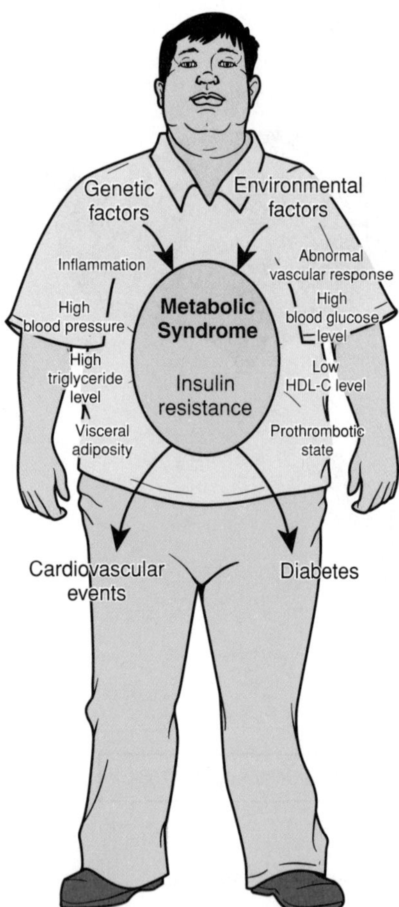

FIGURE **21-2** Mechanisms of metabolic syndrome.

The latest report from the Academy of Sciences (2002) stresses the importance of balancing diet with physical activity to improve circulation, increase HDL levels, and burn calories. Muscles are the primary storage and utilization site for glucose, and as exercise leads to more muscle and less fat, blood glucose levels tend to return to normal levels. The report makes recommendations about daily maximum caloric intake of food to be consumed based on height, weight, and gender for four different levels of physical activity (sedentary, low active, active, and very active). The report also illustrates how difficult it is to lose weight based just on reduction of calories alone, and how important it is to maintain a level a physical activity to prevent reduction in lean body mass (protein wasting). It recommends 60 minutes of moderate-intensity physical activity (e.g., walking at a rate of 4 to 5 miles per hour), or high-intensity activity (e.g., jogging at a rate of 4 to 5 miles in 20 to 30 minutes) four to seven times weekly, in addition to the activities of daily living, to maintain body weight (in adults) in the recommended body mass index range (18 to 25 kg/m^2). The exercise does not have to be completed at the same time, but can be worked into a person's daily activities.

If after lifestyle modifications and diet and exercise the patient is not able to meet the therapeutic goals in treating metabolic syndrome, then drug therapy may be necessary. Patient education is vitally important in making patients aware of and treating metabolic syndrome.

Box 21-2 ***General Treatment Goals for Patients with Metabolic Syndrome***

Blood Pressure Goals
<130/80 mm Hg
<125/75 mm Hg if 1 g/day of proteinuria is present
Blood pressure should be measured at every visit

Lipid Goals
Low-density lipoprotein (LDL)
<100 mg/dL (primary goal)
<70 mg/dL (alternative goal for patients with cardiovascular disease)
OR,
Non–high-density lipoproteins (non-HDL) <130 mg/dL
Triglycerides <150 mg/dL
High-density lipoprotein (HDL)
Men >40 mg/dL
Women >50 mg/dL

Blood Glucose Goals
Hemoglobin A_{1c} <7%
Fasting plasma glucose <120 mg/dL
Postprandial plasma glucose <180 mg/dL

This education should be emphasized and reiterated frequently by the physician, pharmacist, and nurse.

Drug Therapy for Metabolic Syndrome

Drug therapy must be individualized for each patient's underlying diseases.

Hypertension

A combination of a thiazide diuretic plus an angiotensin-converting enzyme inhibitor or a beta blocker will be necessary. Other combinations of therapy may be used depending on the person's race and the presence of other diseases. (See Chapter 23 for a discussion of the treatment of hypertension.)

Dyslipidemia

The treatment of dyslipidemia is generally to lower the triglycerides and LDL cholesterol and raise the HDL cholesterol. After lifestyle changes, medicines most commonly used are the 3-hydroxy-methylglutaryl coenzyme A reductase inhibitors (also known as statins), fibric acid derivatives, and niacin. (See Chapter 22 for a discussion of the treatment of dyslipidemias.)

Type 2 Diabetes Mellitus

Several different classes of medicines may be used to treat insulin resistance and type 2 diabetes. The thiazolidinediones reduce insulin resistance in peripheral tissues; metformin decreases production of glucose by the liver, and to a lesser extent, reduces insulin resistance in peripheral tissues; alpha-glycosidase inhibitors reduce the absorption of glucose from the intestine, reducing postprandial hyperglycemia; and sulfonylureas and meglitinides stimulate the beta cells of the pancreas to release more insulin. Insulin injections also benefit patients who do not secrete adequate amounts of insulin. (See Chapter 36 for a discussion of the treatment of type 2 diabetes mellitus.)

NURSING PROCESS *for Metabolic Syndrome*

See the nursing process for each of the primary cardiovascular diseases:

Dyslipidemias, Chapter 22, p. 354
Hypertension, Chapter 23, p. 367
Dysrhythmias, Chapter 24, p. 393
Angina Pectoris, Chapter 25, p. 409
Peripheral Vascular Disease, Chapter 26, p. 420
Thromboembolic Disorders, Chapter 27, p. 431
Heart Failure, Chapter 28, p. 452

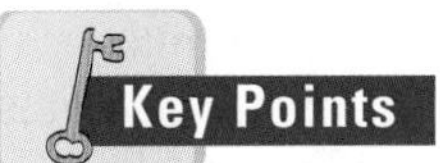

Key Points

- Cardiovascular diseases are a major cause of premature death in the United States.
- More than 20% of the U.S. adult population has metabolic syndrome, and is at much greater risk for cardiovascular diseases. The key characteristics of metabolic syndrome (also known as insulin resistance syndrome and syndrome X) are type 2 diabetes mellitus, abdominal obesity, hypertriglyceridemia, low HDL cholesterol, and hypertension.
- The most cost-effective and successful forms of treatment are smoking cessation, weight reduction, exercise, stress reduction, and dietary modification. If change in diet and exercise do not produce an acceptable decrease in blood lipid levels, blood glucose levels, and hypertension, antilipemic agents, antihyperglycemic agents, and antihypertensive agents may be added to the patient's regimen.

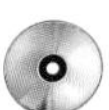

Go to your Companion CD-ROM for appendices, an Audio Glossary, animations, Drug Dosage Calculators, customizable Patient Self-Assessment forms, and Review Questions for the NCLEX® Examination.

evolve Be sure to visit the companion Evolve site at http://evolve.elsevier.com/Clayton for WebLinks and additional online resources.

MEDICATION SAFETY REVIEW

MATH REVIEW QUESTIONS

1. Order: Lipitor 20-mg tab
   Available: Atorvastatin 10-mg tablets
   Give ____ tablets.
2. Order: Mevacor 10-mg tab daily
   Available: Lovastatin 20-mg tab
   Give ____ tablets.
3. Order: Nicardipine 1 mg IV stat
   Available: Nicardipine 2.5 mg/mL
   Give ____ mL.
4. Order: Verapamil 5 mg IV
   Available: Verapamil 2.5 mg/mL
   Give ____ mL.

CRITICAL THINKING QUESTIONS

1. Develop a teaching plan for the patient who is at risk for metabolic syndrome. Be specific with your interventions. Include the following topics: smoking reduction, exercise, proper diet, and stress reduction.
2. List the key characteristics of metabolic syndrome and the role they play in development.
3. Explain how the BMI is figured.

CONTENT REVIEW QUESTIONS

1. Which of the following would be an acceptable BMI?
   1. 20.3
   2. 17.5
   3. 26
   4. 35
2. Which of the following is not used as an evaluation tool for metabolic syndrome?
   1. Blood pressure
   2. Lipid profile
   3. Blood glucose
   4. Liver enzymes
3. Recommendations about daily maximum caloric intake of food to be consumed should be based on which of the following? *(Select all that apply.)*
   1. Height and weight
   2. Gender
   3. Race
   4. Levels of physical activity
4. If lifestyle changes are not effective for metabolic syndrome, the client may need drug therapy. Select all of the following drugs that may be used in treating metabolic syndrome.
   1. Thiazide diuretics
   2. Beta blockers
   3. Statins
   4. Analgesics

CHAPTER

22 Drugs Used to Treat Dyslipidemias

evolve http://evolve.elsevier.com/Clayton

Chapter Content

Objectives

1. Identify the four major types of lipoproteins.
2. Describe the primary treatment modalities for lipid disorders.
3. State the oral administration instructions for antilipemic agents.

Key Terms

atherosclerosis
hyperlipidemia
dyslipidemias
triglycerides
lipoproteins
chylomicrons
metabolic syndrome

ATHEROSCLEROSIS

(For an introduction to cardiovascular diseases, see Chapter 21.) Coronary artery disease (CAD) (also called coronary heart disease [CHD]) is a major cause of premature death in the United States and most other industrialized nations. Major treatable causes of CAD are hypertension, cigarette smoking, type 2 diabetes mellitus, and atherosclerosis. **Atherosclerosis** (ath er oh skle ro′ sis) is characterized by the accumulation of fatty deposits on the inner walls of arteries and arterioles throughout the body that reduces the blood supply to vital organs resulting in strokes, angina pectoris, myocardial infarction, and peripheral vascular disease. A primary cause of atherosclerosis is the abnormal elevation of cholesterol and triglycerides in the blood in a disease known as **hyperlipidemia** (hi per lip id e′ me ah). **Dyslipidemias** are defined as abnormalities with one or more of the blood fats (lipids). Dyslipidemias can be caused by genetic abnormalities, secondary causes (e.g., lifestyle, drugs, or underlying diseases), or both. A diet high in saturated fats, cholesterol, carbohydrates, total calories, and alcohol, as well as a sedentary lifestyle, contribute significantly to dyslipidemias.

Cholesterol is a naturally occurring substance that is essential for synthesizing body steroids used by the endocrine system, synthesizing bile acids needed for food absorption, and cell wall synthesis. The body is able to manufacture enough cholesterol to meet metabolic needs. However, the body also converts excess dietary carbohydrates into **triglycerides** (try glis′ er eyds) (a precursor of cholesterol) and dietary fat into cholesterol. Once absorbed from the gastrointestinal (GI) tract, fats (lipids), triglycerides, and cholesterol are bound to circulating proteins called **lipoproteins** for transport through the body. Lipoproteins are subdivided into five categories based on composition: chylomicrons, very low-density lipoproteins (VLDLs), intermediate-density lipoproteins (IDLs), low-density lipoproteins (LDLs), and high-density lipoproteins (HDLs). The five types differ in concentration of triglycerides, cholesterol, and proteins. Clinically, the IDL is included in the LDL measurement. **Chylomicrons** (ky lo my′ kronz) consist of about 90% triglycerides and 5% cholesterol; VLDL represents about 15% to 20% of total serum cholesterol and most of the total blood triglyceride concentration, whereas HDL contains about 20% to 30% cholesterol and 1% to 7% triglycerides. The purpose of HDL appears to be to transport cholesterol from peripheral cells to the liver for metabolism. HDL is sometimes referred to as a "good" lipoprotein because high levels indicate that cholesterol is being removed from vascular tissue, where it may participate in the development of CAD. Low levels of HDL are considered a positive risk factor in the development of CAD; high levels of HDL are a negative risk factor in CAD. LDL accounts for 60% to 70% of total serum cholesterol and is the major contributor to atherosclerosis. The probability that atherosclerosis will develop is related directly to the concentration of LDL cholesterol (LDL-C) in the blood circulation. LDL is the primary target of cholesterol-lowering therapy. High triglycerides are also associated with an increased risk of CAD. Consequently, patient assessment and cholesterol-lowering treatment goals are based on the total cholesterol, LDL-C, HDL-C, and triglyceride levels (Table 22-1). Other markers that are being tested to see whether they are better predictors of the risk for impending heart disease are the apolipoprotein A-1

Table 22-1 ***Classification of Cholesterol and Triglyceride Levels Based on NCEP Guidelines***

	OPTIMAL	NEAR OPTIMAL	BORDERLINE HIGH RISK	HIGH RISK	VERY HIGH RISK
Total cholesterol (mg/dL)	<200		200-239	≥240	
LDL cholesterol	<100	100-129	130-159	160-189	≥190
HDL cholesterol*	≥60†				
Triglycerides	<150		150-199	200-499	≥500

Expert Panel on Detection, Evaluation, and Treatment of High Blood Cholesterol in Adults: *Third Report of the National Cholesterol Education Program (NCEP)*, National Heart, Lung, and Blood Institute, National Institutes of Health, NIH Publication No. 02-5215, September, 2002.
*Low HDL cholesterol = <40 mg/dL.
†<70 mg/dL for people at very high risk for cardiovascular disease.

Table 22-2 ***Lipoprotein Disorders Treatable with Diet and Drug Therapy****

DYSLIPIDEMIA	ABNORMAL LIPIDS	SINGLE DRUG TREATMENT	COMBINATION DRUG TREATMENT
Familial hypercholesterolemia	↑ LDL-C	Statin Bile acid resin, niacin	Bile acid resin + niacin; bile acid resin + statin; niacin + statin
Polygenic hypercholesterolemia	↑ LDL-C	Bile acid resin, niacin, statin	Bile acid resin + niacin; bile acid resin + statin; niacin + statin
Familial hypertriglyceridemia	↑ Triglycerides	Fibrate, niacin	Fibrate + niacin
Mixed hyperlipidemia	↑ LDL-C, ↑ triglycerides	Niacin, statin, fibrate†	Niacin + statin; niacin + bile acid resin; niacin + fibrate

LDL-C, Low-density lipoprotein cholesterol.
*Diet, exercise, and weight loss are primary treatments; the primary drug treatment is listed first, followed by other treatments in decreasing order.
†Combined fibrate and statin therapy are not recommended due to increased risk of myopathy.

concentration (the major protein component of HDL), apolipoprotein B concentration (a measure of the total number of atherogenic particles), C-reactive protein (an indicator of inflammation), and non-HDL cholesterol, the sum of cholesterol in both LDL-C and triglyceride-rich lipoproteins.

TREATMENT OF HYPERLIPIDEMIAS

An estimated 105 million American adults have total blood cholesterol levels 200 mg/dL and higher, and of these, about 37 million American adults have levels of 240 mg/dL or greater. Some of the most common hyperlipidemias of *genetic* origin are treatable with medicines (Table 22-2). It is becoming recognized, however, that our lifestyles may be the greatest contributor to causing hyperlipidemia. A cluster of risk factors that relate directly to excesses in lifestyle is now recognized as **metabolic syndrome** (see Chapter 21).

The National Cholesterol Education Program (NCEP) recommends that treatment regimens be based on the presence of CAD, the level of total cholesterol, level of HDL-C, and the success of appropriate diet intervention. The primary treatment for hyperlipidemia is what is termed as therapeutic lifestyle changes (TLCs), which includes weight reduction, exercise, and a diet low in cholesterol and fat. Studies show that with reduction in elevated cholesterol and triglycerides, the frequency of heart attacks and strokes is substantially reduced. The NCEP recommends reduced intake of saturated fatty acids (<7% of total calories) with the remainder of total fats from polyunsaturated and monounsaturated fatty acids (25% to 35% of total calories), and intake of less than 200 mg cholesterol per day. The addition of plant stanols and sterols (2 g per day) and soluble fiber (10 to 15 g per day) can further reduce LDL-C by approximately 10%. Carbohydrates should be limited to 60% of the total daily caloric intake. Weight reduction can substantially reduce LDL-C while raising HDL levels. Regular exercise can also raise HDL levels, promote weight loss, lower blood pressure, reduce the risk of diabetes mellitus, and improve coronary blood flow. If a good trial of change in diet and exercise does not produce an acceptable decrease in blood lipid levels, antilipemic agents may be added to the patient's regimen. In general, for every 1% reduction in LDL, there is a 1% reduction in the rate of coronary artery disease events.

DRUG THERAPY FOR HYPERLIPIDEMIAS

Actions

Antilipemic agents may be used to treat hyperlipidemias only if diet, exercise, and weight reduction are not successful in adequately lowering LDL-C levels. (See individual monographs for mechanisms of action of antilipemic agents.)

Uses

The NCEP recognizes bile acid–binding resins (cholestyramine, colestipol, colesevelam), niacin, and the hydroxymethylglutaryl coenzyme A (HMG-CoA) reductase inhibitors (statins) (atorvastatin, fluvastatin, lovastatin, pravastatin, rosuvastatin, simvastatin) as the primary drugs for lowering serum cholesterol levels. The fibric acids (gemfibrozil, fenofibrate) are effective triglyceride-lowering agents but are not first-line drugs to treat hyperlipidemias because they do not usually produce substantial reductions in LDL-C. Omega-3 fatty acids have recently been approved by the U.S. Food and Drug Administration (FDA) for treatment of very high (>500 mg/dL) triglyceride levels in adults.

Selection of initial antilipemic therapy depends on the type of dyslipidemia present. Pharmacologic antilipemic therapy is often started with the bile acid resins because of their safety record and success in lowering cholesterol levels. Prescription-strength niacin is effective in lowering total cholesterol and triglyceride levels and raising HDL-C levels. The statins are the most potent and highly effective in lowering LDL-C and appear to be relatively safe, but are substantially more expensive than other treatments.

After starting drug therapy, the LDL-C level should be measured at 4 to 6 weeks and again at 3 months. If the response to initial drug therapy is inadequate, the patient should be switched to another drug or to a combination of two drugs. The combination of a bile acid resin with either niacin or a statin has the potential of lowering LDL-C levels by 40% to 50%. In rare cases of particularly high cholesterol levels, triple therapy with a bile acid–binding resin, niacin, and a statin may be required. Drug therapy is likely to continue for many years or a lifetime; plasma lipid levels return to pretreatment levels in 2 to 3 weeks if therapy is discontinued.

NURSING PROCESS *for Hyperlipidemia Therapy*

Assessment

History of Risk Factors. Ask age, note gender and race, and take family history of incidence of elevated cholesterol and lipids. Ask if any other first-generation family members have a history of or have died from CAD. Obtain ages and details of individuals with a history of CAD. Are there any living relatives with elevated cholesterol or elevated triglycerides?

Hypertension. Ask whether the individual has ever been informed of having an elevated blood pressure. If yes, obtain details. Ask about medications that have been prescribed. Are the medications being taken regularly? If not, why not? Take blood pressure in lying, sitting, and standing positions daily.

Smoking. Obtain a history of the number of cigarettes or cigars smoked daily. How long has the person smoked? Has the patient ever tried to stop smoking? Ask what effect smoking has on the patient's vascular system. How does the individual feel about modifying his or her smoking habit?

Dietary Habits

- Obtain a dietary history. Ask specific questions to obtain data relating to foods eaten that are high in fat, cholesterol, refined carbohydrates, and sodium. Discuss the amount of "fast foods," snack foods, and restaurant dining that is done because any of these tends to increase fat intake. Using a calorie counter, ask the person to estimate the number of calories eaten per day. How much meat, fish, and poultry is eaten daily (size and number of servings)? Estimate the percentage of total daily calories provided by fat.
- Discuss food preparation, for example, baked, broiled, or fried foods. How many servings of fruits and vegetables are eaten daily? What types of oils or fats are used in food preparation? See a nutrition text for further dietary history questions.
- What is the frequency and volume of alcoholic beverages consumed?

Glucose Intolerance. Ask specific questions regarding whether the individual now has or ever had an elevated serum glucose (blood sugar)? If yes, what dietary modifications have been made? How successful are they? What medications are being taken for the elevated serum glucose (e.g., oral hypoglycemic agents or insulin)?

Elevated Serum Lipids. Find out whether the patient is aware of having elevated lipids, triglycerides, or cholesterol. If elevated, what measures has the patient tried for reduction and what effect have the interventions had on the blood levels at subsequent examinations? Review laboratory data available (e.g., LDL, VLDL). A fasting lipoprotein profile that includes total cholesterol, LDL cholesterol, HDL cholesterol, and triglycerides is recommended for all adults 20 years of age or older at least once every 5 years.

Obesity. Weigh the patient. Ask about any recent weight gain or loss and whether intentional or unintentional. Using the person's height and weight, determine the person's body mass index (BMI) (see Chapter 21). If obesity is present, what strategies for weight reduction have been tried?

Psychomotor Functions

- *Type of lifestyle:* Ask the patient to describe the exercise level in terms of amount (e.g., walking 3 miles), intensity (e.g., walking 3 mph), and frequency (e.g., walking every other day). Is the patient's job physically demanding or of a sedentary nature?
- *Psychological stress:* How much stress does the individual estimate having in life? How does the patient cope with stressful situations at home and in the work setting?

Nursing Diagnoses

- Tissue perfusion, ineffective (indication)
- Health maintenance, ineffective (indication)
- Knowledge, deficient (side effects)

Planning

History of Risk Factors

- Review the modifiable risk factors and plan interventions and health teaching needed for appropriate alterations in lifestyle.
- Review ordered medications to be used concurrently with lifestyle modifications to identify health teaching needed.
- Order baseline laboratory studies (e.g., lipid profile studies, liver function tests, clotting time).

Medication Administration. Plan drug administration in accordance with recommendations in individual drug monographs to avoid possible interference with the absorption of other drugs ordered.

Implementation

Nursing interventions must be individualized and based on patient assessment data.

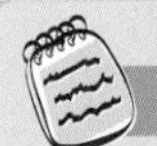

Patient Education and Health Promotion

Nutrition. Patients who take bile acid–sequestering resins may require supplemental vitamins. (The fat-soluble vitamins [D, E, A, and K] may become deficient with long-term resin therapy.)

- Encourage intake of high-bulk foods (e.g., whole grains, raw fruits and vegetables) and intake of eight to ten 8-ounce glasses of water per day to minimize constipating effects of resins.
- Arrange a dietary consultation with the nutritionist to address dietary modifications needed (e.g., low fat, low cholesterol). Nurses should enhance and reinforce this teaching on a continuum. Stress the importance of attaining a normal weight as a major treatment of hyperlipidemia. See information on the American Heart Association's (AHA) step 1 diet and step 2 diet recommendations for CAD.

Vitamin K Deficiency. If the patient is receiving a prescription for a bile acid resin, teach the patient the signs and symptoms of vitamin K deficiency including bleeding gums, bruising, dark tarry stools, and "coffee ground" emesis. This interaction is rare, but if symptoms occur, they should be reported immediately to the health care provider.

Follow-up Care. Stress the need for long-term regular assessment of the required serum levels (e.g., lipid profile values, liver studies, bleeding times) to track progress, to identify need for modifications in therapeutic interventions, and to detect possible side effects to the medications. To do so, blood studies and regular visits to the health care provider are necessary.

Relating to Medication Regimen. Examine the individual drug monographs for details on mixing and scheduling medication administration and techniques to improve compliance of these medications.

Fostering Health Maintenance

- Throughout the course of treatment, discuss medication information and how it will benefit the patient.
- Drug therapy is one component in the management of hyperlipemia. TLCs are equally important to drug therapy; therefore the need to modify dietary habits and control obesity, glucose levels, serum cholesterol, lipids, and hypertension must be strongly emphasized. Teach the patient about which high-cholesterol foods to avoid (e.g., liver, egg yolks, meats, fried foods, fatty desserts, and nuts [cashews, macadamia, Brazil]). Cholesterol is an animal product and not found in plants. Encourage switching to skim or 1% fat milk, egg whites, and fruits and vegetables, especially grapefruit and the use of unsaturated vegetable oils such as corn, olive, and soybean oils. Cessation of smoking and an increase in daily exercise (30 minutes of moderate-intensity exercise most days of the week) is strongly recommended. People having metabolic syndrome must recognize the importance of weight reduction and increased exercise to modify the insulin resistance that can dramatically affect the management of the disorder.
- Provide the patient and significant others with important information contained in the specific drug monograph for the drugs prescribed. Additional health teaching and nursing interventions for side effects to expect and report are described in each drug monograph that follows.
- Seek cooperation and understanding of the following points so that medication compliance is increased: name of medication, dosage, route and times of administration, side effects to expect, and side effects to report.

Written Record. Enlist the patient's aid in developing and maintaining a written record of monitoring parameters (e.g., daily serum glucose levels, blood pressure, and weight) (see Patient Self-Assessment Form on p. 455). An individualized nutritional diary should also be kept while instituting and learning the diet modifications (e.g., reduction in fats, refined carbohydrates, low-cholesterol foods). Complete the Premedication Data column for use as a baseline to track response to drug therapy. Ensure that the patient understands how to use the form and instruct the patient to bring the completed form to follow-up visits. During follow-up visits, focus on issues that will foster adherence with the therapeutic interventions prescribed.

DRUG CLASS: Bile Acid–Binding Resins

Actions

Cholestyramine, colestipol, and colesevelam are resins that bind bile acids in the intestine. After oral administration, the resin forms a nonabsorbable complex with bile acids, preventing enterohepatic recirculation of the bile acids. Because of the removal of bile acids, liver cells compensate by increasing metabolism of cholesterol to produce more bile acids, resulting in a net reduction in total cholesterol levels. Bile acid–binding resins can reduce LDL-C by 15% to 30% and increase HDL up to 5%. Some patients also have a 5% to 10% increase in triglyceride levels.

Uses

Cholestyramine, colestipol, and colesevelam are used in conjunction with dietary therapy to decrease elevated cholesterol concentrations in hyperlipidemia and to reduce the risks of atherosclerosis leading to CAD. These agents may also be used with the statins to further lower LDL-C. They are generally not used in patients who already have elevated triglyceride levels.

Other uses of the bile acid–binding resins include treatment of pruritus secondary to partial biliary stasis, diarrhea secondary to excess fecal bile acids or pseudomembranous colitis, and digitalis glycoside toxicity.

Therapeutic Outcomes

The primary therapeutic outcome expected from bile acid–binding resin therapy is reduction of LDL and total cholesterol levels.

Nursing Process for Bile Acid–Binding Resins

Premedication Assessment

1. Serum triglyceride and cholesterol levels should be determined before initiation of therapy and periodically thereafter.
2. Obtain data relating to any GI alterations before initiation of therapy (e.g., presence of abdominal pain, nausea, flatus).

Planning

Availability. Cholestyramine: 4-g powder packets; colestipol: 1 g tablets, granules in 5-g packets, 300 and 500 g containers; colesevelam: 625 mg tablets.

Implementation

Dosage and Administration

Cholestyramine—PO: 4 g one to six times daily. Initial dosage is 4 g daily. Maintenance dosage is 8 to 16 g per day. Maximum daily dose is 24 g.

Colestipol—PO: granules: 5 to 30 g of granules per day in divided doses; initial dose is 5 g once or twice daily. Tablets: 2 to 16 g tablets per day; initial dose 2 g once or twice daily.

Colesevelam—PO: 6 tablets once daily or in two divided doses with liquid at meals.

- The powder resin must be mixed with 2 to 6 ounces of water, juice, soup, applesauce, or crushed pineapple, and should be allowed to stand for a few minutes to allow absorption and dispersion. Do not attempt to swallow the dry powder. Follow administration with an additional glass of water.
- Recommended time of administration is with meals but may be modified to avoid interference with absorption of other medications.
- Tablets should be swallowed whole; do not crush, chew, or cut. Tablets should be taken with liquids.
- Taste may become a reason for noncompliance. Place the powder in a favorite beverage, or opt for tablets to minimize objectionable taste.

Evaluation

Side Effects to Expect

Constipation, Bloating, Fullness, Nausea, and Flatulence. These adverse effects can be minimized by starting with a low dose; mixing the resin with noncarbonated, pulpy juices or sauces; and swallowing without gulping air. Maintain adequate fiber in the diet and drink sufficient water.

Drug Interactions

Digoxin, Warfarin, Thyroid Hormones, Thiazide Diuretics, Phenobarbital, Nonsteroidal Antiinflammatory Agents, Tetracycline, Beta Blocking Agents, Gemfibrozil, Glipizide, Phenytoin. The resins may bind these medicines, which reduces absorption. The interaction can usually be minimized by administering these medicines 1 hour before or 4 hours after administration of resins.

Amiodarone. The resins significantly decrease absorption of amiodarone. The resins also block the enterohepatic recirculation of amiodarone. Consequently, amiodarone and the resins should not be used concurrently.

Fat-Soluble Vitamins (D, E, A, K), Folic Acid. High doses of resins may reduce absorption of these agents, but this interaction is not usually significant in normally nourished patients.

DRUG CLASS: Niacin

Actions

Niacin, also known as nicotinic acid, is a water-soluble B vitamin (also known as vitamin B_3). The mechanisms of action as an antilipemic agent are not completely known but are not related to its effects as a vitamin. Niacin inhibits VLDL synthesis by liver cells, which causes a decrease in LDL and triglyceride production. Triglyceride levels are reduced by 20% to 50% and total cholesterol and LDL-C can be reduced by 5% to 25%. Niacin may also reduce the metabolism of HDL, causing a 15% to 35% increase in HDL levels. Niacin also causes the release of histamine, causing peripheral vasodilation and increased blood flow (flushing of the skin).

Uses

Nicotinic acid is the only form of vitamin B_3 that is approved by the FDA for treatment of dyslipidemias. Niacin is used in conjunction with dietary therapy to decrease elevated cholesterol concentrations in dyslipidemias and to reduce the risks of atherosclerosis leading to CAD. It can be used in combination with bile acid–binding resins or the statins (niacin + lovastatin = Advicor) for greater combined lowering of cholesterol levels. Another benefit to niacin therapy is its significantly lower cost in comparison with the other antilipemic agents. Niacin should be used with caution in patients with diabetes because of glucose intolerance.

Different forms of vitamin B_3 cannot be used interchangeably. Other forms of vitamin B_3 are niacinamide and inositol hexaniacinate, which do not lower elevated cholesterol levels. Immediate-release niacin products cause more facial and skin flushing, and the sustained release products have a higher possibility of causing hepatotoxicity than the immediate release products. Dietary supplements of niacin should not be used to treat dyslipidemia. The recommended Dietary Reference Intake for nutritional supplementation is less than 20 mg per day. Doses of niacin required to treat dyslipidemias is 1 to 6 g per day.

Therapeutic Outcomes

The primary therapeutic outcomes expected from niacin are reduction of LDL (5% to 25%) and total cholesterol levels, reduction in triglyceride levels (20% to 50%), and an increase in HDL levels (15% to 35%).

Nursing Process for Niacin

Premedication Assessment

1. Serum triglyceride and cholesterol levels should be determined before initiation of therapy and periodically thereafter.
2. Liver function tests (bilirubin, aspartate aminotransferase [AST], alanine aminotransferase [ALT], gamma-glutamyltransferase [GGT], alkaline phosphatase, prothrombin time) should be determined before initiating therapy and every 6 to 8 weeks during the first year of therapy.
3. Baseline uric acid and blood glucose levels should be determined before initiating therapy. Niacin therapy may induce hyperuricemia, gout, and hyperglycemia in susceptible patients.
4. Baseline blood pressure and heart rate should be determined before initiating therapy.
5. Obtain data relating to any GI alterations before initiating therapy (e.g., presence of abdominal pain, nausea, flatus).

Planning

Availability. 50, 100, 250, or 500 mg tablets; 125, 250, 400, or 500 mg time-release capsules; 250, 500, 750, or 1000 mg time-release tablets.

Implementation

Dosage and Administration. PO: Initially, 100 mg three times daily with meals. Increase by 300 mg weekly until the therapeutic level or the maximum level is attained. Usual daily doses range from 1 to 6 g daily, but some patients require 9 g daily.

Hepatotoxicity. There appears to be a higher incidence of hepatotoxicity associated with the extended release products. Some clinicians recommend limiting the extended release products to 1500 mg daily to reduce the risk of hepatotoxicity.

Evaluation

Side Effects to Expect

Flushing, Itching, Rash, Tingling, Headache. These symptoms are common at the beginning of therapy, especially with the immediate release products. Tolerance develops quickly. Administer niacin with food. Patients can also reduce symptoms by taking aspirin (325 mg) or ibuprofen (200 mg) 30 minutes before each dose of niacin. Side effects can also be minimized by taking with food.

Nausea, Gas, Abdominal Discomfort, Pain. GI upset can be minimized by starting with low doses and administering all doses with food.

Dizziness, Faintness, Hypotension. Niacin is a vasodilator and may cause hypotension, especially if a patient is receiving other antihypertensive agents. Anticipate the development of hypotension, and take measures to prevent an occurrence. Teach the patient to rise slowly from a supine or sitting position and to sit or lie down if feeling faint. Monitor blood pressures in both the supine and sitting positions.

Side Effects to Report

Fatigue, Anorexia, Nausea, Malaise, Jaundice. These are the early symptoms associated with hepatotoxicity. Report to the health care provider for further evaluation.

Myopathy. Symptoms of muscle aches, soreness, and weakness may be early signs of myopathy. Serum creatine phosphokinase levels more than 10 times the upper limit of normal confirm the diagnosis.

Drug Interactions

HMG-CoA Reductase Inhibitors. The potential of developing myopathy is increased when niacin is added to the treatment regimen. The incidence is less than 1%.

DRUG CLASS: HMG-CoA Reductase Inhibitors

Actions

HMG-CoA reductase enzyme inhibitors (Table 22-3) are the most potent antilipemic agents available. They are also known as the statins. The statins competitively

Drug Table 22-3 HMG-CoA REDUCTASE INHIBITORS (STATINS)

GENERIC NAME	BRAND NAME	AVAILABILITY	DAILY DOSE	MAXIMUM DAILY DOSE
HMG-CoA REDUCTASE INHIBITORS (STATINS)				
atorvastatin	Lipitor	Tablets: 10, 20, 40, 80 mg	10-40 mg daily at any time	Up to 80 mg daily
fluvastatin	Lescol Lescol XL	Capsules: 20, 40 mg Tablets, extended release: 80 mg	20 mg at bedtime 80 mg at bedtime	Up to 80 mg at bedtime
lovastatin	Mevacor Altoprev	Tablets: 10, 20, 40 mg Tablets, extended release: 10, 20, 40, 60 mg	20-40 mg with evening meal 10-60 mg daily at bedtime	80 mg daily 60 mg daily at bedtime
pravastatin	Pravachol	Tablets: 10, 20, 40, 80 mg	40 mg daily at anytime	Up to 80 mg daily
rosuvastatin	Crestor	Tablets: 5, 10, 20, 40 mg	5-40 mg daily at any time	Up to 40 mg daily
simvastatin	Zocor	Tablets: 5, 10, 20, 40, 80 mg	5-20 mg daily at bedtime	Up to 80 mg at bedtime
HMG-CoA REDUCTASE INHIBITOR COMBINATION PRODUCTS				
atorvastatin-amlodipine	Caduet	atorvastatin/amlodipine (10/5 to 80/10)		atorvastatin 80 mg amlodipine 10 mg
lovastatin-niacin (extended release)	Advicor	lovastatin/niacin (20/500, 20/750, 20/1000)		lovastatin 40 mg niacin 2000 mg
pravastatin-aspirin	Pravigard PAC	pravastatin/aspirin (20/81 to 80/325)		pravastatin 80 mg aspirin 325 mg
simvastatin-ezetimibe	Vytorin	simvastatin/ezetimibe (10/10 to 80/10)		simvastatin 80 mg ezetimibe 10 mg

inhibit the enzyme responsible for converting HMG-CoA to mevalonate in the biosynthetic pathway to cholesterol in the liver. The reduction in liver cholesterol increases the removal of LDL from the circulating blood. Levels of LDL-C may be reduced by as much as 50%. The statins also cause a reduction in VLDL and triglyceride levels (20% to 30%) and mild increases (5% to 15%) in HDL. These agents are more effective if administered at night because of peak production of cholesterol at this time. Statins also have other beneficial effects unrelated to their lipid-lowering capacity. They reduce inflammation, platelet aggregation, thrombin formation, and plasma viscosity, thus reducing factors that contribute to heart attacks and strokes.

Uses

The statins are used in conjunction with dietary therapy to decrease elevated cholesterol concentrations in hyperlipidemias and to reduce the risks of atherosclerosis leading to CAD. The statins listed are similar in effectiveness at recommended starting doses and times.

Therapeutic Outcomes

The primary therapeutic outcome expected from HMG-CoA reductase inhibitors is reduction of LDL and total cholesterol levels.

Nursing Process for HMG-CoA Reductase Inhibitors

Premedication Assessment

1. Serum triglyceride and cholesterol levels should be determined before initiating therapy and periodically thereafter.
2. Liver function tests (AST, ALT) should be obtained before initiating therapy, every 4 to 6 weeks during the first 3 months of therapy, every 6 to 12 months during the next 12 months or after dose elevation, and every 6 months thereafter.
3. Obtain data relating to any GI alterations before initiating therapy (e.g., presence of abdominal pain, nausea, or flatus).
4. Confirm that the patient is not pregnant before initiating a statin. Inform the patient to notify her health care provider should she contemplate conception or become pregnant while receiving statin therapy.

Planning

Availability. See Table 22-3.

Implementation

Dosage and Administration. See Table 22-3. Lovastatin should be administered with food to enhance absorption. The other statins may be administered without food.

Evaluation

Side Effects to Expect

Headaches, Nausea, Abdominal Bloating, Gas. These symptoms are usually mild and disappear with continued therapy.

Side Effects to Report

Liver Dysfunction. Liver function tests should be monitored as described previously. If the transaminases (AST, ALT) rise to three times the upper limit of normal and are persistent, the medicine should be discontinued.

Myopathy. Symptoms of muscle aches, soreness, and weakness may be early signs of myopathy. Serum creatine phosphokinase levels more than 10 times the upper limit of normal confirm the diagnosis. Myopathy is most common with lovastatin (at <1%). Myopathy is more common (5%) if statins are used in combination with niacin, gemfibrozil, or cyclosporine.

Rhabdomyolysis and Myoglobinuria. Renal failure has been rarely reported; this is an extension of severe, progressive myopathy.

Drug Interactions

Cyclosporine, Itraconazole, Ketoconazole, Fluconazole, Fibrates, Niacin, Nefazodone, Verapamil, Erythromycin, Ranolazine. The incidence of myopathy is increased when lovastatin, simvastatin, or atorvastatin is prescribed in conjunction with these medicines. These medicines inhibit the metabolism of the statins, inducing toxicity.

Cimetidine, Ranitidine, Omeprazole. Coadministration with fluvastatin results in significantly increased fluvastatin levels. Dosage reductions of fluvastatin may be necessary.

Propranolol. Concurrent administration of propranolol and simvastatin results in a significantly lower serum level of simvastatin. Either increase the dose of simvastatin or switch to another statin.

Rifampin. Concurrent administration of rifampin and fluvastatin results in significantly lower levels of fluvastatin. Either increase the dose of fluvastatin or switch to another statin.

Warfarin. When lovastatin or simvastatin and warfarin are prescribed together, the prothrombin time (International Normalized Ratio [INR]) may be prolonged. Observe for possible overanticoagulation and bleeding.

Grapefruit Juice. Grapefruit juice inhibits the metabolism of atorvastatin, lovastatin, and simvastatin, increasing their plasma concentrations and a greater potential for myopathy. People taking these medicines should avoid grapefruit juice.

DRUG CLASS: Fibric Acids

Actions

The mechanism of action of the fibric acids (e.g., gemfibrozil, fenofibrate) is unknown; however, they do lower triglyceride levels by 20% to 40%. In patients with hypertriglyceridemia they raise HDL levels by 10% to 15%. They also reduce LDL-C by 10% to 15% in patients with elevated cholesterol. Fenofibrate may lower LDL-C more effectively than gemfibrozil. However, in patients with concurrent hypertriglyceridemia, gemfibrozil may have no effect on or may slightly increase LDL-C levels.

Uses

The fibrates are the most effective triglyceride-lowering agents. Gemfibrozil and fenofibrate are used in conjunction with dietary therapy to decrease elevated triglyceride levels in patients who are at risk for pancreatitis. Gemfibrozil can also be used in patients with hyperlipidemia who have low HDL levels and elevated LDL-C and triglycerides and who have not responded to weight loss, dietary therapy, and other pharmacologic therapy such as resins, statins, or niacin. Fibric acids must be used with caution in combination with statins due to the risk of myopathy and rhabdomyolysis.

Therapeutic Outcomes

The primary therapeutic outcome expected from fibric acid therapy is a 20% to 40% reduction in triglyceride levels and a 10% to 15% increase in HDL levels.

Nursing Process for Fibric Acids

Premedication Assessment

1. Serum triglyceride and cholesterol levels should be obtained before initiating therapy and periodically thereafter.
2. Liver function tests should be determined before initiating therapy and then every 6 months thereafter.
3. Baseline blood glucose levels should be determined before gemfibrozil therapy. Gemfibrozil may cause moderate hyperglycemia.
4. Obtain data relating to any GI alterations before initiating therapy (e.g., presence of abdominal pain, nausea, flatus).

Planning

Availability. Gemfibrozil (Lopid): 600 mg tablets. Fenofibrate (Tricor): 48, 50, 54, 145, 160 mg tablets; 43, 67, 130, 134, and 200 mg capsules.

Implementation

Dosage and Administration

Gemfibrozil—1200 mg per day in two divided doses, 30 minutes before the morning and evening meals.

Fenofibrate—Initially, 45 to 160 mg per day, given with meals. Increase dosage every 4 to 8 weeks up to 160 mg daily with a meal. Dosages of fenofibrate need to be reduced in older adult patients and patients with renal insufficiency. See the manufacturer's recommendations.

Evaluation

Side Effects to Expect

Nausea, Diarrhea, Flatulence, Bloating, Abdominal Distress. These are relatively common adverse effects. Starting with a lower dose taken between meals can help minimize these effects. If symptoms persist, notify the health care provider. Potentially more serious complications may be developing.

Side Effects to Report

Fatigue, Anorexia, Nausea, Malaise, and Jaundice. These are the early symptoms associated with gallbladder disease and hepatotoxicity. Report to the health care provider for further evaluation.

Myopathy. Symptoms of muscle aches, soreness, and weakness may be early signs of myopathy. Serum creatine phosphokinase levels more than 10 times the upper limit of normal confirm the diagnosis. Myopathy is most common with lovastatin and gemfibrozil. Myopathy is more common (5%) if statins are used in combination with niacin, gemfibrozil, or cyclosporine.

Drug Interactions

Warfarin. The fibric acids may enhance the pharmacologic effect of warfarin. Reduce the dosage of warfarin using the prothrombin time (INR) as an indicator to prevent bleeding.

Sulfonylureas, Insulin. Gemfibrozil may increase the pharmacologic effect of these agents. Monitor for signs of hypoglycemia and reduce the dose of the insulin or sulfonylurea as needed.

Bile Acid–Binding Resins. The resins may bind to fenofibrate, reducing absorption. The interaction can usually be minimized by administering fenofibrate 1 hour before or 4 hours after administration of resins.

HMG-CoA Reductase Inhibitors. The potential of developing myopathy is increased when the fibric acids are added to the treatment regimen. The incidence is less than 5%.

DRUG CLASS: Miscellaneous Antilipemic Agents

ezetimibe (ehz et' tih meeb)
▶ ZETIA (zeh' te ah)

Actions

Ezetimibe is the first of a new class of agents used to reduce atherosclerosis. Ezetimibe acts by blocking the absorption of cholesterol from the small intestine. It does not bind to cholesterol and reduce absorption as the bile acid resins do, but instead acts on the small intestine to inhibit the absorption of cholesterol present in the small intestine that derives from cholesterol secreted in the bile and from the diet. Early studies indicate that ezetimibe reduces total cholesterol by about 12%, LDL-C by 18%, and triglycerides by 7%, while having a minimal effect on raising HDL levels.

Uses

Ezetimibe is used in conjunction with dietary therapy to decrease elevated cholesterol concentrations in hyperlipidemia and to reduce the risks of atherosclerosis leading to CAD. This agent may also be used with the statins to further lower cholesterol. Combined therapy with fibric acid derivatives is not recommended. Ezetimibe may have an advantage over the bile acid resins because it does not elevate triglyceride levels.

Therapeutic Outcomes

The primary therapeutic outcome expected from ezetimibe therapy is reduction of LDL and total cholesterol levels.

Nursing Process for Ezetimibe

Premedication Assessment

1. Serum triglyceride and cholesterol levels should be determined before initiating therapy and periodically thereafter.
2. Obtain data relating to any GI alterations before initiating therapy (e.g., presence of abdominal pain, nausea, flatus).

Planning

Availability. PO: 10 mg tablets.

Implementation

Dosage and Administration. Adult: PO: 10 mg once daily. It may be taken with or without meals.

Evaluation

Side Effects to Expect

Abdominal Pain, Diarrhea. These adverse effects are mild and generally do not require discontinuation of therapy.

Drug Interactions

Bile Acid Resins. The resins may bind to ezetimibe, reducing absorption. The interaction can usually be minimized by administering ezetimibe 1 hour before or 4 hours after administering resins.

omega-3 fatty acids
▶ OMACOR (oh' mah cor)

Actions

Omacor is the first of a new class of agents used to reduce atherosclerosis. Omacor is a combination product containing two omega-3 fatty acids: eicosapentaenoic acid (EPA) and docosahexaenoic acid (DHA). Omega-3 fatty acids are sometimes referred to as "fish oils" because of higher concentrations of these fatty acids in fish oils. The mechanism of action is not known, but the end result is that the omega-3 fatty acids reduce synthesis of triglycerides in the liver. Early studies indicate that Omacor reduces triglyceride levels 20% to 50%, with small increases in HDL-C. In some cases, LDL-C also increased.

Uses

Omacor is used in conjunction with dietary therapy to decrease very elevated triglyceride levels (>500 mg/dL) in adult patients. This agent may also be used with the statins to further lower cholesterol. Omacor may have an advantage over the fibrates and niacin because it does not cause myositis or rhabdomyolysis, particularly when combined with statins. Omacor should be used with caution in patients with sensitivity or allergy to fish. Omacor should be discontinued in patients who have not shown an adequate response after 2 months of treatment.

Therapeutic Outcomes

The primary therapeutic outcome expected from Omacor therapy is reduction of elevated triglyceride levels.

Nursing Process for Omega-3 Fatty Acids

Premedication Assessment

1. Serum triglyceride, total cholesterol, HDL-C, and LDL-C levels should be determined before initiating therapy and periodically thereafter.
2. Liver function tests (AST, ALT) should be determined before initiating therapy and every 6 to 8 weeks during the first year of therapy.
3. Obtain data relating to any GI alterations before initiating therapy (e.g., presence of abdominal pain, nausea, flatus).

Planning

Availability. PO: 1 g capsules

Implementation

Dosage and Administration. *Adult:* PO: 4 g one time daily or 2 g two times daily.

Evaluation

Side Effects to Expect and Report. In 2004, Omacor was approved for use and reports of side effects are quite limited. If any of the following adverse effects occur, report to the health care provider immediately: arm, back, or jaw pain; chest pain or discomfort; chest tightness or heaviness; difficult or labored breathing; fast or irregular heartbeat; nausea; shortness of breath; sweating; tightness in chest; or wheezing.

Other minor adverse effects reported during clinical studies include back pain; unusual or unpleasant (after)taste; belching; bloated full feeling; change in taste; chills; cough; diarrhea; excess air or gas in stomach; fever; general feeling of discomfort or illness; headache; hoarseness; joint pain; loss of appetite; lower back or side pain; muscle aches and pains; pain; painful or difficult urination; rash; runny nose; shivering; sore throat; sweating; trouble sleeping; unusual tiredness or weakness; or vomiting. Symptoms should be reported to the health care provider if they persist.

Drug Interactions. No drug interactions have been reported to date.

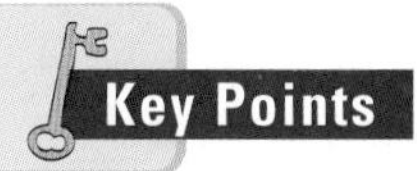

Key Points

- Coronary artery disease (CAD) is a major cause of premature death in the United States.
- Major treatable causes of CAD are hypertension, cigarette smoking, and atherosclerosis.
- A primary cause of atherosclerosis is the abnormal elevation of cholesterol and triglycerides in the blood in a disease known as *hyperlipidemia.* A diet high in saturated fats, cholesterol, carbohydrates, total calories, and alcohol, as well as a sedentary lifestyle are the most common and treatable causes of hyperlipidemia.
- The most cost-effective and successful forms of treatment are smoking cessation, weight reduction, exercise, and dietary modification. If change in diet and exercise do not produce an acceptable decrease in blood lipid levels, an antilipemic agent may be added to the patient's regimen.
- Patients should be fully informed of the significance of hyperlipidemias, the potential complications of not modifying lifestyles, and drug therapy. Drug therapy is likely to continue for many years or a lifetime.
- The primary medicines used to lower elevated cholesterol levels are the bile acid–binding resins, niacin, ezetimibe, and the statins. The fibric acid derivatives and omega-3 fatty acids lower triglyceride levels.

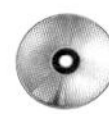

Go to your Companion CD-ROM for Appendices, an Audio Glossary, animations, Drug Dosage Calculators, customizable Patient Self-Assessment forms, and Review Questions for the NCLEX® Examination.

evolve Be sure to visit the companion Evolve site at http://evolve.elsevier.com/Clayton for WebLinks and additional online resources.

MEDICATION SAFETY REVIEW

MATH REVIEW QUESTIONS

1. Order: Nicotinic acid (niacin) 1.5 g PO in three divided doses, daily
   Available: Nicotinic acid (niacin) 500-mg tablets
   Give: _______ tablets per dose.
   A total of _______ mg daily.
2. Order: Lovastatin (Mevacor) 80 mg PO daily
   Available: Lovastatin (Mevacor) 20-mg tablets
   Give: _______ tablets.
   A total of _______ mg daily.
3. Order: Lipitor 40 mg PO bid
   Available: Lipitor 20-mg tablets
   Give: _______ tablets per dose.
   A total of _______ mg daily.

CRITICAL THINKING QUESTIONS

1. Why is it essential to monitor a patient taking a bile acid–binding resin medication for a fat-soluble vitamin deficiency?
2. Why would bleeding problems be a potential side effect of bile acid–binding resin drugs?
3. What effect do HMG-CoA reductase inhibitors have on LDL, HDL, and VLDL cholesterol and plasma triglycerides?
4. What type of premedication assessments are required before administering bile acid–binding resins, niacin, HMG-CoA reductase inhibitors, fibric acids, omega-3-fatty acids, and ezetimibe?

CONTENT REVIEW QUESTIONS

1. A common side effect of niacin that the patient should be educated on how to avoid is:
   1. headache and hypertension.
   2. nausea, diarrhea, and flatulence.
   3. flushing, itching, and headache.
   4. constipation.
2. Fibric acids are used to lower:
   1. triglycerides.
   2. cholesterol.
   3. fatty acids.
   4. insulin resistance.
3. HMG-CoA reductase drugs are also known as:
   1. nicotinic acid.
   2. statins.
   3. hypoglycemics.
   4. cholesterol potentiators.
4. Liver function studies are not required/recommended before:
   1. fibric acids.
   2. HMG-CoA reductase inhibitors.
   3. niacin.
   4. bile acid–binding resins.
5. Grapefruit juice should not be taken with:
   1. fibric acids.
   2. HMG-CoA reductase inhibitors.
   3. niacin.
   4. bile acid–binding resins.
6. Omega-3 fatty acids are often referred to as:
   1. fish oils.
   2. statins.
   3. water-soluble vitamins.
   4. bile-acid resins.
7. Which of the following statements is/are true about Omacor? *(Select all that apply.)*
   1. Omacor is used to decrease very elevated triglyceride levels.
   2. Omacor is often used with statins to further lower cholesterol levels.
   3. Omacor may cause myositis or rhabdomyolysis.
   4. Omacor should be used with caution in patients with allergies to fish.

CHAPTER

23 Drugs Used to Treat Hypertension

evolve http://evolve.elsevier.com/Clayton

Chapter Content

Objectives

1. Summarize nursing assessments and interventions used for the treatment of hypertension.
2. State recommended lifestyle modifications for a diagnosis of hypertension.
3. Identify 10 classes of drugs used to treat hypertension.
4. Review Figure 23-2 to identify options and progression of treatment for hypertension.
5. Identify specific factors the hypertensive patient can use to assist in managing the disease.
6. Develop patient education objectives for individuals with hypertension.
7. Summarize the action of each drug class used to treat hypertension.

Key Terms

arterial blood pressure
systolic blood pressure
diastolic blood pressure
pulse pressure
mean arterial pressure (MAP)
cardiac output (CO)
hypertension
primary hypertension
secondary hypertension
systolic hypertension

HYPERTENSION

(For an introduction to cardiovascular diseases, see Chapter 21.) A primary function of the heart is to circulate blood to the organs and tissues of the body. When the heart contracts (systole) (sis' tahl e), blood is pumped out through the pulmonary artery to the lungs and out through the aorta to the other organs and peripheral tissues. The pressure with which the blood is pushed from the heart is referred to as the **arterial blood pressure** or **systolic blood pressure.** When the heart muscle relaxes between contractions (diastole) (dy as' tahl e), the blood pressure drops to a lower level, the **diastolic blood pressure.** When recorded in the patient's chart, the systolic pressure is recorded first, followed by the diastolic pressure (e.g., 120/80 mm Hg). The difference between the systolic and diastolic pressure is called the **pulse pressure,** which is an indicator of the tone of the arterial blood vessel walls. The **mean arterial pressure (MAP)** is the average pressure throughout each cycle of the heartbeat and is significant because it is the pressure that actually pushes the blood through the circulatory system to perfuse tissue. It is calculated by adding one third of the pulse pressure to the diastolic pressure or by using the following equation:

$$\text{MAP} = \frac{\text{systolic pressure} - \text{diastolic pressure}}{3} + \text{diastolic pressure}$$

Under normal conditions, the arterial blood pressure stays within narrow limits. It reaches its peak during high physical or emotional activity and is usually at its lowest level during sleep.

Arterial blood pressure (BP) can be defined as the product of **cardiac output (CO)** and peripheral vascular resistance (PVR):

$$\text{BP} = \text{CO} \times \text{PVR}$$

CO is the primary determinant of systolic pressure; peripheral vascular resistance determines the diastolic pressure. CO is determined by the stroke volume (the volume of blood ejected in a single contraction of the left ventricle), heart rate (controlled by the autonomic nervous system), and venous capacitance (capability of veins to return blood to the heart). Systolic blood pressure is thus increased by factors that increase heart rate or stroke volume. Venous capacitance affects the volume of blood (or preload) that is returned to the heart through the central venous circulation. Venous constriction decreases venous capacitance, increasing preload and systolic pressure, and venous dilation increases venous capacitance and decreases preload and systolic pressure. Peripheral vascular resistance is regulated primarily by contraction and dilation of arterioles. Arteriolar constriction increases peripheral vascular resistance and thus diastolic blood pressure. Other factors that affect vascular resistance include the elasticity of the blood vessel walls and the viscosity of the blood.

Hypertension is a disease characterized by an elevation of the systolic blood pressure, the diastolic blood pressure, or both. Statistics in North America show that blood pressures above 140/90 mm Hg are associated with premature death, which results from accelerated vascular disease of the brain, heart, and kidneys. **Primary hypertension** accounts for 90% of all clinical cases of high blood pressure. The cause of primary hypertension is unknown. At present, it is incurable but controllable. It is estimated that more than 50 million people in the United States have hypertension. The prevalence increases steadily with advancing age such that people who are normotensive at age 55 have a 90% lifetime risk of developing hypertension. In every age-group, the incidence of hypertension is higher for African Americans than whites of both sexes. Other major risk factors associated with high blood pressure are listed in Box 23-1. **Secondary hypertension** occurs after the development of another disorder within the body (Box 23-2).

The Seventh Report of the Joint National Committee on Detection, Evaluation and Treatment of High Blood Pressure 2003 (JNC 7) has classified blood pressure by stages that represent the degree of risk of nonfatal and fatal cardiovascular disease events and renal disease (Table 23-1). The category of "prehypertension" was added to the classification system in the 2003 report because of the very high likelihood of people with a blood pressure in this range of having a heart attack, heart failure, stroke, and/or kidney disease. People with blood pressure in this range are in need of increased education and lifestyle modification to gain control of their blood pressure to prevent cardiovascular disease.

The JNC 7 guidelines consider an elevation in both systolic and diastolic blood pressure readings when making a diagnosis of hypertension. The individual should be seated quietly for at least 5 minutes in a chair (rather than an examination table), with feet on the floor, and the arm supported at heart level. An appropriately sized cuff (cuff bladder encircling at least 80% of the arm) should be used for accuracy. A person must have two or more elevated readings on two or more separate occasions after initial screening to be classified as having hypertension. When systolic and diastolic readings fall into two different stages, the higher of the two stages is used to classify the degree of hypertension present. Table 23-2 lists follow-up recommendations based on the initial set of blood pressure measurements. Measurement of blood pressure in the standing position is indicated periodically, especially in those at risk for postural hypotension.

In 2000, the Coordinating Committee of the National High Blood Pressure Education Program updated the JNC-VI guidelines and urged health practitioners to use the systolic blood pressure as the major criterion for the diagnosis and management of hypertension in middle-aged and older Americans. Prior to this time, the diastolic blood pressure had been the major determinant for the control of blood pressure. Recent evidence indicates that **systolic hypertension** is the most common form of hypertension and is present in about two thirds of hypertensive individuals older than 60 years of age.

When a person has been diagnosed with hypertension, further evaluation through medical history, physical examination, and laboratory tests should be completed to (1) identify causes of the high blood pressure, (2) assess the presence or absence of target organ damage and cardiovascular disease (see Box 23-1), and (3) identify other cardiovascular risk factors that may guide treatment (see Table 23-1).

Box 23-1 *Major Risk Factors Associated with Hypertension and Target Organ Damage*

Major Risk Factors

Hypertension*
Cigarette smoking
Obesity* (body mass index ≥30 kg/m^2)
Physical inactivity
Dyslipidemia*
Diabetes mellitus*
Microalbuminuria or estimated glomerular filtration rate (GFR) <60 mL/min
Age (older than 55 for men, 65 for women)
Family history of premature cardiovascular disease (men younger than age 55; women, age 65)

Target Organ Damage

Heart
- Left ventricular hypertrophy
- Angina or prior myocardial infarction
- Prior coronary revascularization
- Heart failure

Brain
- Stroke or transient ischemic attack

Chronic kidney disease
Peripheral arterial disease
Retinopathy
Glomerular filtration rate (GFR)
Components of the metabolic syndrome

From The Seventh Report of the Joint National Committee on Prevention, Detection, Evaluation, and Treatment of High Blood Pressure, National Institutes of Health, Publication No. 03-5233, May 2003.

Box 23-2 *Identifiable Causes of Hypertension*

Sleep apnea
Drug-induced or related causes
Chronic kidney disease
Primary aldosteronism
Renovascular disease
Chronic steroid therapy and Cushing's syndrome
Pheochromocytoma
Coarctation of the aorta
Thyroid or parathyroid disease

From The Seventh Report of the Joint National Committee on Prevention, Detection, Evaluation, and Treatment of High Blood Pressure, National Institutes of Health, Publication No. 03-5233, May 2003.

Table 23-1 ***Classification and Management of Blood Pressure for Adults****

	BLOOD PRESSURE (mm Hg)				INITIAL DRUG THERAPY	
BP CLASSIFICATION	**SYSTOLIC**		**DIASTOLIC**	**LIFESTYLE MODIFICATION**	**WITHOUT COMPELLING INDICATION**	**WITH COMPELLING INDICATION**
Normal	<120	and	<80	Encourage	No antihypertensive drug indicated	Drug(s) for compelling indications
Prehypertension	120-139	or	80-89	Yes	No antihypertensive drug indicated	Drug(s) for compelling indications†
Stage 1 hypertension	140-159	or	90-99	Yes	Thiazide-type diuretics for most; may consider ACEI, ARB, BB, CCB, or combination	Drug(s) for the compelling indications† Other antihypertensive drugs (diuretics, ACEI, ARB, BB, CCB) as needed
Stage 2 hypertension	≥160	or	≥100	Yes	Two-drug combination for most‡ (usually thiazide-type diuretic and ACEI or ARB, or BB, or CCB)	Drug(s) for the compelling indications Other antihypertensive drugs (diuretics, ACEI, ARB, BB, CCB) as needed

From The Seventh Report of the Joint National Committee on Prevention, Detection, Evaluation, and Treatment of High Blood Pressure, National Institutes of Health, Publication No. 03-5233, May 2003.
*Treatment determined by highest BP category.
†Treat patients with chronic kidney disease or diabetes to BP goal of <130/80 mm Hg.
‡Initial combined therapy should be used cautiously in those at risk for orthostatic hypotension.
ACEI, Angiotensin-converting enzyme inhibitor; *ARB,* angiotensin-receptor blocker; *BB,* beta blocker; *CCB,* calcium channel blocker.

Table 23-2 ***Recommended Follow-Up Schedule After Initial Blood Pressure Measurement***

INITIAL BLOOD PRESSURE (mm Hg)*		
SYSTOLIC	**DIASTOLIC**	**FOLLOW-UP RECOMMENDED†**
<130	<85	Recheck in 2 years
130-139	85-89	Recheck in 1 year‡
140-159	90-99	Confirm within 2 months‡
160-179	100-109	Evaluate or refer to source of care within 1 month
≥180	≥110	Evaluate or refer to source of care immediately or within 1 week, depending on clinical situation

*If systolic and diastolic categories are different, follow recommendations for shorter time follow-up (e.g., 160/86 mm Hg should be evaluated or referred to source of care within 1 month).
†Modify the scheduling of follow-up according to reliable information about past blood pressure measurements, other cardiovascular risk factors, or target organ disease.
‡Provide advice about lifestyle modifications.

TREATMENT OF HYPERTENSION

The primary purpose for controlling hypertension is to reduce the frequency of cardiovascular disease (angina, myocardial infarction, heart failure, stroke, renal failure, retinopathy). To accomplish this goal, the blood pressure must be reduced and maintained below 140/90 mm Hg, if possible. Patients who also have conditions such as diabetes mellitus, heart failure, or renal disease should have a goal of less than 130/80 mm Hg. Major lifestyle modifications shown to lower blood pressure include weight reduction in those who are overweight or obese, adoption of the Dietary Approaches to Stop Hypertension (DASH) diet, dietary sodium reduction, physical activity, and moderation of alcohol consumption (Table 23-3). Treatment schedules should interfere as little as possible with the patient's lifestyle; however, nonpharmacologic therapy must include elimination of smoking, weight control, routine activity, restriction of alcohol intake, stress reduction, and sodium control. If this therapy is successful in controlling high blood pressure, drug therapy is not necessary. Even if lifestyle changes are not adequate to control hypertension, they may reduce the number and doses of antihypertensive medications needed to manage the condition.

Patient education is vitally important in treating hypertension. This education should be emphasized and reiterated frequently by the physician, pharmacist, and nurse.

DRUG THERAPY FOR HYPERTENSION

Actions

Drugs used in the treatment of hypertension can be subdivided into several categories of therapeutic agents based on site of action (Figure 23-1). Clinical studies classify antihypertensive agents into *preferred agents* (diuretics and beta-adrenergic blockers), *alternative agents* (angiotensin-converting enzyme [ACE] inhibitors, angiotensin II receptor antagonists [ARBs], calcium ion antagonists, and alpha-1 adrenergic blockers), and *adjunctive agents* (central-acting alpha-2 agonists,

Table 23-3 ***Lifestyle Modifications to Manage Hypertension****

MODIFICATION	RECOMMENDATION	APPROXIMATE SYSTOLIC BLOOD PRESSURE REDUCTION (RANGE)
Weight reduction	Maintain normal body weight (body mass index 18.5-24.9 kg/m^2)	5-20 mm Hg/10 kg weight loss
Adopt DASH eating plan	Consume a diet rich in fruits, vegetables, and low-fat dairy products with a reduced content of saturated and total fat	8-14 mm Hg
Dietary sodium reduction	Reduce dietary sodium intake to no more than 100 mmol per day (2.4 g sodium or 6 g sodium chloride)	2-8 mm Hg
Physical activity	Engage in regular aerobic physical activity such as brisk walking (at least 30 minutes per day, most days of the week)	4-9 mm Hg
Moderation of alcohol consumption	Limit consumption to no more than two drinks (1 oz or 30 mL ethanol [e.g., 24 oz beer, 10 oz wine, or 3 oz 80-proof whiskey]) per day in most men and no more than one drink per day in women and lighter weight persons	2-4 mm Hg

From The Seventh Report of the Joint National Committee on Prevention, Detection, Evaluation, and Treatment of High Blood Pressure, National Institutes of Health, Publication No. 03-5233, May 2003.
*For overall cardiovascular risk reduction, stop smoking.
The effects of implementing these modifications are dose and time dependent and could be greater for some individuals.
DASH, Dietary Approaches to Stop Hypertension.

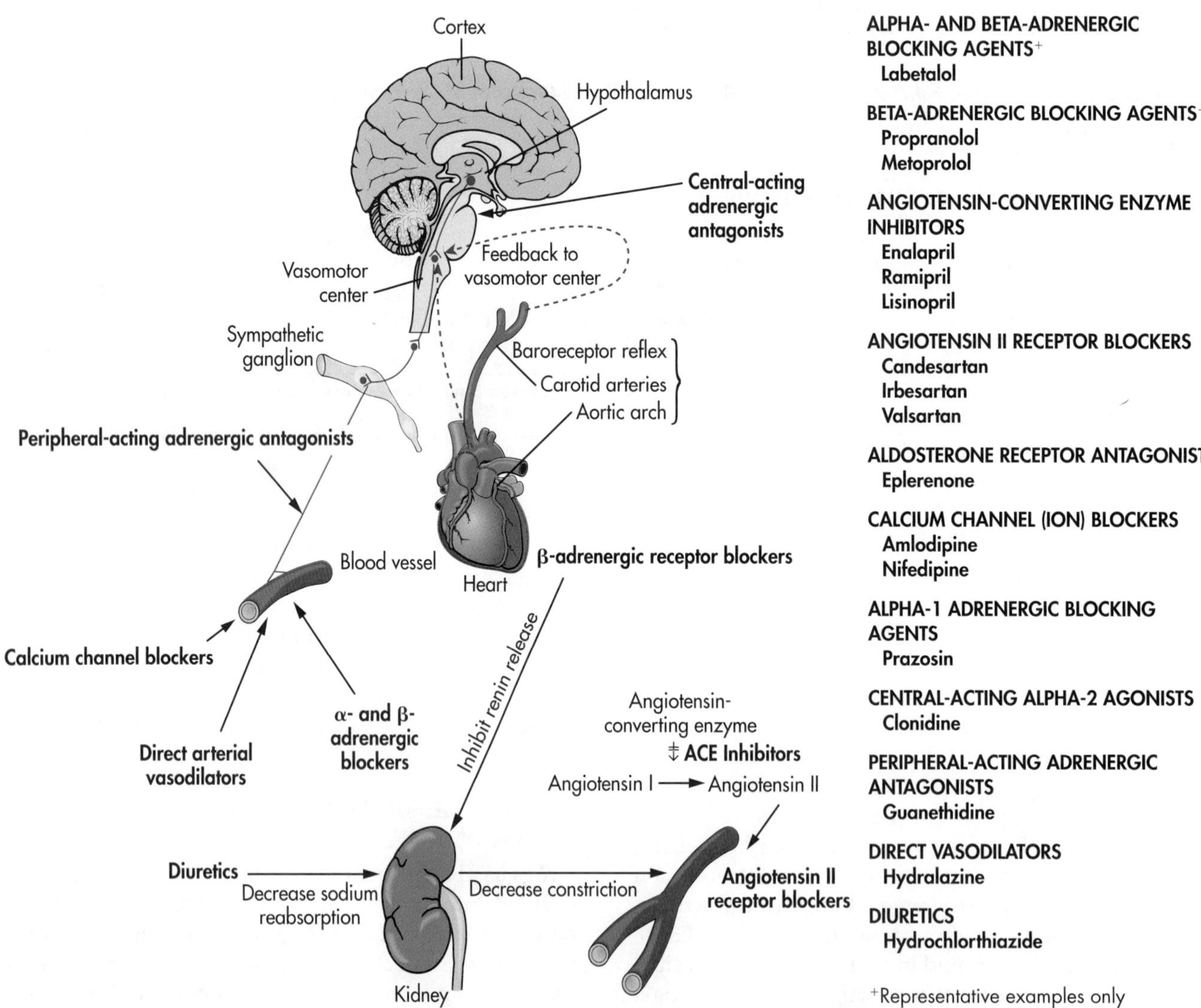

FIGURE **23-1** Sites of action of antihypertensive agents. *β-blockers,* Beta-adrenergic blockers; *CCB,* calcium channel blockers; *ACE,* angiotensin-converting enzyme inhibitors; *ARB,* angiotensin II receptor blocker; *α_1 blockers,* alpha-1 adrenergic blocking agents; *central α_2 agonists,* central-acting alpha-2 agonists.

peripheral-acting adrenergic antagonists, and direct vasodilators). Both preferred agents and alternative agents can be used alone, or in combination, to treat hypertension, but adjunctive agents should be used only in combination with a preferred or an alternative agent.

The guidelines also provide recommendations for specific groups of patients. For example, older patients with isolated systolic hypertension should first be treated with diuretics. Patients with diabetes and high blood pressure should be treated with the ACE inhibitors. Patients who have hypertension and have suffered a myocardial infarction should be treated with a beta-adrenergic blocking agent, and in most cases, an ACE inhibitor. Other studies have demonstrated that if a patient has heart failure, a diuretic and an ACE inhibitor may be beneficial. If a patient has angina pectoris, dihydropyridine calcium ion antagonists (e.g., amlodipine, nifedipine) may be added to other therapy because they have been proven to relieve chest pain and reduce the incidence of stroke. Other combinations of therapy found to be particularly effective are an ACE inhibitor plus a diuretic or calcium ion antagonist, or an ARB plus a diuretic. See individual monographs for mechanisms of action of each class of antihypertensive agent.

Uses

A key to long-term success with antihypertensive therapy is to individualize therapy for a patient based on demographic characteristics (e.g., age, gender, race), coexisting diseases and risk factors (e.g., migraine headaches, dysrhythmias, angina, diabetes mellitus), previous therapy (what has or has not worked in the past), concurrent drug therapy for other illnesses, and cost. As outlined in Figure 23-2, the JNC 7 recommends that if lifestyle modifications do not lower blood pressure adequately for patients with stage 1 or 2 hypertension, a diuretic or an alternative agent should be the initial treatment of choice. A low dose should be selected to protect the patient from adverse effects, although it may not immediately control the blood pressure. It must be recognized that it may take months to control hypertension adequately while avoiding adverse effects of therapy. If, after 1 to 3 months, the first drug is not effective, the dosage may be increased, another agent from another class may be substituted, or a second drug from another class with a different mechanism of action may be added (Figure 23-3). The guidelines also recommend that if the first drug started was not a diuretic, a diuretic should be initiated as the second drug, if needed, because the majority of patients will respond to a two-drug regimen if it includes a diuretic. In general, most patients with hypertension will require two or more antihypertensive medications to achieve goal blood pressure (<140/90 mm Hg, or <130/80 mm Hg for patients who have diabetes or chronic kidney disease). After blood pressure is reduced to the goal level and maintenance doses of medicines are stabilized, it may be appropriate to change a patient's medication to a combination antihypertensive product to simplify the regimen and enhance compliance. See Table 23-4 for a list of the ingredients of antihypertensive combination products.

Patients with stage 2 hypertension may require more aggressive therapy with a second or third agent added if control is not achieved by monotherapy in a relatively short time. Patients with an average diastolic blood pressure of greater than 120 mm Hg require immediate therapy and, if significant organ damage is present, may require hospitalization for initial control.

Patients who have modified their lifestyles with appropriate exercise, diet, weight reduction, and control of hypertension for at least 1 year may be candidates for "step-down" therapy. The dosage of antihypertensive medications may be gradually reduced in a slow, deliberate manner. Most patients may still require some therapy, but occasionally, the medicine can be discontinued. Patients whose drugs have been discontinued should have regular follow-up examination because blood pressure often rises again to hypertensive levels, sometimes months or years later, especially if lifestyle modifications are not continued.

NURSING PROCESS *for Hypertensive Therapy*

Assessment

History of Risk Factors

- Make note of patient's gender, age, and race. People who are older, male, and of the African American race have a higher incidence of hypertension.
- Has the client been told previously about the elevated blood pressure readings? If so, under what circumstances were the blood pressure readings taken?
- Is there a family history of hypertension, coronary heart disease, stroke, diabetes mellitus, or dyslipidemia?

Smoking. Obtain a history of the number of cigarettes or cigars smoked daily. How long has the person smoked? Has the person ever tried to stop smoking? Ask if the person knows what effect smoking has on the vascular system. How does the individual feel about modifying the smoking habit?

Dietary Habits. Obtain a dietary history. Ask specific questions to obtain data relating to the amount of salt used in cooking and at the table, as well as foods eaten that are high in fat, cholesterol, refined carbohydrates, and sodium. Using a calorie counter, ask the person to estimate the number of calories eaten per day. How much meat, fish, and poultry are eaten daily (size and number of servings)? Estimate the percent of total daily calories provided by fats. Discuss food preparation (e.g., baked, broiled, fried foods). How many servings of fruits and vegetables are eaten daily? What types of oils/fats are used in food preparation? See a nutrition text for further dietary history questions. What is the frequency and volume of alcoholic beverages consumed?

Elevated Serum Lipids. Ask whether the patient is aware of having elevated lipids, triglycerides, or

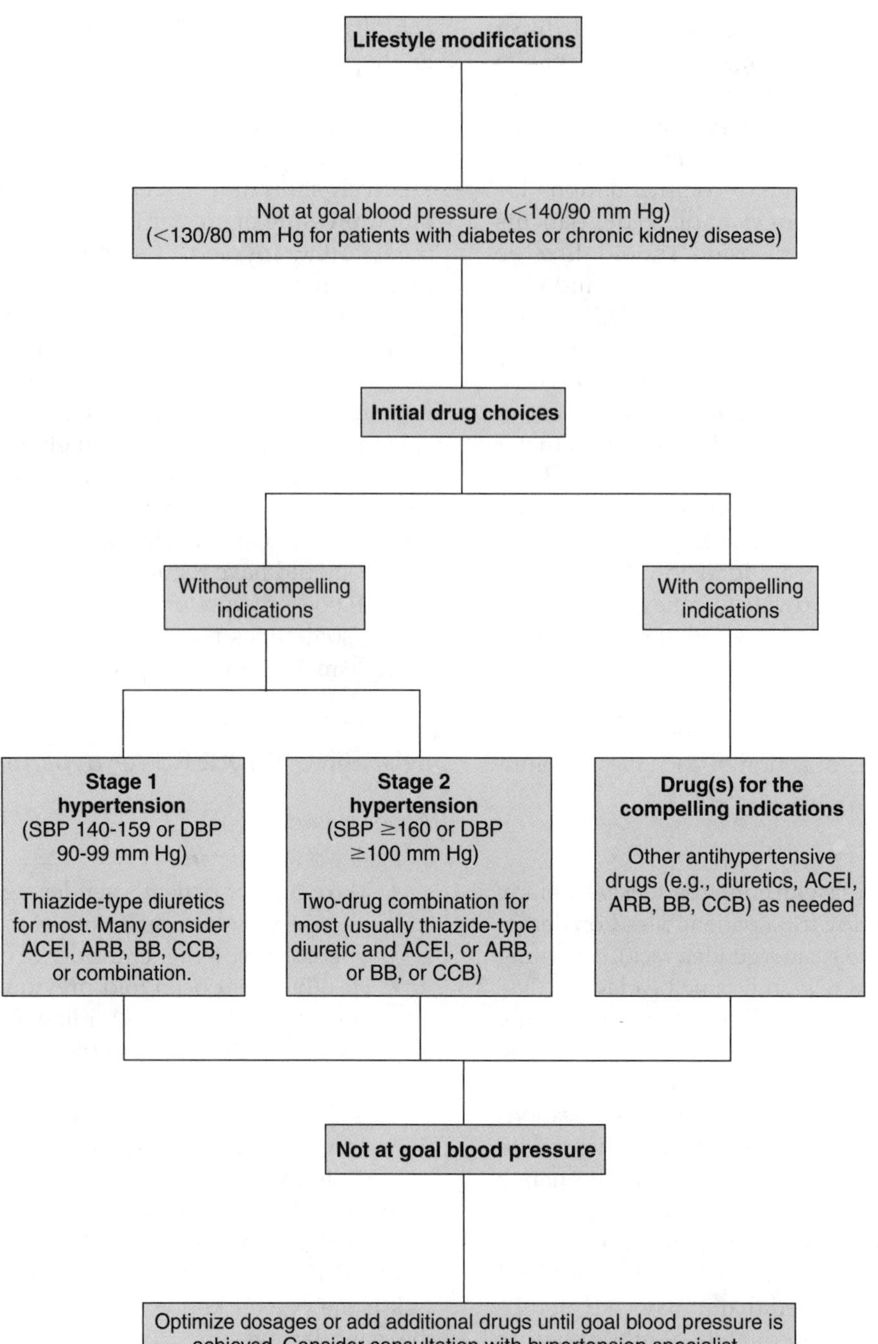

FIGURE **23-2** Treatment algorithm for hypertension.

cholesterol. If elevated, what measures has the person tried for reduction and what effect have the interventions had on the blood levels at subsequent examinations? Review laboratory data available (e.g., cholesterol, triglycerides, low-density lipoprotein [LDL], very low-density lipoprotein [VLDL]).

Renal. Has the patient had any laboratory tests to evaluate renal function (e.g., urinalysis: microalbuminuria, proteinuria, microscopic hematuria) or blood analysis showing an elevated blood urea nitrogen (BUN) or serum creatinine? Does the patient have nocturia?

Obesity. Weigh and measure the patient. Measure the waist circumference 2 inches above the navel. Ask about any recent weight gains or losses and whether intentional or unintentional. Note abnormal waist-hip ratio.

Psychomotor Functions

- Determine type of lifestyle. Ask the patient to describe exercise level in terms of amount (walking 3 miles), intensity (walking 3 mph), and

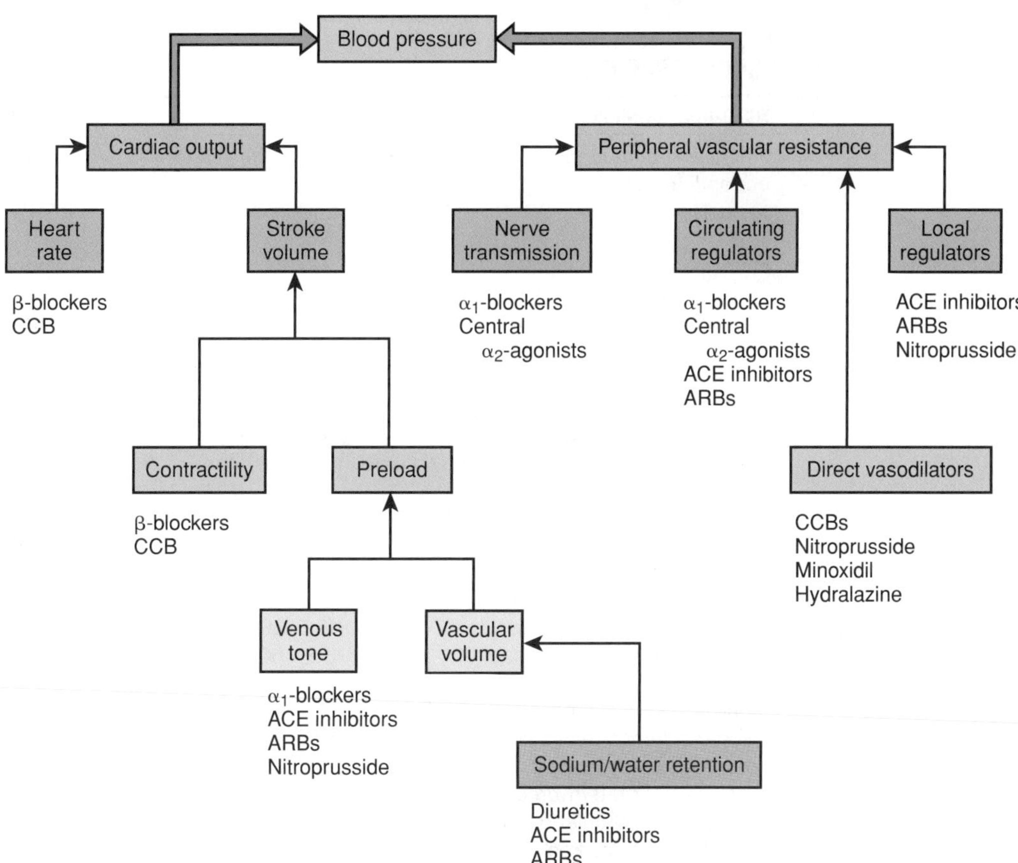

FIGURE **23-3** Effects of antihypertensive agents.

frequency (walking every other day). Is the patient's job physically demanding or of a sedentary nature?

- Determine psychological stress. How much stress does the individual estimate having in life? How does the person cope with stressful situations at home and in the workplace?
- Has the client experienced any fatigue or reduction in activity level due to intolerance or palpitations, angina, or dyspnea? When walking, does the individual experience severe leg cramps (claudication) that force him/her to stop and rest or to severely limit ambulation?

Medication History

- Has the patient ever taken or is the patient currently taking any medications for the treatment of high blood pressure? If blood pressure medications have been prescribed but are not being taken, why was the medicine discontinued? Were any side effects noticed while receiving the medications, and how did the patient manage them?
- Obtain a listing of all medications being taken, including prescribed, over-the-counter, herbal preparations, and street drugs. Research these medications in the drug monographs to determine potential drug-to-drug interactions that may affect the individual's blood pressure or the effectiveness of the medicines prescribed.
- If the patient is female, ask if she is now or has been taking oral contraceptives or is receiving hormone replacement therapy (HRT).

Physical Assessments

Blood Pressure. Obtain two or more blood pressure measurements.

- The individual should be seated quietly for at least 5 minutes in a chair with back supported (rather than an examination table), with feet on the floor, and arm supported at heart level.
- An appropriately sized cuff (cuff bladder encircling at least 80% of the arm) should be used for accuracy.
- When measuring blood pressure, the cuff should be inflated to 30 mm Hg above the point at which the radial pulse disappears. The sphygmomanometer pressure should then be reduced at 2 to 3 mm/second. Two readings should be performed at least 1 minute apart.
- Verify the readings in the opposite arm. A difference in blood pressure between the two arms can be expected in about 20% of patients. The higher value should be the one used in treatment decisions.
- People must have two or more elevated readings on two or more separate occasions after initial screening to be classified as having hypertension.
- Orthostatic hypotension is defined by a decrease in systolic blood pressure of 20 mm Hg

Drug Table 23-4 COMBINATION DRUGS FOR HYPERTENSION

COMBINATION TYPE	FIXED-DOSE COMBINATION (mg)*	TRADE NAME
ACEIs and CCBs	amlodipine/benazepril hydrochloride (2.5/10, 5/10, 5/20, 10/20)	Lotrel
	enalapril maleate/felodipine (5/2.5,5/5)	Lexxel
	trandolapril/verapamil (2/180, 1/240, 2/240, 4/240)	Tarka
CCBs and statin	amlodipine/atorvastatin (2.5/10 to 10/80)	Caduet
ACEIs and diuretics	benazepril/hydrochlorothiazide (5/6.25, 10/12.5, 20/12.5, 20/25)	Lotensin HCT
	captopril/hydrochlorothiazide (25/15, 25/25, 50/15, 50/25)	Capozide
	enalapril maleate/hydrochlorothiazide (5/12.5, 10/25)	Vaseretic
	lisinopril/hydrochlorothiazide (10/12.5, 20/12.5, 20/25)	Prinzide
	moexipril HCl/hydrochlorothiazide (7.5/12.5, 15/12.5, 15/25)	Uniretic
	quinapril HCl/hydrochlorothiazide (10/12.5, 20/12.5, 20/25)	Accuretic
ARBs and diuretics	candesartan cilexetil/hydrochlorothiazide (16/12.5, 32/12.5)	Atacand HCT
	eprosartan mesylate/hydrochlorothiazide (600/12.5, 600/25)	Teveten/HCT
	irbesartan/hydrochlorothiazide (150/12.5, 300/12.5, 300/25)	Avalide
	losartan potassium/hydrochlorothiazide (50/12.5, 100/25)	Hyzaar
	telmisartan/hydrochlorothiazide (40/12.5, 80/12.5, 80/25)	Micardis/HCT
	valsartan hydrochlorothiazide (80/12.5, 160/12.5, 160/25)	Diovan/HCT
BBs and diuretics	atenolol/chlorthalidone (50/25, 100/25)	Tenoretic
	bisoprolol fumarate/hydrochlorothiazide (2.5/6.25, 5/6.25, 10/6.25)	Ziac
	propranolol LA/hydrochlorothiazide (40/25)	Inderide
	metoprolol tartrate/hydrochlorothiazide (50/25, 100/25)	Lopressor HCT
	nadolol/bendrofluthiazide (40/5, 80/5)	Corzide
	timolol maleate/hydrochlorothiazide (10/25)	Timolide
Central-acting drug and diuretic	methyldopa/hydrochlorothiazide (250/15, 250/25, 500/30, 500/50)	Aldoril
	reserpine/chlorothiazide (0.125/250, 0.125/500)	
	reserpine/hydrochlorothiazide (0.125/25, 0.125/50)	
Diuretic and diuretic	amiloride HCl/hydrochlorothiazide (5/50)	Moduretic
	spironolactone/hydrochlorothiazide (25/25, 50/50)	Aldactazide
	triamterene/hydrochlorothiazide (37.5/25, 50/25, 75/50)	Dyazide, Maxzide

From The Seventh Report of the Joint National Committee on Prevention, Detection, Evaluation, and Treatment of High Blood Pressure, National Institutes of Health, Publication No. 03-5233, May 2003.
*Some drug combinations are available in multiple fixed doses. Each drug dose is reported in milligrams.
ACEI, Angiotensin-converting enzyme inhibitor; *ARB,* angiotensin-receptor blocker; *BB,* beta blocker; *CCB,* calcium channel blocker.

or more, or diastolic blood pressure of 10 mm Hg or more after 3 minutes of quiet standing. Food ingestion, time of day, age, and hydration can affect this form of hypotension, as can a history of parkinsonism, diabetes, or multiple myeloma.

- Ensure that the patient has not ingested caffeine within the past 2 to 3 hours.

Height and Weight. Weigh and measure the patient. What has the person's weight been? Ask about any recent weight gains or losses and whether intentional or unintentional. Calculate the body mass index (BMI) (see Chapter 21 for more discussion and classification of BMI):

$$\frac{\text{Weight (in kilograms)}}{\text{Height (in square meters [m}^2\text{])}} = \text{BMI (kg/m}^2\text{)}$$

or

$$\frac{\text{Weight (in pounds)}}{\text{Height (in square inches [in}^2\text{])}} \times 703 = \text{BMI (lb/in}^2\text{)}$$

Bruits. Check neck, abdomen, and extremities for the presence of bruits.

Peripheral Pulses. Palpate and record femoral, popliteal, and pedal pulses bilaterally.

Eyes. As appropriate to the level of education, perform a funduscopic examination of interior eye, noting arteriovenous nicking, hemorrhages, exudates, or papilledema.

Nursing Diagnoses

- Knowledge, deficient, related to hypertension (indication)
- Noncompliance with drug therapy (indication, side effects)
- Sexual dysfunction (side effects)

Planning

History of Risk Factors

- Examine data to determine the individual's extent of understanding of hypertension and its control.

- Using the patient's history, analyze lifestyle elements to determine health teaching needs of the individual and significant others.

Medication History. Plan patient education needed to implement or reinforce prescribed medication therapy.

Physical Assessment. Schedule physical assessments at specific intervals as appropriate to the patient's status and clinical site policies (e.g., vital signs taken every 4 hours or 8 hours; intake and output, daily weights).

Baseline and Diagnostic Studies. Review the chart and reports available that are used to build baseline information (e.g., electrocardiogram; urinalysis; blood glucose and hematocrit, serum potassium, creatinine and calcium levels; a lipid profile [total cholesterol, LDL cholesterol, high-density lipoprotein (HDL) cholesterol, triglycerides] after a 9- to 12-hour fast).

Implementation

- Perform nursing assessments on a scheduled basis.
- Make referrals as indicated for stress management, smoking cessation, dietary counseling, and for an exercise program appropriate for the individual's needs.
- When initiating antihypertensive therapy in the hospitalized patient, protect from possible falls secondary to hypotension by assisting during ambulation and carefully assessing for faintness. Take blood pressure in supine, sitting, and standing positions to identify hypotensive responses.

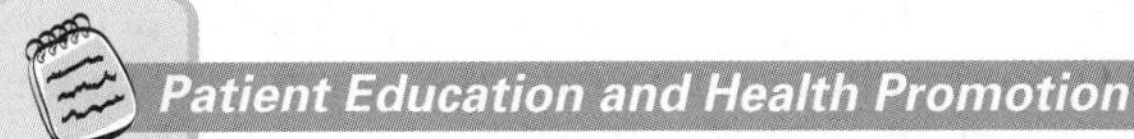

Patient Education and Health Promotion

Smoking. Suggest that the patient stop smoking. Explain the increased risk of coronary artery disease if the habit is continued. It may be necessary to settle for a drastic decrease in smoking in some people, although abstinence should be the goal.

Nutritional Status. Dietary counseling is essential in the treatment of hypertension. Control of obesity alone may be sufficient to alter the hypertensive condition. Most patients are placed on a reduced-sodium diet (2.3 g sodium or <6 g table salt per day). The goal of dietary therapy is a reduction of cholesterol, lipids saturated fat, and alcohol consumption. Foods high in potassium and calcium are encouraged to decrease blood pressure. See the DASH diet for further information (see Table 23-3).

Dietary planning should always involve the patient in menu planning so that personal preferences, availability of food products, and costs are discussed. Include the person who purchases and prepares the meals in the dietary counseling.

Show the patient various food labels and explain what ingredients indicate a high sodium content (e.g., salt, sodium, sodium chloride, sodium bicarbonate, sodium aluminum sulfate). Suggest the use of a variety of spices as substitutes for sodium when cooking. Explain foods that should be avoided in large quantities (e.g., bacon, smoked meats, crab meat, tuna, crackers, processed cheeses, ham).

Teach the individual to record weights in the same clothing, at the same time daily, and using the same scale. Generally, a weight gain or loss of more than 2 pounds is reported to the health care provider; however, specific parameters may vary and should be discussed during initiation of therapy.

Stress Management

- Identify stress-producing situations in the patient's life and seek means to significantly reduce these factors. In some cases, referral for training in stress management, relaxation techniques, meditation, or biofeedback may be necessary. If stress is produced in the work setting, it may be appropriate to involve the industrial nurse.
- Stress within the family is often significant and may require professional counseling for the family and patient.

Exercise and Activity. Develop a plan for moderate exercise to improve the patient's general condition. Consult the health care provider for any individual modifications deemed appropriate. Suggest including activities that the patient finds helpful in reducing stress. Nurses can help an individual increase physical activity throughout the day by encouraging them to:

- Play active games with their children
- Engage in a sport
- Find a friend with whom to walk or jog
- Take a class in yoga or tai chi
- Walk a dog
- Garden on the weekends
- Walk or bicycle to school or work
- Take the stairs, never the elevator
- Park the car at the farthest point in the parking lot at work, school, or when shopping

Blood Pressure Monitoring. Demonstrate the correct procedure for taking blood pressure. It is best to have the patient or family bring in the blood pressure equipment that will be used at home to perform the blood pressure measurement. Validate the patient's and family's understanding by having them perform this task on several occasions under supervision. Monitor blood pressure, pulse, and respirations at least every shift while hospitalized and upon discharge in accordance with the health care provider's orders, usually daily. The patient should be given some numerical guidelines, as established by the health care provider, for a desired goal of therapy and what to do if this is not being achieved. Normal home blood pressure should be at least lower than 137/85 mm Hg. Nighttime home blood pressure is usually lower than daytime pressure.

Medication Regimen

- Caution the patient that for the first 2 weeks of antihypertensive therapy drowsiness may occur. Patients should be told that this side effect is self-limiting. They should be cautious in operating power equipment and motor vehicles while this symptom exists.

- A common side effect of antihypertensive medications is hypotension. Instruct the patient to rise slowly from a sitting or supine position. Tell the patient to avoid standing for long periods, especially within 2 hours of taking antihypertensive medication. Weakness, dizziness, or faintness can usually be relieved by increasing muscular activity or by sitting or lying down.
- Teach the person to perform exercises that prevent blood pooling in the extremities when sitting or standing for long periods. These exercises include flexing the calf muscles, wiggling the toes, rising on the toes, and then returning to the feet in a flat position.
- Teach the person and significant other how to take and record blood pressure at prescribed intervals.
- The patient should always report a lack of response to the medication prescribed and/or a blood pressure that *continues to rise* after medications have been taken. (Ask the health care provider to state specific parameters.)

Fostering Health Maintenance

- Throughout the course of treatment, discuss medication information and how it will benefit the patient.
- Drug therapy is one component in the management of hypertension. Lifestyle changes are equally important to drug therapy; therefore the need to maintain an exercise program and modify dietary habits to control obesity and serum cholesterol is crucial. Cessation of smoking and minimal alcoholic intake are strongly recommended.
- Provide the patient and significant others with the important information contained in the specific drug monograph for the drugs prescribed. Additional health teaching and nursing interventions for drug side effects to expect and report will be found in each drug monograph.
- Seek cooperation and understanding of the following points so that medication compliance is increased: name of medication, dosage, routes and times of administration, side effects to expect, and side effects to report.
- The most effective therapy prescribed by the health care provider will control hypertension only if the patient is motivated. Motivation improves when the patient has a positive experience with and trust in the health care providers. Empathy builds trust and is an excellent motivator.

Written Record. Enlist the patient's aid in developing and maintaining a written record of monitoring parameters (e.g., blood pressures, weight, exercise) (see p. 455 and Appendix I). Complete the Premedication Data column for use as a baseline to track response to drug therapy. Ensure that the patient understands how to use the form and instruct the patient to bring the completed form to follow-up visits. During follow-up visits, focus on issues that will foster adherence with the therapeutic interventions prescribed.

DRUG CLASS: Diuretics

Actions

The diuretics act as antihypertensive agents by causing volume depletion, sodium excretion, and vasodilation of peripheral arterioles. The mechanism of peripheral arteriolar vasodilation is unknown.

Uses

There are four classes of diuretic agents: carbonic anhydrase inhibitors, thiazide and thiazide-like agents, loop diuretics, and potassium-sparing diuretics (see Chapter 29). The carbonic anhydrase inhibitors are weak antihypertensive agents and therefore are not used for this purpose. The potassium-sparing diuretics are rarely used alone but are commonly used in combination with the thiazide and loop diuretics for added antihypertensive effect and to counteract the potassium-excreting effects of these more potent diuretic-antihypertensive agents.

The diuretics are the most commonly prescribed antihypertensive agents because they are one of the classes of agents that have been shown to reduce cardiovascular morbidity and mortality associated with hypertension. The thiazides are most effective if the renal creatinine clearance is greater than 30 mL per minute; however, as renal function deteriorates, the more potent loop diuretics are needed to continue excretion of sodium and water.

Diuretics are also commonly prescribed in combination therapy. They potentiate the hypotensive activity of the nondiuretic antihypertensive agents, have a low incidence of adverse effects, and are often the least expensive of the antihypertensive agents.

Diuretics are used (often with other classes of antihypertensive therapy) to treat all stages of hypertension. The agents are discussed more extensively in Chapter 29.

Nursing Process for Diuretic Agents

Premedication Assessment

1. Obtain baseline blood pressure readings in supine and standing positions.
2. Obtain baseline weight, blood pressure, and apical pulse.
3. Initiate laboratory studies requested by the health care provider (e.g., electrolytes).
4. Obtain baseline assessments of patient's state of hydration.

Planning

Availability. See Chapter 29.

Implementation

Dosage and Administration. See Chapter 29.

Evaluation

See Chapter 29.

DRUG CLASS: Beta-Adrenergic Blocking Agents

Actions

The beta-adrenergic blocking agents (beta blockers) (see Table 13-3) inhibit cardiac response to sympathetic nerve stimulation by blocking the beta receptors. As a result, the heart rate, cardiac output, and consequently, the blood pressure, are reduced. The beta blockers also inhibit renin release from the kidneys, diminishing the cascade of the renin-angiotensin-aldosterone system that would induce vasoconstriction and sodium reabsorption aggravating hypertension.

Uses

The beta-adrenergic blocking agents are agents of another class that have been shown to reduce morbidity and mortality associated with hypertension; therefore they are widely used as antihypertensive agents. The clinical advantages of the beta-adrenergic blocking agents in treating hypertension include minimal postural or exercise hypotension, minimal effect on sexual function, blood pressure reduction in the supine position, and little or no slowing of the central nervous system (CNS).

The JNC 7 recommends beta blockers as initial therapy for stages 1 and 2 hypertension. However, beta blockers are not as effective in African American patients and should be avoided in patients with asthma, type 1 diabetes mellitus, heart failure caused by systolic dysfunction, and peripheral vascular disease.

Nursing Process for Beta-Adrenergic Blocking Agents

Premedication Assessment

1. Check history for respiratory conditions that could be aggravated by bronchoconstriction, type 1 diabetes mellitus, heart failure, or peripheral vascular disease. If any of these conditions are present, contact the health care provider to discuss the situation before initiation of beta-adrenergic blocking agent therapy.
2. Obtain baseline blood pressure readings and apical pulse.

Planning

Availability. See Table 13-3.

Implementation

Dosage and Administration. See Table 13-3.

Individualization of Dosage. Although the onset of activity is rapid, it may often take several days to weeks for a patient to show optimal improvement and become stabilized on an adequate maintenance dosage. Patients must be periodically reevaluated to determine the lowest effective dosage necessary to control the disorder being treated.

Sudden Discontinuation. Patients must be counseled against poor compliance or sudden discontinuation of therapy without a health care provider's advice. Sudden discontinuation of therapy has resulted in an exacerbation of anginal symptoms followed in some cases by myocardial infarction. When discontinuing long-term treatment with beta blockers, the dosage should be gradually reduced over a period of 1 to 2 weeks with careful monitoring of the patient. If anginal symptoms develop or become more frequent, beta blocker therapy should be restarted at least temporarily.

Evaluation

Most of the adverse effects associated with beta-adrenergic blocking agents are dose related. Response by individual patients is highly variable. Many of these side effects may occur but may be transient. Strongly encourage patients to see their health care provider before discontinuing therapy. Minor dosage adjustment may be all that is required for most side effects.

Side Effects to Expect and Report

Bradycardia, Peripheral Vasoconstriction (Purple Mottled Skin). Withhold additional doses until the patient is evaluated by a health care provider.

Bronchospasm, Wheezing. Withhold additional doses until the patient has been evaluated by a health care provider.

Diabetic Patients. Monitor for hypoglycemia: headache, weakness, decreased coordination, general apprehension, diaphoresis, hunger, or blurred or double vision. Many of these symptoms may be masked by the beta-adrenergic blocking agents. Notify the health care provider if any of the above mentioned symptoms are appearing intermittently.

Heart Failure. Monitor patients for an increase in edema, dyspnea, crackles, bradycardia, and orthopnea. Notify the health care provider if these symptoms develop.

Drug Interactions

Antihypertensive Agents. All the beta blockers have hypotensive properties that are additive with antihypertensive agents (e.g., guanethidine, methyldopa, hydralazine, clonidine, prazosin, minoxidil, captopril, diltiazem, verapamil, reserpine).

If it is decided to discontinue therapy in patients receiving beta blockers and clonidine concurrently, the beta blocker should be withdrawn gradually and discontinued several days before the gradual withdrawal of the clonidine. Severe rebound hypertension may occur if the beta blocker is not gradually discontinued first.

Beta-Adrenergic Agents. Depending on the doses used, the beta stimulants (e.g., isoproterenol, metaproterenol, terbutaline, albuterol [see Table 13-2]) may inhibit the action of the beta blockers, and vice versa.

Lidocaine, Procainamide, Phenytoin, Disopyramide, Digoxin. Although these drugs are occasionally used concurrently, monitor patients carefully for additional dysrhythmias, bradycardia, and signs of heart failure.

Enzyme-Inducing Agents. Enzyme-inducing agents such as cimetidine, phenobarbital, pentobarbital, and phenytoin enhance the metabolism of propranolol, metoprolol, pindolol, and timolol. This reaction probably does not occur with nadolol or atenolol because they are not metabolized but excreted unchanged. The dosage of the beta blocker may have to be increased to provide therapeutic activity. If the enzyme-inducing agent is discontinued, the dosage of the beta blocking agent will also require reduction.

Nonsteroidal Antiinflammatory Drugs (NSAIDs). Indomethacin, and possibly other prostaglandin inhibitors, inhibit the antihypertensive activity of the beta blockers, resulting in loss of hypertensive control.

The dosage of the beta blocker may have to be increased to compensate for the antihypertensive inhibitory effect of NSAIDs.

DRUG CLASS: Angiotensin-Converting Enzyme Inhibitors

Actions

Angiotensin-converting enzyme (ACE) inhibitors represent a major breakthrough in the treatment of hypertension. The renin-angiotensin-aldosterone system plays a major role in the regulation of blood pressure. When there is a reduction in blood pressure, sodium concentration, or renal blood flow, renin is secreted by the kidneys. The renin converts angiotensinogen, which is secreted by the liver, to angiotensin I. Angiotensin I is then converted by angiotensin I–converting enzyme to angiotensin II. Angiotensin II produces potent vasoconstriction by acting on receptors within blood vessels. It also promotes aldosterone secretion, which causes sodium retention by stimulation of mineralocorticoid receptors in the adrenal cortex. These actions result in increased blood pressure secondary to the vasoconstriction and enhanced cardiac output secondary to sodium retention. The ACE inhibitors inhibit angiotensin I–converting enzyme, the enzyme responsible for the conversion of angiotensin I to angiotensin II, thus reducing serum levels of this potent vasoconstrictor and aldosterone stimulant.

Uses

The ACE inhibitors reduce blood pressure, preserve cardiac output, and increase renal blood flow. They are effective as single therapy for stage 1 or 2 hypertension, severe accelerated hypertension, and renal hypertension. The JNC 7 considers them an alternative to diuretic or beta blocker therapy. Although they may be used alone, they tend to be more effective when combined with diuretic therapy. They are not as effective in lowering blood pressure in African Americans unless used with a diuretic. Advantages of ACE inhibitors are the infrequency of orthostatic hypotension; lack of CNS depression and sexual dysfunction side effects; lack of aggravation of asthma, obstructive pulmonary disease, gout, cholesterol levels, or diabetes; and an additive effect with diuretics. The ACE inhibitors are also effective in the treatment of heart failure and post-myocardial infarction, and routinely used to slow the progression of diabetic nephropathy.

Therapeutic Outcomes

The primary therapeutic outcome expected from the ACE inhibitors is reduction in blood pressure.

Nursing Process for Angiotensin-Converting Enzyme Inhibitors

Premedication Assessment

1. Obtain baseline blood pressure readings in supine and standing positions and apical pulse.
2. Obtain a history of bowel elimination patterns.
3. Initiate laboratory studies as requested by the health care provider (e.g., renal function tests such as blood urea nitrogen [BUN] and serum creatinine, electrolytes, and complete blood count [CBC] to serve as a baseline for future comparison).
4. Ask whether the patient is pregnant or likely to become pregnant. If so, discuss with the health care provider before initiating ACE inhibitor therapy.
5. Ask if the patient has a persistent cough.

Planning

Availability. See Table 23-5.

Implementation

Dosage and Administration. See Table 23-5. Captopril should be administered without food and requires twice-daily dosing. All of the other agents are administered once daily.

NOTE: The initial doses of ACE inhibitors may cause hypotension with dizziness, tachycardia, and fainting; these adverse effects occur more commonly in patients also receiving diuretics. Symptoms occur within 3 hours after the first several doses. This effect may be minimized by discontinuing the diuretic 1 week before initiating ACE inhibitor therapy. Patients should be warned that this side effect may occur, that it is transient, and that they should lie down immediately if symptoms develop.

Evaluation

Side Effects to Expect

Nausea, Fatigue, Headache, Diarrhea. These side effects are usually mild and tend to resolve with continued therapy. Encourage the patient not to discontinue therapy without first consulting a health care provider.

Orthostatic Hypotension (Dizziness, Weakness, Faintness). Although these side effects are infrequent and usually mild, certain patients, particularly those also receiving diuretics, may suffer some degree of orthostatic hypotension, particularly when therapy is initiated. Observe the patient closely for at least 2 hours after the initial dose and for at least an additional hour until blood pressure has stabilized.

Drug Table 23-5 ANGIOTENSIN-CONVERTING ENZYME (ACE) INHIBITORS

GENERIC NAME	BRAND NAME	AVAILABILITY	APPROVED USES	DOSAGE RANGE
benazepril	Lotensin	Tablets: 5, 10, 20, 40 mg	Hypertension	PO: Initial—10 mg once daily Maintenance—20-40 mg daily
captopril	Capoten	Tablets: 12.5, 25, 50, 100 mg	Hypertension; heart failure; diabetic nephropathy	PO: Initial—25 mg two or three times daily 1 hr before meals Maintenance—75-450 mg daily 1 hr before meals
enalapril	Vasotec	Tablets: 2.5, 5, 10, 20 mg	Hypertension; heart failure	PO: Initial—2.5-5 mg once daily Maintenance—10-40 mg daily
enlaprilat	Vasotec IV	Inj: 1.25 mg/mL	Hypertension	IV: 1.25 mg over 5 min every 6 hr
fosinopril	Monopril	Tablets: 10, 20, 40 mg	Hypertension; heart failure	PO: Initial—10 mg once daily Maintenance—20-80 mg daily
lisinopril	Prinivil, Zestril	Tablets: 2.5, 5, 10, 20, 40 mg	Hypertension; heart failure; post-myocardial infarction	PO: Initial—5-10 mg once daily Maintenance—20-40 mg daily
moexipril	Univasc	Tablets: 7.5, 15 mg	Hypertension	PO: Initial—with diuretic, 3.75 mg; without diuretic, 7.5 mg Maintenance—7.5-30 mg in one or two divided doses 1 hr before meals
perindopril	Aceon	Tablets: 2, 4, 8 mg	Hypertension	PO: Initial—4 mg daily Maintenance—4-16 mg daily
quinapril	Accupril	Tablets: 5, 10, 20, 40 mg	Hypertension, heart failure	PO: Initial—1 mg daily Maintenance—20-80 mg daily
ramipril	Altace	Capsules: 1.25, 2.5, 5, 10 mg	Hypertension; heart failure	PO: Initial—1.25-2.5 mg daily Maintenance—2.5-20 mg daily
trandolapril	Mavik	Tablets, 1, 2, 4, mg	Hypertension; heart failure	PO: Initial—1 mg daily Maintenance—4-8 mg daily

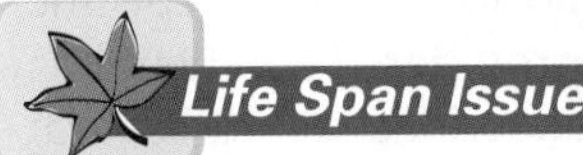

Life Span Issues

Antihypertensive Therapy

Older adults are more likely to develop orthostatic hypotension with antihypertensive therapy. The nurse should monitor the patient's blood pressure in the supine and sitting positions during the initiation of antihypertensive therapy or when the drug dosage is adjusted. Safety precautions should be initiated to prevent accidental injury. Teach the patient to rise slowly from a supine to a sitting and then standing position.

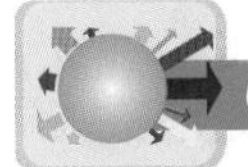

Clinical Landmine

Hypotension with ACE Inhibitors

The initial doses of ACE inhibitors may cause hypotension with dizziness, tachycardia, and fainting; these adverse effects occur more commonly in patients also receiving diuretics. Symptoms occur within 3 hours after the first several doses. This effect may be minimized by discontinuing the diuretic 1 week before initiating ACE inhibitor therapy. Patients should be warned that this side effect may occur, that it is transient, and that they should lie down immediately if symptoms develop.

Monitor the blood pressure in both the supine and standing positions. Anticipate the development of postural hypotension and take measures to prevent an occurrence. Teach the patient to rise slowly from a supine or sitting position and to sit or lie down if feeling faint.

Side Effects to Report

Swelling of the Face, Eyes, Lips, Tongue; Difficulty Breathing. Angioedema has been reported to occur in a small number of patients, especially after the first dose. Patients should be cautioned to discontinue further therapy and seek medical attention immediately.

Neutropenia. Neutropenia (300 neutrophils/mm^3) and agranulocytosis (drug-induced bone marrow suppression) have rarely been observed in patients receiving ACE inhibitors. The neutropenia appears within the first 3 to 12 weeks of therapy and develops slowly; the white count falls to its nadir in 10 to 30 days. The white count returns to normal about 2 weeks after discontinuation of ACE inhibitor therapy.

The patients most susceptible are those receiving captopril who also have impaired renal function or serious autoimmune diseases, such as lupus erythematosus, or who are exposed to drugs known to affect the white cells or immune response, such as corticosteroids.

Patients at risk should have differential and total white cell counts before initiation of therapy and then every 2 weeks thereafter for the first 3 months of therapy. Stress the importance of returning for this laboratory work. Patients should be told to notify their health care provider promptly if any evidence of infection such as sore throat or fever, which may be an indicator of neutropenia, should develop.

Nephrotoxicity. A small number of hypertensive patients who are receiving ACE inhibitors, particularly those with preexisting renal impairment and those also taking NSAIDs, have developed increases in BUN and serum creatinine. These elevations have usually been minor and transient, especially when the ACE inhibitor was administered concomitantly with a diuretic. Renal function should be monitored during the first few weeks of therapy. Report an increasing BUN and creatinine level. Dosage reduction of the ACE inhibitor or possible discontinuation of the NSAID or diuretic may be required.

Hyperkalemia. Because ACE inhibitors inhibit aldosterone, patients may develop slight increases in serum potassium. Approximately 1% of patients may develop hyperkalemia (greater than 5.7 mEq/L). Most cases resolve without discontinuation of therapy. Patients most susceptible to the development of hyperkalemia are those with renal impairment or diabetes mellitus and those already receiving a potassium supplement or a potassium-sparing diuretic. Many symptoms associated with altered fluid and electrolyte balance are subtle and interspersed with general symptoms of drug toxicity or the disease process itself.

Gather data relative to *changes* in the patient's mental status (e.g., alertness, orientation, and confusion), muscle strength, muscle cramps, tremors, nausea, and general appearance (e.g., drowsy, anxious, or lethargic).

Always check the electrolyte reports for early indications of electrolyte imbalance. Keep accurate records of intake and output, daily weights, and vital signs.

Chronic Cough. As many as one third of patients receiving ACE inhibitors may develop a chronic, dry, nonproductive, persistent cough. This is thought to be due to an accumulation of bradykinin. It may appear from 1 week to 6 months after initiation of ACE inhibitor therapy. Women appear to be more susceptible than men. Patients should be told to contact their health care provider if the cough becomes troublesome. The cough resolves within 1 to 30 days after discontinuation of therapy. An angiotensin II receptor–blocking (ARB) agent may be substituted for the ACE inhibitor if the frequency of cough is excessive.

Pregnancy. Medicines that act directly on the renin-angiotensin system can cause fetal and neonatal harm. There is concern about the potential for birth defects in neonates whose mothers received ACE inhibitors, especially during the second and third trimesters of pregnancy. Women who wish to become pregnant or become pregnant while receiving ACE inhibitors should discuss alternative therapies with their health care provider as soon as possible.

Drug Interactions

Drugs That Enhance Therapeutic and Toxic Effects. Diuretics, phenothiazines, alcohol, beta adrenergic–blocking agents (e.g., propranolol, atenolol, pindolol), and other antihypertensive agents. Probenecid blocks the excretion of captopril, causing an increased antihypertensive effect. Monitor the blood pressure response to the cumulative effects of antihypertensive agents. Take the blood pressure in supine and standing positions.

Drugs That Reduce Therapeutic Effects. Antacids may diminish absorption of ACE inhibitors. Separate the administration times by 2 hours. NSAIDs may reduce the antihypertensive effects of the ACE inhibitors. Rifampin may decrease the antihypertensive effects of enalapril. Monitor carefully for poor blood pressure control or a gradually increasing blood pressure.

Digoxin. ACE inhibitors may increase the serum levels of digoxin. Monitor the patient for symptoms of anorexia, nausea, vomiting, headaches, blurred or colored vision, and bradycardia. A digoxin serum level may be ordered by the health care provider.

Lithium. ACE inhibitors may induce lithium toxicity. Monitor for lithium toxicity manifested by nausea, anorexia, fine tremors, persistent vomiting, profuse diarrhea, hyperreflexia, lethargy, and weakness.

Hyperkalemia. ACE inhibitors may cause small increases in potassium levels by inhibiting aldosterone secretion. Patients should not take dietary supplements of potassium or potassium-sparing diuretics (e.g., triamterene, spironolactone, amiloride) without specific approval from the health care provider. If a patient has received spironolactone or eplerenone up to several months before ACE inhibitor therapy, the serum potassium level should be monitored closely, because the potassium-sparing effect of spironolactone or eplerenone may persist.

Capsaicin. Capsaicin may cause or aggravate coughing associated with ACE inhibitor therapy. Monitor for increased frequency of dry, persistent cough. Report to the health care provider.

DRUG CLASS: Angiotensin II Receptor Blockers

Actions

The angiotensin II receptor blockers (also known as ARBs) are a class of antihypertensive agents that act by binding to angiotensin II receptor sites, blocking the very potent vasoconstrictor from binding to the receptor (also called AT_1 receptor) sites in the vascular smooth muscle, brain, heart, kidneys, and adrenal glands. The blood pressure–elevating and sodium-retaining effects of angiotensin II are thus blocked. The angiotensin II receptor antagonists have no effect on renal function, prostaglandin levels, triglycerides, cholesterol, or blood glucose levels. These agents do not affect bradykinin and therefore do not cause a dry cough.

Uses

The angiotensin II receptor antagonists have been found to be as effective in lowering blood pressure as the ACE inhibitors and beta blockers. Men and women usually have similar responses; however, African American patients do not respond as well to monotherapy. The angiotensin II receptor antagonists are indicated for the treatment of hypertension and may be used alone or in combination with other antihypertensive agents. The blood pressure–lowering effect is seen within 1 week, but may take 3 to 6 weeks for full therapeutic effect. If the antihypertensive effect is not controlled by angiotensin II receptor antagonists alone, a low dose of a diuretic, usually hydrochlorothiazide, may be added.

Therapeutic Outcomes

The primary therapeutic outcome expected from angiotensin II receptor antagonists is reduction in blood pressure.

Nursing Process for Angiotensin II Receptor Antagonists

Premedication Assessment

1. Obtain baseline blood pressure readings in supine and standing positions and apical pulse.
2. Initiate laboratory studies requested by the health care provider (e.g., renal function tests such as BUN, serum creatinine, electrolytes, and CBC) to serve as a baseline for future comparison.
3. Ask whether the patient is pregnant or likely to become pregnant. If so, discuss with the health care provider before initiating angiotensin II receptor antagonist therapy.
4. Obtain a history of bowel elimination patterns and any gastrointestinal (GI) symptoms.

Planning

Availability. See Table 23-6.

Implementation

Dosage and Administration. See Table 23-6.

Evaluation

Side Effects to Expect

Headache, Dyspepsia, Cramps, Diarrhea. These side effects are usually mild and tend to resolve with continued therapy. Encourage the patient not to discontinue therapy without first consulting the health care provider.

Orthostatic Hypotension (Dizziness, Weakness, Faintness). Although these side effects are infrequent and usually mild, certain patients, particularly those also receiving diuretics, may suffer some degree of orthostatic hypotension, particularly when therapy is initiated. Observe the patient closely for at least 2 hours after the initial dose and for at least 1 additional hour until blood pressure has stabilized.

Drug Table 23-6 ANGIOTENSIN II RECEPTOR BLOCKERS (ARBs)

GENERIC NAME	BRAND NAME	AVAILABILITY	DOSAGE RANGE
candesartan	Atacand	Tablets: 4, 8, 16, 32 mg	PO: Initial—16 mg once daily; adjust over 4-6 weeks with total daily dosage from 8-32 mg. Dose may be administered once or twice daily for optimal control.
eprosartan	Teveten	Tablets: 600 mg	PO: Initial—600 mg once daily; adjust over 2-3 weeks with total daily dose of 400-800 mg daily. Dose may be administered once or twice daily for optimal control.
irbesartan	Avapro	Tablets: 75, 150, 300 mg	PO: Initial—150 mg once daily; adjust over 3-4 weeks with a total daily dose of 300 mg daily.
losartan	Cozaar	Tablets: 25, 50, 100 mg	PO: 50 mg once daily; adjust over 4-6 weeks with a total daily dose from 25-100 mg administered once or twice daily for optimal control.
olmesartan	Benicar	Tablets: 5, 20, 40 mg	PO: Initial—20 mg once daily; adjust over 2 weeks with total daily dose of 20-40 mg daily. Twice daily dosing offers no benefit.
telmisartan	Micardis	Tablets: 20, 40, 80 mg	PO: Initial—40 mg once daily; adjust over 4-6 weeks with total daily dose from 20-80 mg.
valsartan	Diovan	Capsules: 40, 80, 160, 320 mg	PO: Initial—80 mg once daily; adjust over 4-6 weeks with total daily dose from 80-320 mg.

Monitor the blood pressure in both the supine and standing positions. Anticipate the development of postural hypotension and take measures to prevent an occurrence. Teach the patient to rise slowly from a supine or sitting position and to sit or lie down if feeling faint.

Side Effects to Report

Pregnancy. Medicines that act directly on the renin-angiotensin system can cause fetal and neonatal harm. There is potential for birth defects in neonates whose mothers received ACE inhibitors, especially during the second and third trimesters of pregnancy. Women who wish to become pregnant or who become pregnant while receiving angiotensin II receptor antagonists should discuss alternative therapies with their health care provider as soon as possible.

Hyperkalemia. Because angiotensin II receptor antagonists inhibit aldosterone secretion, patients may develop slight increases in serum potassium. Most cases resolve without discontinuation of therapy. Patients most susceptible to the development of hyperkalemia are those with renal impairment or diabetes mellitus and those already receiving a potassium supplement, eplerenone, or potassium-sparing diuretic. Many symptoms associated with altered fluid and electrolyte balance are subtle and interspersed with general symptoms of drug toxicity or the disease process itself.

Gather data relative to *changes* in the patient's mental status (e.g., alertness, orientation, confusion), muscle strength, muscle cramps, tremors, nausea, and general appearance (e.g., being drowsy, anxious, lethargic).

Always check the electrolyte reports for early indications of electrolyte imbalance. Keep accurate records of intake and output, daily weights, and vital signs.

Drug Interactions

Drugs That Enhance Therapeutic and Toxic Effects. Diuretics, phenothiazines, alcohol, beta-adrenergic blocking agents (e.g., propranolol, atenolol, pindolol), and other antihypertensive agents. Cimetidine and fluconazole inhibit the metabolism of losartan, causing an increased antihypertensive effect. Monitor the blood pressure response to the cumulative effects of antihypertensive agents. Take the blood pressure readings in supine and standing positions.

Drugs That Reduce Therapeutic Effects. Rifampin increases the metabolism of losartan, reducing its antihypertensive effects. The dosage of losartan may need to be increased, or the patient may be switched to another angiotensin II receptor antagonist.

Hyperkalemia. Angiotensin II receptor antagonists may cause small increases in potassium levels by reducing aldosterone secretion. Patients should not take dietary supplements of potassium or potassium-sparing diuretics (e.g., triamterene, spironolactone, amiloride) without specific approval from the health care provider. If a patient has received spironolactone or eplerenone up to several months before angiotensin II receptor antagonist therapy, the serum potassium level should be monitored closely because the potassium-sparing effect of spironolactone and eplerenone may persist.

DRUG CLASS: Aldosterone Receptor Antagonist

eplerenone (ep lehr′ en own)
INSPRA (in′ sprah)

Actions

Eplerenone represents the first of a new class of antihypertensive agents known as aldosterone receptor blocking agents. The renin-angiotensin-aldosterone system plays a major role in the regulation of blood pressure. When there is a reduction in blood pressure, sodium concentration or renal blood flow, renin is secreted by the kidneys. The renin converts angiotensinogen, which is secreted by the liver, to angiotensin I. Angiotensin I is converted by angiotensin I–converting enzyme to angiotensin II. Angiotensin II produces potent vasoconstriction by acting on receptors within blood vessels. It also promotes aldosterone secretion, which causes sodium retention by stimulation of mineralocorticoid receptors in the adrenal cortex, blood vessels, and brain. These actions result in increased blood pressure secondary to the vasoconstriction and enhanced cardiac output secondary to sodium retention. Eplerenone, the aldosterone receptor–blocking agent, blocks stimulation of the mineralocorticoid receptors by aldosterone, thus preventing sodium reabsorption.

Uses

Eplerenone is used in treating hypertension either alone or in combination with other antihypertensive agents.

Therapeutic Outcomes

The primary therapeutic outcome expected from eplerenone is reduction in blood pressure.

Nursing Process for Eplerenone

Premedication Assessment

1. Obtain baseline blood pressure readings in supine and standing positions.
2. Obtain a history of bowel elimination patterns.
3. Initiate laboratory studies as requested by the health care provider (e.g., renal function tests such as BUN and serum creatinine, electrolytes, triglycerides, cholesterol, liver function tests, (e.g., bilirubin, aspartate aminotransferase [AST], alanine aminotransferase [ALT], gamma-glutamyltransferase [GGT], alkaline phosphatase, prothrombin time) and uric acid) to serve as a baseline for future comparison.
4. Ask whether the patient is pregnant or likely to become pregnant. If so, discuss with the health care provider before initiating eplerenone therapy.

Planning

Availability. PO: 25- and 50-mg tablets.

Implementation

Dosage and Administration. PO: Initial: 50 mg once daily with or without food. The full therapeutic effect should be apparent within 4 weeks. For patients with an inadequate blood pressure response, the dosage may be increased to 50 mg two times daily.

NOTE: For patients older than the age of 65, or patients with mild to moderate hepatic failure, dosages greater than 50 mg daily are not recommended. For patients taking metabolism inhibitors such as cimetidine, erythromycin, saquinavir, verapamil, diltiazem, or fluconazole, the starting dose should be reduced to 25 mg once daily.

NOTE: Eplerenone therapy is contraindicated in patients with:

- Serum potassium greater than 5.5 mEq/L
- Type 2 diabetes with microalbuminuria
- Serum creatinine greater than 2.0 mg/dL in males or 1.8 mg/dL in females
- Creatinine clearance less than 50 mL/min
- Patients taking potassium-sparing diuretics (amiloride, spironolactone, or triamterene)
- Patients taking strong metabolic inhibitors (e.g., ketoconazole, itraconazole)

Evaluation

Side Effects to Expect

Nausea, Fatigue, Headache, Diarrhea. These side effects are usually mild and tend to resolve with continued therapy. Encourage the patient not to discontinue therapy without first consulting a health care provider.

Orthostatic Hypotension (Dizziness, Weakness, Faintness). Although these side effects are infrequent and usually mild, certain patients, particularly those also receiving diuretics, may suffer some degree of orthostatic hypotension, particularly when therapy is initiated.

Monitor the blood pressure in both the supine and standing positions. Anticipate the development of postural hypotension and take measures to prevent an occurrence. Teach the patient to rise slowly from a supine or sitting position and to sit or lie down if feeling faint.

Side Effects to Report

Hyperkalemia. Because eplerenone inhibits aldosterone, patients may develop slight increases in serum potassium. Patients most susceptible to the development of hyperkalemia (greater than 5.5 mEq/L) are those with renal impairment or diabetes mellitus. Many symptoms associated with altered fluid and electrolyte balance are subtle and interspersed with general symptoms of drug toxicity or the disease process itself.

Gather data relative to *changes* in the patient's mental status (e.g., alertness, orientation, confusion), muscle strength, muscle cramps, heart rate and rhythm, tremors, nausea, and general appearance (e.g., drowsy, anxious, lethargic).

Always check the electrolyte reports for early indications of electrolyte imbalance. Keep accurate records of intake and output, daily weights, and vital signs.

Nephrotoxicity. A small number of hypertensive patients who are receiving eplerenone, particularly those with preexisting renal impairment, have developed increases in BUN and serum creatinine. Renal function should be monitored during the first few weeks of therapy. Report an increasing BUN and creatinine level. Dosage reduction or discontinuation of eplerenone may be required. Eplerenone therapy is not recommended in patients with creatinine clearances less than 50 mL/min.

Hypertriglyceridemia, Hypercholesterolemia, Hyperuricemia. Increases in serum triglyceride, cholesterol, and uric acid levels have been reported during eplerenone therapy. Report rising levels to the health care provider.

Hepatotoxicity. The symptoms of hepatotoxicity are anorexia, nausea, vomiting, jaundice, hepatomegaly, splenomegaly, and abnormal liver function tests (e.g., elevated bilirubin, AST, ALT, GGT, alkaline phosphatase, prothrombin time).

Gynecomastia, Vaginal Bleeding. A small number of men have developed gynecomastia and a small number of women have developed vaginal bleeding while receiving eplerenone therapy. Report these conditions to a health care provider.

Drug Interactions

Drugs That Enhance Therapeutic and Toxic Effects. Diuretics, phenothiazines, alcohol, beta adrenergic–blocking agents (e.g., propranolol, atenolol, pindolol), and other antihypertensive agents. Monitor the blood pressure response to the cumulative effects of antihypertensive agents. Take the blood pressures in supine and standing positions. Assess the patient for hypotension, lightheadedness, dizziness, and bradycardia. Provide for patient safety; prevent falls.

Drugs That May Induce Hyperkalemia. Concurrent use of eplerenone and the following agents may induce hyperkalemia: ACE inhibitors (e.g., lisinopril, captopril, enalapril, ramipril), angiotensin II receptor blockers (e.g., losartan, candesartan, valsartan), potassium-sparing diuretics (e.g., triamterene, amiloride, spironolactone), salt substitutes (often contain higher concentrations of potassium for flavoring), foods marketed as "low sodium" often have higher concentrations of potassium for flavoring.

Lithium. Eplerenone may induce lithium toxicity. Monitor for lithium toxicity manifested by nausea, anorexia, fine tremors, persistent vomiting, profuse diarrhea, hyperreflexia, lethargy, and weakness.

Grapefruit Juice, St. John's Wort. Grapefruit juice and St. John's wort slow the metabolism of eplerenone in a minor way. If the patient develops orthostatic hypotension, a dosage reduction in eplerenone may be required.

DRUG CLASS: Calcium Ion Antagonists

Actions

Calcium ion antagonists are known variously as calcium antagonists, calcium channel blockers, slow channel blockers, and calcium ion influx inhibitors. These agents inhibit the movement of calcium ions across a cell membrane. This results in fewer dysrhythmias, a slower rate of contraction of the heart, and relaxation of smooth muscle of blood vessels, resulting in vasodilation and reduced blood pressure. The calcium ion antagonists are classified by structure: benzothiazepines—diltiazem; diaminopropanol ether—bepridil; diphenylalkylamine—verapamil; and dihydropyridines—amlodipine, felodipine, isradipine, nicardipine, nifedipine, nimodipine, and nisoldipine.

Uses

Although each of these agents act by calcium ion inhibition, there are significant differences in clinical use because they act somewhat differently on coronary blood vessels, systemic blood vessels, the pacemaker cells of the heart, and the conducting tissue of the heart. Their clinical effects are also dependent on the type and severity of the patient's disease. All of the available calcium channel blockers are effective antihypertensive agents, but clinicians tend to use the dihydropyridine group more often because they have better peripheral vasodilating effects, reducing afterload. Calcium channel blockers are more effective in patients with higher pretreatment blood pressures. They increase renal sodium excretion and are usually well tolerated. Calcium channel blockers are ideal as first- or second-line medicines in patients with hypertension and coexisting angina and are an alternative to the use of beta blockers in patients with asthma or diabetes mellitus. They are particularly effective in African Americans and elderly hypertensive patients, who are more likely to have low-renin hypertension. The calcium channel blockers also do not affect gout or peripheral vascular disease.

Therapeutic Outcomes

The primary therapeutic outcome expected from calcium ion antagonist therapy is reduction in blood pressure.

Nursing Process for Calcium Ion Antagonist Therapy

Premedication Assessment

1. Obtain baseline blood pressure readings in the supine and standing positions and apical pulse.
2. Obtain baseline weight.
3. If the patient is taking digoxin concurrently, initiate close monitoring for potential digitalis toxicity.

Planning

Availability. See Table 23-7.

Implementation

Dosage and Administration. See Table 23-7.

Dosage Adjustments. See individual drugs for dosage parameters. Adjustments are made based on the individual patient's response to therapy.

Evaluation

Side Effects to Report

Hypotension and Syncope. Caution the patient that hypotension and syncope may occur during the first week. These side effects decline once the dosage is stabilized.

Take blood pressure readings every shift in the hospitalized patient and stress the need for the patient to monitor blood pressure after discharge.

Prevent hypotensive episodes by instructing the patient to rise slowly from a supine or sitting position and perform exercises to prevent blood pooling when standing or sitting in one position for prolonged periods. If faintness occurs, instruct the patient to sit or lie down.

Edema. Assess the patient for development of edema. Perform daily weights at the same time, in similar clothing, and on the same scale. Report increases in weight to the health care provider for further evaluation.

Drug Interactions

Drugs That Enhance Therapeutic and Toxic Effects. Diuretics, phenothiazines, alcohol, beta adrenergic–blocking agents (e.g., propranolol, atenolol, pindolol), histamine H_2 antagonists (e.g., cimetidine, ranitidine), and other antihypertensive agents. Monitor the blood pressure response to the cumulative effects of antihypertensive agents. Take the blood pressures in supine and standing positions. Assess the patient for hypotension, lightheadedness, dizziness, and bradycardia. Provide for patient safety; prevent falls.

Digoxin. Calcium ion antagonists may increase serum levels of digoxin. Monitor the patient for symptoms of anorexia, nausea, vomiting, headaches, blurred or colored vision, and bradycardia. The health care provider may order a digitalis serum level.

Glucose Metabolism. The dosage of oral hypoglycemic agents may require adjustment in patients with type 2 diabetes mellitus. Assess for signs of hyperglycemia. Perform blood glucose testing on a regular basis.

Verapamil, Disopyramide. DO NOT administer disopyramide 48 hours before or 24 hours after the administration of verapamil.

DRUG CLASS: Alpha-1 Adrenergic Blocking Agents

Actions

The alpha-1 blockers—doxazosin, prazosin, and terazosin—act by blocking postsynaptic alpha-1 adrenergic receptors to produce arteriolar and venous vasodilation, reducing peripheral vascular resistance without reducing cardiac output or inducing a reflex tachycardia.

Drug Table 23-7 **CALCIUM ION ANTAGONISTS USED TO TREAT HYPERTENSION**

GENERIC NAME	BRAND NAME	AVAILABILITY	DOSAGE RANGE
amlodipine	Norvasc	Tablets: 2.5, 5, 10 mg	PO: Initial—5 mg once daily; adjust over 7-14 days to a maximum of 10 mg/day
diltiazem	Cardizem	Tablets: 30, 60, 90, 120 mg Tablets, extended release: 120, 180, 240, 300, 360, 420 mg Capsules, sustained release: 60, 90, 120, 180, 240, 300, 360, 420 mg IV: 5 mg/mL in 5- and 10-mL vials Powder for injection: 25 mg	PO: Initial—60-120 mg sustained release capsule twice daily; adjust as needed after 14 days Maintenance—240-360 mg daily Maximum—480 mg once daily
felodipine	Plendil	Tablets: 5, 10 mg Tablets, extended release: 2.5 mg	PO: Initial—5 mg daily; adjust after 14 days Maintenance—5-10 mg daily Maximum—10 mg daily
isradipine	DynaCirc	Capsules: 2.5, 5 mg Tablets, extended release: 5, 10 mg	PO: Initial—2.5 mg twice daily. Maximal response may require 2-4 weeks. Maintenance—10 mg daily Maximum—20 mg daily
nicardipine	Cardene	Capsules: 20, 30 mg Capsules, extended release: 30, 45, 60 mg IV: 2.5 mg/mL in 10-mL vials	PO: Initial—20 mg three times daily Maximal response may require 2 weeks of therapy Adjust dose by measuring blood pressure about 8 hours after last dose. Peak effect is determined by measuring blood pressure 1-2 hours after dosage administration. Maintenance—20-40 mg three times daily
nifedipine	Procardia	Capsules: 10, 20 mg Tablets, sustained release: 30, 60, 90 mg	PO: Initial—10 mg three times daily Adjust over 7-14 days to balance antianginal and hypotensive activity Maintenance—10-20 mg three to four times daily Sustained release tablets are administered once daily Maximum—capsules—180 mg daily; sustained release tablets—120 mg daily
nisoldipine	Sular	Tablets: Sustained release: 10, 20, 30, 40 mg	PO: Initial—20 mg once daily; adjust over 7-14 days by 10 mg/week Maintenance: 20-60 mg once daily
verapamil	Calan, Isoptin	Tablets: 40, 80, 120 mg Tablets, sustained release: 120, 180, 240, 360 mg Capsules, sustained release: 100, 120, 180, 200, 240, 300, 360 mg IV: 2.5 mg/mL in 2- and 4-mL ampules and syringes	PO: Initial—80 mg three or four times daily Sustained release tablets and capsules: 120-240 mg once daily in the morning Maintenance—240-480 mg daily Administer with food

They produce a decrease in standing blood pressure slightly greater than in supine blood pressure. These agents also have a modest positive effect on serum lipids, increasing HDL cholesterol and reducing LDL cholesterol, total cholesterol, and triglyceride concentrations.

The alpha-1 blockers do not increase catecholamines; therefore there is no increase in heart rate or myocardial oxygen consumption. They also have no effect on uric acid concentrations.

Because of the presence of alpha-1 receptors on the prostate gland and certain areas of the bladder, terazosin and doxazosin are also able to reduce urinary outflow resistance in men with enlarged prostate glands.

Uses

These agents may be used alone or in combination with other antihypertensive agents in the treatment of stage 1 or 2 hypertension. They have additive effects with beta blockers and diuretics. The JNC 7 lists these agents as alternative drugs if beta blockers, diuretic therapy, or other alternative therapy is not successful or not tolerated. Blood pressure response with alpha-1 blockers appears to be similar in African American and white patients. They can be used safely in patients with angina, gout, and hyperlipidemia. The three alpha-1 blockers have similar antihypertensive effects and adverse effects. Doxazosin and terazosin have a longer duration of action and can be administered once daily. Prazosin is often used with diuretic therapy because of its tendency to cause sodium and water retention.

Doxazosin and terazosin are also used to reduce mild to moderate urinary obstruction manifestations (e.g., hesitancy, terminal dribbling of urine, interrupted stream, impaired size and force of stream, sensation of incomplete bladder emptying) in men with benign prostatic hyperplasia.

Therapeutic Outcomes

The primary therapeutic outcomes expected from alpha-1 adrenergic receptor blocker therapy are reduction of blood pressure and reduced symptoms and improvement in urine flow associated with prostatic enlargement.

Nursing Process for Alpha-1 Adrenergic Blocking Agents

Premedication Assessment

1. Obtain baseline blood pressure readings in supine and standing positions and apical pulse.
2. Check if patient is pregnant or has a history of severe cerebral or coronary arteriosclerosis, gastritis, or peptic ulcer disease. (Reduction of blood pressure may diminish blood flow to these regions, which causes therapy to worsen the condition.)

Planning

Availability. See Table 23-8.

Implementation

Dosage and Administration. See Table 23-8.

NOTE: The initial doses of doxazosin, prazosin, and terazosin may cause hypotension with dizziness, tachycardia, and fainting; these adverse effects occur in less than 1% of patients starting therapy. Symptoms occur 15 to 90 minutes after initial doses and occur most often in patients who are already receiving propranolol (and presumably other beta-adrenergic blocking agents). This effect may be minimized by giving the first doses with food and limiting the initial dose to 1 mg. Patients should be warned that this side effect may occur, that it is transient, and that they should lie down immediately if symptoms develop.

Evaluation

Side Effects to Expect

Drowsiness, Headache, Dizziness, Weakness, Lethargy. Tell the patient that these side effects may occur but that they tend to be self-limiting. Tell the patient not

Drug Table 23-8 ALPHA-1 ADRENERGIC BLOCKING AGENTS

GENERIC NAME	BRAND NAME	AVAILABILITY	DOSAGE RANGE
doxazosin	Cardura	Tablets: 1, 2, 4, 8 mg	Hypertension: PO: Initial—1 mg daily AM or PM. Hypotensive effects are most likely within 2-6 hours. Monitor standing blood pressure Maintenance—Increase to 2 mg, then, if needed, 4, 8, and 16 mg to achieve desired reduction in blood pressure Benign prostatic hyperplasia: PO: Initial—as for hypertension. Increase dosage at weekly intervals to 2 mg, then 4 and 8 mg once daily Maintenance—8 mg daily; monitor blood pressure
prazosin	Minipress	Capsules: 1, 2, 5 mg	Hypertension: PO: Initial—1 mg two or three times daily with first dose at bedtime to reduce syncopal episodes. Maintenance—6-15 mg/day in two or three divided doses Maximum dose—20-40 mg/day
terazosin	Hytrin	Capsules: 1, 2, 5, 10 mg Tablets: 1, 2, 5, 10 mg	Hypertension: PO: Initial—1 mg at bedtime. Measure blood pressure 2-3 hours after dosing and evaluate for symptoms of dizziness or tachycardia; if response is substantially diminished at 24 hours, increase dosage. Maintenance—1-5 mg daily Maximum dose—20 mg/day Benign prostatic hyperplasia: PO: Initial—as for hypertension; gradually increase dosage in stepwise fashion to 2, 5, or 10 mg daily for acceptable urinary output Maintenance—10 mg daily for 4-6 weeks to assess urinary response Maximum dose—20 mg/day

to stop taking the medication and to consult a health care provider if the problem becomes unacceptable.

Dizziness, Tachycardia, Fainting. These side effects occur in about 1% of patients when therapy is initiated. They develop 15 to 90 minutes after the first dose is taken. To decrease the incidence, administer the first dose with food and limit the initial dose to 1 mg.

Instruct the patient to lie down immediately if these symptoms start to occur, and provide for the patient's safety.

Drug Interactions

Drugs That Enhance Therapeutic and Toxic Effects. Diuretics, tranquilizers, alcohol, barbiturates, antihistamines, beta-adrenergic blocking agents (e.g., propranolol, atenolol, pindolol), and other antihypertensive agents. Monitor the blood pressure response to the cumulative effects of antihypertensive agents. Take the blood pressures in supine and standing positions.

Monitor for an increase in severity of side effects such as sedation, hypotension, and bradycardia or tachycardia.

DRUG CLASS: Central-Acting Alpha-2 Agonists

Actions

The central-acting alpha-2 agonists (e.g., clonidine, guanabenz, guanfacine, methyldopa) act by stimulating the alpha-adrenergic receptors in the brainstem, resulting in reduced sympathetic outflow from the CNS with a decrease in heart rate and peripheral vascular resistance, resulting in a drop in both systolic and diastolic blood pressure.

Uses

The alpha-2 agonists are considered to be adjunctive antihypertensive agents and are recommended for use only in combination with preferred or alternative antihypertensive agents. Clonidine is available as a transdermal therapeutic system (TTS) that is applied once weekly. These drugs cause more frequent side effects such as sedation, dizziness, dry mouth, fatigue, and sexual dysfunction. When used alone, methyldopa often causes fluid retention. They can safely be used in combination with other agents such as diuretics, vasodilators, and beta blockers.

Therapeutic Outcomes

The primary therapeutic outcome expected from the alpha-2 agonists is reduction in blood pressure.

Nursing Process for Central-Acting Alpha-2 Agonists

Premedication Assessment

1. Obtain baseline blood pressure readings in supine and standing positions and apical pulse.
2. Assess the patient's mental status; affective and cognitive behaviors should be used as a baseline for subsequent comparison. If depression is suspected, report to the health care provider.
3. Obtain baseline data relating to usual sleep pattern.

Planning

Availability. See Table 23-9.

Drug Table 23-9 CENTRAL-ACTING ALPHA-2 AGONISTS

GENERIC NAME	BRAND NAME	AVAILABILITY	DOSAGE RANGE
clonidine	Catapres Catapres-TTS	Tablets: 0.1, 0.2, 0.3 mg Transdermal patch: 2.5, 5, 7.5 mg	PO: Initial—0.1 mg twice daily Maintenance—0.2-0.8 mg daily in divided doses Maximum—2.4 mg daily Transdermal—Apply to a hairless area of intact skin on upper arm or torso once every 7 days; use a different site each week Initial—Start with 2.5-mg patch; after second week, add another 2.5-mg patch or use a larger system Maximum—two 7.5-mg patches per week NOTE: Antihypertensive effect starts 2-3 days after initiation of therapy
guanabenz	Wytensin	Tablets: 4, 8 mg	PO: Initial—4 mg twice daily; increase 4-8 mg daily every 1-2 weeks Maximum—32 mg twice daily
guanfacine	Tenex	Tablets: 1, 2 mg	PO: Initial—1 mg daily at bedtime Maintenance—1-2 mg Maximum—3 mg daily
methyldopa	Aldomet	Tablets: 250, 500 mg IV: 250 mg/5 mL in 5- and 10-mL vials	PO: Initial—250 mg two or three times daily Maintenance—500 mg to 2 g daily in 2-4 doses

Implementation

Dosage and Administration. See Table 23-9.

Sudden Discontinuation. Never suddenly discontinue clonidine or guanabenz because it may cause a rebound effect with a rapid increase in blood pressure, manifested by nervousness, agitation, restlessness, tremors, headache, nausea, and increased salivation.

Rebound symptoms are most pronounced after 1 to 2 months of therapy and may begin to appear within a few hours of a missed dose. Within 8 to 24 hours, severe symptoms may develop.

When therapy is to be discontinued, a gradual reduction in dosage is necessary over 2 to 4 days, during which blood pressure must be carefully monitored.

If the clonidine transdermal patch becomes loose, the adhesive overlay should be applied directly over the patch to ensure good adhesion.

Evaluation

Side Effects to Expect

Drowsiness, Dry Mouth, Dizziness. Tell the patient that these symptoms may occur but that they tend to be self-limiting. Tell the patient not to discontinue the medication and to consult a health care provider if the side effects become an unacceptable problem.

Altered Urine Color. Methyldopa or its metabolites may discolor the urine, causing it to darken on exposure to air. It is to be expected and is not harmful.

Altered Test Reactions. A false-positive urine glucose test may occur when using Clinitest. Diastix is not affected by methyldopa.

Methyldopa may cause up to 20% of patients to develop a positive reaction to the direct Coombs' test. Less than 0.2% of these patients will develop hemolytic anemia, however. Blood counts should be determined annually during therapy to detect hemolytic anemia.

Side Effects to Report

Depression. Assess the patient's affect (e.g., loneliness, sadness, anxiety, anger), cognition (e.g., confusion, ambivalence, loss of interest), and other behavioral responses (e.g., agitation, irritability, altered activity level, withdrawal) before starting therapy. After starting therapy with clonidine, carefully monitor the patient for changes in usual response patterns. Assess otherwise normal emotions for an increase in duration or intensity.

Note the patient's degree of socialization, response to stimulation, and changes in interactions with others. All individuals taking this drug should be monitored for development of depression, especially those with a history of depression.

Rash. About 10% to 15% of patients using the clonidine patch develop contact dermatitis. Patients who develop moderate or severe erythema or vesicle formation at the site of application of clonidine transdermal patches should consult a health care provider about the possible need to remove the patch and use alternative therapy.

Drug Interactions

Drugs That Enhance Therapeutic and Toxic Effects. Guanethidine, digoxin, barbiturates, tranquilizers, antihistamines, alcohol, beta-adrenergic blocking agents (e.g., propranolol, atenolol, pindolol), verapamil, and other antihypertensive agents. Monitor the blood pressure response to the cumulative effects of antihypertensive agents. Take the blood pressure in supine and standing positions.

Monitor for an increase in severity of side effects such as sedation, hypotension, and bradycardia or tachycardia.

Drugs That Reduce Therapeutic Effects. Tricyclic antidepressants (e.g., amitriptyline, imipramine, desipramine), trazodone, and prazosin may block the antihypertensive effects of clonidine and methyldopa. The beta-adrenergic blocking agents (e.g., propranolol, atenolol, pindolol) may cause potentially life-threatening increases in blood pressure when taken with clonidine. Monitor carefully for poor blood pressure control or a gradually increasing blood pressure.

Sedative Effects. Alcohol, barbiturates, phenothiazines, benzodiazepines, and antihistamines all potentiate the sedative effects of guanabenz. Patients should be warned that their tolerance to alcohol and other depressants may be diminished.

Haloperidol. Methyldopa used concurrently with haloperidol may produce irritability, aggressiveness, abusive behavior, and dementia. Concurrent use is usually not recommended.

DRUG CLASS: Peripheral-Acting Adrenergic Antagonists

guanadrel (gwan' a drel)

HYLOREL (hi lor' el)

Actions

Guanadrel is similar to guanethidine as an antihypertensive agent in that it causes a release and subsequent depletion of norepinephrine from adrenergic nerve endings. This causes a relaxation of vascular smooth muscle, which decreases total peripheral resistance and venous return. A hypotensive effect results that is greater in the standing than in the supine position. Heart rate is slightly decreased, but there is no significant change in cardiac output. Fluid retention often occurs.

Uses

Guanadrel is recommended for use in refractory hypertension uncontrolled by other agents with fewer side effects. Guanadrel is used in combination with a thiazide diuretic.

Therapeutic Outcomes

The primary therapeutic outcome of guanadrel is reduction in blood pressure.

Nursing Process for Guanadrel

Premedication Assessment

1. Obtain baseline blood pressure readings in the supine and standing positions and apical pulse.
2. Obtain baseline weight.

Planning

Availability. PO: 10 mg tablets.

Implementation

Dosage and Administration. *Adult:* PO: Initially 10 mg daily in two divided doses. Adjust the dosages weekly to monthly until the therapeutic goal has been attained. The usual dosage range is 20 to 75 mg divided into two or three daily doses.

Evaluation

Side Effects to Expect

Orthostatic Hypotension. Orthostatic hypotension occurs often, especially with sudden changes in posture. Patients can usually avoid this complication by rising slowly from supine and sitting positions. Patients should also be cautioned not to stand in one position for prolonged periods. These orthostatic effects are increased with alcohol consumption or prolonged standing with little movement.

Sedation. Sedation and lethargy commonly occur when guanadrel therapy is initiated or during adjustment to higher doses. These effects are most notable during the first few days and tend to subside with time.

Side Effects to Report

Edema. Some patients will develop significant salt and water retention, causing edema and heart failure. Weigh patients daily, using the same scale, at the same time of day, in similar clothing. Report increases of 2 pounds or more per week. Report edema of the extremities and increase in dyspnea, pallor, tachycardia, wheezing, and frothy or blood-tinged sputum.

Drug Interactions

Drugs That Enhance Therapeutic and Toxic Effects. Guanethidine, barbiturates, disopyramide, quinidine, diuretics, tranquilizers, antihistamines, alcohol, and beta-adrenergic blocking agents (e.g., propranolol, atenolol, pindolol), diuretics, and other antihypertensive agents. Monitor the blood pressure response to the cumulative effects of antihypertensive agents. Take the blood pressures in supine and standing positions. Monitor for an increase in severity of side effects such as sedation, hypotension, and bradycardia or tachycardia.

Drugs That Reduce Therapeutic Effects. Tricyclic antidepressants (e.g., amitriptyline, imipramine), amphetamines, ephedrine, phenothiazines, monoamine oxidase inhibitors (MAOIs), haloperidol. Monitor carefully for poor blood pressure control or a gradually increasing blood pressure.

guanethidine sulfate (gwan eth′ i deen)
ISMELIN (is′ meh lin)

Actions

Guanethidine depletes norepinephrine from postganglionic sympathetic nerve terminals. It also inhibits the release of norepinephrine in response to sympathetic nerve stimulation. Blood pressure decreases because of a reduction in cardiac output and peripheral vascular resistance. Because reflex-mediated vasoconstriction is blocked by guanethidine, a much greater hypotensive effect occurs when standing, and postural hypotension is common.

Uses

Guanethidine is recommended for use in refractory hypertension uncontrolled by other agents with fewer side effects. Guanethidine is used in combination with a diuretic.

Therapeutic Outcomes

The primary therapeutic outcome of guanethidine is reduction in blood pressure.

Nursing Process for Guanethidine

Premedication Assessment

1. Obtain baseline blood pressure readings in the supine and standing positions and apical pulse.
2. Obtain baseline weight.

Planning

Availability. PO: 10 and 25 mg tablets.

Implementation

Dosage and Administration. *Adult:* PO: Initially 10 mg daily. Increase the dose 10 mg every 5 to 7 days, if the blood pressure measurements so indicate and side effects are tolerable. Maintenance doses range between 25 and 50 mg daily; however, much higher doses are occasionally required.

Evaluation

Side Effects to Expect

Lightheadedness, Weakness. Guanethidine causes arteriolar and venous dilation that permits pools of blood to collect in the lower extremities, causing a reduction in cerebral blood flow. These symptoms often disappear during the day and can be lessened by rising slowly, sitting on the edge of the bed for a few minutes, and performing leg, foot, and toe exercises before standing. These orthostatic effects are increased with alcohol consumption or prolonged standing with little movement.

Side Effects to Report

Edema. Some patients will develop significant salt and water retention, causing edema and heart failure. Weigh patients daily, using the same scale, at the same time of day, in similar clothing. Report increases of 2 pounds or more per week.

Report edema of the extremities, as well as increase in dyspnea, pallor, tachycardia, wheezing, and frothy or blood-tinged sputum.

Drug Interactions

Drugs That Enhance Therapeutic and Toxic Effects. Barbiturates, disopyramide, quinidine, diuretics, tranquilizers, antihistamines, alcohol, beta-adrenergic blocking agents (e.g., propranolol, atenolol, pindolol), and other antihypertensive agents. Monitor the blood pressure response to the cumulative effects of antihypertensive agents. Take the blood pressure in supine and standing positions. Monitor for an increase in severity of side effects, such as sedation, hypotension, and bradycardia or tachycardia.

Drugs That Reduce Therapeutic Effects. Tricyclic antidepressants (e.g., amitriptyline, imipramine), amphetamines, ephedrine, phenothiazines, and haloperidol. Monitor carefully for poor blood pressure control or a gradually increasing blood pressure.

Insulin and Oral Hypoglycemic Agents. Guanethidine may increase the hypoglycemic effects of insulin and oral hypoglycemic agents. Monitor patients with diabetes mellitus for headache, weakness, decreasing muscle coordination, and diaphoresis. (Onset of hypoglycemic symptoms may be rapid.) Give orange juice with 2 teaspoons of sugar if the patient is still alert and responsive.

reserpine (res' er peen)
SERPASIL (ser' pah sil)

Actions

Reserpine is an alkaloid obtained from the root of a species of *Rauwolfia*. It is one of the oldest antihypertensive agents available. Reserpine acts as an antihypertensive agent by reducing norepinephrine levels in peripheral nerve endings, which slows heart rate and reduces peripheral vascular resistance. It also stimulates the vagus nerve, causing a further reduction in heart rate. Reserpine also depletes norepinephrine from various other organs, including the brain. Depletion of norepinephrine and serotonin in the brain may be the cause of the sedative and depressant actions of reserpine. Reserpine's strong inhibition of sympathetic activity allows increased parasympathetic activity to occur, which is responsible for some of its side effects, including nasal stuffiness, increased gastric acid secretion, diarrhea, and bradycardia.

Uses

Reserpine has an extremely long duration of action; it may take 2 to 6 weeks before the maximum effect of the drug is seen. It is used to treat stage 1 hypertension. It is relatively inexpensive when compared with other antihypertensive agents and is thus preferred by funding agencies, but the side effects associated with therapy often lead to noncompliance.

Therapeutic Outcomes

The primary therapeutic outcome of reserpine is reduction in blood pressure.

Nursing Process for Reserpine

Premedication Assessment

1. Obtain baseline blood pressure readings in the supine and standing positions and apical pulse.
2. Obtain baseline weight.
3. Assess the patient's mental status; affective and cognitive behaviors should be used as a baseline for subsequent comparison. If depression is suspected, report to the health care provider.
4. Obtain baseline data relating to usual sleep pattern.

Planning

Availability. PO: 0.1 and 0.25 mg tablets.

Implementation

Dosage and Administration. Adult: PO: Initially 0.5 mg daily for 1 to 2 weeks. Maintenance: 0.1 to 0.25 mg daily.

Evaluation

Side Effects to Expect

Nasal Stuffiness. Encourage the patient not to treat this symptom with over-the-counter nasal decongestants because they aggravate the hypertension. Fortunately, this side effect tends to be self-limiting, but tell the patient to consult the health care provider if it becomes a serious problem.

Diarrhea. Diarrhea and stomach cramps may be associated with depressed sympathetic activity. These side effects tend to be self-limiting, but if they persist or if there is an increase in abdominal pain, the health care provider should be notified.

Side Effects to Report

Depression. Depression caused by this medication may progress to the point of the patient becoming suicidal.

Assess the patient's affect (e.g., loneliness, sadness, anxiety, anger), cognition (e.g., confusion, ambivalence, loss of interest), and other behavioral responses (e.g., agitation, irritability, altered activity level, withdrawal) before starting therapy. After starting medication therapy with reserpine, carefully monitor the patient for changes in usual response patterns. Assess otherwise normal emotions for an increase in duration or intensity.

Note the patient's degree of socialization, responses to stimulation, and changes in interactions with others. All individuals taking this drug should be monitored for development of depression, especially those with a history of depression.

Nightmares, Insomnia. If these symptoms occur, report them to the health care provider for evaluation. Drug therapy may need to be changed.

Gastric Symptoms. Patients experiencing gastric symptoms such as burning, pain, nausea, or vomiting should report them immediately because this medication can cause formation of new ulcers or exacerbation of old ulcers.

Drug Interactions

Drugs That Enhance Therapeutic and Toxic Effects. Phenothiazines, procainamide, disopyramide, thiothixene, quinidine, diuretics, tranquilizers, antihistamines, alcohol, beta-adrenergic blocking agents (e.g., propranolol, atenolol, pindolol), and other antihypertensive agents. Monitor the blood pressure response to cumulative effects of antihypertensive agents. Take blood pressure readings in supine and standing positions. Monitor for an increase in severity of side effects such as sedation, hypotension, and bradycardia or tachycardia.

Drugs That Reduce Therapeutic Effects. Tricyclic antidepressants (e.g., amitriptyline, imipramine, doxepin). Monitor carefully for poor blood pressure control or a gradually increasing blood pressure.

DRUG CLASS: Direct Vasodilators

hydralazine (hy dral′ ah zeen)

APRESOLINE (ah pres′ o leen)

Actions

Hydralazine causes direct arteriolar smooth muscle relaxation, resulting in reduced peripheral vascular resistance. The reduction in peripheral resistance causes a reflex increase in heart rate, cardiac output, and renin release with sodium and water retention. Consequently, the hypotensive effectiveness is reduced unless the patient is also taking a sympathetic inhibitor (e.g., beta blockers) and a diuretic.

Uses

This antihypertensive agent is used to treat stage 2 hypertension and hypertension associated with renal disease and toxemia of pregnancy. It may also be used to provide symptomatic relief in patients with heart failure by reducing resistance (afterload) to left ventricular output. Because of the reflex increase in cardiac rate, hydralazine is often used in combination with a drug that inhibits tachycardia (e.g., beta blockers, clonidine, methyldopa).

A combination product (BiDil) containing hydralazine and isosorbide dinitrate has recently been approved by the U.S. Food and Drug Administration (FDA). This combination has been shown to reduce hospitalizations, improve quality of life, and reduce mortality among African Americans with hypertension and heart failure.

Therapeutic Outcomes

The primary therapeutic outcome of hydralazine is reduction in blood pressure.

Nursing Process for Hydralazine

Premedication Assessment

Obtain baseline blood pressure readings in the supine and standing positions and apical pulse.

Planning

Availability. PO: 10, 25, 50, and 100 mg tablets; intramuscular (IM), intravenous (IV): 20 mg/mL in 1-mL ampules.

Implementation

Dosage and Administration. *Adult:* PO: Initially, 10 mg four times daily for the first 2 to 4 days, then 25 mg four times daily. The second week, increase the dosage to 50 mg four times daily as the patient tolerates the dosage and the blood pressure is brought under control. IM, IV: 20 to 40 mg repeated as necessary. Monitor blood pressure often. Results usually become evident within 10 to 20 minutes.

Evaluation

Side Effects to Expect

Nausea, Dizziness, Palpitations, Tachycardia, Numbness and Tingling in the Legs, Nasal Congestion. Although these symptoms may be anticipated, they require monitoring. If severe, they should be reported so that the dosage can be adjusted appropriately. Nasal congestion can be treated with an antihistamine, such as chlorpheniramine.

Orthostatic Hypotension. This may occur particularly during initiation of therapy. Patients can usually avoid this complication by rising slowly from supine and sitting positions.

Side Effects to Report

Fever, Chills, Joint and Muscle Pain, Skin Eruptions. Tell patients to report the development of these symptoms. Monitor laboratory reports for leukocyte counts and the antinuclear antibody (ANA) titer.

Drug Interactions

Drugs That Enhance Therapeutic and Toxic Effects. Diuretics, alcohol, beta-adrenergic blocking agents (e.g., propranolol, atenolol, pindolol), and other antihypertensive agents. Monitor the blood pressure response to the cumulative effects of antihypertensive agents. Take the blood pressure in supine and standing positions.

Monitor for an increase in severity of side effects, such as sedation, hypotension, and bradycardia or tachycardia.

minoxidil (min ox′ i dil)

LONITEN (lon′ i ten)

Actions

Minoxidil acts by direct relaxation of the smooth muscle of arterioles, reducing peripheral vascular resistance. Because of the decrease in peripheral vascular resistance, there is a compensatory increase in heart rate and sodium and water retention. For this reason, minoxidil is usually administered in conjunction with a beta-adrenergic blocking agent and a potent diuretic such as furosemide or bumetanide.

Uses

Minoxidil is used only for severely hypertensive patients who do not respond adequately to maximum therapeutic doses of a diuretic and two other antihypertensive agents.

Therapeutic Outcomes

The primary therapeutic outcome of minoxidil is reduction in blood pressure.

Nursing Process for Minoxidil

Premedication Assessment

1. Obtain baseline blood pressure reading in the supine and standing positions and apical pulse.
2. Obtain baseline weight.
3. Obtain resting pulse rate to serve as a baseline for subsequent comparisons.

Planning

Availability. PO: 2.5 and 10 mg tablets.

Implementation

Dosage and Administration. *Adult:* PO: Initially 5 mg daily. Dosage may be gradually increased after at least 3-day intervals to 10 mg, 20 mg, and then 40 mg daily in one or two doses. Maintenance: 10 to 40 mg daily. Maximum dosage is 100 mg daily.

Evaluation

Side Effects to Expect

Hair Growth. Within 3 to 6 weeks after starting therapy, about 80% of patients will start developing *hypertrichosis*, an elongation, thickening, and increased pigmentation of fine body hair. It is usually noticed first on the face and later extends to the back, arms, legs, and scalp.

Growth may be controlled by shaving or by depilatory creams. After discontinuation, new hair growth stops, but it may take up to 6 months for a complete return to pretreatment appearance.

Side Effects to Report

Gynecomastia. Swelling or tenderness of the breasts may develop in men.

Salt and Water Retention. This drug is usually administered with a diuretic and a beta-adrenergic blocking agent to reduce the incidence of fluid retention and for additive antihypertensive effects.

Perform daily weights using the same scale, in similar clothing, and at approximately the same time of day. Report gains of more than 2 pounds per week and swelling or puffiness of the face, ankles, or hands to a health care provider.

Increased Resting Pulse. Instruct and validate the patient's ability to take own pulse. A resting pulse that increases 20 or more beats per minute above normal should be reported.

Lightheadedness, Fainting, Dizziness. These symptoms should be reported to a health care provider. If possible, the patient's blood pressure during these episodes should be taken and reported.

Orthostatic Hypotension. This may occur, particularly during initiation of therapy. Patients can usually avoid this complication by rising slowly from supine and sitting positions.

Heart Failure. Assess for development of dyspnea, orthopnea, edema, and weight gain.

Drug Interactions

Drugs That Enhance Therapeutic and Toxic Effects. Diuretics, alcohol, beta-adrenergic blocking agents (e.g., propranolol, atenolol, pindolol), guanethidine, guanadrel, and other antihypertensive agents. Monitor the blood pressure response caused by the cumulative effects of antihypertensive agents. Take the blood pressure in supine and standing positions. Monitor for increase in severity of side effects, such as sedation, hypotension, and bradycardia or tachycardia.

nitroprusside sodium (ny tro prus' ide)
NITROPRESS (ny' tro pres)

Actions

Nitroprusside is a potent vasodilator that acts directly on the smooth muscle of blood vessels. It produces both arterial and venous vasodilation, thus reducing both preload and afterload on the heart.

Uses

Nitroprusside is used in patients with sudden severe hypertensive crisis and in those with refractory heart failure.

Therapeutic Outcomes

The primary therapeutic outcomes of nitroprusside are reduction in blood pressure and improvement in symptoms associated with heart failure.

Planning

Availability. IV: 50 mg per vial in 2- and 5-mL vials.

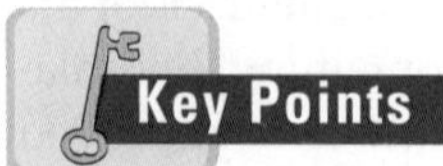

- The public has made significant strides in the past two decades in recognizing the risk factors associated with cardiovascular disease. This awareness has led to reduction in the incidence of heart attacks and strokes. Hypertension, however, is still a national health problem. Nurses can play a significant role in public education efforts, monitor for nonadherence, monitor blood pressure response to therapy, and encourage patients to make changes in lifestyle to reduce the severity of hypertension.

- Nonadherence to hypertensive therapy is a major problem, and nurses need to understand that educating the patient regarding the consequences of discontinuing therapy is not enough; rather the nurse must investigate the "whys" for discontinuing the therapy. Many of the reasons the patient gives may be overcome or reduced by proper interventions or a change in the type of antihypertensive agents prescribed.
- Because hypertension is a "silent killer," it is important that nurses and other health professionals extend public screening programs to the community.

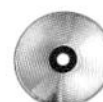
Go to your Companion CD-ROM for Appendices, an Audio Glossary, animations, Drug Dosage Calculators, customizable Patient Self-Assessment forms, and Review Questions for the NCLEX® Examination.

evolve Be sure to visit the companion Evolve site at http://evolve.elsevier.com/Clayton for WebLinks and additional online resources.

MEDICATION SAFETY REVIEW

MATH REVIEW QUESTIONS

1. Order: Clonidine hydrochloride (Catapres) 0.6 mg PO daily in two divided doses.
   Available: Clonidine hydrochloride (Catapres) 0.1- and 0.2-mg tablets
   Give: ____ tablets of ____ mg, and ____ tablets of ____ mg.
   (Catapres is also available in 0.3-mg tablets. What nursing action would be appropriate?)
2. Order: Enalapril (Vasotec) 10 mg bid
   Available: Vasotec 5-mg tablets
   Give: _____ tablets bid.
3. Order: Captopril (Capoten) 25 mg daily
   Available: Capten 12.5 mg
   Give: _____ tablets daily.
4. Order: Carvedilol (Coreg) 12.5 mg daily
   Available: Coreg 6.25 mg
   Give: _____ tablets daily.
5. Order: Propranolol (Inderal) 3 mg IV stat
   Available: Inderal 1 mg/mL in 1-mL ampules
   Give: _____ mL.
   (What must be monitored when administering this medication IV?)

CRITICAL THINKING QUESTIONS

1. A male patient is receiving methyldopa 3 g per day. Sexual dysfunction is a possible nursing diagnosis related to methyldopa therapy manifested by impotence or failure to ejaculate. Address the health teaching needed and how the nurse could approach this subject.
2. Discuss the essential patient education needed regarding the initiation of therapy with captopril.
3. State the nursing assessments needed to monitor therapeutic response and the development of side effects to expect or report from beta adrenergic–blocking agents and calcium ion antagonists.
4. Review beta adrenergic–blocking agent information in the monograph and develop patient education objectives for a patient receiving this class of drugs for treatment of hypertension.
5. A female patient is being started on a drug regimen for hypertension that includes the use of losartan. Initially her blood pressure (BP) is 160/100 mm Hg, pulse is 64, respirations are 20 per minute, and weight is 148 pounds. She seems quiet and introspective and contributes little information other than "yes" or "no" responses during an initial assessment. What further nursing actions would be appropriate?
6. Lifestyle modifications are extremely important for the treatment of hypertension, but habits can be difficult to change for patients. What should be the nurse's approach?

Continued

CONTENT REVIEW QUESTIONS

1. With this type of antihypertensive agent, the premedication assessment should include checking for respiratory conditions that are present because this class of drug may cause a chronic cough:
   1. angiotensin II receptor antagonists.
   2. diuretics.
   3. angiotensin-converting enzyme inhibitors.
   4. beta-adrenergic blocking agents.

2. The generic drug names of all but one drug in this classification end in "pril."
   1. Angiotensin II receptor antagonists
   2. Diuretics
   3. Angiotensin-converting enzyme inhibitors
   4. Beta-adrenergic blocking agents

3. Angiotensin II receptor antagonists act by:
   1. binding to angiotensin I receptor sites.
   2. binding to angiotensin II receptor sites.
   3. altering renal function.
   4. altering calcium ion movement across the cells.

4. Initial therapy for hypertension is most often:
   1. diuretics and alpha blockers.
   2. beta blockers and calcium ion antagonists.
   3. diuretics and angiotensin II receptor blockers.
   4. diuretics or beta-adrenergic blocking agents.

5. A drug that reduces peripheral vascular resistance will:
   1. decrease the heart rate.
   2. decrease cardiac output.
   3. reduce blood pressure.
   4. increase blood pressure.

6. All antihypertensive agents in this class end in "sartan."
   1. Angiotensin II receptor antagonists
   2. Diuretics
   3. Angiotensin-converting enzyme inhibitors
   4. Beta-adrenergic blocking agents

7. The aldosterone receptor blocker, eplerenone, acts by:
   1. blocking conversion of angiotensin I to angiotensin II.
   2. reducing sodium reabsorption.
   3. volume depletion, sodium excretion, and vasodilation of peripheral arterioles.
   4. blocking calcium ion movement across the cell membrane.

CHAPTER

24 Drugs Used to Treat Dysrhythmias

evolve http://evolve.elsevier.com/Clayton

Chapter Content

Objectives

1. Describe the therapeutic response that should be observable when an antidysrhythmic drug is administered.
2. Identify baseline nursing assessments that should be implemented during the treatment of dysrhythmias.
3. List the dosage forms and precautions needed when preparing IV lidocaine for the treatment of dysrhythmias.
4. Cite common side effects that may be observed with the administration of amiodarone, bretylium tosylate, disopyramide, lidocaine, flecainide, mexiletine, procainamide, and quinidine.
5. Identify the potential effects of muscle relaxants used during surgical intervention when combined with antidysrhythmic drugs.

Key Terms

electrical system
dysrhythmia
atrial flutter
atrial fibrillation
paroxysmal supraventricular tachycardia
atrioventricular blocks
tinnitus

DYSRHYTHMIAS

The function of the heart is to sustain life by rhythmically pumping blood to itself through the coronary arteries and to the rest of the body's tissues. The **electrical system** or conduction system of the heart is the anatomical structure that controls the sequence of muscle contractions so that an optimal volume of blood is pumped from the heart with each beat (Figure 24-1). The electrical system is composed of nerve fibers that conduct electrical impulses to cardiac muscle, causing it to contract.

In the normal heart, a contraction of the heart muscle begins in the pacemaker cells of the sinoatrial (SA) node. The electrical wave passes through the electrical system in the atrial muscle and causes it to contract, forcing blood in the atrial chambers into the ventricles below. The electrical current then enters the atrioventricular (AV) node, which focuses and conducts an electrical current through the bundle of His and the Purkinje fibers to the ventricular muscle tissue. The muscle contracts from the apex upward, causing blood to be pumped from the ventricles into the pulmonary artery to the lungs and into the aorta to the rest of the body.

A **dysrhythmia** (sometimes called an *arrhythmia*) occurs when there is a disturbance of the normal electrical conduction, resulting in an abnormal heart muscle contraction or heart rate. All people have an occasional irregular contraction of the heart. The danger is the frequency with which the dysrhythmia occurs because the heart muscle loses its efficiency in pumping an adequate volume of blood. Thus certain types of dysrhythmias can produce additional dysrhythmias that can stop the heart from pumping even though it continues to beat for a short time (fibrillation). A person may "sense" an abnormal contraction (dysrhythmia) because of a "flip-flop" or "racing" of the heart. A nurse may also suspect that a patient is having dysrhythmia because of an irregular pulse. Dysrhythmias, however, must be identified with the aid of an electrocardiogram (ECG), which provides a tracing of the electrical activity of the heart.

Dysrhythmias are caused by the firing of abnormal pacemaker cells, or the blockage of normal electrical pathways, or a combination of both. Normally, the rate and rhythm of electrical activity and muscle contraction are regulated by the pacemaker cells of the SA node. High emotional stress, ischemia (see Chapter 25), or heart failure (see Chapter 28) may trigger normally quiet pacemaker cells in areas of the heart other than the SA or AV nodes to fire. This sends an electrical impulse out of sequence with those from the normal pacemaker cells, causing an irregular muscular contraction, sometimes sensed as a "flip-flop" of the heart. The second cause of a dysrhythmia is a partial obstruction of the normal conduction pathway, causing an irregular flow of electrical impulses that results in an irregular pattern of muscle contractions. This is sometimes called a "reentrant" dysrhythmia. Normally, healthy heart tissue has mechanisms that protect against reentrant dysrhythmias. Various forms of heart disease cause changes in

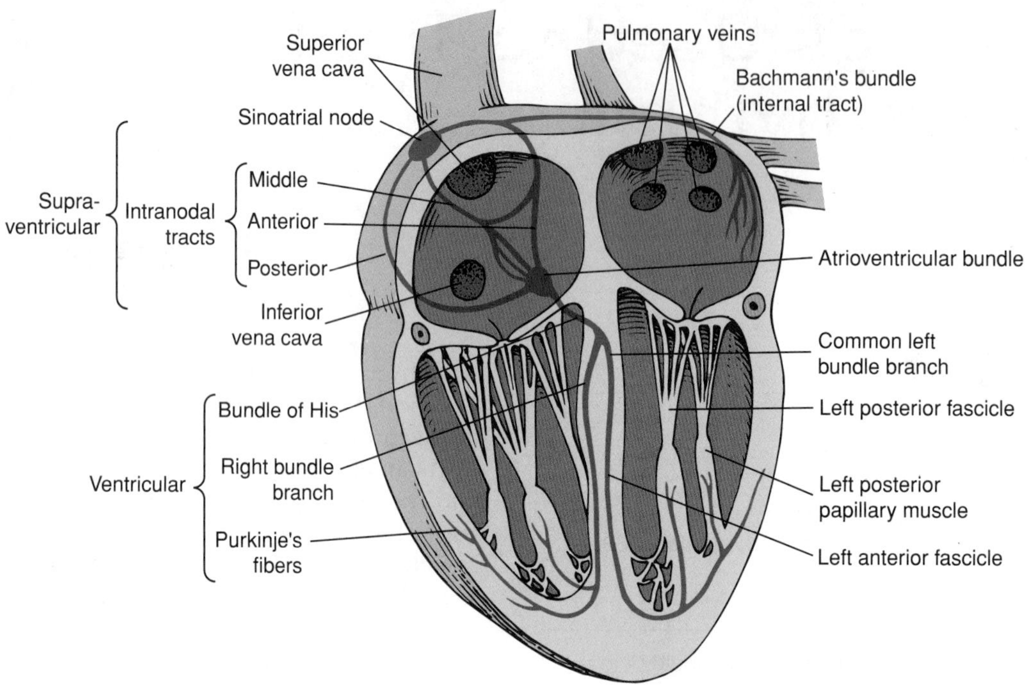

FIGURE **24-1** Schematic diagram of the heart, illustrating the conduction system.

the conduction pathways that allow continuous reentrant dysrhythmias.

Dysrhythmias are most commonly classified by origin within the heart tissues. Those that develop above the bundle of His (see Figure 24-1) are called *supraventricular.* Examples of supraventricular dysrhythmias are atrial flutter, atrial fibrillation, premature atrial contractions (PAC), sinus tachycardia, sinus bradycardia, and paroxysmal supraventricular tachycardia. Dysrhythmias developing below the bundle of His are referred to as *ventricular dysrhythmias.* These include premature ventricular contractions (PVCs), ventricular tachycardia (VT), and ventricular fibrillation (VF). Dysrhythmias that result from obstruction of conduction pathways are described by location (e.g., supraventricular or ventricular, left or right bundle branches). Atrioventricular blocks can be subclassified by degree of block: first degree = partial block, delayed AV conduction; second degree = partial block with occasional blocked beats; and third degree = complete block, the atria and ventricles function independently of each other. Another method of classification is based on heart beat rate: bradyarrhythmia (<60 beats/minute) or tachyarrhythmia (>100 beats/minute).

The tissues of the electrical system can be classified by conduction rate depending on whether calcium or sodium ions create the stimulus for muscle contraction. The SA and AV nodes depend on calcium ions for electrical conduction and are referred to as *slow conduction fibers.* The atrial muscle, His-Purkinje system, and the ventricular muscle depend on sodium for contraction and are sometimes referred to as *fast conduction fibers.*

TREATMENT FOR DYSRHYTHMIAS

When a dysrhythmia is suspected, a patient is often admitted to a coronary care unit, where wire leads are placed in appropriate locations to provide continuous ECG monitoring (telemetry). A combination of the physical examination, patient history, and ECG pattern is used to diagnose the underlying cause of the dysrhythmia. The goal of treatment is to restore normal sinus rhythm and normal cardiac function and to prevent recurrence of life-threatening dysrhythmias.

DRUG THERAPY FOR DYSRHYTHMIAS

Actions

Antidysrhythmic agents are complex agents with multiple mechanisms of action. They are classified according to their effects on the electrical conduction system of the heart (Table 24-1). Class I agents act as myocardial depressants by inhibiting sodium ion movement. The Class Ia agents prolong the duration of the electrical stimulation on cells and the refractory time between electrical impulses. Class Ib agents shorten the duration of the electrical stimulation and the time between the electrical impulses. Class Ic antidysrhythmics are the most potent myocardial depressants and slow conduction rate through the atria and the ventricles.

Class II agents are beta-adrenergic blocking agents. Many dysrhythmias are caused by stimulation of the beta cells of the sympathetic nervous system of the heart. Class III agents slow the rate of electrical conduction and prolong the time interval between contractions by blocking potassium channels. Class IV agents block calcium ion flow, prolonging duration of the electrical stimulation and slowing AV node conduction.

Table 24-1 Classification of Antidysrhythmic Agents

CLASS	DRUGS	MECHANISM	EFFECT CV	RP	AM
Ia	quinidine (Quinadine) procainamide (Procanbid) disopyramide (Norpace)	Na channel blockers (intermediate acting)	↓	↑	↓
Ib	lidocaine (Xylocaine) mexiletine (Mexitil) tocainide (Tonocard)	Na channel blockers (quick acting)	↓/↔	↓	↓
Ic	flecainide (Tambocor) propafenone (Rythmol) moricizine (Ethomozine)	*Na channel blockers* (slow acting)	↓	↔	↓
II	propranolol (Inderal) esmolol (Brevibloc) metoprolol (Lopressor)	Beta blockers	↓	↑	↓
III	amiodarone (Cordarone) bretylium (Bretylol) sotalol (Betapace) ibutilide (Corvert) dofetilide (Tikosyn)	*K channel blockers*	↑/↔	↑	↔
IV	verapamil (Calan) diltiazem (Cardizem)	Ca channel blockers	↓	↑	↓
Misc.	digoxin (Lanoxin) adenosine (Adenocard)	Vagal stimulation Slows conduction	↓	↓/↔	↓

CV, Conduction velocity; *RP*, refractory period; *AM*, automaticity.

Uses

See individual monographs for uses of antidysrhythmic agents.

NURSING PROCESS *for Antidysrhythmic Agents*

The information that nurses assess relative to the cardinal signs of cardiovascular disease can provide a basis for subsequent evaluation of the patient's response to the therapeutic modalities prescribed.

Assessment

Dysrhythmias are initially assessed by ECG monitoring. There are a variety of types of telemetry monitoring equipment available. It is vitally important for the nurse not to rely completely on computerized systems, but rather to perform frequent patient assessments while viewing the telemetry system as an adjunct to astute nursing observations. A 24-hour ambulatory ECG (Holter monitor), electrophysiologic studies (EPS), exercise electrocardiography, and laboratory values are used to analyze and diagnose the patient's myocardial status.

Patients are usually admitted to the coronary care unit where specialized monitoring equipment is available for continuous surveillance of the patient. The nurses have advanced education in cardiac physiology and the nursing care of these individuals. (See a general medical-surgical nursing text for an in-depth explanation of care of the patient with a dysrhythmia.)

Medication History. Obtain details of all medications prescribed and being taken. Tactfully find out if the prescribed medications are being taken regularly and if not, why.

History of Six Cardinal Signs of Cardiovascular Disease

- *Dyspnea (difficulty in breathing):* Record if dyspnea occurs while resting or during exertion. Is the patient affected by position such as lying down, or do they awaken from sleep at night?
- *Chest pain:* Record data as to the time of onset, frequency, duration, and quality of the chest pain. Note any conditions the patient has found that either aggravate or relieve the chest pain. Are there any associated symptoms with the pain such as sweating, ashen gray or pale skin, heart skipping a beat, shortness of breath, nausea or vomiting, or racing of the heart? (Not all patients with a dysrhythmia have chest pain.)
- *Fatigue:* Determine whether fatigue occurs only at specific times of the day, such as evening. Ask the patient if fatigue decreases in relation to a decrease in activity level or if it is present at about the same time daily. Are they able to keep up with family and co-workers?
- *Edema:* Record the presence or absence of edema. If present, record location of edema, assessment data (e.g., degree of pitting present; ankle, midcalf, or thigh circumference) and any measures the patient has used to eliminate edema. Chart the time of day that the edema is present, (e.g., when rising in the morning, later in the evening)

and the specific parts on the body where present. When performing daily weights, use the same scale, at the same time of day, with the patient in a similar type of clothing.

- *Syncope:* Ask the patient about conditions surrounding any episodes of syncope. Record the degree of symptoms such as general muscle weakness, inability to stand upright, feeling of faintness, or loss of consciousness. Record what activities, if any, bring on these syncopal episodes.
- *Palpitations:* Record the patient's description of palpitations, such as "my heart skips some beats" or "it began to feel as if it were racing." Ask if these conditions are preceded by mild or strenuous exercise and how long the palpitations last.

Basic Mental Status. Identify the person's level of consciousness and clarity of thought. Both of these factors are indicators of adequate or inadequate cerebral perfusion. Subsequent regular observations for this data should be made so that apparent improvement or deterioration can be assessed.

Vital Signs. Vital signs should be taken as often as necessary to monitor the patient's status.

- *Blood pressure:* Blood pressure readings should be performed at least two times daily in stable cardiac patients and more often if indicated by the patient's symptoms or the health care provider's orders. Be sure to use the proper-sized blood pressure cuff and have the patient's arm at heart level.
- Record the blood pressure in both arms. A systolic pressure variance of 5 to 10 mm Hg is normal; readings reflecting a variance of more than 10 mm Hg should be reported for further evaluation. ***Always report a narrowing pulse pressure*** (difference between systolic and diastolic readings).
- *Pulse:* Assess bilaterally the rhythm, quality, equality, and strength of the pulses (carotid, brachial, radial, femoral, popliteal, posterior tibial, and dorsalis pedis). If any pulse is diminished or absent, record the level at which initial changes are noted. The usual words to describe the pulse are "absent," "weak," "normal," "increased," or "bounding." Report irregular rate, rhythm and reported palpitations. Check for delayed capillary refill.
- *Respirations:* Observe and chart the rate and depth of respirations. Check breath sounds at least every shift, making specific notations regarding the presence of abnormal breath sounds such as crackles, wheezes, rales. Observe the degree of dyspnea that occurs and whether it happens with or without exertion.
- *Temperature:* Record the patient's temperature at least every shift.

Auscultation and Percussion. Nurses with advanced skills can perform auscultation and percussion to note changes in heart size and heart and lung sounds. (See a medical-surgical nursing text for details of performing these advanced skills.) As appropriate to nursing skills, note changes in cardiac rhythm, heart rate, changes in heart sounds, or murmurs.

Laboratory Tests. Review laboratory tests and report abnormal results to the health care provider promptly. Such tests may include serum electrolytes, especially potassium, calcium, magnesium, and sodium; arterial blood gases such as pH, pO_2, pCO_2, HCO_3; coagulation studies to evaluate the blood clotting; serum enzymes aspartate aminotransferase (AST), creatine kinase (CK-MB), troponin levels, lactic dehydrogenase (LDH); serum lipids (e.g., cholesterol, triglycerides); ECG; radiographic examinations; nuclear cardiography; cardiac catheterization; electrophysiology (EPS) testing; and exercise treadmill.

Examine urinalysis reports and perform hourly monitoring of intake and output (I&O) as ordered. Report output that is less than intake or is below 30 to 50 mL per hour. Monitor other renal function tests such as the blood urea nitrogen (BUN) and serum creatinine. Abnormalities of these tests or insufficient hourly output may indicate inadequate renal perfusion.

Nursing Diagnoses

- Cardiac output, decreased (indication)
- Activity intolerance (indication)
- Tissue perfusion, ineffective (indication)
- Fatigue (indication)

Planning

Medication. Order medications prescribed and schedule these on the medication administration record (MAR).

History of Six Cardinal Signs of Cardiovascular Disease. Individualize the care plan to address the patient's degree of dyspnea, chest pain, fatigue, edema, syncope, and palpitations.

Basic Mental Status. Schedule basic neurologic checks at least once per shift.

Vital Signs, Auscultation, and Percussion. Schedule measurement of vital signs and auscultation and percussion of the heart and chest in a manner consistent with the patient's status.

Laboratory Tests. Order stat and subsequent laboratory studies.

Emergency Treatment. The nurse should be aware of the policy for calling "codes," location of the emergency cart, and procedures used to check the emergency cart supplies. Know the procedure for defibrillation and cardioversion.

Implementation

- Monitor electrocardiographic tracings on a continuum (telemetry).

- Perform physical assessments of the patient in accordance with the clinical setting policies (e.g., every 4 to 8 hours, depending on the patient's status).
- Assist the patient, as needed, to perform activities of daily living (ADLs). Make note of the degree of impairment or dyspnea seen with and without exertion.
- Administer oxygen as ordered and as necessary (PRN).
- Administer prescribed medications and treatments that can best alleviate the patient's symptoms and provide maximum level of comfort.
- Encourage physical activity as prescribed. Do not allow the patient to overexert or become fatigued.
- Institute measures to reduce anxiety. Support the patient in a calm manner even if the patient responds in a hostile or confrontational way.

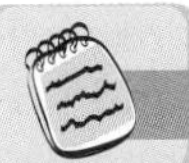

Patient Education and Health Promotion

- Review the patient's history to identify modifiable coronary artery disease factors. Design an individualized approach to assist the patient to modify factors that are within the patient's control.
- Cooperatively discuss and practice using coping mechanisms to handle the individual's anxiety.
- Teach the patient to take own pulse and blood pressure, and stress signs and symptoms that should be reported.

Fostering Health Maintenance. Throughout the course of treatment, discuss medication information and how it will benefit the patient.

Drug therapy is one component of the treatment of dysrhythmias, and it is critical that the medications be taken as prescribed. Provide the patient and significant others with the important information contained in the specific drug monograph for the drugs prescribed. Additional health teaching and nursing interventions for drug side effects to expect and report will be found in each drug monograph.

Seek cooperation and understanding of the following points so that medication compliance is increased: name of medication, dosage, route and times of administration, side effects to expect, and side effects to report.

Written Record. Enlist the patient's aid in developing and maintaining a written record of monitoring parameters (e.g., pulse rate, blood pressure, degree of dyspnea and what precipitates it, chest pain, edema) (see Patient Self-Assessment Form on p. 455). Complete the Premedication Data column for use as a baseline to track response to drug therapy. Ensure that the patient understands how to use the form and instruct the patient to bring the completed form to follow-up visits. During follow-up visits, focus on issues that will foster adherence with the therapeutic interventions prescribed. ■

DRUG CLASS: Antidysrhythmic Agents

adenosine (aden' oh seen)
ADENOCARD (aden' oh card)

Actions

Adenosine is a naturally occurring chemical found in every cell within the body. It is not related to other antidysrhythmic agents. It has a variety of physiologic roles, including energy transfer, promotion of prostaglandin release, inhibition of platelet aggregation, antiadrenergic effects, coronary vasodilation, and suppression of heart rate.

Uses

Because of its strong depressant effects on the SA and AV nodes, adenosine is recommended for the treatment of paroxysmal supraventricular tachycardia that involves conduction in the SA node, atrium, or AV node.

Therapeutic Outcomes

The primary therapeutic outcome expected from adenosine therapy is conversion of supraventricular tachycardias to normal sinus rhythm.

Nursing Process for Adenosine

Premedication Assessment

Obtain data relating to the six cardinal signs of cardiovascular disease to be used as a baseline for subsequent evaluation of response to therapy.

Planning

Availability. IV: 3 mg/mL in 2 mL and 4 mL vials, 2 and 5 mL syringes.

Implementation

Dosage and Administration. IV: 6 mg administered by rapid IV bolus injection (over 1 to 2 seconds) followed by a saline flush. A follow-up dose of 12 mg by rapid IV bolus is recommended if the initial dose is unsuccessful in restoring a normal heart rate. The 12-mg dose may be repeated once if required.

Evaluation

Side Effects to Expect. The most commonly reported adverse reactions with adenosine include flushing of the face (18%), shortness of breath (12%), chest pressure (7%), nausea (3%), and headache and light-headedness (2%). Because the half-life of adenosine is less than 10 seconds, adverse effects are very short-lived. Treatment of any prolonged adverse effect would include oxygen and possibly other antidysrhythmic agents.

Drug Interactions

Drugs That Enhance Therapeutic and Toxic Effects. Dipyridamole and carbamazepine potentiate the effects of adenosine. Smaller doses of adenosine should be used if therapy is required.

Drugs That Reduce Therapeutic Effects. Theophylline, aminophylline, and caffeine competitively antagonize adenosine, thus larger doses of adenosine are required with concurrent use.

amiodarone hydrochloride (am e o′ dahr own)
CORDARONE (cor′ dahr own)

Actions

Amiodarone is an antidysrhythmic agent unrelated to other medicines used to treat dysrhythmias. Although its mechanism of action is unknown, it is a class III agent that acts by prolonging the action potential of atrial and ventricular tissue and by increasing the refractory period without altering the resting membrane potential, thus delaying repolarization. In addition, amiodarone has been shown to antagonize noncompetitively both alpha- and beta-adrenergic receptors, causing systemic and coronary vasodilation.

Uses

Amiodarone is being used in the management of life-threatening supraventricular tachyarrhythmias, atrial fibrillation and flutter, bradycardia-tachycardia syndromes, ventricular tachycardia and fibrillation, and hypertrophic cardiomyopathy resistant to currently available therapy.

Side Effects

Adverse reactions are very common with the use of amiodarone, particularly in patients receiving more than 400 mg/day. Approximately 15% to 20% of patients discontinue therapy because of adverse effects.

Therapeutic Outcomes

The primary therapeutic outcome expected from amiodarone therapy is conversion to and maintenance of normal sinus rhythm.

Nursing Process for Amiodarone

Premedication Assessment

1. Obtain data relating to the six cardinal signs of cardiovascular disease to be used as a baseline for subsequent evaluation of response to therapy.
2. Initiate requested laboratory tests to be used for evaluation of pulmonary, ophthalmic, thyroid, and liver function.
3. Record data relating to the patient's usual sleep pattern and any gastrointestinal (GI) symptoms present before initiation of therapy.

Planning

Availability. PO: 100, 200, and 400 mg tablets; IV: 50 mg/mL in 3-mL ampules.

Implementation

Dosage and Administration. Note: Amiodarone is contraindicated in patients with severe sinus-node dysfunction that causes sinus bradycardia, with second- and third-degree AV block, and when episodes of bradycardia have caused syncope (except in the presence of a pacemaker).

The difficulty of using amiodarone effectively and safely is that it poses a significant risk to patients. Patients must be hospitalized while the loading dose is given, and the response often requires 2 weeks or more. Because absorption and elimination are variable, maintenance-dose selection is difficult, and it is not unusual to require a reduction in dosage or a discontinuation of treatment. The time at which a previously controlled life-threatening dysrhythmia will recur after discontinuation or dosage adjustment is unpredictable, ranging from weeks to months. Attempts to substitute other antidysrhythmic agents when amiodarone is discontinued are made difficult by the gradually but unpredictably changing amiodarone body store. A similar problem exists when amiodarone is not effective; it still poses the risk of a drug interaction with whatever subsequent treatment is tried. PO: Loading dose: 800 to 1600 mg daily in divided doses for 1 to 3 weeks until an initial therapeutic response occurs. After the loading dose, a dosage of 600 to 800 mg daily is given for approximately 1 month. Maintenance: The lowest effective dose should be used, usually 400 mg daily.

Baseline Tests. Before start of therapy, baseline pulmonary, ophthalmic, thyroid, and liver function tests should be completed.

Gastric Irritation. If gastric irritation occurs, administer with food or milk. If symptoms persist or increase in severity, report for health care provider evaluation.

Evaluation

Side Effects to Report

Fatigue, Tremors, Involuntary Movements, Sleep Disturbances, Numbness and Tingling, Dizziness, Ataxia, Confusion. Many of these symptoms are dose related and resolve with reduction of dosage or discontinuation of therapy. Peripheral neuropathy may be associated with long-term therapy, although the onset and presentation of symptoms are variable. Symptoms usually resolve 1 to 4 months after the discontinuation of therapy.

Teach the patient to rise slowly from a supine or sitting position, and encourage the patient to sit or lie down if feeling faint.

Perform a baseline assessment of the patient's degree of alertness and orientation to name, place, and time before starting therapy. Make regularly scheduled subsequent mental status evaluations and compare findings. Report development of alterations. Provide for patient safety during episodes of dizziness.

Exertional Dyspnea, Nonproductive Cough, Pleuritic Chest Pain. Pulmonary interstitial pneumonitis/alveolitis has been reported in 10% to 15% of patients. Particular care should be taken not to assume that such symptoms are related to cardiac failure. Tests for diffusion capacity are most likely to show abnormality. Symptoms gradually resolve after discontinuation of therapy. Periodic chest x-rays and clinical evaluation are recommended every 3 to 6 months.

Thyroid Disorders. Administration of amiodarone has been associated with the development of hypothyroidism (2% to 10%) and hyperthyroidism (1% to 3%). Patients with a history of thyroid disorders appear to be more susceptible to this complication. Baseline and periodic thyroid function tests should be completed in all patients.

Yellow-Brown Pigmentations in the Cornea, Blurred Vision, Halos. Corneal microdeposits have been observed by slit lamp examination as early as 2 weeks after the initiation of therapy. Symptoms of blurred vision, narrowing peripheral vision, or visual halos develop in about 10% of patients. This complication is reversible after drug withdrawal. Use of methylcellulose ophthalmic solution and a minimization of the maintenance doses may limit this complication. Provide for patient safety during temporary visual impairment. Instruct the patient not to rub the eyes with force when tearing.

Nausea, Vomiting, Constipation, Abdominal Pain, Anorexia. GI complaints occur in about 25% of patients but rarely require discontinuation of therapy. These adverse effects commonly occur during high-dosage administration and usually respond to dosage reduction or divided dosages.

Dysrhythmias. Amiodarone can cause an exacerbation of the preexisting dysrhythmia and in 2% to 4% of patients induce others as well.

Photosensitivity. Amiodarone has produced photosensitivity in approximately 10% of patients. The severity of the rash may depend on the degree of sun exposure. Symptoms such as burning, tingling, erythema, and blistering may occur as early as 2 hours after exposure to the sun. The use of sunscreens may minimize this adverse effect. Patients should be encouraged to wear long-sleeved shirts and to avoid wearing shorts outdoors. Photosensitivity may persist for up to 4 months after discontinuation of therapy. With long-term treatment, a blue-gray discoloration of the exposed skin may occur. The risk is increased in patients of fair complexion and those with excessive sun exposure and may be related to cumulative dose and duration of therapy. This effect gradually subsides after discontinuation of therapy. The patient should also be instructed not to use artificial tanning lamps.

Hepatotoxicity. Abnormal liver function tests (e.g., aspartate aminotransferase [AST], alanine aminotransferase [ALT]) occur in 4% to 9% of patients. Liver enzymes in patients on relatively high maintenance doses should be monitored on a regular basis. Persistent significant elevations in the liver enzymes or hepatomegaly are indications for considering a reduction in dosage or discontinuation of therapy. Hepatitis and other liver abnormalities may develop in 1% to 3% of patients. The symptoms of hepatotoxicity are anorexia, nausea, vomiting, jaundice, hepatomegaly, splenomegaly, and abnormal liver function tests.

Drug Interactions

Cimetidine, Fluoroquinolones. Administration of cimetidine or the fluoroquinolones (e.g., sparfloxacin, moxifloxacin) with amiodarone significantly increases serum levels of amiodarone. Reduce the dose of amiodarone and monitor closely for dysrhythmias if administered concurrently.

Rifampin. Rifampin significantly reduces the serum levels of amiodarone. The dose of amiodarone may need to be increased for therapeutic effect.

Digoxin. Administration of amiodarone to patients receiving digoxin therapy regularly results in an increase in the serum digoxin concentration. The dose of digoxin should be reduced by 50% or discontinued. Digoxin serum levels should be closely monitored and patients observed for clinical evidence of toxicity (e.g., anorexia, nausea, fatigue, blurred or colored vision, bradycardia, dysrhythmia).

Warfarin. Potentiation of warfarin is almost always seen within 3 to 4 days in patients receiving concomitant therapy. The dose of the anticoagulant should be reduced by one-third to one-half, and prothrombin times (INR) should be monitored closely. Observe for the development of petechiae; ecchymoses; nosebleeds; bleeding gums; dark, tarry stools; and bright-red or "coffee-ground" emesis.

Quinidine. Elevation of quinidine serum levels (32% to 50%) is often observed within 2 to 3 days. The dosage of quinidine should be reduced by one third to one half or discontinued.

Procainamide. Elevation of procainamide serum levels (50%) is often observed in less than 7 days. The dosage of procainamide should be reduced by one third or discontinued.

Phenytoin. Elevation of phenytoin serum levels (200% to 300%) is observed over several weeks. The dosage of phenytoin must be gradually reduced, based on patient response. Monitor patients undergoing concurrent therapy for signs of phenytoin toxicity: nystagmus, sedation, and lethargy. Serum levels should be monitored periodically. Phenytoin may also reduce amiodarone levels. Monitor closely for loss of therapeutic effects.

Beta Blockers, Calcium Ion Antagonists. Amiodarone should be used with caution in patients receiving beta-adrenergic blocking agents (e.g., propranolol, timolol, nadolol, pindolol) or calcium ion antagonists (e.g., diltiazem, verapamil, nifedipine) because of the possible potentiation of bradycardia, sinus arrest, and AV block. If necessary, amiodarone can be used after insertion of a pacemaker in patients with severe bradycardia or sinus arrest.

Theophylline. Amiodarone may increase theophylline serum levels, resulting in toxicity. Effects may not be observed until after at least 1 week of concurrent therapy. Toxicity may persist for more than 1 week after amiodarone has been discontinued.

DRUG CLASS: Beta-Adrenergic Blocking Agents

Actions

The beta-adrenergic blocking agents (e.g., acebutolol, esmolol, propranolol) are widely used as antidysrhythmic agents. These agents inhibit cardiac response to sympathetic nerve stimulation by blocking the beta receptors. As a result, the heart rate, systolic blood pressure, and cardiac output are reduced.

Uses

These agents are effective in the treatment of various ventricular dysrhythmias, sinus tachycardia, paroxysmal supraventricular tachycardia, premature ventricular contractions, and tachycardia associated with atrial flutter or fibrillation because atrioventricular conduction is diminished.

Therapeutic Outcomes

The primary therapeutic outcome expected from beta blocker therapy is conversion to and maintenance of normal sinus rhythm.

Nursing Process for Beta-Adrenergic Blocking Agents

See Chapter 13 for further discussion of nursing process associated with beta-adrenergic inhibition.

bretylium tosylate (bret il′ ee um tahs′ e layt)

▸ BRETYLOL (bret′ il ol)

Actions

Bretylium, an adrenergic blocking agent, inhibits the release of norepinephrine.

Uses

Bretylium is a class III antidysrhythmic agent used for short-term suppression of life-threatening ventricular dysrhythmias, primarily tachycardia and fibrillation, that have not responded to other widely used antidysrhythmic drugs. Bretylium is not a cardiac depressant, so it is particularly useful in patients with poor myocardial contractility and low cardiac output.

Therapeutic Outcomes

The primary therapeutic outcome expected from bretylium therapy is conversion of dysrhythmia to normal sinus rhythm.

Nursing Process for Bretylium Tosylate

Premedication Assessment

1. Obtain data relating to the six cardinal signs of cardiovascular disease to be used as a baseline for subsequent evaluation of response to therapy.
2. Schedule blood pressure readings at intervals appropriate to the patient's status.

Planning

Availability. IV: 50 mg/mL in 10-mL ampules, vials, and syringes; 2 mg/mL and 4 mg/mL in 250-mL containers of dextrose 5%.

Implementation

Dosage and Administration. For ventricular fibrillation after failure of electrical cardioversion, 5 mg/kg IV undiluted. Repeat cardioversion. If fibrillation persists, the dosage may be increased to 10 mg/kg and repeated every 15 to 30 minutes. Dosages up to 40 mg/kg/day have been reported. For other ventricular dysrhythmias, administer 5 to 10 mg/kg IV over 8 to 10 minutes. The dose may be repeated in 1 to 2 hours if the dysrhythmia persists. IV: Continuous infusion; recommended dosage is 1 to 2 mg/minute. IM: 5 to 10 mg/kg undiluted. Do not give more than 5 ml at one site. Dosage may be repeated in 1 to 2 hours if the dysrhythmia persists. Thereafter repeat every 6 to 8 hours. Observe injection site for signs of inflammation and necrosis.

Evaluation

Side Effects to Expect

Dizziness, Lightheadedness. These symptoms are transient and may be reduced by keeping the patient in a supine position. When changing positions, encourage the patient to move slowly and to lie down if feeling faint.

Hypertension, Hypotension. Transient hypertension followed by hypotension is often observed when therapy is initiated. Avoid the use of subtherapeutic doses (less than 5 mg/kg), because hypotension often occurs. Systolic blood pressures below 75 mm Hg may be treated with infusions of dopamine or norepinephrine. Initiate at low doses and titrate as needed based on frequent blood pressure readings.

Drug Interactions

Digoxin. Bretylium is not recommended in the treatment of dysrhythmias associated with digoxin toxicity. The sudden release of norepinephrine caused by the initiation of bretylium therapy may seriously aggravate the digitalis toxicity.

disopyramide (die so peer′ ah myd)
▶ NORPACE (nor′ pace)

Actions

Disopyramide is a class Ia antidysrhythmic agent.

Uses

Disopyramide is used to treat atrial fibrillation, Wolff-Parkinson-White syndrome, paroxysmal supraventricular tachycardia, premature ventricular tachycardia, and ventricular tachycardia. It may be used in both digitalized and nondigitalized patients. It is a useful drug alternative to quinidine or procainamide when patients develop an intolerance to or serious side effects from these agents.

Therapeutic Outcomes

The primary therapeutic outcome expected from disopyramide therapy is conversion of dysrhythmia to normal sinus rhythm.

Nursing Process for Disopyramide

Premedication Assessment

1. Obtain data relating to the six cardinal signs of cardiovascular disease to be used as a baseline for subsequent evaluation of response to therapy.
2. Assess usual pattern of urination and defecation.

Planning

Availability. PO: 100 and 150 mg capsules; 100 and 150 mg controlled release capsules.

Implementation

Dosage and Administration. PO: Dosage is individualized, but is usually 400 to 800 mg/day. Recommended adult dosage schedule is 150 mg every 6 hours. If body weight is less than 110 lb (50 kg), the recommended dose is 100 mg every 6 hours. Therapeutic blood level is 2 to 6 mg/L.

Evaluation

Side Effects to Expect

Dry Mouth, Nose, Throat. Suggest frequent mouth rinses or sucking on ice chips or hard candy to relieve symptoms.

Side Effects to Report

Myocardial Toxicity. Report bradycardia or increasing signs of heart failure. Monitoring of the ECG for various types of dysrhythmias may be indicated as ordered by the physician.

Urinary Hesitancy. Tell the patient that hesitancy in starting to urinate may occur. Suggest running tap water or immersing hands in water as means to stimulate urination. Report decreased urinary output and bladder distention. In the hospitalized patient, record input and output. Palpate the area of the symphysis pubis to assess for distention.

Constipation with Distention and Flatus. Report difficulties in defecation to the physician. Assess distention by measuring abdominal girth, as appropriate. Assess ability to expel flatus.

Drug Interactions

Drugs That Enhance Therapeutic and Toxic Effects. Procainamide, quinidine, digoxin, erythromycin, and beta-adrenergic blocking agents (e.g., propranolol, atenolol, timolol). Monitor for increases in severity of drug effects such as bradycardia and hypotension.

Drugs That Reduce Therapeutic Effects. Phenytoin, barbiturates, glutethimide, primidone, and rifampin. Monitor for an increase in frequency of the patient's dysrhythmia.

Drugs That Increase Hypotensive Effects. Diuretics and antihypertensive agents. Instruct patients to rise slowly from a supine position. If symptoms become more severe, report to the health care provider.

flecainide acetate (fleh kayn′ ayd)
▶ TAMBOCOR (tam boh′ kor)

Actions

Flecainide acetate is a class Ic antidysrhythmic agent that may be taken orally.

Uses

Flecainide may be used in the treatment of sustained ventricular tachycardia, nonsustained ventricular tachycardia, paroxysmal supraventricular tachyarrhythmia, and frequent premature ventricular contractions. Flecainide is usually used for more serious ventricular dysrhythmias that have not responded to more traditional therapy. In addition to its therapeutic activity, a particular advantage is its twice daily dosing schedule. Flecainide has a negative inotropic effect and may cause or worsen heart failure, particularly in patients with preexisting severe heart failure. This adverse effect may take hours to months to develop. New or worsened heart failure occurs in approximately 5% of patients. Flecainide may also aggravate an existing dysrhythmia and precipitate new ones, especially in patients with underlying heart disease.

Therapeutic Outcomes

The primary therapeutic outcome expected from flecainide therapy is conversion of dysrhythmia to normal sinus rhythm.

Nursing Process for Flecainide

Premedication Assessment

1. Obtain data relating to the six cardinal signs of cardiovascular disease to be used as a baseline for subsequent evaluation of response to therapy.
2. If any symptoms of heart failure are present, notify the health care provider before starting therapy.

Planning

Availability. PO: 50, 100, and 150 mg tablets.

Implementation

Dosage and Administration. NOTE: Flecainide should not be used in patients with second- or third-degree atrioventricular block in the absence of an artificial ventricular pacemaker and must be used with caution in patients with known heart failure. Monitor the ECG before and during initiation of therapy. Adult: Sustained ventricular tachycardia: PO: Initially, 100 mg every 12 hours; increase in 50 mg increments twice daily every 4 days. Most patients respond at 150 mg twice daily. Maximum daily dose is 400 mg.

Evaluation

Side Effects to Expect. The more frequent adverse effects that occur with flecainide therapy are dizziness, lightheadedness, faintness, and unsteadiness (19%); visual disturbances such as blurred vision, difficulty in focusing, and spots before the eyes (16%); dyspnea (1%); headache (10%); nausea (9%); fatigue (8%); constipation (5%); edema (3%); and abdominal pain.

Dizziness, Headache, Constipation, Nausea. These side effects are usually mild and tend to resolve with continued therapy. Encourage the patient not to discontinue therapy without first consulting a health care provider.

Side Effects to Report

Visual Disturbances. Provide for patient safety during temporary visual impairment. Caution the patient to temporarily avoid any tasks that require visual acuity, such as driving or operating power machinery. Instruct the patient not to rub the eyes with force when tearing. These side effects are usually mild and tend to resolve with continued therapy. Encourage the patient not to discontinue therapy without first consulting the health care provider.

Increasing Dyspnea, Exercise Intolerance, Edema. Flecainide may induce or aggravate preexisting heart failure. If these symptoms become more pronounced, the patient should be instructed to contact the health care provider for further evaluation.

Dysrhythmias. Flecainide may induce or aggravate preexisting dysrhythmias. The patient should be instructed to contact the health care provider for further evaluation if sensations of a "jumping" or "racing" heart develop.

Drug Interactions

Drugs That Enhance Therapeutic and Toxic Effects. Amiodarone, cimetidine, verapamil, and disopyramide. Monitor for increases of drug effects such as dysrhythmias, heart failure, and bradycardia.

Digoxin. When multiple doses of flecainide are administered to patients stabilized on a dose of digoxin, there is a 10% to 20% increase in serum digoxin concentrations. This increase may result in signs of digitalis toxicity, such as anorexia, nausea, fatigue, blurred or colored vision, bradycardia, and dysrhythmias. Monitor serum digoxin levels, ECG readings, and the clinical course of the patient closely.

Propranolol. When flecainide and propranolol are administered concurrently, there is a 20% increase in serum flecainide levels and a 30% increase in propranolol levels, with additive pharmacologic effects from each. Monitor serum levels, ECG readings, and the clinical course of the patient closely. Dosage reductions of either one or both agents may be required.

Urinary Acidifiers. These agents (e.g., ascorbic acid, ammonium chloride) may lower the urine pH, causing an increase in the urinary excretion of flecainide. Patients should be observed for redevelopment of dysrhythmias, which may require an increase in dosage of flecainide.

lidocaine (li′ do kayn)
▶ XYLOCAINE (zi′ lo kayn)

Actions

Lidocaine is a class Ib agent.

Uses

Lidocaine is used in the treatment of premature ventricular contractions, ventricular tachycardia, and ventricular fibrillation.

Therapeutic Outcomes

The primary therapeutic outcome expected from lidocaine therapy is conversion of dysrhythmia to normal sinus rhythm.

Nursing Process for Lidocaine

Premedication Assessment

1. Obtain data relating to the six cardinal signs of cardiovascular disease to be used as a baseline for subsequent evaluation of response to therapy.
2. Assess and record data relating to the patient's basic mental status (e.g., orientation, agitation, confusion).

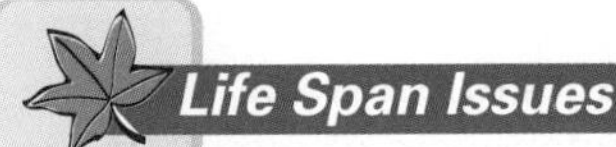

Life Span Issues

Lidocaine

Lidocaine for IV use to treat dysrhythmias, often used for older adults, is different from lidocaine used as a local anesthetic. For use with dysrhythmias, check the label carefully to ensure that it says "lidocaine (or Xylocaine) for cardiac dysrhythmia." Serious dysrhythmias may result if lidocaine with preservatives or lidocaine with epinephrine are administered intravenously to the patient.

3. Label the container for IV use: *Lidocaine for Dysrhythmia.*

Planning

Availability. IM: 300 mg per 3 mL; 10% (100 mg/mL) in 5-mL ampules. Direct IV: 1% (10 mg/mL) in 5-mL ampules and disposable syringes, and 20-, 30-, and 50-mL vials; 2% (20 mg/mL) in 5-mL disposable syringes and ampules, and 20-, 30-, and 50-mL vials. IV admixtures: 4% (40 mg/mL) in 5-mL ampules and 25- and 50-mL vials; 10% (100 mg/mL) in 10-mL additive vials; 20% (200 mg/mL) in 5-mL and 10-mL additive syringes, and 10-mL vials. IV infusion: 0.2% (2 mg/mL) in 500 and 1000 mL of 5% dextrose; 0.4% (4 mg/mL) in 250 and 500 mL of 5% dextrose; 0.8% (8 mg/mL) in 250 and 500 mL of 5% dextrose.

Implementation

Dosage and Administration. NOTE: Lidocaine for IV use for dysrhythmia is *different* from lidocaine used as a local anesthetic. For use with dysrhythmia, check the label carefully to be certain it says *Lidocaine for Dysrhythmia* or *Lidocaine without Preservatives.* Severe dysrhythmia could result if lidocaine with preservatives or lidocaine with epinephrine are administered to these patients. Lidocaine should *not* be used in patients with complete heart block.

Adult: IM: 200 to 300 mg in the deltoid muscle. The IM route should be used only in emergency situations until an IV can be established. IV: Initial dose (bolus) is 50 to 100 mg (1 mg/kg) at a rate of 25 to 50 mg per minute. Boluses of 50 to 100 mg may be given every 3 to 5 minutes until the desired effect is achieved or side effects appear. Do not exceed 300 mg by intermittent bolus. To maintain the antidysrhythmic effect, an IV infusion must be initiated. The usual rate of administration is 1 to 4 mg per minute. For routine lidocaine administration for cardiac dysrhythmias, add 50 mL of 40 mg/mL (2 g) of lidocaine to 5% dextrose. Therapeutic blood levels are 1 to 5 mg/L.

Pediatric: IV, initial bolus: 1 mg/kg up to 15 mg if under 25 kg (55 lb); up to 25 mg if over 25 kg (55 lb). Continuous infusion: 20 to 40 mcg/kg per minute (maximum total dose 5 mg/kg).

Evaluation

Side Effects to Report

Lightheadedness, Muscle Twitching, Hallucinations, Agitation, Euphoria. Monitor patients carefully for progressive symptoms of restlessness, agitation, anxiety, hallucinations, and euphoria.

Act calmly with the excited, anxious, or euphoric patient. Provide for safety and fulfillment of patient's needs. Report patient's alteration in response to the health care provider as soon as possible.

Respiratory Depression. Observe the rate and depth of respiratory effort. Monitor for cyanosis and increasing frequency of dysrhythmia.

Drug Interactions

Drugs That Enhance Therapeutic and Toxic Effects. Phenytoin, cimetidine, procainamide, tocainide and beta-adrenergic blocking agents (e.g., nadolol, atenolol, timolol, propranolol). Monitor for an increase in severity of side effects such as bradycardia and hypotension.

Neuromuscular Blocking Action. When lidocaine is administered in conjunction with succinylcholine, observe for respiratory depression. Patients who are on respirators may require additional time to be weaned off ventilatory assistance.

mexiletine (mehx ihl′ et een)
▶ MEXITIL (mehx it′ ihl)

Actions

Mexiletine is a class Ib antidysrhythmic agent similar in many respects to lidocaine.

Uses

Mexiletine has the advantage of good oral absorption with minimal initial hepatic metabolism, thus allowing it to be administered orally. Mexiletine can be effective therapy in the treatment of unifocal and multifocal premature ventricular contractions, couplets, and ventricular tachycardia but is usually ineffective in the therapy of drug-resistant ventricular tachycardia. It is usually more effective against drug-resistant ventricular tachycardia when used in combination with other antidysrhythmic agents.

Therapeutic Outcomes

The primary therapeutic outcome expected from mexiletine therapy is conversion of dysrhythmia to normal sinus rhythm.

Nursing Process for Mexiletine

Premedication Assessment

1. Obtain data relating to the six cardinal signs of cardiovascular disease to be used as a baseline for subsequent evaluation of response to therapy.

2. Record data relating to any GI symptoms present before initiation of therapy.
3. Assess and record data relating to the patient's mental status (e.g., orientation, agitation, confusion).

Planning

Availability. PO: 150-, 200-, and 250-mg capsules.

Implementation

Dosage and Administration. NOTE: Mexiletine should not be used in patients with second- or third-degree heart block if a pacemaker is not present. Dosage adjustment is necessary in patients with severe renal dysfunction (creatinine clearance less than 10 mL/min) and in patients with severe heart failure or acute MI.

PO: 200 to 400 mg every 8 hours, or 10 to 14 mg/kg/day.

Administration with food or antacids may minimize gastric irritation without significantly inhibiting absorption. If symptoms persist or increase in severity, report for health care provider evaluation.

Evaluation

Side Effects to Expect

Nausea, Vomiting, Dyspepsia. Mexiletine may cause GI adverse effects in approximately 40% of patients. These adverse effects are usually not serious and do not correlate well with high serum levels but are more prevalent with large orally administered doses.

Side Effects to Report

Dysrhythmias. Mexiletine may induce or aggravate dysrhythmias. This is uncommon in patients with less serious dysrhythmias, such as frequent, premature beats or nonsustained ventricular tachycardia. Patients with more serious dysrhythmias, such as sustained ventricular tachycardia, are more susceptible to myocardial toxicity.

Neurotoxicity, Seizures. Mexiletine has dose-related effects on the central nervous system (CNS). At higher serum levels (greater than 2.0 mcg/mL) mexiletine may precipitate neurologic toxicity and occasionally paradoxical seizure activity.

The initial manifestation of mexiletine neurotoxicity is usually a fine hand tremor, but ataxia, dizziness, lightheadedness, nystagmus, paresthesia, blurred vision, diplopia, dysarthria, confusion, and drowsiness are other signs of impending toxicity. Provide for patient safety during these episodes.

Confusion. Some patients have been reported to experience serious side effects such as seizures, severe ataxia, or mental confusion without manifestation of early warning signs. Perform a baseline assessment of the patient's degree of alertness and orientation to name, place, and time before starting therapy. Make regularly scheduled subsequent mental status evaluations and compare findings. Report development of alterations.

Drug Interactions

Drugs That Reduce Therapeutic Effects. Phenytoin, rifampin. The hepatic metabolism of mexiletine is enhanced by rifampin and phenytoin. Patients should be observed for redevelopment of dysrhythmia, which may require an increase in dosage of mexiletine.

Urinary Acidifiers. These agents (e.g., ascorbic acid, ammonium chloride) may lower the urine pH, causing an increase in the urinary excretion of mexiletine. Patients should be observed for redevelopment of dysrhythmia, which may require an increase in dosage of mexiletine.

moricizine (mor is′ ih zeen)

▶ ETHMOZINE (eth moh′ zeen)

Actions

Moricizine is an antidysrhythmic agent chemically unrelated to other medicines used to treat dysrhythmias. It acts by inhibition of influx of sodium ions into myocardial cells, slowing conduction velocity. It is classified as a type Ic antidysrhythmic, but it demonstrates characteristics of the other type I agents.

Uses

Moricizine is used for the treatment of life-threatening ventricular dysrhythmias. Because of its ability to cause additional dysrhythmia, its use is reserved for those patients in whom the benefits outweigh the potential risks.

Therapeutic Outcomes

The primary therapeutic outcome expected from moricizine therapy is conversion of dysrhythmia to normal sinus rhythm.

Nursing Process for Moricizine

Premedication Assessment

1. Obtain data relating to the six cardinal signs of cardiovascular disease to be used as a baseline for subsequent evaluation of response to therapy.
2. Record data relating to any GI symptoms present before initiation of therapy.
3. Assess and record data relating to the patient's mental status (e.g., orientation, agitation, confusion).

Planning

Availability. PO: 200, 250, and 300 mg tablets.

Implementation

Dosage and Administration. PO: Initially, 200 mg every 8 hours. Dosages may be adjusted every 3 days in increments of 150 mg per day. The usual adult dosage is between 600 and 900 mg daily. Administer in divided doses around the clock. If gastric irritation is a problem, administer with food or milk.

Evaluation

Side Effects to Expect

Hypotension, Dizziness. These may occur, particularly during initiation of therapy. They usually subside within a few days. Instruct the patient to rise slowly from a supine position. Monitor the patient's blood pressure.

Nausea. GI complaints occur in about 10% of patients, but discontinuation of therapy is rarely required. Administer with food or milk to alleviate nausea. Encourage the patient not to discontinue therapy without first consulting a health care provider.

Side Effects to Report

Dysrhythmias. Moricizine may induce or aggravate dysrhythmias. Patients with more serious dysrhythmias such as sustained ventricular tachycardia are more susceptible to myocardial toxicity. The patient should be instructed to contact the health care provider for further evaluation if sensations of a jumping or "racing" heart develop.

Euphoria, Confusion. Perform a baseline assessment of the patient's degree of alertness and orientation to name, place, and time before starting therapy. Make regularly scheduled subsequent mental status evaluations and compare findings. Report development of alterations. Provide for patient safety during episodes of dizziness. After discharge, caution the patient about operating machinery or driving if dizziness, euphoria, or confusion is a recurrent problem.

Drug Interactions

Drugs That Enhance Therapeutic and Toxic Effects. Digoxin, cimetidine, and propranolol. Monitor for an increase in severity of side effects such as emesis, lethargy, hypotension, dysrhythmias, and bradycardia.

Theophylline. Moricizine, when given with theophylline, may result in theophylline toxicity. Observe for vomiting, dizziness, restlessness, and cardiac dysrhythmias. Monitor theophylline serum levels. The dosage of theophylline may have to be reduced.

procainamide hydrochloride (pro kane' ah myd)
PROCANBID (pro kahn' bid)

Actions

Procainamide is an effective synthetic class Ia antidysrhythmic agent that has many cardiac effects similar to those of quinidine but generally with fewer side effects.

Uses

Procainamide is used to treat a wide variety of ventricular and supraventricular dysrhythmias, atrial fibrillation, and flutter. It is usually not as effective in the last two disorders as quinidine.

Therapeutic Outcomes

The primary therapeutic outcome expected from procainamide therapy is conversion of dysrhythmia to normal sinus rhythm.

Nursing Process for Procainamide

Premedication Assessment

Obtain data relating to the six cardinal signs of cardiovascular disease to be used as a baseline for subsequent evaluation of response to therapy.

Planning

Availability. PO: 250, 375, and 500 mg capsules; 250, 500, 750, and 1000 mg sustained release tablets. IV: 500 mg/mL in 2 mL vials.

Implementation

Dosage and Administration. NOTE: Do not use in complete atrioventricular (AV) block, and use with extreme caution in partial AV block. *Adult:* PO, loading dose: 1 to 1.25 g; follow with 750 mg 1 hour later if the dysrhythmia is still present. Maintain the dosage at 0.5 to 1 g every 4 to 6 hours. Some patients may require maintenance doses every 3 to 4 hours to maintain adequate control of dysrhythmias. Administer in divided doses around the clock. If gastric irritation is a problem, administer with food or milk. IM: 0.5 to 1 g every 6 hours until PO therapy is possible. IV: 100 mg every 5 minutes at 25 to 50 mg/min until the dysrhythmia is suppressed, a maximum of 1 g has been administered, or side effects develop.

Patients should have ECG and blood pressure monitoring when receiving intravenous doses of procainamide. Once the dysrhythmia is suppressed, a continuous infusion may be started at 25 to 30 mg/kg/min. If dysrhythmia recurs, suppress the dysrhythmia with bolus therapy as above and increase the rate of infusion.

Serum levels of procainamide are performed to measure the amount of procainamide in the bloodstream. Blood should be drawn before the daily dose of medication or at least 6 hours after administration. It is important to be consistent in the time of drawing the blood and administering the dose if more than one serum level is to be drawn in the same patient. Therapeutic blood levels are 4 to 8 mg/L.

Evaluation

Side Effects to Expect

Drowsiness, Sedation, Dizziness. Tell patients they may experience these symptoms early in therapy, as the dosage is being adjusted. Instruct patients to use caution in operating power equipment or driving.

Hypotension. Hypotension may be observed while therapy is being initiated, particularly by the IV route. Hypotension is usually transient and can be avoided by rising slowly from supine and sitting positions.

Side Effects to Report

Fever, Chills, Joint and Muscle Pain, Skin Eruptions. Tell patients to report the development of these symptoms. Monitor laboratory reports for leukocyte counts and the antinuclear antibody (ANA) titer.

Drug Interactions

Drugs That Enhance Therapeutic and Toxic Effects. Digoxin, cimetidine, ranitidine, quinidine, trimethoprim, and beta-adrenergic blocking agents (e.g., timolol, nadolol, propranolol). Monitor for an increase in severity of side effects such as bradycardia and hypotension.

Neuromuscular Blockade, Respiratory Depression. Surgical muscle relaxants (tubocurarine and succinylcholine) and aminoglycoside antibiotics (e.g., gentamicin, streptomycin, amikacin, kanamycin, netilmicin). Monitor the patient's respiratory rate and depth. Observe for signs of cyanosis and additional dysrhythmia.

Patients who are on respirators may require additional time to be weaned off ventilatory assistance.

Hypotension with Diuretics and Antihypertensive Agents. Instruct patients to rise slowly from a supine position. If symptoms begin to recur more frequently, report to the physician.

propafenone (pro pah' fen own)
RYTHMOL (rith' mohl)

Actions

Propafenone is classified as a class 1c antidysrhythmic agent. It also has weak beta-blocking and calcium channel blocking effects.

Uses

Propafenone is used for the treatment of paroxysmal atrial fibrillation and life-threatening ventricular dysrhythmias such as ventricular tachycardia. Because of its ability to cause additional dysrhythmias, its use is reserved for those patients in whom the benefits outweigh the potential risks.

Therapeutic Outcomes

The primary therapeutic outcome expected from propafenone therapy is conversion of dysrhythmia to normal sinus rhythm.

Nursing Process for Propafenone

Premedication Assessment

1. Obtain data relating to the six cardinal signs of cardiovascular disease to be used as a baseline for subsequent evaluation of response to therapy.
2. Record data relating to any GI symptoms present before initiation of therapy.

Planning

Availability. PO: 150, 225, and 300 mg tablets; 225, 325, and 425 extended release capsules.

Implementation

Dosage and Administration. NOTE: Because propafenone has mild beta-adrenergic blocking properties, it should not be used in patients with asthma. PO: Initially, 150 mg every 8 hours. At 3- or 4-day intervals the dosage may be increased to 225 mg every 8 hours, then 300 mg every 8 hours (900 mg/day).

Administer in divided doses around the clock. If a patient misses a dose of propafenone, the next dose should not be doubled because of an increased risk of adverse reactions.

Evaluation

Side Effects to Expect

Dizziness. This may occur, particularly during initiation of therapy. It usually subsides within a few days. Instruct the patient to rise slowly from a supine position. Monitor the patient's blood pressure.

Nausea, Vomiting, Constipation. GI complaints occur in approximately 11% of patients, but discontinuation of therapy is rarely required. Administer with food or milk to alleviate nausea. Encourage the patient not to discontinue therapy without first consulting a health care provider.

Side Effects to Report

Dysrhythmias. Propafenone may induce or aggravate dysrhythmias. Patients with more serious dysrhythmias such as sustained ventricular tachycardia are more susceptible to myocardial toxicity. The patient should be instructed to contact the health care provider for further evaluation if sensations of a jumping or "racing" heart develop.

Drug Interactions

Drugs That Enhance Therapeutic and Toxic Effects. Quinidine and cimetidine. Monitor for an increase in severity of side effects from propafenone such as hypotension, somnolence, bradycardia, and dysrhythmias.

Drugs That Decrease Therapeutic Effects. Rifampin. Monitor patients with concurrent therapy for increased frequency of dysrhythmias.

Digoxin. Propafenone produces dose-related increases in serum digoxin levels. Measure plasma digoxin levels and reduce digoxin dosage when propafenone is started.

Propranolol, Metoprolol. Propafenone appears to inhibit the metabolism of these beta blockers. A reduction in beta blocker dosage may be necessary during concurrent therapy with propafenone.

Warfarin. Propafenone increases plasma warfarin concentrations by inhibiting warfarin metabolism, thus prolonging prothrombin time. Observe for the development of petechiae, ecchymoses, nosebleeds, bleeding gums, dark tarry stools, and bright red or "coffee-ground" emesis. Monitor the prothrombin time (INR) and reduce the dosage of warfarin if necessary.

quinidine (kwin' i deen)

Actions

Quinidine, originally obtained from cinchona bark, has been used as an antidysrhythmic agent for several decades. It is classified as a class 1a antidysrhythmic agent, working on the muscle of the heart and stabilizing the rate of conduction of impulses. It slows the heart and changes a rapid, irregular pulse to a slow, regular pulse.

Uses

Quinidine is used most often to suppress atrial fibrillation, atrial flutter, paroxysmal supraventricular and ventricular tachycardia, and premature ventricular contractions. Use with extreme caution in patients with digitalis intoxication or heart block.

Therapeutic Outcomes

The primary therapeutic outcome expected from quinidine therapy is conversion of dysrhythmia to normal sinus rhythm.

Nursing Process for Quinidine

Premedication Assessment

1. Obtain data relating to the six cardinal signs of cardiovascular disease to be used as a baseline for subsequent evaluation of response to therapy.
2. Assess and record data relating to the patient's usual pattern of bowel elimination.

Planning

Availability. *Quinidine sulfate:* PO: 200 and 300 mg tablets; 300 mg sustained release tablets. *Quinidine gluconate:* PO: 324 mg sustained release tablets; IM, IV, 80 mg/mL in 10-mL vials.

Implementation

Dosage and Administration. *Adult:* Quinidine sulfate: PO: 200 to 400 mg three to five times daily. Higher doses may be used, but the maximum single dose should not exceed 600 to 800 mg. Administer with food or milk if gastric irritation develops. Quinidine gluconate: IM: 600 mg initially, then 400 mg every 2 hours as needed. Quinidine gluconate: IV: 800 mg diluted to 40 mL with 5% dextrose and infused at a rate of 1 mL/minute. NOTE: IV administration is *extremely hazardous*. Blood pressure and ECG readings should be monitored continuously because hypotension and dysrhythmia may occur. Therapeutic blood levels are 1.5 to 3 mg/L.

Pediatric: Quinidine sulfate: PO: 30 mg/kg per 24 hours divided into four to six doses. Quinidine gluconate: IM: as for PO administration.

Serum levels of quinidine are performed to measure the amount of quinidine in the bloodstream. Blood should be drawn before the daily dose of medication is given or at least 6 hours after administration. It is important to be consistent in the time of drawing the blood and administering the dose if more than one serum level is to be drawn in the same patient.

Evaluation

Side Effects to Expect

Diarrhea. Diarrhea is common during initiation of therapy. It usually subsides, but occasionally a different medication may need to be administered because of this adverse effect. Chart the frequency and consistency of the diarrhea, and monitor the patient for dehydration and electrolyte imbalance.

Dizziness, Faintness. This may occur, particularly during initiation of therapy. They usually subside within a few days. Instruct the patient to rise slowly from a supine position. Monitor the patient's blood pressure.

Side Effects to Report

Cinchonism. Monitor patients for signs of *cinchonism* and report the development of rash, chills, fever, ringing in the ears (tinnitus), and increasing mental confusion.

Hypotension with Diuretics and Antihypertensive Agents. Instruct the patient to rise slowly from a supine position. If symptoms become excessive, report to the health care provider.

Drug Interactions

Drugs That Enhance Therapeutic and Toxic Effects. Cimetidine, phenothiazines, procainamide, digoxin, verapamil, amiodarone, and beta-adrenergic blocking agents (e.g., propranolol, atenolol, timolol). Monitor for increases in severity of drug effects such as bradycardia, tachycardia, and hypotension.

Drugs That Reduce Therapeutic Effects. Rifampin, barbiturates, nifedipine, phenytoin, sucralfate, and disopyramide. Monitor for an increase in dysrhythmia.

Neuromuscular Blockade, Respiratory Depression. Quinidine may prolong the effects of the surgical muscle relaxants (e.g., tubocurarine, succinylcholine) and aminoglycoside antibiotics (e.g., gentamicin, streptomycin, kanamycin, netilmicin). Monitor the patient's respiratory rate and depth. Observe for signs of cyanosis and additional dysrhythmias.

Patients who are on respirators may require additional time to be weaned from ventilatory assistance.

Digoxin. Quinidine may increase the effects of digoxin. Monitor the patient for symptoms of anorexia, nausea, vomiting, headaches, blurred or colored vision, and bradycardia. A digoxin serum level and quinidine serum level may be ordered by the health care provider.

Warfarin. Quinidine may increase the anticoagulant effects of warfarin. Monitor for signs of increased bleeding: bleeding gums, increased menstrual flow, petechiae, and bruises.

Monitor the laboratory report and notify the physician immediately if the prothrombin time or the internationalized ratio (INR) is abnormally high.

Key Points

- Dysrhythmias are complex in origin, severity, and treatment for control.
- Many of the agents used to treat dysrhythmias have serious adverse effects and must be monitored closely.
- Nurses need to check references carefully in advance of administering these drugs for the correct method of preparation, preadministration assessments needed, rate of administration of drugs given IV, and monitoring parameters essential during drug administration.
- Nurses can play a significant role in public education efforts, monitor patient response to therapy, monitor for noncompliance, and encourage patients to participate in their own therapy.

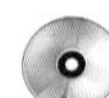

Go to your Companion CD-ROM for Appendices, an Audio Glossary, animations, Drug Dosage Calculators, customizable Patient Self-Assessment forms, and Review Questions for the NCLEX® Examination.

evolve Be sure to visit the companion Evolve site at http://evolve.elsevier.com/Clayton for WebLinks and additional online resources.

MEDICATION SAFETY REVIEW

MATH REVIEW

1. Order: Quinidine 0.8 g PO TID.
   Available: Quinidine 200-mg tablets.
   Give: ____ tablets per dose.
   Give: ____ total grams in 24 hours.
2. Order: Procainamide hydrochloride (Pronestyl) 1 g q6h.
   Available: Procainamide hydrochloride (Pronestyl) 250-mg capsules.
   Give: ____ capsules per dose.
3. Order: Adenosine 12 mg IV
   Available: Adenosine 3 mg/mL
   Give: ____ mL

CRITICAL THINKING QUESTIONS

Situation: Adenosine (Adenocard) 6 mg IV bolus was given stat to a patient being treated in the emergency room today for paroxysmal supraventricular tachycardia. The instructor discusses this case with the student nurses. Using any reference book, answer the following questions:

1. What is the normal conduction of impulses through the heart?
2. What is paroxysmal supraventricular tachycardia, and why is this dangerous to the patient?
3. The instructor requests the students to look up the following information for the drug adenosine:
   Drug action:
   Dosage:
   Preparation of drug for IV use:
   Dilution: Yes No
   Solutions that can be used to dilute the IV medication:
   Rate of administration:
   Incompatibility:
   Side effects to expect/report:

Situation: The health care provider orders quinidine sulfate 200 mg PO TID.

4. What time schedule would be used to fulfill this order? When a quinidine serum level is ordered, based on the time schedule established, when would the laboratory draw the blood sample?
5. What nursing assessments should be made during the administration of quinidine sulfate? What health teaching should be done?

Situation: The health care provider orders disopyramide (Norpace) 150 mg PO q6h.

6. What time schedule would be used to administer the drug?
7. After a week of therapy the therapeutic blood level report from the laboratory is 8 mg/L. What nursing actions should be initiated?

CONTENT REVIEW QUESTIONS

1. A patient taking disopyramide (Norpace) develops a productive cough. The nurse should:
   1. disregard the symptom.
   2. perform a respiratory assessment.
   3. call the physician for an increase in dosage.
   4. check daily laboratory clotting test results.
2. Adenosine (Adenocard) is ordered for the patient; the nurse knows this drug must be administered with ______ only.
   1. 1.5% dextrose and water
   2. 5% dextrose and 0.9% sodium chloride
   3. 0.9% sodium chloride
   4. May be given with any other drug or IV solution
3. The health care provider asks you to get lidocaine for use in the treatment of a patient with a heart irregularity. You would select:
   1. 1% lidocaine with epinephrine.
   2. 2% lidocaine with epinephrine.
   3. 1% lidocaine.
   4. lidocaine for cardiac dysrhythmias.
4. When administering quinidine the nurse should be aware that the drug may increase the effects of which two drugs?
   1. Digoxin and warfarin
   2. Propranolol and warfarin
   3. Cimetidine and theophylline
   4. Prednisone and theophylline
5. Which of the following is true about amiodarone? *(Select all that may apply.)*
   1. Amiodarone is used for the treatment of life-threatening supraventricular tachyarrhythmias.
   2. It can be used in patients with heart block.
   3. Patients should be hospitalized when treatment is initiated.
   4. GI complaints occur in 25% of patients.
6. If the Purkinje system is damaged, conduction of the electrical impulse is impaired through the:
   1. atria.
   2. AV node.
   3. ventricles.
   4. bundle of His.

CHAPTER

25 Drugs Used to Treat Angina Pectoris

evolve http://evolve.elsevier.com/Clayton

Chapter Content

Objectives

1. Describe the actions of nitrates, beta-adrenergic blockers, calcium channel blockers, and angiotensin-converting enzyme inhibitors on the myocardial tissue of the heart.
2. Explain the rationale for the use of HMG-CoA reductase inhibitors (statins) to treat anginal attacks.
3. Identify assessment data needed to evaluate an anginal attack.
4. Implement medication therapy health teaching for an anginal patient in the clinical setting.

Key Terms

angina pectoris
ischemic heart disease
chronic stable angina
unstable angina
variant angina

ANGINA PECTORIS

Coronary heart disease (CAD) is the leading cause of disability, socioeconomic loss, and death in the United States, and angina pectoris is the first clinical indication of underlying disease in many patients. **Angina pectoris** is the name given to a feeling of chest discomfort arising from the heart because of lack of oxygen to heart cells. It is a symptom of coronary artery disease, also called ischemic heart disease. **Ischemic heart disease** develops when the supply of oxygen needed by heart cells is inadequate. The lack of oxygen is caused by reduced blood flow through the coronary arteries caused by atherosclerosis or spasm of the arteries. Atherosclerosis can develop as localized plaques or as a generalized narrowing of the coronary arteries. Patients are usually asymptomatic until there is at least 50% narrowing of the artery. Coronary artery disease caused by atherosclerosis is a progressive disease; however, progression can be slowed by diet control and by use of cholesterol-lowering agents (see Chapter 22).

The presentation of angina pectoris is highly variable. The sensation of discomfort is often described variously as a squeezing, tightness, choking, pressure, burning, or heaviness. This discomfort may radiate to the neck, lower jaw, shoulder, and arm. The usual anginal attack begins gradually, reaches peak intensity over the next several minutes, and then gradually subsides after the person stops activity and rests. Attacks can last from 30 seconds to 30 minutes. Anginal episodes are usually precipitated by factors that require an increased oxygen supply (e.g., physical activity such as climbing a flight of stairs or lifting). Other precipitating factors include exposure to cold temperatures, emotional stress, sexual intercourse, and eating a large meal.

Angina pectoris is classified as chronic stable, unstable, or variant angina. **Chronic stable angina** is precipitated by physical exertion or stress, lasts only a few minutes, and is relieved by rest or nitroglycerin. It is usually caused by fixed atherosclerotic obstruction in the coronary arteries. **Unstable angina** is unpredictable; it changes in ease of onset, frequency, duration, and intensity. It is probably caused by a combination of atherosclerotic narrowing, vasospasm, and thrombus formation. **Variant angina** occurs while the patient is at rest, is characterized by specific electrocardiographic changes, and is caused by vasospasm of a coronary artery reducing blood flow. The type of angina pectoris is diagnosed by a combination of history, electrocardiographic changes during an anginal attack, and exercise tolerance testing with or without thallium-201 scintigraphy.

TREATMENT OF ANGINA PECTORIS

The goals in treating angina pectoris are to prevent myocardial infarction and death, thereby prolonging life, and to relieve anginal pain symptoms, improving the quality of life. In many cases, coronary angioplasty or coronary artery bypass surgery will first be considered because they have been proven to save lives over time. The choice of therapy often depends on the clinical response to initial medical therapy.

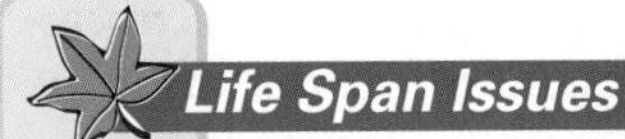

Life Span Issues

Anginal Attacks

The goal of treatment of an anginal attack, which most often occurs in older adults, is relief of pain, not simply a reduction of pain. If pain relief is not achieved with the use of nitroglycerin, the patient should immediately contact the health care provider or be seen in the emergency department. Do not administer analgesics in an attempt to eliminate the pain.

All patients should receive extensive patient education to help them reduce the risks of coronary artery disease. Avoidance of activities that can precipitate attacks (e.g., strenuous exercise, exposure to cold weather, drinking caffeine-containing beverages, cigarette smoking, eating heavy meals, and emotional stress) should be attempted. Risk factors, such as diabetes mellitus, hypertension, and dyslipidemia, must also be treated. A structured exercise program designed for each patient can be successful in weight reduction in overweight patients and improving cardiovascular health. Healthy muscle tissue requires less oxygen. Medications are effective in preventing ischemic attacks and myocardial infarction.

DRUG THERAPY FOR ANGINA PECTORIS

Actions

The underlying pathophysiology of ischemic heart disease is an imbalance between the oxygen demands of the heart and the ability of coronary arteries to deliver the oxygen, spasticity of coronary arteries, platelet aggregation, and thrombus formation. The oxygen demand of the heart is determined by the heart rate, contractility, and ventricular volume. Therefore the pharmacologic treatment of angina is aimed at decreasing oxygen demand by decreasing heart rate, myocardial contractility, and ventricular volume without inducing heart failure. Because platelet aggregation, blood flow turbulence, and blood viscosity also play a role, especially in unstable angina, platelet-active agents are also prescribed to prevent anginal attacks (see Chapter 27). Because atherosclerosis causes narrowing and closure of coronary arteries, inducing angina and myocardial infarction, the use of the HMG-CoA reductase inhibitors (statins) has also become standard therapy in treating angina pectoris (see Chapter 22).

Uses

Six groups of drugs may be used to treat angina pectoris: nitrates, beta-adrenergic blocking agents, angiotensin-converting enzyme (ACE) inhibitors, calcium ion antagonists, statins, and platelet-active agents. Combination therapy is beneficial in many patients.

Drug therapy for patients with angina must be individualized. Most patients will be given prescriptions (e.g., nitroglycerin sublingual tablets or translingual spray) for treating acute attacks and prescriptions for therapy to prevent further ischemia and myocardial infarction (and possible death). Therapy to prevent myocardial infarction consists of the statins to lower low-density lipoprotein (LDL) cholesterol levels and reduce inflammation, platelet aggregation, thrombus formation, and an ACE inhibitor that helps dilate coronary blood vessels and reduce thrombus formation. The most effective agents for relieving ischemia and angina are beta blockers, calcium ion antagonists, and nitrates. A new drug, ranolazine, a fatty oxidase enzyme inhibitor, modifies metabolism within the myocardial cells to reduce oxygen demand of the contracting heart muscles, thus reducing symptoms of angina. The decision of which medicine to use depends on other conditions the patient may have and the expected adverse effects of therapy. Aspirin, clopidogrel, or ticlopidine (see Chapter 27), which are platelet-active agents, may also be considered to slow platelet aggregation.

NURSING PROCESS *for Anginal Therapy*

Assessment

History of Anginal Attacks. Ask specific questions to identify the onset, duration, and intensity of the pain. Ask the patient to describe the chest sensation and the pattern of occurrence (e.g., under the sternum; in the jaw, neck, and shoulder; radiation down left arm, right arm, or both; into the wrist, hand, and fingers). What activities precipitate an attack? Does the pain occur with or without exertion? Is the pain relieved by rest? Does the chest pain occur shortly after eating? Does the individual experience fatigue, shortness of breath, indigestion, or nausea in relation to the anginal attack?

Medication History

- What medications, prescription and nonprescription, are being taken? Does the patient take any herbal or dietary supplements? What medications are being used for the treatment of the angina? What effect does taking nitroglycerin have on the anginal pain? How many nitroglycerin tablets are required to obtain pain relief during an attack? How many nitroglycerin tablets are being taken per day? How old is the nitroglycerin being used sublingually? Is it stored properly?
- Have the prescribed medications been taken regularly? If not, determine reasons for nonadherence.

Central Nervous System

- *Mental status:* Identify the individual's level of consciousness and clarity of thought. Check for orientation to date, time, and place, as well as level of confusion, restlessness, or irritability. Ask the patient if he or she has noticed any changes in

memory or level of awareness. These factors are indicators of cerebral perfusion.
- *Syncope:* Ask the patient to describe the conditions surrounding any episodes of syncope. Record the degree of presenting symptoms, such as general mental weakness, inability to stand upright, feeling faint, or loss of consciousness. Record what activities, if any, bring on these episodes.
- *Anxiety:* What degree of apprehension is present? Did stressful events precipitate the attack?

Cardiovascular System
- *Palpitations:* Record the patient's description of palpitations, such as "my heart skips some beats" or "it began to feel as if it were racing." Ask if these conditions are preceded by mild or strenuous exercise and how long the palpitations last.
- *Heart rate:* Count and record the rate, rhythm, and quality of the pulse.
- *Blood pressure:* Record the blood pressure. It may be increased or decreased during an attack. Compare with previous baseline readings.
- *Respirations:* The patient may be dyspneic. Ask whether the attack occurred while at rest or during exertion.
- *Cardiovascular history:* What concurrent cardiovascular disease does the patient have (e.g., hypertension, dyslipidemia)?
- *Peripheral perfusion:* Check for peripheral perfusion by taking pedal pulses and checking skin color and temperature. Check hair pattern on feet and lower legs.
- *Smoking:* Does the patient smoke? How much? Does the patient understand the effects of smoking on the cardiovascular system?

Nutritional History
- *Diet:* Is the patient on a special diet (e.g., low sodium, low fat)? Is the patient being treated for high cholesterol? Does eating cause fatigue or shortness of breath?
- *Fluids:* Does the patient have any edema, especially in the ankles?

Nursing Diagnoses
- Pain, acute (indication)
- Tissue perfusion, ineffective (indication)
- Activity intolerance related to myocardial ischemia (indication)
- Injury, risk for (side effects)
- Lifestyle, sedentary (risk factor)

Planning

History of Anginal Attacks. Review the history of anginal attacks to identify precipitating factors. Work with the patient to plan interventions that will minimize factors that trigger attacks.

As ordered by the health care provider, complete requisitions and establish patient teaching needed to implement tests that may be ordered (e.g., stress electrocardiogram [ECG], echocardiogram, nuclear scan of the heart's function, and blood studies including lipid profile and cardiac enzymes). Mutually establish goals with the patient to alter risk factors that are modifiable.

Medication History. Review medications being taken and establish whether they are being taken correctly. Analyze nonadherence issues, and plan interventions with the patient. Plan to review drug administration as needed.

Central Nervous System. Plan for stress reduction education and discussion of effective means of coping with stressful events.

Cardiovascular System. Identify the degree of cardiovascular symptoms produced by the anginal attack. Develop a plan to intervene to improve tissue oxygenation and provide for patient safety. Ask what, if any, activities of daily living (ADLs) have been altered to cope with the symptoms.

Take vital signs and include an assessment of the individual's pain rating.

Nutritional History. Examine the dietary history to establish whether a referral to a nutritionist would benefit the individual's understanding of the diet regimen. Plan interventions needed to deal with dietary nonadherence.

Implementation
- Adequate tissue perfusion is essential. Instruct the patient to take measures to avoid fatigue and cold weather, which can cause vasoconstriction, and provide for personal safety when symptoms of hypoxia are present (e.g., lightheadedness, dyspnea, chest pain).
- When pain is present, comfort measures and prescribed pain medications must be implemented to allow the individual to decrease the pain. Fatigue may increase pain perception; spacing activities so that fatigue does not occur is recommended. Administer oxygen as prescribed and check oxygen saturation.

For medication administration see individual monographs.

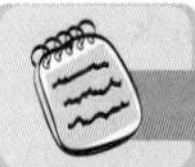

Patient Education and Health Promotion

Medications
- Teach the signs and symptoms of hypotension, which may occur when nitrates are taken. Weakness, dizziness, or faintness can usually be relieved by increasing muscular activity (alternately flexing and relaxing muscles in legs) or by sitting or lying down. Resting for 10 to 15 minutes after taking medication may also assist in managing hypotension. Because lightheadedness or fainting is a possibility when taking nitroglycerin, safety measures to prevent injury from the transient orthostatic hypotension must be stressed.

- Explain that a headache may occur with the use of nitroglycerin, but it should subside within 20 to 30 minutes.
- Teach specific administration techniques to the patient for the type of medication prescribed, for example, sublingual, transmucosal tablets, translingual spray, topical ointment, and transdermal disks.

Lifestyle Modifications

- Lifestyle modifications are essential for many individuals with angina. Teach appropriate behavioral changes, such as stress management (e.g., relaxation techniques, meditation, three-part breathing).
- The patient must resume ADLs within the boundaries set by the health care provider. Encourage activities such as regular moderate exercise; meal preparation; resumption of usual sexual activity; and social interactions.
- Individuals unable to attain the degree of activity hoped for through drug therapy may become frustrated. Allow for verbalization of feelings, and then implement actions appropriate to the circumstances.
- Participation in regular exercise is essential. Follow guidelines of the American Heart Association regarding an exercise program. Increase exercise demands gradually, and monitor effects on the cardiovascular system. Changes in the level of exercise may require participation in a supervised program, that is, cardiac rehabilitation. Tell the patient to avoid overexertion. Anginal pain may occur with exercise, and taking nitroglycerin before exercise or performing certain activities may be recommended. Instruct the patient to always *stop exercising* or performing any activity *when chest pain is present.*
- Discuss the need for smoking cessation and make referrals to available self-help programs in the area. Smoking causes vasoconstriction; encourage drastic reduction and preferably elimination of smoking. Encourage the patient to set a date to stop smoking.
- Dietary modification aimed at decreasing the cholesterol level and a reducing program to maintain ideal weight are usually prescribed by the physician. Depending on coexisting conditions, other dietary modifications, such as a diet low in sodium, may be suggested. Discourage the use of caffeine-containing products because they may precipitate an anginal attack when taken in excess.
- If hypertension accompanies the angina, stress the importance of following prescribed emotional, dietary, and medicinal regimens to control the disease.
- Instruct the patient not to ingest alcohol while receiving nitroglycerin therapy. Alcohol causes vasodilation, potentially resulting in postural hypotension.
- Teach proper storage of medication in a dark, airtight container, especially sublingual nitroglycerin.
- Always *report poor pain control* to the health care provider.

Fostering Health Maintenance

- Throughout the course of treatment, discuss medication information and how it will benefit the patient.
- Drug therapy is essential to maintain adequate oxygenation of the myocardial cells and body tissues. Although medications can control the anginal attacks, lifestyle changes to deal with the management of precipitating factors must also occur.
- Provide the patient and significant others with the important information contained in the specific drug monograph for the drugs prescribed. Additional health teaching and nursing interventions for side effects to expect and report are described in the drug monographs that follow.
- Seek cooperation and understanding of the following points so that medication adherence is increased: name of medication; dosage, route, and times of administration; side effects to expect; and side effects to report.

Written Record. Enlist the patient's aid in developing and maintaining a written record of monitoring parameters (e.g., blood pressure, pulse, degree of pain relief, exercise tolerance, side effects experienced) (see Patient Self-Assessment Form in Chapter 28, on p. 455). Complete the Premedication Data column for use as a baseline to track response to drug therapy. Ensure that the patient understands how to use the form and instruct the patient to bring the completed form to follow-up visits. During follow-up visits, focus on issues that will foster adherence with the therapeutic interventions prescribed.

DRUG CLASS: Nitrates

Actions

The nitrates are the oldest effective therapy for angina pectoris. Although they have been termed *coronary vasodilators,* these agents do not increase total coronary blood flow. First, nitrates relieve angina pectoris by inducing relaxation of peripheral vascular smooth muscles, resulting in dilatation of arteries and veins. This reduces venous blood return (reduced preload) to the heart, which in turn leads to decreased oxygen demands on the heart. Second, nitrates increase myocardial oxygen supply by dilating large coronary arteries and redistributing blood flow, enhancing oxygen supply to ischemic areas.

Uses

Nitroglycerin is currently the drug of choice for treating angina pectoris. It is available in different doses for adjustment to the patient's needs. Sublingual tablets dissolve quite rapidly and are used primarily for acute attacks of angina. The sustained release tablets and capsules, ointment, transmucosal tablets, and transdermal patches are used prophylactically to prevent anginal attacks. All long-acting nitrates, including isosorbide dinitrate and mononitrate, appear to be equally effective when a sufficient nitrate-free interval (see below) is incorporated into the medicine regimen. The translingual spray may be used for both acute treatment and prophylaxis of anginal attacks.

Amyl nitrite is a volatile liquid, available in small glass ampules. The ampules are encased in a loosely woven material so that the ampule can be crushed easily under the patient's nostrils for inhalation. The onset of action is less than 1 minute, but the duration is only about 10 minutes.

With continued use of transdermal nitroglycerin patches and frequent doses of oral nitrates and sustained release nitrates, tolerance and loss of antianginal response develop. The best way to avoid tolerance is to have periodic nitrate-free periods. An 8- to 12-hour nitrate-free period will eliminate the development of tolerance. Depending on the type of angina, patients will be told when not to use nitrates (e.g., bedtime) unless they have an acute attack. When used with beta blockers or calcium antagonists, nitrates produce greater antianginal and antiischemic effects than when used alone. These agents also help provide prophylaxis against attacks during nitrate-free periods.

Therapeutic Outcomes

The primary therapeutic outcomes from nitrate therapy are as follows:

- Relief of anginal pain during an attack.
- Reduced frequency and severity of anginal attacks.
- Increased tolerance of activities.

Nursing Process for Nitrates

Premedication Assessment

1. Assess pain level, location, duration, intensity, and pattern.
2. Ask when the last dose of nitrates was taken and what degree of relief was obtained.

Planning

Availability. See Table 25-1.

Implementation

Dosage and Administration. See Table 25-1.

Sublingual Administration

1. Instruct the patient to sit or lie down at the first sign of an oncoming anginal attack.
2. Instruct the patient to place a tablet under the tongue and allow it to dissolve; encourage the patient not to swallow the saliva immediately.
3. The American Heart Association (2005) now recommends that if chest pain is not relieved by one sublingual nitroglycerin tablet within 5 minutes, seek medical attention (call 9-1-1).
4. One or two tablets may be taken prophylactically a few minutes before engaging in activities that may trigger an anginal attack.
5. Chart the patient's ability to place the sublingual medication under the tongue correctly.

Medication Deterioration. Every 3 months the nitroglycerin prescription should be refilled and the old tablets safely discarded. (Be sure the patient knows how to have the prescription refilled.)

Medication Storage. Store nitroglycerin in the original dark-colored glass container with a tight lid.

Medication Accessibility. Nonhospitalized patients should carry nitroglycerin at all times but not in a pocket directly next to the body because heat hastens the deterioration of the medication. When taken, the drug should produce a slight stinging or burning sensation, which usually indicates that it is still potent.

Allow the hospitalized patient to keep the nitroglycerin at bedside or on the person, if ambulatory. Check hospital policy to see if a fresh supply of medicine should be issued, rather than using the agents brought from home. (Remember that the nurse is still responsible for gathering and charting relevant data regarding all medication taken by the patient when the medication is left at bedside.)

Sustained Release Tablet Administration. Sustained release nitroglycerin is usually taken on an empty stomach every 8 to 12 hours. If gastritis develops, it may be necessary to take the sustained release tablet with food.

Transmucosal Tablet Administration. When placed under the upper lip or buccal pouch, transmucosal tablets release nitroglycerin for absorption by the oral mucosa over the next 3 to 5 hours. Patients may eat, drink, and talk while the tablet is in place. The usual initial dose is one tablet three times daily: one on arising, one after lunch, and one after the evening meal. Do not administer more than one tablet every 2 hours.

Translingual Spray Administration. Patients should be instructed to familiarize themselves with the position of the spray orifice, which can be identified by the finger rest on top of the valve. This can be particularly helpful for administration at night.

The spray is *highly flammable.* Instruct the patient not to use it where it might be ignited.

1. At the time of administration, the patient should preferably be in a sitting position.
2. The canister should be held vertically with the valve head uppermost and the spray orifice as close to the mouth as possible. Do not shake the container because bubbles formed may slow the release of nitroglycerin.
3. The dose should be sprayed onto or under the tongue by pressing the button firmly.

Drug Table 25-1 **NITRATES**

GENERIC NAME	BRAND NAME	AVAILABILITY	ONSET	DURATION	DOSAGE RANGE
amyl nitrite		Inhalation: 0.3 mL ampules in a woven sack for crushing	0.5 min	3-5 min	Inhalation: 1 ampule crushed in sack and placed under patient's nostrils for inhalation at time of acute attack
isosorbide dinitrate	Isordil	Sublingual tablets: 2.5, 5, 10 mg	2-3 min	1-3 hr	Sublingual: 2.5-10 mg for acute attack
		Oral tablets: 5, 10, 20, 30, 40 mg	30-60 min	4-6 hr	PO: 2.5-30 mg three or four times daily on empty stomach
		Sustained release tablets and capsules: 40 mg	30-60 min	6-8 hr	PO: 20-40 mg q6-8h or 80 mg q8-12h
isosorbide mononitrate	Monoket	Oral tablets: 10 mg	30-60 min	NA	PO: 20 mg twice daily, 7 hr apart
	ISMO	Oral tablets: 20 mg			
	Imdur	Sustained release tablets: 30, 60, 120 mg	3-4 hr	8-12 hr	PO: 30-240 mg once daily; do not crush or chew tablets
nitroglycerin	Nitrostat	Sublingual tablets: 0.3, 0.4, 0.6 mg	1-2 min	>30 min	Sublingual: 0.3-0.6 mg for prophylactic use before activity that may induce angina pectoris or at time of acute attack
	Nitrong	Oral sustained release capsules: 2.5, 6.5, 9 mg	30-45 min	3-8 hr	PO: 2.5-9 mg two to four times daily for prophylaxis
	Nitro-Bid	Ointment: 2%	30 min	3 hr	Topical: 0.5-4 inches of ointment using special applicator q4-6h
	Nitrogard	Transmucosal: 2, 3 mg tablets	2-3 min	3-5 hr	Buccal: place 1-3 mg between cheek and gum q3-5h
	Nitro-Dur	Transdermal: 0.1, 0.2, 0.3, 0.4, 0.6, 0.8 mg/hr patches	30-60 min	<24 hr	Topical: 1 patch applied for 12 hr; patient should wait 12 hr after removing old patch before applying new patch
	Nitrolingual	Translingual: 0.4 mg metered spray	2 min	30-60 min	Spray: 1-2 sprays onto or under tongue for acute attack; repeat if needed in 3-5 min; may be used prophylactically 5-10 min before exercise
	Nitro-Bid IV	Intravenous: 5 mg/mL in 1, 5, 10 mL vials; 25, 50, 100, 200 mg in 5% dextrose 250 and 500 mL	1-2 min	3-5 min	IV: initially, 5 mcg/min through an infusion pump; adjust dosage as needed

4. The mouth should be closed immediately after each dose. ***The spray should not be swallowed or inhaled.***

The American Heart Association (2005) now recommends that if chest pain is not relieved by one sublingual nitroglycerin dose within 5 minutes, seek medical attention (call 9-1-1).

Topical Ointment Administration

1. Position the dose-measuring applicator paper with the printed side down.
2. Squeeze the proper amount (usually 1 to 2 inches) of ointment onto the applicator paper.
3. Place the measuring applicator on the skin, ointment down, spreading in a thin, uniform layer. Do not massage or rub in. Any area without hair may be used; however, many people prefer the chest, flank, or upper arm. The lower extremities are not used, especially if there is reduced peripheral perfusion. (Because of the potential for skin irritation, do not shave an area to apply the medication.)
4. Help the patient develop a site rotation schedule to prevent skin irritation. Tell the patient not to apply the ointment to an area that still shows signs of irritation. Use of the applicator allows measuring of the proper dose and prevents absorption through the fingertips.
5. Cover the area where the patch is placed with a clear plastic wrap, and tape in place. (Alert the patient that the medication may discolor clothing.)
6. Close the tube tightly and store in a cool place.
7. When terminating the use of the topical ointment, gradually reduce the dose and frequency of application over 4 to 6 weeks.

Transdermal Disk Administration. The transdermal disk provides a controlled release of nitroglycerin through a semipermeable membrane for 24 hours when applied to intact skin. The dosage released depends on the surface area of the disk. Therapeutic effect can be observed in about 30 minutes after attachment and continues for about 30 minutes after removal.

1. The disk should be applied to a clean, dry, hairless area of skin. Do not apply to shaved areas because skin irritation may alter drug absorption. If hair is likely to interfere with patch adhesion or removal, trim the hair but do not shave. Optimal locations for patch placement are the upper chest or side; pelvis; and inner, upper arm. Avoid scars, skinfolds, and wounds. Rotate skin sites daily. (Help the patient develop a rotation chart.)
2. Wash hands before applying and after removing the product.
3. See individual product information to determine whether a patch can be worn while swimming, bathing, or showering.
4. If a disk becomes partially dislodged, discard it and replace with a new disk.
5. Sublingual nitroglycerin may be necessary for anginal attacks, especially while the dosage is being adjusted.
6. Dispose of used patches out of reach of children. Discarded patches still contain enough active ingredient to be dangerous to children.

Intravenous Nitroglycerin Administration. Intravenous nitroglycerin is used in an intensive care setting and requires continuous monitoring of vital signs: blood pressure, pulse, respirations, and central venous pressure.

An infusion pump must be used to monitor the precise delivery of the infusion. Dose is titrated to achieve the desired clinical response. Gradual weaning is needed under controlled conditions to prevent a rebound action.

This medication is never mixed with other medications and is administered only with administration sets made specifically for nitroglycerin because most plastic administration sets absorb the drug. See the manufacturer's literature for exact directions recommended for preparation and administration.

Evaluation

Side Effects to Report

Excessive Hypotension. Excessive hypotension is an extension of the nitrates' pharmacologic activity. Other possible side effects include dizziness, nausea, flushing, and rarely syncope. Report these adverse effects so that more appropriate dosage adjustment may be made.

Prolonged Headache. The most common side effect of nitrate therapy is headache. This can range from a mild sensation of fullness in the head to an intense and severe generalized headache. Most patients develop a tolerance within a few weeks of starting therapy. Analgesics, such as acetaminophen, may be used if needed. Report these adverse effects so that a more appropriate dosage adjustment may be made.

Tolerance (Increasing Dosage to Attain Relief). Tolerance to the nitrate dosages can develop rapidly, particularly if large doses are administered frequently. Tolerance can appear within a few days and may be well established within a few weeks. The smallest dose to give satisfactory results should be used to minimize the development of tolerance. Tolerance is broken by withdrawing the drug for a short period.

Drug Interactions

Alcohol. Alcohol accentuates the vasodilation and postural hypotension of the nitrates. Patients should be warned that drinking alcohol while taking nitrates may cause hypotension.

Calcium Ion Antagonists, Beta-Adrenergic Blocking Agents. Calcium ion antagonists and beta-adrenergic blocking agents may significantly lower blood pressure. Dosage adjustments may be necessary.

Sildenafil, Tadalafil, and Vardenafil. Concurrent use of nitrates and these agents used for erectile dysfunction is ***contraindicated!*** These agents potentiate the vasodilatory effects of the nitrates, resulting in a significant drop in blood pressure that may be fatal.

DRUG CLASS: Beta-Adrenergic Blocking Agents

Actions

The beta-adrenergic blocking agents (beta blockers) (see Table 13-3) reduce myocardial oxygen demand by blocking the beta adrenergic receptors in the heart, preventing stimulation from norepinephrine and epinephrine that would normally cause an increased heart rate. Beta blockers also reduce blood pressure (see Chapter 23).

Uses

The goal of beta blocker therapy is to reduce the number of anginal attacks, reduce nitroglycerin use, and improve exercise tolerance while minimizing side effects. All beta blockers are effective in treating angina pectoris, so product selection should be based on other conditions the patient may have (e.g., diabetes, chronic obstructive airway disease, peripheral vascular disease) and adherence issues. The cardioselective agents (see Chapter 13) will have less effect on the beta-2 receptors of the lungs and peripheral vasculature, minimizing side effects from these body systems. Acebutolol, atenolol, betaxolol, and metoprolol are examples of beta blockers that can be administered once daily to minimize anginal attacks if adherence is a problem. Dosages of beta blockers needed to control angina are extremely patient-specific; therefore therapy should start at low doses and work upward, depending on the patient's need. Optimally, exercise stressing should be used to determine the most appropriate dosage. Combination therapy with nitrates and beta blockers appears to be more effective than nitrates or beta blockers alone. Beta blockers may also be combined with calcium antagonists such as the slow-release dihydropyridines or the long-acting dihydropyridines (see later).

Therapeutic Outcomes

The primary therapeutic outcomes expected from beta blocker therapy are as follows:

- Decreased frequency and severity of anginal attacks.
- Increased tolerance of activities.
- Reduced use of nitroglycerin for acute anginal attacks.

Nursing Process for Beta-Adrenergic Blocking Agents

Premedication Assessment

1. Take blood pressure in supine and standing positions.
2. Check history for respiratory disorders, such as bronchospasm, chronic bronchitis, emphysema, and asthma.
3. Check for history of diabetes. If present, determine baseline serum glucose before starting therapy.

See Chapter 13 for further discussion of patient education and the nursing process associated with beta adrenergic inhibition.

DRUG CLASS: Calcium Ion Antagonists

Actions

These agents are known variously as calcium antagonists, calcium channel blockers, slow channel blockers, and calcium ion influx inhibitors. Regardless of their names, they all share the ability to inhibit the movement of calcium ions across a cell membrane.

Calcium ion antagonists (Table 25-2) may be used to treat angina pectoris by decreasing myocardial oxygen demand (decreasing workload) and increasing myocardial blood supply by coronary artery dilation. By inhibiting smooth muscle contraction, the calcium ion antagonists dilate blood vessels and decrease resistance to blood flow. Dilation of peripheral vessels reduces the workload of the heart. Coronary artery dilation improves coronary blood flow.

Drug Table 25-2 CALCIUM ION ANTAGONISTS USED TO TREAT ANGINA PECTORIS

GENERIC NAME	BRAND NAME	AVAILABILITY	DOSAGE RANGE
amlodipine	Norvasc	Tablets: 2.5, 5, 10 mg	PO: initial—5 mg once daily; adjust over 7-14 days to a maximum of 10 mg/day
diltiazem	Cardizem	Tablets: 30, 60, 90, 120 mg Tablets, extended release: 120, 180, 240, 300, 360, 420 mg	PO: initial—30 mg four times daily, gradually increasing dosage to 180-360 mg in three or four divided doses
		Sustained release capsules: 60, 90, 120, 180, 240, 300 mg	PO: initial—120-180 mg sustained release capsule once daily; adjust as needed after 14 days Maintenance—240-480 mg daily
bepridil	Vascor	Tablets: 200, 300 mg	PO: initial—200 mg daily; adjust after 10 days, depending on response Maintenance—300 mg daily Maximum—400 mg daily
nicardipine	Cardene	Capsules: 20, 30 mg	PO: initial—20 mg three times daily Maximal response may require 2 wk of therapy Allow at least 3 days between dosage adjustments Maintenance—20-40 mg three times daily
		Sustained release capsules: 30, 45, 60 mg	PO: initial—30 mg twice daily Maintenance—30-60 mg twice daily
nifedipine	Procardia, Adalat	Capsules: 10, 20 mg	PO: initial—10 mg three times daily; adjust over 7-14 days to balance antianginal and hypotensive activity Maintenance—10-20 mg three times daily
		Sustained release tablets: 30, 60, 90 mg	Sustained release tablets are administered once daily—30-60 mg Maximum—capsules: 180 mg daily; sustained release tablets: 120 mg daily
verapamil	Calan, Isoptin	Tablets: 40, 80, 120 mg Sustained release tablets and capsules: 120, 180, 200, 240, 300, 360 mg	PO: initial—40-120 mg three times daily Maintenance—120-480 mg daily Administer with food

Uses

Although each of these agents acts by calcium ion inhibition, there are significant differences in clinical use. Their clinical effects also depend on the type and severity of the patient's disease. The primary calcium ion antagonists used to treat angina are the long-acting dihydropyridines (e.g., amlodipine, felodipine) and the sustained release products of non-dihydropyridine diltiazem and verapamil. The overall effect of calcium ion antagonists will be the combined effects of vasodilator and myocardial actions with reflex-mediated adrenergic activity. Nifedipine, a potent peripheral arterial vasodilator, reduces peripheral vascular resistance, which may cause a reflex tachycardia. Verapamil and diltiazem also have myocardial depressant effects that prevent tachycardia. They must, however, be used with extreme caution in patients who may be developing heart failure.

Therapeutic Outcomes

The primary therapeutic outcomes expected from calcium ion antagonists are as follows:

- Decreased frequency and severity of anginal attacks.
- Increased tolerance of activities.

Nursing Process for Calcium Ion Antagonists

Premedication Assessment

1. Take blood pressure in supine and standing positions.
2. Check for history of heart failure; withhold drug and consult physician if heart failure is present.
3. Check laboratory values for hepatotoxicity.

Planning

Availability. See Table 25-2.

Implementation

Dosage and Administration. See Table 25-2. See Chapter 23 for a further discussion of patient education and the nursing process associated with calcium ion antagonist therapy.

DRUG CLASS: Angiotensin-Converting Enzyme Inhibitors

Actions

ACE inhibitors represent a major breakthrough in the treatment of cardiovascular disease. Their action is more completely described in Chapter 23, pp. 374-376, but through inhibition of the angiotensin-converting enzyme, these drugs have very significant action on the endothelial wall of coronary arteries that promote vasodilation and minimize platelet cell aggregation, preventing thrombus formation.

Uses

The ACE inhibitors have been proven to reduce the incidence of myocardial infarction and should be used as routine secondary prevention for patients with known coronary artery disease, particularly in patients with diabetes mellitus without renal failure.

Therapeutic Outcomes

The primary therapeutic outcome expected from the ACE inhibitors is reduction in frequency of recurrent myocardial infarction.

Nursing Process for Angiotensin-Converting Enzyme Inhibitors

Premedication Assessment

1. Obtain baseline blood pressure readings in supine and standing positions and apical pulse.
2. Obtain a history of bowel elimination patterns.
3. Initiate laboratory studies as requested by the physician (e.g., ECG, renal function tests such as blood urea nitrogen [BUN] and serum creatinine, electrolytes, and complete blood count [CBC] to serve as a baseline for future comparison).
4. Ask if the patient has a persistent cough.

Planning

Availability. See Chapter 23, Table 23-5.

Implementation

Dosage and Administration. See Chapter 23 and Table 23-5 for further discussion of patient education and the nursing process associated with ACE inhibitor therapy.

NOTE: The initial doses of ACE inhibitors may cause hypotension with dizziness, tachycardia, and fainting; these adverse effects occur more commonly in patients also receiving diuretics. Symptoms occur within 3 hours after the first several doses. This effect may be minimized by discontinuing the diuretic 1 week before initiating ACE inhibitor therapy. Patients should be warned that this side effect may occur, that it is transient, and that they should lie down immediately if symptoms develop.

DRUG CLASS: Fatty Oxidase Enzyme Inhibitor

ranolazine (ran ol ah zeen)

▶ RANEXA (ran x ah)

Actions

Ranolazine, a fatty oxidase inhibitor, is an enzyme modulator. Its exact mechanism of action is unknown, but it shifts the metabolism within myocardial cells to reduce the oxygen required to generate energy for muscle contractions. As the demand for oxygen is reduced, the imbalance between oxygen supply and demand will diminish, reducing myocardial ischemia and symptoms of angina.

Uses

Ranolazine is the first new agent in over 20 years to be used to treat chronic stable angina. It is used in combination with a dihydropyridine calcium channel blocker (e.g., amlodipine), beta-blockers, and/or nitrates. Unlike other antianginal medicines, ranolazine does not affect blood pressure or heart rate. Because ranolazine prolongs the QT interval (a potentially life-threatening event), it should only be used to treat angina in patients who have not achieved an antianginal response from other agents. Ranolazine will not reduce the symptoms of an acute anginal episode.

Therapeutic Outcomes

The primary therapeutic outcomes expected from ranolazine therapy are as follows:

- Reduced frequency and severity of anginal attacks.
- Increased tolerance of activities.
- Reduced use of nitroglycerin in acute anginal attacks.

Nursing Process for Ranolazine

Premedication Assessment

1. Initiate laboratory studies as requested by the health care provider (e.g., ECG; renal function tests such as blood urea nitrogen [BUN] and serum creatinine; electrolytes; and complete blood count [CBC]) to serve as a baseline for future comparison.

Planning

Availability: PO: 500 mg extended-release tablets

Implementation

NOTE: It is recommended that ranolazine NOT be taken concurrently with other medicines known to prolong the QT interval: quinidine, dofetilide, sotalol, erythromycin, and antipsychotics (e.g., thioridazine, ziprasidone). Baseline and follow-up ECGs should be obtained to evaluate effects on the patient's QT interval.

Dosage and administration: 500 mg twice daily. May be increased to 1000 mg twice daily. Ranolazine may be taken with or without meals. Tablets should be swallowed whole and not crushed, broken, or chewed.

Evaluation

Side Effects to Expect and Report

Dizziness, Headache, Constipation, and Nausea. These side effects are usually mild, occurring in fewer than 6% of patients. Patients should not operate an automobile or machinery, or engage in activities requiring mental alertness until it is known how they will react to the medicine. Patients should withhold medicine and contact their health care provider if they experience palpitations or fainting spells while taking ranolazine.

Drug Interactions

Drugs That Enhance Therapeutic and Toxic Effects. Ketoconazole, diltiazem, and verapamil significantly increase the serum levels and potential toxicity of ranolazine. In general, these agents should not be used concurrently with ranolazine. If used concurrently, monitor closely for development of dizziness, nausea, asthenia, constipation, and headache.

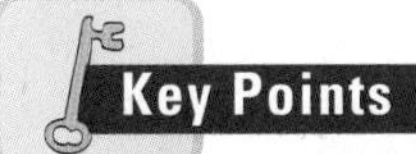

- Coronary heart disease is the leading cause of disability, socioeconomic loss, and death in the United States.
- Angina pectoris is the first clinical indication of underlying coronary artery disease in many patients.
- The frequency of anginal attacks can be reduced by controlling risk factors and avoiding precipitating causes, such as stress.
- Medicines such as nitrates, beta blockers, ACE inhibitors, statins, platelet inhibitors, and calcium ion antagonists can help control symptoms.
- Nurses can play a significant role in public education efforts, monitoring for noncompliance, monitoring patient response to therapy, and encouraging patients to make changes in lifestyle to reduce the severity of angina pectoris.

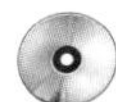

Go to your Companion CD-ROM for Appendices, an Audio Glossary, animations, Drug Dosage Calculators, customizable Patient Self-Assessment forms, and Review Questions for the NCLEX® Examination.

evolve Be sure to visit the companion Evolve site at http://evolve.elsevier.com/Clayton for WebLinks and additional online resources.

MEDICATION SAFETY REVIEW

MATH REVIEW QUESTIONS

1. Order: Nitroglycerin 0.3 mg sublingual PRN for chest pain

   Available: Nitroglycerin 0.15-mg sublingual tablets

   Give: ____ tablets.

   Explain the procedure for sublingual administration of nitroglycerin.

Continued

MATH REVIEW QUESTIONS—cont'd

2. Order: Nifedipine (Procardia) 30 mg PO q6h
   Available: Nifedipine 10-mg capsules
   Give: ___ capsules per dose.
   Give: ___ mg nifedipine in 24 hours.

3. Order: Propranolol hydrochloride (Inderal) 160 mg PO daily
   Available: Propranolol hydrochloride (Inderal) concentrated oral solution 80 mg/mL
   Give: ___ mL.

CRITICAL THINKING QUESTIONS

Situation: A 64-year-old man comes to the emergency department with acute chest pain. He is holding his chest with his fist directly over the sternum. He appears diaphoretic. He is in work clothes and has been mowing the lawn. It is 98° F outside.

1. What nursing actions would be appropriate immediately?
2. What drugs would likely be ordered if this is acute angina pectoris?
3. Describe the correct procedure for administering sublingual nitroglycerin.
4. If a stat dose of nitroglycerin sublingual spray is ordered, what instructions would you give the patient for administering it?

Situation: When giving morning medications in the nursing home, the nurse comes to an order to apply a Nitro-Dur patch 2.5 mg to a patient. The medication administration record (MAR) indicates that the previous patch was applied to the right scapular area, but the patch is not there.

5. How would you proceed to execute the order?
6. Summarize the actions of each major classification of drugs used to treat angina pectoris.
7. Identify preassessment data that should be obtained before initiating drug therapy for angina.

CONTENT REVIEW QUESTIONS

1. Premedication assessments for calcium ion antagonist drugs include checking:
   1. laboratory values for nephrotoxicity.
   2. laboratory values for hepatotoxicity.
   3. potassium level.
   4. for respiratory diseases/disorders.

2. Transmucosal tablets administered for angina release nitroglycerin over the next:
   1. 3 to 5 hours.
   2. 6 to 10 hours.
   3. 10 to 12 hours.
   4. 12 to 18 hours.

3. Following the administration of a nitrate the patient may experience:
   1. bradycardia.
   2. tachycardia.
   3. hypotension.
   4. prolonged palpitations.

4. Patients using Nitro-Dur patches should wait ___ hours after removing an old patch before applying a new patch.
   1. 3 to 5
   2. 6 to 10
   3. 8 to 12
   4. 12 to 24

5. The most effective agents for relieving ischemia and angina are:
   1. beta blockers, calcium antagonists, and nitrates.
   2. HMG-CoA reductase inhibitors and nitrates.
   3. nitrates and antiplatelet agents.
   4. beta blockers and HMG-CoA reductase inhibitors.

6. During assessment of a patient with chest pain, the nurse recognizes that chest pain associated with angina is:
   1. always sudden in onset and is accompanied by a feeling of doom.
   2. usually precipitated by stress and relieved by rest.
   3. aggravated by inspiration, coughing, and movement of the upper body.
   4. accompanied by a residual soreness in the chest that lasts for several days.

7. The nurse determines that outcomes from teaching regarding precipitating factors of angina have been met when the patient states:
   1. "I will stop my sexual activities."
   2. "I will rest for 1 to 2 hours after every meal."
   3. "I will avoid outdoor activities when it is very hot or very cold."
   4. "I will limit my coffee intake, but I may substitute regular cola products."

CHAPTER

26 Drugs Used to Treat Peripheral Vascular Disease

evolve http://evolve.elsevier.com/Clayton

Chapter Content

Objectives

1. List the baseline assessments needed to evaluate a patient with peripheral vascular disease.
2. Identify specific measures the patient can use to improve peripheral circulation and prevent complications from peripheral vascular disease.
3. Identify the systemic effects to expect when peripheral vasodilating agents are administered.
4. Explain why hypotension and tachycardia occur frequently with the use of peripheral vasodilators.
5. Develop measurable objectives for patient education for patients with peripheral vascular disease.
6. State both pharmacologic and nonpharmacologic goals of treatment for peripheral vascular disease.

Key Terms

arteriosclerosis obliterans
intermittent claudication
paresthesias
Raynaud's disease
vasospasm

PERIPHERAL VASCULAR DISEASE

The classification "peripheral vascular disease" can be applied to a variety of illnesses associated with blood vessels outside the heart, but it generally refers to diseases of the blood vessels of the arms and legs (the extremities). These illnesses can be subdivided into two types based on arterial or venous origin: peripheral arterial disease and venous disorders, such as acute deep vein thrombosis (see Chapter 27). The arterial disorders are subdivided into those that result from arterial narrowing and occlusion (obstructive) and those caused by arterial spasm (vasospastic).

The most common form of obstructive arterial disease is **arteriosclerosis obliterans,** also called atherosclerosis obliterans. It results from atherosclerotic plaque formation with narrowing of the lower aorta and the major arteries that provide circulation to the legs. As with atherosclerosis of the coronary arteries, the risk factors that play an important role in the development of this disease are high levels of low-density lipoprotein cholesterol (LDL-C), hypertension, cigarette smoking, low levels of high-density lipoprotein cholesterol (HDL-C), and diabetes mellitus.

Patients tend to remain symptom-free until there is significant narrowing (75% to 90%) in key locations of the major arteries and arterioles of the legs. The typical pain pattern described is one of aching, cramping, tightness, or weakness that occurs during exercise. The primary pathophysiology is obstruction of blood flow through the arteries resulting in ischemia to the tissues supplied by those arteries. A term commonly applied to this condition is **intermittent claudication,** the symptom of which is pain secondary to lack of oxygen to muscles during exercise. In the early stages of symptoms, the patient finds relief by stopping the exercise for a few minutes. As the disease progresses over time without treatment, the arteries become obstructed, resulting in thrombosis and the potential for gangrene. Additional symptoms that develop are pain at rest, numbness, and **paresthesias** (numbness with a tingling sensation). The disease is often accompanied by increased blood viscosity. Physical findings are reduced arterial pulsations on palpation; systolic bruits over the involved arteries; waxy, pale, dry coloration; lower temperature of the skin of the extremity; edema; and numbness to sensation.

Peripheral vascular disease caused by arterial vasospasm is known as **Raynaud's disease,** named after the man who first described the illness in 1862. It is unfortunate that more than one century later, the pathophysiology and treatment are still not well defined. Raynaud's disease is classified as primary, in which the cause is unknown, or secondary, in which other conditions contribute to the symptoms. Secondary causes are frequent exposure to cold weather, obstructive arterial disease, occupational trauma (e.g., pneumatic hammer users, pianists) and certain drugs (e.g., beta blockers, imipramine, nicotine, bromocriptine, vinblastine, clonidine). Heredity may also play a role in this disease. The onset of Raynaud's disease is usually during the teen years to the 40s, and it occurs four times more frequently in women.

Raynaud's disease is thought to be caused by vasospasm (vasoconstriction of blood vessels) and subsequent ischemia of the arteries of the skin of the hands, fingers, and sometimes toes. The physiologic mechanisms that trigger the vasospasm are unknown. Sudden coldness applied to the extremity, such as cold water, will induce an attack. The signs and symptoms associated with Raynaud's disease are numbness, tingling, and a sense of skin tightness in the affected area, and blanching of the skin because of sudden vasoconstriction followed by cyanosis. As the attack subsides, vasodilation causes a redness, or rubor, to the pale skin. The skin appears normal except during spasm. In the early years of the illness, only the tips of fingers of both hands are involved, but as the disease progresses the skin on the hands is also affected by the arteriospasm.

TREATMENT OF PERIPHERAL VASCULAR DISEASE

The goals of treatment of arteriosclerosis obliterans are reversal of the progression of the atherosclerosis, improved blood flow, pain relief, and prevention of skin ulceration and gangrene. An important concept that must be stressed to most patients is that other diseases they may have (e.g., diabetes, hypertension, angina, and dyslipidemia) are all interrelated. Control of diet, high blood pressure, smoking, weight, and diabetes will significantly help all these diseases. Implementation of the American Heart Association's diet An Eating Plan for Healthy Americans can arrest the progression of atherosclerosis. Lipid-lowering agents can be started if diet is not successful in treating the hypercholesterolemia. A daily exercise program (usually walking) can significantly improve collateral blood circulation around areas of obstruction and reduce the frequency of intermittent claudication. Proper foot care (e.g., keeping feet warm and dry, with properly fitting shoes), especially if the patient has diabetes, is also extremely important in preventing ulcerative complications. Other nonpharmacologic treatments that may improve blood flow to the extremities are avoidance of cold, elevation of the head of the bed 12 to 16 inches, and arterial angioplasty and surgery.

Most vasospastic attacks of Raynaud's disease can be stopped by avoiding cold temperatures, emotional stress, tobacco, and drugs known to induce attacks. Keeping the hands and feet warm with gloves and socks and using foam "wrap-arounds" when handling iced beverages can reduce exposure to cold.

DRUG THERAPY FOR PERIPHERAL VASCULAR DISEASE

Actions

As the causes of peripheral vascular disease have become better understood, clinical studies have defined which pharmacologic therapies are truly successful. It has been shown that nonpharmacologic treatment of arteriosclerosis obliterans is substantially more successful in treating the underlying pathologic condition. Pentoxifylline has had modest success. Pentoxifylline is classified as a hemorrheologic agent. It acts by enhancing red blood cell flexibility, which reduces blood viscosity, thus providing better oxygenation to muscle tissue to stop intermittent claudication. Vasodilator therapy, the mainstay of treatment until the 1980s, has little long-term benefit in most cases. A new approach to treatment became available with the availability of the platelet aggregation inhibitor cilostazol. When drug therapy for Raynaud's disease is required, such as when the disease interferes with the ability to work, medicines with a vasodilating effect are used.

Uses

Pentoxifylline and cilostazol are the only agents approved by the U.S. Food and Drug Administration (FDA) that are specifically indicated for the treatment of intermittent claudication caused by chronic occlusive arterial disease of the limbs.

Classes of drugs that have been somewhat successful in treating Raynaud's disease are the calcium ion antagonists, adrenergic antagonists, angiotensin-converting enzyme (ACE) inhibitors, and direct vasodilators.

The three calcium ion antagonists studied for the treatment of Raynaud's disease are diltiazem, verapamil, and nifedipine. Of the three, nifedipine has had the greatest success in reducing the frequency of vasospastic attack in about two thirds of patients.

Adrenergic antagonists (e.g., prazosin, reserpine, guanethidine, methyldopa) have been used for many years in the treatment of Raynaud's disease. Unfortunately, treatment has been only moderately successful, and many side effects are associated with these drugs.

The ACE inhibitors cause an increase in bradykinin, a potent vasodilator. Captopril has been most extensively tested and causes a reduction in both frequency and severity of attacks.

For more than 50 years, nitroglycerin, a direct vasodilator, has been applied as an ointment base to the hands of patients with Raynaud's disease. The treatment reduces the frequency and severity of attacks, but the side effects of dizziness, headache, and postural hypotension limit its use. Other vasodilators (e.g., papaverine, isoxsuprine, cyclandelate) have been used extensively over the years but have not been tested in controlled studies. They are, however, still occasionally used as adjunctive therapy to treat peripheral vascular diseases.

NURSING PROCESS *for Peripheral Vascular Disease Therapy*

Assessment

A baseline assessment of the patient should be completed that includes the following data to evaluate the history and degree of oxygenation that exists in the extremities.

Subsequent regular assessments should be performed for comparison and analysis of therapeutic effectiveness or lack of response to all treatments initiated.

History of Risk Factors. Ask age, note gender and race, and take family history of incidence of symptoms of peripheral vascular disease, hypertension, and cardiac disease.

Impotence. Has the male patient experienced impotence?

Hypertension. Take blood pressure in sitting and supine positions daily. Ask about medications that have been prescribed. Are the medications being taken regularly? If not, why not?

Smoking. Obtain a history of the number of cigarettes or cigars smoked daily. How long has the person smoked? Has the person ever tried to stop smoking? Ask if the patient understands the effect of smoking on the vascular system. How does the individual feel about modifying the smoking habit?

Dietary Habits

- Obtain a dietary history. Ask specific questions to obtain data relating to foods eaten that are high in fat, cholesterol, refined carbohydrates, and sodium. Using a calorie counter, ask the person to estimate the number of calories eaten per day. How much meat, fish, and poultry is eaten daily (size and number of servings)? Estimate the percent of total daily calories provided by fats.
- Discuss food preparation, for example, baked, broiled, and fried foods. How many servings of fruits and vegetables are eaten daily? What types of oils and fats are used in food preparation? See a nutrition text for further dietary history questions.
- What is the frequency and volume of alcoholic beverages consumed?

Glucose Intolerance. Ask specific questions regarding whether the individual has now or ever had an elevated serum glucose (blood sugar). If yes, what dietary modifications have been made? How successful are they? What medications are being taken for the elevated serum glucose (e.g., oral hypoglycemic agents, insulin)?

Elevated Serum Lipids. Find out whether the patient is aware of having elevated lipids, triglycerides, or cholesterol. If any of these are elevated, what measures has the patient tried for reduction and what effect have the interventions had on the blood levels at subsequent examinations? Review laboratory data available (e.g., LDL, very low-density lipoprotein [VLDL]).

Infection. Has the individual developed any slow-to-heal or nonhealing sores?

Obesity. Weigh the patient. Ask about any recent weight gains or losses and whether intentional or unintentional.

Psychomotor Functions

Type of Lifestyle. Ask the patient to describe the exercise level in terms of amount (e.g., walking three blocks), intensity (e.g., how long does it take to walk three blocks), and frequency (e.g., walking every other day). Is the patient's job physically demanding or sedentary?

Psychological Stress. How much stress does the individual estimate having in life? How does the individual cope with stressful situations at home and at work?

Assessment of Tissue

Oxygenation. Observe the color of each hand, finger, leg, and foot; report cyanosis or reddish blue locations. Does the patient have dependent cyanosis (cyanosis when the legs are in the dependent position)? Examine the skin of the extremities for any signs of ulceration.

Temperature. Feel the temperature in each hand, finger, leg, and foot. Report paleness and coldness. (NOTE: these symptoms will be increased if the limb is elevated above the level of the heart.)

Edema. Assess, record, and report edema and its extent, and determine whether it is relieved or unchanged when the limb is dependent.

Peripheral Pulses. Record the pedal and radial pulses at least every 4 hours if circulatory impairment is found in that limb. Compare findings among the extremities; report diminished or absent pulses immediately. When pulses are difficult to palpate or are absent, a Doppler ultrasound device may aid in determining peripheral blood flow.

Limb Pain. Assess pain in the patient carefully. Pain during exercise that is relieved by rest may be from claudication. Conversely, pain when the patient is at rest may be from sudden obstruction by a thrombus or an embolus. Check the apprehension level of the patient, pedal and radial pulses, details of onset and location of pain, and vital signs, and determine whether pain is increased by dorsiflexion of the foot (positive Homans' sign). Until status of patient's limb pain is established, have the patient remain on bed rest and administer an analgesic if ordered. Notify physician of findings.

Nursing Diagnoses

- Tissue perfusion, ineffective (indication)
- Pain, acute or chronic (indication)
- Activity intolerance, risk for (indication)
- Injury, risk for (indication)

Planning

History of Risk Factors

- Review the modifiable risk factors and plan interventions and health teaching needed for appropriate alterations in lifestyle.
- Review ordered medications to be used concurrently with lifestyle modifications for health teaching needed regarding their use.
- Order baseline laboratory studies requested by the physician (e.g., lipid profile studies, liver function tests, clotting time).

Assessment of Tissue. Schedule assessment of pertinent data on the care plan and Kardex at regular intervals that correlate with the patient's status.

Psychomotor Function and Lifestyle Pattern. Examine assessment data to determine an appropriate teaching plan that will incorporate changes in lifestyle issues (e.g., control of hypertension, smoking cessation, dietary alterations, stress-related factors, the disease process itself) and drug therapy prescribed.

Medication Administration. Plan drug administration in accordance with recommendations in individual drug monographs to avoid possible interference with the absorption of other drugs ordered.

Implementation

- Prepare the patient for diagnostic tests (e.g., ultrasonography, pulse volume recordings, segmental limb pressure, exercise testing) and possible invasive procedures, such as arteriography.
- Do not place pillows in the popliteal space or flex the knee rest on the bed. Use a cradle or footboard to prevent bed sheets from constricting the circulation.
- Always check with the health care provider before initiating elevation of the extremities. It is *contraindicated* in patients with *arterial* insufficiency.
- Perform baseline assessments of tissue perfusion (e.g., skin temperature, peripheral pulses) at intervals appropriate to the patient's status (at least every 4 hours).
- Implement pain management measures.

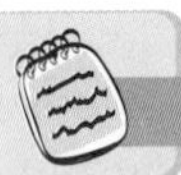

Patient Education and Health Promotion

Promoting Tissue Perfusion

- Teach self-care measures that promote peripheral circulation.
- Smoking causes vasoconstriction of the blood vessels. Therefore, encourage drastic reduction and preferably total abstinence from smoking.
- Encourage patients to wear nothing that constricts peripheral blood flow (e.g., tight-fitting anklets, socks, garters). Tell the patient *not* to elevate the extremities above the level of the heart without specific orders to do so from the health care provider. The physician *may* order the patient's bed elevated at night.
- Meticulous foot and hand care is essential. Teach proper self-care of the limbs including visual inspection techniques, and explain how to take femoral, popliteal, and pedal pulses.
- Stress the need to inspect the extremities for possible skin breakdown or signs of infection. The patient should notify the physician immediately of sudden changes in color, such as mottling or a more purplish color. Cold temperatures will increase pain or decrease sensations in the extremities. Conversely, hot tubs or showers may cause additional vasodilatation that adds to the drug's effects.
- Areas of discoloration in nails, cracking of skin, calluses, or blisters on the extremities require complete follow-up. Listen to the patient's description of changes noted. Tell the patient that going barefoot can be dangerous because of potential injuries to the feet.
- Because of the possible decrease in sensation in the extremities, encourage the patient to test the water temperature before immersing the hands or feet. After bathing, gently pat (do not vigorously rub) the feet and hands to dry them.
- To avoid skin breakdown, the patient should alternate pairs of shoes to allow for thorough drying between wearings, change socks or hose daily, and avoid rubber-soled shoes.
- Standing or sitting for prolonged periods should be avoided. Patients who must sit for extended periods of time must have a properly fitting chair. The seat should be of the correct depth so that no pressure is exerted on the popliteal space. Encourage individuals not to sit with knees or ankles crossed and to take frequent short breaks for walks. Further, people who must stand for long periods should seek aspects of the job that can be performed sitting down in a properly fitting chair or other alternatives.

Psychomotor Functions

- Maximum mobility should be maintained. Devise a daily activity plan that includes walks and usual activities of daily living (ADLs), such as shopping and housework.
- Pain management and the psychological aspects of dealing with a prolonged illness with persistent symptoms are a major challenge to the patient and the nurse (see Chapter 20).

Environment. During periods of exposure to cold temperature, the patient should wear several layers of lightweight clothing. Caution should be exercised during exposure to the cold to avoid frostbite. Because of decreased sensations in the extremities, frostbite can occur without the patient's awareness.

Nutritional Aspects

- Dietary education is strongly indicated in the treatment of peripheral vascular disease. It is particularly important to control obesity and cholesterol and triglyceride levels.
- When ulcerations are present, encourage a high-protein diet with adequate intake of vitamins to promote the healing process.
- Unless other medical conditions contraindicate, instruct the patient to drink eight 8-ounce glasses of water daily to promote adequate hydration of body tissues. Maintaining blood volume will

help reduce peripheral vasoconstriction. Check with the physician regarding recommendations for fluid or caffeine restriction.

Medication Regimen

- Certain medications for the treatment of peripheral vascular disease cause vasodilatation of blood vessels. As a result, orthostatic hypotension may occur. Teach patients to rise slowly from a sitting or lying position, steady themselves, flex the leg muscles, and then proceed with movement.
- Teach the individual to take and record own blood pressure.
- Administer prescribed medicines, and consult the health care provider before discontinuing medications.

Fostering Health Maintenance

- Throughout the course of treatment, discuss medication information and explain how the medication will benefit the patient.
- Drug therapy is not a total solution for atherosclerosis. The patient may not be committed to the lifestyle changes needed to control the modifiable aspects of the disease. Often, setting short-term goals to control the pain and finding other interventions that will allow the patient to view efforts positively will help encourage permanent adoption of the needed changes.
- Patients who are unresponsive to lifestyle modifications and drug therapy may require surgical interventions to reestablish blood flow to the affected area. Procedures such as a bypass graft, endarterectomy, or angioplasty may be appropriate. Failure to reestablish blood flow to an extremity may result in amputation.
- Provide the patient and significant others with important information contained in the specific drug monographs for the drugs prescribed. Additional health teaching and nursing interventions for side effects to expect and report are described in each drug monograph.
- Seek cooperation and understanding of the following points so that medication compliance is increased: name of medication, dosage, route and times of administration, side effects to expect, and side effects to report.

Written Record. Enlist the patient's aid in developing and maintaining a written record of monitoring parameters (e.g., color of limb, pain in limb, temperature and pulses in limb, amount of edema present) (see Patient Self-Assessment Form in Chapter 28, on p. 455). Complete the Premedication Data column for use as a baseline to track response to drug therapy. Ensure that the patient understands how to use the form and instruct the patient to bring the completed form to follow-up visits. During follow-up visits, focus on issues that will foster adherence with the therapeutic interventions prescribed. ■

DRUG CLASS: Hemorrheologic Agent

pentoxifylline (pen tox e′ fi leen)
TRENTAL (tren′ tahl)

Actions

Pentoxifylline is not an anticoagulant, but it is thought to increase erythrocyte flexibility, decrease the concentration of fibrinogen in blood, and prevent aggregation of red blood cells and platelets. These actions decrease the viscosity of blood and improve its flow properties, resulting in increased blood flow to the affected microcirculation to enhance tissue oxygenation.

Uses

Pentoxifylline is the agent approved for the treatment of intermittent claudication. Pentoxifylline therapy should be considered an adjunct to, and not a replacement for, smoking cessation, weight loss, exercise therapy, surgical bypass, or removal of arterial obstructions in the treatment of peripheral vascular disease.

Therapeutic Outcomes

The primary therapeutic outcome expected from pentoxifylline is improved tissue perfusion with a reduced frequency of pain, improved tolerance to exercise, and improved peripheral pulses.

Nursing Process for Pentoxifylline

Premedication Assessment

1. Perform baseline gastrointestinal assessments to determine if nausea, vomiting, dyspepsia, or intolerance to caffeine products exists.
2. Assess for the presence of dizziness or headache.
3. Ask specifically about any cardiac symptoms. Report to health care provider if present.
4. Obtain baseline data on degree of pain present.

Planning

Availability. PO: 400 mg extended release tablets.

Implementation

Dosage and Administration. PO: 400 mg three times daily. If adverse gastrointestinal (GI) or central nervous system (CNS) effects develop, dosage should be reduced to 400 mg twice daily. If adverse effects persist, therapy should be discontinued. Symptomatic relief may start within 2 to 4 weeks, but treatment should be continued for at least 8 weeks to determine maximal efficacy.

Evaluation

Side Effects to Expect

Nausea, Vomiting, Dyspepsia. Dyspepsia, nausea, and vomiting occur in about 1% to 3% of patients. Belching and flatus occur in less than 1% of patients.

These side effects are usually mild and tend to resolve with continued therapy. Administration with food or milk may help minimize discomfort. Encourage the patient not to discontinue therapy without first consulting a physician.

Dizziness, Headache. CNS disturbances characterized by dizziness occur in about 2% of patients, and headache and tremor occur less frequently. These side effects are usually mild and tend to resolve with continued therapy. Provide for patient safety during episodes of dizziness. Encourage the patient to sit down if feeling faint. Encourage the patient not to discontinue therapy without first consulting a physician.

Side Effects to Report

Chest Pain, Dysrhythmias, Shortness of Breath. Without causing undue alarm, strongly encourage the patient to seek a physician's attention for further evaluation.

Intolerance to Caffeine, Theophylline, Theobromine. Pentoxifylline is a xanthine derivative. Patients should be asked specifically about intolerance to xanthine derivatives before starting therapy.

Drug Interactions

Antihypertensive Agents. Although pentoxifylline is not an antihypertensive agent, patients receiving pentoxifylline therapy frequently display a small reduction in systemic blood pressure. Blood pressure should be monitored to observe for hypotension. The dosage of antihypertensive therapy may have to be reduced to minimize adverse effects.

Theophylline. Concurrent use of pentoxifylline and theophylline-containing drugs leads to increased theophylline levels and theophylline toxicity in some individuals. Monitor patients closely for signs of toxicity (e.g., nausea, tachycardia) and adjust theophylline dosage as necessary.

DRUG CLASS: Vasodilators

isoxsuprine hydrochloride (i sok′ su preen)

VASODILAN (vas o dy′ lan)

Actions

Isoxsuprine hydrochloride is an alpha-adrenergic antagonist and a beta-adrenergic stimulant that causes vasodilatation of the smooth muscles of the blood vessels.

Uses

Isoxsuprine is used to treat the symptoms of peripheral vascular spasm, cerebral vascular insufficiency, Raynaud's and Buerger's diseases, and arteriosclerosis obliterans.

Therapeutic Outcomes

The primary therapeutic outcome expected from isoxsuprine therapy is improved tissue perfusion with a reduced frequency of pain, improved tolerance to exercise, and improved peripheral pulses.

Nursing Process for Isoxsuprine

Premedication Assessment

1. Obtain baseline assessment of degree of pain present and symptoms of peripheral vascular constriction.
2. Take baseline vital signs.

Planning

Availability. PO: 10 and 20 mg tablets.

Implementation

Dosage and Administration. PO: 10 to 20 mg three or four times daily. IM: 5 to 10 mg two or three times daily. Intramuscular administration may be used initially in acute conditions.

Evaluation

Side Effects to Expect

Flushing, Tingling, Sweating, Nausea, Vomiting. Explain to the patient that these side effects may occur during the initial phase of therapy; however, they resolve with continued therapy.

Side Effects to Report

Hypotension, Tachycardia. Monitor blood pressure and pulse throughout the course of therapy. Prevent hypotensive episodes by having the patient rise slowly from a supine or sitting position and perform exercises to prevent blood pooling when standing or sitting in one position for prolonged periods. Have the patient sit or lie down if feeling faint.

Severe Rash. Discontinue medication if a severe rash develops. Notify the physician so that appropriate alternate agents may be prescribed.

Nervousness, Weakness. As therapy progresses, these symptoms may develop. Tell the patient to discuss them with the health care provider if they become a problem.

Drug Interactions

Drugs That Enhance Therapeutic and Toxic Effects. Antihypertensive agents: The vasodilating action of isoxsuprine and antihypertensive agents may result in excessive hypotensive effects. Assess the blood pressure at regular intervals to monitor the combined effects. Monitor the patient for hypotension, lightheadedness, dizziness, and tachycardia. Provide for patient safety; prevent falls.

Drugs That Reduce Therapeutic Effects. Warn the patient against taking over-the-counter cough and cold preparations without first consulting the physician or pharmacist. Many of these products will counteract the effects of isoxsuprine.

papaverine hydrochloride (pah pav′ er in)
PAVAGEN TD (pah vah′ jen TD)

Actions

Papaverine relaxes smooth muscle, vasodilates cerebral and coronary blood vessels, and inhibits atrial and ventricular premature contractions and ventricular dysrhythmias.

Uses

Papaverine is a drug that has been tried for many illnesses for many years, but there is little objective evidence to indicate that it has any therapeutic value. Papaverine is used orally as a smooth muscle relaxant to treat cerebral and peripheral ischemia associated with arterial spasm and myocardial ischemia complicated by dysrhythmias.

Therapeutic Outcomes

The primary therapeutic outcome expected from papaverine is improved tissue perfusion with a reduced frequency of pain, improved tolerance to exercise, and improved peripheral pulses.

Nursing Process for Papaverine

Premedication Assessment

1. Obtain baseline assessment of degree of pain present and symptoms of peripheral vascular constriction.
2. Take baseline vital signs.

Planning

Availability. PO: 150 mg timed release capsules; IV: 30 mg/mL in 2-mL ampules and 10-mL vials.

Implementation

Dosage and Administration. PO: 60 to 300 mg one to five times daily; timed release products: 150 mg every 12 hours. In difficult cases, increase to 150 mg every 8 hours or 300 mg every 12 hours.

Evaluation

Side Effects to Expect and Report

Flushing, Sweating, Nausea, Abdominal Distress, Tachycardia, Vertigo, Drowsiness, Headache. These side effects are usually mild and are dose related. Monitor vital signs (blood pressure, pulse, respirations) and report deviations from baseline data for the physician's evaluation.

Drug Interactions

Drugs That Enhance Therapeutic and Toxic Effects. Antihypertensive agents: the vasodilating action of papaverine and antihypertensive agents may result in excessive hypotensive effects. Assess the blood pressure at regular intervals to monitor the combined effects. Monitor the patient for hypotension, lightheadedness, dizziness, and tachycardia. Provide for patient safety; prevent falls.

Drugs That Reduce Therapeutic Effects. Warn the patient against taking over-the-counter cough and cold preparations without first consulting the health care provider. Many of these products will counteract the effects of papaverine.

phenoxybenzamine hydrochloride
(fen ok se ben′ zah meen)
DIBENZYLINE (di ben′ zi leen)

Actions

Phenoxybenzamine is an alpha-adrenergic blocking agent that relaxes the smooth muscle of blood vessels, resulting in vasodilatation and improved blood flow to peripheral tissues.

Uses

Phenoxybenzamine is used in blood vessel disorders (e.g., Raynaud's disease, leg ulceration, complications of frostbite).

Therapeutic Outcomes

The primary therapeutic outcome expected from phenoxybenzamine is improved tissue perfusion with a reduced frequency of pain, improved tolerance to exercise, and improved peripheral pulses.

Nursing Process for Phenoxybenzamine

Premedication Assessment

1. Obtain baseline assessment of degree of pain present and symptoms of peripheral vascular constriction.
2. Take baseline vital signs.

Planning

Availability. PO: 10 mg capsules.

Implementation

Dosage and Administration. PO: Initially 10 mg per day. After determining response for 4 or more days, increase the dose by 10-mg increments every few days to a maximum of 60 mg per day. Several weeks of therapy are usually required to observe full therapeutic benefits.

Evaluation

Side Effects to Expect and Report

Nasal Stuffiness, Miosis, Hypotension, Tachycardia. Monitor blood pressure and pulse. Prevent hypotensive episodes by instructing the patient to rise slowly from a supine or sitting position and perform exercises to prevent blood pooling when standing or sitting in one position for prolonged periods. Have the patient sit or lie down if feeling faint. Report increasing episodes so that dosage is adjusted accordingly.

Drug Interactions

Drugs That Enhance Therapeutic and Toxic Effects. Antihypertensive agents and alcohol: the vasodilating action of phenoxybenzamine and antihypertensive agents may result in excessive hypotensive effects. Assess the blood pressure at regular intervals to monitor the combined effects. Monitor the patient for hypotension, lightheadedness, dizziness, and tachycardia. Provide for patient safety; prevent falls.

Drugs That Reduce Therapeutic Effects. Warn the patient against taking over-the-counter cough and cold preparations without first consulting the health care provider. Many of these products will counteract the effects of phenoxybenzamine.

DRUG CLASS: Platelet Aggregation Inhibitor

cilostazol (sigh lo stay' zohl)
PLETAL (pleh' tahl)

Actions

Cilostazol is a selective inhibitor of cellular cyclic adenosine monophosphate (cAMP) phosphodiesterase III (PDE III). Suppression of this enzyme causes increased levels of cAMP, resulting in vasodilatation and inhibition of platelet aggregation. Other mechanisms in addition to vasodilatation are thought to play a role but are not fully known at this time.

Uses

Cilostazol is approved for the treatment of intermittent claudication. Cilostazol therapy should be considered an adjunct to, and not a replacement for, smoking cessation, weight loss, exercise therapy, surgical bypass, or removal of arterial obstructions in the treatment of peripheral vascular disease.

Therapeutic Outcomes

The primary therapeutic outcome expected from cilostazol is improved tissue perfusion with a reduced frequency of pain, improved tolerance to exercise, and improved peripheral pulses.

Nursing Process for Cilostazol

Premedication Assessment

1. Assess for the presence of dizziness or headache.
2. Obtain baseline assessment of degree of pain present and symptoms of peripheral vascular disease.
3. Ask specifically about any cardiac symptoms. Report to a health care provider if present.

Planning

Availability. PO: 50 and 100 mg tablets.

Implementation

Dosage and Administration. PO: 100 mg two times daily, taken 30 minutes before or 2 hours after breakfast and dinner. Symptomatic relief may start within 2 to 4 weeks, but treatment should be continued for at least 12 weeks to determine maximal efficacy.

NOTE: Do not administer to patients with heart failure. Phosphodiesterase inhibitors have been reported to significantly worsen heart failure.

Evaluation

Side Effects to Expect

Dyspepsia, Diarrhea. Dyspepsia and diarrhea occur in about 2% to 5% of patients. These side effects are usually mild and tend to resolve with continued therapy. Encourage the patient not to discontinue therapy without first consulting a health care provider.

Dizziness, Headache. CNS disturbances characterized by dizziness occur in about 2% of patients. Headache severe enough to cause discontinuation occurred in 3% of patients. These side effects are usually mild and tend to resolve with continued therapy. Provide for patient safety during episodes of dizziness. Encourage the patient to sit down if feeling faint. Encourage the patient not to discontinue therapy without first consulting a health care provider.

Side Effects to Report

Chest Pain, Palpitations, Dysrhythmias, Shortness of Breath. Without causing undue alarm, strongly encourage the patient to seek a health care provider's attention for further evaluation.

Drug Interactions

Diltiazem, Erythromycin, Omeprazole, Fluconazole, Fluvoxamine, Sertraline, Ketoconazole, Grapefruit Juice. These substances may inhibit the metabolism of cilostazol. If cilostazol therapy is necessary for patients already receiving any of the preceding drugs, the starting dose of cilostazol should be one half the normal starting dose. Monitor patients closely for an increased incidence of adverse effects.

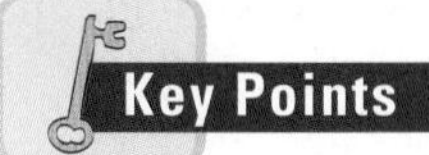

Key Points

- Peripheral vascular disease is a cause of significant morbidity in the United States. Major treatable causes of peripheral vascular disease are hypertension, cigarette smoking, and atherosclerosis.
- The most cost-effective and successful forms of treatment are smoking cessation, weight reduction, exercise, and dietary modification.
- Patients should be fully informed of the significance of peripheral vascular disease, the potential complications of not modifying lifestyles, and the use of drug therapy.

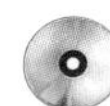

Go to your Companion CD-ROM for Appendices, an Audio Glossary, animations, Drug Dosage Calculators, customizable Patient Self-Assessment forms, and Review Questions for the NCLEX® Examination.

evolve Be sure to visit the companion Evolve site at http://evolve.elsevier.com/Clayton for WebLinks and additional online resources.

MEDICATION SAFETY REVIEW

MATH REVIEW QUESTIONS

1. Order: pentoxifylline (Trental) 400 mg PO daily for 4 days, then 400 mg daily bid

   Available: pentoxifylline (Trental) 400-mg tablets

   How many 400 mg tablets would be needed to administer the first 4 days of dosages?

   How many 400 mg tablets would be needed to administer the next 5 days of dosages?

2. Order: papaverine hydrochloride (Pavagen) 300 mg q12h

   Available: papaverine hydrochloride (Pavagen) 150-mg timed release capsules

   Give: ____ capsules per dose.

CRITICAL THINKING QUESTIONS

Situation: A patient tells you that when she and her husband go for their daily walks, he can only go two blocks and then must sit down because of pain in the calves of his legs. They rest awhile, walk another two blocks, and the pain is back. She asks your advice.

1. What would you say?

Two days later, the patient's husband is assigned to you for nursing care. His primary nursing diagnosis is ineffective tissue perfusion related to insufficient oxygenation of the lower limbs manifested by pain on walking two blocks and diminished popliteal pulses, bilaterally.

2. What nursing assessments would you make?
3. His health care provider prescribes cilostazol (Pletal) 100 mg, bid. Review the drug monograph and discuss the drug's action and side effects to anticipate.
4. What health teaching would be needed in relation to his prescribed drug therapy?

Situation: A 76-year-old patient has been experiencing arteriosclerosis obliterans with intermittent claudication. He refuses to give up smoking. At his last office visit, he was given a prescription for pentoxifylline (Trental) 400 mg PO tid with meals. After leaving the examination room he tells you (the office nurse) that the health care provider did not explain how this would work to improve his "leg pain."

5. Give the patient a simple explanation of what is thought to be the mechanism of action of pentoxyfylline and draw a diagram that depicts "erythrocyte flexibility." Use the visual aid to help him understand how the drug could improve his leg pain.
6. One week later, the patient calls the office and says, "That new medication you gave me for my leg pain isn't working." How should you respond?

Continued

CONTENT REVIEW QUESTIONS

1. The physician orders phenoxybenzamine hydrochloride and the patient asks you what side effects to expect from this medication. The main point to make when responding is:
   1. that the side effects are a rapid pulse, nasal congestion, and episodes of low blood pressure.
   2. that most of the side effects you've explained will resolve with continued therapy.
   3. if the side effects occur, the drug should be stopped immediately.
   4. to decrease the dose when the side effects explained occur.

2. Pentoxifylline (Trental) acts:
   1. to increase the flexibility of the erythrocytes.
   2. as an anticoagulant.
   3. to increase the viscosity of blood flow.
   4. to break down the plaque in the blood vessels.

3. Premedication assessments with peripheral vascular disease should include:
   1. checking for renal disease.
   2. obtaining a pain rating.
   3. checking mentation.
   4. assessing respiratory function.

4. The usual medical treatment of Raynaud's disease involves:
   1. transluminal balloon angioplasty.
   2. amputation of the affected digits.
   3. calcium ion antagonists.
   4. pentoxifylline and cilostazol.

5. The most significant risk factors in the development of peripheral vascular disease are *(select all that apply)*:
   1. hypertension.
   2. cigarette smoking.
   3. low LDL levels.
   4. high HDL levels.

6. A patient with chronic arterial occlusive disease has a nursing diagnosis of *Tissue perfusion, altered.* Appropriate teaching for the patient includes instructions to:
   1. rest and sleep with the legs elevated.
   2. soak the feet in warm water 30 minutes a day.
   3. walk at least 30 minutes per day.
   4. use alternative forms of nicotine as a substitute for smoking.

7. The nurse teaches the patient with any venous disorder that the best way to prevent venous stasis and increase venous return is to:
   1. ambulate.
   2. sit with the legs elevated.
   3. frequently rotate ankles.
   4. continuously wear compression gradient stockings.

CHAPTER 27

Drugs Used to Treat Thromboembolic Disorders

evolve http://evolve.elsevier.com/Clayton

Chapter Content

Objectives

1. State the primary purposes of anticoagulant therapy.
2. Analyze Figure 27-1 to identify the site of action of warfarin, heparin, and fibrinolytic agents.
3. Identify the effects of anticoagulant therapy on existing blood clots.
4. Describe conditions that place an individual at risk for developing blood clots.
5. Identify specific nursing interventions that can prevent clot formation.
6. Explain laboratory data used to establish dosing of anticoagulant medications.
7. Describe specific monitoring procedures to detect hemorrhage in the patient taking anticoagulants.
8. Describe procedures used to ensure that the correct dose of an anticoagulant is prepared and administered.
9. Explain the specific procedures and techniques used to administer heparin subcutaneously (subcut), via intermittent administration through a heparin lock, and via intravenous (IV) infusion.
10. Identify the purpose, dosing determination, and scheduling factors associated with the use of protamine sulfate.
11. State the nursing assessments needed to monitor therapeutic response and the development of side effects to expect or report from anticoagulant therapy.
12. Develop objectives for patient education for patients receiving anticoagulant therapy.

Key Terms

thromboembolic diseases
thrombosis
thrombus
embolus
intrinsic clotting pathway
extrinsic clotting pathway
platelet inhibitors
anticoagulants
thrombolytic agents

THROMBOEMBOLIC DISEASES

Diseases associated with abnormal clotting within blood vessels are known as **thromboembolic diseases** and are major causes of morbidity and mortality. **Thrombosis** is the process of formation of a fibrin blood clot **(thrombus)**. An **embolus** is a small fragment of a thrombus that breaks off and circulates until it becomes trapped in a capillary, causing either ischemia or infarction to the area distal to the obstruction (e.g., cerebral embolism, pulmonary embolism).

Major causes of thrombus formation are immobilization with venous stasis; surgery and the postoperative period; trauma to lower limbs; certain illnesses (e.g., heart failure, vasospasm, ulcerative colitis); cancers of the lung, prostate, stomach, and pancreas; pregnancy and oral contraceptives; and heredity.

Normally, blood clot formation and dissolution constitute a fine balance within the cardiovascular system. The clotting proteins normally circulate in an inactive state and must be activated to form a fibrin clot. When there is a trigger, such as increased blood viscosity from bed rest and stasis or damage to a blood vessel wall, the *clotting cascade* is activated. For example, if a blood vessel is injured and collagen in the vessel wall is exposed, platelets first adhere to the site of injury and release adenosine diphosphate (ADP), leading to additional platelet aggregation that forms a "platelet plug." At the same time platelets are forming a plug, the **intrinsic clotting pathway** is triggered by the presence of collagen activating factor XII. Activated factor XIIa activates factor XI to XIa, which activates factor IX to IXa. Factor IXa, in the presence of calcium, platelet factor 3 (PF3), and factor VIII, activates factor X. Activated factor Xa, in the presence of calcium, PF3, and factor V, stimulates the conversion of prothrombin to thrombin (see Figure 27-1).

Sources outside the blood vessels, such as tissue extract or thromboplastin (tissue factor), can trigger the **extrinsic clotting pathway** by activating factor VII to VIIa. Factor VIIa can also activate factor X, which results in the formation of thrombin. After stimulation from either the intrinsic or extrinsic pathway, thrombin, in the presence of calcium, activates fibrinogen to soluble fibrin. With time and the presence of factor XIII, the loose fibrin mesh is converted to a tight, insoluble fibrin mesh clot. Thrombin also stimulates

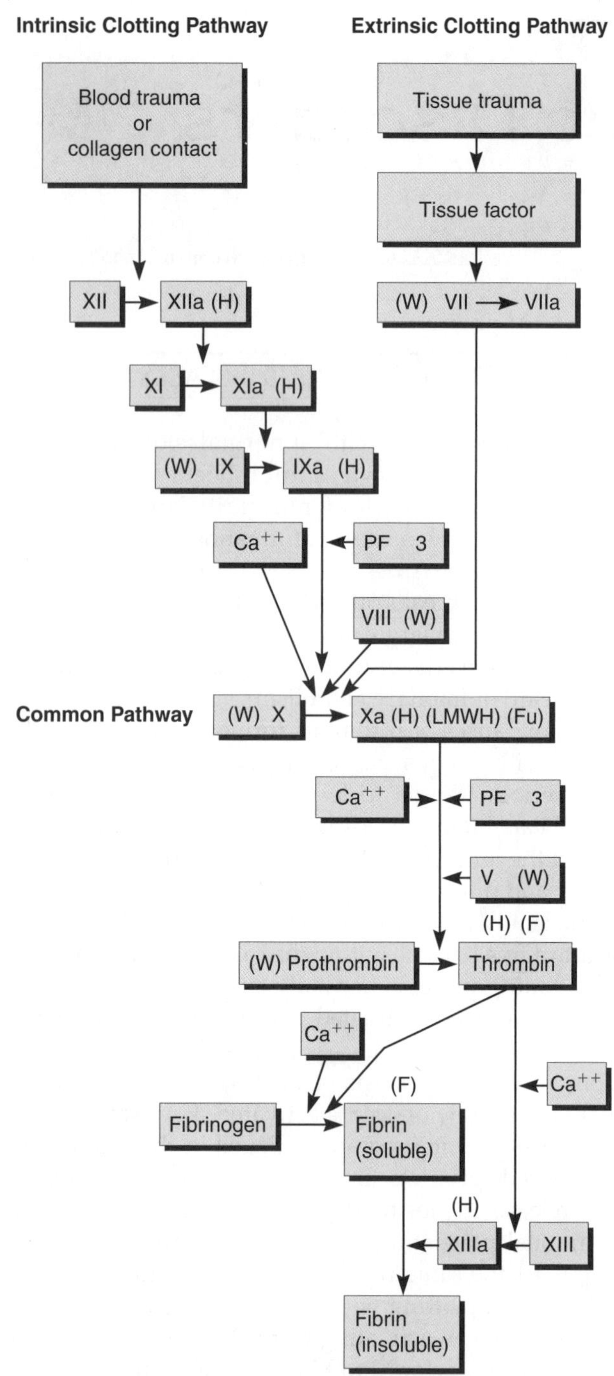

FIGURE **27-1** The clotting cascade. *F,* Site of fibrinolytic action; *H,* site of heparin action; *PF3,* platelet factor 3; *W,* site of warfarin action; *LMWH,* site of low-molecular-weight heparins; *Fu,* fondaparinux.

platelet aggregation and stimulates further activity of factors V, VIIa, VII, and Xa. As the fibrin clot is being formed, it also triggers the release of fibrinolysin, an enzyme that dissolves fibrin, preventing the clot from spreading.

Historically, thrombi have been classified into red and white blood clots. A red thrombus is actually a venous thrombus and is composed almost entirely of fibrin and erythrocytes (red blood cells) with a few platelets. Venous thrombi generally form in response to venous stasis after immobility or surgery. The poor circulation prevents dilution of activated coagulation factors by rapidly circulating blood. The most common cause of red thrombus formation is deep vein thrombosis of the lower extremities. These thrombi may extend upward into the veins of the thigh and have the potential of fragmenting to cause life-threatening pulmonary emboli. White thrombi develop in arteries and are composed of platelets and fibrin. This type of thrombus forms in areas of high blood flow in response to injured vessel walls. Coronary artery occlusion leading to myocardial infarction is an example of a white thrombus.

TREATMENT OF THROMBOEMBOLIC DISEASES

Diseases caused by intravascular clotting (e.g., deep vein thrombosis, myocardial infarction, dysrhythmias with clot formation, coronary vasospasm leading to thrombus formation) are major causes of death. When thrombosis is suspected, patients are admitted to the hospital and often placed in an intensive care unit, where they can be closely observed for further signs and symptoms of thrombosis formation and progression and anticoagulant and thrombolytic therapy can be started. A combination of physical examination, patient history, Doppler ultrasound, phlebography, radiolabeled fibrinogen studies, and angiograms is used to diagnose the presence and etiology of a thrombus and an embolism. Routine laboratory tests that are run to assess the clotting process and ensure that occult bleeding is not present are platelet count, hematocrit, prothrombin time (PT), activated partial thromboplastin time (APTT), activated clotting time (ACT), urinalysis, and stool guaiac test.

Nonpharmacologic prevention and treatment of thromboembolic disease include patient education on how to prevent venous stasis (e.g., leg exercises, leg elevation), the use of properly fitted thromboembolic disease (TED) deterrent stockings, and sequential compression devices (SCDs). If a patient suffering a heart attack (myocardial infarction, acute coronary syndrome) is able to be transported to a cardiac intensive care facility soon after symptoms develop, revascularization treatment to reopen the coronary arteries may be performed. Thrombolytic agents may be used to dissolve the clot before it is permanently formed. Revascularization procedures used may be a percutaneous coronary intervention (PCI) or coronary artery bypass graft (CABG). Percutaneous coronary intervention, also known as angioplasty, is the insertion of a catheter into the femoral artery with advancement up the aorta into the coronary artery obstruction. Different types of devices on the tip of the catheter, such as a balloon, dilate the artery obstruction, or blades or lasers "Roto-root" out the obstruction. A vascular stent is then often placed in the artery to keep the formerly obstructed area open. If a patient has multiple narrowed or obstructed arteries, a CABG procedure is ordered wherein a segment of the saphenous vein from the leg is harvested and attached to the coronary artery above and below the obstruction, forming a bypass for perfusion to the myocardial tissues below. The internal mammary artery can also be used in this procedure. The major pharmacologic treatments used in the prevention and treatment of thromboembolic diseases are the platelet inhibitors, anticoagulants, the glycoprotein IIb/IIIa inhibitors, and thrombolytic agents.

DRUG THERAPY FOR THROMBOEMBOLIC DISEASES

Actions

The pharmacologic agents used to treat thromboembolic disease act either to prevent platelet aggregation or inhibit a variety of steps in the fibrin clot formation cascade (see Figure 27-1). See individual monographs for a more detailed discussion of mechanisms of action.

Uses

Agents used in the prevention and treatment of thromboembolic disease can be divided into **platelet inhibitors, anticoagulants,** glycoprotein IIb/IIIa inhibitors, and **thrombolytic agents.** Antiplatelet agents (e.g., aspirin) are used preventively to reduce arterial clot formation (white thrombi) by inhibiting platelet aggregation. The anticoagulants (e.g., warfarin, heparin, and heparin derivatives [ardeparin, enoxaparin, dalteparin]) are also used prophylactically to prevent formation of arterial and venous thrombi in predisposed patients. The heparin derivatives are also known as low-molecular-weight heparins (LMWHs). The primary purpose of anticoagulants is to prevent new clot formation or the extension of existing clots. They cannot dissolve an existing clot. The thrombolytic agents (e.g., streptokinase, alteplase) are used to dissolve thromboemboli once formed.

NURSING PROCESS *for Anticoagulant Therapy*

Assessment

History. Ask specific questions to determine whether the patient or family members have a history of any type of vascular difficulty. Patients at greater risk for clot formation are those with a history of clot formation, those with recent abdominal, thoracic, or orthopedic surgery, and those on prolonged bed rest or anticoagulant therapy.

Current Symptoms

- Ask the patient to describe the symptoms. Is the patient now taking or has the patient recently taken anticoagulants? Individualize further questioning to obtain data that would support or rule out thrombosis formation or progression of thrombosis.
- Collect data about reduced tissue perfusion (e.g., symptoms relating to cerebral, cardiopulmonary, or peripheral vascular disease, depending on underlying pathophysiology).

Medications

- Obtain a thorough medication history of both prescribed and over-the-counter medications being taken.
- Ask specific questions relating to medicines being taken that affect clotting.
- Ask whether the patient has been complying with medication regimens and if any dosage adjustment has taken place. If anticoagulants are being taken, has the patient reported for scheduled laboratory studies? Has the patient had any reactions to the medication?

Basic Assessment

- Obtain vital signs and auscultation of breath sounds. Observe for dyspnea at rest or with exertion.
- Check mental status (e.g., orientation to date, time, and place; alertness; confusion). Use as a baseline for future comparison.
- Assess for specific signs of reduced tissue perfusion. Perform a focused assessment depending on the underlying pathologic condition (e.g., cardiopulmonary, cerebral, or peripheral vascular disease).
- Collect data about any pain experienced.
- Ask specific questions about the patient's state of hydration. Review intake and output.

Diagnostic Studies. Review completed diagnostic studies and laboratory data (e.g., PT, APTT, hematocrit, platelet count, Doppler studies, exercise testing, serum triglycerides, arteriogram, cardiac enzyme studies).

Nursing Diagnoses

- Tissue perfusion, ineffective (indication)
- Gas exchange, impaired (indication)

Planning

History of Causative Disorder or Factors. Review the patient's history to identify the diagnosis for which the anticoagulant or thrombolytic therapy was prescribed.

History of Current Symptoms. Plan to perform a focused assessment at appropriate intervals consistent with the patient's status to detect further signs and symptoms of thrombosis formation or progression. Does the patient have any concurrent disease processes that may increase the risk of bleeding (e.g., ulcer disease, concurrent chemotherapy, or radiation therapy)?

Medications. Schedule prescribed anticoagulant medications on the medication administration record (MAR). Remember to *mark the one-time dosages clearly* because some medicines prescribed are based on the results of laboratory data completed daily or more frequently.

Hydration. Schedule intake and output (I&O) every shift or more frequently depending on the patient's status. Place information to be assessed for status of hydration on the Kardex.

Laboratory and Diagnostic Studies

- Order requested laboratory and diagnostic studies relating to the disease process (e.g., platelet count, hematocrit, PT, APTT, arteriogram, Doppler studies).
- Mark the Kardex or enter data in computer when additional laboratory studies are ordered (e.g., collection of stools for guaiac testing).

Prevention of Clot Formation or Extension

- Record activity level permitted on the Kardex or in the computer. Place the patient on a turning schedule if on complete bed rest, or schedule activities for mobility.
- Mark the Kardex or enter data in computer with orders for use of TED hose. Schedule times for removal and inspection of the legs every shift.
- Sequential compression devices (SCDs) are used to promote venous return from the legs. SCDs inflate and deflate plastic sleeves around the legs to promote venous flow. These are removed when ambulating, and discontinued when the patient resumes full activity.

Implementation

Techniques for Preventing Clot Formation

- Provide early, regular ambulation after surgery. Use active or passive leg exercises for patients on bed rest or restricted activity.
- Develop and follow a specific turning schedule for patients on complete bed rest to prevent tissue breakdown and blood stasis. Implement good back care and deep breathing and coughing exercises as part of general nursing care.
- Do not flex the knees or place pressure against the popliteal space with pillows.
- Do not allow the patient to stand or sit motionless for prolonged periods.
- Use elastic hose, such as TED stockings. Remove stockings and inspect the skin on every shift. Make sure they are being worn properly and not becoming bunched around the knees or ankles.
- Apply SCDs as ordered and indicated. Make sure they are applied properly.

Patient Assessment. Monitor vital signs and mental status every 4 to 8 hours or more frequently, depending on the patient's status. Observe for signs and symptoms of bleeding due to medications (e.g., blurred vision, hematuria, ecchymosis, occult blood in the stools, change in mentation).

Nutritional Status

- The dietary regimen will depend on the patient's diagnosis and clinical status.
- Adequate hydration to promote fluidity of the blood is important. Unless coexisting diagnoses prohibit, give at least six to eight 8-ounce glasses of liquid daily.

Laboratory and Diagnostic Data. Monitoring and reporting laboratory results to the health care provider are essential during anticoagulant therapy. Coagulation tests that might be ordered include the following: whole blood clotting time (WBCT), PT, APTT, and activated coagulation time (ACT). The PT, reported as the International Normalized Ratio (INR), is routinely used to monitor warfarin therapy, and the APTT is most commonly used to monitor heparin therapy.

Medication Administration. Never administer an anticoagulant without first checking the chart for the most recent laboratory results. Be certain that the anticoagulant to be administered is ordered *after* the most recent results have been reported to the health care provider. Follow policy statements regarding checking of anticoagulant doses with other qualified professionals. Reduce localized bleeding at the injection site by using the smallest needle possible for injections and rotate injection sites. See individual monographs for specific administration techniques related to a particular medicine.

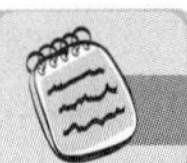

Patient Education and Health Promotion

Nutritional Status

- While receiving anticoagulant therapy, patients must limit intake of green leafy vegetables that contain vitamin K. (Vitamin K inhibits the action of warfarin.)
- Instruct the patient to drink six to eight 8-ounce glasses of liquid daily, unless the physician has prescribed fluid restrictions.

Exercise and Activity

- For peripheral vascular disease, Buerger-Allen exercises may be recommended. Teach procedure and frequency.
- Discuss the level of exercise prescribed by the physician. Walking may be prescribed to promote venous blood flow. Elevation of the legs when seated may be encouraged to promote venous blood flow.
- Stress the need to prevent body injury while taking anticoagulants. Tell the patient to avoid using power equipment, use care in stepping up or down from curbs, not participate in contact sports, use only an electric razor, and brush teeth gently with a soft-bristled toothbrush.

Medication Regimen

- Instruct the patient to take the dosage of the medication exactly as prescribed. Explain the importance of returning for laboratory blood tests to determine effectiveness and the need to adjust medicine dosages. Tell the patient to resume a regular schedule if one dose of warfarin is missed.

PATIENT SELF-ASSESSMENT FORM Anticoagulants

MEDICATIONS	COLOR	TO BE TAKEN

Patient ______

Health Care Provider ______

Health Care Provider's phone ______

Next appt.* ______

What I Should Monitor		Premedication Data	Date	Date	Date	Date	Date	Date	Comments
Weight									
Blood pressure									
Pulse									
Color of urine	Normal								
	Red								
	Orange								
Mouth	Gums bleed with brushing								
Shaving	Bleeding: difficulty stopping blood								
Bruising	Nosebleeds: (____) of times?								
	Bruising to light touch								
Pain relief	Name limb (e.g., left leg, right leg)								
	Color of limb								
	Temperature								
Activities of daily living	Able to do								
	Done with difficulty								
	Too difficult to do								
Bowel movements	Normal								
	Diarrhea								
	Color: normal or black, tarry								
	Smell: normal or foul								
Report immediately	Chest pain								
	Faintness								
	Dizziness								
	Red vomitus								
	Black stools								
Other									

*Please bring this record with you to your next appointment.
Use the back of this sheet for additional information.

If two or more doses are missed, the patient should consult a physician.

- Tell the patient to wear a medication alert bracelet.
- Explain symptoms the patient should report, such as nosebleeds, tarry stools, "coffee ground" or blood-tinged vomitus, petechiae (tiny purple or red spots occurring in various sites on the skin), ecchymoses (bruises), hematuria (blood in the urine), bleeding from the gums or any other body opening, or cuts or injuries from which the bleeding is difficult to control. Check dressings periodically for bleeding. Report excessive menstrual flow.
- In some cases the health care provider may want the patient to perform guaiac testing to detect blood in the stool. If ordered, specific patient education should be done to teach the patient or support person how to perform the test.
- Tell patients that because not all bleeding is clearly visible, they should report immediately a rapid, weak pulse; deep, rapid respirations; moist, clammy skin; and a general feeling of weakness or faintness.
- Tell the patient *not* to take any medication, including over-the-counter medications, without first consulting a health care provider, because many drugs interact with warfarin to either increase or decrease its effectiveness. Never discontinue anticoagulant therapy without health care provider agreement.
- Patients should always inform any health care provider (e.g., physician, home health care provider, dentist) that anticoagulant therapy is being taken whenever seeking care.

Fostering Health Maintenance

- Throughout the course of treatment, discuss medication information and how it will benefit the patient.
- Provide the patient and significant others with important information contained in the specific drug monograph for the medicines prescribed. Additional health teaching and nursing interventions for the side effects to expect and report are described in the drug monographs that follow. Teach the patient to avoid power equipment, to use an electric razor, and to use a soft-bristled toothbrush. Use caution in cutting with a knife or using any other sharp objects.
- Seek cooperation and understanding of the following points so that medication compliance is increased: name of medication, dosage, route and times of administration, side effects to expect, and side effects to report.

Written Record. Enlist the patient's aid in developing and maintaining a written record of monitoring parameters (see the Patient Self-Assessment Form on p. 433). Complete the Premedication Data column for use as a baseline to track response to drug therapy. Ensure that the patient understands how to use the form and instruct the patient to bring the completed form to follow-up visits. During follow-up visits, focus on issues that will foster adherence with the therapeutic interventions prescribed.

DRUG CLASS: Platelet Inhibitors

aspirin (as' per in)

Actions

Aspirin is well known as a salicylate and a nonsteroidal antiinflammatory agent. A unique property of aspirin, when compared with other salicylates, is platelet aggregation inhibition with prolongation of bleeding time. The platelet loses its ability to aggregate and form clots for the duration of its lifetime (7 to 10 days). The mechanism of action is acetylation of the cyclooxygenase enzyme, which inhibits the synthesis of thromboxane A_2, a potent vasoconstrictor and inducer of platelet aggregation.

Uses

Aspirin is used to reduce the risk of recurrent transient ischemic attacks (TIAs) and stroke. There is controversy in the literature as to whether aspirin is equally effective in women. Aspirin is also used to reduce the risk of myocardial infarction in patients with previous myocardial infarction or unstable angina pectoris.

Therapeutic Outcomes

The primary therapeutic outcomes expected from aspirin therapy when used for antiplatelet therapy are as follows:

- Reduced frequency of TIAs or stroke.
- Reduced frequency of myocardial infarction.

Nursing Process for Aspirin

Premedication Assessment

1. Perform baseline neurologic assessment: orientation to date, time, and place; mental alertness; bilateral hand grip; motor functioning (balance and hearing).
2. Monitor for gastrointestinal (GI) symptoms before and during therapy. Stool guaiac testing may be ordered if GI tract bleeding is suspected.
3. Check on concurrent use of anticoagulant agents.
4. If the patient is receiving oral hypoglycemic agents, review baseline serum glucose levels.

Planning

Availability. See Tables 20-4 and 20-5.

Implementation

Dosage and Administration. *For prevention of blood clots:* PO: 80 to 1300 mg daily. The dosage depends on whether the patient has a previous history of clot formation and other medications the patient may be receiving. The larger doses are usually subdivided into 325-mg doses two to four times daily. Administer with meals to minimize gastric irritation.

Evaluation

See Chapter 20, Drugs Used for Pain Management.

dipyridamole (dye per id′ a mole)
PERSANTINE (per sahn′ teen)

Actions

Dipyridamole is a platelet-adhesiveness inhibitor that is thought to work by inhibiting thromboxane A_2, increasing cyclic adenosine monophosphate (cAMP) in platelets, potentiating prostacyclin-mediated inhibition, and possibly reducing red blood cell uptake of adenosine, which also inhibits platelets.

Uses

Dipyridamole has been used extensively in combination with warfarin to prevent thromboembolism after cardiac valve replacement. It has also been prescribed in combination with aspirin to prevent myocardial infarction, TIAs, and stroke. Recent studies, however, indicate that the combination is no more effective than aspirin alone.

Therapeutic Outcomes

The primary therapeutic outcome from dipyridamole therapy is preventing blood clots secondary to artificial valve placement.

Nursing Process for Dipyridamole

Premedication Assessment

Obtain baseline vital signs.

Planning

Availability. PO: 25, 50, and 75 mg tablets.

Implementation

Dosage and Administration. *Adult:* PO: 75 to 100 mg four times daily with warfarin to prevent thromboembolism secondary to valve replacement.

Evaluation

Side Effects to Expect and Report

Dizziness, Abdominal Distress. Dizziness and abdominal distress are transient and disappear with continued therapy. Encourage the patient not to discontinue therapy.

Monitor the blood pressure daily in both the supine and standing positions.

Anticipate the development of postural hypotension and take measures to prevent an occurrence. Teach the patient to rise slowly from a supine or sitting position, and encourage the patient to sit or lie down if feeling faint.

Drug Interactions. No clinically significant drug interactions have been reported with dipyridamole.

clopidogrel (clo pid′ oh grel)
PLAVIX (plah′ vix)

Actions

Clopidogrel is chemically related to ticlopidine. Clopidogrel is a prodrug; one of its metabolites, as yet unknown, is thought to act by inhibiting the ADP pathway required for platelet aggregation. The full antiplatelet activity is seen after 3 to 7 days of continuous therapy. The antiaggregatory effect persists for approximately 5 days after discontinuation of therapy. Clopidogrel also prolongs bleeding time.

Uses

Clopidogrel is used to reduce the risk of additional atherosclerotic events (e.g., myocardial infarction, stroke, vascular death) in patients who have had a recent stroke, recent myocardial infarction, or established peripheral arterial disease. The medical histories of those patients at greatest risk include TIAs, atrial fibrillation, angina pectoris, and carotid artery stenosis. Because clopidogrel has a different mechanism of action from aspirin, it is anticipated that health care providers may use both drugs concurrently. The overall safety profile of clopidogrel appears to be at least as good as that of medium-dose aspirin and better than 250 mg of ticlopidine twice daily.

Therapeutic Outcomes

The primary therapeutic outcomes expected from clopidogrel therapy are reduced frequency of TIAs, stroke, myocardial infarctions, or complications from peripheral vascular disease.

Nursing Process for Clopidogrel

Premedication Assessment

1. Obtain baseline vital signs.
2. Order baseline laboratory studies requested by the health care provider (e.g., complete blood count [CBC]).
3. Assess and record any GI symptoms.

Planning

Availability. PO: 75 mg tablets.

Implementation

Dosage and Administration. *Adult:* PO: 75 mg once daily with food or on an empty stomach.

Evaluation

Side Effects to Expect

Nausea, Vomiting, Anorexia, Diarrhea. These effects tend to occur most frequently with early dosages and tend to resolve with continued therapy over the next 2 weeks. They can also be minimized by taking the medicine with food. Encourage the patient not to discontinue therapy without first consulting a health care provider.

Side Effects to Report

Neutropenia, Agranulocytosis. Neutropenia (absolute neutrophil count <1200 neutrophils/mm^3) was discovered in 0.4% of patients in clinical trials. While neutropenic, patients are very susceptible to infection. Encourage the patient to report symptoms of infection (e.g., sore throat, fever, excessive fatigue) to the physician as soon as possible.

Bleeding. A normal physiologic effect of clopidogrel is prolongation of bleeding time. Patients should report any incidents of bleeding as soon as possible. Incidents to be reported include nosebleeds, easy bruising, bright red or "coffee ground" emesis, hematuria, and dark tarry stools.

Patients should inform other health care practitioners (e.g., other physicians, dentist) that they are receiving platelet inhibitor therapy.

Drug Interactions

Phenytoin, Tamoxifen, Tolbutamide, Warfarin, Torsemide, Fluvastatin, Nonsteroidal Antiinflammatory Drugs (NSAIDs). At higher doses, clopidogrel may inhibit the metabolism of these agents. Caution should be used when any of these drugs is coadministered with clopidogrel.

ticlopidine (ty cloh' ped een)
▶ TICLID (ty' clid)

Actions

Ticlopidine is thought to act by inhibiting the ADP pathway required for platelet aggregation. The antiplatelet activity is seen after 3 to 5 days of continuous therapy. The antiaggregatory effect persists for up to 10 days after discontinuation of therapy. Ticlopidine also prolongs bleeding time. The maximal effect is seen after 5 or 6 days of continuous therapy.

Uses

Ticlopidine is used to reduce the risk of additional strokes in patients who have had a stroke and those who are at risk for a stroke. The medical histories of those patients at greatest risk include TIAs, atrial fibrillation, and carotid artery stenosis. Studies indicate that it is equally effective in men and women.

Early studies indicate that ticlopidine is more effective in reducing the risk of strokes than aspirin, but the potential for side effects (e.g., neutropenia/agranulocytosis) limits its use to patients who cannot tolerate aspirin therapy (GI bleeding or hypersensitivity) or who should not take aspirin.

Therapeutic Outcomes

The primary therapeutic outcome expected from ticlopidine therapy is reduced frequency of TIAs and stroke.

Nursing Process for Ticlopidine

Premedication Assessment

1. Obtain baseline vital signs.
2. Order baseline laboratory studies requested by the physician (e.g., CBC).
3. Assess and record any GI symptoms.

Planning

Availability. PO: 250 mg tablets.

Implementation

Dosage and Administration. *Adult:* PO: 250 mg two times daily with meals.

Evaluation

Side Effects to Expect

Nausea, Vomiting, Anorexia, Diarrhea. These effects tend to occur most frequently with early dosages and tend to resolve with continued therapy over the next 2 weeks. They can also be minimized by taking the medicine with food. Encourage the patient not to discontinue therapy without first consulting a physician.

Side Effects to Report

Neutropenia, Agranulocytosis. Neutropenia (absolute neutrophil count <1200 neutrophils/mm^3) was discovered in 2.4% of patients in clinical trials. While neutropenic, patients are susceptible to infection. The neutropenic effects occur within 3 weeks to 3 months after start of therapy. The manufacturer recommends that blood counts be taken every 2 weeks for the first 3 months of therapy. Stress the importance of returning for this laboratory work. Encourage the patient to report symptoms of infection (e.g., sore throat, fever, excessive fatigue) to the health care provider as soon as possible.

Bleeding. A normal physiologic effect of ticlopidine is prolongation of bleeding time. Patients should report any incidents of bleeding as soon as possible. Incidents to be reported include nosebleeds, easy bruising, bright red or "coffee ground" emesis, hematuria, and dark tarry stools.

Patients should inform other health care practitioners (e.g., another physician, dentist) that they are receiving platelet inhibitor therapy.

Drug Interactions

Cimetidine. Cimetidine significantly reduces the metabolism of ticlopidine. Monitor patients closely for signs of toxicity from the ticlopidine.

Ginkgo Biloba, Danshen. These herbal medicines increase the risk for bleeding as a result of decreased platelet aggregation. Concurrent therapy with ticlopidine is not recommended.

DRUG CLASS: Anticoagulants

dalteparin (dalt eh′ pair in)
▶ FRAGMIN (frag′ min)

Actions

Dalteparin is the second (after enoxaparin) of the LMWHs that are essentially the active components of the heparin protein molecule. The LMWHs have the advantage of specific action at certain steps of the coagulation pathway, resulting in less potential for hemorrhage and longer duration of action. Dalteparin enhances antithrombin activity against factor Xa and thrombin, which prevents completion of the coagulation cascade. Dalteparin has no antiplatelet activity and has only minimal effect on the PT and APTT.

Uses

Dalteparin is used to prevent deep vein thrombosis after hip replacement surgery or abdominal surgery. It may also be used for systemic anticoagulation and in combination with aspirin to prevent clot formation in patients with unstable angina pectoris and non–Q-wave myocardial infarction. Dalteparin is manufactured from heparin derived from pigs and should not be used in patients allergic to pork by-products.

Therapeutic Outcomes

The primary therapeutic outcomes from dalteparin therapy are prevention of deep vein thrombosis after abdominal or hip replacement surgery and prevention of angina pectoris and myocardial infarction.

Nursing Process for Dalteparin

Premedication Assessment

1. Perform scheduled laboratory tests, including CBC, platelet count, and stool occult blood tests before starting dalteparin therapy.
2. Obtain baseline vital signs.

Planning

Availability. Subcutaneously: 2500, 5000, 7500, and 10,000 units of anti–factor Xa in prefilled syringes with a 27-gauge, ½-inch needle (preservative-free); 10,000 units in 9.5-mL multidose vials that also contain benzyl alcohol preservative; 25,000 units/mL multidose vial that also contains benzyl alcohol preservative.

Implementation

Dosage and Administration. NOTE: *Do not inject intramuscularly!* To prevent loss of drug, do not expel air bubble from syringe before injection.

Adult: Subcutaneously: Administer by deep subcutaneous injection into a U-shaped area around the navel, the upper outer side of the thigh, or the upper outer quadrangle of the buttock. When the area around the navel or the thigh is used, lift up a fold of skin with the thumb and forefinger while giving the injection. Insert the entire length of the needle at a 45- to 90-degree angle. The skinfold should be held throughout the injection. Inject the drug slowly, leaving the needle in place for 10 seconds after injection. To minimize bruising, do not rub the injection site after completion of the injection. Alternate sites every 24 hours. Periodic CBCs, including platelet count, and stool occult blood tests, are recommended during the course of treatment with dalteparin. No special monitoring of clotting times (e.g., APTT) is required.

Dosage Range

Angina/Myocardial Infarction. Subcutaneously: 120 units/kg (but no more than 10,000 units) every 12 hours with concurrent oral aspirin (75 to 165 mg/day) therapy.

Hip Replacement Surgery. Subcutaneously: 2500 to 5000 before surgery. At 4 to 8 hours after surgery, 2500 units. Postoperative days: 5000 units daily. The usual duration of administration is 5 to 10 days after surgery.

Deep Vein Thrombosis Prophylaxis. *Abdominal surgery:* Subcutaneously: 2500 units once daily, starting 1 to 2 hours before surgery and repeat once daily for 5 to 10 days postoperatively. *High-risk patients:* In abdominal surgery patients at high risk for thromboembolic complications (e.g., malignancy), administer 5000 units subcutaneously the evening before surgery and repeat once daily for 5 to 10 days postoperatively. Alternatively, in patients with malignancy, administer 2500 units subcutaneously 1 to 2 hours before surgery with an additional 2500 units subcutaneously 12 hours later and then 5000 units once daily for 5 to 10 days postoperatively. *Medical patients:* Subcutaneously: In medical patients with severely restricted mobility during acute illness, 5000 units administered by subcutaneous injection once daily.

Evaluation

Side Effects to Expect

Hematoma Formation, Bleeding at Injection Site. Inappropriate administration techniques lead to hematoma formation at the site of injection. USE PROPER TECHNIQUE!

Side Effects to Report

Bleeding. Inspect the skin and mucous membranes for petechiae, ecchymoses, or hematomas. Also monitor for hematuria, bleeding gums, and melena.

Assess and record vital signs at regular intervals. Report signs and symptoms of internal bleeding (e.g., decreasing blood pressure; increasing pulse; cold, clammy skin; feeling faint; disoriented sensorium).

Check urine and stools for blood. Urine may appear red, smoke-colored, or brownish. Stools may appear to be dark and tarry. Perform a Hemoccult test on the stool if necessary.

Vomitus may contain bright red blood or may have a "coffee ground" appearance.

Assessment of dressings or drainage tubes for any signs of bleeding is necessary for postoperative patients.

Thrombocytopenia. Dalteparin may induce type I or type II heparin-induced thrombocytopenia (HIT) (see the section on heparin later in this chapter). Monitor platelet counts daily.

Drug Interactions. No clinically significant drug interactions have been reported, but dalteparin should be used cautiously in patients receiving antiplatelet or warfarin therapy.

enoxaparin (en ox a pair′ in)
LOVENOX (lo′ vehn ox)

Actions

Enoxaparin is the first of the LMWHs that are essentially the active components of the heparin protein molecule. The LMWHs have the advantage of specific action at certain steps of the coagulation pathway, resulting in less potential for hemorrhage and longer duration of action. Enoxaparin is specifically active against factor Xa and thrombin; it prevents completion of the coagulation cascade. Enoxaparin has no antiplatelet activity and does not affect the PT or APTT.

Uses

Enoxaparin is used to prevent deep vein thrombosis following hip replacement surgery, knee replacement surgery, or abdominal surgery. It is also approved for use in conjunction with warfarin to treat acute deep vein thrombosis with or without pulmonary embolus and for the prevention of ischemic complications of unstable angina and non–Q-wave myocardial infarction when coadministered with aspirin. Enoxaparin is manufactured from heparin derived from pigs and should not be used in patients allergic to pork by-products.

Therapeutic Outcomes

The primary therapeutic outcome from enoxaparin therapy is prevention of deep vein thrombosis after hip replacement surgery and ischemic complications of angina and myocardial infarction.

Nursing Process for Enoxaparin

Premedication Assessment

1. Perform scheduled laboratory tests, including CBCs, platelet count, and stool occult blood tests, before starting enoxaparin therapy.
2. Obtain baseline vital signs.

Planning

Availability. Subcutaneous: 30 mg in 0.3 mL; 40 mg in 0.4 mL; 60 mg in 0.6 mL; 80 mg in 0.8 mL; 100 mg in 1 mL; 120 mg in 0.8 mL; and 150 mg in 1 mL. Each concentration is packaged in a prefilled syringe (preservative free) with a 27-gauge, ½-inch needle.

The 300 mg/3 mL multidose vial contains benzyl alcohol preservative.

Implementation

Dosage and Administration. NOTES:

- *Do not inject intramuscularly!* To prevent loss of drug, do not expel air bubble from syringe before injection.
- Dosage adjustment is required in patients with a creatinine clearance of less than 30 mL per minute.
- Men less than 57 kg (125 lb) and women less than 45 kg (99 lb) who receive standard doses of 30 to 40 mg one or two times daily of enoxaparin should be more carefully observed for signs and symptoms of bleeding.

Adult: Subcutaneously: Do not expel the air bubble from the prefilled syringe before administration. Administer by deep subcutaneous injection into the anterolateral or posterolateral abdominal wall every 12 to 24 hours. The entire length of the needle should be introduced into a skinfold held between the thumb and forefinger; the skinfold should be held throughout the injection. Inject the drug slowly, leaving the needle in place for 10 seconds after injection. To minimize bruising, do not rub the injection site after completion of the injection. Alternate sites every 12 hours. Use the right side in the morning and the left side in the evening. Periodic CBCs, including platelet count, and stool occult blood tests are recommended during the course of treatment with enoxaparin. No special monitoring of clotting times (e.g., APTT) is required.

Dosage Range. Subcutaneously: *Prophylaxis:* 30-40 mg one or two times daily, depending on the medical and surgical condition. *Therapeutic:* 1 mg/kg every 12 hours or 1.5 mg/kg every 24 hours, administered at the same time daily.

Evaluation

Side Effects to Expect

Hematoma Formation, Bleeding at Injection Site. Inappropriate administration techniques lead to hematoma formation at the site of injection. USE PROPER TECHNIQUE!

Side Effects to Report

Bleeding. Inspect the skin and mucous membranes for petechiae, ecchymoses, or hematomas. Also monitor for hematuria, bleeding gums, and melena.

Assess and record vital signs at regular intervals. Report signs and symptoms of internal bleeding (e.g., decreasing blood pressure; increasing pulse; cold, clammy skin; feeling faint; disoriented sensorium).

Check urine and stools for blood. Urine may appear red, smoke-colored, or brownish. Stools may appear to be dark and tarry. Perform a Hemoccult test on the stool if necessary.

Vomitus may contain bright red blood or may have a "coffee ground" appearance.

Assessment of dressings or drainage tubes for any signs of bleeding is necessary for postoperative patients.

Thrombocytopenia. Enoxaparin may induce type I or type II HIT (see the section on heparin later in this chapter). Monitor platelet counts on a daily basis.

Drug Interactions. No clinically significant drug interactions have been reported, but enoxaparin should be used cautiously in patients receiving antiplatelet or warfarin therapy.

fondaparinux (fon dah pair′ in oo)
ARIXTRA (ahr iks′ trah)

Actions

Fondaparinux is a selective factor Xa inhibitor. Fondaparinux binds to antithromin III, potentiating its action against factor Xa, preventing completion of the coagulation cascade. Fondaparinux has no antiplatelet activity and has no effect on the PT and APTT.

Uses

Fondaparinux is used to prevent deep vein thrombosis in patients undergoing hip fracture or hip replacement surgery or knee replacement surgery, and to treat patients with acute deep vein thrombosis. When discontinued, fondaparinux-mediated anticoagulation remains for 2 to 4 days in patients with normal renal function, and longer in patients with renal impairment. Fondaparinux cannot be used interchangeably (unit for unit) with heparin or LMWHs because they differ in manufacturing process, anti-Xa and anti-IIa activity, units, and dosage.

Therapeutic Outcomes

The primary therapeutic outcomes from fondaparinux therapy are prevention of deep vein thrombosis in patients after hip or knee surgery, and treatment of acute deep vein thrombosis.

Nursing Process for Fondaparinux

Premedication Assessment

1. Perform scheduled laboratory tests, including serum creatinine, CBC, platelet count, and stool occult blood tests before start of fondaparinux therapy.
2. Obtain baseline vital signs.
3. Inspect the skin and mucous membranes for petechiae, ecchymoses, or hematomas. Also monitor for hematuria, bleeding gums, and melena before administering each dose of medication.

Planning

Availability. Subcutaneous: 2.5 mg in 0.5 mL; 5 mg in 0.4 mL; 7.5 mg in 0.6 mL; 10 mg in 0.8 mL single-dose prefilled syringes (preservative free) with 27-gauge, ½-inch needles.

Implementation

Dosage and Administration. NOTES:

- *Do not inject intramuscularly!*
- Use with caution in patients with a creatinine clearance of 30 to 50 mL per minute. Do not use in patients with a creatinine clearance less than 30 mL per minute.

Adult: Subcutaneously: Do not expel the air bubble from the syringe before administration. Administer by deep subcutaneous injection, rotating the injection site between the left and right anterolateral and left and right posterolateral abdominal wall. The administration site should vary with each injection. Using the thumb and forefinger, a fold of skin must be lifted for giving the injection. Insert the entire length of the needle at a 45- to 90-degree angle. The skinfold should be held throughout the injection. Inject the drug slowly, leaving the needle in place for 10 seconds after injection. To minimize bruising, do not rub the injection site after completion of the injection. Periodic serum creatinine, CBCs, including platelet count, and stool occult blood tests are recommended during the course of treatment with fondaparinux. No special monitoring of clotting times (APTT) is required.

Dosage Range

Deep Vein Thrombosis Prophylaxis. Subcutaneously: 2.5 mg daily at least 6 to 8 hours after hip fracture, hip replacement, or knee replacement surgery. The usual duration of administration is 5 to 9 days, and up to 11 days of administration has been tolerated. In patients undergoing hip fracture surgery, an extended prophylaxis course of up to 24 additional days is recommended.

Acute Deep Vein Thrombosis and Pulmonary Embolism Treatment. Subcutaneously: 5 mg (body weight <50 kg), 7.5 mg (body weight 50 to 100 kg), or 10 mg (body weight >100 kg) once daily. Continue for at least 5 days until a therapeutic oral anticoagulant effect is established (INR 2 to 3). Initiate concomitant treatment with warfarin as soon as possible, usually within 72 hours. The usual duration of administration of fondaparinux is 5 to 9 days.

Evaluation

Side Effects to Expect

Hematoma Formation, Bleeding at Injection Site. Inappropriate administration techniques lead to hematoma formation at the site of injection. USE PROPER TECHNIQUE!

Side Effects to Report

Bleeding. Inspect the skin and mucous membranes for petechiae, ecchymoses, or hematomas. Also monitor for hematuria, bleeding gums, and melena.

Assess and record vital signs at regular intervals. Report signs and symptoms of internal bleeding (e.g., decreasing blood pressure; increasing pulse; cold, clammy skin; feeling faint; disoriented sensorium).

Check urine and stools for blood. Urine may appear red, smoke-colored, or brownish. Stools may appear to be dark and tarry. Perform an occult blood test on the stool if necessary.

Vomitus may contain bright red blood or may have a "coffee ground" appearance.

Assessment of dressings or drainage tubes for any signs of bleeding is necessary for postoperative patients.

Thrombocytopenia. Fondaparinux may cause type I or type II HIT (see the section on heparin later in this chapter). Monitor platelet counts on a daily basis.

Drug Interactions. No clinically significant drug interactions have been reported, but fondaparinux should be used cautiously in patients receiving antiplatelet or warfarin therapy.

heparin (hep' ahr in)

Actions

Heparin is a natural substance extracted from gut and lung tissue of pigs and cattle. In full therapeutic doses, heparin acts as a catalyst to accelerate the rate of action of a naturally occurring inhibitor of thrombin, antithrombin III (sometimes called the heparin cofactor). In the presence of heparin, antithrombin III rapidly neutralizes thrombin; activated factors IXa, Xa, XI, and XII; and plasmin. Heparin also inhibits activation of factor VIII, the fibrin stabilizing factor, preventing soluble fibrin clots from becoming insoluble clots (see Figure 27-1). Heparin has no fibrinolytic activity and cannot lyse established fibrin clots.

In low doses, heparin causes the neutralization of only factor Xa, preventing the conversion of prothrombin to thrombin. This allows lower dosages to be used with fewer complications from therapy. This is the rationale routinely used in prophylaxis with subcutaneous heparin to prevent the postoperative thrombi.

Uses

Heparin is used to treat deep venous thrombosis, pulmonary embolism, cerebral embolism, and acute peripheral arterial embolism. It is used in the treatment of patients with heart valve prostheses. It is also used prophylactically before and during cardiovascular surgery; in postoperative, immobilized patients; and during hemodialysis to prevent active coagulation and clot formation.

Therapeutic Outcomes

The primary therapeutic outcomes from heparin therapy are as follows:

- When used in low doses, prophylactically, heparin prevents deep venous thrombosis.
- In full doses, heparin is used to treat a thromboembolism and promote neutralization of activated clotting factors, thus preventing the extension of thrombi and the formation of emboli. If therapy is started shortly after the formation of a thrombus, heparin will minimize tissue damage by preventing it from developing into an insoluble, stable thrombus.

Nursing Process for Heparin

Premedication Assessment

1. Take baseline vital signs.
2. Always check the most recent laboratory data (APTT) to ensure that the results are within the recommended range for heparin therapy.
3. Inspect the skin and mucous membranes for petechiae, ecchymoses, or hematomas. Also monitor for hematuria, bleeding gums, and melena before administering each dose of medication.

Planning

Availability. Subcutaneous, intravenous (IV): 1000, 2000, 2500, 5000, 10,000, 20,000, and 40,000 units/mL in various sizes of ampules and vials.

Implementation

Dosage and Administration. Accuracy of dose: always confirm the dosage calculations with two nurses before subcutaneous or IV administration. Be certain the strength is correct. There is a *drastic difference* in clinical response between 1 mL of 1:1000 units and 1 mL of 1:10,000 units of heparin.

Dosage adjustment: blood samples for laboratory studies (APTT) are usually drawn 4 to 6 hours after each subcutaneous dose or just before each IV dose. Blood may be drawn every 6 to 8 hours during a continuous IV infusion. Do not draw blood samples from the same arm being used for heparin infusion.

Heparin dosage is considered to be in the normal therapeutic range if the APTT is 1.5 to 2.5 times the control APTT value (e.g., if control is 30 seconds, the patient receiving full-dose heparin should have an APTT of 45 to 75 seconds for optimal therapy).

Subcutaneous: *Prophylactic:* 5000 units every 8 to 12 hours. Therapeutic: initially 10,000 to 15,000 units. *Maintenance:* loading dose: 10,000 to 20,000 units followed by 8000 to 10,000 units every 8 hours, or 15,000 units every 12 hours.

Subcutaneous injection is usually made into the tissue over the abdomen (Figure 27-2). Do not inject within 2 inches of the umbilicus. The injection site should not be massaged before or after injection, and sites should be rotated for each dose to prevent the development of a massive hematoma.

Needle length and angle need to be adapted to the patient's size so that the drug will be deposited into the

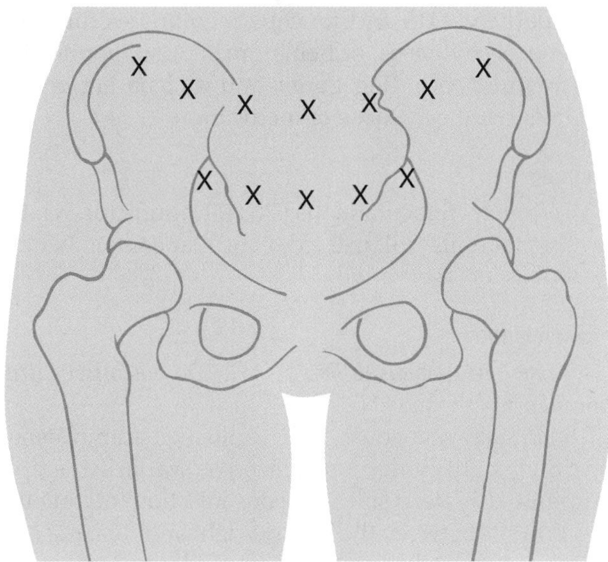

FIGURE **27-2** Sites of heparin administration.

subcutaneous tissue. (Usually a 26- or 27-gauge, ½-inch needle is used.) The injection is usually made at a 90-degree angle to the skin. Always use a tuberculin syringe so that the dosage can be accurately measured. DO NOT aspirate. This will increase local tissue damage and create the possibility of hematoma formation. DO NOT inject into a hematoma or an area with any infection present. Follow a planned site rotation schedule.

After injection, apply gentle pressure for 1 or 2 minutes to control local bleeding, but do not massage the area. Ice packs on the site after injection may be used; check the hospital policy. At this time, there is little documented evidence that ice packs prevent hematoma formation or affect drug absorption.

Intramuscular (IM): Not recommended because of the development of hematomas.

IV (intermittent): Initially 10,000 unit bolus; maintenance: 5000 to 10,000 units every 4 to 6 hours.

A heparin lock, consisting of a 22- to 29-gauge scalp vein needle attached to a 3½-inch tubing ending in a resealing rubber diaphragm, may be used to administer intermittent IV doses of heparin (see Figure 12-3). Advantages of a heparin lock are the mobility that it provides the patient and fewer venipunctures.

After injecting a bolus of heparin through the rubber diaphragm, flush the line with 1 mL of saline solution. The heparin flush solution ensures that the patient will receive the entire heparin bolus, and it prevents the formation of a clot in the scalp vein needle.

IV (continuous infusion): Initially 70 to 100 units/kg bolus; maintenance 15 to 25 units/kg/hr.

Continuous infusions of heparin provide the advantage of steady heparin levels in the blood. Periodic dosage adjustment is required based on the response of the patient. Loading doses are often rounded to the nearest 500 units and maintenance infusion rates to the nearest 100 units for administration.

When making a solution for infusion, always have two nurses confirm your calculations and the strength of the heparin to be used. As a safety measure, never make infusions that run more than 6 to 8 hours. This protects patients from receiving massive doses of heparin should the infusion "run away." Always use an electronic control device for infusion. However, the infusion should be monitored at least every 30 to 60 minutes.

Antidote. Protamine sulfate, 1 mg, will neutralize approximately 100 units of heparin. If protamine sulfate is given more than 30 minutes after the heparin was administered, give only half the dose of protamine sulfate. Because excessive doses of protamine may also cause excessive anticoagulation, it must be used judiciously.

Evaluation

Patients receiving full-dose heparin therapy should be monitored for hematocrit, platelet counts, APTT, and signs of bleeding.

Adverse effects of heparin therapy are most commonly caused by inappropriate administration technique or overdosage. Factors that can influence the incidence of complications include age, weight, gender, and recent trauma. The most common signs of overdosage are petechiae, hematomas, hematuria, bleeding gums, and melena.

Side Effects to Expect

Hematoma Formation, Bleeding at Injection Site. Inappropriate administration techniques lead to hematoma formation at the site of injection. USE PROPER TECHNIQUE!

Side Effects to Report

Bleeding. Inspect the skin and mucous membranes for petechiae, ecchymoses, or hematomas. Also monitor for hematuria, bleeding gums, and melena.

Always monitor menstrual flow to be certain that it is not excessive or prolonged.

Assess and record vital signs at regular intervals. Report signs and symptoms of internal bleeding (e.g., decreasing blood pressure; increasing pulse; cold, clammy skin; feeling faint; disoriented sensorium).

Check urine and stools for blood. Urine may appear red, smoke-colored, or brownish. Stools may appear to be dark and tarry. Perform a Hemoccult test on the stool if necessary.

Vomitus may contain bright red blood or may have a "coffee ground" appearance.

Assessment of dressings or drainage tubes for any signs of bleeding is necessary for postoperative patients.

Thrombocytopenia. Heparin therapy may induce two types of thrombocytopenia. Type I HIT results from a direct effect of heparin on platelets, causing sequestration and a fall in the platelet count to as low as $100,000/mm^3$. This reversible form of thrombocytopenia occurs within the first several days of heparin therapy. The patient is asymptomatic, and heparin therapy should be continued if therapeutically indicated. The platelet count should return to normal.

Type II HIT should be suspected when the platelet count falls below 100,000/mm^3. This type of thrombocytopenia is an allergic reaction to heparin that causes aggregation of platelets. The onset of falling platelet counts is immediate after heparin therapy is started if the patient has previously received heparin, or it occurs after 5 to 22 days in the previously unexposed patient. Type II HIT occurs in about 3% of patients. Patients are at risk for white thrombus formation caused by sudden aggregation of platelets. Heparin therapy should be immediately discontinued if patients develop signs of clot formation, such as pain in an extremity, symptoms of a stroke, or chest pain resembling angina. Warfarin therapy may be initiated or continued, and antiplatelet therapy (aspirin) may also be started. Thrombin inhibitors such as argatroban or lepirudin may also be used. LMWHs are contraindicated because of the potential for cross-allergenicity. Platelet counts should be monitored daily.

Drug Interactions

Increased Therapeutic and Toxic Effects. Concurrent use of NSAIDs, aspirin, danshen, ginkgo biloba, dipyridamole, clopidogrel, and ticlopidine may predispose the patient to hemorrhage.

tinzaparin (tin zah pair′ in)
▶ INNOHEP (in′ noh hep)

Actions

Tinzaparin is an LMWH that is essentially the active component of the heparin protein molecule. The LMWHs have the advantage of specific action at certain steps of the coagulation pathway, resulting in less potential for hemorrhage and longer duration of action. Tinzaparin enhances antithrombin activity against factor Xa and thrombin, which prevents completion of the coagulation cascade. Tinzaparin has no antiplatelet activity and has no effect on the PT and APTT.

Uses

Tinzaparin is used to treat acute deep vein thrombosis. Tinzaparin is manufactured from heparin derived from pigs. Tinzaparin should not be used in patients allergic to pork by-products.

Therapeutic Outcomes

The primary therapeutic outcome from tinzaparin therapy is resolution of deep vein thrombosis.

Nursing Process for Tinzaparin

Premedication Assessment

1. Perform scheduled laboratory tests, including CBCs, platelet count, and stool occult blood tests before start of tinzaparin therapy.
2. Obtain baseline vital signs.
3. Inspect the skin and mucous membranes for petechiae, ecchymoses, or hematomas. Also monitor for hematuria, bleeding gums, and melena before administering each dose of medication.

Planning

Availability. Subcutaneous: 20,000 antifactor Xa international units/mL in 2-mL vials that contain benzyl alcohol as a preservative.

Implementation

Dosage and Administration. NOTE: *Do not inject intramuscularly!*

Adult: Subcutaneously: 175 units/kg administered once daily until patient is stabilized on warfarin therapy. Administer by deep subcutaneous injection rotating the injection site between the left and right anterolateral and posterolateral abdominal wall. The administration site should vary with each injection. Using the thumb and forefinger, a fold of skin must be lifted for giving the injection. Insert the entire length of the needle at a 45- to 90-degree angle. The skinfold should be held throughout the injection. Inject the drug slowly, leaving the needle in place for 10 seconds after injection. To minimize bruising, do not rub the injection site after completion of the injection. Periodic CBCs, including platelet count, and stool occult blood tests are recommended during the course of treatment with tinzaparin. No special monitoring of clotting times (APTT) is required.

Evaluation

Side Effects to Expect

Hematoma Formation, Bleeding at Injection Site. Inappropriate administration techniques lead to hematoma formation at the site of injection. USE PROPER TECHNIQUE!

Side Effects to Report

Bleeding. Inspect the skin and mucous membranes for petechiae, ecchymoses, or hematomas. Also monitor for hematuria, bleeding gums, and melena.

Assess and record vital signs at regular intervals. Report signs and symptoms of internal bleeding (e.g., decreasing blood pressure; increasing pulse; cold, clammy skin; feeling faint; disoriented sensorium).

Check urine and stools for blood. Urine may appear red, smoke-colored, or brownish. Stools may appear to be dark and tarry. Perform an occult blood test on the stool if necessary.

Vomitus may contain bright red blood or may have a "coffee ground" appearance.

Assessment of dressings or drainage tubes for any signs of bleeding is necessary for postoperative patients.

Thrombocytopenia. Tinzaparin may cause type I or type II HIT (see the section on heparin later in this chapter). Monitor platelet counts on a daily basis.

Drug Interactions. No clinically significant drug interactions have been reported, but tinzaparin should be used cautiously in patients receiving antiplatelet or warfarin therapy.

warfarin (war′ fah rin)
COUMADIN (koo′ mah din)

Actions

Warfarin is a potent anticoagulant that acts by inhibiting the activity of vitamin K, which is required for the activation of clotting factors II, VII, IX, and X and proteins C and S in the blood. Blockade of the activation of these factors prevents clot formation (see Figure 27-1).

Uses

Warfarin is used to treat or prophylactically prevent venous thrombosis, embolism associated with atrial fibrillation or heart valve replacement, pulmonary embolism, and coronary occlusion.

Therapeutic Outcomes

The primary therapeutic outcomes from warfarin therapy are as follows:

- Prevention and treatment of venous thrombosis and embolism.
- Prevention and treatment of thromboemboli associated with atrial fibrillation.
- Reduced risk of death, recurrent myocardial infarction, and thromboembolic events, such as stroke, after myocardial infarction.
- Prevention and treatment of thromboemboli associated with cardiac valve replacement.

Nursing Process for Warfarin

Premedication Assessment

1. Obtain baseline vital signs.
2. Always check most recent PT or INR results to determine if within the recommended range for warfarin therapy.
3. Inspect the skin and mucous membranes for petechiae, ecchymoses, or hematomas. Also monitor for hematuria, bleeding gums, and melena before administering each dose of medication.
4. The pregnancy category for warfarin is X. Ensure that patients of childbearing age are not pregnant at the time warfarin therapy is initiated. Warfarin therapy should be avoided during pregnancy, particularly in weeks 6 through 12 and at term. Warfarin may be administered during pregnancy in patients with prosthetic heart valves after discussing the risks and benefits of therapy with the patient.

Planning

Availability. PO: 1, 2, 2.5, 4, 5, 6, 7.5, and 10 mg tablets. IV: 2 mg/mL in 2.5-mL vials.

Implementation

Dosage and Administration. Dosage adjustment, adult: Dosage during therapy is based on the prothrombin times. The PT is expressed as the INR, an internationally accepted standard for adjusting for variability in the PT assay. The optimal dosage is that which prolongs the PT and maintains the INR at 2 to 3. Certain medical conditions (e.g., mechanical prosthetic valves, recurrent systemic embolism) require an INR of 2.5 to 3.5 and concurrent antiplatelet therapy.

When warfarin therapy is initiated, the patient should be monitored closely for evidence of hemorrhage because of the drug's cumulative effects.

Stress the need to comply with the prescribed regimen and the need for laboratory data to determine the correct maintenance dose. Instruct the patient to resume a regular schedule if one dose is missed. If two or more doses are missed, the patient should consult a health care provider.

PO and IV: 10 mg daily for 2 to 4 days. Maintenance: 2 to 10 mg daily as determined by the PT reported as the INR. When administered IV, inject as a slow bolus injection over 1 to 2 minutes into a peripheral vein. *Do not inject intramuscularly!*

Antidote. Vitamin K is a specific antidote for warfarin-induced hemorrhage but is rarely needed. Most cases of bleeding induced by warfarin overdose can be controlled by discontinuing warfarin therapy. An alternative in severe hemorrhage is a transfusion with plasma or whole blood.

Evaluation

Side Effects to Report

Bleeding. Inspect the skin and mucous membranes for petechiae, ecchymoses, or hematomas. Also monitor for hematuria, bleeding gums, and melena.

Always monitor menstrual flow to be certain that it is not excessive or prolonged.

Assess and record vital signs at regular intervals. Report signs and symptoms of internal bleeding (e.g., decreasing blood pressure; increasing pulse; cold, clammy skin; feelings of faintness; disoriented sensorium).

Check urine and stools for blood. Urine may appear red, smoke-colored, or brownish. Stools may appear to be dark and tarry. Perform a Hemoccult test on the stool if necessary.

Vomitus may contain bright red blood or may have a "coffee ground" appearance.

Assessment of dressings or drainage tubes for any signs of bleeding is necessary for postoperative patients.

Drug Interactions

Drugs That Enhance Therapeutic and Toxic Effects. The following drugs, when used concurrently with warfarin, may enhance the therapeutic and toxic effects of warfarin:

acetaminophen	fluoxetine	ofloxacin
allopurinol	flutamide	omeprazole
amiodarone	fluvastatin	papaya
anabolic steroids	ginkgo biloba	phenytoin
aspirin	ifosfamide	piroxicam
beta blockers	isoniazid	propafenone
capecitabine	itraconazole	propoxyphene
chloral hydrate	ketoconazole	propranolol
cimetidine	levofloxacin	quinidine
ciprofloxacin	lovastatin	salicylates
cisapride	lyceum	simvastatin
co-trimoxazole	methyl salicylate (oil of wintergreen)	sulfinpyrazone
danshen	metronidazole	sulfonamides
devil's claw	miconazole	tamoxifen
disulfiram	moricizine	tetracyclines
dong quai	norfloxacin	thyroid hormones
erythromycin	NSAIDs	tramadol
ethanol		valproate
fluconazole		zafirlukast

Drugs That Decrease the Therapeutic Effect. The following drugs, when used concurrently with warfarin, may decrease the therapeutic activity of warfarin:

acerola	coenzyme Q_{10}	smartweed
aprepitant	dicloxacillin	St. John's wort
barbiturates	etretinate	sucralfate
black psyllium	griseofulvin	terbinafine
blond psyllium	nafcillin	trazodone
cabbage	rifampin	vitamin C
carbamazepine	rose hip	vitamin K
chlordiazepoxide		
cholestyramine		

All Prescription and Nonprescription Medications. Caution the patient *not* to take *any* over-the-counter (including herbal medicines) or prescription medication without first consulting the physician or pharmacist.

DRUG CLASS: Glycoprotein IIb/IIIa Inhibitors

During percutaneous coronary intervention procedures, it was found that patients were quite susceptible to new blood clots forming from the debris often released from atherosclerotic plaque disruption. Antiplatelet and antithrombotic agents such as aspirin and heparin were initially used, but new agents, called glycoprotein IIb/IIIa inhibitors, have been developed. Three of these inhibitors are now available: abciximab (ReoPro), eptifibatide (Integrilin), and tirofiban (Aggrastat).

Actions

The glycoprotein IIb/IIIa inhibitors act by blocking the glycoprotein IIb/IIIa receptor on platelets, preventing platelet aggregation and clot formation. Platelet aggregation inhibition persists during continuous infusion and is reversible on discontinuing the infusion.

Uses

Glycoprotein IIb/IIIa inhibitors are administered intravenously during the PCI procedure and for 12 to 24 hours afterward, significantly reducing the risk of acute myocardial infarction and death. Other antiplatelet and antithrombotic agents such as aspirin, clopidogrel, and heparin are used in conjunction with the glycoprotein IIb/IIIa inhibitors. Major complications of therapy include bleeding and thrombocytopenia. The hematocrit, platelet counts, and activated clotting time (ACT) must be monitored closely during and after therapy.

Therapeutic Outcomes

The primary therapeutic outcome from glycoprotein IIb/IIIa inhibitor therapy is prevention of clot formation during percutaneous intervention procedures.

DRUG CLASS: Fibrinolytic Agents

Over the past two decades there have been significant advances in the treatment of thromboemboli. Enzymes have been discovered that work within the clotting system to dissolve recently formed thrombi. The agents used are called fibrinolytic agents because of their ability to cause the dissolution of fibrin clots.

All thrombolytic agents increase the risk of bleeding, including intracranial bleeding, and should be used only in eligible patients. In addition, thrombolytic therapy increases the risk of stroke, including hemorrhagic stroke, in older adult patients.

The goals of fibrinolytic therapy are to lyse the thrombi during the early phase of clot formation, limit the damage to surrounding tissues by restoring circulation to the area distal to the thrombus, and reduce the morbidity and mortality after the formation of a thromboembolism.

Actions

Fibrinolytic agents work by stimulating the body's own clot-dissolving mechanism, converting plasminogen, a naturally occurring substance secreted by endothelial cells in response to injury to the artery, to plasmin (also known as fibrinolysin), which digests fibrin. The clot is then dissolved, restoring blood flow to the area. There are currently five fibrinolytic agents available: streptokinase, urokinase, alteplase, reteplase, and tenecteplase.

Streptokinase (Kabikinase) has the advantages of having proven clinical effectiveness, relative ease of administration, and relatively low cost. Disadvantages are the potential for allergenicity if additional doses must be given in the future and the potential for hemorrhage in other parts of the body.

Urokinase (Abbokinase) is effective and nonallergenic, but it is expensive and has the potential for causing hemorrhage in other parts of the body. Urokinase can also be used to dissolve clots to open IV catheters, including central venous lines.

Alteplase (recombinant plasminogen activator [rtPA]) (Activase) is of proven clinical effectiveness, more clot specific (a lower potential for hemorrhage elsewhere in the body), and nonantigenic.

Disadvantages are a 10- to 20-fold higher cost, a prolonged administration time, and the need for concurrent heparin therapy.

Reteplase (rtPA) (Retavase) is administered as two boluses to dissolve clots. It is of proven clinical effectiveness, more clot specific (a lower potential for hemorrhage elsewhere in the body), and nonantigenic. Disadvantages are high cost and the need for concurrent heparin therapy.

Tenecteplase (rtPA) (TNKase) is approved for use to treat clots associated with myocardial infarction. It is the first "clot buster" that can be administered over 5 seconds in a single dose, offering health care providers the fastest administration of a thrombolytic to date in the treatment of heart attack. Tenecteplase is a bioengineered variant of alteplase. The ease of administration may allow this drug to be administered outside the hospital while the patient is being transported to a cardiovascular center, buying potentially lifesaving time.

Uses

The fibrinolytic agents are used to dissolve clots secondary to coronary artery occlusion (myocardial infarction, also known as acute coronary syndrome), pulmonary emboli, cerebral emboli (stroke), and deep venous thrombosis. The decision for use and selection of the agent depend on the location of the thrombus, clinical condition and age of the patient, preference of the patient care team, and the availability of alternative therapies, such as angioplasty or bypass graft surgery. A key factor in the successful treatment of these conditions is the early treatment with fibrinolytic agents. Fibrinolytic agents tend to be much more successful against the "soluble" fibrin clot because they restore circulation to the obstructed area.

Urokinase and streptokinase may also be used to reopen IV catheters, including central venous catheters, obstructed by blood clots.

Therapeutic Outcomes

The primary therapeutic outcome from fibrinolytic therapy is reperfusion of the tissues obstructed by the thrombus.

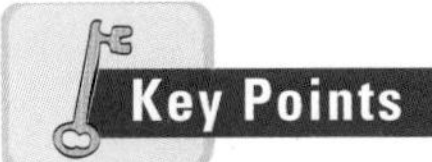

- Diseases caused by intravascular clotting are major causes of death and must be treated rapidly to reduce tissue damage associated with thrombosis.
- The major pharmacologic treatments are platelet inhibitors, anticoagulants, glycoprotein IIb/IIIa inhibitors, and fibrinolytic agents.
- Nurses can play a significant role, especially in the nonpharmacologic prevention and treatment of thromboembolic disease, which includes patient education on how to prevent venous stasis, the use of properly fitted support stockings, and appropriate use of prescribed medicines.

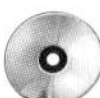
Go to your Companion CD-ROM for Appendices, an Audio Glossary, animations, Drug Dosage Calculators, customizable Patient Self-Assessment forms, and Review Questions for the NCLEX® Examination.

evolve Be sure to visit the companion Evolve site at http://evolve.elsevier.com/Clayton for WebLinks and additional online resources.

MEDICATION SAFETY REVIEW

MATH REVIEW QUESTIONS

1. Order: heparin 2000 units subcutaneously stat
   Available: heparin 10,000 units/mL
   Give ____ mL.
2. Order: 100 mL D5W with 30,000 units heparin
   Infuse at a rate of 800 units per hour IV. Set the infusion pump, calibrated in mL per hour, at ____ mL per hour.
   Three hours after the infusion is started, the physician changes the order to 1200 units per hour.
   How much heparin has already been infused? ____ units.
   What rate would the infusion pump be adjusted to?
   Set infusion pump at ____ mL per hour.
3. Order: Persantine 75 mg qid
   With how many 75-mg tablets should the patient be dismissed in order to take the medication for the next 7 days?
   ____ tablets.

Continued

CRITICAL THINKING QUESTIONS

1. A patient comes from surgery after a femoral bypass with a heparin drip running through a pump. What nursing assessments should be made to monitor this patient's postoperative progress? The operative record indicates that the patient has had a total of 50,000 units of heparin during the operative procedure. The postoperative orders do not state a specific rate of flow for the heparin drip that is currently running through the pump at 8 mL per hour. What actions should be taken by the nurse?
2. Review the procedure for administration of enoxaparin and fondaparinux subcutaneously. What monitoring of the patient should be done during therapy with this drug?
3. Identify laboratory tests used to monitor different types of anticoagulant drugs.
4. Summarize premedication assessments that should be completed before administering any anticoagulant drug.
5. Research the clinical guidelines regarding precautions used for checking dosages of anticoagulant drugs.

CONTENT REVIEW QUESTIONS

1. How long does the antiplatelet activity of fondaparinux (Arixtra) remain in a (nonrenal compromised) patient after it is discontinued?
   1. Unknown
   2. 2 to 4 days
   3. 4 to 6 days
   4. 7 to 12 days
2. The laboratory test used to monitor the dosage of warfarin is:
   1. INR and PT.
   2. INR and WBCT.
   3. INR and ACT.
   4. PT and APTT.
3. The action of aspirin on clotting is to:
   1. prevent the clotting cascade.
   2. prevent thrombus formation.
   3. prevent platelet aggregation.
   4. decrease bleeding time.
4. Fibrinolytic agents have the action of:
   1. preventing the clotting cascade.
   2. preventing thrombus formation.
   3. preventing platelet aggregation.
   4. dissolving recently formed thrombi.
5. A nurse has initiated discharge teaching for a patient who is to be maintained on warfarin (Coumadin) following hospitalization for thrombophlebitis. The nurse determines that additional teaching is needed when the patient says:
   1. "I should change my diet to include more green leafy vegetables."
   2. "I will check with my physician or pharmacist before I begin or stop any medication."
   3. "I should wear a Medic-Alert bracelet to indicate I am on anticoagulant therapy."
   4. "I will need to have my blood drawn routinely to monitor the effects of the Coumadin."
6. Which of the following is correct when administering enoxaparin subcutaneously?
   1. Aspirate before administering the medication.
   2. Hold the needle in place for 10 seconds after administration.
   3. Massage the site after administration.
   4. Administer in the upper arms and rotate sites.
7. A nurse instructs a patient discharged with warfarin therapy to:
   1. limit intake of vitamin C.
   2. report symptoms of nausea to the physician.
   3. have blood drawn routinely to check electrolytes.
   4. be aware of and report signs or symptoms of bleeding.

CHAPTER

28 Drugs Used to Treat Heart Failure

evolve http://evolve.elsevier.com/Clayton

Chapter Content

Objectives

1. Summarize the pathophysiology of heart failure, including the body's compensatory mechanisms.
2. Identify the goals of treatment of heart failure.
3. Explain the process of digitalizing a patient, including the initial dosage, preparation, and administration of the medication, as well as the nursing assessments needed to monitor therapeutic response and digoxin toxicity.
4. Describe safety precautions associated with the preparation and administration of digoxin.
5. State the primary actions on cardiac output of digoxin, angiotensin-converting enzyme inhibitors, nitrates, and calcium channel blockers.
6. Identify essential assessment data, nursing interventions, and health teaching needed for a patient with heart failure.

Key Terms

systolic dysfunction
diastolic dysfunction
inotropic agents
digitalis toxicity
positive inotropy
negative chronotropy
digitalization

HEART FAILURE

The incidence of heart failure (previously known as *congestive heart failure*), unlike that of other cardiovascular diseases, continues to increase because of population aging and improved survival after acute myocardial infarction (AMI). It is estimated that 1% of individuals older than age 65 and 10% of those older than age 75 experience heart failure. Some 5 million Americans experience this disabling condition; more than 500,000 patients develop symptoms annually; and more than 200,000 people die from heart failure each year. The 5-year mortality rate for heart failure is approximately 50%.

Heart failure is a cluster of signs and symptoms that arise when the left or right ventricle or both ventricles lose the ability to pump enough blood to meet the body's circulatory needs. It is the common pathway for several causes of heart failure, the most common of which is **systolic** (sis tahl' ik) **dysfunction** (or contracting dysfunction). Normally the heart pumps at a rate to support the body's need for blood flow and oxygenation of the vital organs and muscles. Systolic heart failure results when the heart lacks sufficient force to pump all the blood (decreased cardiac output) with which it is presented to meet the body's oxygenation needs (decreased tissue perfusion). Early clinical symptoms are decreased exercise tolerance and poor perfusion to peripheral tissues. As the condition progresses, the left ventricle chamber enlarges (left ventricular hypertrophy) and an increase in blood volume is required to fill the expanding ventricle to maintain cardiac output. Causes of systolic dysfunction are those that cause damage to heart muscle itself. The most common is coronary artery disease leading to MI. Other causes are dysrhythmias, cardiomyopathies and congenital heart disease. Usually the left ventricle fails first, but with progression of the disease, the right ventricle also enlarges because of increased pulmonary resistance and eventually fails.

Diastolic (dy as tahl' ik) **dysfunction** (or filling dysfunction) causes heart failure because the left ventricle develops a "stiffness" and fails to relax enough between contractions to allow adequate filling before the next contraction. Symptoms of diastolic dysfunction are pulmonary congestion and peripheral edema. There are many causes for the development of diastolic dysfunction, such as constrictive pericarditis, ventricular muscle hypertrophy caused by chronic hypertension, valvular heart disease causing flow resistance, and aortic stenosis.

The general pathogenesis of heart failure is diagrammed in Figure 28-1. When the vital organs and peripheral tissues are not adequately perfused, compensatory mechanisms begin to overcome the inadequate heart output. The sympathetic nervous system releases epinephrine and norepinephrine, producing tachycardia and increasing contractility. The increased

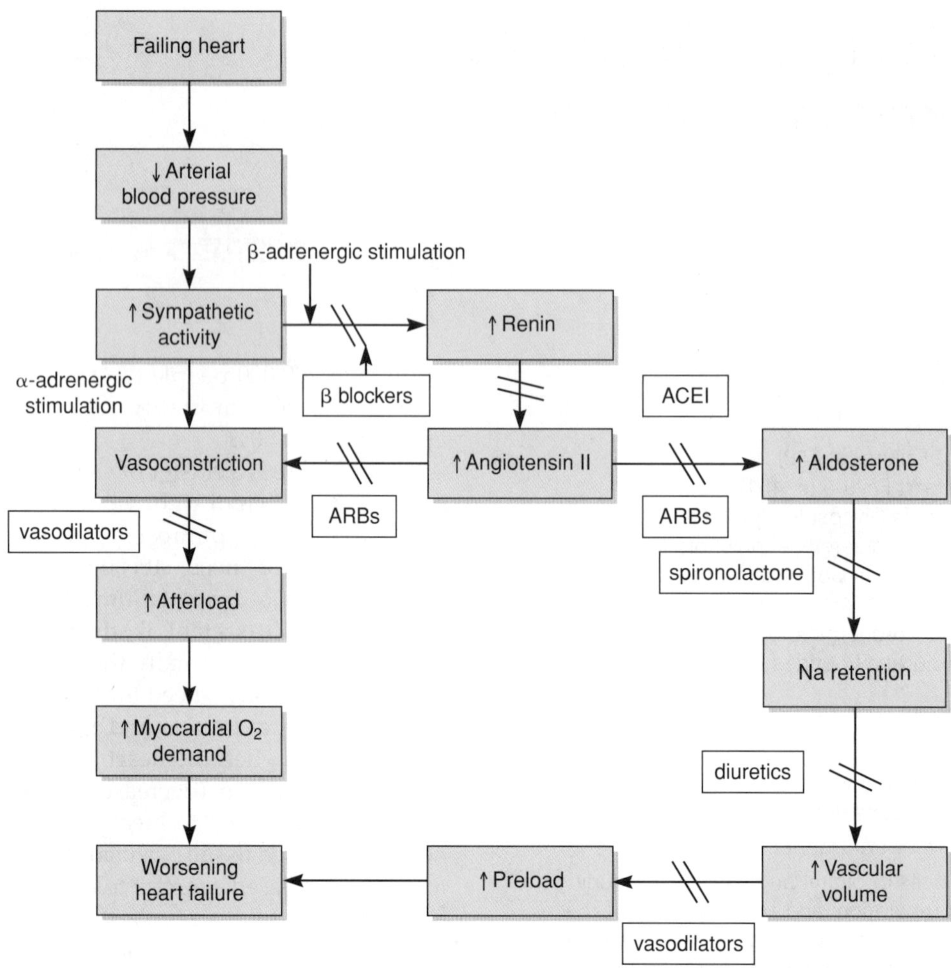

FIGURE **28-1** Pathway by which heart failure develops and how specific classes of medicines block physiologic mechanisms to reduce worsening of failure. Cardiac glycosides and phosphodiesterase inhibitors are also used to increase myocardial contractility. *ARBs,* Angiotensin II receptor blockers; *ACEI,* angiotensin-converting enzyme inhibitors; *β blockers,* beta-adrenergic blocking agents.

sympathetic stimulation also increases peripheral vasoconstriction, resulting in an increased afterload against which the heart must pump, causing a further decrease in cardiac output (Figure 28-1). The renin-angiotensin-aldosterone system stimulates renal distal tubule sodium and water retention in an effort to increase circulating blood volume, which increases preload to the heart. There is also an increased production of vasopressin (antidiuretic hormone) from the pituitary gland that increases water recovery from the kidneys and increases intravascular volume and preload. With decreased perfusion secondary to low cardiac output, the kidneys also increase sodium reabsorption in the proximal tubules to help expand circulating blood volume. The increased intravascular volume initially improves tissue perfusion, but over time, excessive amounts of sodium and water are retained, causing increased pressure within the capillaries, resulting in edema formation.

The early symptoms of heart failure are variable depending on the underlying cause of the disease. Traditionally, the signs and symptoms of heart failure have been classified based on whether failure is developing in the right ventricle or left ventricle. But it has been found that the symptoms overlap to such an extent due to the complexity of the syndrome that it is difficult to attribute a particular clinical indicator to a specific ventricle. It is also important to recognize that the clinical indicators vary considerably over time based on treatments being applied (Box 28-1).

TREATMENT OF HEART FAILURE

The goals of treatment of heart failure are reduction of signs and symptoms associated with fluid overload, increased exercise tolerance, and prolongation of life. If the heart failure is acute, the patient must be hospitalized for a diagnostic workup to determine the underlying cause. The New York Heart Association Functional Classification System is commonly used to group patients with heart failure according to degree of impairment (Table 28-1). Figure 28-2 illustrates an updated classification with treatment guidelines from

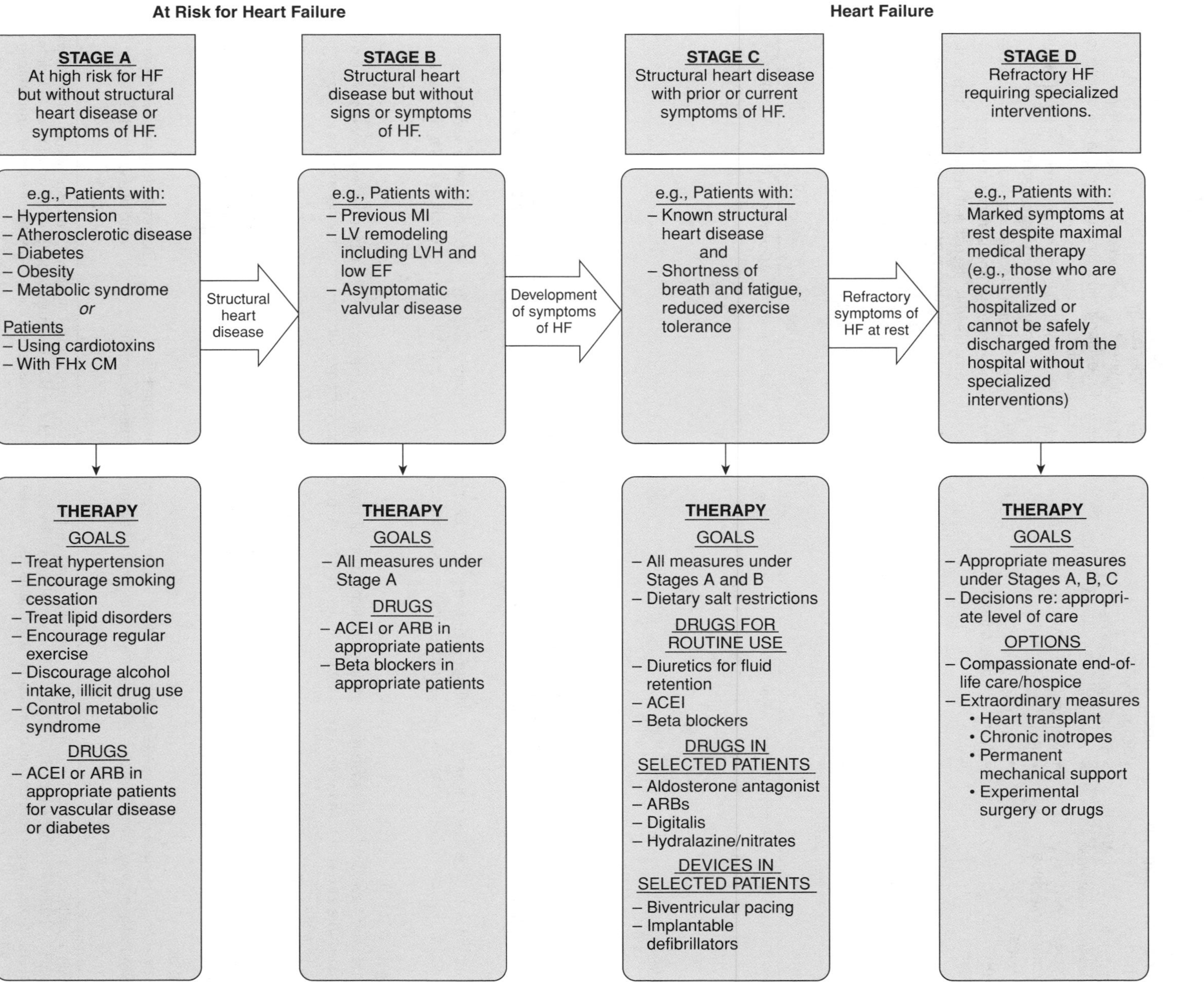

FIGURE **28-2** Stages in the development of heart failure/recommended therapy by stage. *FHx CM,* Family history of cardiomyopathy; *ACEI,* angiotensin-converting enzyme inhibitors; *ARB,* angiotensin receptor blocker.

Box 28-1 *Clinical and Laboratory Presentation of Heart Failure*

General

Patient presentation may range from asymptomatic to cardiogenic shock.

Symptoms

- Dyspnea, particularly on exertion
- Orthopnea
- Paroxysmal nocturnal dyspnea
- Exercise intolerance
- Tachypnea
- Cough
- Fatigue
- Nocturia
- Hemoptysis
- Abdominal pain
- Anorexia
- Nausea
- Bloating
- Ascites
- Mental status changes

Signs

- Pulmonary rales
- Pulmonary edema
- S_3 gallop
- Pleural effusion
- Cheyne-Stokes respiration
- Tachycardia
- Cardiomegaly
- Peripheral edema
- Jugular venous distention
- Hepatojugular reflux
- Hepatomegaly

Laboratory Tests

- B-type natriuretic peptide >100 picogram/mL
- Electrocardiogram: May be normal or could show numerous abnormalities including acute ST-T–wave changes from myocardial ischemia, atrial fibrillation, bradycardia, and left ventricular hypertrophy
- Serum creatinine: May be increased owing to hypoperfusion. Preexisting renal dysfunction can contribute to volume overload
- Complete blood count: Useful to determine if heart failure is due to reduced oxygen-carrying capacity
- Chest radiograph: Useful for detection of cardiac enlargement, pulmonary edema, and pleural effusions
- Echocardiogram: Used to assess left ventricular size, valve function, pericardial effusion, wall motion abnormalities, and ejection fraction

From Parker RB, Patterson JH, Johnson JA: Heart failure. In DiPiro JP, et al. [eds.]: *Pharmacotherapy, a pathophysiologic approach,* ed 6, New York, 2005, McGraw-Hill.

Table 28-1 *New York Heart Association Functional Classification System**

FUNCTIONAL CAPACITY	OBJECTIVE ASSESSMENT
CLASS I	
Patients who have cardiac disease but without resulting limitation of physical activity. Ordinary physical activity does not cause undue fatigue, palpitation, dyspnea, or anginal pain.	No objective evidence of cardiovascular disease.
CLASS II	
Patients who have cardiac disease resulting in slight limitation of physical activity. They are comfortable at rest. Ordinary physical activity results in fatigue, palpitation, dyspnea, or anginal pain.	Objective evidence of minimal cardiovascular disease.
CLASS III	
Patients who have cardiac disease resulting in marked limitation of physical activity. They are comfortable at rest. Less than ordinary activity causes fatigue, palpitation, dyspnea, or anginal pain.	Objective evidence of moderately severe cardiovascular disease.
CLASS IV	
Patients who have cardiac disease resulting in inability to carry on any physical activity without discomfort. Symptoms of heart failure or the anginal syndrome may be present even at rest. If any physical activity is undertaken, discomfort is increased.	Objective evidence of severe cardiovascular disease.

NOTE: "Functional Capacity" and "Objective Assessment" are independent categories. "Functional Capacity" is an estimate of what the patient's heart will allow the patient to do and should not be influenced by the character of the structural lesions, or an opinion as to treatment or prognosis. "Objective Assessment" is based on measurements such as electrocardiograms, stress tests, x-ray studies, echocardiograms, and radiologic images.

*The Criteria Committee of the New York Heart Association: *Nomenclature and criteria for diagnosis of diseases of the heart and great vessels,* ed 9, Boston, 1994, Little, Brown.

Requests for reprints should be sent to the Office of Scientific Affairs, American Heart Association, 7272 Greenville Avenue, Dallas, TX 75231-4596.

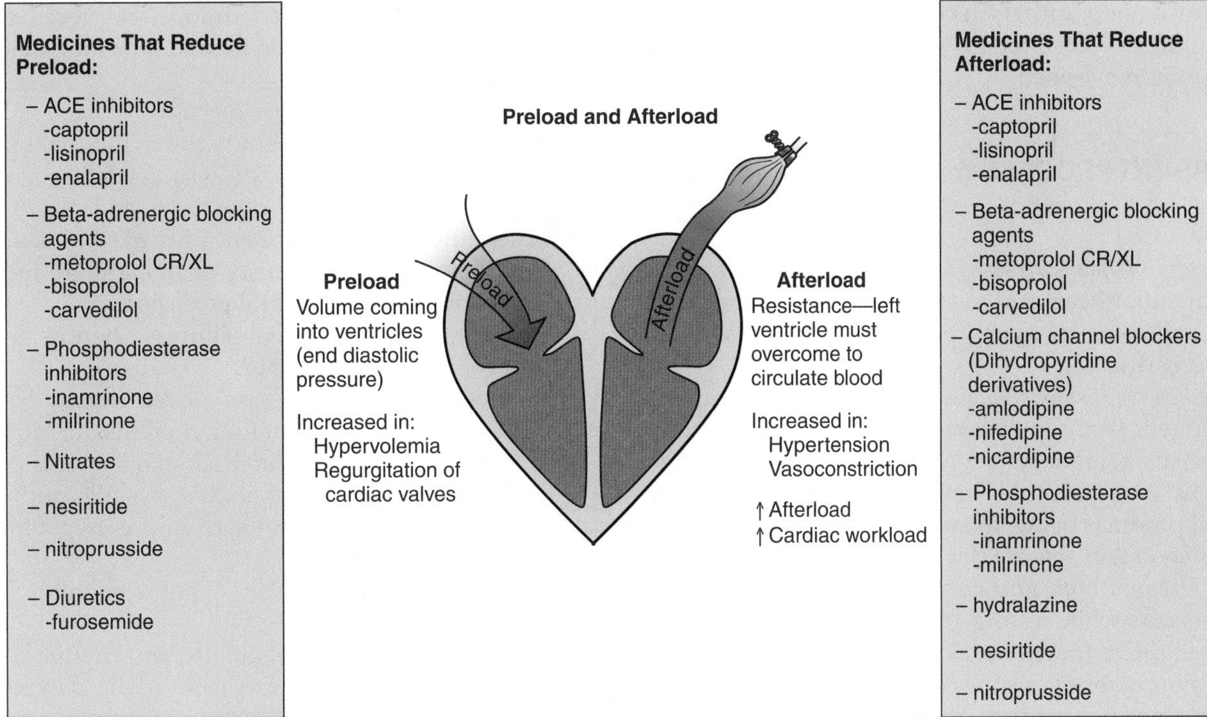

FIGURE **28-3** Medicines that reduce preload and afterload to reduce heart failure.

the American College of Cardiology and the American Heart Association. Heart failure is treated by correcting the underlying disease (e.g., coronary artery disease, hypertension, dyslipidemia, or thyroid disease), smoking cessation, regular exercise when able, bed rest when necessary, sodium-restricted diet, and controlling symptoms with a combination of pharmacologic agents.

DRUG THERAPY FOR HEART FAILURE

Actions

Heart failure is treated with a combination of vasodilator, inotropic, and diuretic therapy (see Figure 28-1). If the failure is acute, most therapy will be administered intravenously (IV) in an intensive care unit. Vasodilators are used to reduce the strain on the left ventricle by reducing systemic vascular resistance (afterload) against which the left ventricle is working. The reduced vascular resistance will also increase tissue perfusion to vital organs and muscles. The second goal of vasodilator use is to reduce preload so that the high volume of blood returning to the heart is decreased. The reduction in preload decreases pulmonary congestion and allows the patient to breathe more easily (Figure 28-3).

Inotropic (in oh troh' pik) **agents** stimulate the heart to increase the force of contractions, thus boosting cardiac output. This also helps reduce pulmonary congestion and improve tissue perfusion. As renal perfusion is improved, potent diuretics are administered to enhance sodium and water excretion. This provides substantial symptomatic relief to the patient in addition to reducing the workload on the heart.

Uses

IV nitroglycerin (see Chapter 25), nitroprusside (see Chapter 23), and nesiritide are used as vasodilators to reduce preload and afterload in critically ill patients. Angiotensin-converting enzyme (ACE) inhibitors are the mainstays of oral vasodilator therapy for treating chronic heart failure. Recent studies indicate that certain patients will also benefit from the use of beta-adrenergic blocking agents. A major component of the pathophysiologic causes of heart failure is increased sympathetic activity. Carvedilol, a noncardioselective beta blocker and an alpha-1 blocker, blocks the adrenergic activity while lowering systemic vascular resistance as a vasodilator (see Chapters 13 and 23). Other vasodilators used are minoxidil, hydralazine (see Chapter 23), and nesiritide. The calcium ion antagonists (e.g., nifedipine, amlodipine, and nicardipine) may be used to reduce afterload in patients with heart failure; however, the calcium ion antagonists also have negative inotropic properties that can aggravate heart failure in certain patients (see Chapters 23 and 25). A combination product containing hydralazine and isosorbide dinitrate (BiDil) has recently been approved by the U.S. Food and Drug Administration (FDA). This combination has been shown to reduce hospitalizations, improve quality of life, and reduce mortality among African Americans with hypertension and heart failure.

Inotropic agents used to treat acute failure are IV dobutamine (see Chapter 13), inamrinone, or milrinone. Digoxin, a digitalis glycoside, has been used for decades to treat heart conditions when an oral inotropic agent is needed. Most patients with heart failure require a loop diuretic such as furosemide or bumetanide (see Chapter 29) to assist in reducing fluid and sodium overload.

NURSING PROCESS *for Heart Failure Therapy*

Assessment

History of Heart Disease. Obtain a history of prior treatment for heart and related cardiovascular disease (e.g., hypertension, hyperlipidemia), diabetes mellitus, and lung disease.

Medication History. Obtain details of all medications prescribed. Tactfully determine if the prescribed medications are being taken regularly and if not, why? Ask for a list of all over-the-counter medications and any herbal products being taken.

History of Six Cardinal Signs of Heart Disease

- *Dyspnea (difficulty breathing):* Record if dyspnea occurs while resting, on exertion, or while asleep at night (paroxysmal nocturnal dyspnea). Are symptoms of dyspnea accompanied by a productive or nonproductive cough? Ask the patient to describe sputum. (With heart failure, it is frothy and may be blood-tinged.) How has the patient been coping with any orthopneic problems?
- *Chest pain:* Because heart failure results in decreased cardiac output and lower oxygenation of tissue, the heart may experience inadequate tissue perfusion, resulting in chest pain.
- Record data as to the time of onset, frequency, duration, and quality of chest pain. Note any conditions the patient has found that either aggravate or relieve the chest pain.
- *Fatigue:* Determine whether fatigue occurs only at specific times of the day, such as toward evening. Ask the patient if fatigue subsides in relation to a decrease in activity level or is present at about the same time daily.
- *Edema:* Record the presence or absence of edema. If present, record location of edema, assessment data (e.g., degree of pitting present; ankle, midcalf, or thigh circumference), appearance of the skin (e.g., shiny, weeping with pressure), and any measures the patient has used to eliminate edema. Chart the time of day that the edema is present (e.g., when rising in the morning, before bedtime) and the specific parts on the body where present. When performing daily weights, use the same scale, at the same time of day, with the patient in a similar type of clothing.
- *Syncope:* Ask the patient about conditions surrounding any episodes of syncope. Record the degree of symptoms, such as general muscle weakness, inability to stand upright, feeling faint, or loss of consciousness. Record what activities, if any, bring on these syncopal episodes.
- *Palpitations:* Record the patient's description of palpitations, such as, "my heart skips some beats." Ask if these conditions are preceded by strenuous or mild exercise and how long the palpitations last.

Indications of Altered Cardiac Function

- *Basic mental status:* Identify the individual's level of consciousness (e.g., drowsiness, lethargy, confusion; orientation to date, time, and place). Assess the clarity of thought present. Both level of consciousness and clarity of thought are indicators of adequate cerebral perfusion.
- *Vital signs:* Obtain vital signs as often as necessary to monitor the patient's status.
- *Blood pressure:* Obtain baseline readings and a history of prior treatment for hypertension. Monitor at specific intervals and report a narrowing pulse pressure (difference between systolic and diastolic readings). With heart failure, hypotension may be present.
- *Temperature:* Record every 8 hours; monitor more frequently if elevated.
- *Pulse:* Record the rate, quality, and rhythm of the pulse. With heart failure, tachycardia may represent an attempt by the body to compensate for decreased cardiac output. Tachycardia is often the first clinical symptom of heart failure.
- *Heart and lung sounds:* Nurses with advanced skills can perform auscultation and percussion to note changes in heart size and heart and lung sounds. Lung fields are assessed in a sitting position to detect abnormal lung sounds (e.g., wheezes, crackles). (Refer to a medical-surgical nursing textbook for details of performing these skills.)
- *Skin color:* Note the color of the skin, mucous membranes, tongue, earlobes, and nail beds. Chart the exact location of any pallor or cyanosis present.
- *Neck veins:* Record jugular vein distention.
- *Clubbing:* Inspect the fingernails and toenails for clubbing. Perform the blanching test on fingernails and toenails.
- *Central venous pressure:* If ordered, obtain baseline and subsequent readings at specified intervals. Report alterations within parameters indicated by the physician.
- *Abdomen:* Inspect abdomen, noting size, shape, softness, or distention. Read history to obtain data relating to liver enlargement.
- *Fluid volume status:* Continue to assess intake and output at intervals appropriate to the patient's condition (every hour during acute, severe status). Report intake that exceeds output. Ask about the frequency of nocturia. This often occurs with heart failure because renal perfusion is improved when the patient lies down and fluid moves from the interstitial spaces back into the general circulation.
- *Diagnostic tests:* Review laboratory/diagnostic tests and report abnormal results to the physician promptly. Tests include serum electrolytes, especially potassium, calcium, magnesium, and sodium; arterial blood gases (ABGs); serum lipids;

electrocardiogram (ECG); echocardiogram; nuclear imaging studies; chest x-ray; urinalysis and kidney function; and hemodynamic assessments.
- *Nutrition:* Take a history of the diet that has been prescribed and assess adherence to the diet. Obtain data regarding appetite and the presence of nausea and vomiting.
- *Activity and exercise:* Ask questions to gather information about the effect of exercise on the patient's functioning. Is the person normally sedentary or moderately or very active? Has there been a reduction in activity level to handle associated fatigue or dyspnea? Are the activities of daily living (ADLs) being performed by the person?
- *Anxiety level:* Patients experiencing cardiac disorders exhibit varying degrees of anxiety. Note the level of anxiety or depression present.

Nursing Diagnoses
- Cardiac output, decreased (indication)
- Gas exchange, impaired (indication)
- Activity intolerance (indication)
- Tissue perfusion, impaired (indication)
- Fluid volume, excess (indication)

Planning
Medication. Order medications prescribed and schedule these on the medication administration record (MAR). Perform focused assessments to determine effectiveness and side effects of pharmacologic interventions.

History of Six Cardinal Signs of Cardiovascular Disease. Individualize the care plan to address the patient's degree of dyspnea, chest pain, fatigue, edema, syncope, and palpitations.

Altered Cardiac Functions. Plan interventions to address indicators of altered cardiac functions that will stabilize the patient's condition. Educate the patient with heart failure to the physiologic and psychological changes that occur, and plan with the patient for the needed interventions and lifestyle changes.

Diagnostic Tests. Order stat and subsequent laboratory studies.

Implementation
- Obtain baseline ABGs or monitor pulse oximeter as ordered. Administer oxygen therapy as prescribed and periodically review results.
- Position the patient in Fowler's or semi-Fowler's position to maximize lung expansion and oxygenation. Reposition the patient at least every 2 hours; use alternate mattress and provide skin care to prevent breakdown.
- Auscultate lung sounds at specified intervals consistent with the patient's condition. Assess for neck vein distention.
- Weigh the patient daily, using the same scale, in similar clothing, at the same time—usually before breakfast. Record and report significant weight changes. (Weight gains and losses are the single best indicator of fluid gain or loss.) As appropriate to patient's condition, obtain and record abdominal girth measurements.
- When fluid restrictions are prescribed, half of fluids is usually given with meals and the other half is given on a per-shift basis.
- Maintain degree of dietary sodium restriction prescribed.
- Avoid using salt substitutes when potassium-sparing diuretics are given.
- Administer medications prescribed (e.g., bronchodilators, ACE inhibitors, nitrates, digoxin, diuretics, antianxiety agents) on schedule or as needed. Monitor degree of response achieved and report ineffectiveness.
- Pace nursing activities to avoid undue fatigue; implement exercise gradually while monitoring vital signs before and after ambulation. Assess for signs and symptoms of fatigue or poor oxygenation before, during, and after exercise.
- Do not plan exercise or ambulation within 1 hour after eating to avoid excessive oxygen depletion.
- Monitor vital signs and perform focused assessment of heart and respiratory functions at specified intervals.
- Perform neurologic assessment to determine changes in mental status.
- Deal calmly with an anxious patient, offer explanations of procedures being performed, and listen to concerns and intervene appropriately.
- Monitor the rate of IV infusions carefully; contact primary care provider regarding concentration of admixtures of drugs to IV infusion solution when limitation of fluids is indicated.
- Give stool softeners to avoid Valsalva maneuver.

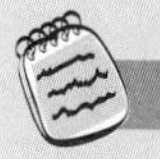

Patient Education and Health Promotion
- Teach the patient and significant others the functional changes caused by heart failure. Emphasize the need for lifelong treatment and adherence to drug therapy, diet, and exercise regimens to obtain maximum control of the disease process.
- Assess understanding of symptoms that indicate when to call the health care provider: dyspnea; a productive cough; worsening fatigue; edema in the feet, ankles, or legs; weight gain of 2 pounds or more in a 2-day period; and development of angina or chest pain, palpitation, or confusion.
- Provide instructions for taking the blood pressure, pulse, and respirations, and give the acceptable parameters for each, as prescribed by the health care provider.
- Explain oxygen therapy that is prescribed and, if being discharged on oxygen, where to obtain oxygen equipment and supplies, rate of administration, and the care and maintenance of the equipment.

- Demonstrate how to put the patient in a Fowler's position. Discuss adaptations needed at home to use these positions for relief of dyspnea. Explain that an upright position provides maximum oxygenation.
- Teach good skin care and the need to change positions at least every 2 hours, especially when edema is present. Have the patient inspect ankles, feet, and abdomen daily for edema. If using a recliner or bed, the sacral area should also be checked regularly for edema.
- Discuss the importance of spacing ADLs to conserve energy and avoid fatigue. Review the prescribed activity level and stress monitoring pulse, dyspnea, and fatigue levels as a guide to when the patient is overexerting.
- Explore coping mechanisms the person uses in response to stress. Discuss how the patient is adapting to the needed changes in lifestyle to manage the disease process. Address depression issues if present.
- Diet therapy is an integral part of the treatment of heart failure. Schedule meetings with the nutritionist to enable the patient to learn how to manage specific dietary modifications prescribed (usually a low-sodium, high-potassium diet with weight reduction parameters for obese patients). If possible, have the patient practice food selections using the daily menus while still in the hospital. Take cultural food preferences into consideration and offer guidance from the nutrition staff as well as the nurses. Teach about foods low in sodium and high in potassium. Potassium restrictions may be indicated if the patient is taking a potassium-sparing diuretic. Salt substitutes are high in potassium, so use must be limited. Alcohol intake should be limited to no more than one drink per day or eliminated from the diet.
- Teach the patient the importance of maintaining a regular, mild exercise routine as prescribed by the physician. At one time it was felt exercise was harmful, but mild, regular exercise is now prescribed, with limitations defined by the physician.
- Fluid restrictions may be imposed, usually in moderate to advanced heart failure; discuss specific ways to manage these limitations.
- Teach the signs and symptoms of potassium deficiency or excess, depending on medications prescribed.

Medication Regimen

- Heart failure requires lifelong treatment, and adherence to prescribed therapy is imperative to gain control of the disease.
- Teach the signs and symptoms of digitalis toxicity (e.g., anorexia, nausea, vomiting, bradycardia, visual disturbances, psychiatric disturbances). Explain medication administration parameters: if the pulse is less than 60 or more than 100, do not administer digoxin until checking with a physician. (An antidote is available for digoxin toxicity.) Instruct the patient that it is important to report for blood draws to check serum levels of the drug at the specific times scheduled.
- Diuretics should be taken in the morning to avoid nighttime diuresis. Depending on the type of diuretic prescribed, potassium supplements may be necessary. However, if a potassium-sparing diuretic is ordered, limiting potassium intake may be appropriate. Salt substitutes should be avoided because they are high in potassium.
- Tell the patient to perform daily weights using the same scale, in similar clothing, at the same time—usually before breakfast. Record and report significant weight changes because weight gains and losses are the best indicators of fluid gain or loss. Usually a gain of 2 pounds in 2 days should be reported.
- When ACE inhibitors are ordered, hypotension, hyperkalemia, and a persistent cough are possible. Discuss management of these side effects.

Fostering Health Maintenance

- Throughout the course of treatment, discuss medication information and how it will benefit the patient.
- Drug therapy is one component of the treatment of heart failure, and it is critical that the medications be taken as prescribed. Provide the patient and significant others with the important information contained in the specific drug monograph for the drug prescribed. Additional health teaching and nursing interventions for drug side effects to expect and report will be found in each drug monograph.
- It is important to control the underlying condition causing the heart failure (e.g., hypertension, hyperlipidemia). The patient and family must understand the importance of complying with diet, exercise, and other prescribed treatments designed to maximize the patient's degree of oxygenation.
- Seek cooperation and understanding of the following points so that medication adherence is increased: name of medication, dosage, route and times of administration, side effects to expect, and side effects to report.

Written Record. Enlist the patient's aid in developing and maintaining a written record of monitoring parameters (e.g., pulse rate, blood pressure, degree of dyspnea and what precipitates it, chest pain, edema) (see Patient Self-Assessment Form on p. 455). Complete the Premedication Data column for use as a baseline to track response to drug therapy. Ensure that the patient understands how to use the form, and instruct the patient to bring the completed form to follow-up visits. During follow-up visits, focus on issues that will foster adherence with the therapeutic interventions prescribed. ■

PATIENT SELF-ASSESSMENT FORM **Cardiovascular Agents**

MEDICATIONS	COLOR	TO BE TAKEN

Patient ______________________

Health Care Provider ______________________

Health Care Provider's phone ______________________

Next appt.* ______________________

What I Should Monitor		Premedication Data	Date	Date	Date	Date	Date	Date	Comments
Weight	AM PM								
Blood pressure	AM PM								
Pulse	AM PM								
Chest pain	Activity Lasting how long? How many nitroglycerin taken?								
Bowel movements	Normal (times) Diarrhea (times) Constipation								
Fatigue All day / After exercise / Normal 10 / 5 / 1									
Edema	Morning								
	Evening								
	Other								
	Can wear shoes, slippers?								
Visual changes	Clear, hazy, blurred, colored halos?								
Fainting and dizziness	Standing, sitting, or lying								
Heart beat ("skips a beat," "racing" feeling, or irregular)	Times per day At rest Activity Asleep								
Difficulty breathing	Times per day At rest Activity Asleep (____) of pillows								
Exercise: Degree of tiredness	Walk across room Walk (____) stairs Walk (____) blocks								
Extremely / Very / Normal 10 / 5 / 1									
Sexual activity (note any pain experienced in comments section). Very tired / Tired / Normal 10 / 5 / 1									
Other									

*Please bring this record with you to your next appointment.
Use the back of this sheet for additional information.

DRUG CLASS: Digitalis Glycosides

digoxin (di joks′ in)

LANOXIN (lah noks′ in)

Actions

The digitalis glycosides are among the oldest therapeutic agents used for the treatment of heart failure. Their use in medicine dates to the eighteenth century. In 1785, William Withering, an English physician and botanist, published excellent observations on the treatment of various ailments with digoxin. Once derived naturally from the dried leaves of *Digoxin purpurea* (purple foxglove), the drug is now synthetically prepared. Digoxin is the only digitalis glycoside currently available in the United States.

Digoxin glycosides have two primary actions on the heart: digoxin increases the force of contraction (positive inotropy) (in oh troh′ pe), and it slows the heart rate (negative chronotropy) (kron oh troh′ pe), reducing the conduction velocity and prolonging the refractory period at the atrioventricular (AV) node. The exact mechanisms of these actions are unknown, but the net result is that the heart is able to fill and empty more completely, thus improving circulation. With improved circulation, there is a reduction in systemic and pulmonary congestion, in heart size toward normal, and in peripheral edema because of better perfusion of blood through the kidneys.

Uses

Digoxin is used to treat mild to severe systolic heart failure not responding to diuretics, beta blockers, and ACE inhibitors. Digoxin may also be used in to treat atrial fibrillation, atrial flutter, and paroxysmal tachycardia. Digoxin is not used to treat diastolic heart failure and may indeed worsen this condition.

The goal of treatment for heart failure is to give adequate doses of digoxin so that the most optimal cardiac effects are achieved and cardiac output is increased, pulse rate is slowed, and vasoconstriction decreases, resulting in the disappearance of many of the signs and symptoms of heart failure (i.e., dyspnea, orthopnea, edema). The once-standard approach to giving loading doses (digitalization) of the drug over a period of hours or days is no longer thought to be necessary in most cases to produce the desired cardiac effect. A maintenance dose is now given, usually once daily. Many patients must continue to take digoxin preparations for the remainder of their lives.

Therapeutic Outcomes

The primary therapeutic outcomes expected from digoxin therapy are improved cardiac output, resulting in improved tissue perfusion, and improved tolerance to activity, as demonstrated by the ability to perform ADLs without supplemental oxygen therapy or fatigue.

Nursing Process for Digoxin

Premedication Assessment

1. Take *apical* pulse for *1 full minute;* follow institution guidelines for withholding drug, for example, if pulse less than 60 or greater than 100 beats per minute. NOTE: In the long-term care setting, radial pulse may be acceptable.
2. Before initiating therapy, obtain baseline data such as vital signs, lung sounds, weight, laboratory studies (e.g., serum electrolytes, liver and kidney function studies).
3. As therapy progresses, monitor for development of digoxin toxicity, hypokalemia, hypomagnesemia, or sudden increase in pulse rate that previously had been normal or low.

Planning

Availability. PO: 0.125 and 0.25 mg tablets; 0.05, 0.1, and 0.2 mg gelcaps; pediatric elixir, 0.05 mg/mL. IV: 0.25 mg/mL in 1- and 2-mL vials and ampules, and 0.1 mg/mL in 1-mL ampules.

Implementation

Digitalization. Digitalization is the administration of a larger dose of digoxin for an initial period of 24 hours. Following this initial "loading" period, the patient is switched to a daily maintenance dose. Be sure to monitor the patient carefully for signs of digoxin toxicity.

Pulse Variations. Always take the apical pulse 1 *full* minute *before* administering any digoxin preparation. Do not administer the drug when the pulse rate in an adult is less than 60 beats per minute until the physician is consulted. In a child, report findings less than 90 beats per minute. The physician may decide to withhold the medication.

Accurate Identification. Digoxin is often given in minute amounts. *Always* have mathematical computations checked by another professional nurse.

Use the correct type of syringe to facilitate accuracy in dosage measurement. Always question any order that is unusual *before* administration. Read the medication label carefully for proper drug and strength.

Dosage and Administration. Give digoxin after meals to minimize gastric irritation.

NOTE: It is recommended that a baseline ECG be obtained before initiation of therapy. Assuming the patient has not ingested digoxin in the preceding 2 weeks, the following dosages apply:

- *Adult:* PO: Digitalizing: 0.25 to 0.50 mg initially followed by 0.125 mg every 6 hours until adequate digitalization is achieved. Maintenance: 0.125 to 0.25 mg daily. Some patients may require 0.375 to 0.5 mg daily. IV: Digitalizing: 0.25 to 0.5 mg initially followed by 0.125 mg every 6 hours until adequate digitalization is achieved. Administer at a rate of 0.5 to 1 mL per minute.

Maintenance: Same as for PO administration. Adult therapeutic blood levels are 0.5 to 1.8 ng/mL.
- *Pediatric (premature):* Intramuscular (IM) or intravenous (IV): Digitalizing: 0.0075 to 0.0125 mg/kg initially followed by 0.00375 to 0.006 mg/kg every 6 to 8 hours for two doses (total digitalizing dose: 0.015 to 0.025 mg/kg). Maintenance: 0.003 to 0.0075 mg/kg once daily.
- *Pediatric (age 1 to 24 months):* IM or IV: Digitalizing: 0.015 to 0.025 mg/kg initially followed by 0.0075 to 0.0125 mg/kg every 6 to 8 hours for two doses (total digitalizing dose: 0.03 to 0.05 mg/kg). Maintenance: 0.007 to 0.016 mg/kg once daily. PO: Digitalizing: 0.0175 to 0.03 mg/kg initially, followed by 0.00875 to 0.015 mg/kg every 6 to 8 hours for two doses (total digitalizing dose: 0.035 to 0.06 mg/kg). Maintenance: 0.00875 to 0.021 mg/kg once daily.
- *Pediatric (ages 2 to 5 years):* PO: Digitalizing: 0.015 to 0.02 mg/kg initially, followed by 0.0075 to 0.01 mg every 6 to 8 hours for two doses (total digitalizing dose: 0.03 to 0.04 mg/kg). Maintenance: 0.0075 to 0.012 mg/kg once daily. IM or IV: Digitalizing: 0.0125 to 0.0175 mg/kg initially, followed by 0.006 to 0.009 mg/kg every 6 to 8 hours for two doses (total digitalizing dose: 0.025 to 0.035 mg/kg). Maintenance: 0.006 to 0.012 mg/kg once daily.
- *Pediatric (ages 5 to 10 years):* PO: Digitalizing: 0.01 to 0.0175 mg/kg initially, followed by 0.005 to 0.009 mg every 6 to 8 hours for two doses (total digitalizing dose: 0.02 to 0.035 mg/kg). Maintenance: 0.005 to 0.012 mg/kg once daily.
- *Pediatric (older than 10 years):* PO: Digitalizing: 0.005 to 0.007 mg/kg initially, followed by 0.0025 to 0.0035 mg/kg every 6 to 8 hours for two doses (total digitalizing dose: 0.010 to 0.015 mg/kg). Maintenance: 0.0025 to 0.005 mg/kg daily.

Serum Levels. Serum levels of digoxin are obtained to measure the amount of digoxin in the bloodstream. Blood should be drawn before the daily dose of medication is given or at least 6 hours after administration. It is important to be consistent in the time of drawing the blood and administering the dose if more than one serum level is to be obtained from the same patient.

Treatment of Digoxin Toxicity. Basic treatment of digoxin-induced dysrhythmias consists of stopping the digoxin and any potassium-depleting diuretics, checking the potassium level (administering potassium as indicated), and administering antidysrhythmic drugs (e.g., phenytoin, lidocaine). In some instances, atropine may be prescribed for sinus bradycardia. A pacemaker may be necessary to correct continuing bradycardia.

Antidote for Severe Digoxin Intoxication. In cases of severe digoxin intoxication as indicated by life-threatening dysrhythmias such as ventricular tachycardia, fibrillation or severe sinus bradycardia, steady-state digoxin serum concentrations greater than 10 ng/mL, or a serum potassium concentration greater than 5 mEq/L in a known case of digoxin ingestion, treatment with an antidote, digoxin immune Fab (ovine) (Digibind), is usually indicated. This product contains antigen-binding fragments from sheep that have been injected with a digoxin-human albumin complex, against which the sheep make antibodies. The antibodies are harvested and purified into the antigen-binding fragments that have a strong binding affinity for digoxin. When injected into humans who have received digoxin, the fragments bind to molecules of digoxin, making them unavailable for binding at the site of action. The fragment-digoxin complex accumulates in the blood and is excreted by the kidneys. Improvement in signs and symptoms of digoxin intoxication begins less than 30 minutes after injection of the antigen-binding fragments.

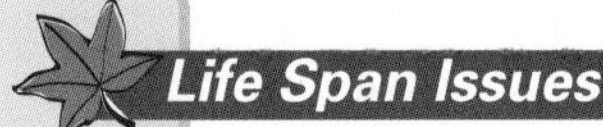

Life Span Issues

Digoxin Dosage

Pediatric dosages for digoxin are extremely small and should be measured in a tuberculin syringe using the metric scale. All dosage calculations should be checked with a second qualified nurse in accordance with the institutional policy.

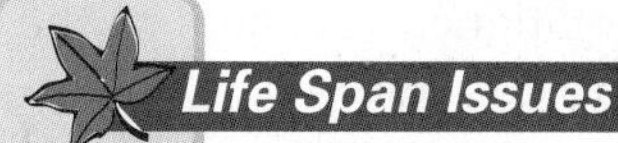

Life Span Issues

Digoxin Toxicity

Older adults frequently experience digoxin toxicity because of digoxin's long half-life. Early symptoms of toxicity are anorexia and mild nausea, but they are frequently overlooked or are not associated with drug toxicity. Any change in pulse rhythm and rate or CNS signs (e.g., mental status, orientation, change in color vision, hallucinations, behavioral changes) should be investigated and reported. In children, digoxin toxicity is often first detected by the development of atrial dysrhythmias.

Evaluation

Side Effects to Report

Digoxin Toxicity

Cardiac Effects. Always observe the patient for the development of a pulse deficit, bradycardia (heart rate <60 beats per minute), tachycardia (heart rate >100 beats per minute), or bigeminy. These may be signs of developing heart block. Whenever the individual is attached to a monitor, the pattern should be closely watched for any type of abnormal cardiac dysrhythmia.

In children, digoxin toxicity is often first detected by the development of atrial dysrhythmias.

Noncardiac Effects. Noncardiac symptoms of digoxin toxicity are often vague and difficult to separate from symptoms of heart disease. Any patient taking digoxin products who develops loss of appetite, nausea, vomiting, diarrhea, extreme fatigue, weakness of the arms and legs, psychiatric disturbances (e.g., nightmares, agitation, listlessness, hallucinations), or visual disturbances (e.g., hazy or blurred vision, difficulty in reading, difficulty in red-green color perception) should be evaluated for digoxin toxicity.

Other Diseases. The patient's other clinical conditions may also induce digoxin intoxication. Patients who suffer from hypothyroidism, acute myocardial infarction, renal disease, severe respiratory disease, or far-advanced heart failure may require lower than normal doses of digoxin. Monitor closely.

Electrolyte Balance. Adverse effects of digoxin may also be induced by electrolyte imbalance, resulting in hypokalemia, hypomagnesemia, and hypocalcemia (see Drug Interactions, following).

Monitor laboratory reports and notify the physician of deviations from the normal range of 4 to 5.4 mEq/L of potassium. Always monitor the pulse carefully if the potassium level is abnormal. Hypokalemia is especially likely to occur when the patient exhibits nausea, vomiting, diarrhea, or heavy diuresis.

Drug Interactions

Drugs That Enhance Therapeutic and Toxic Effects. Nefazodone, quinidine, nifedipine, verapamil, ranolazine, macrolide antibiotics (clarithromycin, erythromycin), propafenone, beta-adrenergic blocking agents (e.g., atenolol, esmolol, timolol, nadolol, propranolol), succinylcholine, calcium gluconate, and calcium chloride. Monitor for signs and symptoms of digoxin toxicity.

Drugs That Reduce Therapeutic Effects. St. John's wort, aminoglycoside antibiotics (e.g., gentamicin, tobramycin, neomycin), cholestyramine, colestipol, rifampin, and antacids. Monitor patient symptoms for response to therapy; recurrence or intensification of the patient's disease should be reported to the physician.

Drugs That May Alter Electrolyte Balance, Altering Digoxin Response. Drugs that may alter digoxin response and the incidence of any of the side effects by alteration of electrolyte balance include the following:

May Cause Hypokalemia

amphotericin B (Fungizone)
bumetanide (Bumex)
chlorthalidone (Hygroton)
corticosteroids
ethacrynic acid (Edecrin)
furosemide (Lasix)
metolazone (Zaroxolyn)
thiazide diuretics

May Cause Hyperkalemia

amiloride (Midamor)
angiotensin-converting enzyme (ACE) inhibitors
angiotensin receptor–blocking agents (ARBs)
beta-adrenergic blockers
eplerenone
heparin
mannitol infusions
potassium chloride
potassium gluconate
potassium penicillin G
potassium supplements (K-Lyte, Kaon, K-Lore, others)
salt substitutes
spironolactone
succinylcholine
triamterene

May Cause Hypomagnesemia

bumetanide
chlorthalidone (Hygroton)
ethacrynic acid (Edecrin)
ethanol
furosemide (Lasix)
metolazone (Zaroxolyn)
neomycin (Mycifradin)
thiazide diuretics

DRUG CLASS: Phosphodiesterase Inhibitors

inamrinone (in am′ rhin own)

Actions

Inamrinone (formerly amrinone) is an inotropic agent that increases the force and velocity of myocardial contractions by inhibiting cyclic adenosine monophosphate (cAMP) phosphodiesterase activity and increases cellular levels of cAMP in the heart muscle. It also is a vascular smooth muscle relaxant that causes vasodilation, reducing preload and afterload.

Uses

Inamrinone is used for the short-term management of systolic dysfunction heart failure in patients who have not responded adequately to digoxin, diuretics, or vasodilator therapy. The inotropic effects of inamrinone are additive to those of digoxin, and it can be used in fully digitalized patients. Inamrinone is usually not used in treating diastolic heart failure and may indeed worsen this condition.

Therapeutic Outcomes

The primary therapeutic outcomes expected from inamrinone therapy are improved cardiac output resulting in improved tissue perfusion and reduced dyspnea, orthopnea, and fatigue.

Nursing Process for Inamrinone

Premedication Assessment

1. Take baseline vital signs including pain rating.
2. Obtain baseline laboratory studies ordered by the physician (e.g., complete blood count [CBC], bilirubin, aspartate aminotransferase [AST], alanine aminotransferase [ALT], gamma-glutamyltransferase [GGT], alkaline phosphatase, prothrombin time).
3. Record any gastrointestinal (GI) symptoms present before initiating therapy.

Planning

Availability. IV: 5 mg/mL in 20-mL ampules.

Implementation

Dosage and Administration

Incompatibility with Dextrose Solutions. Do not dilute inamrinone with dextrose solutions. With time, the inamrinone loses potency. Inamrinone may be injected into running dextrose infusions through a Y connector or directly into the tubing.

Adult: IV: Initiate therapy with a bolus of 0.75 mg/kg given slowly over 2 to 3 minutes. Continue therapy with a maintenance infusion between 5 and 10 mcg/kg/minute. This should place the inamrinone serum level at approximately the 3 mcg/mL level.

Based on clinical response, an additional bolus injection of 0.75 mg/kg may be given 30 minutes after the initial bolus. In general, the total daily dose should not exceed 18 mg/kg/24 hours.

Evaluation

Side Effects to Expect

Nausea, Vomiting, Abdominal Discomfort. These side effects are usually transient and subside with continued therapy. If discomfort becomes severe, reduce the dosage rate and call a health care provider immediately.

Side Effects to Report

Dysrhythmias, Hypotension. As would be expected, the cardiovascular side effects of dysrhythmias (3%) and hypotension (1.3%) are the most commonly reported adverse effects. Monitor blood pressure and heart rate and rhythm closely during therapy. These adverse effects are often dose related and will respond to a reduction in infusion rate. Contact a health care provider immediately if dysrhythmias or significant hypotension develop.

Thrombocytopenia. Thrombocytopenia with platelet counts of less than 100,000/mm^3 has been reported in 2.4% of patients. It appears to be dose dependent, occurring within 48 to 72 hours after initiation of therapy. It is more common with higher-than-recommended doses. Platelet counts should be performed before and periodically during therapy. If thrombocytopenia does occur, discontinuation of therapy should be considered, especially when platelet counts decrease to less than 50,000/mm^3. The nadir in platelet count appears to be variable but occurs within 1 to 4 weeks.

Hepatotoxicity. Hepatotoxicity has been reported in approximately 0.2% of patients after IV therapy. The symptoms of hepatotoxicity are anorexia, nausea, vomiting, jaundice, hepatomegaly, splenomegaly, and abnormal liver function tests (e.g., elevated bilirubin, AST, ALT, alkaline phosphatase, prothrombin time). If these symptoms appear, it is recommended that inamrinone therapy be discontinued.

Drug Interactions

Digoxin. Concurrent administration of inamrinone and digoxin produces additive inotropic effects.

Furosemide. Inamrinone and furosemide are chemically incompatible. When furosemide is mixed with inamrinone, a precipitate forms immediately. Do not infuse into the same IV line.

milrinone (mihl' rhin own)

PRIMACOR (pry' mah cohr)

Actions

Milrinone is an inotropic agent that increases the force and velocity of myocardial contractions by inhibiting phosphodiesterase enzymes in heart muscle. It also is a vascular smooth muscle relaxant that causes vasodilation, reducing preload and afterload.

Uses

Milrinone is used for the short-term management of severe systolic dysfunction heart failure in patients who have not responded adequately to digoxin, diuretics, or vasodilator therapy. It has the advantages of fewer GI side effects and a substantially lower frequency of thrombocytopenia and hepatotoxicity when compared with inamrinone. Milrinone does, however, cause a higher incidence of supraventricular and ventricular dysrhythmias than does inamrinone.

The inotropic effects of milrinone are additive to those of digoxin, and it can be used in fully digitalized patients. Milrinone is usually not used in treating diastolic heart failure and may indeed worsen this condition.

Therapeutic Outcomes

The primary therapeutic outcomes expected from milrinone therapy are improved cardiac output resulting in improved tissue perfusion and reduced dyspnea, orthopnea, and fatigue.

Nursing Process for Milrinone

Premedication Assessment

1. Take baseline vital signs including pain rating.
2. Obtain baseline laboratory studies ordered by the physician (e.g., CBC).

Planning

Availability. IV: 1 mg/mL in 10- and 20-mL vials. Premixed injection: 200 mcg/mL in 5% dextrose injection in 100 mL.

Implementation

Dosage and Administration

- Diluents: 0.45% or 0.9% sodium chloride or dextrose 5% for injection may be used to prepare dilutions of milrinone for IV infusion.
- *Adult:* IV: Initiate therapy with a loading dose of 50 mcg/kg given slowly over 10 minutes.
- Continue therapy with a maintenance infusion between 0.375 and 0.75 mcg/kg per minute.

In general, the total daily dose should not exceed 1.13 mg/kg/24 hours.

Evaluation

Side Effects to Report

Dysrhythmias, Hypotension. The cardiovascular side effects of dysrhythmias (12%) and hypotension (1.3%) are the most commonly reported adverse effects.

Monitor blood pressure and heart rate and rhythm closely during therapy. These adverse effects are often dose related and will respond to a reduction in infusion rate. Contact a physician immediately if dysrhythmias or significant hypotension develops.

Thrombocytopenia. Thrombocytopenia with platelet counts of less than 100,000/mm^3 has been reported in 0.4% of patients. See previous monograph, *Inamrinone,* on p. 458 for additional information regarding thrombocytopenia.

Drug Interactions

Furosemide. Milrinone and furosemide are chemically incompatible. When furosemide is mixed with milrinone, a precipitate forms immediately. Do not infuse into the same IV line.

DRUG CLASS: Angiotensin-Converting Enzyme Inhibitors

Actions

ACE inhibitors represent a major breakthrough in the treatment of heart failure. Large studies show that ACE inhibitors reduce morbidity and mortality associated with heart failure. The ACE inhibitors reduce afterload by blocking angiotensin II–mediated peripheral vasoconstriction and help reduce circulating blood volume (preload) by inhibiting the secretion of aldosterone. (See Chapter 23 for a more complete description of the mechanism of action of ACE inhibitors.)

Uses

The ACE inhibitors reduce blood pressure (afterload), preserve cardiac output, and increase renal blood flow. Captopril, enalapril, fosinopril, lisinopril, ramipril, trandolapril, and quinapril are now recommended as the drugs of choice over digoxin for the treatment of mild to moderate systolic dysfunction heart failure.

Therapeutic Outcomes

The primary therapeutic outcomes expected from ACE inhibitors are improved cardiac output resulting in improved tissue perfusion and improved tolerance to activity, as demonstrated by the ability to perform ADLs without supplemental oxygen therapy or fatigue.

Nursing Process for Angiotensin-Converting Enzyme Inhibitors

See Chapter 23 for a more complete description of the nursing process for ACE inhibitors.

DRUG CLASS: Beta-Adrenergic Blocking Agents

Actions

The beta-adrenergic blocking agents (beta blockers) (see Table 13-3) inhibit cardiac response to sympathetic nerve stimulation by blocking the beta receptors. As a result, the heart rate, cardiac output, aggravating hypertension, and consequently, the blood pressure, are reduced. The beta blockers also inhibit renin release, diminishing the cascade of the renin-angiotensin-aldosterone systems that would induce vasoconstriction and sodium reabsorption.

Uses

The beta-adrenergic blocking agents are agents of another class that have been shown to reduce morbidity and mortality associated with heart failure. The exact mechanism by which beta blockers increase survival in heart failure patients is unknown, but it is thought to include inhibition of renin release, suppression of the effect of elevated circulating catecholamines, and secondary prevention of angina and myocardial infarction. Because beta-adrenergic blocking agents and ACE inhibitors act through different mechanisms, beta blockers and ACE inhibitors are commonly used together to treat heart failure. There is a question of whether all beta blockers have the same clinical effect. Those most well studied and shown to be effective in treating heart failure are bisoprolol, long-acting metoprolol (Toprol XL), and carvedilol.

Nursing Process for Beta-Adrenergic Blocking Agents

See Chapter 23 for a more complete description of the nursing process for beta-adrenergic blocking agents.

DRUG CLASS: Natriuretic Peptides

nesiritide (nes ear′ it ayd)

NATRECOR (naht′ reh cor)

Actions

Nesiritide is the first of a new class of drugs, the human B-type natriuretic peptides (hBNPs). It is a hormone normally secreted by the cardiac ventricles in response to fluid and pressure overload. It helps the heart recover from deteriorating cardiac function by reducing preload and afterload pressures, increasing diuresis and sodium excretion, suppressing the renin-angiotensin-aldosterone system, and reducing secretion of norepinephrine.

Uses

Nesiritide is used as a vasodilator in patients with severe heart failure who have dyspnea at rest or with minimal activity.

Therapeutic Outcomes

The primary therapeutic outcomes of nesiritide are reduction of workload on the heart and improvement in symptoms associated with heart failure.

Planning

Availability

IV: 1.5 mg single-use vials.

Key Points

- Heart failure is a cluster of signs and symptoms that arise when the left or right ventricle or both ventricles lose the ability to pump enough blood to meet the body's circulatory needs. It is an illness that is growing in frequency as the general population ages.
- The morbidity and mortality associated with heart failure can be reduced through medication, diet, activity and symptom monitoring.
- Nurses can play a significant role in discussion of treatment options, planning for lifestyle changes, counseling before discharge, and reinforcement of key points during office visits. Best results are attained when the patient, family, and nurse work together in developing the care plan.

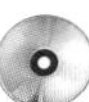

Go to your Companion CD-ROM for Appendices, an Audio Glossary, animations, Drug Dosage Calculators, customizable Patient Self-Assessment forms, and Review Questions for the NCLEX® Examination.

evolve Be sure to visit the companion Evolve site at http://evolve.elsevier.com/Clayton for WebLinks and additional online resources.

MEDICATION SAFETY REVIEW

MATH REVIEW QUESTIONS

1. A 64-year-old, 165-pound male patient, is in emergency department with stat orders:

   Order: Digoxin 6 mcg/kg IV stat

   Available: Digoxin 0.1 mg/mL

   165 lb = ____ kg

   Based on this order, what dose of digoxin would be given stat? ____ mcg or ____ mg

   Use any drug reference to determine the following:

   - Is digoxin given IV diluted or undiluted?
   - What rate of IV injection is recommended?
   - With what IV solutions is digoxin compatible?

2. The patient above is transferred from the emergency department to the coronary unit for 24 hours. The following orders exist for medications:

   Order: Digoxin 0.125 mg IV every 6 hours after stat dose

   Available: Digoxin 0.1 mg/mL and digoxin 0.25 mg/mL

   Give: Digoxin ____ mL of ____ mg/mL

3. After digitalization, a maintenance dose is prescribed:

   Order: Digoxin 0.375 mg PO daily

   Available: Digoxin 0.125- and 0.25-mg tablets

   Give: ____ tablets of ____-mg tablet

CRITICAL THINKING QUESTIONS

1. When initiating digoxin therapy, what assessments should be made on a continuum? Discuss the rationale for these observations.
2. In addition to the medications listed in the Medication Safety Review, the patient is started on furosemide 60 mg daily. What is the action of furosemide? Explain the nursing assessments that should be made to evaluate the effectiveness of the diuretic therapy.
3. Describe the purpose of drug therapy for heart failure when administering vasodilator drugs such as nitroprusside or nifedipine, a calcium channel blocker.
4. Why is it usually necessary to use a combination of drugs to treat heart failure?
5. What are the actions of each drug classification used to treat heart failure?
6. Describe precautions in the preparation of inamrinone for IV use.

CONTENT REVIEW QUESTIONS

1. When an explanation of heart failure says that the sympathetic nervous system is activated, what actions occur?
   1. Hypertrophy of the cardiac wall
   2. Dilation of the chambers of the heart
   3. Increased heart rate, contractility, and peripheral vascular resistance
   4. Blood flow to kidneys decreases; kidneys increase release of renin
2. Inamrinone should be mixed for IV administration with:
   1. 5% dextrose/0.9% saline.
   2. 5% dextrose/0.2% water.
   3. 0.9% saline.
   4. 5% dextrose/0.2% sodium chloride and 20 mEq potassium chloride.

Continued

CONTENT REVIEW QUESTIONS—cont'd

3. ACE inhibitors:
   1. reduce blood pressure (afterload).
   2. decrease renal flow.
   3. increase peripheral vascular resistance.
   4. cause vasoconstriction.

4. Digitalis toxicity symptoms are:
   1. increased renal output.
   2. anorexia, nausea, vomiting, blurred vision.
   3. increased potassium level.
   4. peripheral edema, pulse deficit, nocturnal leg cramps.

5. A patient with chronic heart failure tells the nurse at the clinic that he has gained 5 pounds in the past 3 days, even though he has continued to follow a low-sodium diet. The nurse recognizes that the patient:
   1. may be consuming hidden sources of sodium that are not obvious in prepared foods.
   2. should be instructed about a low-calorie, low-fat diet in addition to the sodium restriction.
   3. should have the sodium restriction increased because it appears the patient has excessive sodium retention.
   4. should be evaluated for other symptoms that would indicate an exacerbation of heart failure.

6. The nurse monitors the patient receiving treatment for acute heart failure with the knowledge that marked hypotension is most likely to occur with the intravenous administration of:
   1. amrinone.
   2. furosemide.
   3. nitroprusside.
   4. digoxin.

7. Most patients with heart failure need medications to:
   1. reduce afterload.
   2. increase contractility.
   3. reduce preload.
   4. reduce heart rate.

CHAPTER

29 Drugs Used for Diuresis

evolve http://evolve.elsevier.com/Clayton

Chapter Content

Objectives

1. Cite nursing assessments used to evaluate a patient's state of hydration.
2. Review possible underlying pathologic conditions that may contribute to the development of excess fluid volume in the body.
3. State which electrolytes may be altered by diuretic therapy.
4. Cite nursing assessments used to evaluate renal function.
5. Identify the effects of diuretics on blood pressure, electrolytes, and diabetic or prediabetic patients.
6. Review the signs and symptoms of electrolyte imbalance and normal laboratory values of potassium, sodium, and chloride.
7. Identify the action of diuretics.
8. Explain the rationale for administering diuretics cautiously to older adults and individuals with impaired renal function, cirrhosis of the liver, or diabetes mellitus.
9. Describe the goal of administering diuretics to treat hypertension, heart failure, or increased intraocular pressure or before vascular surgery in the brain.
10. List side effects that can be anticipated whenever a diuretic is administered.
11. Cite alterations in diet that may be prescribed concurrently with loop, thiazide, or potassium-sparing diuretic therapy.
12. State the nursing assessments needed to monitor therapeutic response or the development of side effects to expect or report from diuretic therapy.
13. Develop objectives for patient education for patients taking loop, thiazide, and potassium-sparing diuretics.

Key Terms

aldosterone
tubule
loop of Henle
orthostatic hypotension
electrolyte imbalance
hyperuricemia

DRUG THERAPY WITH DIURETICS

Actions

Diuretics are drugs that act to increase the flow of urine. The purpose of diuretics is to increase the net loss of water. To achieve this, they act on the kidneys in different locations to enhance the excretion of sodium. The methylxanthines increase glomerular filtration, spironolactone inhibits tubular reabsorption of sodium by inhibiting **aldosterone**, and the thiazides and loop diuretics act directly on the kidney tubules to inhibit the reabsorption of sodium and chloride from the lumen of the **tubule.** Sodium and chloride that are not reabsorbed are excreted into the collecting ducts and then into the ureters to the bladder, taking large volumes of water to be excreted from the body through urination (Figure 29-1).

Uses

Diuretics are mainstays of treatment in two major diseases affecting the cardiovascular system: heart failure and hypertension. They are routinely used in heart failure to remove excessive sodium and water to relieve symptoms associated with pulmonary congestion and edema. The Seventh Report of the Joint National Committee on Detection, Evaluation and Treatment of High Blood Pressure (JNC 7) recommends that, after lifestyle modifications, diuretics (often in addition to other antihypertensive agents) be used as primary agents to treat hypertension because they have been shown to reduce cardiovascular morbidity and mortality associated with hypertension.

Diuretics have a variety of other medical uses as well. Mannitol reduces cerebral edema, acetazolamide is used to reduce intraocular pressure associated with glaucoma, spironolactone can be effective in reducing ascites associated with liver disease, and furosemide may be used to treat hypercalcemia.

NURSING PROCESS *for Diuretic Therapy*

The information the nurse assesses about the patient's general clinical symptoms is important to the physician when analyzing data for diagnosis and success of therapy. In addition to assessing overall clinical symptoms, the nurse should include the following data for subsequent evaluation of the patient's response to prescribed therapeutic modalities that act on the urinary system.

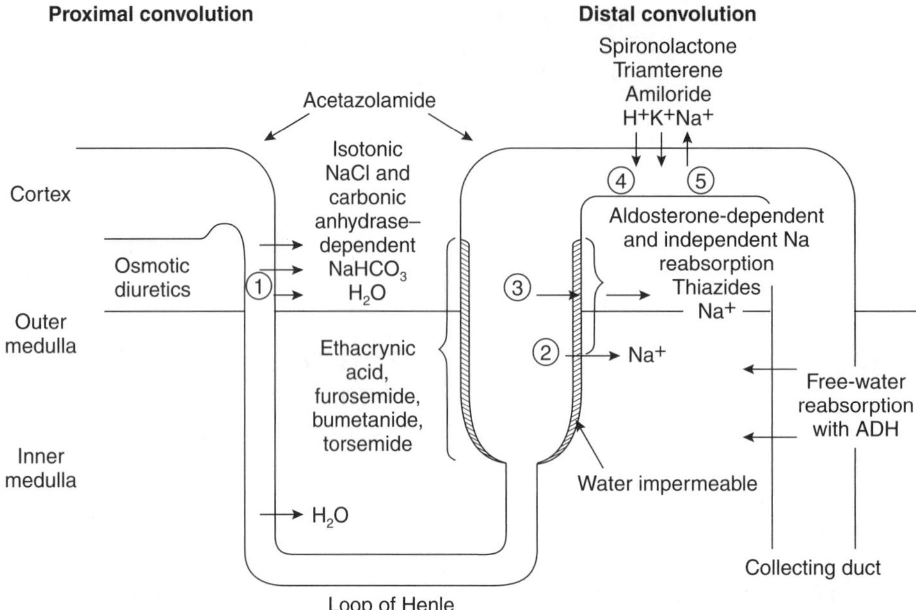

FIGURE **29-1** Sites of actions of diuretics within the nephron.

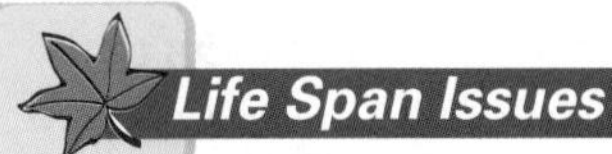

Diuretic Therapy

During the use of diuretic therapy, the patient, often an older adult, must be monitored for hydration status and electrolyte balance as well as for the response of the presenting symptoms to the therapy. Patients taking digoxin are particularly susceptible to digitalis toxicity as a result of electrolyte imbalance.

Assessment

History of Related Causative Disorders/Factors. Ask questions relating to any history of disorders that contribute to fluid volume excess: heart disorders (e.g., myocardial infarction, heart failure, valvular disease, dysrhythmias); liver disease (e.g., ascites, cirrhosis, cancer); renal disease (e.g., renal failure); and factors such as immobility, hypertension, pregnancy, and use of corticosteroid agents.

History of Current Symptoms. Ask questions to ascertain information relating to the onset, duration, and progression of specific symptoms relating to edema, weakness, fatigue, dyspnea, productive cough, and weight gain.

Pattern of Urination. Ask the patient to describe his or her current urination pattern and to cite changes. Such details as frequency, dysuria, incontinence, changes in the stream, hesitancy in starting to void, hematuria, nocturia, and urgency are all significant.

Medication History. Obtain information on all prescribed and over-the-counter medications being taken. Tactfully ask questions regarding compliance.

Hydration Status. Obtain baseline vital signs; note pulse that is bounding and full or irregular (indicating possible dysrhythmias); check respiratory rate and quality; listen to lung sounds to detect presence of crackles or rhonchi; ask for a history of recent weight gain or loss; assess for edema of the extremities, and assess for neck vein distention. Blood pressure may be elevated.

Dehydration. Assess, report, and record significant signs of dehydration in the patient. Observe for poor skin turgor, sticky oral mucous membranes, a shrunken or deeply furrowed tongue, crusted lips, weight loss, deteriorating vital signs, soft or sunken eyeballs, weak pedal pulses, delayed capillary filling, excessive thirst, high urine specific gravity (or no urine output), and possible mental confusion.

Skin Turgor. Check skin turgor by *gently* pinching the skin together over the sternum, on the forehead, or on the forearm. Elasticity is present and the skin rapidly returns to a flat position in the well-hydrated patient. In dehydrated patients, the skin will remain in a peaked or pinched position and return very slowly to the flat, normal position.

Skin turgor is not a reliable indicator in older adults, because the natural aging changes of the skin. See assessments under Dehydration.

Oral Mucous Membranes. With adequate hydration, the membranes of the mouth feel smooth and glisten. With dehydration, they appear dull and are sticky. Assess skin turgor, oral mucosa, and firmness of eyeballs.

Laboratory Changes. The values of the hematocrit, hemoglobin, blood urea nitrogen (BUN), and electrolytes will appear to fluctuate, based on the state of hydration. When a patient is overhydrated, the values appear to drop as a result of hemodilution. A dehydrated patient will show higher values because of hemoconcentration.

Overhydration. Increases in abdominal girth, weight gain, neck vein engorgement, and circumference of the medial malleolus indicate overhydration. Measure the abdominal girth daily at the umbilical level. Measure the extremities bilaterally daily at a level approximately 5 cm above the medial malleolus. Weigh the patient daily using the same scale, at the same time, and in similar clothing.

Edema. *Edema* is a term used to describe excess fluid accumulation in the extracellular spaces. Edema is considered "pitting" when an indentation remains in the tissue after pressure is exerted against a bony part, such as the shin, ankle, or sacrum. The degree is usually recorded as +1 (slight) to +4 (deep).

Pale, cool, tight, shiny skin is another sign of edema. Also listen to lung sounds to detect the presence of excess fluid (crackles).

Assess for the presence of edema (record degree of pitting), obtain baseline measurement of abdominal girth when edema is present, and check for the presence of fluid waves in the abdomen.

Electrolyte Imbalance. Because the symptoms of most electrolyte imbalances are similar, the nurse should gather information relative to changes in the patient's mental status (alertness, orientation, confusion), muscle strength, muscle cramps, tremors, nausea, and general appearance.

Susceptible People. Those who are particularly susceptible to the development of electrolyte disturbances frequently have a history of renal or cardiac disease, hormonal disorders, or massive trauma or burns or are receiving diuretic or steroid therapy. Review available electrolyte studies.

Hypokalemia. Serum potassium (K^+) levels less than 3.5 mEq/L. Hypokalemia is especially likely to occur when a patient exhibits vomiting, diarrhea, or heavy diuresis. All diuretics, except the potassium-sparing type, are likely to cause hypokalemia.

Hyperkalemia. Serum potassium (K^+) levels greater than 5.5 mEq/L. Hyperkalemia occurs most commonly when a patient is given excessive amounts of potassium supplementation, either intravenously or orally. It may also occur as an adverse effect of potassium-sparing diuretics.

Hyponatremia. Serum sodium (Na^+) less than 135 mEq/L. Remember the phrase, "Where sodium goes, water goes." Because diuretics act by excreting sodium, monitor the patient for hyponatremia during and after diuresis.

Hypernatremia. Serum sodium (Na^+) greater than 145 mEq/L. Hypernatremia occurs most frequently when a patient is given intravenous (IV) fluids in excess of fluid excreted.

Nursing Diagnoses

- Fluid volume, excess (indication)
- Cardiac output, decreased (indication)
- Fluid volume, risk for deficient (side effect)
- Injury, risk for, related to diuretic therapy (side effect)

Planning

History of Causative Disorder/Factors. Review the patient's history to identify the underlying diagnosis for which the diuretic is prescribed. Also review drug monographs for conditions that contradict or suggest precautions when used (e.g., potassium-sparing diuretics with renal failure).

History of Current Symptoms. Plan to perform a focused assessment at least every shift to identify any changes in the patient's status.

Pattern of Urination. Schedule appropriate nursing interventions for identified problems relating to the pattern of urinary elimination. Be sure to provide assistance with voiding for people with impaired mobility, fatigue, or other impairments.

Medications. Schedule prescribed medications on the medication administration record (MAR). Remember to administer diuretics in the morning whenever possible to prevent nocturia.

Hydration. Schedule intake and output (I&O) every shift or more frequently depending on patient status. Place information to be assessed for status of hydration on the Kardex (e.g., measure abdominal girth every shift, record degree of edema present in legs every shift) or computerized method of charting used for daily planning.

Renal Diagnostics. Many laboratory tests are ordered throughout the treatment of renal dysfunction (e.g., BUN, serum creatinine, creatinine clearance, serum osmolalities, urine osmolalities). Plan schedules for appropriate timing of collections of blood and urine samples.

Nutrition. *Edema:* Patients with edema are routinely placed on a restricted sodium diet to help control edema associated with heart failure. Depending on the type of diuretic prescribed (potassium-sparing or non–potassium-sparing), the patient may be placed on potassium restrictions or potassium supplements.

Diet therapy for renal disease is directed at keeping a normal equilibrium of the body while decreasing the excretory load on the kidneys. See a nutrition text for modifications specific to acute and chronic renal failure.

Implementation

Intake and Output. I&O should be recorded accurately every shift and totaled every 24 hours for all patients having renal evaluations or receiving diuretics.

Intake. Measure and record *accurately* all fluids taken (e.g., oral, parenteral, rectal, via tubes). Ice chips and foods, such as gelatin, that turn to a liquid state must be included. Irrigation solutions should be carefully measured so that the difference between that instilled and that returned can be recorded as intake.

Remember to enlist the help of the patient, family, and other visitors in this process. Ask them to keep a record of how many glasses or cups of liquids (e.g., water, juice, soda, tea, coffee) are consumed. The nurse then converts the household measurements to milliliters.

Output. Record all output from the mouth, urethra, rectum, wounds, and tubes (i.e., surgical drains, nasogastric tubes, indwelling catheters).

Liquid stools should be recorded according to consistency, color, and quantity.

Urine output should include information on quantity, color, pH, odor, and specific gravity.

All other secretions should be characterized by color, consistency, volume, and changes from previous collections, if possible.

Daily output is usually 1200 to 1500 mL, or 30 to 50 mL per hour. Always report urine output below this hourly rate. Low hourly output may indicate dehydration, renal failure, or cardiac disease.

Keep the urinal or bedpan readily available. Tell patients and their visitors the importance of not dumping the bedpan or urinal. Instruct them to use the call light and allow the hospital personnel to empty and record all output.

Serum Electrolytes. Monitor serum electrolyte reports; notify health care provider of deviations from normal values.

Nutrition. Order prescribed special diet depending on underlying pathologic condition. If fluid restrictions are prescribed, state the amount of fluid to be taken on each tray and the amount that may be taken orally each shift on the Kardex or in the computer and have this information posted at the head of the patient's bed.

Laboratory Diagnostics. Order requested laboratory studies relating to the disease process.

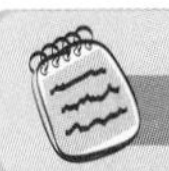

Patient Education and Health Promotion

Purposes of Diuresis

- If the disease process is hypertension, stress the importance of following the prescribed ways to deal with emotions and the dietary and medicinal regimens that can control the disease (see discussion of nursing process for hypertensive therapy, Chapter 23).
- Teach the patient and significant others the functional changes that hypertension and heart failure cause. Emphasize the need for lifelong treatment and adherence to drug therapy, diet, and exercise regimens to obtain maximum control of the disease process.
- Diuretics are used in the treatment of several disease processes, for example, hypertension, glaucoma, ascites, hypercalcemia, heart failure, and renal disease. Be certain the patient understands the medication administration schedule and desired therapeutic outcome for the prescribed therapy.

Medication Considerations

- Diuretics should be taken in the morning to avoid nocturia.
- When the diuretic is prescribed on a scheduled pattern other than daily, assist the patient with the development of ways to remember when to take the medication (e.g., using a calendar on which to mark dosages or using a medication holder that is marked with the days of the week and is loaded weekly with the medications to be taken).
- Instruct the patient to perform daily weights using the same scale, in similar clothing, at the same time daily—usually before breakfast. Record and report significant weight changes because weight gains and losses are the best indicator of fluid loss or gain. Usually a gain of 2 pounds in 2 days should be reported.
- Potassium supplements may be prescribed concurrently with diuretics other than potassium-sparing diuretics.
- Diuretic therapy may produce postural hypotension. Teach the patient to rise slowly from a supine or sitting position, and encourage the patient to sit or lie down if feeling faint.

Nutrition

- The health care provider usually prescribes dietary modifications appropriate to the underlying pathologic condition, such as weight reduction or sodium restriction.
- Patients receiving potassium-sparing diuretics should be taught which foods are high in potassium content. These foods should be moderately restricted but not withheld from the diet. Salt substitutes should be avoided because they are high in potassium.
- When taking diuretics, other than the potassium-sparing type, the patient is required to eat potassium-rich foods.

Fostering Health Maintenance

- Throughout the course of treatment, discuss medication information and how it will benefit the patient. Stress the importance of nonpharmacologic interventions and the long-term effects that compliance with the treatment regimen can provide.
- Provide the patient and significant others with important information contained in the specific drug monograph for the medicines prescribed. Additional health teaching and nursing interventions for the side effects to expect and report are described in the drug monographs that follow.
- Seek cooperation and understanding of the following points so that medication compliance is increased: name of medication, dosage, route and times of administration, side effects to expect, and side effects to report.

Written Record. Enlist the patient's aid in developing and maintaining a written record of monitoring parameters (see Patient Self-Assessment Form on p. 467). Complete the Premedication Data column for use as a baseline to track response to drug therapy. Ensure that the patient understands how to use the form and instruct the patient to bring the completed form to follow-up visits. During follow-up visits, focus on issues that will foster adherence with the therapeutic interventions prescribed.

PATIENT SELF-ASSESSMENT FORM Diuretics or Urinary Antibiotics

MEDICATIONS	COLOR	TO BE TAKEN

Patient ____________

Health Care Provider ____________

Health Care Provider's phone ____________

Next appt.* ____________

What I Should Monitor			Premedication Data	Date	Date	Date	Date	Date	Date	Comments
Weight										
Blood pressure										
Pulse										
Faintness, dizziness	At rest									
	On exertion									
	No. of occurrences									
Muscle weakness	With exertion									
	When at rest									
Pain pattern and severity Severe 10 — Moderate 5 — Low 1										
Description: On urination Without urination Flank area Suprapubic area										
Voiding and frequency	___ times voiding per day									
	___ times voiding per hour									
Fluid intake	___ glasses per day									
	___ cups per day									
Urine	Color (check one)	Straw								
		Dark								
		Red								
	Odor: usual or unusual									
Other										

*Please bring this record with you to your next appointment.
Use the back of this sheet for additional information.

DRUG CLASS: Carbonic Anhydrase Inhibitor

acetazolamide (ah see tah zol′ a myd)

▶ DIAMOX (dy′ ah moks)

Actions

Acetazolamide is a weak diuretic that acts by inhibiting the enzyme carbonic anhydrase within the kidney, brain, and eye. As a diuretic, it promotes the excretion of sodium, potassium, water, and bicarbonate.

Uses

Acetazolamide is not used frequently as a diuretic because of the availability of more effective medications. However, it is used to reduce intraocular pressure in patients with glaucoma and to reduce seizure activity in patients with certain types of epilepsy (see Chapters 19 and 43).

DRUG CLASS: Methylxanthines

aminophylline (ah mi noff′ ih lin)

Actions

Aminophylline is a methylxanthine derivative used for its diuretic effects in cardiorenal disease and as a bronchodilator in patients with pulmonary disease. The methylxanthine derivatives include theophylline, caffeine, and theobromine, all of which display weak diuretic properties. All act by improving blood flow to the kidneys.

Uses

Aminophylline is rarely used as a diuretic because of the availability of more effective diuretic agents. However, a diuresis is occasionally noted when aminophylline is used in the treatment of asthma. For a discussion of aminophylline as a bronchodilator, see Chapter 31.

DRUG CLASS: Loop Diuretics

bumetanide (bu met′ an eyd)
BUMEX (bu′ mex)

Actions

Bumetanide is a potent diuretic that acts primarily by inhibiting sodium and chloride reabsorption from the ascending limb of the loop of Henle in the kidneys. It also acts by increasing renal blood flow into the glomeruli and inhibits electrolyte absorption in the proximal tubule, enhancing sodium, chloride, phosphate, and bicarbonate excretion into the urine. Its diuretic activity starts 30 to 60 minutes after administration; peak activity is within 1 to 2 hours and lasts 4 to 6 hours.

Uses

Bumetanide is used to treat edema resulting from heart failure, cirrhosis of the liver, and renal disease, including nephrotic syndrome.

Therapeutic Outcomes

The primary therapeutic outcome associated with bumetanide therapy is diuresis with reduction of edema and improvement in symptoms related to excessive fluid accumulation.

Nursing Process for Bumetanide

Premedication Assessment

1. Obtain baseline data before initiation of therapy, such as vital signs, lung sounds, weight, degree of edema present, laboratory studies (e.g., serum electrolytes, liver and renal function tests).
2. Obtain data relating to the patient's mental status (orientation, alertness, confusion), muscle strength, muscle cramps, tremors, nausea, and general appearance.
3. Patients with diabetes require baseline measurement of blood glucose levels.
4. Check for symptoms of acute gout. If present, notify the health care provider.

Planning

Availability. PO: 0.5, 1, and 2 mg tablets. IV: 0.25 mg/mL in 2, 4, and 10 mg ampules.

Implementation

Dosage and Administration. *Adult:* PO: Initially 0.5 to 2 mg is administered as a single, daily dose. If additional diuresis is required, additional doses may be administered at 4- to 5-hour intervals. Do not exceed a maximum daily dose of 10 mg. Administer with food or milk to reduce gastric irritation. DO NOT administer after midafternoon, to prevent nocturia. IM or IV: Initially, 0.5 to 1 mL is administered over 1 to 2 minutes. Additional doses may be administered at 2- to 3-hour intervals as necessary. Do not exceed 10 mg per 24 hours.

Evaluation

Side Effects to Expect

Oral Irritation, Dry Mouth. Start regular oral hygiene measures when the therapy is initiated. Suggest the use of 1 teaspoon of hydrogen peroxide in 6 to 8 ounces of water as a mouthwash. Commercial mouthwashes contain alcohol, which may cause further drying and oral irritation.

Another method to alleviate dryness is sucking on ice chips or hard candy.

Orthostatic Hypotension. Although orthostatic hypotension (e.g., dizziness, weakness, faintness) is infrequent and generally mild, all diuretics may cause it to some degree, particularly when therapy is being initiated. Monitor the blood pressure daily in both the supine and standing positions.

Anticipate the development of postural hypotension, and take measures to prevent an occurrence. Teach the patient to rise slowly from a supine or sitting position, and encourage the patient to sit or lie down if feeling faint.

Side Effects to Report

Gastric Irritation, Abdominal Pain. If gastric irritation occurs, administer with food or milk. If symptoms persist or increase in severity, report for physician evaluation.

Electrolyte Imbalance, Dehydration. The electrolytes most commonly altered are potassium (K^+), sodium (Na^+), and chloride (Cl^-). *Hypokalemia* is most likely to occur.

Many symptoms associated with altered fluid and electrolyte balance are subtle and interspersed with general symptoms of drug toxicity or the disease process itself.

Gather data about *changes* in the patient's mental status (alertness, orientation, confusion), muscle strength, muscle cramps, tremors, nausea, and general appearance.

Always check the electrolyte reports for early indications of electrolyte imbalance. Keep accurate records of I&O, daily weights, and vital signs.

Hives, Pruritus, Rash. Report symptoms for further evaluation by the physician. Pruritus may be relieved by adding baking soda to the bath water.

Drug Interactions

Alcohol, Barbiturates, Narcotics. Orthostatic hypotension associated with bumetanide therapy may be aggravated by these agents.

Digoxin. Bumetanide may cause excessive potassium excretion, leading to hypokalemia. If the patient is also receiving digoxin, monitor closely for digitalis toxicity (anorexia, nausea, fatigue, blurred or colored vision, bradycardia, dysrhythmias).

Aminoglycosides. The potential for ototoxicity from the aminoglycosides (e.g., gentamicin, amikacin, netilmicin) is increased. Assess the patient for gradual, often subtle, changes in hearing. Note if the patient seems to speak more loudly, asks for statements to be repeated, or turns the television or radio progressively louder.

Cisplatin. The potential for ototoxicity from the combination of cisplatin and bumetanide is increased. Assess the patient for gradual, often subtle changes in hearing. Note if the patient seems to speak more loudly, asks for statements to be repeated, or turns the television or radio progressively louder.

Nonsteroidal Antiinflammatory Drugs (NSAIDs). NSAIDs (e.g., indomethacin, ibuprofen, naproxen) inhibit the diuretic activity of bumetanide. The dose of bumetanide may have to be increased or the NSAID discontinued. Maintain accurate I&O records and monitor for a decrease in diuretic activity.

Corticosteroids. Corticosteroids (e.g., prednisone) may enhance the loss of potassium. Check potassium levels and monitor more closely for hypokalemia when these two agents are used concurrently.

Probenecid. Probenecid inhibits the diuretic activity of bumetanide. In general, do not use concurrently.

ethacrynic acid (eth ah krin′ ik)
▶ EDECRIN (eh′ deh krin)

Actions

Ethacrynic acid is another diuretic that acts primarily on the ascending limb of the loop of Henle to prevent sodium and chloride reabsorption. Ethacrynic acid does not appear to affect renal blood flow or glomerular filtration rate. Its diuretic activity begins within 30 minutes, peaks in approximately 2 hours, and lasts 6 to 8 hours.

Uses

Ethacrynic acid is used to treat edema resulting from heart failure, cirrhosis of the liver, renal disease, and malignancy and for hospitalized pediatric patients with congenital heart disease. It is thought that because ethacrynic acid inhibits the reabsorption of sodium to a much greater extent than other diuretics, it may be more effective in patients with significant renal failure. It is also used in conjunction with 0.9% sodium chloride infusions to enhance excretion of calcium in patients with hypercalcemia.

Therapeutic Outcomes

The primary therapeutic outcome associated with ethacrynic acid therapy is diuresis with reduction of edema and improvement in symptoms related to excessive fluid accumulation.

Nursing Process for Ethacrynic Acid

Premedication Assessment

1. Obtain baseline data before initiation of therapy, such as vital signs, lung sounds, weight, degree of edema present, and laboratory studies (e.g., serum electrolytes, liver and renal function tests).
2. Obtain data relating to the patient's mental status (orientation, alertness, confusion), muscle strength, muscle cramps, tremors, nausea, and general appearance.
3. Patients with diabetes require baseline measurement of blood glucose levels.

Planning

Availability. PO: 25 and 50 mg tablets. IV: 50 mg per vial.

Implementation

Dosage and Administration. *Adult:* PO: 50 to 100 mg initially followed by 50 to 200 mg daily. Do not exceed 400 mg per day. Administer with food or milk to reduce gastric irritation. DO NOT administer after midafternoon, to prevent nocturia. IV: 50 mg or 0.5 to 1 mg/kg. Add 50 mL of dextrose 5% or saline solution to 50 mg of ethacrynic acid. This solution is stable for 24 hours. Administer over several minutes through the tubing of a running infusion or by direct IV line. Occasionally the addition of a diluent may result in an opalescent solution. These solutions should not be used. Do not mix with blood derivatives.

Pediatric: PO: Initially 25 mg daily. Increase the dosage in increments of 25 mg to the desired effect. IV: 1 mg/kg. Dilute with dextrose 5%, and administer over 5 minutes through a running infusion. DO NOT use IV solution if it turns opalescent when the diluent is added.

Always monitor vital signs and I&O at regular intervals when administering this agent intravenously.

Report blood pressure that decreases steadily or a narrowing pulse pressure, which may indicate hypovolemia.

Evaluation

Side Effects to Expect

Orthostatic Hypotension. Although this effect is infrequent and generally mild, all diuretics may cause some degree of orthostatic hypotension (dizziness, weakness, faintness), particularly when therapy is initiated or dosages are increased. Monitor the blood pressure daily in both the supine and standing positions.

Anticipate the development of postural hypotension and take measures to prevent its occurrence. Teach the patient to rise slowly from a supine or sitting position, and encourage the patient to sit or lie down if feeling faint.

Side Effects to Report

Electrolyte Imbalance, Dehydration. The electrolytes most commonly altered are potassium (K^+), sodium (Na^+), and chloride (Cl^-). *Hypokalemia* is most likely to occur.

Many symptoms associated with electrolyte imbalance are subtle and interspersed with general symptoms of drug toxicity or the disease process itself.

Gather data about *changes* in the patient's mental status (alertness, orientation, confusion), muscle strength, muscle cramps, tremors, nausea, and general appearance.

Always check the electrolyte reports for early indications of electrolyte imbalance. Keep accurate records of I&O, daily weights, and vital signs.

Gastrointestinal Bleeding. Observe for "coffee ground" vomitus or dark, tarry stools, particularly in patients receiving IV therapy.

Dizziness, Deafness, Tinnitus. People with impaired renal function may experience these symptoms. Assess the patient for gradual, often subtle changes in balance and hearing. Note if the patient seems more unsteady when standing, speaks loudly, asks for statements to be repeated, or turns the television or radio progressively louder.

Diarrhea. Diarrhea may become severe. Report to the health care provider, and monitor the patient for dehydration and fluid and electrolyte imbalance.

Hyperglycemia. Diabetic or prediabetic patients must be monitored for the development of hyperglycemia, particularly during the early weeks of therapy. Assess regularly for glycosuria, and report if it occurs with any frequency. Patients receiving oral hypoglycemic agents or insulin may require an adjustment in dosage.

Drug Interactions

Aminoglycosides. The potential for ototoxicity from the aminoglycosides (e.g., gentamicin, amikacin, netilmicin, tobramycin) is increased. Assess the patient for gradual, often subtle changes in hearing. Note if the patient seems to speak loudly, asks for statements to be repeated, or turns the television or radio progressively louder.

Cisplatin. The potential for ototoxicity from the combination of cisplatin and ethacrynic acid is increased. Assess the patient for gradual, often subtle changes in hearing. Note if the patient seems to speak more loudly, asks for statements to be repeated, or turns the television or radio progressively louder.

Nonsteroidal Antiinflammatory Drugs. NSAIDs (e.g., indomethacin, ibuprofen, naproxen) inhibit the diuretic activity of ethacrynic acid. The dose of ethacrynic acid may have to be increased or the NSAID discontinued. Maintain accurate I&O records, and monitor for a decrease in diuretic activity.

Digoxin. Ethacrynic acid may cause excess potassium excretion, leading to hypokalemia. If the patient is also receiving digoxin, monitor closely for digitalis toxicity (anorexia, nausea, fatigue, blurred or colored vision, bradycardia, dysrhythmias).

Corticosteroids. Corticosteroids (e.g., prednisone) may enhance the loss of potassium. Check potassium levels and monitor more closely for hypokalemia when these two agents are used concurrently.

furosemide (fuhr oh' sah myd)
▶ LASIX (lay' siks)

Actions

Furosemide acts primarily on the ascending limb of the loop of Henle but also on the proximal and distal portions of the tubule to prevent sodium and chloride reabsorption. Furosemide diuresis results in enhanced excretion of sodium, chloride, potassium, hydrogen, calcium, magnesium, ammonium, bicarbonate, and possibly phosphate. Maximum diuretic effect occurs 1 to 2 hours after oral administration and lasts 4 to 6 hours. Diuresis occurs 5 to 10 minutes after IV administration, peaks within 30 minutes, and lasts approximately 2 hours.

Uses

Furosemide is one of the most potent and effective diuretics currently available. In addition to treating edema caused by heart failure, renal disease, and cirrhosis of the liver, furosemide may be used for the treatment of hypertension, alone or in combination with other antihypertensive therapy. It is also used in conjunction with 0.9% sodium chloride infusions to enhance excretion of calcium in patients with hypercalcemia.

Therapeutic Outcomes

The primary therapeutic outcome associated with furosemide therapy is diuresis with reduction of edema and improvement in symptoms related to excessive fluid accumulation.

Nursing Process for Furosemide

Premedication Assessment

1. Obtain baseline data before initiation of therapy, such as vital signs, lung sounds, weight, degree of edema present, and laboratory studies (e.g., serum electrolytes, liver and renal function tests).
2. Obtain data relating to the patient's mental status (orientation, alertness, confusion), muscle strength, muscle cramps, tremors, nausea, and general appearance.
3. Patients with diabetes require baseline measurement of blood glucose levels.
4. Note any reduction in hearing.
5. Check for symptoms of acute gout. If present, notify the physician.

Planning

Availability. PO: 20, 40, and 80 mg tablets; 10 mg/mL and 40 mg/5 mL oral solution. IV: 10 mg/mL in 2, 4, and 10 mL vials.

Implementation

NOTE: Patients who are allergic to sulfonamides may also be allergic to furosemide.

Dosage and Administration. *Adult:* PO: 20 to 80 mg as a single dose given preferably in the morning. If a second dose is necessary, administer 6 to 8 hours later. Increase in increments of 20 to 40 mg per day. Administer with food or milk to reduce gastric irritation. DO NOT administer after midafternoon, to prevent nocturia. IV: 20 to 40 mg given over 1 to 2 minutes. Much larger doses are frequently administered intravenously. The rate of administration should not exceed 4 mg per minute. Do not exceed 1000 mg per day. Always monitor vital signs and I&O at regular intervals with the IV administration of this agent. Report blood pressure that decreases steadily or a narrowing pulse pressure, which may indicate hypovolemia.

Pediatric: PO: Initially 1 to 2 mg/kg. If the response is not satisfactory, increase by 1 to 2 mg/kg every 6 hours. IV: Initially 1 mg/kg. If diuresis is not satisfactory, increase by 1 mg/kg every 2 hours to a maximum of 6 mg/kg.

Evaluation

Side Effects to Expect

Oral Irritation, Dry Mouth. Start regular oral hygiene measures when therapy is initiated. Suggest the use of 1 teaspoon of hydrogen peroxide in 6 to 8 ounces of water as a mouthwash. Commercial mouthwashes contain alcohol and may cause further drying and oral irritation. Another measure to alleviate dryness is sucking on ice chips or hard candy.

Orthostatic Hypotension. Although orthostatic hypotension (dizziness, weakness, faintness) is infrequent and generally mild, all diuretics may cause some degree of orthostatic hypotension, particularly when therapy is being initiated or dosages are increased. Monitor the blood pressure daily in both the supine and standing positions.

Anticipate the development of postural hypotension and take measures to prevent an occurrence. Teach the patient to rise slowly from a supine or sitting position, and encourage the patient to sit or lie down if feeling faint.

Side Effects to Report

Electrolyte Imbalance, Dehydration. The electrolytes most commonly altered are potassium (K^+), sodium (Na^+), and chloride (Cl^-). *Hypokalemia* is most likely to occur.

Many symptoms associated with altered fluid and electrolyte balance are subtle and interspersed with general symptoms of drug toxicity or the disease process itself.

Gather data about *changes* in the patient's mental status (alertness, orientation, confusion), muscle strength, muscle cramps, tremors, nausea, and general appearance.

Always check the electrolyte reports for early indications of electrolyte imbalance. Keep accurate records of I&O, daily weights, and vital signs.

Hyperuricemia. Furosemide may inhibit the excretion of uric acid, resulting in **hyperuricemia.** Patients who have had previous attacks of gouty arthritis are particularly susceptible to additional attacks as a result of hyperuricemia. Monitor the laboratory reports for early indications of hyperuricemia. Report to the health care provider, who may then add a uricosuric agent or allopurinol to the patient's medication regimen.

Hyperglycemia. Diabetic or prediabetic patients must be monitored for the development of hyperglycemia, particularly during the early weeks of therapy. Assess regularly for glycosuria, and report if it occurs with any frequency. Patients receiving oral hypoglycemic agents or insulin may require an adjustment in dosage.

Hives, Pruritus, Rash. Report symptoms for further evaluation by the physician. Pruritus may be relieved by adding baking soda to the bath water.

Drug Interactions

Digoxin. Furosemide may cause excessive excretion of potassium, resulting in hypokalemia. If the patient is also receiving digoxin, monitor closely for digitalis toxicity (anorexia, nausea, fatigue, blurred or colored vision, bradycardia, dysrhythmias).

Propranolol. The action of propranolol may be increased. Monitor for hypotension and bradycardia. Dosage adjustment may be necessary.

Theophylline Derivatives. The action of theophylline derivatives may be increased. Assess patients for signs of theophylline toxicity (restlessness, irritability, insomnia, nausea, vomiting, tachycardia, dysrhythmias). Serum levels of theophylline may be beneficial in dosage adjustment.

Aminoglycosides. The potential for ototoxicity from the aminoglycosides (e.g., gentamicin, amikacin, netilmicin, tobramycin) is increased. Assess the patient for gradual, often subtle, changes in balance and hearing. Note if the patient seems more unsteady when standing, speaks loudly, asks for statements to be repeated, or turns the television or radio progressively louder.

Cisplatin. The potential for ototoxicity from the combination of cisplatin and furosemide is increased. Assess the patient for gradual, often subtle changes in hearing. Note if the patient seems to speak more loudly, asks for statements to be repeated, or turns the television or radio progressively louder.

Nonsteroidal Antiinflammatory Drugs. NSAIDs (e.g., indomethacin, ibuprofen, naproxen) inhibit the diuretic activity of furosemide. The dose of furosemide may have to be increased or the NSAID discontinued. Maintain accurate I&O records, and monitor for a decrease in diuretic activity.

Salicylates. The potential for salicylate toxicity may be increased if taken concurrently for several days. Monitor patients for nausea, tinnitus, fever, sweating, dizziness, mental confusion, lethargy, and impaired hearing. Serum levels of salicylates may be beneficial in determining the amounts of salicylate dosage reduction.

Metolazone. When used concurrently, there is a considerably greater diuresis than when either agent is used alone. Monitor closely for dehydration and electrolyte imbalance.

Phenytoin. Phenytoin may inhibit the absorption of orally administered furosemide. The dosage of furosemide may have to be increased based on the clinical response of the patient to normal doses.

torsemide (tohr sah' myd)
DEMADEX (dehm' ah dex)

Actions

Torsemide is a sulfonamide type of loop diuretic similar to furosemide. It acts on the ascending limb of the loop of Henle to prevent sodium and chloride reabsorption. Torsemide does not appear to affect glomerular filtration rate or renal blood flow. Maximum diuretic effect occurs 1 to 2 hours after oral administration and lasts 6 to 8 hours. Diuresis occurs 5 to 10 minutes after IV administration, peaks within 60 minutes, and lasts up to 6 hours.

Uses

Torsemide is used to treat edema caused by heart failure, renal disease, and cirrhosis of the liver. Torsemide may also be used for the treatment of hypertension, alone or in combination with other antihypertensive therapy.

Therapeutic Outcomes

The primary therapeutic outcome associated with torsemide therapy is diuresis with reduction of edema and improvement in symptoms related to excessive fluid accumulation.

Nursing Process for Torsemide

Premedication Assessment

1. Obtain baseline data before initiation of therapy, such as vital signs, lung sounds, weight, degree of edema present, laboratory studies (e.g., serum electrolytes, liver and renal function tests).
2. Obtain data relating to the patient's mental status (orientation, alertness, confusion), muscle strength, muscle cramps, tremors, nausea, and general appearance.
3. Patients with diabetes require baseline measurement of blood glucose levels.
4. Note any reduction in hearing.

Planning

Availability. PO: 5, 10, 20, and 100 mg tablets. IV: 10 mg/mL in 2 and 5 mL ampules.

Implementation

NOTE: Patients who are allergic to sulfonamides may also be allergic to torsemide.

Dosage and Administration. PO: Initially 5 to 20 mg once daily. If the dose is inadequate, increase the dose upward by doubling it until the desired diuretic response is achieved. IV: Same as for PO dosages. Administer slowly over 2 or more minutes.

Evaluation

Side Effects to Expect

Oral Irritation, Dry Mouth. Start regular oral hygiene measures when therapy is initiated. Suggest the use of 1 teaspoon of hydrogen peroxide in 6 to 8 ounces of water as a mouthwash. Commercial mouthwashes contain alcohol and may cause further drying and oral irritation. Another measure to alleviate dryness is sucking on ice chips or hard candy.

Orthostatic Hypotension. Although orthostatic hypotension (dizziness, weakness, faintness) is infrequent and generally mild, all diuretics may cause some degree of orthostatic hypotension, particularly when therapy is initiated or dosage is increased. Monitor the blood pressure daily in both the supine and standing positions.

Anticipate the development of postural hypotension and take measures to prevent it. Teach the patient to rise slowly from a supine or sitting position, and encourage the patient to sit or lie down if feeling faint. Provide for patient safety.

Side Effects to Report

Electrolyte Imbalance, Dehydration. The electrolytes most commonly altered are potassium (K^+), sodium (Na^+), and chloride (Cl^-). *Hypokalemia* is most likely to occur.

Many symptoms associated with altered fluid and electrolyte balance are subtle and interspersed with general symptoms of drug toxicity or the disease process itself.

Gather data about *changes* in the patient's mental status (alertness, orientation, confusion), muscle strength, muscle cramps, tremors, nausea, and general appearance.

Always check the electrolyte reports for early indications of electrolyte imbalance. Keep accurate records of I&O, daily weights, and vital signs.

Hyperuricemia. Torsemide may inhibit the excretion of uric acid, resulting in hyperuricemia. Patients who have had previous attacks of gouty arthritis are particularly susceptible to additional attacks as a result of hyperuricemia. Monitor the laboratory reports for early indications of hyperuricemia. Report to the health care provider, who may then add a uricosuric agent or allopurinol to the patient's medication regimen.

Hyperglycemia. Diabetic or prediabetic patients must be monitored for the development of hyperglycemia, particularly during the early weeks of therapy. Assess regularly for glycosuria, and report if it occurs with any frequency. Patients receiving oral hypoglycemic agents or insulin may require an adjustment in dosage.

Hives, Pruritus, Rash. Report symptoms for further evaluation by the physician. Pruritus may be relieved by adding baking soda to the bath water.

Drug Interactions

Digoxin. Torsemide may cause excessive excretion of potassium, resulting in hypokalemia. If the patient is also receiving digoxin, monitor closely for digitalis toxicity (anorexia, nausea, fatigue, blurred or colored vision, bradycardia, dysrhythmias).

Theophylline Derivatives. The action of theophylline derivatives may be increased. Assess patients for signs of theophylline toxicity (e.g., restlessness, irritability, insomnia, nausea, vomiting, tachycardia, dysrhythmias). Serum levels of theophylline may be beneficial in dosage adjustment.

Aminoglycosides. The potential for ototoxicity from the aminoglycosides (e.g., gentamicin, amikacin, netilmicin, tobramycin) is increased. Assess the patient for gradual, often subtle, changes in balance and hearing. Note if patient seems more unsteady when standing, speaks loudly, asks for statements to be repeated, or turns the television or radio progressively louder.

Cisplatin. The potential for ototoxicity from the combination of cisplatin and torsemide is increased. Assess the patient for gradual, often subtle changes in hearing. Note if the patient seems to speak more loudly, asks for statements to be repeated, or turns the television or radio progressively louder.

Nonsteroidal Antiinflammatory Drugs. NSAIDs (e.g., indomethacin, ibuprofen, naproxen) inhibit the diuretic activity of torsemide. The dose of torsemide may have to be increased or the NSAID discontinued. Maintain accurate I&O records, and monitor for a decrease in diuretic activity.

Salicylates. The potential for salicylate toxicity may be increased if taken concurrently for several days. Monitor patients for nausea, tinnitus, fever, sweating, dizziness, mental confusion, lethargy, and impaired hearing. Serum levels of salicylates may be beneficial in determining the amounts of salicylate dosage reduction.

Metolazone. When torsemide and metolazone are used concurrently, there is a considerably greater diuresis than when either agent is used alone. Monitor closely for dehydration and electrolyte imbalance.

DRUG CLASS: Thiazide Diuretics

Actions

The benzothiadiazides, more commonly called the thiazides, have been an important and useful class of diuretic and antihypertensive agents for the past three decades. As diuretics, thiazides act primarily on the distal tubules of the kidney to block the reabsorption of sodium and chloride ions from the tubule. The unreabsorbed sodium and chloride ions are passed into the collecting ducts, taking molecules of water with them, thus resulting in a diuresis.

Uses

The thiazides are used as diuretics in the treatment of edema associated with heart failure, renal disease, hepatic disease, pregnancy, obesity, premenstrual syndrome, and administration of adrenocortical steroids. The antihypertensive properties of the thiazides result from a direct vasodilatory action on the peripheral arterioles (see Chapter 23).

Therapeutic Outcomes

The primary therapeutic outcomes associated with thiazide therapy are as follows:

- Diuresis with reduction of edema and improvement in symptoms related to excessive fluid accumulation
- Reduction in elevated blood pressure

Nursing Process for Thiazide Diuretics

Premedication Assessment

1. Obtain baseline data before initiation of therapy, such as vital signs, lung sounds, weight, degree of edema present, laboratory studies (e.g., serum electrolytes, liver and renal function tests).

2. Obtain data relating to the patient's mental status (orientation, alertness, confusion), muscle strength, muscle cramps, tremors, nausea, and general appearance.
3. Patients with diabetes require baseline measurement of blood glucose levels.
4. Note any reduction in hearing.
5. Check for any symptoms of acute gout. If present, notify the physician.

Planning

Availability. Tables 29-1 and 29-2 list thiazide diuretics and those diuretics chemically related to the thiazides. Most of the diuretics listed are administered in divided daily doses for the treatment of hypertension. However, single daily dosages may be most effective for mobilization of edema fluid.

Implementation

DO NOT administer after midafternoon, to prevent nocturia.

Dosage and Administration. See Tables 29-1 and 29-2. Administer with food or milk to reduce gastric irritation.

Evaluation

Side Effects to Expect

Orthostatic Hypotension. Although orthostatic hypotension (dizziness, weakness, faintness) is infrequent and generally mild, all diuretics may cause some degree of orthostatic hypotension, particularly when therapy is being initiated. Monitor the blood pressure daily in both the supine and standing positions.

Anticipate the development of postural hypotension, and take measures to prevent it. Teach the patient to rise slowly from a supine or sitting position, and encourage the patient to sit or lie down if feeling faint.

Side Effects to Report

Gastric Irritation, Nausea, Vomiting, Constipation. If gastric irritation occurs, administer with food or milk. If symptoms persist or increase in severity, report to the health care provider for evaluation.

Electrolyte Imbalance, Dehydration. Use of thiazides may cause or aggravate electrolyte imbalance; therefore patients should be observed regularly for signs such as dry mouth, drowsiness, confusion, muscular weakness, and nausea. The electrolytes most commonly altered are potassium (K^+), sodium (Na^+), and chloride (Cl^-). *Hypokalemia* is most likely to occur, and supplementary potassium is often prescribed to prevent or treat it.

Many symptoms associated with altered fluid and electrolyte balance are subtle and interspersed with general symptoms of drug toxicity or the disease process itself.

Gather data about *changes* in the patient's mental status (alertness, orientation, confusion), muscle

Drug Table 29-1 THIAZIDE DIURETIC PRODUCTS

GENERIC NAME	BRAND NAME	DOSAGE FORMS AVAILABLE	DOSAGE RANGE
bendroflumethiazide	Naturetin	Tablets: 5, 10 mg	2.5-15 mg
chlorothiazide	Diuril	Tablets: 250, 500 mg Oral suspension: 250 mg/5 mL Injection: 500 mg/20 mL	1000-2000 mg
hydrochlorothiazide	Esidrix, HydroDiuril, Oretic	Tablets: 25, 50, 100 mg Capsules: 12.5 mg Solution: 50 mg/5 mL	12.5-100 mg
hydroflumethiazide		Tablets: 50 mg	25-100 mg
methyclothiazide	Enduron	Tablets: 2.5, 5 mg	2.5-5 mg
polythiazide		Tablets: 1, 2, 4 mg	1-4 mg
trichlormethiazide	Naqua, Metahydrin, Diurese	Tablets: 4 mg	1-4 mg

Drug Table 29-2 THIAZIDE-RELATED DIURETICS

GENERIC NAME	BRAND NAME	DOSAGE FORMS AVAILABLE	DOSAGE RANGE
chlorthalidone	Hygroton, Thalitone	Tablets: 15, 25, 50, 100 mg	50-200 mg
indapamide	Lozol	Tablets: 1.25, 2.5 mg	2.5-5 mg
metolazone	Zaroxolyn, Mykrox	Tablets: 0.5, 2.5, 5, 10 mg	2.5-10 mg

strength, muscle cramps, tremors, nausea, and general appearance.

Always check the electrolyte reports for early indications of electrolyte imbalance. Keep accurate records of I&O, daily weights, and vital signs.

Hyperuricemia. The plasma uric acid is frequently elevated by the thiazides, which inhibit the excretion of uric acid. Patients who have had previous episodes of hyperuricemia or attacks of gouty arthritis are particularly susceptible to additional attacks when receiving thiazide therapy. Monitor the laboratory reports for early indications of hyperuricemia. Report to the health care provider, who may then add a uricosuric agent or allopurinol to the patient's medication regimen.

Hyperglycemia. The thiazides may induce hyperglycemia and aggravate cases of preexisting diabetes mellitus. Diabetic or prediabetic patients must be monitored for the development of hyperglycemia, particularly during the early weeks of therapy. Assess regularly for glycosuria, and report if it occurs with any frequency. Dosages of oral hypoglycemic agents and insulin may need adjustment in patients with diabetes mellitus who also require diuretic therapy.

Hives, Pruritus, Rash. Report symptoms for further evaluation by the health care provider. Pruritus may be relieved by adding baking soda to the bath water.

Drug Interactions

Digoxin. Thiazide diuretics may cause excessive excretion of potassium, resulting in hypokalemia. If the patient is also receiving digoxin, monitor closely for signs of digitalis toxicity (e.g., anorexia, nausea, fatigue, blurred or colored vision, bradycardia, dysrhythmias).

Corticosteroids. Corticosteroids (e.g., prednisone) may enhance the loss of potassium. Check potassium levels and monitor more closely for hypokalemia when these two agents are used concurrently.

Lithium. Thiazide diuretics may induce lithium toxicity. Monitor patients for lithium toxicity manifested by nausea, anorexia, fine tremors, persistent vomiting, profuse diarrhea, hyperreflexia, lethargy, and weakness.

Nonsteroidal Antiinflammatory Drugs. NSAIDs (e.g., indomethacin, ibuprofen, naproxen) inhibit the diuretic activity of this agent. The dose of thiazide may have to be increased or the NSAID discontinued. Maintain accurate I&O records, and monitor for a decrease in diuretic activity.

Oral Hypoglycemic Agents, Insulin. Because of the hyperglycemic effects of the thiazide diuretics, dosage adjustments of insulin and oral hypoglycemic agents are often required.

DRUG CLASS: Potassium-Sparing Diuretics

amiloride (ah mihl' or eyd)

MIDAMOR (my' da mor)

Actions

Amiloride is a potassium-sparing diuretic that also has weak antihypertensive activity. Its mechanism of action is unknown, but it acts at the distal renal tubule to retain potassium and excrete sodium, resulting in a mild diuresis.

Uses

Amiloride is usually used in combination with other diuretics in patients with hypertension or heart failure to help prevent hypokalemia that may result from other diuretic therapy.

Therapeutic Outcomes

The primary therapeutic outcome associated with amiloride therapy is diuresis with reduction of edema and improvement in symptoms related to excessive fluid accumulation.

Nursing Process for Amiloride

Premedication Assessment

1. Obtain baseline data before initiating therapy, such as vital signs, lung sounds, weight, degree of edema present, and laboratory studies (e.g., serum electrolytes, liver and renal function tests).
2. Obtain data relating to the patient's mental status (orientation, alertness, confusion), muscle strength, muscle cramps, tremors, nausea, and general appearance.

Planning

Availability. PO: 5 mg tablets.

Implementation

Dosage and Administration. *Adult:* PO: Initially 5 mg daily. Dosages may be increased in 5-mg increments up to 20 mg daily with close monitoring of electrolytes. Administer with food or milk to reduce gastric irritation. DO NOT administer after midafternoon, to prevent nocturia.

Evaluation

Side Effects to Expect

Anorexia, Nausea, Vomiting, Flatulence. These side effects should be mild, particularly if the dose is administered with food. Persistent nausea and vomiting should be evaluated for other causes, as well as for the development of electrolyte imbalance.

Headache. Monitor the blood pressure at regularly scheduled intervals because amiloride is used for hypertension. Additional readings should be taken during headaches to determine if headaches are caused by the agents or by hypertension. Report persistent headaches.

Side Effects to Report

Electrolyte Imbalance, Dehydration. The electrolytes most commonly altered are potassium (K^+), sodium (Na^+), and chloride (Cl^-). *Hyperkalemia* is most likely to occur. Report potassium levels greater than 5 mEq/L.

Many symptoms associated with altered fluid and electrolyte balance are subtle and interspersed with general symptoms of drug toxicity or the disease process itself.

Gather data about *changes* in the patient's mental status (alertness, orientation, confusion), muscle strength, muscle cramps, tremors, nausea, and general appearance.

Always check the electrolyte reports for early indications of electrolyte imbalance. Keep accurate records of I&O, daily weights, and vital signs.

Drug Interactions

Lithium. Amiloride may induce lithium toxicity. Monitor patients for lithium toxicity as manifested by nausea, anorexia, fine tremors, persistent vomiting, profuse diarrhea, hyperreflexia, lethargy, and weakness.

Potassium Supplements, Salt Substitutes. Amiloride inhibits potassium excretion. DO NOT administer with potassium supplements or use salt substitutes high in potassium because of the potentially dangerous effects of hyperkalemia.

Hyperkalemia. ACE inhibitors (e.g., captopril, lisinopril, ramipril), angiotensin II receptor blockers (ARBs) (e.g., losartan, candesartan) and the aldosterone receptor blocking agent (e.g., eplerenone) inhibit aldosterone. Patients may develop hyperkalemia (>5.7 mEq/L). Most cases resolve without discontinuation of therapy. Patients most susceptible to the development of hyperkalemia are those with renal impairment or diabetes mellitus and those already receiving a potassium supplement. In general, potassium-sparing diuretics (e.g., amiloride, triamterene) should not be taken concurrently with these antihypertensive agents.

Nonsteroidal Antiinflammatory Drugs. NSAIDs (e.g., indomethacin, ibuprofen, naproxen) inhibit the diuretic activity of amiloride. The dose of amiloride may have to be increased or the NSAID discontinued. Maintain accurate I&O records and monitor for a decrease in diuretic activity.

spironolactone (spy ro no lak' tone)
ALDACTONE (al dak' tone)

Actions

Spironolactone blocks the sodium-retaining and potassium- and magnesium-excreting properties of aldosterone, resulting in a loss of water with the increased sodium excretion.

Uses

Spironolactone is a diuretic that is particularly useful in relieving edema and ascites that do not respond to the usual diuretics. It may be given with thiazide diuretics to increase its effect and reduce the hypokalemia often induced by the thiazides. Spironolactone has also been shown to further reduce morbidity and mortality for patients with heart failure who are also being treated with an ACE inhibitor and a loop diuretic.

Therapeutic Outcomes

The primary therapeutic outcome associated with spironolactone therapy is diuresis with reduction of edema and improvement in symptoms related to excessive fluid accumulation and heart failure.

Nursing Process for Spironolactone

Premedication Assessment

1. Obtain baseline data before initiating therapy, such as vital signs, lung sounds, weight, degree of edema present, and laboratory studies (e.g., serum electrolytes, liver and renal function tests).
2. Obtain data relating to the patient's mental status (orientation, alertness, confusion), muscle strength, muscle cramps, tremors, nausea, and general appearance.
3. Tactfully ask about any preexisting problems with libido.

Planning

Availability. PO: 25, 50, and 100 mg tablets.

Implementation

Dosage and Administration. *Adult:* PO: Initially 50 to 100 mg daily. Maintenance dosage is usually 100 to 200 mg daily, but doses up to 400 mg may be prescribed. Administer with food or milk to reduce gastric irritation. DO NOT administer after midafternoon, to prevent nocturia.

Pediatric: PO: 1.5 to 3.5 mg/kg/day in divided doses every 6 to 24 hours. Readjust the dosage every 3 to 5 days.

Evaluation

Side Effects to Expect and Report

Mental Confusion. Perform a baseline assessment of the patient's alertness, drowsiness, lethargy, and orientation to time, date, and place before starting drug therapy. Compare subsequent mental status, and analyze on a regular basis.

Headache. Monitor blood pressure at regularly scheduled intervals because this agent is used for hypertension. Additional readings should be taken during headaches to determine if headaches are caused by the agent or the hypertension. Report persistent headaches.

Diarrhea. The onset of new symptoms occurring after initiating the drug therapy requires evaluation if persistent.

Electrolyte Imbalance, Dehydration. The electrolytes most commonly altered are potassium (K^+), sodium (Na^+), and chloride (Cl^-). *Hyperkalemia* is most likely to occur. Report potassium levels greater than 5 mEq/L.

Many symptoms associated with altered fluid and electrolyte balance are subtle and interspersed with general symptoms of drug toxicity or the disease process itself.

Gather data about *changes* in the patient's mental status (alertness, orientation, confusion), muscle strength, muscle cramps, tremors, nausea, and general appearance.

Always check the electrolyte reports for early indications of electrolyte imbalance. Keep accurate records of I&O, daily weights, and vital signs.

Gynecomastia, Reduced Libido, Breast Tenderness. Because the chemical structure of spironolactone is similar to that of estrogenic hormones, an occasional male patient will report gynecomastia, reduced libido, and diminished erection. Women may complain of breast soreness and menstrual irregularities. These effects are reversible after therapy is discontinued.

Drug Interactions

Potassium Supplements, Salt Substitutes. Spironolactone inhibits potassium excretion. DO NOT administer with potassium supplements or use salt substitutes high in potassium because of potentially dangerous effects from hyperkalemia.

Hyperkalemia. ACE inhibitors (e.g., captopril, lisinopril, ramipril), ARBs (e.g., losartan, candesartan), and the aldosterone receptor–blocking agent (e.g., eplerenone) inhibit aldosterone. Patients may develop hyperkalemia (>5.7 mEq/L). Most cases resolve without discontinuation of therapy. Patients most susceptible to the development of hyperkalemia are those with renal impairment or diabetes mellitus and those already receiving a potassium supplement. In general, potassium-sparing diuretics should not be taken concurrently with these antihypertensive agents.

Nonsteroidal Antiinflammatory Drugs. NSAIDs (e.g., indomethacin, ibuprofen, naproxen) inhibit the diuretic activity of spironolactone. The dosage of spironolactone may have to be increased or the NSAID discontinued. Maintain accurate I&O records and monitor for a decrease in diuretic activity.

triamterene (try am′ ter een)
▶ DYRENIUM (dy reen′ ee um)

Actions

Triamterene is a very mild diuretic that acts by blocking the exchange of potassium for sodium in the distal tubule of the kidney, resulting in retention of potassium with excretion of sodium and water.

Uses

Triamterene is an effective agent to use in conjunction with the potassium-excreting diuretics, such as the thiazides, and the loop diuretics.

Therapeutic Outcomes

The primary therapeutic outcome associated with triamterene therapy is diuresis with reduction of edema and improvement in symptoms related to excessive fluid accumulation.

Nursing Process for Triamterene

Premedication Assessment

1. Obtain baseline data before initiating therapy, such as vital signs, lung sounds, weight, degree of edema present, laboratory studies (e.g., serum electrolytes, liver and renal function tests).
2. Obtain data relating to the patient's mental status (orientation, alertness, confusion), muscle strength, muscle cramps, tremors, nausea, and general appearance.

Planning

Availability. PO: 50 and 100 mg capsules.

Implementation

Dosage and Administration. *Adult:* PO: 50 to 150 mg two times daily.

Evaluation

Side Effects to Expect and Report

Electrolyte Imbalance, Dehydration, Leg Cramps, Nausea, Vomiting, Weakness. The electrolytes most commonly altered are potassium (K^+), sodium (Na^+), and chloride (Cl^-). *Hyperkalemia* is most likely to occur. Report potassium levels greater than 5 mEq/L.

Many symptoms associated with altered fluid and electrolyte balance are subtle and interspersed with general symptoms of drug toxicity or the disease process itself.

Gather data about *changes* in the patient's mental status (alertness, orientation, confusion), muscle strength, muscle cramps, tremors, nausea, and general appearance (drowsy, anxious, lethargic).

Always check the electrolyte reports for early indications of electrolyte imbalance. Keep accurate records of I&O, daily weights, and vital signs.

Hives, Pruritus, Rash. Report symptoms for further evaluation by the physician. Pruritus may be relieved by adding baking soda to the bath water.

Drug Interactions

Salt Substitutes, Potassium Supplements. Triamterene inhibits potassium excretion. DO NOT administer with potassium supplements or use salt substitutes high in potassium because of the potentially dangerous effects from hyperkalemia.

Hyperkalemia. ACE inhibitors (e.g., captopril, lisinopril, ramipril), ARBs (e.g., losartan, candesartan), and the aldosterone receptor–blocking agent (e.g., eplerenone) inhibit aldosterone. Patients may develop hyperkalemia (>5.7 mEq/L). Most cases resolve without discontinuation of therapy. Patients most susceptible to

Drug Table 29-3 COMBINATION DIURETICS

GENERIC NAME	BRAND NAME	DOSAGE RANGE
spironolactone 25 mg, hydrochlorothiazide 25 mg	Aldactazide	1-8 tablets daily
spironolactone 50 mg, hydrochlorothiazide 50 mg	Aldactazide	1-4 tablets daily
triamterene 37.5 mg, hydrochlorothiazide 25 mg	Dyazide	1 or 2 capsules twice daily after meals
triamterene 37.5 mg, hydrochlorothiazide 25 mg	Maxzide 25 mg	1 or 2 tablets daily after meals
triamterene 75 mg, hydrochlorothiazide 50 mg	Maxzide	1 tablet daily
amiloride 5 mg, hydrochlorothiazide 50 mg	Moduretic	1 or 2 tablets daily with meals

the development of hyperkalemia are those with renal impairment or diabetes mellitus and those already receiving a potassium supplement. In general, potassium-sparing diuretics should not be taken concurrently with these antihypertensive agents.

Nonsteroidal Antiinflammatory Drugs. NSAIDs (e.g., indomethacin, ibuprofen, naproxen) inhibit the diuretic activity of triamterene. The dosage of triamterene may have to be increased or the NSAID discontinued. Maintain accurate I&O records and monitor for a decrease in diuretic activity.

DRUG CLASS: Combination Diuretic Products

A common problem associated with thiazide diuretic therapy is hypokalemia. In an attempt to minimize this adverse effect, several products have been manufactured that contain a potassium-sparing diuretic with a thiazide diuretic (Table 29-3). The goal of the combination products is to promote diuresis and antihypertensive effect through different mechanisms of action while maintaining normal serum potassium levels. Patients receiving a combination product are at risk for side effects resulting from any of the component drugs. Many cases of *hyperkalemia* and hyponatremia have been reported after the use of the combination products.

Combination products should not be used as initial therapy for edema or hypertension. Therapy with individual products should be adjusted for each patient. If the fixed combination represents the appropriate dosage for each component, the use of a combination product may be more convenient for patient compliance. Patients must be reevaluated periodically for appropriateness of therapy and to prevent electrolyte imbalance.

- Diuretics are drugs that act to increase the flow of urine.
- The purpose of diuretics is to increase the net loss of water.
- Diuretics are mainstays in the symptomatic treatment of heart failure, hypertension, and renal disease.
- Diuretics also have a variety of other medical uses, such as reducing cerebral edema, intraocular pressure, ascites, and hypercalcemia.
- The information the nurse obtains about the patient's general clinical symptoms is important to the health care provider when analyzing data for diagnosis and success of therapy.

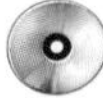
Go to your Companion CD-ROM for Appendices, an Audio Glossary, animations, Drug Dosage Calculators, customizable Patient Self-Assessment forms, and Review Questions for the NCLEX® Examination.

evolve Be sure to visit the companion Evolve site at http://evolve.elsevier.com/Clayton for WebLinks and additional online resources.

MEDICATION SAFETY REVIEW

MATH REVIEW QUESTIONS

1. Order: Ethacrynic acid 50 mg IV in 50 mL D5W. The patient has an IV pump running that is calibrated in milliliters per hour. Infuse the medication over 30 minutes.

   Set the pump at ____ mL/hr.

2. Order: Furosemide 40 mg PO, stat

   Available: Furosemide 20 mg tablets

   Give ____ tablet(s).

3. Order: Furosemide 40 mg IV daily

   Available: Furosemide 10 mg/mL

   Give ____ mL.

CRITICAL THINKING QUESTIONS

1. The health care provider orders furosemide 60 mg stat in an IV push. The drug resource book states, "The rate of administration should not exceed 4 mg/minute." Based on this information, how long would it take to administer the furosemide? What other facts should be checked before starting an IV push of the drug?

2. A patient being treated for hypertension with diuretic therapy calls the health care provider's office to report feeling weak, light-headed, and fatigued. What additional information would be useful before discussing the symptoms with the health care provider?

3. Identify specific precautions associated with the use of ACE inhibitors and certain diuretics.

4. Research precautions in using diuretics when the patient's urinary output is reduced or renal disease is present.

CONTENT REVIEW QUESTIONS

1. Lasix (furosemide) is a commonly prescribed diuretic with an onset of action of ________ orally; and ____________ minutes after IV administration.
   1. 30 minutes; 5 to 15
   2. 1 to 2 hours; 5 to 10
   2. 3 hours; 25
   4. 4 to 6 hours; 5 to 10

2. Thiazide diuretics may cause:
   1. nephrotoxicity.
   2. ototoxicity.
   3. hyperuricemia.
   4. hypertension.

3. NSAIDs taken concurrently with certain diuretics (e.g., bumetanide, furosemide, and ethacrynic acid) can:
   1. increase diuresis.
   2. decrease diuresis.
   3. have no effect on diuresis.
   4. require a decreased dosage of the diuretic.

4. Potassium supplements and salt substitutes should not be given with the following class of diuretic:
   1. thiazide.
   2. loop.
   3. potassium-sparing.
   4. carbonic anhydrase inhibitors.

5. The main purpose of using diuretics in treating heart failure is to:
   1. relieve symptoms associated with pulmonary congestion and edema.
   2. reduce cerebral edema.
   3. reduce ascites.
   4. increase preload.

6. Which of the following are ways to assess for hydration? *(Select all that apply.)*
   1. Skin turgor
   2. Oral mucous membranes
   3. Vital signs
   4. Laboratory changes

7. Why are diuretics usually not administered after midafternoon?
   1. They are irritating to the GI lining
   2. They cause orthostatic hypotension
   3. To prevent nocturia
   4. To prevent polyuria

CHAPTER 30 Drugs Used to Treat Upper Respiratory Disease

evolve http://evolve.elsevier.com/Clayton

Chapter Content

Objectives

1. State the causes of allergic rhinitis and nasal congestion.
2. Explain the major actions (effects) of sympathomimetic, antihistaminic, and corticosteroid decongestants and cromolyn.
3. Define *rhinitis medicamentosa,* and describe the patient education needed to prevent it.
4. Review the procedure for administration of medications by nose drops, sprays, and inhalation.
5. Explain why all decongestant products should be used cautiously in people with hypertension, hyperthyroidism, diabetes mellitus, cardiac disease, increased intraocular pressure, or prostatic disease.
6. State the premedication assessments and nursing assessments needed during therapy to monitor therapeutic response and side effects to expect or report from using decongestant drug therapy.
7. Identify essential components involved in planning patient education that will enhance adherence with the treatment regimen.

Key Terms

rhinitis
sinusitis
allergic rhinitis
antigen-antibody
histamine
rhinorrhea
decongestants
rhinitis medicamentosa
antihistamines
antiinflammatory agents

UPPER RESPIRATORY TRACT ANATOMY AND PHYSIOLOGY

The respiratory system is a series of airways that start with the nose and mouth and end at the alveolar sacs within the lungs. The upper respiratory tract is composed of the nose and its turbinates, sinuses, nasopharynx, pharynx, tonsils, eustachian tubes, and larynx (Figure 30-1). The nose and its structures serve two functions: olfactory (smell) and respiratory. The olfactory region is located in the upper part of each nostril. It is an area of specialized tissue cells (olfactory cells) containing microscopic hairs that react to odors in the air and then stimulate the olfactory cells. The olfactory cells in turn send signals to the brain, which processes the sensation that people perceive as a particular smell.

The respiratory function of the nose is to warm, humidify, and filter the air inhaled to prepare it for the lower respiratory airways. Both nasal passages have folds of skin called turbinates that significantly increase the surface area of the passages and contain massive numbers of blood vessels. The blood circulating through the membranes lining the turbinates warms and humidifies inhaled air. The inhaled air is also filtered of particulate matter. The hairs at the entrance to the nostrils remove large particles, and the turbinates and the narrowness of the nasal passages cause turbulence of the airflow passing through from each inhalation. All the surfaces of the nose are coated with a thin layer of mucus secreted by goblet cells. Because of the turbulence of airflow, particles are thrown against the walls of the nasal passages and become trapped in the mucosal secretions. The epithelial cells lining the posterior two thirds of the nasal passages contain cilia that sweep the particulate matter back toward the nasopharynx and pharynx. Once in the pharynx the particulate matter is either expectorated or swallowed. The warming, humidification, and filtration processes continue as the air passes into the trachea, bronchi, and bronchioles.

The nasal structures are innervated by the autonomic nervous system. Cholinergic stimulation causes vasodilation of the blood vessels lining the nasal mucosa, and sympathetic (primarily alpha adrenergic) stimulation causes vasoconstriction. The cholinergic fibers also innervate the secretory glands. When stimulated, they produce serous and mucous secretions within the nostrils.

The paranasal sinuses are hollow air-filled cavities in the cranial bones on both sides and behind the nose. There are eight sinuses, four on each side. The purpose of the paranasal sinuses appears to be to act as resonating chambers for the voice and as a means of lightening the bones of the head. The sinuses are lined with the same mucous membranes and ciliated epithelia as those of the upper respiratory tract. The sinuses are

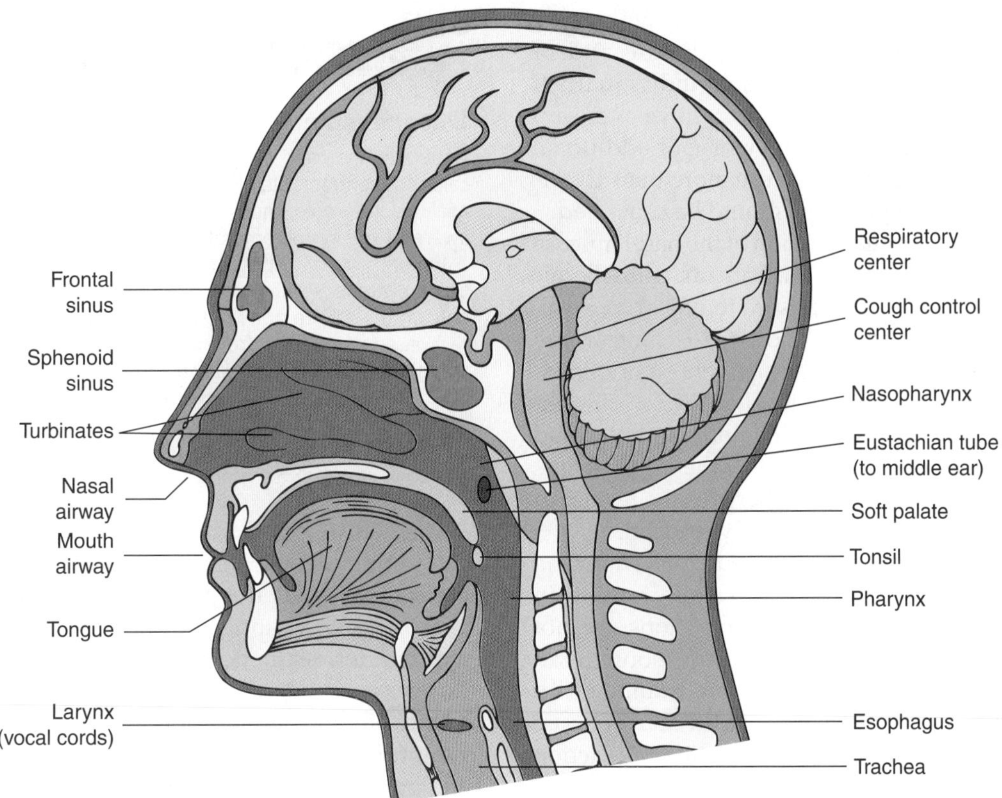

FIGURE **30-1** The upper respiratory tract.

connected to the nasal passages by ducts and drain into the nasal cavity by activity from ciliated cells.

On either side of the oral pharynx is the pharyngeal tonsil, a collection of lymphoid tissue that is called the adenoids when enlarged. The tonsils are located in an area where mucus laden with particulate matter, such as virus particles and bacteria, accumulates from the ciliary action of cells in the nasopharynx above. The lymphoid tissue is rich in immunoglobulins and is thought to play a role in the immunologic defense mechanisms of the upper airway.

Sneezing is a physiologic reflex used by the body to clear the nasal passages of foreign matter. The sneeze reflex is initiated by irritation of the nasal mucosa by foreign particulate matter. It is quite similar to the cough reflex that clears the lower respiratory airways of secretions and foreign matter.

COMMON UPPER RESPIRATORY DISEASES

Rhinitis is inflammation of the nasal mucous membranes. Signs and symptoms are sneezing, nasal discharge, and nasal congestion. Rhinitis is often subclassified into acute and chronic based on the duration of the signs and symptoms. The most common causes of acute rhinitis are the common cold (e.g., viral infection), bacterial infection, presence of a foreign body, and drug-induced congestion (rhinitis medicamentosa). Common causes of chronic rhinitis are allergy, nonallergic perennial rhinitis, chronic sinusitis, and a deviated septum.

The common cold is actually a viral infection of the upper respiratory tissues. When considering the amount of time lost from school and work and the number of health care provider office visits annually, it is probably the single most expensive illness in the United States. Seasons in which viral infections reach near-epidemic proportions are midwinter, spring, and early fall, a few weeks after school starts. Six different virus families (including 120 to 200 subtypes) cause coldlike symptoms; the most common are the rhinoviruses and the coronaviruses. Viruses are spread from person to person by direct contact and sneezing. The earliest symptoms of a cold are a clear, watery nasal discharge and sneezing. Nasal congestion from engorgement of the nasal blood vessels and swelling of nasal turbinates quickly follows. Over the next 48 hours, the discharge becomes cloudy and much more viscous. Other symptoms include coughing, a "scratchy" or mildly sore throat (pharyngitis), and hoarseness (laryngitis). Other symptoms that occur less frequently are headache, malaise, chills, and fever. A few patients may develop a fever up to 100° F. Symptoms should subside over 5 to 7 days.

Complications occasionally develop secondary to the challenge to the body's immune system by cold viruses. Complications also arise from thick, tenacious mucus obstructing sinus ducts or the eustachian tubes to the middle ears. Bacteria are easily trapped behind these obstructions in the sinuses and the ears, resulting in bacterial **sinusitis,** or otitis media (infection of the middle ear). Viral infections are also a common cause of exacerbations of obstructive lung disease and of acute asthmatic attacks in susceptible individuals. If symptoms of the cold do not start to resolve over several days, or if symptoms become worse or additional symptoms appear (e.g., temperature more than 100° F, earache), a health care provider should be consulted.

Allergic rhinitis is inflammation of the nasal mucosa secondary to an allergic reaction. Patients with allergic rhinitis have had previous exposure to one or more allergens (e.g., pollens, grasses, house dust mites) and have developed antibodies to the allergen. After this exposure, when a person inhales the allergen, an **antigen-antibody** reaction occurs, causing inflammation and swelling of the nasal passages. One of the major causes of symptoms associated with an allergy is the release of histamine during the antigen-antibody reaction.

Histamine is a compound derived from an amino acid called *histidine.* It is stored in small granules in most body tissues. Its physiologic functions are not completely known, but it is released in response to allergic reactions and tissue damage from trauma or infection. When histamine is released in the area of tissue damage or at the site of an antigen-antibody reaction (e.g., a pollen inhaled into the nose of a patient allergic to that specific pollen), it reacts with the H_1 receptors in the area and the following reactions take place: arterioles and capillaries in the region dilate, allowing increased blood flow to the area that results in redness; capillaries become more permeable, resulting in the outward passage of fluid into the extracellular spaces, causing edema (manifested by congestion in the mucous membranes and turbinates of the patient's nose); and nasal, lacrimal, and bronchial secretions are released, resulting in the running nose **(rhinorrhea)** and watery eyes (conjunctivitis) noted in patients with allergies. Patients with allergic rhinitis also complain of itching of the palate, ears, and eyes. Most patients with asthma have an allergic component to the disease that triggers acute attacks of asthma.

When large amounts of histamine are released, such as in a severe allergic reaction, there is extensive arteriolar dilatation. Blood pressure drops (hypotension), skin becomes flushed and edematous, and severe itching (urticaria) develops. Constriction and spasm of the bronchial tubes make respiratory effort more difficult (dyspnea), and copious amounts of pulmonary and gastric secretions are released.

Allergies may be seasonal or perennial. Seasonal allergies occur when the allergen is abundant: tree pollen is prevalent from late March to early June; ragweed is abundant from early August until the first hard freeze in October; grasses pollinate from mid-May to mid-July. Weather conditions, such as rainfall, humidity, and temperature, affect the amount of pollen produced in a particular year but not the actual onset or termination of the specific allergen's season. It is common for a person to be allergic to more than one allergen simultaneously, so seasons may overlap or may occur more than once per year. People who have allergies to multiple antigens, such as smoke, molds, animal dander, feathers, house dust mites, and pollens, have varying degrees of symptoms year-round and are said to have perennial allergies. It is important that the symptoms of allergy be treated, not only for symptomatic relief but also to prevent irreversible changes within the nose. These changes include thickening of the mucosal epithelium, loss of cilia, loss of smell, recurrent sinusitis and otitis media, growth of connective tissue, and the development of nasal or sinus polyps that aggravate rhinitis and secondary infections.

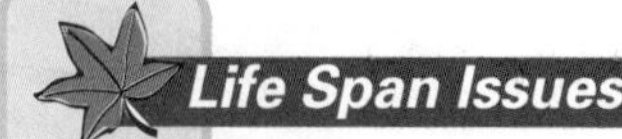

Life Span Issues

Decongestants

Antihistamines and sympathomimetic amines, more commonly called decongestants, are frequently used in combination with analgesics in cold and flu remedies. People are often not fully aware of the ingredients of OTC combination products.

Patients with diabetes mellitus, hypertension, or ischemic heart disease should use products containing decongestants only on the advice of a physician or pharmacist.

A paradoxical effect from antihistamines often seen in children and older adults is CNS stimulation rather than sedation, which may cause insomnia, nervousness, and irritability. Antihistamines may also cause urinary retention and should be used with caution in older men who have an enlarged prostate gland.

Overuse of topical **decongestants** may lead to a rebound of nasal secretions known as **rhinitis medicamentosa.** This secondary congestion (rhinitis medicamentosa) is thought to be caused by excessive vasoconstriction of the blood vessels and by direct irritation of the nasal membranes by the solution. When the vasoconstrictor effects wear off, the irritation causes excessive blood flow to the passages, causing swelling and engorgement to reappear; the nose feels more stuffy and congested than before treatment. (Over the next few weeks, a vicious cycle develops, with more frequent use of the topical decongestant needed to relieve nasal passage swelling and obstruction.) Rhinitis medicamentosa may develop as early as 3 to 5 days after use of long-acting topical decongestants (e.g., oxymetazoline, xylometazoline) but usually does not develop until after 2 to 3 weeks of regular use of short-acting topical decongestants (e.g., phenylephrine).

TREATMENT OF UPPER RESPIRATORY DISEASES

Common Cold

Treatment of the common cold is limited to relieving the symptoms associated with rhinitis and, if present, pharyngitis and laryngitis; reducing the risk of complications; and preventing spread of viral infection to others. Decongestants are the most effective agent in relieving nasal congestion and rhinorrhea.

The use of antihistamines (H_1 receptor antagonists) in the symptomatic relief of cold symptoms has been controversial. Studies indicate that preschool-aged children do not benefit from use of antihistamines but older children, adolescents, and adults receive some benefit.

Depending on whether a fever, pharyngitis, or a cough is present, patients may also benefit from the use of analgesics, antipyretics (see Chapter 20), expectorants, and antitussive agents (see Chapter 31). Laryngitis should be treated by resting the vocal cords as much as possible. Inhaling cool mist vapor several times daily to humidify the larynx may be beneficial, but putting medication in the inhaled vapor is of no value. Lozenges and gargles do nothing to relieve hoarseness because they do not reach the larynx.

Allergic Rhinitis

The first step in treating allergic rhinitis is to identify the allergens, usually through skin testing, to avoid exposure if possible. Unfortunately it is often not possible to eliminate exposure to many allergens without severely restricting lifestyle. Medicines must then be used to block the allergic reaction or treat the symptoms. The pharmacologic agents used include antihistamines, decongestants, and intranasal corticosteroid antiinflammatory agents. Saline nasal spray can be quite effective in reducing nasal irritation between doses of other pharmacologic agents. If the patient is physically able, vigorous exercise for 15 to 30 minutes once or twice daily increases sympathetic output and induces vascular vasoconstriction.

Mild allergic rhinitis can be well treated by either an oral second-generation antihistamine (loratadine, desloratadine, cetirizine, fexofenadine) or a nasal corticosteroid alone. Patients with moderate to severe symptoms of allergic rhinitis with nasal congestion often require both an oral second-generation antihistamine and nasal corticosteroids. If symptoms are only partially controlled, if high doses of intranasal or oral corticosteroids are required, or if the allergic rhinitis is complicated by asthma or sinusitis, immunotherapy may be required. Therapy should be started before the anticipated appearance of allergens and continue during the time of exposure.

Rhinitis Medicamentosa

The best treatment of rhinitis medicamentosa is prevention. Unfortunately, most patients are not aware of the condition until it becomes a problem. Following the directions for a daily dosage and limiting the duration of therapy to that which is described on the topical decongestant product are the best ways to avoid the condition.

Several treatment strategies have been successful in treating rhinitis medicamentosa. Regardless of the approach used, the patient must understand what caused the rebound congestion and why it is important to eliminate the problem. One strategy is to completely withdraw the topical decongestant at once. The patient is likely to be congested and uncomfortable for the next week, but use of a saline nasal spray can help moisturize irritated nasal tissues. Nasal steroid solutions can also be used, but it will take several days to reduce inflammation and congestion. Probably the most successful approach, although the longest to complete, is to have the patient work to clear one nostril at a time. Start by reducing the strength and frequency of the decongestant used in the left nostril, while continuing with the normal dosage in the right nostril. Saline or corticosteroid nasal spray can be used every other dose in the left nostril. Eventually the saline can be used more frequently and the decongestant can be discontinued in the left nostril. Once the patient can breathe normally through the left nostril, the same approach of reduced strength and frequency of decongestant can be started in the right nostril. Frequent follow-up with the patient and reinforcement of progress made are important to the success of this treatment.

DRUG THERAPY FOR UPPER RESPIRATORY DISEASES

Actions and Uses

Antihistamines, or H_1 receptor antagonists, are the drugs of choice in treating allergic rhinitis. Because they are administered orally and thus distributed systemically, they also reduce the symptoms of nasal itching, sneezing, rhinorrhea, lacrimation, and conjunctival itching. The antihistamines do not, however, reduce nasal congestion.

Decongestants are alpha adrenergic stimulants that cause vasoconstriction to the nasal mucosa, which significantly reduces nasal congestion. When treating allergic rhinitis, decongestants are often administered in conjunction with antihistamines to reduce nasal congestion and counteract the sedation caused by many antihistamines.

Antiinflammatory agents administered intranasally are used to treat nasal symptoms resulting from mild to moderate allergic rhinitis. In general, antiinflammatory agents are not used to treat symptoms associated with a cold because the symptoms start to resolve before the antiinflammatory agents can become effective. The antiinflammatory agents used to treat allergic rhinitis are corticosteroids and cromolyn sodium.

NURSING PROCESS *for Upper Respiratory Diseases*

Nasal congestion, allergic rhinitis, and sinusitis are treated by prescription or over-the-counter (OTC) medicine. The nurse's role in the health care provider's office is to perform the initial assessment of symptoms and then focus on teaching the proper techniques of self-administering and monitoring the medication therapy. Always review the patient's history for other diseases being treated (e.g., hypertension, glaucoma, asthma, prostatic hyperplasia), which may contraindicate the concurrent use of some upper respiratory medications used as OTC or prescribed treatments.

Assessment

Description of Symptoms

- What symptoms are present; for example, frequency of sneezing or coughing, hoarseness, nasal congestion, nasal secretions, and type (watery, viscous, color)?
- When did the symptoms start?
- Does the patient have a history of allergies? If yes, what are the known allergens? Are the symptoms associated with a particular time of year or the release of pollen from plants? Are the symptoms triggered by exposure to household environmental factors (e.g., exposure to animal dander, dust, molds, or foods)?
- Has the individual recently been exposed to someone with a common cold?
- Is the individual having pain or discomfort? What is the specific area affected and the degree of pain?

History of Treatment

- What prescribed or OTC medicines have been used? Are any effective?
- When allergies are suspected, has skin testing been completed to determine what specific allergens are initiating the attacks?
- If pain is present, how has pain relief been obtained? Is the degree of pain relief satisfactory?

History of Concurrent Medical Problems. Ask specific questions to determine if the patient has concurrent medical problems such as glaucoma, prostatic hyperplasia, asthma, hypertension, and/or diabetes mellitus as described in the drug monograph preassessments.

Nursing Diagnoses

- Breathing pattern, ineffective (indication)
- Airway clearance, ineffective (indication)
- Knowledge, deficient (side effects, treatment)

Planning

Symptoms and Treatment. Establish the educational needs of the patient related to the underlying cause of the upper respiratory symptoms and the assistance needed to understand self-medication, treatments prescribed, and details of when to consult a health care provider because of lack of response to therapy or increasing symptoms.

Implementation

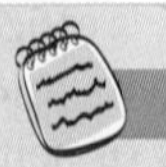

Patient Education and Health Promotion

- Make sure that the patient understands the importance of adequate rest, hydration, and personal hygiene in preventing spread of infection, when present.
- Discuss the specific medications prescribed, the therapeutic effects that can be expected, and when to contact a health care provider if therapy does not yield the expected benefit. Explain symptoms that should be reported to the health care provider that would indicate a poor response to therapy (e.g., escalation of symptoms, pain, or temperature with sinusitis).
- Make sure that the patient understands when to take the medicine; for example, if treating symptoms of allergy, antihistamines should be taken 45 to 60 minutes before exposure to the allergen.
- Proper technique is important to therapy success. Explain the procedures for proper installation of nose drops or nasal sprays associated with the prescribed treatment regimen. Document and verify that the patient can self-administer the medication as recommended.
- Teach the patient to monitor temperature, pulse, respirations, and blood pressure as appropriate to the underlying diagnosis and the medicines used to treat the diagnosis.

Fostering Health Maintenance

- Throughout the course of treatment, discuss medication information and how it will benefit the patient. Recognize that nonadherence may occur, especially when treatment response is not immediate.
- Seek cooperation and understanding of the following points so that medication adherence is increased: name of medication, dosage, route and times of administration, side effects to expect, and side effects to report. Numerous OTC preparations may be contraindicated when other medications or coexisting diseases are present. For example, patients taking antihypertensive medicines should not take decongestants. (See individual drug monographs for details.)

DRUG CLASS: Sympathomimetic Decongestants

Actions

Sympathomimetic nasal decongestants (Table 30-1) stimulate the alpha adrenergic receptors of the nasal mucous membranes, causing vasoconstriction. This constriction reduces blood flow in the engorged nasal area, resulting in shrinkage of the engorged turbinates and mucous membranes, thus promoting sinus drainage, improving nasal air passage, and relieving the feeling of stuffiness and obstruction.

Uses

Decongestants are the drugs of choice in relieving congestion associated with rhinitis caused by the common cold. They are also often used in conjunction with antihistamines when treating allergic rhinitis to reduce nasal congestion and to counteract the sedation caused by many antihistamines.

Drug Table 30-1 **NASAL DECONGESTANTS**

GENERIC NAME	BRAND NAME	AVAILABILITY	ADULT DOSAGE RANGE
ephedrine	Ephedrine Pretz-D	Solution: 0.25%	Nasal: 2 or 3 drops two or three times daily
epinephrine	Adrenalin	Solution: 0.1%	Nasal: 1 or 2 drops in each nostril q4-6h
naphazoline	Privine	Solution: 0.05%	Nasal: 2 or 3 drops or sprays no more than q3h (drops) or q4-6h (spray)
oxymetazoline	Afrin, Duration	Solution: 0.05%	Nasal: 2 or 3 drops or sprays of 0.05% solution twice daily
phenylephrine	Neo-Synephrine, Sinex	Solution: 0.125%, 0.25%, 0.5%, 1%	Nasal: 0.25% q3-4h
pseudoephedrine	Sudafed, Efidac/24	Tablets or capsules: 15, 30, 60, 120, 240 mg Liquid: 15, 30 mg/5 mL Drops: 7.5 mg/0.8 mL	PO: 60 mg q6h; do not exceed 240 mg/24 hr
tetrahydrozoline	Tyzine	Solution: 0.05%, 0.1%	Nasal: 2-4 drops of 0.1% solution q4-6h
xylometazoline	Otrivin	Solution: 0.05%, 0.1%	Nasal: 2 or 3 sprays q8-10h

Decongestants can be administered orally or applied directly to the nose (topically) in the form of nasal spray or drops to treat rhinitis. An advantage of topical administration is essentially no systemic effects. Disadvantages to the nasal sprays and drops are lack of effect on conjunctival symptoms, inconvenience, and the potential to cause rhinitis medicamentosa.

Nasal decongestants provide temporary relief of symptoms, but it is important for the patient to follow directions on the label carefully. Initially the stuffiness or blocked sensation is relieved. However, misuse, including excessive use or frequency of administration, may cause a rebound swelling (rhinitis medicamentosa) of the nasal passages.

Alpha adrenergic agents used as nasal decongestants have the ability to stimulate alpha receptors at other sites in the body as well. Therefore they should be used with caution when taken orally in patients with hypertension, hyperthyroidism, diabetes mellitus, cardiac disease, increased intraocular pressure, or prostatic hyperplasia.

Therapeutic Outcomes

The primary therapeutic outcome associated with sympathomimetic decongestant therapy is reduced nasal congestion with easier breathing.

Nursing Process for Sympathomimetic Decongestants

Premedication Assessment

1. Check the patient's history for evidence of hypertension, hyperthyroidism, diabetes mellitus, cardiac dysrhythmias, glaucoma, or prostatic hyperplasia. If any one of these conditions is present, consult the health care provider before initiating therapy.
2. Take baseline vital signs.

Planning

Availability. See Table 30-1.

Implementation

Dosage and Administration. See Table 30-1. See also Chapter 8 for techniques to administer nose drops and nasal spray.

Evaluation

Side Effects to Expect

Mild Nasal Irritation. Burning or stinging may be experienced when sympathomimetic decongestants are administered to the nasal membranes. This may be avoided by using a weaker solution.

Side Effects to Report

Hypertension. Excessive use of decongestants may result in significant hypertension. Patients already receiving antihypertensive therapy should avoid using decongestants. When sympathomimetic decongestants are used, blood pressure monitoring should be initiated and the health care provider contacted if blood pressures become elevated.

Drug Interactions

Drugs That Enhance Toxic Effects. Excessive use of beta-adrenergic blocking agents (e.g., propranolol, timolol, atenolol, nadolol) and monoamine oxidase inhibitors (e.g., tranylcypromine, phenelzine, isocarboxazid) may result in significant hypertension. Patients already receiving antihypertensive therapy should avoid using decongestants.

Methyldopa, Reserpine. Frequent decongestant use inhibits the antihypertensive activity of methyldopa and reserpine. Concurrent therapy is not recommended.

DRUG CLASS: Antihistamines

Actions

Antihistamines, or H_1-receptor antagonists, are chemical agents that act by competing with the allergy-liberated histamine for H_1-receptor sites in the patient's arterioles, capillaries, and secretory glands in mucous membranes. Antihistamines do not prevent histamine release, but they will reduce the symptoms of an allergic reaction if the concentration of the antihistamine exceeds the concentration of histamine at the receptor site. Antihistamines are therefore more effective if taken before histamine is released or when symptoms first appear.

Uses

Antihistamines are the drugs of choice for the systemic treatment of allergic rhinitis and conjunctivitis. These agents reduce rhinorrhea, lacrimation, nasal and conjunctival pruritus, and sneezing. The antihistamines do not, however, stop nasal congestion. The antihistamines shown in Table 30-2 have similar histamine-blocking effects when taken in recommended dosages, but they vary in duration of action, sedative effects, and anticholinergic effects. Occasionally a patient may develop a tolerance to the antihistaminic effects. Changing to another antihistamine is usually quite effective.

Antihistamines are best taken on a scheduled, rather than PRN, basis during the allergy season. These agents are much more effective if taken before exposure to the allergen, such as 45 to 60 minutes before going outdoors during the pollen season.

There is no evidence that one agent is particularly better at treating symptoms of allergic rhinitis over another, although there is a difference between products in their frequency and type of side effects. The most common side effect of many antihistaminic agents is sedation. Most patients acquire a tolerance to this adverse effect with continued therapy. Reduction in dosage or a change to another antihistamine may occasionally be necessary. The most sedating antihistamines are diphenhydramine, cyproheptadine, clemastine, and doxylamine (doxylamine and diphenhydramine are the active ingredient in OTC sleep aids). The least sedating are fexofenadine, loratadine, and desloratadine. Although some patients do not feel a sense of sedation after taking an antihistamine, their cognitive functions such as attention, memory, coordination, and psychomotor performance can be significantly impaired. A disturbing observation by these patients is that they often are not aware that their cognitive abilities are impaired. This is particularly important

Drug Table 30-2 ANTIHISTAMINES*

GENERIC NAME	BRAND NAME	AVAILABILITY	SEDATION†	ADULT DOSAGE RANGE	MAXIMUM DAILY DOSE
azelastine	Astelin	Nasal spray	–	2 sprays per nostril twice daily	—
cetirizine	Zyrtec	Tablets, syrup	±	5-10 mg once daily	20 mg
chlorpheniramine maleate	Chlor-Trimeton	Tablets, capsules, syrup	+	4 mg three to six times daily	24 mg
clemastine fumarate	Tavist	Tablets, syrup	+++	1.34-2.68 mg twice daily	8 mg
cyproheptadine hydrochloride		Tablets, syrup	+	4 mg three times daily	32 mg
desloratidine	Clarinex	Tablets, syrup	±	5 mg once daily	5 mg
diphenhydramine hydrochloride	Benadryl, AllerMax	Injection, capsules, tablets, syrup, elixir	+++	25-50 mg three or four times daily	300 mg
fexofenadine	Allegra	Tablets	±	60 mg twice daily	180 mg
ipratropium	Atrovent	Nasal spray	–	2 sprays per nostril two or three times daily	—
loratadine	Claritin	Tablets, syrup	±	10 mg daily	10 mg
promethazine hydrochloride‡	Phenergan	Injection, tablets, syrup, suppository	+++	12.5-25 mg three or four times daily	100 mg

*Many of these antihistamines are also available in combination with decongestants.
†Sedation index: +++, high; ++, moderate; +, low; ±, low to none; –, none.
‡Promethazine is a phenothiazine with antihistaminic properties.

when patients taking antihistamines perform potentially dangerous activities such as driving.

All antihistamines display anticholinergic side effects, particularly when higher dosages are used. Symptoms include dry mouth, stuffy nose, blurred vision, constipation, and urinary retention. Patients with asthma, prostatic enlargement, or glaucoma should take antihistamines only with a health care provider's supervision. The drying effects may also make respiratory mucus more viscous and tenacious. Use antihistamines with caution in patients who have a productive cough. If the cough continues but becomes nonproductive, consider additional hydration, and discontinue the antihistamine.

Therapeutic Outcomes

The primary therapeutic outcome associated with antihistamine therapy is reduced symptoms of allergic rhinitis (e.g., rhinorrhea, lacrimation, itching, conjunctivitis).

Nursing Process for Antihistamines

Premedication Assessment

1. Review the patient's history for evidence of glaucoma, prostatic hyperplasia, or asthma. If any one of these is present, consult the health care provider before initiating therapy.
2. Assess the patient's work environment, and consider whether drowsiness will affect safety and work performance.
3. Because antihistamines are prescribed for a variety of symptoms, such as hay fever, dermatologic reactions, drug hypersensitivity, rhinitis, and transfusion reactions, it is necessary for the nurse to individualize the patient assessments with the underlying pathologic condition.

Planning

Availability. See Table 30-2.

Implementation

Dosage and Administration. See Table 30-2.

Evaluation

Side Effects to Expect

Sedative Effects. The types of antihistamines ordered can produce varying degrees of sedation. Tolerance may be produced over time, thus diminishing the effect.

Operating power equipment or driving may be hazardous. Caution patients.

Cognitive Impairment. Even though newer antihistamines are less sedating, patients should still be cautioned against impaired memory, coordination, and psychomotor performance. Many states make it a crime to operate a motor vehicle while under the influence of medicines (in addition to alcohol).

Operating power equipment or driving may be hazardous. Caution patients to watch closely for signs of impairment (forgetfulness, poor coordination) in these situations.

Drying Effects. Monitor the patient's cough and degree of sputum production when antihistamines are administered. Because of their drying effects, antihistamines may impair expectoration.

Fluid Intake. Give adequate fluids concurrently with the use of antihistamines. Maintain fluid intake at eight to ten 8-ounce glasses daily.

Blurred Vision; Constipation; Urinary Retention; Dryness of Mouth, Throat, and Nose Mucosa. These symptoms are the anticholinergic effects produced by antihistamines. Patients taking these medications should be monitored for these effects.

Mucosa dryness may be alleviated by sucking hard candy or ice chips or by chewing gum.

Caution the patient that blurred vision may occur, and make appropriate suggestions for personal safety of the individual.

Drug Interactions

Central Nervous System (CNS) Depressants. CNS depressants, including sleep aids, analgesics, tranquilizers, and alcohol, will potentiate the sedative effects of antihistamines. People who work around machinery, drive a car, pour and give medicines, or perform other duties in which they must remain mentally alert should not take these medications while working.

DRUG CLASS: Respiratory Antiinflammatory Agents

Intranasal corticosteroids

Actions

The exact mechanism by which corticosteroids reduce inflammation is not known.

Uses

Patients with allergic seasonal rhinitis who do not respond to antihistamines and sympathomimetic agents may be given corticosteroids to relieve symptoms of the allergy. Corticosteroids, whether applied topically or administered systemically, have been shown to be highly effective for the treatment of allergic rhinitis. Intranasal corticosteroids are successful in controlling nasal symptoms associated with mild to moderate allergic rhinitis, but systemic steroids are required for severe cases.

The newer, topically active aerosol steroids, such as beclomethasone, budesonide, fluticasone, and flunisolide, are highly effective with few side effects. The therapeutic effect (reduction of sneezing, nasal itching, stuffiness, and rhinorrhea) is usually observed by the third day, although maximal effects may not be evident for 2 weeks. If symptoms do not improve within 3 weeks, therapy is discontinued. Dexamethasone intranasal aerosol has a higher incidence of systemic side effects and is generally not used unless therapy with the other intranasal corticosteroids is not effective. To minimize the development of adrenal suppression, these corticosteroids should be used only for short courses of therapy for acute seasonal allergies.

Therapeutic Outcomes

The primary therapeutic outcome associated with intranasal corticosteroid therapy is reduced rhinorrhea, rhinitis, itching, and sneezing.

Nursing Process for Intranasal Corticosteroid Therapy

Premedication Assessment

1. Blocked nasal passages should be treated with a topical decongestant just before beginning intranasal corticosteroids.
2. Ask the patient to blow the nose thoroughly before administering nasal therapy.

Planning

Availability. See Table 30-3.

Implementation

Dosage and Administration. See Table 30-3. See also Chapter 8 for techniques to administer nasal spray.

Counseling. The therapeutic effects, unlike those of sympathomimetic decongestants, are not immediate. This should be explained to the patient in advance to ensure cooperation and continuation of treatment with the prescribed dosage regimen. Full therapeutic benefit requires regular use and is usually evident within a few days, although a few patients may require up to 3 weeks for maximum benefit.

Preparation Before Administration. Patients with blocked nasal passages should be encouraged to use a decongestant just before intranasal corticosteroid administration to ensure adequate penetration. Patients should also be advised to clear their nasal passages of secretions before use.

Maintenance Therapy. After the desired clinical effect is obtained, the maintenance dose should be reduced to the smallest amount necessary to control the symptoms.

Evaluation

Side Effects to Expect

Nasal Burning. Nasal burning is usually mild and tends to resolve with continued therapy. Encourage the patient not to discontinue therapy without first consulting the health care provider.

cromolyn sodium (kro′ mo lin)
NASALCROM (nay zal krom′)

Actions

Cromolyn sodium is an antiinflammatory agent that inhibits the release of histamine and other mediators of inflammation, but its mechanism of action is unknown. It must be administered before the body receives a stimulus to release histamine, such as an antigen that initiates an antigen-antibody allergic reaction.

Uses

Cromolyn is recommended for use in conjunction with other medications in treating patients with severe allergic rhinitis to prevent the release of histamine that results in symptoms of allergic rhinitis.

Cromolyn has no direct bronchodilatory, antihistaminic, or anticholinergic activity and does not relieve nasal congestion. The concomitant use of antihistamines or nasal decongestants may be necessary during initial treatment with cromolyn. A 2- to 4-week course of therapy is usually required to determine clinical

Drug Table 30-3 INTRANASAL CORTICOSTEROIDS

GENERIC NAME	BRAND NAME	AVAILABILITY	ADULT DOSAGE RANGE
beclomethasone dipropionate, monohydrate	Beconase AQ	Nasal spray: 180 doses/canister	1 or 2 sprays (42-84 mcg) in each nostril twice daily
budesonide	Rhinocort Aqua	Nasal aerosol: 120 doses/canister	2 (64 mcg) inhalations in each nostril morning and evening
flunisolide	Nasarel	Nasal spray: 200 doses/bottle	2 sprays (58 mcg) in each nostril twice daily; maximum daily dose is 8 sprays (400 mcg) in 24 hr
fluticasone	Flonase	Nasal spray: 120 actuations/bottle	2 (100 mcg) sprays in each nostril once daily
mometasone	Nasonex	Nasal spray: 120 actuations/bottle	2 sprays (100 mcg) in each nostril once daily
triamcinolone	Nasacort AQ Nasacort HFA	Nasal spray: 30 and 120 actuations/bottle Nasal aerosol: 100 actuations/canister	2 sprays (110 mcg) in each nostril once daily; maximum daily dose is 4 sprays in 24 hr

response. Therapy should be continued only if there is a decrease in the severity of allergic symptoms during treatment.

Therapeutic Outcomes

The primary therapeutic outcome associated with cromolyn therapy is reduced rhinorrhea, itching, and sneezing.

Nursing Process for Cromolyn

Premedication Assessment

1. Cromolyn must be taken before exposure to the stimulus that initiates an attack or allergic rhinitis.
2. Check to see if the concurrent use of antihistamines or nasal decongestants has been ordered by the health care provider, especially during initiation of cromolyn therapy.
3. Have the patient blow the nose before nasal instillation.

Planning

Availability. Nasal spray: 40 mg/mL in 13 mL (100 sprays) and 26 mL (200 sprays) metered-spray device. Inhalation with nebulizer: 20 mg/2 mL; aerosol spray: 800 mcg delivered from 8.1 g container (112 metered sprays), and a 14.2 g container (200 metered sprays). Oral concentrate: 100 mg/5 mL.

Implementation

Dosage and Administration. See Chapter 8 for techniques to administer nasal spray.

Counseling. The therapeutic effects, unlike those of sympathomimetic amines, are not immediate. This should be explained to the patient in advance to ensure cooperation and continuation of treatment with the prescribed dosage regimen. Full therapeutic benefit requires regular use and is usually evident within 2 to 4 weeks. Therapy must be continued even though the patient is symptom-free.

Nasal Spray. Adult patients with blocked nasal passages should be encouraged to use a decongestant just before intranasal cromolyn administration to ensure adequate penetration. Patients should also be advised to clear their nasal passages of secretions and then inhale through the nose during administration. One spray is placed in each nostril three or four times daily at regular intervals. Maximum is six sprays in each nostril daily.

Evaluation

Side Effects to Expect

Nasal Irritation. The most common side effect is irritation manifested by sneezing, nasal itching, burning, and stuffiness. Patients usually develop a tolerance to the irritation. Rarely is this a cause for discontinuing intranasal therapy.

Side Effects to Report

Bronchospasm, Coughing. Notify the health care provider if inhalation causes bronchospasm or coughing.

Drug Interactions. No significant drug interactions have been reported.

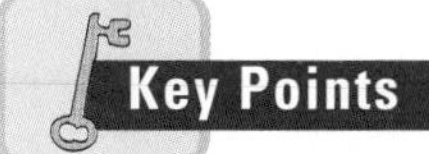

- Rhinitis is defined as inflammation of the nasal mucous membranes.
- Signs and symptoms are sneezing, nasal discharge, and nasal congestion. The most common causes of acute rhinitis are the common cold, allergies, bacterial infection, presence of a foreign body, and drug-induced congestion (rhinitis medicamentosa).
- The nurse's role in working with patients with rhinitis is to perform the initial assessment of symptoms and then focus on teaching the proper techniques of self-administering and monitoring the medication therapy. Frequent follow-up with the patient and reinforcement of gains made are important to the success of these treatments.

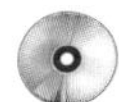

Go to your Companion CD-ROM for Appendices, an Audio Glossary, animations, Drug Dosage Calculators, customizable Patient Self-Assessment forms, and Review Questions for the NCLEX® Examination.

evolve Be sure to visit the companion Evolve site at http://evolve.elsevier.com/Clayton for WebLinks and additional online resources.

MEDICATION SAFETY REVIEW

CRITICAL THINKING QUESTIONS

1. A patient has been using phenylephrine nasal drops two or three times daily for the past 3 weeks. He comes to the health care provider's office complaining that his symptoms are worse than when he initiated treatment. What assessments should the nurse make?
2. A patient has been using chlorpheniramine maleate tablets three times per day and is having considerable sedation. Her once-productive cough has become nonproductive. What nursing actions should be considered?

Continued

CRITICAL THINKING QUESTIONS—cont'd

3. Explain how to properly administer a medication by inhalation such as fluticasone, two sprays in each nostril once daily.
4. Perform health teaching for the proper administration of nose drops.
5. Research OTC products available at the local pharmacy for treatment of upper respiratory disorders (e.g., common cold, influenza, allergies). For each product:
   - Prepare a list of the active ingredients listed.
   - Read the contraindications or precautions listed on the labels.

   Based on above research, develop a teaching plan to be used when these drugs are prescribed or found to be present when an intake assessment is performed.
6. Describe safety issues associated with the use of antihistamines.

CONTENT REVIEW QUESTIONS

1. The reason that intranasal corticosteroids are used for short periods to treat seasonal allergies is:
   1. bronchospasm/chronic cough may occur with prolonged therapy.
   2. to prevent elevated blood sugar.
   3. to minimize adrenal suppression.
   4. to prevent central nervous system depression.
2. Premedication assessment for sympathomimetic decongestants (e.g., oxymetazoline, phenylephrine) includes checking the history for:
   1. evidence of hypertension, hyperthyroidism, diabetes mellitus, glaucoma, or prostatic hyperplasia.
   2. gastrointestinal symptoms that are present before initiating therapy.
   3. any diseases or disorders of the hepatobiliary system.
   4. urinary retention, constipation, or blurred vision.
3. Before initiating antihistamine medications, the history should be checked for:
   1. evidence of hypertension, hyperthyroidism, diabetes mellitus, glaucoma, or prostatic hyperplasia.
   2. urinary retention, constipation, or blurred vision.
   3. glaucoma, prostatic hyperplasia, asthma, and concurrent use of sedating drugs.
   4. hypertension, hyperthyroidism, and concurrent use of nasal decongestants.
4. The action of cromolyn sodium is:
   1. bronchodilation.
   2. antihistamine.
   3. antiinflammatory agent.
   4. decongestant.
5. Blurred vision, constipation, urinary retention, and dryness of oral mucosa are anticholinergic effects produced by:
   1. steroids.
   2. decongestants.
   3. diuretics.
   4. antihistamines.
6. Patients using intranasal corticosteroids should be counseled about which of the following?
   1. Therapeutic effects are not immediate.
   2. Dosages must continue to be increased over time.
   3. Avoiding the operation of equipment.
   4. Regular use is not necessary with this medication.
7. Which of the following classes of medicines is more beneficial if given before exposure to allergens?
   1. Decongestants
   2. Antihistamines
   3. Steroids
   4. Beta-adrenergic agents

CHAPTER

31 Drugs Used to Treat Lower Respiratory Disease

evolve http://evolve.elsevier.com/Clayton

Chapter Content

Objectives

1. Compare the physiologic responses of the respiratory system to emphysema, chronic bronchitis, and asthma.
2. Describe the physiology of respirations.
3. Identify components of blood gases.
4. Cite nursing assessments used to evaluate the respiratory status of a patient.
5. Implement patient education for patients receiving drug therapy for lower respiratory disease.
6. Distinguish the mechanisms of action of expectorants, antitussives, and mucolytic agents.
7. Review the procedures for administration of medication by inhalation.
8. State the nursing assessments needed to monitor therapeutic response and the development of side effects to expect or report from expectorant, antitussive, and mucolytic therapy.
9. State the nursing assessments needed to monitor therapeutic response and the development of side effects to expect or report from sympathomimetic bronchodilator therapy.
10. State the nursing assessments needed to monitor therapeutic response and the development of side effects to expect or report from anticholinergic bronchodilator therapy.
11. State the nursing assessments needed to monitor therapeutic response and the development of side effects to expect from xanthine-derivative therapy.
12. State the nursing assessments needed to monitor therapeutic response and the development of side effects to expect or report from corticosteroid inhalant therapy.

Key Terms

ventilation	arterial blood gases (ABGs)
perfusion	oxygen saturation
diffusion	spirometry
goblet cells	cough
obstructive airway diseases	asthma
bronchospasm	bronchitis
chronic obstructive pulmonary disease (COPD)	emphysema
chronic airflow limitation disease (CALD)	bronchodilation
restrictive airway diseases	expectorants
	antitussives
	mucolytic agents
	bronchodilators
	antiinflammatory agents
	immunomodulators

LOWER RESPIRATORY TRACT ANATOMY AND PHYSIOLOGY

The respiratory system is a series of airways that start with the nose and mouth and end at the alveolar sacs. The nose and mouth airways connect at the pharynx. Passing out of the pharynx the airways divide into the esophagus of the gastrointestinal tract and the larynx (voice box) and trachea of the respiratory tract. The trachea divides into the right and left mainstem bronchi, which enter the lungs. The bronchi subdivide in each lung into many smaller bronchioles, which further subdivide into many smaller airways called alveolar ducts that terminate in alveolar sacs. The alveolar sacs are surrounded by capillaries of the blood circulatory system. Human lungs contain 300 to 500 million sacs for gaseous exchange and have a surface area approximately equal to that of a tennis court. The anatomic parts of the body associated with the lower respiratory system are the larynx, trachea, bronchi, bronchioles, and alveolar sacs (Figure 31-1).

The primary function of the lower respiratory tract is the ventilatory cycle. **Ventilation** is the movement of air in and out of the lungs. It is the process of transport

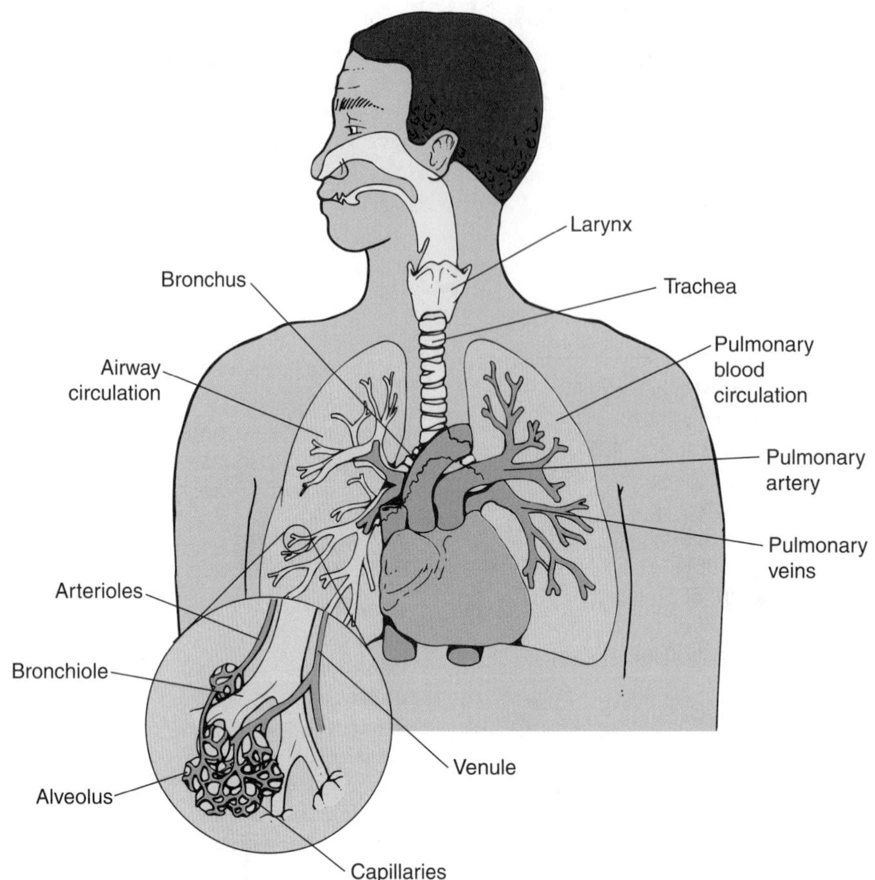

FIGURE 31-1 The respiratory tract and the alveoli.

(inhalation) of air containing oxygen to the alveolar sacs, exchange of oxygen for carbon dioxide across the alveolar membranes containing blood capillaries, and exhalation of "stale air," including carbon dioxide. Ventilation of the lungs is accomplished by contraction and relaxation of the diaphragmatic and intercostal muscles (muscles between the ribs). During inspiration, the diaphragmatic and intercostal muscles contract, creating a vacuum in the lungs and pulling air in through the mouth and nose. During exhalation, relaxation of the muscles allows the chest to return to its unexpanded position, forcing air out of the lungs.

Blood flow through the pulmonary arteries to the capillaries surrounding the alveoli to the pulmonary veins is called **perfusion. Diffusion** is the process by which oxygen (O_2) passes across the alveolar membrane to the blood in the capillaries and carbon dioxide (CO_2) passes from the blood to the alveolar sacs. Oxygen is transported by combining with hemoglobin in red blood cells or by dissolving in the blood plasma. Blood circulation provides distribution of oxygen to the body's cells for the sustenance of life. Ventilation and perfusion must be equal to maintain homeostasis.

The fluids of the respiratory tract originate from specialized mucous glands **(goblet cells)** and serous glands that line the respiratory tract. The goblet cells produce a gelatinous mucus that forms a thin layer over the interior surfaces of the trachea, bronchi, and bronchioles. Mucus secretion is increased by exposure to irritants, such as smoke, airborne particulate matter, and bacteria. The serous glands are controlled by the cholinergic nervous system. When stimulated, the serous glands secrete a watery fluid to the interior surface of the bronchial tree. There, the mucous secretions of the goblet cells and the watery secretions of the serous glands combine to form respiratory tract fluid.

Normally, respiratory tract fluid forms a protective layer over the trachea, bronchi, and bronchioles. Foreign bodies, such as smoke particles and bacteria, are caught in the respiratory tract fluid and are swept upward by ciliary hairs that line the bronchi and trachea to the larynx, where they are removed by the cough reflex. The expectorated (coughed up) material contains pulmonary mucous secretions, foreign particulate matter such as smoke and bacteria, and epithelial cells sloughed from the lining of the airways. Common names given to the expectorated mass are sputum and phlegm. If too much mucus is secreted as a result of chronic irritation, cilia are destroyed by chronic inhalation of smoke, dehydration dries the mucus, or anticholinergic agents inhibit watery secretions from the serous glands; the mucus becomes viscous, forming

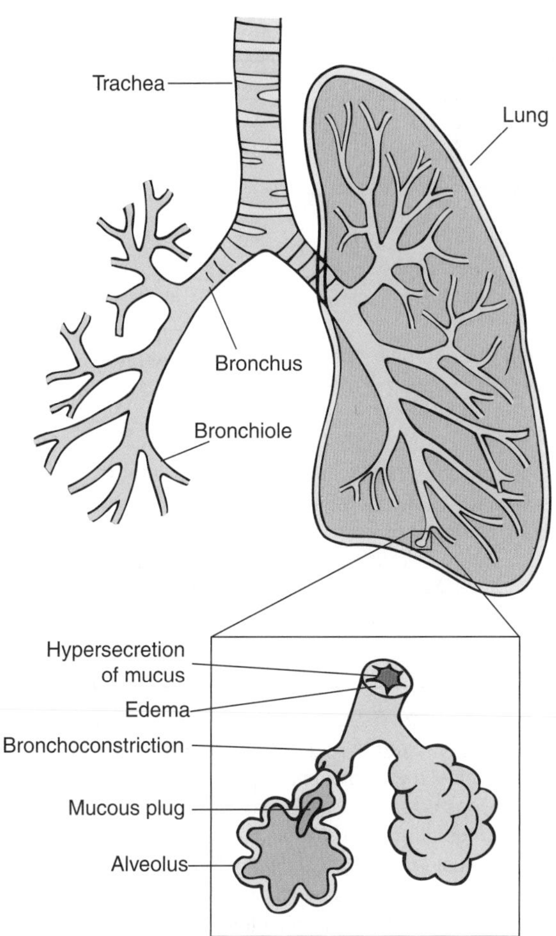

FIGURE **31-2** Factors restricting the airway. Major factors include hypersecretion of mucus, mucosal edema, and bronchoconstriction. Mucous plugs may form in the alveoli.

thick plugs in the bronchiolar airways (Figure 31-2). These thick plugs are difficult to eliminate. Colonization of pathogenic microorganisms in the lower respiratory tract results, which causes additional mucous secretions and the possible development of pneumonia from trapped bacteria.

The smooth muscle of the tracheobronchial tree is innervated by the parasympathetic and sympathetic branches of the autonomic nervous system. Stimulation of the cholinergic nerves causes bronchial constriction and increased mucus secretion. Sympathetic stimulation of adrenergic nerves causes dilatation of bronchial and bronchiolar airways and inhibition of respiratory tract fluids. Both beta-1 and beta-2 adrenergic receptors are present, but the beta-2 receptors predominate.

COMMON LOWER RESPIRATORY DISEASES

Respiratory diseases are often divided into two types: obstructive and restrictive. **Obstructive airway diseases** are those that narrow air passages, create turbulence, and increase resistance to airflow. Diseases cause narrowing of the airways through smooth muscle constriction **(bronchospasm)**, edema, inflammation of the bronchial walls, or excess mucus secretion. Examples of obstructive lung disease are asthma and acute bronchitis. Chronic obstructive illnesses are also referred to as **chronic obstructive pulmonary disease (COPD)**, and **chronic airflow limitation disease (CALD)**; the terms are used interchangeably. **Restrictive airway diseases** are those in which lung expansion is limited from loss of elasticity (e.g., pulmonary fibrosis) or physical deformity of the chest (e.g., kyphoscoliosis). Chronic bronchitis and emphysema are examples of both a restrictive and an obstructive lung disease.

Pulmonary function tests have been developed to assess both the ventilation and diffusion capacity of the lungs to assist in diagnosis and to give an objective assessment of improvement or deterioration of the patient's clinical condition. The best indicators of overall pulmonary function (ventilation and diffusion) are the **arterial blood gases (ABGs)**, such as Pa_{O_2}, Pa_{CO_2}, and pH (Table 31-1). To determine ABGs, a sample of arterial blood must be drawn and immediately analyzed to measure the pH and partial pressures of oxygen and carbon dioxide in the blood. Another measure that is more readily available and noninvasive is the oxygen saturation of hemoglobin. **Oxygen saturation** (Sa_{O_2}) is the ratio, expressed as a percent, of the oxygen actually bound to hemoglobin compared with the maximum amount of oxygen that could be bound to hemoglobin (see Table 31-1). Oxygen saturation is routinely used because a transcutaneous monitor (oximeter) is easily attached to the skin to continuously measure and report oxygen saturation.

Spirometry studies are routinely used to assess the capabilities of the patient's lungs, thorax, and respiratory muscles in moving volumes of air during inhalation and exhalation. A spirometer measures volumes of air. Terms used with spirometry are listed in Table 31-2. Patients with obstructive disease have difficulty with expiration and usually have a normal total lung capacity (TLC), a decreased vital capacity (VC), and an increased residual capacity (RC). Patients with restrictive disease have a decrease in all measured lung volumes. The forced expiratory volume in 1 second (FEV_1) and the forced vital capacity (FVC) are the most commonly used pulmonary function tests. The FEV_1 is used to determine the reversibility of airway disease and the effectiveness of bronchodilator therapy. The peak expiratory flow rate (PERF) meter is not as accurate but is much less costly and more readily available than other pulmonary function tests. This meter is routinely used by patients at home and by health care providers to assess the benefits of therapy in treating acute and chronic asthmatic symptoms. A patient is considered to have significant reversibility of airway obstruction if there is a 15% to 20% improvement in the FEV_1 or PEFR after bronchodilator therapy.

One of the first symptoms of a respiratory disease is the presence of a **cough**, a reflex initiated by irritation of

Table 31-1 Laboratory Tests Used to Assess Respiratory Function

TEST	NORMAL VALUE	RESULTS
pH	7.35-7.45 (arterial)	>7.45 = Alkalosis <7.35 = Acidosis
$PaCO_2$	35-45 mm Hg	Abnormalities indicate respiratory acid-base imbalance. ↑ = Hypercapnia = respiratory acidosis ↓ = Hypocapnia = respiratory alkalosis
HCO_3	21-28 mEq/L	Abnormalities indicate metabolic acid-base imbalance. ↑ = Metabolic alkalosis ↓ = Metabolic acidosis
PaO_2	80-100 mm Hg	Measures the amount of oxygen moving through pulmonary alveoli into blood for transport to other tissues; depends on the amount of inspired oxygen. ↓ = Hypoxemia, hypoventilation ↑ = Hyperventilation
SaO_2	95%	Measures the ratio of actual oxygen content of hemoglobin compared with the hemoglobin's oxygen-carrying capacity. When decreased, either there is an impairment of oxygen binding to hemoglobin (e.g., metabolic acidosis) or inadequate amounts of oxygen are being inspired.

Table 31-2 Terminology Used with Spirometry

TERM	DEFINITION
Tidal volume (TV)	Volume of air inspired or expired during normal breathing
Vital capacity (VC)	Volume of air exhaled after maximal inspiration to full expiration
Residual volume (RV)	Volume of air left in lungs after maximal exhalation
Functional residual capacity (FRC)	Volume of air left in lungs after normal exhalation
Total lung capacity (TLC)	Vital capacity plus residual volume (VC + RV) = TLC
Forced expiratory volume (FEV)	Volume of air forced out of the lungs by maximal exhalation
Forced expiratory volume in 1 second (FEV_1)	Volume of air forced out in 1 second to give the rate of flow
Forced vital capacity (FVC)	Maximal volume of air exhaled with maximal forced effort after maximal inhalation
Peak expiratory flow rate (PEFR)	Maximal rate of airflow produced during forced expiration

the airway. It is a protective, beneficial mechanism for clearing excess secretions from the tracheobronchial tree. The same irritants responsible for asthma or allergy may stimulate the cough receptors, or congestion of the nasal mucosa from a cold may cause a postnasal drip into the back of the throat that stimulates the cough.

A cough is productive if it helps remove accumulated secretions and phlegm from the tracheobronchial tree. A nonproductive cough results when irritants repeatedly stimulate the cough receptors but are not removed by the coughing reflex. Excessive coughing, particularly if it is dry and nonproductive, is not only discomforting but also tends to be self-perpetuating because the rapid air expulsion further irritates the tracheobronchial mucosa.

Asthma is a common chronic airway disease that affects more than 17 million people of all ages in the United States. It is the most common chronic illness of children and accounts for about 50% of emergency department visits by children younger than 18 years of age. It accounts for 100 million days of restricted activity, 500,000 hospitalizations, and 5000 deaths annually. Asthma is a highly variable disease in terms of onset and frequency of attacks, length of remission, and stimuli that cause attacks. For unknown reasons, the prevalence of asthma is increasing in the United States. Mortality rates have declined overall since 1995, but a disparity among ethnic groups remains: asthma mortality is nearly 3 times higher in African American males than in white males and is 2.5 times higher in African American females than in white females.

Asthma is an inflammatory disease of the bronchi and bronchioles. There are intermittent periods of acute, reversible airflow obstruction (bronchoconstriction) caused by bronchiolar inflammation and overresponsiveness to a variety of stimuli. Examples of stimuli that trigger bronchospasm and inflammation are respiratory viral infections, inhaled allergens, cold air, dry air, emotional stress, and smoke. Symptoms of asthma include cough, wheezing, shortness of breath, tightness of the chest, and increased mucus production. The exact causes of asthma are unknown. Asthmatic patients are often subdivided into categories based on severity of disease: mild intermittent, mild persistent, moderate persistent, and severe persistent (Figure 31-3).

Table 31-3 *Classification, Characteristics, and Therapies for COPD*

	0: AT RISK	I: MILD	II: MODERATE	III: SEVERE	IV: VERY SEVERE
Characteristics	• Chronic symptoms • Exposure to risk factors • Normal spirometry	• FEV_1/FVC <70% • FEV_1 ≥80% • With or without symptoms	• FEV_1/FVC <70% • 50% ≤FEV_1 <80% • With or without symptoms	• FEV_1/FVC <70% • 30% ≤FEV_1 <50% • With or without symptoms	• FEV_1/FVC <70% • FEV_1 <30% or FEV_1 <50% predicted plus chronic respiratory failure
	Avoidance of risk factor(s); influenza vaccination				
		Add short-acting bronchodilator when needed			
			Add regular treatment with one or more long-acting bronchodilators		
			Add rehabilitation		
				Add inhaled glucocorticosteroids if repeated exacerbations	
					Add long-term oxygen if chronic respiratory failure
					Consider surgical treatments

From Global Initiative for Chronic Obstructive Lung Disease: Global strategy for the diagnosis, management, and prevention of chronic obstructive pulmonary disease. 2005 Update. Based on an April 1998 NHLBL/WHO Workshop. Available at www.goldcopd.com/GuidelinesResources.asp?l1=2&l2=0.

Chronic **bronchitis** is a condition in which chronic irritation causes inflammation and edema with excessive mucus secretion leading to airflow obstruction. Common causes of chronic irritation are cigarette smoke, grain and coal dust exposure, and air pollution. A persistent, productive cough present on most days is one of the earliest signs of the disease. The classic patient with chronic bronchitis has a chronic productive cough and moderate dyspnea, is often obese, and suffers from significant hypoxia with cyanosis. The ABGs will confirm hypoxia and respiratory acidosis. This type of patient is often called a "blue bloater." Because of mucus overproduction and formation of mucous plugs, these patients are prone to recurrent respiratory infections. As this disease progresses, patients often develop polycythemia (increased red blood cell production) to transport oxygen and right-sided heart failure (cor pulmonale) secondary to the lung disease and pulmonary hypertension.

Emphysema is a disease of alveolar tissue destruction without fibrosis. Alveolar sacs lose elasticity and collapse during exhalation, trapping air within the lung. The classic patient with emphysema is short of breath with minimal exertion (dyspneic), breathes through pursed lips, is thin because of weight loss, is barrel chested from increased use of accessory muscles, and has only scanty sputum production with a minimal cough. These patients are often called "pink puffers" because they maintain normal oxygenation by increased breathing rate. Table 31-3 classifies the severity of each stage of COPD based on symptoms and spirometry tests.

TREATMENT OF LOWER RESPIRATORY DISEASES

Cough

Treatment of the cough is of secondary importance; primary treatment is aimed at the underlying disorder. If the air is dry, a vaporizer or humidifier may be used to liquefy secretions so that they do not become irritating. A dehydrated state thickens respiratory secretions; therefore drinking large amounts of fluids will help reduce secretion viscosity (thickness). Patients can also suck on hard candies to increase saliva flow to coat the throat, thereby reducing irritation. If these simple measures do not reduce the cough, an expectorant or a cough suppressant (antitussive) may be used. The therapeutic objective is to decrease the intensity and frequency of the cough yet permit adequate elimination of tracheobronchial phlegm. In severe cases of pulmonary congestion, a mucolytic agent may be required.

Asthma

The National Heart, Lung, and Blood Institute: National Asthma Education and Prevention Program (NAEPP) has published *Guidelines for the Diagnosis and Management of Asthma—Report 2*, with updates—2002, which recommends the following goals of therapy for asthma: maintain normal activity levels; maintain near-normal pulmonary function rates; prevent chronic and troublesome symptoms (e.g., coughing or breathlessness in the night, in the early morning, or after exertion); prevent recurrent exacerbations; and avoid adverse effects from asthma medications. The guidelines describe four components to asthma therapy: patient education, environmental control,

Management of asthma in adults

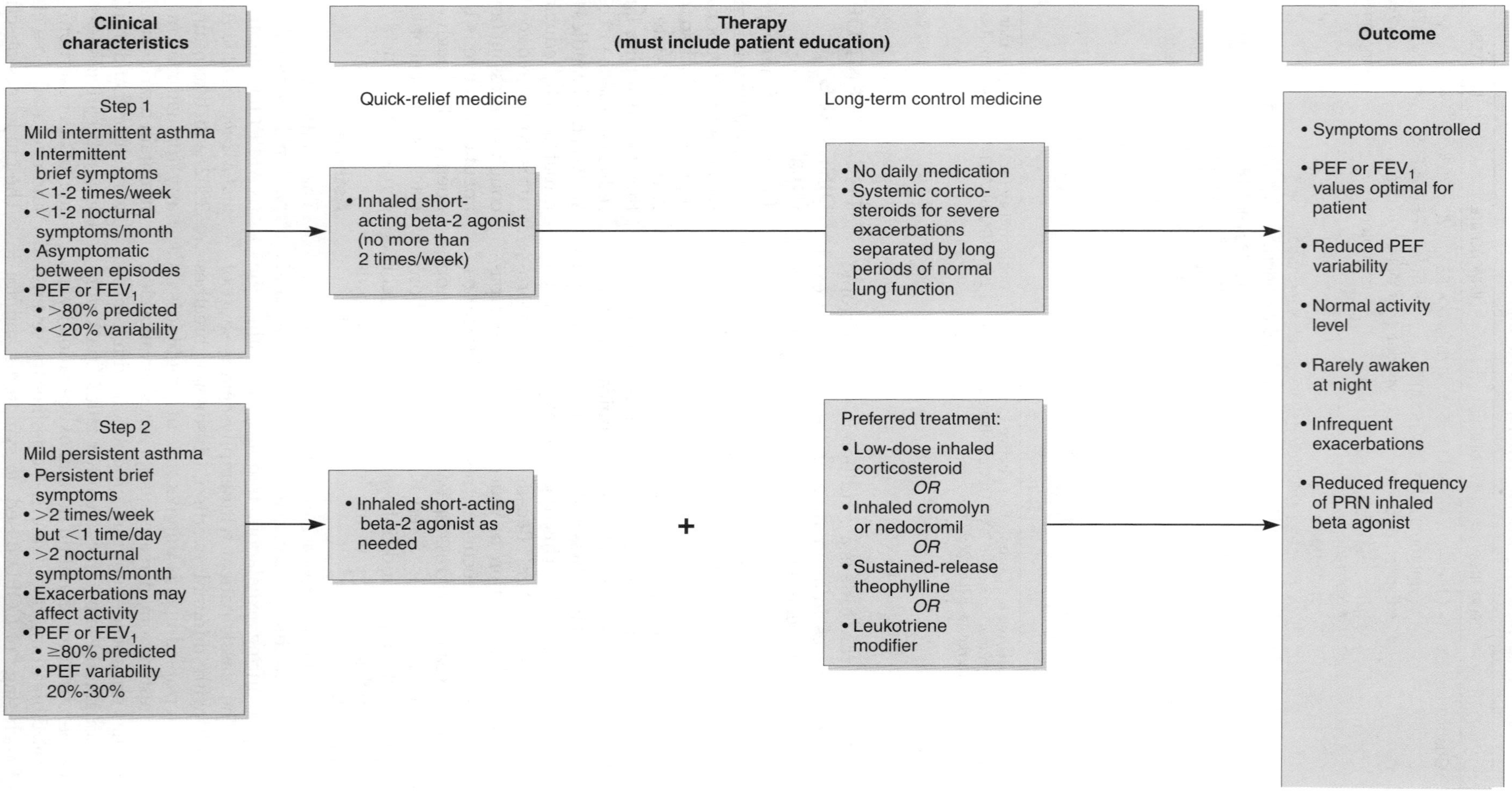

Clinical characteristics	Therapy (must include patient education): Quick-relief medicine		Therapy (must include patient education): Long-term control medicine	Outcome

Step 1
Mild intermittent asthma
• Intermittent brief symptoms <1-2 times/week
• <1-2 nocturnal symptoms/month
• Asymptomatic between episodes
• PEF or FEV_1
  • >80% predicted
  • <20% variability
	• Inhaled short-acting beta-2 agonist (no more than 2 times/week)		• No daily medication
			• Systemic cortico-steroids for severe exacerbations separated by long periods of normal lung function
				• Symptoms controlled
				• PEF or FEV_1 values optimal for patient
				• Reduced PEF variability
				• Normal activity level
				• Rarely awaken at night
				• Infrequent exacerbations
				• Reduced frequency of PRN inhaled beta agonist

Step 2
Mild persistent asthma
• Persistent brief symptoms
• >2 times/week but <1 time/day
• >2 nocturnal symptoms/month
• Exacerbations may affect activity
• PEF or FEV_1
  • ≥80% predicted
  • PEF variability 20%-30%
	• Inhaled short-acting beta-2 agonist as needed	+	Preferred treatment:
			• Low-dose inhaled corticosteroid
			OR
			• Inhaled cromolyn or nedocromil
			OR
			• Sustained-release theophylline
			OR
			• Leukotriene modifier	

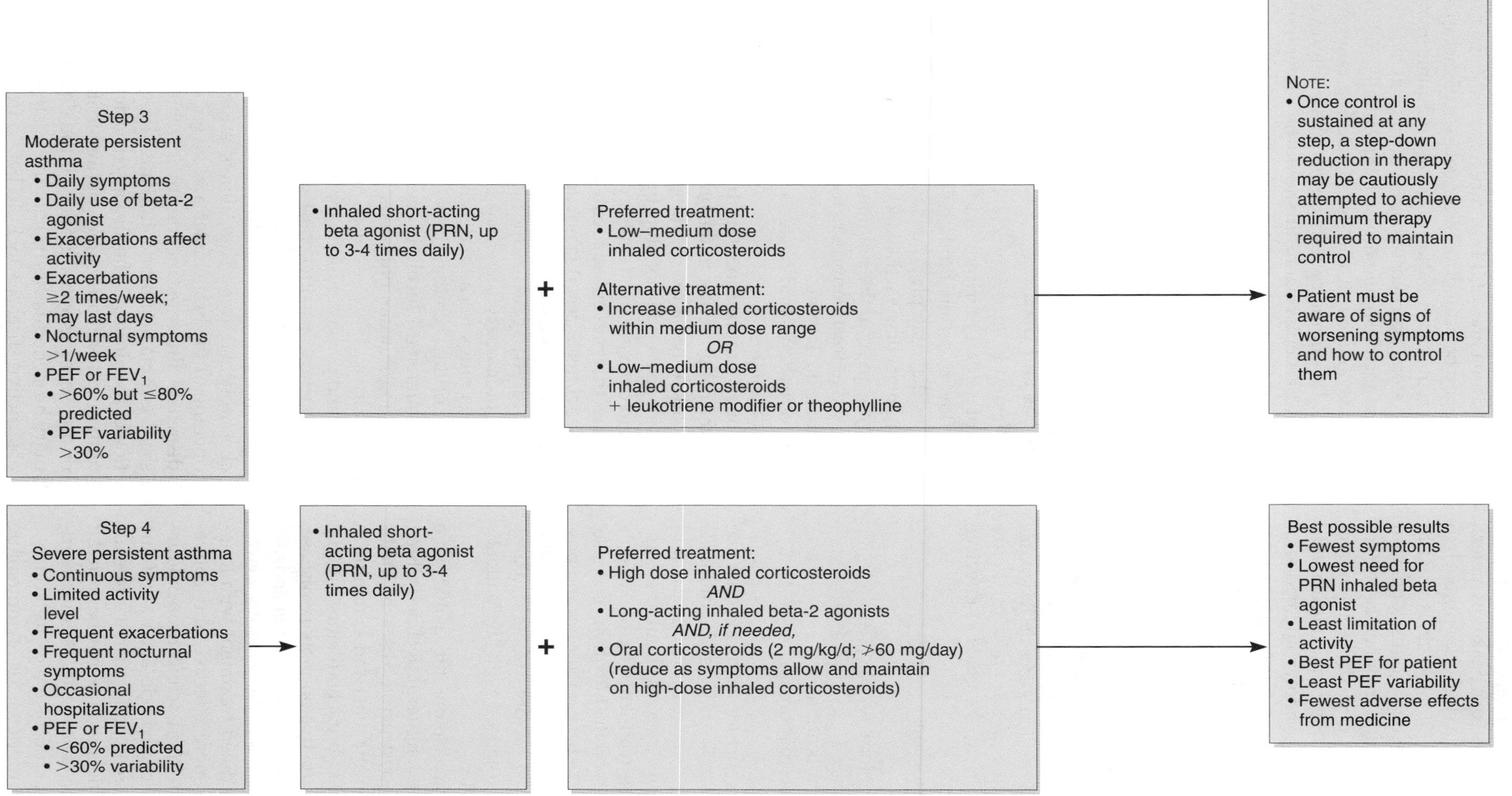

FIGURE 31-3 Stepwise management of chronic asthma in adults. Therapy is "stepped up" to the next level of therapy if control is not achieved at the current step with proper use of medication. "Step-down," or reduction of dosages, should be considered when the desired outcomes have been achieved and sustained for several weeks at the current step. Step-down therapy is desired to identify the minimum dosages of therapy required to maintain the desired outcomes. *FEV,* Forced expiratory volume; *PEF,* peak expiratory flow; *PRN,* as needed.

comprehensive pharmacologic therapy, and objective monitoring measures (regular use of a peak flowmeter). The guidelines also recommend a stepwise approach to asthma therapy (see Figure 31-3). Medicines used to treat asthma can be divided into two groups: long-term control medications to achieve and maintain control of persistent asthma and quick-relief medications to treat symptoms and exacerbations. Long-term control medications are the corticosteroids, cromolyn and nedocromil, long-acting beta-2 agonists, xanthines, and leukotriene modifiers. The quick-relief medications are short-acting beta-2 agonists, anticholinergic agents, and systemic corticosteroids.

Bronchitis and Emphysema

It is common for patients with obstructive lung disease to have symptoms of more than one of these diseases, but one usually predominates, and overall treatment is similar. According to the *Global Strategy for the Diagnosis, Management, and Prevention of Chronic Obstructive Pulmonary Disease, 2005 Update,* the goals of effective COPD management are to:

- Prevent disease progression
- Relieve symptoms
- Improve exercise tolerance
- Improve health status
- Prevent and treat complications
- Prevent and treat exacerbations
- Reduce mortality

Management principles include ensuring that the patient understands the disease process, the rationale for various procedures used to treat the disease, and the goals of therapy. Spirometry tests should be completed periodically to assess treatment success. Patients must also be taught appropriate nutrition, exercise, proper coughing techniques, chest percussion and postural drainage to mobilize mucous secretions and plugs, and elimination of risk factors such as smoking. All these efforts must be balanced with the patient's perceptions of quality of life.

None of the existing medications for COPD have been shown to modify the long-term decline in lung function associated with obstructive disease. Medicines are used for symptomatic relief and to minimize frequency of complications. Bronchodilators are the cornerstone of chronic obstructive pulmonary disease, but the extent to which they are effective depends on how much reversibility there is to the patient's airway narrowing. Regularly scheduled treatment with long-acting bronchodilators is more effective and convenient than treatment with short-acting bronchodilators. Ipratropium, an anticholinergic agent, and the beta adrenergic agonists are equally effective to start therapy. Oral long-acting theophylline may be added if additional bronchodilation is necessary. Adding regular treatment with inhaled corticosteroids to bronchodilator treatment is appropriate for symptomatic COPD patients who are classified as having stage III or stage IV disease. In some patients, such as those with both asthma and COPD, a corticosteroid (e.g., prednisone) may be added for short courses of therapy during an acute exacerbation of asthma. Chronic treatment with systemic corticosteroids should be avoided. Each of these agents should be used sequentially and the patient reevaluated at each step before a new drug is added. If spirometry tests do not show improvement with a particular agent, it should be discontinued to avoid side effects of the medicine.

Oxygen therapy may also be used if the patient is chronically hypoxemic, has nocturnal or exercise-induced hypoxemia, or has an acute exacerbation of obstructive disease and the Po_2 drops below 55 mm Hg. Normal doses are 2 to 3 L per minute.

DRUG THERAPY FOR LOWER RESPIRATORY DISEASES

Actions and Uses

Expectorants liquefy mucus by stimulating the secretion of natural lubricant fluids from the serous glands. The flow of serous fluids helps liquefy thick mucous masses that may plug the narrow bronchioles. A combination of ciliary action and coughing will then expel the phlegm from the pulmonary system. Expectorants are used to treat nonproductive cough, bronchitis, and pneumonia, in which mucous plugs inhibit the expulsion of irritants and bacteria that cause bronchitis or pneumonia.

Cough suppressants (antitussives) act by suppressing the cough center in the brain. They are used when the patient has a dry, hacking, nonproductive cough. These agents will not stop the cough completely but should decrease the frequency and suppress the severe spasms that prevent adequate rest at night. Under normal circumstances, it is not appropriate to suppress a productive cough.

Mucolytic agents reduce the stickiness and viscosity of pulmonary secretions by acting directly on the mucous plugs to cause dissolution. This eases the removal of the secretions by suction, postural drainage, and coughing. Mucolytic agents are most effective in removing mucous plugs obstructing the tracheobronchial airway. They are used in treating patients with acute and chronic pulmonary disorders, before and after bronchoscopy, after chest surgery, and as part of the treatment of tracheostomy care.

Bronchodilators relax the smooth muscle of the tracheobronchial tree. This allows an increase in the opening of the bronchioles and alveolar ducts, which decreases the resistance to airflow into the alveolar sacs. Asthma and bronchitis cause reversible obstruction of the airways. The airway constriction associated with emphysema is somewhat reversible, depending on the severity and duration of the disease. The primary bronchodilators used in the treatment of airway-obstructive diseases include beta-adrenergic agents, anticholinergic aerosols, and xanthine derivatives.

Antiinflammatory agents play an important role in the treatment of asthma to reduce inflammation. Corticosteroids are the most effective agent. Most commonly used are those administered by inhalation because this places the medicine at the site of inflammation with minimal systemic side effects. Depending on frequency and severity of acute attacks, some asthmatic patients will require short "bursts" of systemic steroids, usually prednisone, for 1 to 2 weeks of therapy. An occasional patient with asthma may require alternate-day or daily steroid administration to control symptoms. All efforts must be made to optimize other forms of treatment before resorting to regular systemic steroid administration because of the potential serious side effects that accompany steroid administration.

Other antiinflammatory agents used are leukotriene modifiers and cromolyn and nedocromil. Leukotriene modifiers are a new class of antiinflammatory agent that block leukotriene formation. Leukotrienes are part of the inflammatory pathway that causes bronchoconstriction. The exact mechanism by which cromolyn and nedocromil help control asthma is not known. These agents have no bronchodilating properties and are useless in patients with chronic obstructive pulmonary disease.

Omalizumab is the first of a new class of agents, known as **immunomodulators,** used to treat patients with asthma exacerbations caused by reaction to airborne allergens.

NURSING PROCESS *for Lower Respiratory Diseases*

The nurse must first understand normal respiratory function before proceeding to the assessment of pathophysiologic conditions of the respiratory tract, such as asthma, chronic bronchitis, and emphysema. COPD and CALD are terms that are used interchangeably. Both emphysema and chronic bronchitis are progressive diseases with little reversibility, whereas asthma is an inflammatory process with reversible airflow obstruction.

Assessment

History of Respiratory Symptoms

- What pulmonary symptoms has the individual had (e.g., childhood or adult allergies, pulmonary infections, pneumonia, tuberculosis, chest trauma, surgeries)? Has the individual had any respiratory problems that have required recent health care provider treatment or emergency department treatment? If yes, get details. When coughing, wheezing, or difficulty breathing occurs, what measures have helped to relieve the symptoms?
- What is the work environment of the individual? Ask about exposure to allergens, dust, and chemicals.
- Ask specifically for details of smoking or exposure to secondhand smoke. History of smoking is usually recorded in pack-years. (Multiply the number of packs of cigarettes smoked per day times the number of years of smoking. For example, if a person smoked $1\frac{1}{2}$ packs of cigarettes per day for 20 years, the patient is said to have a [$1\frac{1}{2} \times 20 = 30$] 30 pack-year history of smoking.)
- Is there a family history of respiratory disease or disorders? If so, obtain details (e.g., diagnosis of disease, people affected).

History of Respiratory Medication

- What prescribed medications, over-the-counter (OTC) medications, or herbal products are being used or have been used for the treatment of the same or similar respiratory problems? Do any medications, such as aspirin or nonsteroidal antiinflammatory drugs (NSAIDs) (e.g., ibuprofen [Advil]), precipitate an asthma attack?
- How effective have the medications been in treating prior or current symptoms?

Description of Current Symptoms

- What is the patient's chief complaint?
- When did the symptoms start? Does the patient have any idea what triggered them?
- Ask the patient to describe the symptoms. What effect do the symptoms have on the patient's ability to carry on activities of daily living (ADLs)?

Respiratory Assessment. NOTE: The extent of the pulmonary examination (inspection, palpation, percussion, auscultation) must be adapted to the nurse's education level and assessment skills (e.g., beginning student, practical nurse, registered nurse).

- Observe the patient's general appearance and degree of respiratory impairment. Adapt the assessment and prioritization of the examination to the degree of respiratory impairment present.
- Take and record baseline vital signs.
- *Respiratory pattern:* Assess the rate, depth, and regularity of the patient's breathing. The normal respiratory rate is approximately 14 to 22 breaths/minute in adults and up to 44 breaths/minute in infants.

Rapid, shallow breathing may be caused by an elevated diaphragm, restrictive lung disease, or pleuritic chest pain.

Rapid, deep breathing may be caused by exercise, anxiety, or metabolic acidosis. *Kussmaul's respiration* is deep breathing associated with metabolic acidosis. It may be fast, normal, or slow. It is most often found in patients with diabetic ketoacidosis.

Breathing associated with obstructive lung disease has a prolonged expiratory phase because of increased airway resistance. If the respiratory rate increases, the patient lacks time for full expiration. The chest overexpands with trapped air and breathing becomes shallow.

Cheyne-Stokes respiration is a cyclic breathing pattern in which periods of deep breathing alternate with periods of apnea. Children and older people normally show this pattern while asleep. Other causes include heart failure, drug-induced respiratory depression, uremia, and stroke.

- *Cough:* Note whether a cough is productive or nonproductive. Record sputum color, consistency, amount, and any appearance of frothiness or blood (hemoptysis). Has the patient experienced any sudden episodes of severe coughing, wheezing, or shortness of breath? Does the patient have coughing or wheezing during certain seasons of the year or when exposed to certain places or conditions (e.g., cats, dogs, smoke, medications, foods)? Does exercise induce coughing?
- *Mental status:* As the oxygen level in the body diminishes and carbon dioxide accumulates, the mental status will deteriorate from alertness to progressively lower levels of functioning (alert → restless → drowsy → unconscious → dead).

Inspection

- *Skin color:* Is the skin color normal or is the patient cyanotic? Where is the cyanosis visible? Peripheral cyanosis is defined as a bluish coloring of an isolated area of the body (e.g., earlobes, toes, feet, fingers). Central cyanosis indicates a general lack of oxygen in the hemoglobin. The entire body has a slight bluish tinge. It is most readily observed on the lips and mucous membranes of the mouth.
- *Dyspnea:* Note whether dyspnea occurs at rest or with exertion. Observe the breathing pattern (e.g., pursed-lip, exertion required to exhale).
- *Muscle involvement:* Elevating the shoulders, retracting the spaces between the ribs, and using the abdominal muscles are associated with advanced respiratory disease.
- *Posture:* Dyspneic patients usually sit upright or lean forward from the waist, resting the elbows on the knees. This helps give the chest maximal expansion.
- *Chest contour:* Note changes in chest contour, such as barrel chest (increased anteroposterior diameter), kyphosis, or scoliosis. Measure and record the chest circumference.
- *Fingernail clubbing:* Assess for flattening or an increase in the angle between the fingernail and the nail base of the fingers. Clubbing has many causes, including hypoxia and lung cancer.

Palpation. Perform palpation of the chest, noting any tender or painful areas, masses, and increased or decreased tactile fremitus. Note diminished expansion of the chest wall on inspiration.

Percussion. Note the presence of dullness, hyperresonance, and diaphragmatic excursion.

Auscultation. Perform auscultation of the chest; note the intensity, pitch, and relative duration of inspiratory and expiratory phases. Identify additional sounds (e.g., crackles, rhonchi, wheezes). Are they inspiratory, expiratory, or both? Where are they located? Do they clear with deep breathing or coughing? Is bronchophony or egophony present?

Cardiovascular Assessment. As appropriate to the symptoms and the diagnosis, perform a cardiovascular assessment (see Chapters 25, 26, and 28). Whenever dyspnea is severe, do not overlook the possibility of cardiovascular involvement—perform a cardiac assessment.

Sleep Pattern. Ask whether the individual has had difficulty sleeping. Obtain details.

Psychosocial Assessment. Ask specifically about the presence and degree of depression, anxiety, and social isolation experienced as a result of the disease process, as well as adaptive or maladaptive responses. Identify support systems in place to assist in providing for the individual's care.

Laboratory and Diagnostic Data. Review pulmonary function tests, ABGs, hematology, sputum tests, and x-ray reports as available and appropriate to the diagnosis. Allergy testing may be appropriate for some individuals. If alpha-1 antitrypsin deficiency is suspected an alpha-1 antitrypsin test and Pi typing may be ordered to determine which type of alpha-1 antitrypsin deficiency is present.

Nursing Diagnoses

- Airway clearance, ineffective (indication)
- Activity intolerance (indication)
- Gas exchange, impaired (indication)
- Breathing pattern, ineffective (indication)

Planning

Description of Current Symptoms. Individualize the care plan to address the patient's degree of dyspnea, cough, pain, fatigue, sleep pattern disturbance, nutritional needs, and other relevant factors.

Medications

- Order medications prescribed, and schedule these on the medication administration record (MAR). Perform focused assessments at regularly scheduled intervals consistent with the patient's status to determine effectiveness and side effects to expect or report.
- Ensure that as-needed (PRN) medications are ordered and readily available for use.
- Plan appropriate teaching for medication administration techniques and drug therapy.

Hydration. Mark the Kardex or enter data into the computer with fluid recommendations to maintain patient hydration consistent with any coexisting diagnoses (e.g., heart failure). Order humidification as prescribed.

Respiratory and Cardiovascular Assessment. Schedule assessments of respiratory and cardiovascular status at least once per shift and more frequently as indicated by the patient's status.

Laboratory and Diagnostic Studies. Order stat and subsequent laboratory studies (e.g., sputum collection, ABGs, pulmonary function tests, hematology, x-ray scans). During an acute asthma attack continual respiratory assessments are performed. Monitor pulse oximetry and oxygen saturation. Compare pulmonary function tests with normal levels and report findings outside the parameters specified by the health care provider.

Implementation

- Perform physical assessments of the patient in accordance with clinical site policies (e.g., every 4 or 8 hours, depending on the patient's status).
- Assist the patient, as needed, to perform self-care activities. Note the degree of impairment or dyspnea seen with and without oxygen.
- Administer oxygen as ordered and as needed. Record spirometer readings as requested.
- Administer prescribed medications and treatments that can best alleviate the patient's symptoms and provide the maximum level of comfort.
- Encourage physical activity as prescribed. Do not allow the patient to overexert or become fatigued.
- Institute measures to reduce anxiety. Support the patient in a calm manner.

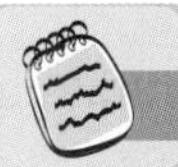

Patient Education and Health Promotion

Peak Flowmeter. People with asthma are routinely taught how to use a peak flowmeter to measure the peak expiratory flow (PEF) to assess the severity of their symptoms. Using the PEF as a guide:

- The green zone is where the PEF is at 80% to 100% of the patient's personal best PEF. When in the green zone, the patient is breathing well and having no cough, wheezing, or chest tightness and should continue therapy as prescribed.
- The yellow zone is where the PEF is at 50% to 80% of the personal best PEF. In the yellow zone, the patient is starting to become symptomatic, having symptoms like coughing, wheezing, or chest tightness. It is time to use quick-relief medicine (inhaled beta-2 agonist).
- The red zone is where the PEF is less than 50% of the personal best PEF. When in the red zone, the patient should contact the health care provider immediately. Quick-relief medicine is continued and corticosteroids are often started at this point.

Avoiding Irritants. Smoking, pollen, and environmental pollutants commonly aggravate respiratory disorders. Check the home and work environment for allergens that may be precipitating or worsening an asthmatic attack. Medicines alone will not alleviate the problem. The control of triggers for the attacks is of paramount importance.

Activity and Exercise. Fatigue and resulting dyspnea may require adjustments in physical activity and employment. Support the patient's concerns. Plan for rest periods to alternate with activity. Provide oxygenation before or during activities as appropriate to the patient's needs.

Initiate the use of an inhaled beta-2 agonist 30 minutes before undertaking exercise known to induce an asthma attack.

Nutritional Status

- A well-balanced diet that prevents excessive weight loss or gain is important.
- Encourage patients with dyspnea to eat several small servings throughout the day and to take small bites. Pulmocare, a nutritional supplement may be prescribed as an adjunct to limited daily food intake. Avoid foods known to increase production of mucus (e.g., milk, chocolate).
- For COPD patients requiring oxygen, administer oxygen via nasal cannula during mealtime.
- Patients who experience asthma attacks during or following the ingestion of processed potatoes, shrimp, or dried fruits or when drinking beer or wine should avoid these items.

Preventing Infections

- Encourage patients to avoid exposure to people with infection; practice good hygiene, such as handwashing; get adequate rest; and dispose of secretions properly.
- Patients should seek medical attention at the earliest sign of suspected infection (e.g., increased cough, increased fatigue, dyspnea, temperature elevation, change in characteristics of secretions).
- Annual influenza vaccinations are recommended for patients having persistent asthma attacks.

Increased Fluid Intake. Unless contraindicated, encourage patients to increase fluid intake. This will aid in decreasing secretion viscosity. Patients should drink 8 to 10 (or more), 8-ounce glasses of water daily as directed by the health care provider.

Environmental Elements. People experiencing difficulty in breathing can benefit from proper temperature, humidification of the air, or ventilation of the immediate surroundings. Moist air from a humidifier can readily relieve nose or throat dryness.

Breathing Techniques. If ordered by the health care provider, teach postural drainage and pursed-lip breathing or abdominal breathing and coughing. Record peak flow readings, and institute prescribed treatments as indicated by the health care provider.

Sleep Patterns. Discuss adaptations that the individual can make in daily routines to ensure adequate rest. As the disease progresses, sleeping in a recliner or in an upright position may be necessary.

Psychosocial Behavior

- Encourage open discussion of the person's fears and expectations regarding therapy.
- Discuss the expectations of therapy (e.g., level of exercise; degree of pain relief, if present; tolerance; frequency of therapy; relief of dyspnea; ability to maintain ADLs and work; other issues as indicated by the underlying pathologic condition).

- Identify support people who can assist the individual during periods of breathlessness and make them, as well as the patient, aware of community resources available, such as the Visiting Nurses Association and home health care agencies.

Medications

- Explain the purpose and method of administration of each prescribed medication. Be certain the individual understands the delivery method for administration of the medication (e.g., aerosol therapy, metered-dose inhalers, nebulizer, peak expiratory flowmeter). The care and cleaning of equipment used for delivery of drugs to the respiratory tract should be explained to prevent bacterial growth.
- When administering medicines by aerosol therapy to a child or to an older patient, make sure that the patient has the strength and dexterity to operate the equipment before discharge. When muscle coordination is not fully developed, as in a younger child, or when dexterity has diminished in an older patient, it may be beneficial to use a spacer device for medicines administered by inhalation (Figure 31-4). Have the patient demonstrate use of the inhaler at each office or emergency department visit. Confirm that the patient exhales completely before initiating the first inhalation of a medication and that the breath is held for approximately 10 seconds during inhalation of the medication. Whenever both a bronchodilator and a steroid are prescribed, administer the bronchodilator as the first puff of medication and then wait a few minutes before administering the second medication. This will allow bronchodilation so that when the second drug, such as a steroid, is given, the drug will have a better chance of reaching the lower portions of the airway. Advise the patient to rinse the mouth (rinse and spit) following inhalation of steroid medications.

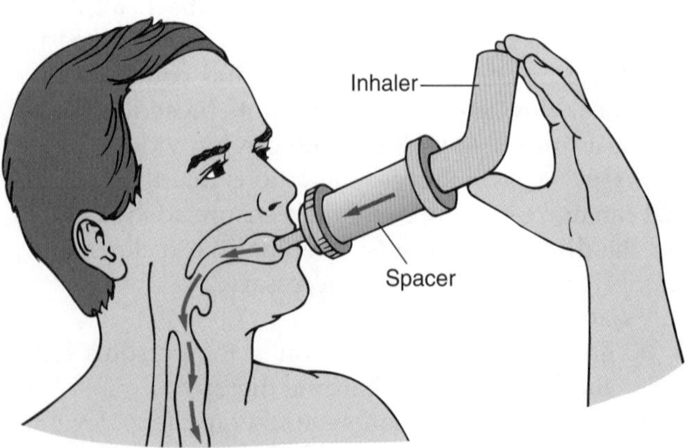

FIGURE **31-4** Use of spacer.

- Oxygen therapy must be explained in detail. The patient who is in a continual hypoxic state must understand that it is not beneficial and may be harmful to increase the oxygen flow above the prescribed rate.
- People receiving theophylline therapy must understand the importance of reporting for laboratory studies to determine the plasma level of the drug. Because cigarette smoking can alter the blood level of this medicine, the individual must understand the ramifications of starting, stopping, or altering level of smoking.
- Be certain the individual understands the proper use of bronchodilators and antiinflammatory agents prescribed. Drugs prescribed for prn use or use during an acute attack of asthma must be thoroughly explained. Teach the patient to check whether an inhaler is full or empty.

Fostering Health Maintenance

- Throughout the course of treatment discuss medication information, the importance of adequate airway clearance, dietary and hydration needs, breathing exercises, physical exercise, pulmonary hygiene, environmental control, the need to balance activities with abilities, and stress reduction and how each of these measures can benefit the patient.
- *Filtration systems:* The use of specialized filtration systems on furnaces and air conditioners can significantly reduce exposure to pollen and fungal spores when used with the windows and outside doors closed. Filters must be changed regularly for full effect. Water-based air-conditioning units must be cleaned regularly to prevent fungal growth that may exacerbate allergy symptoms.
- *Dust mites:* The most common cause of allergy from indoor sources, the dust mite, is found in carpeting and mattresses and is not removed by air cleaners. To kill dust mites, wash bedding frequently in hot water and wash or steam porous surfaces; stuffed animals and pillows can be placed inside a plastic bag and put in the freezer overnight. Encase mattresses, pillows, and box springs in nonallergenic covers. When cleaning, use a damp cloth to remove rather than spread the dust.
- *Pets:* Cats, dogs, and birds are frequently a source of asthma triggers. Pets should be removed from the home or kept outside if at all possible.
- *Smoking:* All smoking must cease.
- *Mold:* Molds are often asthma triggers. Remove houseplants. Do not allow wet clothing to lie around without prompt drying.
- Seek cooperation and understanding of the following points to increase medication adherence: name of medication, dosage, route and times of administration, side effects to expect, and side effects to report.

- It is critical to teach the individual using an inhaler the proper technique of use! Evaluate whether a spacer is needed.
- Teach breathing techniques that will facilitate breathing such as diaphragmatic or abdominal breathing and the pursed-lip technique.
- Humidified air may be required, but when used, it is essential that the humidifier be cleaned thoroughly daily to prevent mold growth.
- Teach the patient to schedule daily activities, including rest, to conserve energy. Eating smaller meals more frequently spaced throughout the day will help provide energy, and less energy will be consumed metabolizing larger meals.
- Teach relaxation therapy to avoid anxiety and stress, known triggers of bronchospasm, and asthma attacks.
- Pulmocare, a specifically designed nutritional supplement for patients with respiratory diseases, may be ordered. Avoid caffeine-containing beverages because caffeine is a weak diuretic. Diuresis promotes thickening of lung secretions, making it more difficult to expectorate them. Milk and chocolate are also known to increase the thickness of secretions and may need to be eliminated from the diet.
- Make the patient and family aware of the community resources available.

Written Record. Enlist the patient's aid in developing and maintaining a written record of monitoring parameters (e.g., respirations, pulse, daily weights, degree of dyspnea relief, exercise tolerance, secretions being expectorated) (see Patient Self-Monitoring Form on p. 504). Complete the Premedication Data column for use as a baseline to track response to drug therapy. Ensure that the patient understands how to use the form and instruct the patient to bring the completed form to follow-up visits. During follow-up visits, focus on issues that will foster adherence with the therapeutic interventions prescribed. Teach the patient to contact the health care provider if the PEF is deteriorating, or if shortness of breath or wheezing persists despite taking prescribed medications.

DRUG CLASS: Expectorants

guaifenesin (gwi feh' neh sin)

Robitussin (row bih tus' sin)

Actions

Guaifenesin is an expectorant that acts by enhancing the output of respiratory tract fluid. The increased flow of secretions decreases mucus viscosity and promotes ciliary action. A combination of ciliary action and coughing then expels the phlegm from the pulmonary system.

Uses

Guaifenesin is used for the symptomatic relief of conditions characterized by a dry, nonproductive cough, as well as to remove mucous plugs from the respiratory tract. Such conditions include the common cold, bronchitis, laryngitis, pharyngitis, and sinusitis. Guaifenesin is often combined with bronchodilators, decongestants, antihistamines, or antitussive agents to aid in making a nonproductive cough more productive. Guaifenesin is more effective if the patient is well hydrated at the time of therapy.

Guaifenesin should not be given to a patient with a dry, persistent cough that lasts more than 1 week; if there is a chronic, persistent cough, such as that which accompanies asthma, bronchitis, and emphysema; or if the cough is accompanied by excessive production of phlegm. These may be indications of more serious conditions for which the patient should seek medical attention.

Therapeutic Outcomes

The primary therapeutic outcome expected from guaifenesin therapy is reduced frequency of nonproductive cough.

Nursing Process for Guaifenesin

Premedication Assessment

Record characteristics of the cough before initiating therapy.

Planning

Availability. PO: 100, 200, 400, and 600 mg tablets; 200 mg capsules; 100 and 200 mg/5 mL liquid. It is also available in individual products in combination with pseudoephedrine, dextromethorphan, codeine phosphate, and phenylpropanolamine.

Implementation

Dosage and Administration. *Adult:* PO: 100 to 400 mg every 4 to 6 hours; do not exceed 2400 mg/day. *Pediatric:* PO: For children 6 to 12 years old, give 100 to 200 mg every 4 hours; do not exceed 1200 mg/day. For children 2 to 6 years old, give 50 to 100 mg every 4 hours; do not exceed 600 mg/day.

Fluid Intake. Maintain fluid intake of eight to twelve 8-ounce glasses of water daily.

Humidification. Suggest the concurrent use of a humidifier.

Evaluation

Side Effects to Expect

Gastrointestinal Upset, Nausea, Vomiting. Development of these side effects is rare.

Drug Interactions. No significant drug interactions have been reported.

PATIENT SELF-ASSESSMENT FORM Respiratory Agents

MEDICATIONS	COLOR	TO BE TAKEN

Patient ______________________

Health Care Provider ______________________

Health Care Provider's phone ______________________

Next appt.* ______________________

What I Should Monitor		Premedication Data	Date	Date	Date	Date	Date	Date	Comments
Peak flow meter	AM L/min								
	Noon								
	PM								
Postural drainage	Times of day performed (e.g., 8 AM, 2 PM)								
Describe cough	Response: productive cough, nonproductive								
	Frequent, intermittent								
	Secretions Color								
	Thickness of secretions: thick, thin								
How do you feel today? (record two times per day) **Awful** 10 — **Improving** 5 — **Good** 1	AM / PM								
Exercise level: degree of tiredness with exercise **Extremely** 10 — **Moderate** 5 — **Normal** 1									
Activities of daily living	Walk (_____) of stairs								
	Walk (_____) of blocks								
	Can perform daily activities (Yes/No)								
Pain pattern	Pain is on *L* (left) or *R* (right) side								
	Pain on inspiration = I								
	Pain on expiration = E								
Difficulty breathing	Sleep with (_____) pillows								
	Difficulty on exertion								
	Difficulty during stress								
	Difficulty when resting								
Appetite **Poor** 10 — **Decreased** 5 — **Normal** 1									
Other									

*Please bring this record with you to your next appointment.
Use the back of this sheet for additional information.

DRUG CLASS: Potassium Iodide

SSKI

Actions

Potassium iodide acts as an expectorant by stimulating increased secretions from the bronchial glands to decrease the viscosity of mucous plugs, making it easier for patients to cough up the dry, hardened plugs blocking the bronchial tubes.

Uses

Potassium iodide is used in the symptomatic treatment of chronic pulmonary diseases, such as bronchial asthma, bronchitis, and pulmonary emphysema in which tenacious mucus is present. It is often used in combination with bronchodilators, sympathomimetic amines, and antitussives for more effective removal of mucus.

Therapeutic Outcomes

The primary therapeutic outcome expected from iodide therapy is reduction of mucus viscosity, allowing a more productive cough to remove accumulated phlegm.

Nursing Process for Potassium Iodide

Premedication Assessment

1. Record characteristics of cough before initiating therapy.
2. Ask if the patient is pregnant before administration. Excessive use of iodine-containing products may result in goiter in the newborn.

Planning

Availability. PO: 1 g/mL solution in 30, 240, and 480 mL containers. Syrup: 325 mg/5 mL in 480 mL containers.

Dosage and Administration. *Adult:* PO: Solution: 0.3 mL (300 mg) to 0.6 mL (600 mg) diluted in one glassful of water, fruit juice, or milk three or four times daily. Syrup: 5 to 10 mL three times daily. Take with food to minimize gastric irritation.

Fluid Intake. Maintain fluid intake of eight to twelve 8-ounce glasses of water daily.

Humidification. Suggest the concurrent use of a humidifier.

Thyroid Function Tests. Long-term use may induce goiter, particularly in children with cystic fibrosis. Always inform the health care provider of the use of this product if thyroid function tests are to be scheduled.

Evaluation

Side Effects to Expect

Nausea, Vomiting, Diarrhea. Symptoms are usually mild. Take with food or milk to minimize gastric irritation. If symptoms become bothersome, report them to the health care provider.

Drug Interactions

Potassium Supplements, Salt Substitutes, Potassium-Sparing Diuretics. DO NOT administer with potassium-sparing diuretics (e.g., amiloride, triamterene, spironolactone). Do not use potassium supplements or salt substitutes high in potassium because of potentially dangerous effects from hyperkalemia.

Lithium, Antithyroid Agents. Concurrent use with lithium and antithyroid medications (e.g., methimazole, propylthiouracil) may result in hypothyroidism.

DRUG CLASS: Saline Solutions

Actions

Saline solutions act by hydrating mucus, reducing its viscosity.

Uses

Saline solutions of varying concentrations can be effective expectorants when administered by nebulization. When administered by inhalation, hypotonic solutions (0.4%, 0.65% sodium chloride) are thought to provide deeper penetration into the more distant airways: a hypertonic solution (1.8% sodium chloride) hydrates and stimulates a productive cough by irritating the respiratory passages. Isotonic saline solutions (0.9% sodium chloride) administered by nebulization are used to hydrate respiratory secretions.

Saline nose drops are sometimes ordered for patients experiencing nasal congestion secondary to low humidity to clear the nasal passage and aid in breathing.

Therapeutic Outcomes

The primary therapeutic outcomes expected from nasal and respiratory saline therapy are moisturized mucous membranes for less irritation from dryness and a more productive coughing because of less viscous mucus.

Nursing Process for Saline Therapy

Premedication Assessment

Record characteristics of cough before initiating therapy.

DRUG CLASS: Antitussive Agents

Actions

Antitussive agents (cough suppressants) act by suppressing the cough center in the brain.

Uses

Antitussive agents are used when the patient has a bothersome dry, hacking, nonproductive cough. These agents will not stop the cough completely but should decrease its frequency and suppress the severe spasms that prevent adequate rest at night. Under normal circumstances it is not appropriate to suppress a productive cough.

Codeine is an effective cough suppressant and the standard against which other antitussive agents are compared. In the relatively low doses and short duration used to suppress cough, addiction is not a problem; dependence may develop, however, after long-term continuous use. Codeine should not be used in patients with chronic pulmonary disease who may have respiratory depression or in patients who have a documented allergy to codeine (rash, pruritus).

Dextromethorphan is almost as effective a cough suppressant as codeine. It does not cause respiratory depression or addiction and is usually the drug of choice for cough suppression in children. Allergy is very rare.

Diphenhydramine is an anticholinergic agent with both antihistaminic and antitussive properties. As with most other antihistamines, diphenhydramine has significant sedative properties. This is often detrimental during the day, especially if the person must be mentally alert, but it is an excellent agent to suppress cough during sleep. Like other anticholinergic agents, diphenhydramine should not be taken by patients with closed-angle glaucoma or prostatic hyperplasia. It also may cause mucus to dry, making it more viscous, especially if the patient is not well hydrated. In addition, it should be used cautiously with other central nervous system (CNS) depressants, such as sedatives, hypnotics, alcohol, or antidepressants.

Therapeutic Outcomes

The primary therapeutic outcome expected from antitussive therapy is reduced frequency of nonproductive cough.

Nursing Process for Antitussive Therapy

Premedication Assessment

Record characteristics of cough before initiating therapy.

Planning

Availability. See Table 31-4.

Implementation

Dosage and Administration. See Table 31-4.

Evaluation

Side Effects to Expect

Drowsiness, Constipation. All the antitussive agents cause some sedation, but diphenhydramine has the most sedative effect. Caution patients about being alert and operating machinery.

Codeine is the most constipating of the antitussive agents. This effect can be minimized by keeping the patient well hydrated and by the use of bulk stool softeners if the patient requires more than 1 or 2 days of codeine therapy.

Drug Interactions

CNS Depressants. The following drugs may enhance the depressant effects of antitussive agents: phenothiazines, antidepressants, sedative-hypnotics, antihistamines, and alcohol.

DRUG CLASS: Mucolytic Agents

acetylcysteine (a see til cist' een)
MUCOMYST (mu' co mist)

Actions

Acetylcysteine acts by dissolving chemical bonds within the mucus itself, causing it to separate and liquefy, thereby reducing viscosity.

Uses

Acetylcysteine is used to dissolve abnormally viscous mucus that may occur in chronic emphysema, emphysema with bronchitis, asthmatic bronchitis, and pneumonia. The reduced viscosity allows easier removal of secretions by coughing, percussion, and postural

Drug Table 31-4 ANTITUSSIVE AGENTS

GENERIC NAME	BRAND NAME	AVAILABILITY	ADULT ORAL DOSAGE RANGE
benzonatate	Tessalon Perles	Capsules: 100, 200 mg	100 mg three times daily
codeine*		Tablets: 15, 30, 60 mg	10-20 mg q4-6h
dextromethorphan	Robitussin CoughGels, Delsym, Benylin Adult	Lozenges: 5, 7.5, 10, 15 mg Syrup: 7.5, 10 mg/5 mL Liquid: 5, 7.5, 10, 15 mg/5 mL Gelcaps: 15, 30 mg	10-30 mg q4-8h; do not exceed 60-120 mg/24 hr
diphenhydramine	Diphen, Tusstat	Syrup: 12.5 mg/5 mL Capsules and tablets: 25, 50 mg	25 mg q4h; do not exceed 150 mg/24 hr
hydrocodone*			5 mg q4-6h

*Often an ingredient in combination antitussive products.

drainage. Acetylcysteine is also used to treat acetaminophen toxicity.

Therapeutic Outcomes

The primary therapeutic outcome expected from acetylcysteine therapy is improved airway flow with more comfortable breathing.

Nursing Process for Acetylcysteine Therapy

Premedication Assessment

1. Record the characteristics of cough and bronchial secretions before starting therapy.
2. Obtain and record baseline vital signs.
3. Observe for and record any gastrointestinal symptoms before starting therapy.
4. Perform a baseline assessment of the patient's mental status (e.g., degree of anxiety, nervousness, alertness).

Planning

Availability. Inhalation: 10% and 20% solutions in 4, 10, 30, and 100 mL vials.

Implementation

Dosage and Administration. *Adult:* Inhalation: The recommended dosage for most patients is 3 to 5 mL of the 20% solution three or four times daily. It may be administered by nebulization, direct application, or by intratracheal instillation.

After administration, the volume of bronchial secretions may increase. Some patients with inadequate cough reflex may require mechanical suctioning to maintain an open airway.

Nebulizer. This solution tends to concentrate as the solution is used. When three fourths of the original amount in the nebulizer is used, dilute the remaining solution with sterile water.

After therapy, wash the patient's face and hands because the drug is sticky and irritating. Thoroughly cleanse equipment used.

Storage. Store the opened solution of the drug in a refrigerator for up to 96 hours. Discard the unused portion.

Discoloration. Use medication stored only in plastic or glass containers. Contact with metals other than stainless steel can cause the solution to discolor.

Evaluation

Side Effects to Expect

Nausea, Vomiting. Acetylcysteine has a pungent odor (similar to rotten eggs) that may cause nausea and vomiting; have an emesis basin available. Do not, however, suggest it by having the basin in clear view.

Side Effects to Report

Bronchospasm. Acetylcysteine may occasionally cause bronchoconstriction and bronchospasm. Concurrent use of a bronchodilator may be necessary.

Drug Interactions

Antibiotics. Acetylcysteine inactivates most antibiotics. Do not mix together for aerosol administration. Schedule administration of inhalation antibiotics 1 hour after administration of acetylcysteine.

DRUG CLASS: Beta-Adrenergic Bronchodilating Agents

Actions

The beta-adrenergic agonists stimulate the beta receptors within the smooth muscle of the tracheobronchial tree to relax, thereby opening the airway passages to greater volumes of air.

Uses

Beta-adrenergic bronchodilators are now the mainstay of all asthma therapy. They are used to reverse airway constriction caused by acute and chronic bronchial asthma, bronchitis, and emphysema. Those agents with more selective beta-2 receptor activity (e.g., albuterol, terbutaline) have more direct bronchodilating activity with fewer systemic side effects. (See Chapter 13 for a discussion of selective beta receptor activity.)

Unfortunately the receptors stimulated by sympathomimetic agents, causing relaxation of the smooth muscle in the tracheobronchial tree, are found in other tissues as well as the pulmonary system. The receptors are also found in the muscles of the heart, blood vessels, uterus, and gastrointestinal, urinary, and central nervous systems. They also help regulate fat and carbohydrate metabolism. For this reason, there are many side effects from these agents, particularly if used too frequently or in higher than recommended doses. Those administered by inhalation generally have fewer systemic effects because inhalation places the drug at the site of action so that smaller dosages may be used.

The short-acting beta agonists (e.g., albuterol, levalbuterol, pirbuterol, terbutaline, metaproterenol) have a rapid onset (a few minutes) and are used to treat acute bronchospasm. During acute exacerbations, these agents can be used every 3 to 4 hours. If a patient is using an increased amount of these inhaled bronchodilators on a daily basis, it is an indication of worsening asthma. Patients then must be reassessed for adherence, inhalation technique, improved environmental control, and the possible addition of corticosteroids to the therapeutic regimen.

Salmeterol and formoterol are long-acting forms of inhaled bronchodilators, sometimes known as long-acting beta agonists (LABA). They are not to be used for acute episodes but for patients with nocturnal asthma and for those who wheeze with exercise. The onset of action is 15 to 30 minutes, but the duration of action is up to 12 hours. Therefore they are used to prevent acute exacerbations of asthma. There is concern that although LABAs decrease the frequency of asthmatic attacks, they may actually make the attacks that do occur more severe.

Patients known to have hypertension, hyperthyroidism, diabetes mellitus, or cardiac disease with dysrhythmias may be particularly sensitive to adverse reactions and must be observed closely.

Therapeutic Outcomes

The primary therapeutic outcome associated with beta adrenergic bronchodilator therapy is easier breathing with reduced wheezing.

Nursing Process for Beta-Adrenergic Bronchodilators

Premedication Assessment

1. Obtain and record baseline vital signs.
2. Assess for the presence of palpitations and dysrhythmias before administration of beta adrenergic agents. If suspected, notify the health care provider and ask whether therapy should be started.
3. Perform an assessment of the patient's baseline mental status (e.g., degree of anxiety, nervousness, alertness).

Planning

Availability. See Table 31-5.

Implementation

Dosage and Administration. See Table 31-5. Patients using inhaled bronchodilators should wait approximately 10 minutes between inhalations. This allows the medicine to dilate the bronchioles so that the second dose can be inhaled more deeply into the lungs for more therapeutic effect.

Make sure that patients understand how to use the inhaler as described in the manufacturer's leaflet for the patient.

Evaluation

Side Effects to Report

Tachycardia, Palpitations. Because most symptoms are dose related, alterations should be reported to the health care provider. Monitor the patient's heart rate and rhythm at regular intervals throughout therapy with bronchodilators. An increase of 20 beats or more per minute after treatment should be reported to the health care provider. Always report palpitations and suspected dysrhythmias.

Tremors. Tell the patient to notify the health care provider if tremors develop after starting any of these medications. A dosage adjustment may be necessary.

Nervousness, Anxiety, Restlessness, Headache. Perform a baseline assessment of the patient's mental status (e.g., degree of anxiety, nervousness, alertness); compare subsequent, regular assessments to the findings obtained. Report escalation of tension.

Nausea, Vomiting. Monitor all aspects of the development of these symptoms. Question the patient concerning other medications being taken and any other symptoms that have also developed. Administer the medication with food and a full glass of water or milk. Report if the symptoms are not relieved.

Dizziness. Provide for patient safety during episodes of dizziness. Report for further evaluation.

Drug Interactions

Drugs That Enhance Toxic Effects. Ticlopidine, tricyclic antidepressants (e.g., imipramine, amitriptyline, nortriptyline, doxepin), monoamine oxidase inhibitors (e.g., tranylcypromine, pargyline), and other sympathomimetic agents (e.g., metaproterenol, isoproterenol) enhance the toxic effects of beta-adrenergic bronchodilators. Monitor for increases in severity of drug effects, such as nervousness, tachycardia, tremors, and dysrhythmias.

Drugs That Reduce Therapeutic Effects. Beta-adrenergic blocking agents (e.g., propranolol, timolol, nadolol, pindolol) reduce the therapeutic effects of beta-adrenergic bronchodilators. Higher dosages or use of another class of bronchodilator may be required.

Antihypertensive Agents. Sympathomimetic agents may reduce the therapeutic effects of antihypertensive agents. Monitor blood pressure for an indication of loss of antihypertensive control.

DRUG CLASS: Anticholinergic Bronchodilating Agents

Anticholinergic agents have been used as bronchodilators in treating obstructive pulmonary disease for more than 200 years, but the potent anticholinergic adverse effects (throat irritation, dry mouth, reduced mucous secretions, increased secretion viscosity, mydriasis, cycloplegia, urinary retention, tachycardia) and the availability of selective sympathomimetic agents have limited their use in pulmonary disorders.

ipratropium bromide (ihp rah trop' eum)
- ATROVENT (at' roh vent)
- ATROVENT HFA

Actions

Ipratropium bromide is administered by aerosol inhalation and produces bronchodilation by competitive inhibition of cholinergic receptors on bronchial smooth muscle. It has minimal effect on ciliary activity, mucus secretion, sputum volume, and viscosity.

Uses

Ipratropium is used as a bronchodilator for long-term treatment of reversible bronchospasm associated with COPD. It may also be used in combination with beta adrenergic bronchodilators in patients with asthma. Initial bronchodilation is evident within the first few minutes after inhalation, but maximal effects are seen in 1 to 2 hours. The duration of significant bronchodilation

Drug Table 31-5 BRONCHODILATORS

GENERIC NAME	BRAND NAME	AVAILABILITY	ADULT DOSAGE RANGE
BETA-ADRENERGIC AGONISTS			
albuterol	Proventil, Ventolin, Volmax	Tablets: 2, 4 mg Aerosol: 90 mcg Syrup: 2 mg/5 mL Tablets, extended release: 4, 8 mg Solution for inhalation	PO: 2-4 mg three or four times daily Inhale: two inhalations q4-6h See manufacturer's recommendations
bitolterol	Tornalate	Solution for inhalation	See manufacturer's recommendations
ephedrine		Capsules: 25 mg Injection: 50 mg/mL	PO: 25-50 mg q3-4h Subcutaneous, IM, IV: 25-50 mg
epinephrine	Primatene Mist	Nebulization: 1:100 Aerosol: 0.2 mg Injection: 0.1, 1 mg/mL	See manufacturer's recommendations
formoterol	Foradil	Inhaler capsule: 12 mcg	Inhale: using aerolizer inhaler, 1 capsule q12h
isoetharine		Solution for inhalation: 1%	See manufacturer's recommendations
isoproterenol	Isuprel	Injection: 0.02, 0.2 mg/mL	See manufacturer's recommendations
levalbuterol	Xopenex Xopenex HFA	Solution for inhalation Aerosol: 45 mcg/puff	See manufacturer's recommendations Inhale: 1-2 inhalations q4-6h
metaproterenol	Alupent	Aerosol: 0.65 mg/puff Nebulization: 0.4%, 0.6%, 5%	See manufacturer's recommendations
pirbuterol	Maxair	Aerosol: 0.2 mg/puff	Inhale: 1-2 inhalations q4-6h
salmeterol	Serevent Diskus	Inhalation powder: 50 mcg	Inhale: 1 inhalation q12h
terbutaline	Brethine	Tablets: 2.5, 5 mg Injection: 1 mg/mL	PO: 5 mg q6h Subcutaneous: 0.25 mg; repeat, if needed, in 30 min
XANTHINE DERIVATIVES			
aminophylline		Tablets: 100, 200 mg Liquid: 105 mg/5 mL Suppositories: 250, 500 mg Injection: 250 mg/10 mL	See manufacturer's recommendations
dyphylline	Dilor, Lufyllin	Tablets: 200, 400 mg Elixir: 100, 160 mg/15 mL Injection: 250 mg/mL	PO: 15 mg/kg, five times daily IM: 250-500 mg slowly
oxtriphylline		Tablets: 100, 200 mg Elixir: 100 mg/5 mL	200 mg four times daily
theophylline	Bronkodyl, Elixophyllin, Theolair, others	Tablets: 100, 125, 200, 300 mg Capsules: 100, 200 mg Elixir: 26.7 mg/5 mL Syrup: 50 mg/5 mL Tablets, extended release: 100, 200, 300 mg Capsules, timed release: 100, 200, 300 mg	9-20 mg/kg/24 hr in four divided doses

is 4 to 6 hours with usual dosages. Because its maximal effects are not seen immediately, the drug is more appropriately used for prophylaxis and maintenance treatment of bronchospasm associated with chronic obstructive lung disease than for acute episodes of bronchospasm associated with asthma.

Ipratropium nasal spray is used for the symptomatic relief of rhinorrhea associated with allergic and nonallergic perennial rhinitis and the common cold. It does not relieve nasal congestion, sneezing, or postnasal drip associated with these conditions.

Therapeutic Outcomes

The primary therapeutic outcomes associated with ipratropium therapy are easier breathing with less effort when the inhaler is used and reduced rhinorrhea when the nasal solution is used.

Nursing Process for Ipratropium

Premedication Assessment

1. Record baseline vital signs.
2. Check the medical record to determine whether the patient has a history of closed-angle glaucoma. If so, reconfirm the administration order with the health care provider before administration of ipratropium.

Planning

Availability. Inhalation: Aerosol canister containing approximately 200 inhalations (18 mcg/metered dose) with metered-dose inhaler mouthpiece. Nasal spray: 0.03% (21 mcg/spray) (30 mL) and 0.06% (42 mcg/spray) (15 mL) nasal spray pumps.

Implementation

NOTE: Ipratropium bromide should not be used in the initial treatment of acute episodes of bronchospasm in which rapid response is required. Use with caution in patients with the potential for closed-angle glaucoma.

Dosage and Administration. Inhalation: The usual dose is two inhalations (36 mcg) four times per day. Patients may take additional inhalations as required but should not exceed 12 inhalations in 24 hours.

Ensure that the patient understands how to inhale the medication:

1. Clear the throat and mouth of sputum.
2. Insert the metal canister into the clear end of the mouthpiece.
3. Remove the protective cap, invert the canister, and shake thoroughly.
4. Enclose the mouthpiece with the lips. The base of the canister should be held vertically. (Keep the eyes closed because temporary blurred vision may result if the aerosol is sprayed into the eyes.)
5. Exhale deeply through the mouth or nose, then inhale slowly through the mouthpiece and at the same time firmly press once on the upended canister base; continue to inhale deeply.
6. Hold breath for a few seconds, then remove the mouthpiece from the mouth and exhale slowly. Wait approximately 15 seconds, and repeat the second inhalation as outlined in steps 4 and 5.
7. Replace the protective cap after use.
8. Keep the mouthpiece clean. Wash with hot water. If soap is used, rinse thoroughly with plain water.

Nasal spray: Rhinorrhea secondary to allergic and nonallergic perennial rhinitis: Two sprays (42 mcg) of 0.3% solution in each nostril two or three times daily. Rhinorrhea secondary to the common cold: Two sprays (84 mcg) of 0.6% solution in each nostril three or four times daily.

Ensure that the patient understands how to prime and use the pump as described in the manufacturer's leaflet.

Evaluation

Side Effects to Expect

Mouth Dryness, Throat Irritation. These side effects are usually mild and tend to resolve with continued therapy. Encourage the patient not to discontinue therapy without first consulting the health care provider.

Ensure that regular oral hygiene measures are continued. Suggest the use of 1 teaspoon of hydrogen peroxide in 6 to 8 ounces of water as a mouthwash. Commercial mouthwashes contain alcohol, which may cause further drying and oral irritation.

Other measures to alleviate dryness include sucking on ice chips or hard candy.

Side Effects to Report

Tachycardia, Urinary Retention, Exacerbation of Pulmonary Symptoms. Instruct the patient to consult a health care provider before continuing with further therapy.

Drug Interactions. No significant interactions have been reported.

tiotropium bromide (ti oh trop′ eum)
SPIRIVA (spy ree′ vah)

Actions

Tiotropium is administered by dry powder inhalation and produces bronchodilation by competitive inhibition of cholinergic receptors on bronchial smooth muscle. It is similar in action to ipratropium, but much longer in duration of action. It has minimal effect on ciliary activity, mucus secretion, sputum volume, and viscosity.

Uses

Tiotroprium is used as a once-daily bronchodilator for long-term treatment of reversible bronchospasm associated with COPD, including bronchitis and emphysema. The bronchodilating effect of the drug does not happen immediately, so it is more appropriately used for maintenance treatment of bronchospasm associated with COPD.

It should not be used as rescue medicine in acute episodes of bronchospasm.

Therapeutic Outcomes

The primary therapeutic outcome associated with tiotropium therapy is easier breathing with less effort.

Nursing Process for Tiotropium

Premedication Assessment

1. Record baseline vital signs.
2. Check the medical record to determine whether the patient has a history of closed-angle glaucoma. If so, reconfirm the administration order with the health care provider before administration of tiotropium.

Planning

Availability. Inhalation: 18 mcg capsules for use in supplied HandiHaler.

Implementation

NOTE: Use with caution in patients with the potential for closed-angle glaucoma, prostatic hyperplasia, or bladder neck obstruction.

Dosage and Administration. Inhalation: The usual dose is one capsule daily administered through the HandiHaler inhaler device.

Ensure that the patient understands how to inhale the medication:

1. Open the dust cover of the inhaler and then open the mouthpiece.
2. Place a capsule in the center chamber.
3. Close the mouthpiece firmly until you hear a click, leaving the dustcover open.
4. Hold the HandiHaler device with the mouthpiece upward and press the piercing button completely in once, and release. This makes holes in the capsule and allows the medication to be released when you breathe in.
5. Clear the throat and mouth of sputum.
6. Breathe out completely. Do not breathe into the mouthpiece at any time.
7. Raise the HandiHaler device to your mouth and close your lips tightly around the mouthpiece.
8. Keep your head in an upright position and breathe in slowly and deeply but at a rate sufficient to hear the capsule vibrate. Breathe in until your lungs are full; then hold your breath as long as is comfortable, and at the same time take the HandiHaler device out of your mouth.
9. Resume normal breathing.
10. After you have finished taking your daily dose, open the mouthpiece again. Tip out the used capsule and dispose of it.
11. Keep the mouthpiece clean. Wash with hot water. If soap is used, rinse thoroughly with plain water.

Evaluation

Side Effects to Expect

Mouth Dryness, Throat Irritation. These side effects are usually mild and tend to resolve with continued therapy. Encourage the patient not to discontinue therapy without first consulting the health care provider.

Other measures to alleviate dryness include sucking on ice chips or hard candy.

Side Effects to Report

Tachycardia, Urinary Retention, Exacerbation of Pulmonary Symptoms. Instruct the patient to consult a health care provider before continuing with further therapy.

Drug Interactions. No significant interactions have been reported.

DRUG CLASS: Xanthine-Derivative Bronchodilating Agents

Actions

Methylxanthines, more commonly known as xanthine derivatives, act directly on the smooth muscle of the tracheobronchial tree to dilate the bronchi, thus increasing airflow in and out of the alveolar sacs.

Uses

Xanthine-derivative bronchodilators are used in combination with sympathomimetic bronchodilators to reverse airway constriction caused by acute and chronic bronchial asthma, bronchitis, and emphysema.

Therapeutic Outcomes

The primary therapeutic outcome associated with xanthine-derivative bronchodilator therapy is easier breathing with less effort.

Nursing Process for Xanthine-Derivative Bronchodilators

Premedication Assessment

1. Check the patient's history for diagnoses of angina pectoris, peptic ulcer disease, hyperthyroidism, glaucoma, or diabetes mellitus.
2. Obtain and record baseline vital signs.
3. Perform baseline assessment of the patient's mental status (e.g., degree of anxiety present, nervousness, alertness).

Planning

Availability. See Table 31-5.

Implementation

Dosage and Administration. See Table 31-5.

Plasma Levels. To maintain consistent plasma levels, administer the medication around the clock.

Evaluation

Side Effects to Expect

Nausea, Vomiting, Epigastric Pain, Abdominal Cramps. These symptoms may occur from irritation caused by increased gastric acid secretions stimulated by these agents. If gastric irritation occurs, administer with food or milk. If symptoms persist or increase in severity, report for health care provider evaluation.

Side Effects to Report

Tachycardia, Palpitations. Because most symptoms are dose related, alterations should be reported to the health care provider. Monitor the patient's heart rate and rhythm at regular intervals throughout therapy with bronchodilators.

Report heart rates significantly higher than baseline values. Always report palpitations and suspected dysrhythmias.

Tremors. Tell the patient to notify the health care provider if tremors develop after starting any of these medications. A dosage adjustment may be necessary.

Nervousness, Anxiety, Restlessness, Headache. Perform a baseline assessment of the patient's mental status (e.g., degree of anxiety, nervousness, alertness); compare subsequent, regular assessments to the findings obtained. Report escalation of tension.

Drug Interactions

Drugs That Enhance Toxic Effects. Cimetidine, erythromycin, diltiazem, nifedipine, verapamil, moricizine, thiabendazole, influenza vaccine, propranolol, zileuton, and allopurinol all enhance the toxic effects of xanthine derivatives. Monitor for increases in severity of drug effects, such as nervousness, agitation, nausea, tachycardia, and dysrhythmias.

Drugs That Reduce Therapeutic Effects. Tobacco or marijuana smoking reduces the therapeutic effects of xanthine derivatives. Increased dosage of the bronchodilator may be required.

Lithium. Xanthine derivatives may increase the renal excretion of lithium carbonate. Increased dosage of lithium is required to maintain therapeutic effects. Monitor for the return of manic or depressive activity. Enlist the aid of family and friends to help identify early symptoms.

Beta-Adrenergic Blocking Agents. Xanthine derivatives and beta-adrenergic blocking agents (e.g., propranolol, timolol, nadolol, atenolol) may have mutually antagonistic actions. Patients must be observed for inhibition of either drug.

DRUG CLASS: Respiratory Antiinflammatory Agents

Corticosteroids Used for Obstructive Airway Disease

Actions

Corticosteroids (see Drugs Affecting the Immune System in Chapter 38), whether applied by aerosol or administered systemically, have been shown to be highly effective in treating obstructive lung disease. The mechanisms of action are not completely known, but corticosteroids have a direct effect on smooth muscle relaxation; they enhance the effect of beta adrenergic bronchodilators and inhibit inflammatory responses that may result in bronchoconstriction.

Uses

Patients with severe asthma or COPD who are unresponsive to sympathomimetic agents or xanthine derivatives may have corticosteroids added to the medication regimen to provide enhanced bronchodilation.

The first course of therapy is often a short course (5 to 7 days) of systemic corticosteroids (e.g., prednisone), with intervals of several weeks or months without steroid treatment. Alternate-day therapy (a single dose every other morning) is the next preferable program. Aerosolized corticosteroids may be used daily by certain patients instead of alternate-day therapy. If the patient has not previously been receiving corticosteroid therapy, several weeks may pass before the full benefits from the aerosolized medication are achieved, but a single aerosol "burst" does produce noticeable benefits in reducing bronchoconstriction. It is important to remember that corticosteroid aerosols should not be regarded as true bronchodilators and should not be used for rapid relief of bronchospasm. (See Chapter 30 for the use of intranasal corticosteroids.)

Therapeutic Outcomes

The primary therapeutic outcome associated with corticosteroid therapy is easier breathing with less effort.

Nursing Process for Corticosteroids

Premedication Assessment

Inspect the oral cavity for the presence of any type of infection.

Planning

Availability. See Table 31-6.

Implementation

Dosage and Administration

Counseling, Adherence. The therapeutic effects, unlike those of sympathomimetic bronchodilators, are not immediate. This should be explained to the patient in advance to ensure cooperation and continuation of treatment with the prescribed dosage regimen, even when the patient is asymptomatic. Full therapeutic benefit requires regular use and may require up to 4 weeks of therapy for maximum benefit.

Preparation before Administration. Patients receiving bronchodilators by inhalation should be advised to use the bronchodilator before the corticosteroid inhalant to enhance penetration of the corticosteroid into the bronchial tree. Wait several

Drug Table 31-6 INHALANT CORTICOSTEROIDS

GENERIC NAME	BRAND NAME	AVAILABILITY	ADULT DOSAGE RANGE
INHALANT CORTICOSTEROIDS			
beclomethasone dipropionate	QVAR	Aerosol: 40 and 80 mcg/actuation; 100 doses/inhaler	One or two inhalations (80 mcg) three to four times daily; maximum of 640 mcg (15 inhalations) daily
budesonide phosphate	Pulmicort Turbuhaler	Aerosol: 200 doses/inhaler	One or two inhalations twice daily; maximum four inhalations twice daily
flunisolide	AeroBid	Aerosol: 100 doses/inhaler	Two inhalations (500 mcg) twice daily; do not exceed 2 mg (eight inhalations) daily
fluticasone	Flovent HFA Flovent Diskus Flovent Rotadisk	Aerosol: 44, 110, 220 mcg/dose Powder: 50, 100, 250 mcg Powder: 50, 100, 250 mg	100-250 mg twice daily; maximum 500 mcg twice daily
mometasone furoate	Asmanex Twisthaler	Powder: 200 mcg/dose	One or two inhalations once daily. Maximum of two doses daily.
triamcinolone acetonide	Azmacort	Aerosol: 240 doses/inhaler	Two inhalations (200 mcg) three to four times daily; do not exceed 1600 mcg (16 inhalations) daily
INHALANT CORTICOSTEROID–BETA-ADRENERGIC BRONCHODILATOR			
fluticasone-salmeterol	Advair Diskus	Powder 100 mcg fluticasone 50 mcg salmeterol 250 mcg fluticasone 50 mcg salmeterol 500 mcg fluticasone 50 mcg salmeterol	One inhalation twice daily for maintenance therapy on a regularly scheduled basis. Not for acute bronchospasm.

minutes before the corticosteroid is inhaled to allow time for the bronchodilator to relax the smooth muscle.

Maintenance Therapy. After the desired clinical effect is obtained, the maintenance dose should be reduced to the smallest amount necessary to control symptoms.

Severe Stress or Asthma Attack. During periods of stress or a severe asthma attack, patients may require treatment with systemic steroids. Exacerbation of asthma that occurs during the course of corticosteroid inhalant therapy should be treated with a short course of systemic steroid. Instruct patients not to use the inhaler because the aerosol not only may cause irritation and exacerbate symptoms but also may not penetrate deeply into the bronchial tree for maximal effect.

Evaluation

Side Effects to Expect

Hoarseness, Dry Mouth. Hoarseness and dry mouth are usually mild and tend to resolve with continued therapy. Encourage the patient not to discontinue therapy without first consulting the health care provider.

Side Effects to Report

Fungal Infections (Thrush). Increased risk factors for the development of oral thrush include concomitant antibiotic use, diabetes, improper aerosol administration, large oral doses of corticosteroids, and poor dental hygiene.

Patients should be instructed on good oral hygiene technique and told to gargle and rinse the mouth after each aerosol treatment with a mouthwash, such as 1 teaspoon of hydrogen peroxide in 6 to 8 ounces of water. Commercial mouthwashes contain alcohol, which may cause further drying and oral irritation.

If thrush develops, it is usually not sufficiently troublesome to require discontinuing steroid aerosol therapy. An antifungal mouthwash such as nystatin (Mycostatin, Nilstat) will generally eradicate the oral candidiasis.

Drug Interactions. No significant drug interactions have been reported.

DRUG CLASS: Antileukotriene Agents

When inflammatory cells are triggered by irritants such as smoke, allergens, or viruses, the phospholipid membrane of the epithelial lining of the airways is disrupted, causing a series of chemical reactions from arachidonic acid that releases leukotrienes, prostaglandins, thromboxanes, and eicosanoids. The leukotrienes produced cause many of the signs and symptoms of asthma, such as bronchoconstriction, vascular permeability leading to edema, and mucus hypersecretion.

montelukast (mon teh lu' cast)
SINGULAIR (sing' yu lair')

Actions

Montelukast is a selective and competitive receptor antagonist of the cysteinyl leukotriene receptor. This is the receptor that leukotriene D_4 stimulates to trigger symptoms of asthma.

Uses

Montelukast is approved for use in conjunction with other medications in the prophylaxis and chronic treatment of asthma. It has been shown to reduce early and late-phase bronchoconstriction, bronchial hyperresponsiveness, daytime asthma symptoms, and nighttime awakening; reduce beta-adrenergic agonist use; and improve pulmonary function tests. The NAEPP recommends antileukotriene agents as alternatives to low-dose inhaled corticosteroids in mild persistent asthma and with low to medium doses of inhaled corticosteroids in moderate persistent asthma.

Montelukast is not a bronchodilator, and it should not be used to treat acute episodes of asthma. However, treatment with montelukast can be continued during acute exacerbations of asthma. Montelukast use should be continual, even during acute asthma exacerbations and symptom-free periods.

Therapeutic Outcomes

The primary therapeutic outcome associated with montelukast therapy is fewer episodes of acute asthmatic symptoms.

Nursing Process for Montelukast

Premedication Assessment

Obtain and record baseline vital signs and pulmonary function tests.

Planning

Availability. 5 and 10 mg tablets; 4 mg chewable tablets; 4 mg granules.

Implementation

Dosage and Administration. *Adult:* PO: 10 mg taken once daily in the evening. Doses greater than 10 mg appear to be of no value. Continue other therapy for asthma as prescribed.

Evaluation

Side Effects to Expect

Headache, Nausea, Dyspepsia. These symptoms are usually mild and disappear with continued therapy. Administration with food or milk may help minimize discomfort. Encourage the patient not to discontinue therapy without first consulting a health care provider.

Drug Interactions. No clinically significant drug interactions have been reported.

zafirlukast (zaf ihr′ lu cast)
▶ ACCOLATE (ak′ oh late)

Actions

Zafirlukast is the first leukotriene receptor antagonist to be introduced in the treatment of asthma. Zafirlukast is a selective and competitive receptor antagonist of the cysteinyl leukotriene receptor. This is the receptor that leukotrienes D_4 and E_4 stimulate to trigger symptoms of asthma.

Uses

Zafirlukast is approved for use in conjunction with other medications in the prophylaxis and long-term treatment of asthma. It has been shown to reduce early and late-phase bronchoconstriction, bronchial hyperresponsiveness, daytime asthma symptoms, and nighttime awakening; reduce beta-adrenergic agonist use; and improve pulmonary function tests. The NAEPP recommends antileukotriene agents as alternatives to low-dose inhaled corticosteroids in mild persistent asthma and with low to medium doses of inhaled corticosteroids in moderate persistent asthma.

Zafirlukast is not a bronchodilator, and it should not be used to treat acute episodes of asthma. However, treatment with zafirlukast can be continued during acute exacerbations of asthma. Zafirlukast use should be continual, even during acute asthma exacerbations and symptom-free periods.

Therapeutic Outcomes

The primary therapeutic outcome associated with zafirlukast therapy is fewer episodes of acute asthmatic symptoms.

Nursing Process for Zafirlukast

Premedication Assessment

Obtain and record baseline vital signs and pulmonary function tests.

Planning

Availability. 20 mg tablets.

Implementation

Dosage and Administration. *Adult:* PO: 20 mg twice daily. Continue other therapy for asthma as prescribed.

Evaluation

Side Effects to Expect

Headache, Nausea. Headache and nausea are usually mild and disappear with continued therapy. Administration with food or milk may help minimize discomfort. Encourage the patient not to discontinue therapy without first consulting a health care provider.

Drug Interactions

Aspirin. Aspirin significantly increases the activity of zafirlukast. If concurrent therapy is required with aspirin, the initial dosage of zafirlukast should be started at half the normal dose. Monitor for therapeutic and toxic effects (e.g., headache, nausea).

Warfarin. Zafirlukast increases the activity of warfarin. If concurrent therapy is required with warfarin, the initial dosage should be started at half the normal dose. Monitor the International Normalized Ratio (INR) for warfarin therapy.

Theophylline, Erythromycin. Theophylline and erythromycin decrease the activity of zafirlukast. The dosage of zafirlukast may need to be increased for therapeutic effect.

DRUG CLASS: Immunomodulator Agent

omalizumab (oh mah lis′ u mab)

XOLAIR (zohl air′)

Actions

One of the causes of acute exacerbations of asthma is airborne allergens that trigger an allergic cascade, resulting in airway inflammation and obstruction. In some patients, when allergens enter the body, immunoglobulin E (IgE) antibodies are produced and circulate in the blood. IgE circulating in the blood binds to mast cells, which contain inflammatory chemicals (e.g., histamine, leukotrienes). When exposed to an allergen, IgE on the mast cell triggers the release of these chemicals, thus causing the inflammation, bronchial constriction, and coughing associated with asthma. Omalizumab, a DNA-derived humanized IgG monoclonal antibody, binds to the circulating IgE antibodies in the blood, decreasing the amount of IgE antibodies available to bind to mast cells, thereby inhibiting the mast cell's release of those inflammatory chemicals that can lead to the symptoms of asthma.

Uses

Omalizumab is used in patients who are at least 12 years old, have moderate to severe persistent asthma, have a positive skin reaction to a perennial airborne allergen, and have symptoms that are not adequately controlled with inhaled corticosteroids. Omalizumab decreases the incidence of asthma exacerbations in these patients. Omalizumab does not stop acute exacerbations of asthma and should not be used to treat acute bronchospasm or status asthmaticus. Systemic or inhaled corticosteroids should not be abruptly discontinued when omalizumab is initiated. Reductions in corticosteroid dosage should be very gradual and only under the supervision of a physician. Patients should be counseled that it may take a few weeks before the omalizumab has a noticeable effect on their asthma, so it is important that they continue taking all other asthma medicines unless otherwise instructed by their health care provider.

Therapeutic Outcomes

The primary therapeutic outcome associated with omalizumab therapy is reduced frequency of acute asthmatic exacerbations.

Nursing Process for Omalizumab

Premedication Assessment

1. Review the patient's medication history to ensure that the patient does not have an allergy to omalizumab. If the patient does, inform the charge nurse and the health care provider immediately. Do not administer the medication without specific approval.
2. Review the patient's medical history to ensure that the patient has positive skin reactions to at least one airborne allergen.
3. Before administering the first dose, ensure that serum IgE levels have been measured; this helps determine the dose of omalizumab to be administered. Following administration of omalizumab, serum total IgE levels become elevated because of formation of omalizumab:IgE complexes. Further measurement of serum IgE levels is not necessary because of inaccuracy of data.
4. Obtain and record baseline vital signs and pulmonary function test results.

Planning

Availability. Subcutaneously: 150-mg single-use vials in powder form.

Implementation

Dissolve the Powder

1. Draw 1.4 mL of sterile water for injection, USP into a 3-mL syringe equipped with a 1-inch, 18-gauge needle.
2. Place the vial upright on a flat surface; using standard aseptic technique, insert the needle and inject the sterile water directly onto the powder.
3. Keeping the vial upright, gently swirl the upright vial for approximately 1 minute to evenly wet the powder. DO NOT SHAKE!
4. After completing step 3, gently swirl the vial for 5 to 10 seconds approximately every 5 minutes to dissolve any remaining solids. There should be no visible gelatinous particles in the solution. Some vials may take longer than 20 minutes to dissolve completely. Repeat step 4 until there are no visible gelatinous particles in the solution. It is acceptable to have small bubbles or foam around the edge of the vial. Do not use if the contents of the vial do not dissolve completely within 40 minutes.

5. Invert the vial for 15 seconds to allow the solution to drain toward the stopper. You will note that it is rather viscous. Using a new 3-mL syringe equipped with a 1-inch, 18-gauge needle, insert the needle into the inverted vial. Position the needle tip at the very bottom of the solution in the vial stopper when drawing the solution into the syringe. Before removing the needle from the vial, pull the plunger all the way back to the end of the syringe barrel to remove all of the solution from the inverted vial.
6. Replace the 18-gauge needle with a 25-gauge needle for subcutaneous injection.
7. Expel air, large bubbles, and any excess solution to obtain the required 1.2-mL dose. A thin layer of small bubbles may remain at the top of the solution in the syringe. Because the solution is slightly viscous, the injection may take 5 to 10 seconds to administer.

Dosage and Administration. *12 years and older:* Subcutaneously: 150 to 375 mg every 2 to 4 weeks, based on patient weight and IgE serum level. Doses greater than 150 mg (1.2 mL) should be divided and administered in more than one site. No dosage adjustments are necessary for age, race, ethnicity, or gender.

NOTE: Allergic reactions and anaphylaxis have occurred within 2 hours of the first or subsequent doses. Symptoms include urticaria and throat and/or tongue edema. Patients should be observed after injection of omalizumab, and medications for the treatment of allergic reactions (e.g., oxygen, epinephrine, diphenhydramine) should be available.

Evaluation

Side Effects to Expect and Report

Injection Site Reactions. The most commonly reported adverse effect is injection site reaction (45%), including bruising, redness, warmth, burning, stinging, itching, hive formation, pain, indurations, mass, and inflammation. Most injection site reactions occur within 1 hour after injection, last less than 8 days, and generally decrease in frequency with subsequent dosing. Immediately report a rash or pruritus with or without fever and withhold additional injections until approved by the health care provider.

Drug Interactions. No drug interactions have been reported.

DRUG CLASS: Miscellaneous Antiiinflammatory Agents

cromolyn sodium (kro′ mo lin)
INTAL (in′ tahl)

Actions

Cromolyn sodium is an antiinflammatory agent with an unknown mechanism of action. It inhibits the release of histamine and other mediators of inflammation. It must be administered before the body receives a stimulus to release histamine, such as an antigen that initiates an antigen-antibody allergic reaction.

Uses

Cromolyn is recommended for use in conjunction with other medications in treating patients with severe bronchial asthma or allergic rhinitis to prevent the release of histamine that results in asthmatic attacks or symptoms of allergic rhinitis.

Cromolyn has no direct bronchodilatory, antihistaminic, or anticholinergic activity. The concomitant use of antihistamines or nasal decongestants may be necessary during initial treatment with cromolyn. A 2- to 4-week course of therapy is usually required to determine clinical response. Therapy should be continued only if there is a decrease in the severity of asthmatic symptoms.

Therapeutic Outcomes

The primary therapeutic outcome associated with cromolyn therapy is reduced frequency of episodes of allergic rhinitis and asthmatic attacks.

Nursing Process for Cromolyn

Premedication Assessment

1. This medication must be taken before exposure to the stimulus that initiates an attack of allergic rhinitis or severe bronchial asthma. Inhalation during an attack of bronchospasm or asthma may exacerbate symptoms.
2. Check to see if the concurrent use of antihistamines or nasal decongestants has been ordered by the health care provider, especially during initiation of cromolyn therapy.

Planning

Availability. Inhalation: 20-mg capsules, 20 mg/2 mL solution for nebulizer, and 112 and 200 metered-dose spray aerosols.

Implementation

Dosage and Administration

Counseling. The therapeutic effects, unlike those of beta adrenergic decongestants, are not immediate. This should be explained to the patient in advance to ensure cooperation and continuation of treatment with the prescribed dosage regimen. Full therapeutic benefit requires regular use and is usually evident within 2 to 4 weeks. Therapy must be continued even if the patient is symptom-free.

Adult: PO: Patients must be advised that the capsules are not absorbed when swallowed and that the drug is inactive when administered by this route. Inhalation: 40 mg (two capsules), via inhaler, four times daily. Inhalation during an acute asthma attack may aggravate symptoms because the powder form of the drug can increase the irritation in the respiratory passage and result in more bronchospasm.

Proper technique is important to the success of therapy. Document and verify that the patient can do the following:

1. Load the inhaler with a capsule and pierce (only once) the capsule immediately before use.
2. Hold the inhaler away from the mouth and exhale, emptying as much air from the lungs as possible.
3. With the head tilted back and teeth apart, close lips around the mouthpiece.
4. Inhale deeply and rapidly through the inhaler with a steady, even breath.
5. Remove the inhaler, hold the breath for a few seconds, and then exhale. (Instruct the patient not to exhale through the inhaler because moisture from the breath will interfere with proper function of the inhaler.)
6. Repeat several times until the powder is inhaled. (A light dusting of powder remaining in the capsule is normal.)

Aerosol: Two metered-dose sprays inhaled four times daily at regular intervals.

For prevention of exercise-induced bronchospasm or bronchospasm associated with cold air or environmental substances, administer two metered-dose sprays 10 to 60 minutes before exposure to the precipitating factor.

Evaluation

Side Effects to Expect

Oral Irritation, Dry Mouth. The most common side effect is irritation of the throat and trachea caused by inhaling the dry powder. This may be manifested by nasal itching and burning, nasal stuffiness, sneezing, coughing, and bronchospasm. Start regular oral hygiene measures when the therapy is initiated. Suggest the use of 1 teaspoon of hydrogen peroxide in 6 to 8 ounces of water as a mouthwash. Commercial mouthwashes contain alcohol, which may cause further drying and oral irritation.

Other measures to alleviate dryness include sucking on ice chips or hard candy.

Side Effects to Report

Bronchospasm, Coughing. Notify the physician if inhalation causes bronchospasm or coughing.

Drug Interactions. No significant drug interactions have been reported.

nedocromil sodium (ned ock′ row mil)
TILADE (ty′ layd)

Actions

Nedocromil sodium is an antiinflammatory agent similar to cromolyn sodium. Its mechanism of action is unknown, but it prevents the release of histamine and other mediators that cause inflammation. It must be administered before the body receives a stimulus to release histamine, such as an antigen that initiates an antigen-antibody allergic reaction.

Uses

Nedocromil is recommended for use in conjunction with other medications in the treatment of patients with mild to moderate bronchial asthma to prevent the release of histamine and other inflammatory mediators that results in asthmatic attacks.

Nedocromil has no direct bronchodilatory, antihistaminic, or anticholinergic activity. The concomitant use of antihistamines or nasal decongestants may be necessary during initial treatment with nedocromil. A 2- to 4-week course of therapy is usually required to determine clinical response. Therapy should be continued only if there is a decrease in the severity of asthmatic symptoms.

Therapeutic Outcomes

The primary therapeutic outcome associated with nedocromil therapy is fewer episodes of acute asthmatic symptoms.

Nursing Process for Nedocromil

Premedication Assessment

1. This medication must be taken before exposure to the stimulus that initiates an attack of allergic rhinitis or severe bronchial asthma. Inhalation during an attack of bronchospasm or asthma may exacerbate symptoms.
2. Check to see if the concurrent use of antihistamines and bronchodilators has been ordered by the physician, especially during the start of nedocromil therapy.

Planning

Availability. Inhalation: 1.75 mg per actuation in 112 metered-dose inhalation aerosol.

Implementation

Dosage and Administration

Counseling. The therapeutic effects, unlike those of beta adrenergic decongestants, are not immediate. This should be explained to the patient in advance to ensure cooperation and continuation of treatment with the prescribed regimen. Full therapeutic benefit requires regular use and is usually evident within 2 to 4 weeks. Therapy must be continued even though the patient is symptom-free.

Adult: Inhalation: Two metered sprays inhaled four times daily at regular intervals. Ensure that the patient understands how to use the inhaler as described in the manufacturer's leaflet. Continue other therapy for asthma as prescribed.

Evaluation

Side Effects to Expect

Oral Irritation, Dry Mouth. The most common side effect is irritation of the throat and trachea caused by inhalation of the medicine. This may be manifested by coughing, sore throat, runny nose, and bronchospasm. Start regular oral hygiene measures when the therapy is initiated. Suggest the use of 1 teaspoon of hydrogen peroxide in 6 to 8 ounces of water as a mouthwash. Commercial mouthwashes contain alcohol, which may cause further drying and oral irritation.

Other measures to alleviate dryness include sucking on ice chips or hard candy.

Side Effects to Report

Bronchospasm, Coughing. Notify the health care provider if inhalation causes bronchospasm or coughing.

Drug Interactions. No significant drug interactions have been reported.

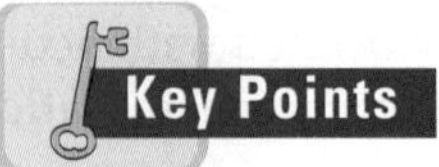

Key Points

- Chronic obstructive pulmonary diseases, also known as chronic airflow limitation disease, include chronic bronchitis and emphysema, both of which are progressive, irreversible diseases that usually cause death after a long debilitating illness.
- Asthma is an inflammatory disease that has airflow limitations; however, the episodes are intermittent and the limitations are reversible.
- Regular use of preventive medicine and removal of triggers such as allergens are key to the long-term treatment of asthma.
- Emphasize taking medications *before* exposure to a suspected trigger of an attack; treat all respiratory infections early.
- Regular use of a peak flowmeter and appropriate use of an inhaler are integral to treating asthma.
- For irreversible chronic airflow disorders, teach measures that can assist the individual to manage the symptoms (e.g., drinking adequate fluid to decrease secretion viscosity; breathing techniques; exercise conditioning to strengthen respiratory muscles; controlled coughing; positioning).
- Nurses can play a significant role in public education efforts, monitoring for nonadherence, and encouraging patients to make changes in lifestyle to reduce the severity of chronic limited airflow disease.
- Help the patient and/or family to identify community resources available in the immediate vicinity.

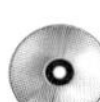

Go to your Companion CD-ROM for Appendices, an Audio Glossary, animations, Drug Dosage Calculators, customizable Patient Self-Assessment forms, and Review Questions for the NCLEX® Examination.

evolve Be sure to visit the companion Evolve site at http://evolve.elsevier.com/Clayton for WebLinks and additional online resources.

MEDICATION SAFETY REVIEW

MATH REVIEW QUESTIONS

1. Ordered: Diphenhydramine (Benadryl) 25 mg q4h
   Available: Diphenhydramine (Benadryl) 13.3 mg/5 mL
   Give ____ mL, or ____ tsp.
2. Ordered: Terbutaline (Brethine) 0.25 mg subcutaneously
   Available: Terbutaline 1 mg/mL
   Give ____ mL.
3. Ordered: Theophylline elixir 9 mg/kg/24 hr in four divided doses. The patient weighs 86 pounds.
   Give ____ mg per individual dose.
   Available: Theophylline elixir 50 mg/5 mL
   Give ____ mL per individual dose.

CRITICAL THINKING QUESTIONS

1. Explain why the action of a beta-adrenergic blocking agent may interfere with the therapeutic effects of bronchodilating agents, such as albuterol (Proventil).
2. Differentiate among the actions of acetylcysteine, guaifenesin, and potassium iodide on mucus in the respiratory tract.
3. Summarize premedication assessments used for each classification of drugs used to treat lower airway disorders.
4. One of the health care provider's patients calls the office about her inhaler medicine. She asks how she can tell if her inhaler canister is almost empty. She had heard about a "float test" and asked you about it. What would your response be?

CONTENT REVIEW QUESTIONS

1. The action of antileukotriene agents (e.g., montelukast [Singulair], zafirlukast [Accolate]) is to:
   1. dilate the bronchi.
   2. inhibit release of histamine.
   3. reduce release of leukotrienes.
   4. dissolve chemical bonds of mucus.
2. Before administering xanthine-derivative bronchodilators (e.g., aminophylline, theophylline), the nurse should assess for:
   1. concurrent use of antihistamines or nasal decongestants.
   2. history of angina pectoris, peptic ulcer, glaucoma, or diabetes mellitus.
   3. liver function test results.
   4. history of closed-angle glaucoma.
3. An antitussive agent acts to:
   1. dissolve mucus.
   2. suppress cough reflex response in the brain.
   3. stimulate increased bronchial gland secretions.
   4. reduce the release of leukotrienes.
4. Guaifenesin (Robitussin) is classified as a(n):
   1. antitussive.
   2. expectorant.
   3. mucolytic.
   4. beta-adrenergic bronchodilator.
5. Whenever administering a beta-adrenergic bronchodilator, preassessment data should include checking for:
   1. liver function tests.
   2. history of glaucoma, diabetes mellitus, or peptic ulcer disease.
   3. palpitations, dysrhythmias, and baseline mental status data.
   4. history of concurrent use of antihistamines or nasal decongestants.
6. Spiriva (tiotropium bromide) is similar to ipratropirum, but has which of the following advantages?
   1. It needs to be used several times a day.
   2. The therapeutic effects last much longer.
   3. It is used to treat acute bronchospasm.
   4. It is taken as an oral capsule.
7. When administering both a bronchodilator and a steroid by inhalation, which medicine should be administered first?
   1. Steroid
   2. Bronchodilator
   3. It does not make a difference
   4. Bronchodilators and steroids should not be taken together
8. Following the inhalation of steroid medications, the patient should do which of the following?
   1. Hold the breath for 30 seconds
   2. Rinse the mouth and swallow
   3. Rinse the mouth and spit out water
   4. Nothing is required

CHAPTER 32 Drugs Used to Treat Oral Disorders

evolve http://evolve.elsevier.com/Clayton

Chapter Content

Objectives

1. Cite the treatment alternatives and associated nursing assessments to monitor response to drug therapy for common mouth disorders.
2. Identify baseline data the nurse should collect on a continual basis for comparing and evaluating drug effectiveness.
3. Identify important nursing assessments and interventions associated with the drug therapy and treatment of diseases of the mouth.

Key Terms

cold sores (fever blisters)	tartar
canker sores	gingivitis
candidiasis	halitosis
mucositis	xerostomia
plaque	dentifrices
dental caries	mouthwashes

MOUTH DISORDERS

Common disorders affecting the mouth are cold sores on the lip; canker sores and candidal infections of soft tissues of the tongue, cheeks, and gums; and plaque and calculus affecting the gums and teeth. Xerostomia, or lack of saliva, originates from nonoral causes. Halitosis can arise from oral or nonoral diseases. A much less common problem, but one that causes significant discomfort, is oral mucositis.

Cold sores (fever blisters) are caused by the herpes simplex type 1 virus (herpes simplex labialis) and are most commonly found at the junction of the mucous membrane and the skin of the lips or nostrils, although they can occur inside the mouth, especially affecting the gums and roof of the mouth. It is estimated that at least one half of all Americans ages 20 to 40 years have had fever blisters. Most victims were infected before 5 years of age. About half of patients will develop recurrent outbreaks of the lesions, often in the same location, separated by latent periods. The recurrence rate and extent of lesions are highly variable. Patients often predict when an outbreak may occur because of predisposing factors, such as systemic illnesses accompanied by fever, cold (hence the names fever blisters and cold sores), or flu; menstruation; extreme physical stress and fatigue; or sun and wind exposure. Chemotherapy or radiation therapy that depresses the immune system also triggers cold sores.

Patients often report that a flare-up of the sores is preceded by a prodrome of burning, itching, and numbness in the area where the lesion develops. The lesions first become visible as small, red papules that develop into fluid-filled vesicles (blisters) 1 to 3 mm in diameter. Smaller lesions often coalesce into larger lesions. Pain is intense, fever may be present, and increased salivation and mouth odor occur. Often the glands in the neck are swollen because of the body's response to infection. Over the next 10 to 14 days, a crust develops over the top of many coalesced, burst vesicles; the base is erythematous. The liquid from the vesicles contains live virus that is contagious if transferred to other people by direct contact (e.g., kissing). If pus develops in the vesicles or under the crust of a cold sore, a secondary bacterial infection may be present and should be evaluated for antibiotic therapy.

Canker sores, also known as recurrent aphthous ulcers (RAS), affect 20% to 50% of people in the United States. The exact cause is unknown, but precipitating factors appear to be stress and local trauma (e.g., chemical irritation, toothbrush abrasion, irritation from orthodontic braces, biting the inside of the cheeks or lips). The lesions are not viral infections as was once thought, and they are not contagious. There appears to be a familial factor, as well as nutritional, emotional, and physiologic factors. They can develop at any age, and they affect both genders in equal numbers. Canker sores can appear as ulcers 0.5 to 2 cm in diameter on surfaces that are not attached to bone, such as the tongue, gums, or inner lining of the cheeks and lips. The lesion is usually gray to whitish yellow with an erythematous halo of inflamed tissue surrounding the ulcer crater. Lesions do not form blisters and usually do not grow together. Patients may experience a single lesion or as many as 30 or more at one time. The lesions can be painful and can inhibit normal eating, drinking, talking, and swallowing, as well as oral hygiene. There are usually no swollen lymph glands or fever unless the sore becomes secondarily infected. Most canker sores last 10 to 14 days and heal without scarring.

Candidiasis is a fungal infection caused by *Candida albicans*, the most common organism associated with oral infections. It is often called "the disease of the diseased" because it appears in debilitated patients and patients taking a variety of medicines. The most common predisposing factors are physiologic (early infancy, pregnancy, old age), diabetes mellitus, malnutrition, malignancies, and radiation therapy. Medicines that predispose a patient to candidiasis are those that depress defense mechanisms (immunosuppressants, corticosteroids, cytotoxics, broad-spectrum antibiotics) and those that cause xerostomia (anticholinergics, antidepressants, antipsychotics, antihypertensives, antihistamines).

There are several forms of candidiasis, but the most common is the acute, pseudomembranous form that is often referred to as thrush. It is characterized by white milk curd–appearing plaques attached to the oral mucosa. These plaques usually can be easily detached, and erythematous, bleeding, sore areas appear beneath them. Thrush is most common in infants, pregnant women, and debilitated patients. Treatment requires local or systemic therapy with antifungal agents, such as nystatin (Mycostatin) suspension, or clotrimazole troches (see discussion of antifungal agents in Chapter 46).

Mucositis is a general term used to describe a painful inflammation of the mucous membranes of the mouth. It is commonly associated with chemotherapy and radiation therapy. Mucositis develops 5 to 7 days after antineoplastic therapy or radiation therapy is administered. The sores are erythematous ulcerations intermixed with white patchy mucous membranes. Candidal infections are often present. Commonly used scales to standardize evaluation of mucositis and therapy are the World Health Organization Oral Mucositis Scale (Box 32-1) and the National Cancer Institute–Common Toxicity Criteria (NCI-CTC). Mucositis is often a primary complaint associated with cancer therapy because it can diminish a patient's perception of quality of life. It can be severely debilitating with pain and difficulty in swallowing, eating, drinking, and talking.

Plaque is the primary cause of most tooth, gum (gingiva), and periodontal disease. Plaque, the whitish yellow substance that builds up on teeth and gumlines around the teeth, is thought to originate from saliva. Plaque forms a sticky meshwork that traps bacteria and food particles. If not removed regularly, it thickens, and bacteria proliferate. The bacteria secrete acids that eat into the enamel of teeth, causing **dental caries** (cavities). If the plaque is not removed within 24 hours, it begins to calcify, forming calculus, or **tartar**. The calculus forms a foundation for additional plaque to form, eventually eroding under the gumline and causing inflammation **(gingivitis)** and periodontal disease.

Halitosis is the term used to describe a very foul mouth odor. A temporary foul odor at certain times is normal in healthy individuals, such as "morning breath" or after eating certain foods (e.g., garlic, onions). Halitosis can also signify an underlying pathologic condition. Halitosis comes from oral and nonoral sources. Nonoral causes of halitosis include sinusitis, tonsillitis, and rhinitis; pulmonary diseases such as tuberculosis or bronchiectasis; and elimination of chemicals from the blood, such as acetone exhaled by patients with diabetic ketoacidosis. Paraldehyde and dimethyl sulfoxide (DMSO) are two medicines excreted primarily through the lungs and leave a characteristic foul odor to the breath. "Smoker's breath" caused by cigarette smoking is a fairly common cause of halitosis. Oral causes of halitosis include decaying food particles, plaque-coated tongue and teeth, dental caries, poor oral or denture hygiene, periodontal disease, and xerostomia.

Xerostomia is a condition in which the flow of saliva is either partially or completely stopped. About 20% of people older than 65 years of age report a change in consistency, a decrease in production, or a discontinuation of salivary flow. Xerostomia causes loss of taste, difficulty in chewing and swallowing food, and difficulty in talking; and it increases tooth decay. Xerostomia can also cause a burning sensation of the tongue, mucositis, and a reduction in the amount of time daily that dentures can be worn. The most common causes of xerostomia are medicines (e.g., anticholinergic agents, diuretics, antidepressants, certain antihypertensive agents), diseases (e.g., diabetes mellitus, depression), and functional conditions (e.g., smoking, mouth breathing).

Box 32-1 World Health Organization Oral Mucositis Scale

GRADE	CLINICAL FEATURES
0	No mucositis present
1	Oral soreness with erythema
2	Oral erythema, ulcers, solid diet tolerated
3	Oral ulcers, liquid diet tolerated
4	Oral feeding not possible

Sonis ST, et al. Perspectives on cancer therapy-induced mucosal injury: pathogenesis, measurement, epidemiology, and consequences for patients, *Cancer* 100(9 Suppl):1995-2025, 2004.

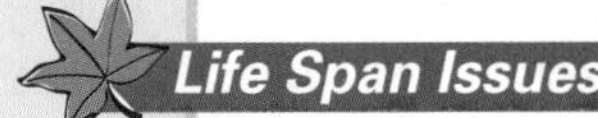

Life Span Issues

Salivary Flow

About 20% of people older than 65 years of age report a change in consistency, a decrease in production, or a discontinuation of salivary flow. The most common causes of xerostomia are medicines, such as anticholinergic agents, diuretics, antidepressants, and certain antihypertensive drugs.

DRUG THERAPY FOR MOUTH DISORDERS

Cold Sores

The goals of treatment are to control discomfort, allow healing, prevent spread to others, and prevent complications. The cold sore should be kept moist to prevent drying and cracking that may make it more susceptible to secondary bacterial infection. Docosanol (Abreva) is the only FDA-approved product clinically proven to shorten healing time as well as the duration of symptoms such as tingling, pain, burning, and itching. It must be applied five times daily starting at the first sign of outbreak (e.g., tingling, redness, itching). Local anesthetics (e.g., benzocaine, dibucaine, lidocaine) in emollient creams, petrolatum, or protectants (e.g., TheraPatch Cold Sore [lidocaine 4%, camphor, eucalyptus oil, glycerin]) can temporarily relieve the pain and itching and prevent drying of the lesion. Topical analgesics (e.g., Blistex [allantoin, menthol, camphor, phenol]) are safe and effective in temporarily reducing pain. Oral analgesics (e.g., aspirin, acetaminophen, ibuprofen, naproxen) may also provide significant pain relief. Broad-brimmed hats and ultraviolet blockers (e.g., Chapstick Lip Moisturizer Ultra, Natural Ice) with a sun protection factor (SPF) of at least 15 can be used for patients whose cold sores occur with sun exposure. Secondary infections can be treated with a topical antibiotic ointment such as Neosporin.

Canker Sores

The goals of treatment are similar to those for cold sores: to control discomfort and promote healing. Topical amlexanox paste 5% (Aphthasol) is an antiinflammatory agent that hastens healing when compared with placebo. The paste should be applied to each lesion as soon as possible after noting the symptoms of a canker sore. The patient should continue to use the paste four times daily, preferably following oral hygiene after breakfast, lunch, and dinner and at bedtime. Protectants such as hydroxypropyl cellulose film (Zilactin) may reduce friction. Topical anesthetics to control discomfort, such as benzocaine (Orabase-B [benzocaine 20% in plasticized hydrocarbon gel]) or butacaine, are particularly effective if applied just before eating or performing oral hygiene. Oral analgesics (e.g., aspirin, acetaminophen, ibuprofen, naproxen) may also provide significant pain relief. Aspirin should not be placed on the lesions because of the high risk of severe chemical burns with necrosis. Oxygen-releasing agents (carbamide peroxide, hydrogen peroxide, perborates) can be used as debriding and cleansing agents up to four times daily for 7 days. Long-term safety has not been established, and tissue irritation and black hairy tongue have been reported. Saline rinses (1 to 3 teaspoons of table salt) in 4 to 8 ounces of warm tap water may be soothing and can be used before topical application of medication. Sustained use of products containing menthol, phenol, camphor, and eugenol should be discouraged because they cause tissue irritation and damage or systemic toxicity if overused. Silver nitrate should not be used to "cauterize" lesions because it may damage healthy tissue surrounding the lesion and predispose the area to later infection.

Mucositis

Basic oral hygiene is an important component of care for any patient with cancer. The purpose is to decrease the complications associated with pain, oral microorganisms, and bleeding. Prior to cancer therapy, a baseline pretreatment oral mucosal assessment should be completed to rule out preexisting conditions or infections that might aggravate impending mucositis. Although it takes 5 to 7 days for mucositis to develop after chemotherapy or radiation therapy, oral hygiene regimens should be started when chemotherapy or radiation therapy is initiated. Oral hygiene, oral irrigations, and methods to relieve dry mouth and lips can be very effective in providing comfort.

Pain associated with oral mucositis can be a major complication that contributes to poor nutrition and hydration. To be effective, topical applications of medications for pain must come in contact with the tissue. Therefore it is advisable to schedule these routines immediately after cleaning the oral cavity. In addition to the previously described protectants, local anesthetics, and analgesics, the following are routine approaches to treating pain in the oral area.

- Lidocaine: Viscous lidocaine 2% before meals to relieve pain. Frequent applications are required, and the sense of taste is diminished. Care must be taken to make sure the patient is not burned by the food because the entire mouth and throat are anesthetized.
- Milk of magnesia can be used to rinse the mouth and coat the mucous membranes.
- Nystatin liquid can be swished in the mouth for 1 minute and then swallowed (swish and swallow routine), or clotrimazole lozenges may be chewed or sucked and then swallowed to reduce candidal oral infections.
- Sucralfate suspensions applied topically have been reported to provide effective pain relief.
- Oral or parenteral analgesics (e.g., morphine) should be administered for severe pain.
- A new medicine—recombinant human keratinocyte growth factor, palifermin (Kepivance)—has been approved specifically for use in preventing and treating the mucositis that develops in leukemia or lymphoma patients undergoing chemotherapy before bone marrow transplantation.

Plaque

Plaque is controlled by toothbrushing, flossing between teeth, and using mouthwashes. If plaque is removed regularly, calculus will not form. Using a dentifrice (toothpaste) and flossing between teeth helps remove dental plaque and stain, resulting in less halitosis and periodontal disease and fewer dental caries. Other devices, such as oral irrigators (WaterPik), sponge-tipped applicators, or electric toothbrushes, can be used for patients who wear orthodontic appliances, are physically or mentally handicapped, or lack manual dexterity and require someone else to clean their teeth. Therapeutic mouthwashes also help reduce plaque accumulated above the gumline.

Halitosis

Halitosis is treated most easily by eliminating causes such as smoking and certain foods. Regularly brushing the teeth or dentures and using dental floss between teeth can remove particles of decaying food. Mouthwashes and breath mints can mask halitosis but usually last less than 1 hour. If halitosis is persistent without a readily identifiable cause, such as smoking or diet, a dentist should be consulted for a thorough examination to ensure that no other pathologic condition is the underlying cause.

Xerostomia

Xerostomia is treated by changing the medicines that cause dry mouth or with artificial saliva. Artificial saliva products do not stimulate natural saliva production but mimic the viscosity, mineral content, and taste. Patients with xerostomia should be seen by a dentist regularly to help avoid additional dental caries and ensure proper denture fit to prevent gum irritation. Commercially available saliva substitutes include Salivart, MouthKote, Saliva Substitute, and Moi-Stir. All are available as sprays for easy administration.

NURSING PROCESS *for Oral Health Therapy*

Assessment

Drug History. Obtain a history of recent drug therapy. Some drugs, such as phenytoin (Dilantin), may cause alterations in the gums, and oral mucositis is common after chemotherapy and radiation therapy.

Dental History

- Obtain a dental history that includes frequency of visits to the dentist and a brief summary of dental procedures that have been performed within the past 1 to 3 years.
- Ask about usual hygiene practices, such as number of times per day brushing or flossing is done, type of toothbrush used, and oral products used (e.g., toothpaste, mouthwashes).
- Ask about tobacco and alcohol use—frequency and amounts.
- Ask about any difficulty chewing, swallowing, or speaking.
- Ask about any recent changes in the taste of foods or alterations within the mouth, such as burning or tingling.

Oral Cavity

- Put on gloves and inspect the oral cavity with the aid of a flashlight and tongue blade. Visually inspect the mucous membranes covering the lips, hard and soft palates, gums, tongue, pharynx, and teeth.
- Note the color of the mucous membranes and the moisture present.
- Inspect the mucous membranes for inflamed or receding gums, ulcerations, crusts, changes in color (e.g., white patches), and sores from poorly fitting dentures. Inquire how well the dentures fit and how long each day they are worn. Assess for the presence of teeth, dental caries, and plaque.
- Observe the amount and consistency of the saliva present.
- Note the presence or absence of halitosis. Presence may indicate poor dental hygiene practices or an oral infection. Some odors occur from a variety of causes (garlic, smoking, ingestion of alcohol) and some systemic diseases (acetone from diabetes, ammonia from liver disease).

Nursing Diagnoses

- Pain, acute or chronic (indication)
- Tissue integrity, impaired (indication)
- Body image, disturbed (indication)
- Deficient knowledge related to hygiene practices, medication regimen (indication)

Planning

- Develop a schedule for oral hygiene measures to be performed consistent with type and severity of mouth disorder.
- Make necessary referrals to the dentist, especially before starting chemotherapy.
- Order prescribed oral hygiene supplies and medications; list medications used as rinses or "swish and swallows" in the medication administration record (MAR).
- Develop a teaching plan to promote maintaining a healthy oral cavity and promote daily hygienic practices.
- For people experiencing cold sores, teach the individual that the lesions are common and may be seen from childhood into adulthood. They are also contagious when an active lesion is present. Avoid contaminating other individuals.

Implementation

Cold Sores

- Cold sores should be kept clean by gentle washing with mild soap solutions. The cold sore should be kept moist to prevent drying and cracking. Cracking may render it more susceptible to secondary bacterial infection, delay healing, and increase discomfort. Therefore products that are highly astringent should be avoided (e.g., tannic acid, zinc sulfate).
- Apply docosanol, local anesthetics, and ultraviolet blockers or oral analgesics as prescribed.
- When secondary infections are present, apply topical antibiotic ointment to the cold sore.

Canker Sores

- Apply topical anesthetics before the patient eats or performs oral hygiene.
- Apply amlexanox (Aphthasol) after meals and oral hygiene, four times daily.
- Administer oral analgesics; apply oxygen-releasing agents for debridement and cleansing agents at appropriate intervals.
- Saline rinses using 1 to 3 teaspoons of table salt in 4 to 8 ounces of warm tap water may be soothing and can be used before topical medications.
- Changes in diet can also reduce irritation to the sores. Avoid sharp-edged foods, such as potato chips and crackers, and spicy foods, pineapple, citrus fruits, and chocolate. Drinking acidic juices and soft drinks through a straw can minimize contact and irritation.

Musositis. Oral hygiene regimens should be started at the time of chemotherapy or radiation therapy. Oral hygiene should include a soft-bristled brush, WaterPik on low setting, or sponge-tipped applicators (in the case of severe lesions). With advanced lesions, pain and discomfort may be severe, and other devices, such as a gravity flow irrigating system or an oral syringe, may be helpful.

Commercially prepared mouthwashes containing alcohol are usually not recommended because they dry the mouth and irritate rather than relieve symptoms of mucositis. Alternative solutions for oral hygiene are 1 tablespoon of salt or hydrogen peroxide in 8 ounces of water or ½ teaspoon of baking soda in 8 ounces of water as a mouthwash. Although each of these solutions has disadvantages, they remain the hallmark of irrigating solutions.

The frequency of oral irrigations is important. Irrigations should be performed immediately before and after meals and at bedtime if symptoms are mild. With moderate lesions, increase the frequency to every 2 hours. In patients with severe symptoms, the mouth may be rinsed hourly. When fungal infections are present, the cleansing regimen should be performed immediately before administering the topical agents (e.g., nystatin liquids as a swish or clotrimazole lozenges). Performing the cleansing routine immediately before the medication is given will improve the contact of the medicine with the denuded surface. Caution the patient not to take food or drink for approximately 15 minutes after the medication.

Mouth dryness can be relieved by chewing gum and sucking on ice chips or Popsicles. Dry lips can be coated with cocoa butter, K-Y jelly, petroleum jelly, or lip balm. Artificial saliva is available.

Administer pain preparations according to prescribed routines using viscous lidocaine 2%, or milk of magnesia rinses, nystatin liquid as a swish and swallow, or sucralfate suspension topically. Use oral or parenteral analgesics for severe pain.

Plaque. Perform toothbrushing and dental flossing and use mouthwashes on a scheduled basis daily to prevent plaque.

Halitosis. Brushing dentures and teeth regularly and using dental floss can remove particles of decaying food. Mouthwashes and breath mints can mask halitosis but usually last less than 1 hour.

Xerostomia. Monitor the medication routine, report xerostomia to the health care provider, and use artificial saliva if prescribed.

Dentures. Dentures should be cleaned each time oral hygiene is performed. For neutropenic patients, dentures should be worn only for eating. Poorly fitting dentures must be repaired to prevent further tissue breakdown.

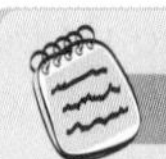

Patient Education and Health Promotion

- Teach the patient proper cleansing techniques for oral hygiene consistent with the conditions present (e.g., normal healthy tissue, mucositis, jaw wiring).
- Instruct people who are to receive radiation or chemotherapy to start oral hygiene on a scheduled regimen immediately rather than waiting until mucositis develops.
- Teach the patient with pain the proper use of prescribed analgesics and comfort measures.
- Discuss dietary practices that may relieve symptoms, such as bland foods. For dry mouth, instruct the person to use gravies or sauces to moisten foods. When mucous membranes are irritated, suggest avoiding hot and spicy foods, alcohol, and tobacco.
- Persistent halitosis that is not relieved by brushing and flossing may have a medical basis. The individual should be told to discuss the matter with the health care provider or dentist to ensure appropriate therapy.
- Fluoride supplements may be recommended in areas of the United States in which the water supply is not fluoridated or the fluoride level is low.

Fostering Health Maintenance

- Discuss hygiene practices and medications prescribed for discomfort, infections, or mucosal breakdown.
- Seek cooperation and understanding of the following points so that medication compliance is increased: name of medication, dosage, route and times of administration, side effects to expect, and side effects to report.
- Discuss a specific schedule for performing oral hygiene measures and include details of products to be used to relieve oral dryness or pain. Discuss basic dietary modifications needed while oral lesions are present (e.g., avoid citrus juices and spicy foods). With severe oral lesions, discuss supplemental nutrition formulas (e.g., Ensure, Boost). Generally cold drinks are more soothing to the oral tissue than hot foods.
- Report to the health care provider conditions that are not relieved by the prescribed therapies.

DRUG CLASS: Dentifrices

Actions

Dentifrices contain one or more abrasive agents, a foaming agent, and flavoring materials. They are available in powder, paste, or gel and are best used with a soft nylon toothbrush. Although dentifrices vary, degree of abrasiveness is an essential property for removing plaque. Some toothpastes contain higher concentrations of abrasive agents (e.g., silicates, dicalcium phosphate, calcium pyrophosphate, calcium carbonate) and are advertised as "smokers' toothpastes" to remove tobacco stains. The most common therapeutic agent added to dentifrices is fluoride for its anticaries activity. Chemicals such as sanguinarine, zinc citrate, triclosan, thymol, and eucalyptol have antibacterial properties that may reduce plaque. Dentifrices advertised as tooth whiteners contain oxidizing ingredients, such as hydrogen peroxide, carbamide peroxide, and perhydrol urea. Zinc chloride, zinc citrate, and soluble pyrophosphates prevent or retard the formation of new calculus from plaque, but will not remove calculus already formed. Potassium nitrate is used for relieving sensitivity to hot and cold liquids and foods in otherwise normal teeth.

Uses

If possible, all people should brush at least twice daily with a fluoride toothpaste. If the teeth and gums are normal, select a fluoride-containing dentifrice that has acceptable taste. All age groups should use toothpastes that are the least abrasive to the teeth while controlling tooth decay and gum disease. This is especially important to patients with receding gums. People who have a sensitivity to hot or cold liquids and foods may want to try a "sensitivity" toothpaste containing potassium nitrate. About 2 weeks of regular use is necessary to eliminate sensitivity to hot or cold beverages and food.

Therapeutic Outcomes

The primary therapeutic outcomes expected from dentifrices are as follows:

- Reduction in plaque formation and cavities.
- A pleasant, refreshing taste.

DRUG CLASS: Mouthwashes

Toothbrushing and flossing are optimal for good oral hygiene; however, they may not be possible for the patient who has undergone oral surgery or who has experienced facial trauma. Mouthwashes may be temporarily effective in removing disagreeable tastes and reducing halitosis. Therapeutic mouthwashes are also available to reduce plaque.

Actions

Mouthwashes are solutions of flavoring, coloring, water, surfactants, and sometimes therapeutic ingredients. Flavoring agents are used to give a pleasant taste and freshen the breath. Coloring helps to imply a certain type of mouthwash: green or blue for minty, red for spicy, and brown for medicinal. Surfactants are foaming agents that aid in removing debris. Alcohol is often present, adding a "bite," enhancing flavor, especially in the medicinal type of product, and solubilizing other ingredients. Therapeutic ingredients include fluoride for anticaries protection and antimicrobial agents (e.g., benzoic acid, thymol, eucalyptol, menthol, cetylpyridinium chloride, domiphen bromide, chlorhexidine) to kill bacteria to reduce plaque formation and decaying food odor. Phenol is a local anesthetic, antiseptic, and antibacterial agent that penetrates and reduces plaque formation. Zinc citrate and zinc chloride are astringents that neutralize sulfur-smelling compounds from decaying debris in the mouth.

Uses

Mouthwashes can be subdivided into cosmetic and therapeutic products based on ingredients. Cosmetic mouthwashes freshen the breath and rinse out some debris, although the odor-reducing effect lasts only 10 to 30 minutes.

Certain mouthwashes are for specific purposes. The most common are the fluoride-containing mouthwashes used to prevent dental caries. Medicinal mouthwashes (e.g., Listerine) reduce plaque accumulation and gingivitis. Chlorhexidine (Peridex) is an antibacterial agent used to treat oral mucositis. Products containing zinc chloride are used as astringents for temporarily decreasing bleeding or irritation. A 0.9% solution of sodium chloride (normal saline) is an effective gargle. It can provide temporary, soothing relief of pharyngeal irritation from nasogastric tubes, endotracheal tubes, sore throat, or oral surgery. Solutions containing hydrogen peroxide cleanse and debride minor lesions; however, use should be limited to 7 to 10 days to prevent further tissue irritation. Lidocaine, a local anesthetic, is available in both an oral spray solution (Xylocaine 10%) and an oral viscous solution (Xylocaine 2%). The spray solution is used as a short-term topical anesthetic for the mucous membranes in the mouth. The viscous solution is a longer-lasting local anesthetic and can be used as a gargle for patients with sore throats or mouth ulcers. This product is frequently used in immunosuppressed patients with painful candidal infections of the mouth and throat.

Unless a mouthwash is being used to treat a specific medical condition (e.g., oral mucositis), it should be remembered that it should not become a substitute for normal oral hygiene. Primary oral hygiene is proper toothbrushing and flossing.

All mouthwashes have specific dosage recommendations. It is important not to exceed these recommendations without a health care provider's order because many of the therapeutic ingredients (e.g., lidocaine, fluoride) can be systemically absorbed, resulting in toxic levels. Most mouthwashes are designed to be used as a rinse (mouthwash is held in the mouth, swished around, and expectorated). Again, prolonged swallowing of mouthwashes may lead to systemic toxicities.

Patients should be advised to refrain from smoking, eating, or drinking for at least 30 minutes after use.

Therapeutic Outcomes

The primary therapeutic outcomes expected from mouthwashes are as follows:

- Temporary reduction in bleeding or irritation.
- Relief of discomfort.
- A refreshing taste.
- Improvement in halitosis.

Key Points

- Common disorders affecting the mouth are cold sores on the lip; canker sores and candidal infections of soft tissues of the tongue, cheeks, and gums; and plaque and calculus affecting the gums and teeth. Xerostomia (lack of saliva) originates from nonoral causes.
- Halitosis can arise from oral or nonoral causes. A much less common problem but one that causes significant discomfort is oral mucositis.
- Health teaching should start with children to promote regular brushing, flossing, and dental care. Stress regular dental checkups, have problems treated promptly when they occur, and if wearing dentures, be certain they fit properly.

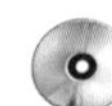

Go to your Companion CD-ROM for Appendices, an Audio Glossary, animations, Drug Dosage Calculators, customizable Patient Self-Assessment forms, and Review Questions for the NCLEX® Examination.

evolve Be sure to visit the companion Evolve site at http://evolve.elsevier.com/Clayton for WebLinks and additional online resources.

MEDICATION SAFETY REVIEW

CRITICAL THINKING QUESTIONS

1. Compare oral hygiene measures appropriate in a healthy mouth with those needed in mild to severe mouth disorders.
2. Research the current oral hygiene practices used in the clinical site when assigned for patients without known oral lesions. What hygiene protocol is used when chemotherapy or radiation therapy is instituted to prevent development of mucositis?

CONTENT REVIEW QUESTIONS

1. When painful oral lesions are present, the best approach to oral hygiene is to:
   1. wait until the lesions are healed.
   2. use commercial mouthwashes for rinsing after meals and at bedtime.
   3. use normal saline, baking soda, or half-strength hydrogen peroxide rinses.
   4. give prescribed oral or parenteral analgesic medications.
2. Mouthwashes given for the purpose of debriding and cleansing minor oral lesions will contain:
   1. dibucaine.
   2. chlorhexidene (Peridex).
   3. hydrogen peroxide.
   4. lidocaine (Xylocaine).
3. Which of the following is true about canker sores? *(Select all that apply.)*
   1. Their exact cause is unknown.
   2. Precipitating factors are stress and local trauma.
   3. The lesions are viral infections.
   4. They are not contagious.
4. Thrush is most common in which of the following? *(Select all that apply.)*
   1. Infants
   2. Pregnant women
   3. Debilitated patients
   4. Teens
5. How soon after chemotherapy or radiation does mucositis develop?
   1. 2 to 3 days
   2. 5 to 7 days
   3. 10 to 12 days
   4. 2 weeks
6. What is the only FDA-approved product clinically proven to shorten healing time as well as duration of symptoms for cold sores?
   1. Docosanol
   2. Triple antibiotic ointment—bacitracin, neomycin, polymyxin B
   3. Lidocaine
   4. Natural Ice
7. Which of the following drugs has been approved specifically for use in preventing and treating the mucositis that develops in leukemia or lymphoma patients undergoing chemotherapy before bone marrow transplantation?
   1. Nystatin
   2. Sucralfate
   3. Viscous lidocaine
   4. Palifermin

CHAPTER 33

Drugs Used to Treat Gastroesophageal Reflux and Peptic Ulcer Diseases

evolve http://evolve.elsevier.com/Clayton

Chapter Content

Objectives

1. Cite common stomach disorders that require drug therapy.
2. Identify factors that prevent breakdown of the body's normal defense barriers resulting in ulcer formation.
3. State the drug classifications and actions used to treat stomach disorders.
4. Develop health teaching for an individual with stomach disorders that incorporates pharmacologic and nonpharmacologic treatment.

Key Terms

parietal cells	heartburn
hydrochloric acid	peptic ulcer disease (PUD)
gastroesophageal reflux disease (GERD)	*Helicobacter pylori*

PHYSIOLOGY OF THE STOMACH

As a major part of the gastrointestinal (GI) tract, the stomach has three primary functions: storing food until it can be used in the lower GI tract; mixing food with gastric secretions until it is a partially digested, semisolid mixture known as chyme; and slowly emptying the stomach at a rate that allows proper digestion and absorption of nutrients and medicine from the small intestine.

Three types of secretory cells line portions of the stomach: chief, parietal, and mucus cells. The chief cells secrete pepsinogen, an inactive enzyme. **Parietal cells** are stimulated by acetylcholine from cholinergic nerve fibers, gastrin, and histamine to secrete **hydrochloric acid**, which activates pepsinogen to pepsin and provides the optimal pH for pepsin to start protein digestion. Normal pH in the stomach ranges from 1 to 5, depending on the presence of food and medications. Hydrochloric acid also breaks down muscle fibers and connective tissue ingested as food and kills bacteria that enter the digestive tract through the mouth. The parietal cells also secrete intrinsic factor needed for absorption of vitamin B_{12}. The mucus cells secrete mucus that coats the stomach wall. The 1-mm-thick coat is alkaline and protects the stomach wall from damage by hydrochloric acid and the digestive enzyme pepsin. It also contributes lubrication for food transport. Small amounts of other enzymes are also secreted in the stomach. Lipases digest fats, and gastric amylase digests carbohydrates. Other digestive enzymes are also carried into the stomach from swallowed saliva.

Prostaglandins also play a major role in protecting the stomach walls from injury by stomach acids and enzymes. Prostaglandins are produced by cells lining the stomach and prevent injury by inhibiting gastric acid secretion, maintaining blood flow, and stimulating mucus and bicarbonate production.

COMMON STOMACH DISORDERS

Gastroesophageal reflux disease (GERD), more commonly referred to as **heartburn**, acid indigestion, or sour stomach, is a common stomach disorder. Approximately one third of the U.S. population experiences heartburn once each month, and 5% to 7% have heartburn daily. Common symptoms are a burning sensation, bloating, belching, and regurgitation. Other symptoms that are reported less frequently are nausea, a "lump in the throat," hiccups, and chest pain.

GERD is the reflux of gastric secretions, primarily pepsin and hydrochloric acid, up into the esophagus. Causes of GERD are a weakened lower esophageal sphincter, delayed gastric emptying, hiatal hernia, obesity, overeating, tight-fitting clothing, and increased acid secretion. Acid secretions are increased by smoking, alcohol, carbonated beverages, coffee, and spicy foods.

Most cases of GERD pass quickly with only mild discomfort, but frequent or prolonged bouts of acid reflux cause inflammation, tissue erosion, and ulcerations in the lower esophagus. Anyone who has recurrent or continuous symptoms of reflux, especially if the symptoms interfere with activities, should be referred

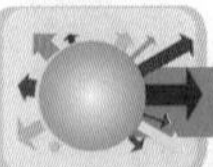

Clinical Landmine

Nurses need to be aware that the symptoms of gastroesophageal reflux disease (GERD) may also accompany more serious conditions, such as ischemic heart disease, scleroderma, and gastric malignancy. It is important to do a thorough physical assessment whenever a patient presents with heartburn or acid indigestion and not simply dismiss the symptoms as gastrointestinal in origin.

to a health care provider. These symptoms may also accompany more serious conditions, such as ischemic heart disease, scleroderma, and gastric malignancy.

Peptic ulcer disease (PUD) is actually several stomach disorders that result from an imbalance between acidic stomach contents and the body's normal defense barriers, causing ulcerations in the GI tract. The most common illnesses are gastric and duodenal ulcers. It is estimated that approximately 10% of all people in the United States will develop an ulcer sometime in their lives. The incidence in men and women is approximately the same. Race, economic status, and psychological stress do not correlate with the frequency of ulcer disease. Often the only symptom that is reported is epigastric pain, described as burning, gnawing, or aching. Patients often report that varying degrees of pain are present for a few weeks and are then gone, only to recur a few weeks later. The pain is most often noted when the stomach is empty, such as at night or between meals, and is relieved by food or antacids. Other symptoms that cause patients to seek medical attention are bloating, nausea, vomiting, and anorexia.

Ulcers appear to be caused by a combination of acid and a breakdown in the body's defense mechanisms that protect the stomach wall. Proposed mechanisms are oversecretion of hydrochloric acid by excessive numbers of parietal cells, injury to the mucosal barrier such as that resulting from prostaglandin inhibitors (including aspirin), and infection of the mucosal wall by ***Helicobacter pylori.*** It had been thought that no bacterium could survive in the highly acidic environment of the stomach; however, *H. pylori* was first isolated from patients with gastritis in 1983. The bacterium seems able to live below the mucus barrier, where it is protected from stomach acid and pepsin. *H. pylori* is now thought to be associated with as many as 90% of duodenal and 70% of gastric ulcers. The exact mechanism by which *H. pylori* contributes to ulcer formation is not known, but several hypotheses are being tested.

Several risk factors increase the likelihood of peptic ulcer disease:

1. There seems to be a genetic predisposition to PUD. Some families have a much greater history of PUD than others.
2. It is a commonly held belief that stress causes ulcers, but no well-controlled studies have supported this.
3. Cigarette smoking increases acid secretion, alters blood flow in the stomach wall, and retards prostaglandin synthesis needed for defense mechanisms.
4. Nonsteroidal antiinflammatory drugs (NSAIDs) have a twofold effect: they inhibit prostaglandins that protect the mucosa and directly irritate the stomach wall. Once ulcerations form, NSAIDs also slow healing.
5. It is commonly thought that certain foods (e.g., spicy foods) and alcohol contribute to ulcer formation. It is true that certain foods increase acid secretion and that alcohol irritates the stomach lining, but results from studies have not corroborated the belief.

TREATMENT OF GASTROESOPHAGEAL REFLUX AND PEPTIC ULCER DISEASES

The goals of treatment of GERD are to relieve symptoms, decrease the frequency and duration of reflux, heal tissue injury, and prevent recurrence. The most important treatment is a change in lifestyle: losing weight (if significantly over the ideal body weight), reducing or avoiding foods and beverages that increase acid production, reducing or stopping smoking, avoiding alcohol, and consuming smaller meals. Additional therapy includes remaining upright for 2 hours after meals, not eating before bedtime, and avoiding tight clothing over the abdominal area. Lozenges may be used to increase saliva production, and antacids and alginic acid therapy may provide relief in patients who experience infrequent heartburn. If the patient's symptoms do not improve within 2 to 3 weeks or if the condition is severe, additional pharmacologic measures should be tried to reduce irritation. About 5% to 10% of patients with GERD require surgery.

The treatment of PUD and GERD is somewhat similar: relieve symptoms, promote healing, and prevent recurrence. Lifestyle changes that eliminate risk factors, such as cigarette smoking, and foods (and alcohol) that increase acid secretion should be initiated. Patients rarely need to be restricted to a bland diet. If NSAIDs are being taken, consideration should be given to switching to acetaminophen if feasible. For decades, ulcer treatment focused on reducing acid secretions (anticholinergic agents, H_2 antagonists, gastric acid pump inhibitors), neutralizing acid (antacids), or coating ulcer craters to hasten healing (sucralfate). Major changes in therapy have come about because the U.S. Food and Drug Administration (FDA) has approved antibiotics to eradicate *H. pylori*. Several large studies are under way to refine the healing and reduce ulcer recurrence rate. Various combinations of antimicrobial agents (e.g., amoxicillin, tetracycline, metronidazole, clarithromycin), bismuth, and antisecretory agents (e.g., H_2 antagonists, proton-pump inhibitors) are used to eradicate *H. pylori.*

DRUG THERAPY FOR GASTROESOPHAGEAL REFLUX AND PEPTIC ULCER DISEASES

Actions

- Antacids neutralize gastric acid, thereby causing the gastric contents to be less acidic.
- Coating agents provide a protective covering over the ulcer crater.
- H_2 antagonists decrease the volume of hydrochloric acid produced, increasing the gastric pH and thereby resulting in decreased irritation to the gastric mucosa.
- Proton pump inhibitors block the formation of hydrochloric acid, reducing irritation of the gastric mucosa.
- Prokinetic agents increase the lower esophageal sphincter muscle pressure and peristalsis, hastening emptying of the stomach to reduce reflux.
- Antispasmodic agents reduce the secretion of saliva, hydrochloric acid, pepsin, bile, and other enzymatic fluids necessary for digestion and decrease GI motility and secretions.

Uses

- Antacids decrease hyperacidity associated with PUD, GERD, gastritis, and hiatal hernia.
- Coating agents provide a protective barrier for the mucosal lining where hydrochloric acid may come in contact with inflamed, eroded areas. They are used to treat existing ulcer craters on the gastric mucosa.
- H_2 antagonists are used to treat acute gastric and duodenal ulcers and gastroesophageal disease and for maintenance to prevent ulcer recurrence.
- Proton pump inhibitors are used to treat hyperacidity conditions (e.g., GERD, Zollinger-Ellison syndrome).
- Prokinetic agents are used to treat GERD.
- Antispasmodic agents decrease gastric secretions by inhibiting vagal stimulation. They are used in treating GI disorders requiring decreased gastric motility or decreased gastric secretions.

NURSING PROCESS *for Agents Used for Stomach Disorders*

Assessment

Nutritional Assessment. Obtain patient data about current height, weight, and any recent weight gain or loss. Identify the normal pattern of eating, including snacking habits. Use a Food Guide Pyramid (MyPyramid at www.mypyramid.gov) as a guide when asking questions to identify the usual foods eaten by the individual. Ask about any nutritional or cultural restrictions associated with dietary practices. Are there any food allergies (obtain details) or foods that particularly cause gastric distress when eaten? Does the individual take any nutritional supplements? How often and how much fast food is eaten?

Esophagus, Stomach. Ask patients to describe symptoms. Question in detail what is meant by the terms *indigestion, heartburn, upset stomach, nausea,* and *belching.*

Pain, Discomfort

- Ask the patient to describe the onset, duration, location, and characteristics of pain or discomfort. Determine whether there is a relationship between the ingestion of certain types of food or drinks and the onset of pain. Ask specifically about coffee, tea, colas, chocolate, and alcohol intake.
- What has the patient done to relieve the pain or discomfort? Have there been any changes in taste (e.g., bitterness, sourness)? Record pain using a rating scale both before and after medications are administered.

Activity, Exercise. Ask specifically what type of work or activities the individual performs that may increase intraabdominal pressure (e.g., lifting heavy objects, bending over frequently).

History of Diseases/Disorders

- What other diagnoses have been made for diseases or disorders (e.g., ulcer, gallbladder, liver, jaundice, irritable bowel syndrome)?
- Have there been any changes in bowel elimination or stool color, consistency, or frequency?

Medication History

- What self-medications have been tried?
- What prescribed medications are being taken?
- What is the schedule of medication administration (e.g., how frequently and when are antacids taken)?

Anxiety/Stress Level. Ask the patient to describe his or her lifestyle. What does the patient think are stressors, and how often do they occur?

Smoking. What is the frequency of smoking?

Nursing Diagnoses

- Pain, acute or chronic (indication)
- Nutrition, risk for imbalanced: less than body requirements, (indication)
- Knowledge, deficient, related to medications and lifestyle changes (indications)

Planning

- Planning should be based on the assessment data, and interventions should be individualized to address patient needs.
- Routine orders: Most health care providers order antacids 1 hour before meals, 2 to 3 hours after meals, and at bedtime. As-needed (PRN) medication dosages also must be discussed.
- Each type of medication used to treat GERD or PUD may require somewhat different scheduling to avoid drug interactions. When developing the time frames for administration of medications on the medication

administration record (MAR), schedule the other prescribed drugs 1 hour before or 2 hours after antacids.
- Changes in diet require careful planning with the patient as well as the person responsible for purchasing and cooking the meals. Schedule teaching sessions appropriately. Not only may some foods need to be altered, but also the number of meals per day may need to be increased with a smaller serving at each meal.

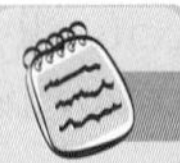

Patient Education and Health Promotion

Nutrition
- Implement prescribed dietary changes: eat small, more frequent meals to support optimal energy requirements and healing; avoid overdistention of the stomach; avoid any seasonings that are intolerable or that aggravate the condition; and avoid coffee, teas, colas, alcoholic beverages (including beer), carbonated beverages, peppermint, spearmint, and citric juices, which may produce discomfort in people who have GERD.
- Avoid late-night snacks or meals that could result in increased gastric secretions.
- Observe for foods that aggravate the condition, and eliminate these from the diet. Drink only small amounts of fluid with the meal and drink mostly between meals. Increase protein foods and decrease fats to about 45 g/day or less; use nonfat milk.

Pain, Discomfort. Keep a written record of the onset, duration, location, and precipitating factors for any pain. Sit upright at the table when eating and do not lie down for at least 2 hours after eating. When a hiatal hernia is present, elevate the head of the bed on 6- to 8-inch blocks to prevent reflux during sleep. Have the patient keep a log of the pain including time of day, any factors that might have precipitated the pain, and degree of pain relief from medications used.

Medications
- Take prescribed medications at recommended times to promote optimal healing. See individual drug monographs for suggested scheduling.
- Avoid NSAIDs and aspirin-containing medicines that irritate the gastric mucosa. Consult the physician or pharmacist regarding scheduling of or discontinuation of these medications.

Lifestyle Changes
- Discuss stress and its effects on the person, and implement needed lifestyle changes.
- Encourage a significant reduction or cessation of smoking.
- Implement plans to gain sufficient rest.

Fostering Health Maintenance
- Discuss medication information and how it will benefit the course of treatment to produce an optimal response. Medications used in the treatment of hyperacidity are important measures to alleviate the irritating effects on the mucosal tissue; stress the importance of not discontinuing treatment, and the need for continued medical follow-up.
- Seek cooperation and understanding of the following points so that medication adherence is increased: name of medication, dosage, route and times of administration, side effects to expect, side effects to report. Stress need to complete a full course of treatment for *H. pylori* so that the organisms are indeed killed and not only suppressed and then regrow because medications were discontinued too early.

Written Record. Enlist the patient's aid in developing and maintaining a written record of monitoring parameters (e.g., a list of foods causing problems, degree of pain relief) (see Patient Self-Assessment form on p. 531). Complete the Premedication Data column for use as a baseline to track response to drug therapy. Ensure that the patient understands how to use the form and instruct the patient to bring the completed form to follow-up visits. During follow-up visits, focus on issues that will foster adherence with the therapeutic interventions prescribed.

DRUG CLASS: Antacids

Actions

Antacids lower the acidity of gastric secretions by buffering the hydrochloric acid (normally pH is 1 or 2) to a lower hydrogen ion concentration. Buffering hydrochloric acid to a pH of 3 or 4 is highly desired because the proteolytic action of pepsin is reduced and the gastric juice loses its corrosive effect.

Uses

Antacid products account for one of the largest sales volumes (more than $1 billion annually) of over-the-counter (OTC) medication. Antacids are commonly used for heartburn, excessive eating and drinking, and PUD. However, nurses and patients must be aware that not all antacids are alike. They should be used judiciously, particularly by certain types of patients (e.g., those with heart failure, hypertension, renal failure). Long-term self-treatment with antacids may also mask symptoms of serious underlying diseases, such as a bleeding ulcer.

The most effective antacids available are combinations of aluminum hydroxide, magnesium oxide or hydroxide, magnesium trisilicate, and calcium carbonate. All act by neutralizing gastric acid. Combinations of these ingredients must be used because any compound used alone in therapeutic quantities may produce severe systemic side effects. Other ingredients found in antacid combination products include simethicone, alginic acid, and bismuth. *Simethicone* is a defoaming agent that breaks up gas bubbles in the stomach, reducing stomach distention and heartburn. It is effective in patients who have overeaten or who have heartburn, but it is not effective in treating PUD. *Alginic acid*

PATIENT SELF-ASSESSMENT FORM Agents Affecting the Digestive System

MEDICATIONS	COLOR	TO BE TAKEN

Patient ______

Health Care Provider ______

Health Care Provider's phone ______

Next appt.* ______

What I Should Monitor		Premedication Data	Date	Date	Date	Date	Date	Date	Comments
Bloating	Time it occurs (night, after eating, midday)								
	Causes (e.g., food eaten)								
Pain: Severity of pain	Time (before/after meals)								
	Location								
Severe 10 — Moderate 5 — Dull 0									
Nausea	Vomiting (describe amount, color, time of day)								
	Nausea (no vomiting)								
Bowels	Color								
	No. of stools per day								
	Soft, watery, or hard								
Diet: List foods that cause problems									
Degree of relief from medications: Great 10 — Good 5 — Poor 1									
Appetite: Excellent 10 — Good 5 — Poor 1									
Other									

*Please bring this record with you to your next appointment.
Use the back of this sheet for additional information.

produces a highly viscous solution of sodium alginate that floats on top of the gastric contents. It may be effective only in the patient being treated for GERD or hiatal hernia and should not be used in the patient with acute gastritis or PUD. *Bismuth* compounds have little acid-neutralizing capacity and are therefore poor antacids.

The following principles should be considered when antacid therapy is planned:

- For indigestion, antacids should not be administered for more than 2 weeks. If after this time the patient is still experiencing discomfort, a health care provider should be contacted.
- Patients with edema, heart failure, hypertension, renal failure, pregnancy, or salt-restricted diets should use low-sodium antacids, such as Riopan, Maalox, and Mylanta II. Therapy should continue only on the recommendation of a health care provider.
- Antacid tablets should be used only for the patient with occasional indigestion or heartburn. Tablets *do not* contain enough antacid to be effective in treating PUD.
- A common complaint of patients consuming large quantities of calcium carbonate or aluminum hydroxide is constipation. Excess magnesium results in diarrhea. If a patient experiences these symptoms and still has stomach discomfort, a health care provider should be consulted.

- Effective management of *acute* ulcer disease requires large volumes of antacids. The selection of an antacid and the quantity to be taken depend on its neutralizing capacity. Any patient with "coffee ground" hematemesis, bloody stools, or recurrent abdominal pain should seek medical attention immediately and not attempt to self-treat the disorder.
- Calcium carbonate and sodium bicarbonate may cause rebound hyperacidity.
- Patients with renal failure should not use large quantities of antacids containing magnesium. The magnesium ions cannot be excreted and may produce hypermagnesemia and toxicity.
- Most antacids have similar ingredients. Selection of an antacid for occasional use should be determined by quantity of each ingredient, cost, taste, and frequency of side effects. Patients may need to try more than one product and weigh the advantages and disadvantages of each.

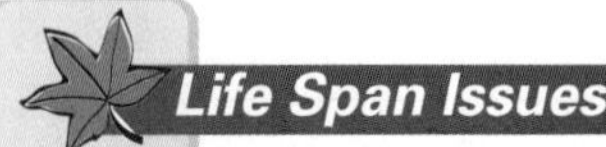

Life Span Issues

Antacids

People older than 65 years of age are the most common purchasers of antacids. Gastrointestinal disorders such as peptic ulcer disease, NSAID-induced ulcers, and gastroesophageal reflux disease occur more often in this age-group. Magnesium-containing antacids are often used as laxatives. Whereas the symptom of ulcer disease in a younger person is usually burning epigastric pain, the symptoms in an older person, if present at all, are usually vague abdominal discomfort, anorexia, and weight loss.

Therapeutic Outcomes

The primary therapeutic outcomes expected from antacid therapy are relief of discomfort, reduced frequency of heartburn, and healing of irritated tissues.

Nursing Process for Antacid Therapy

Premedication Assessment

1. Check renal function studies to ensure that renal function is normal. When renal failure is present, patients should not take large quantities of antacids containing magnesium. Magnesium ions cannot be excreted and may produce hypermagnesemia and toxicity.
2. Check the pattern of bowel elimination for diarrhea or constipation.
3. Record the pattern of gastric pain being experienced; report coffee-ground hematemesis, bloody stools, or recurrent abdominal pain to the health care provider for prompt attention.
4. If the patient is pregnant or has edema, heart failure, hypertension, or salt restrictions, ensure that a low-sodium antacid has been prescribed.
5. Schedule other prescribed medications 1 hour before or 2 hours after antacids are to be administered.

Planning

Availability. See Table 33-1.

- Liquid forms of antacids should be used for treatment of PUD because tablets do not contain enough active ingredients to be effective.
- Antacid tablets may be used for occasional episodes of heartburn. They should be well chewed

Table 33-1 ***Ingredients of Commonly Used Antacids***

PRODUCT	FORM	CALCIUM CARBONATE	ALUMINUM HYDROXIDE	ALUMINUM CARBONATE	MAGNESIUM OXIDE OR HYDROXIDE	MAGNESIUM CARBONATE	SODIUM BICARBONATE	SIMETHICONE	OTHER INGREDIENTS
Aludrox	Tablet, suspension		X		X			X	
Di-Gel	Tablet, liquid		X		X			X	
Gelusil	Tablet		X		X			X	
Maalox TC	Suspension		X		X				
Maalox Extra Strength	Suspension		X		X			X	
Mylanta	Tablet, suspension		X		X			X	
Mylanta Double Strength	Suspension		X		X			X	
Mylanta Supreme	Liquid	X			X				
Phillip's Milk of Magnesia	Tablet, suspension				X				
Riopan	Tablet, suspension								Magaldrate
Riopan Plus	Tablet, suspension							X	Magaldrate
Titralac	Tablet, suspension	X							Glycine
Tums	Tablet	X							

before swallowing for a more rapid onset of action.

Implementation

Dosage and Administration. See Table 33-1. Follow directions on the product container.

Evaluation

Side Effects to Expect

Chalky Taste. A chalky taste is a common problem with antacids. Suggest a change in brands or flavors. Suggest using a liquid instead of tablets.

Side Effects to Report

Diarrhea, Constipation. Diarrhea or constipation is a common problem when antacids are used in therapeutic dosages to treat ulcers. Alternating between calcium- or aluminum-containing compounds and magnesium-containing compounds should help alleviate the problem.

Drug Interactions

Tetracycline Antibiotics, Ciprofloxacin, Ketoconazole, Digoxin, Iron Compounds. The absorption of these medicines is inhibited by antacids. These medications should be administered 1 hour before or 2 to 3 hours after antacids.

Levodopa. Levodopa absorption is increased by antacids. When antacid therapy is added, toxicity may result in the parkinsonian patient who is well controlled taking a certain dosage of levodopa. If the patient's parkinsonism is well controlled on levodopa *and* antacid therapy, withdrawal of antacids may result in a recurrence of parkinsonian symptoms.

Quinidine, Amphetamines. Frequent use of antacid therapy may result in increased urinary pH. Renal excretion of quinidine and amphetamines may be inhibited, and toxicity may occur.

DRUG CLASS: Histamine (H_2)-Receptor Antagonists

Actions

One of the primary mechanisms of hydrochloric acid secretion is histamine stimulation of histamine (H_2) receptors on the stomach's parietal cells. The H_2 antagonists act by blocking H_2 receptors, resulting in a decrease in the volume of acid secreted. The pH of the stomach contents rises as a result of a reduction in acid.

Uses

The H_2 antagonists (cimetidine, ranitidine, nizatidine, famotidine) are used to treat GERD, duodenal ulcers, and pathologic hypersecretory conditions such as Zollinger-Ellison syndrome, and for preventing and treating stress ulcers in critically ill patients. Unapproved uses include prevention of aspiration pneumonitis, acute upper GI bleeding, and hyperparathyroidism.

Famotidine is similar in action and use to cimetidine but has the advantages of one dose daily, fewer drug interactions, and no antiandrogenic effect (which causes gynecomastia).

Ranitidine is similar in action and use to cimetidine but has the advantages of twice-daily dosing, fewer drug interactions, and no antiandrogenic effect.

Nizatidine, in contrast to the other agents, is not available in a parenteral dosage form.

Therapeutic Outcomes

The primary therapeutic outcomes expected from H_2 antagonist therapy are relief of discomfort, reduced frequency of heartburn, and healing of irritated tissues.

Nursing Process for H_2 Antagonists

Premedication Assessment

Perform a baseline assessment of the patient's mental status for comparison with subsequent mental status evaluations to detect central nervous system (CNS) alterations that may occur, particularly with cimetidine therapy.

Planning

Availability. See Table 33-2.

Implementation

Dosage and Administration. See Table 33-2.

- Administer cimetidine, famotidine, and ranitidine with food. Nizatidine may be administered with or without food.
- Because antacid therapy is often continued during early therapy of PUD, administer 1 hour before or 2 hours after the H_2-antagonist dose.

Evaluation

Side Effects to Expect

Dizziness, Headache, Diarrhea, Constipation, Somnolence. Approximately 1% to 3% of patients develop these side effects. They are usually mild and resolve with continued therapy. Encourage the patient not to discontinue therapy without first consulting the health care provider.

Provide patient safety during episodes of dizziness.

If patients develop somnolence and lethargy, encourage them to use caution when working around machinery or driving a car.

Maintain the patient's state of hydration, and obtain an order for stool softeners or bulk-forming laxatives if necessary. Encourage the inclusion of sufficient roughage (fresh fruits, vegetables, whole-grain products) in the diet.

Side Effects to Report

Confusion, Disorientation, Hallucinations. If high dosages (particularly of cimetidine) are used in patients with liver or renal disease or in patients older than 50 years of age, mental confusion, slurred speech, disorientation, and hallucinations may occur. These adverse effects dissipate over 3 or 4 days after therapy has been discontinued.

Drug Table 33-2 HISTAMINE (H_2)-RECEPTOR ANTAGONISTS

GENERIC NAME	BRAND NAME	AVAILABILITY	DOSAGE RANGE
cimetidine	Tagamet, Tagamet HB	Tablets: 200, 300, 400, 800 mg Suspension: 300 mg/5 mL Injection: 300 mg/2 mL	Duodenal and gastric ulcers—PO: 800-1600 mg at bedtime, 400 mg twice daily, or 300 mg four times daily; IM, IV: 300 mg q6-8h GERD—PO: 800 mg twice daily or 400 mg four times daily
famotidine	Pepcid, Pepcid AC	Tablets: 10, 20, 40 mg Tablets, chewable: 10 mg Suspension: 40 mg/5 mL Injection: 10 mg/mL	Duodenal and gastric ulcers—PO: 40 mg once daily at bedtime or 20 mg twice daily GERD—PO: 20 mg twice daily
nizatidine	Axid	Capsules: 150, 300 mg Tablets: 75 mg Oral Solution: 15 mg/mL	Duodenal and gastric ulcers—PO: 300 mg at bedtime or 150 mg twice daily GERD—PO: 150 mg twice daily
ranitidine	Zantac; Zantac 75, 150	Tablets: 75, 150, 300 mg Efferdose tablets: 150 mg Syrup: 15 mg/mL Injection: 1, 25 mg/mL	Duodenal and gastric ulcers—PO: 300 mg at bedtime or 150 mg twice daily GERD—PO: 150 mg twice daily

Perform a baseline assessment of the patient's degree of alertness and orientation to name, place, and time before starting therapy. Make regularly scheduled subsequent mental status evaluations, and compare findings. Report alterations.

Gynecomastia. Mild bilateral gynecomastia and breast soreness may occur with long-term use (longer than 1 month) of cimetidine but will resolve after discontinuing therapy. Report for further observation and possible laboratory tests.

Hepatotoxicity. Although rare, hepatotoxicity has been reported with H_2 antagonists. The symptoms of hepatotoxicity are anorexia, nausea, vomiting, jaundice, hepatomegaly, splenomegaly, and abnormal liver function tests (elevated bilirubin, aspartate aminotransferase [AST], alanine aminotransferase [ALT], gamma-glutamyltransferase [GGT], alkaline phosphatase, prothrombin time).

Drug Interactions

Benzodiazepines. Cimetidine inhibits the metabolism or excretion of the following benzodiazepines: alprazolam, chlordiazepoxide, diazepam, clorazepate, flurazepam, halazepam, prazepam, and triazolam.

Patients taking cimetidine and a benzodiazepine concurrently should be observed for increased sedation; a reduction in dosage of the benzodiazepine may be required. The metabolism of oxazepam, temazepam, and lorazepam does not appear to be affected.

Theophylline Derivatives. Cimetidine inhibits the metabolism or excretion of the following xanthine derivatives: aminophylline, oxtriphylline, dyphylline, and theophylline. Patients at greater risk include those receiving larger doses of theophylline and those with liver disease. Observe for restlessness, vomiting, dizziness, and cardiac dysrhythmias. The dosage of theophylline may need to be reduced.

Beta-Adrenergic Blocking Agents. Beta-adrenergic blocking agents (propranolol, labetalol, metoprolol) may accumulate as a result of inhibited metabolism. Monitor for signs of toxicity, such as hypotension and bradycardia.

Phenytoin. Cimetidine inhibits the metabolism of phenytoin. Monitor patients with concurrent therapy for signs of phenytoin toxicity: nystagmus, sedation, and lethargy. Serum levels may be ordered, and a reduced dosage of phenytoin may be required.

Lidocaine, Quinidine, Procainamide. Cimetidine may inhibit the metabolism of these agents. Monitor patients for signs of toxicity (e.g., bradycardia, additional dysrhythmias, hyperactivity, sedation), and reduce the dosage if necessary.

Antacids. Administer 1 hour before or 2 hours after administration of cimetidine.

Warfarin. Cimetidine may enhance the anticoagulant effects of warfarin. Observe for the development of petechiae, ecchymoses, nosebleeds, bleeding gums, dark tarry stools, and bright red or coffee-ground hematemesis. Monitor the prothrombin time (INR), and reduce the dosage of warfarin if necessary.

Calcium Antagonists. Cimetidine may inhibit the metabolism of diltiazem, nifedipine, and verapamil. Patients should be monitored for increased effects from the calcium antagonists (bradycardia, hypotension, dysrhythmias, fatigue).

Tricyclic Antidepressants. Cimetidine may inhibit the excretion of imipramine, desipramine, and nortriptyline, usually within 3 to 5 days after the start of cimetidine therapy. If anticholinergic effects or toxicity becomes apparent, a decreased dosage of the antidepressant may be required. If cimetidine is discontinued, the patient should be monitored for a decreased response to the antidepressant.

Famotidine, Nizatidine, Ranitidine. In general, there appear to be only minor interactions with these H_2 antagonists. There are conflicting data, however. Studies indicate that patients receiving higher doses of ranitidine may be more susceptible to drug interactions with ranitidine and other drugs. When used concurrently, monitor for toxic effects of warfarin, theophylline, procainamide, and glipizide.

DRUG CLASS: Gastrointestinal Prostaglandins

misoprostol (mis oh pros' tohl)
CYTOTEC (site' oh tech)

Actions

Misoprostol is the first of a new synthetic prostaglandin E series to be used to treat GI disorders. Prostaglandins are normally present in the GI tract to inhibit gastric acid and pepsin secretion to protect the stomach and duodenal lining against ulceration. The prostaglandin E analogs may also induce uterine contractions.

Uses

Misoprostol is used to prevent and treat gastric ulcers caused by NSAIDs, including aspirin. Whereas prostaglandin inhibition is effective in reducing pain and inflammation, especially in arthritis, prostaglandin inhibition in the stomach makes the patient more predisposed to peptic ulcers.

Therapeutic Outcomes

The primary therapeutic outcomes expected from misoprostol therapy are relief of discomfort and healing of irritated tissues.

Nursing Process for Misoprostol Therapy

Premedication Assessment

1. Determine if the patient is pregnant. This drug is a uterine stimulant and may induce miscarriage.
2. Check the pattern of bowel elimination; misoprostol may induce diarrhea.

Planning

Availability. 100 and 200 mcg tablets. WARNING: Misoprostol is contraindicated during pregnancy and in women at risk of becoming pregnant. As a uterine stimulant, it may induce miscarriage.

Implementation

Dosage and Administration. *Adult:* PO: 100 to 200 mcg tablets four times daily with food during NSAID therapy.

Evaluation

Side Effects to Expect

Diarrhea. Diarrhea associated with misoprostol therapy is dose related and usually develops after approximately 2 weeks of therapy. It often resolves after about 8 days, but a few patients require discontinuation of misoprostol therapy. Diarrhea can be minimized by taking misoprostol with meals and at bedtime and avoiding magnesium-containing antacids (e.g., Maalox, Mylanta). Encourage the patient not to discontinue therapy without first consulting the health care provider.

Encourage the inclusion of sufficient roughage (fresh fruits, vegetables, whole-grain products) in the diet.

Side Effects to Report

Pregnancy. Although pregnancy is obviously not a side effect of misoprostol therapy, it is crucial that therapy be discontinued if the patient is pregnant. The patient must receive care from the health care provider who prescribed the misoprostol as well as an obstetrician. The question of alternative therapies to NSAIDs must also be considered.

Drug Interactions. No significant drug interactions have been reported.

DRUG CLASS: Proton Pump Inhibitors

Actions

Proton pump inhibitors (PPI), also known as substituted benzimidazoles, inhibit gastric secretion by inhibiting the gastric acid pump of the stomach's parietal cells. These inhibitors have no anticholinergic or H_2-receptor antagonist actions.

Uses

Proton pump inhibitors are used to treat severe esophagitis, GERD, gastric and duodenal ulcers, and hypersecretory disorders, such as Zollinger-Ellison syndrome. They may also be used in combination with antibiotics (e.g., ampicillin, amoxicillin, clarithromycin) to eradicate *H. pylori,* a common cause of PUD.

Therapeutic Outcomes

The primary therapeutic outcomes expected from proton pump inhibitors are relief of discomfort, reduced frequency of heartburn, and healing of irritated tissues.

Nursing Process for Proton Pump Inhibitor Therapy

Premedication Assessment

Check pattern of bowel elimination; the pump inhibitors may induce diarrhea.

Planning

Availability. See Table 33-3.

Drug Table 33-3 PROTON PUMP INHIBITORS

GENERIC NAME	BRAND NAME	AVAILABILITY	DOSAGE RANGE
esomeprazole	Nexium	Capsules: 20, 40 mg IV: 20, 40 mg	IV, PO: Initial: 20-40 mg once daily for 4 to 8 weeks Maintenance: 20 mg daily
lansoprazole	Prevacid	Capsules: 15, 30 mg Tablets: 15, 30 mg Granules for oral suspension: 15, 30 mg IV: 30 mg	IV, PO: Initial: 15-30 mg once daily 30 minutes before a meal for 4 weeks Maintenance: 15 mg once daily Maximum: 30 mg once daily before a meal
omeprazole	Prilosec	Capsules: 10, 20, 40 mg Tablets: 20 mg Powder for oral suspension: 20, 40 mg	PO: Initial: 20 mg once daily for 4 weeks Maintenance: 20 mg daily Maximum: 120 mg three times daily for Zollinger-Ellison syndrome
pantoprazole	Protonix	Tablets: 20, 40 mg IV: 40 mg/vial	PO: Initial: 40 mg once daily for 8 weeks Maintenance: 40 mg daily IV: Initial: 40 mg once daily for up to 7-10 days; switch to oral dosages
rabeprazole	Aciphex	Tablets: 20 mg	PO: Initial: 20 mg daily after morning meal for up to 4 weeks Maintenance: 20 mg once daily Maximum: 60 mg twice daily

Implementation

Dosage and Administration. See Table 33-3. Capsules and tablets should be swallowed whole; instruct the patient not to open, chew, or crush.

Evaluation

Side Effects to Expect

Diarrhea, Headache, Muscle Pain, Fatigue. These symptoms are relatively mild and rarely result in the discontinuation of therapy. Encourage the patient not to discontinue therapy without first consulting the health care provider.

Maintain the patient's state of hydration. Encourage the inclusion of sufficient roughage (fresh fruits, vegetables, whole-grain products) in the diet.

Side Effects to Report

Rash. Persistent vesicular rash from omeprazole may be cause for discontinuing therapy. Report for further observation and possible laboratory tests.

Drug Interactions

Diazepam, Triazolam, Flurazepam. Omeprazole significantly increases the half-life of diazepam, triazolam, and flurazepam by inhibiting its metabolism. Observe patients for increased sedative effects from these medicines. Caution against hazardous tasks, such as driving and operating machinery. The dosages of diazepam, triazolam, and flurazepam may have to be reduced.

Phenytoin. Omeprazole slows the metabolism of phenytoin. Observe for nystagmus, sedation, and lethargy. The dosage of phenytoin may have to be reduced.

Warfarin. Omeprazole may reduce the rate of metabolism of warfarin. Monitor the patient closely for signs of bleeding tendencies, and monitor the prothrombin time (IHR) closely. Reduction of warfarin dosage may be required.

Sucralfate. Sucralfate inhibits the absorption of proton pump inhibitors. Administer the pump inhibitors at least 30 minutes before sucralfate.

Theophylline. Lansoprazole increases the metabolism of theophylline by approximately 10%. A slight increase in theophylline dosage may be required to maintain therapeutic activity.

Altered Absorption. The reduction in gastric acid secretion may alter absorption of food and drugs as follows:

- *Digoxin:* Monitor for signs of decreased activity (e.g., return of edema, weight gain, heart failure).
- *Ketoconazole, ampicillin, iron:* These medicines require an acid medium for absorption. They should be administered at least 30 to 45 minutes before lansoprazole therapy.
- *Insulin:* The absorption of food may be altered, and an adjustment in timing or dosage of insulin in patients with diabetes may be required.

DRUG CLASS: Coating Agents

sucralfate (sook rahl' fate)

▶ CARAFATE (kair' ah fate)

Actions

Sucralfate is an agent that when swallowed forms a complex that adheres to the crater of an ulcer, protecting it from aggravators such as acid, pepsin, and bile salts. Sucralfate does not inhibit gastric secretions (as do the H_2 antagonists) or alter gastric pH (as do antacids).

Uses

Sucralfate is used to treat duodenal ulcers, particularly in those patients who do not tolerate other forms of therapy.

Therapeutic Outcomes

The primary therapeutic outcomes expected from sucralfate therapy are relief of discomfort and healing of irritated tissues.

Nursing Process for Sucralfate Therapy

Premedication Assessment

Check pattern of bowel elimination; sucralfate may induce constipation.

Planning

Availability. PO: 1 g tablets and 1 g/10 mL suspension.

Implementation

Dosage and Administration. *Adult:* PO: 1 tablet 1 hour before each meal and at bedtime, all on an empty stomach. Because antacid therapy is often continued during early therapy of ulcer disease, administer antacids at least 30 minutes before or after sucralfate.

Evaluation

Side Effects to Expect

Constipation, Dry Mouth, Dizziness. These side effects are usually mild and tend to resolve with continued therapy. Encourage the patient not to discontinue therapy without first consulting the health care provider.

Measures to alleviate dry mouth include sucking on ice chips or hard candy. Avoid mouthwashes that contain alcohol because they cause further drying and irritation.

Maintain the patient's state of hydration, and obtain an order for stool softeners or bulk-forming laxatives if necessary. Encourage the inclusion of sufficient roughage (e.g., fresh fruits, vegetables, whole-grain products) in the diet.

Provide patient safety during episodes of dizziness.

Drug Interactions

Tetracyclines. Sucralfate may interfere with the absorption of tetracycline. Administer tetracyclines 1 hour before or 2 hours after sucralfate.

Omeprazole, Lansoprazole. Sucralfate inhibits the absorption of omeprazole and lansoprazole. Administer omeprazole or lansoprazole at least 30 minutes before sucralfate.

DRUG CLASS: Prokinetic Agents

metoclopramide (met oh klo' prah myd)
REGLAN (reg' lan)

Actions

Metoclopramide is a gastric stimulant whose mechanisms of action are not fully known. It increases lower esophageal sphincter pressure thus reducing reflux, increases stomach contractions, relaxes the pyloric valve, and increases peristalsis in the GI tract, resulting in an increased rate of gastric emptying and intestinal transit. Metoclopramide is an antiemetic that blocks dopamine in the chemoreceptor trigger zone. It inhibits serotonin ($5\text{-}HT_3$) when administered in higher dosages.

Uses

Metoclopramide is used to relieve the symptoms of gastric reflux esophagitis and diabetic gastroparesis, as an aid in small bowel intubation, and to stimulate gastric emptying and intestinal transit of barium after radiologic examination of the upper GI tract. It is also an antiemetic used with cancer chemotherapy.

Therapeutic Outcomes

The primary therapeutic outcomes expected from metoclopramide therapy are relief of discomfort, reduced frequency of heartburn, and healing of irritated tissues.

Nursing Process for Metoclopramide Therapy

Premedication Assessment

1. Determine if other drugs being taken may induce extrapyramidal symptoms; do not administer drug concurrently.
2. Check for a history of epilepsy. If present, check with the health care provider before starting drug therapy.
3. Do not administer to an individual with symptoms of GI perforation, mechanical obstruction, or hemorrhage.
4. For diabetic patients, food absorption may be altered and more frequent monitoring for hypoglycemia may be required.

Planning

Availability. PO: 5 and 10 mg tablets and 5 mg/5 mL syrup. Injection: 5 mg/mL in 2, 10, and 30 mL ampules.

Caution. Approximately 1 in 500 patients may develop extrapyramidal symptoms manifested by restlessness, involuntary movements, facial grimacing, and possibly oculogyric crisis, torticollis, or rhythmic tongue protrusion. Children and young adults are most susceptible, as are those patients receiving higher doses of metoclopramide as an antiemetic. Metoclopramide should not be used in patients with epilepsy or those receiving drugs that are likely to cause extrapyramidal reactions (e.g., phenothiazines) because the frequency and severity of seizures or extrapyramidal reactions may be increased. Metoclopramide must not be used in patients when increased gastric motility may be dangerous, such as with GI perforation, mechanical obstruction, or hemorrhage.

Implementation

Dosage and Administration. *Adult:* PO: Diabetic gastroparesis: 10 mg 30 minutes before each meal and at bedtime. Duration of therapy depends on response and continued well-being after discontinuation of therapy. IV: Antiemesis: Initial two doses: 2 mg/kg. If vomiting is suppressed, follow with 1 mg/kg. Dilute the dose in 50 mL of parenteral solution (D5W, normal saline [0.9%], D5/0.45 saline, Ringer's solution, or lactated Ringer's solution). Infuse over at least 15 minutes, 30 minutes before beginning chemotherapy. Repeat every 2 hours for two doses, followed by one dose every 3 hours for three doses. NOTE: Rapid IV infusion may cause sudden, intense anxiety and restlessness, followed by drowsiness. If extrapyramidal symptoms should develop, treat with diphenhydramine.

Evaluation

Side Effects to Expect

Drowsiness, Fatigue, Lethargy, Dizziness, Nausea. These side effects are usually mild and tend to resolve with continued therapy. Encourage the patient not to discontinue therapy without first consulting the health care provider.

People who work around machinery, drive a car, or perform other duties that require mental alertness should be particularly cautious.

Provide patient safety during episodes of dizziness.

Side Effects to Report

Extrapyramidal Symptoms. Provide patient safety, and then report extrapyramidal symptoms immediately.

Drug Interactions

Drugs That Increase Sedative Effects. Antihistamine, alcohol, analgesics, tranquilizers, and sedative-hypnotics increase the sedative effects of metoclopramide. Monitor the patient for excessive sedation, and reduce dosage if necessary.

Drugs That Decrease Therapeutic Effects. Anticholinergic agents (e.g., atropine, benztropine, antihistamines, dicyclomine) and narcotic analgesics (e.g., meperidine, morphine, oxycodone, and others) decrease the therapeutic effects of metoclopramide. Instruct the patient to try to avoid taking these agents while using metoclopramide.

Altered Absorption. The GI stimulatory effects of metoclopramide may alter absorption of food and drugs as follows:

- Digoxin: Monitor for decreased activity (e.g., return of edema, weight gain, heart failure).
- Levodopa: Monitor for increased activity (e.g., restlessness, nightmares, hallucinations, and additional involuntary movements such as bobbing of head and neck, facial grimacing, and active tongue movements).
- Alcohol: Monitor for signs of sedation and intoxication with smaller amounts of alcohol.
- Insulin: The absorption of food may be altered, and an adjustment in timing or dosage of insulin in patients with diabetes mellitus may be required.

DRUG CLASS: Antispasmodic Agents

Actions

Drugs used as antispasmodic agents are actually anticholinergics. The GI tract is heavily innervated by the cholinergic branch of the autonomic nervous system. Cholinergic fibers stimulate the GI tract, causing secretion of saliva, hydrochloric acid, pepsin, bile, and other enzymatic fluids necessary for digestion; relaxation of sphincter muscles; and peristalsis to move the contents of the stomach and bowel through the GI tract. The antispasmodic agents act by preventing acetylcholine from attaching to the cholinergic receptors in the GI tract. The extent of reduction of cholinergic activity depends on the amount of anticholinergic drug blocking the receptors. Inhibition of cholinergic nerve conduction results in decreased GI motility and reduced secretions.

Because cholinergic fibers innervate the entire body and these agents are not selective in their actions to the GI tract, the effects of blocking this system are seen throughout the body. To provide adequate dosages to inhibit GI motility and secretions, the following effects may also occur: reduced perspiration and oral and bronchial secretions; mydriasis (dilation of the pupils) with blurring of vision; constipation; urinary hesitancy or retention; tachycardia, possibly with palpitations; and mild, transient postural hypotension. Psychiatric disturbances, such as mental confusion, delusions, nightmares, euphoria, paranoia, and hallucinations, may be indications of overdosage.

Uses

Antispasmodic agents are used to treat irritable bowel syndrome, biliary spasm, mild ulcerative colitis, diverticulitis, pancreatitis, infant colic, and, in conjunction with diet and antacids, PUD. Since the advent of the H_2 antagonists, antispasmodic agents are used much less frequently in treating ulcers.

Therapeutic Outcomes

The primary therapeutic outcomes expected from antispasmodic therapy are relief of discomfort, reduced frequency of heartburn, and healing of irritated tissues.

Nursing Process for Antispasmodic Therapy

Premedication Assessment

1. Check the patient's history to screen for presence of closed-angle glaucoma; use of antispasmodic therapy in a patient with this condition could initiate an acute attack.
2. Perform a baseline mental status examination for future comparison of subsequent findings; these medicines may cause confusion, depression, nightmares, or hallucinations. These symptoms should be reported.
3. Obtain a baseline blood pressure, and plan to monitor blood pressure for orthostatic hypotension, a common drug side effect.
4. Use these drugs with caution in older patients and in patients with any condition in which GI transit time is compromised, because anticholinergic agents slow peristalsis.

Planning

Availability. See Table 33-4.

Glaucoma. All patients should be screened for closed-angle glaucoma before initiating therapy. Patients with open-angle glaucoma can safely use anticholinergic agents. Intraocular pressure should be monitored regularly.

Implementation

Dosage and Administration. See Table 33-4. Administer with food or milk to minimize gastric irritation.

Evaluation

Side Effects to Expect

Blurred Vision; Constipation; Urinary Retention; Dryness of the Mouth, Nose, and Throat. These are the anticholinergic effects produced by antispasmodic agents. Patients taking these medications should be monitored for these side effects.

Drug Table 33-4 ANTISPASMODIC AGENTS

GENERIC NAME	BRAND NAME	AVAILABILITY	CLINICAL USES	INITIAL RANGE
atropine	Atropine Sulfate	Injection: 0.05, 0.1, 0.3, 0.4, 0.5, 0.8, 1 mg/mL Tablets: 0.4 mg	Treatment of pylorospasm and spastic conditions of the GI tract	PO: 0.4-0.6 mg
belladonna	Belladonna Tincture	Tincture: 30 mg/dL	Indigestion, peptic ulcer Nocturnal enuresis Parkinsonism	Tincture: PO: 0.6-1 mg three or four times daily
dicyclomine	Bentyl, Di-spaz, ✤ Bentylol	Tablets: 20 mg Capsules: 10, 20 mg Syrup: 10 mg/5 mL Injection: 10 mg/mL	Irritable bowel syndrome Infant colic	Adults: PO: 20-40 mg three or four times daily Infants: PO: 5 mg three or four times daily
glycopyrrolate	Robinul	Tablets: 1, 2 mg Injection: 0.2 mg/mL	Peptic ulcer disease Preanesthetic	PO: 1 mg two or three times daily IM: 0.004 mg/kg 30-60 min before surgery
mepenzolate	Cantil	Tablets: 25 mg	Peptic ulcer disease	PO: 25-50 mg four times daily
methscopolamine	Pamine	Tablets: 2.5, 5 mg	Peptic ulcer disease	PO: 2.5 mg 30 min before meals and 2.5-5 mg at bedtime
propantheline	Pro-Banthine	Tablets: 7.5, 15 mg	Peptic ulcer disease	PO: 15 mg before meals and 30 mg at bedtime
scopolamine	Scopace, Scopolamine, ✤ Transderm-V	Tablets: 0.4 mg Injection: 0.3, 0.4, 0.86, 1 mg/mL	GI hypermotility, pylorospasm, irritable colon syndrome	PO: 0.4 to 0.8 mg Subcutaneously or IM: 0.32-0.65 mg

✤ Available in Canada.

Mucosa dryness may be alleviated by sucking hard candy or ice chips or by chewing gum.

If patients develop urinary hesitancy, assess for bladder distention. Report to the health care provider for further evaluation.

Give stool softeners as prescribed. Encourage adequate fluid intake and foods that provide sufficient bulk.

Caution the patient that blurred vision may occur, and make appropriate suggestions for patient safety.

Side Effects to Report

Confusion, Depression, Nightmares, Hallucinations. Perform a baseline assessment of the patient's degree of alertness and orientation to name, place, and time *before* initiating therapy. Make regularly scheduled subsequent mental status evaluations, and compare findings. Report alterations. Provide patient safety during these episodes. Reducing the daily dosage may control these adverse effects.

Orthostatic Hypotension. All antispasmodic agents may cause some degree of orthostatic hypotension, although it is infrequent and generally mild. It is manifested by dizziness and weakness, particularly when therapy is initiated. Monitor the blood pressure daily in both the supine and standing positions.

Anticipate the development of postural hypotension, and take measures to prevent it. Teach the patient to rise slowly from a supine or sitting position. Encourage the patient to sit or lie down if feeling faint.

Palpitations, Dysrhythmias. Report for further evaluation.

Drug Interactions

Amantadine, Tricyclic Antidepressants, Phenothiazines. These agents may potentiate the anticholinergic side effects. Confusion and hallucinations characterize excessive anticholinergic activity.

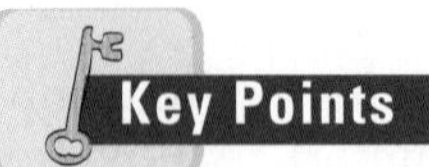

- GERD and PUD continue to be common illnesses that are often initially self-treated. Once medication therapy is instituted, it is important to thoroughly explain the medications prescribed and side effects that should be expected or reported. Some medications taken for GERD and ulcer disease can have significant adverse side effects that will need health care provider management.
- The nurse should solicit information about whether symptoms have decreased and whether the patient is experiencing adverse effects from therapy. Have the patient maintain a record of the pain using a standard pain rating scale. Also have the patient record the degree of relief obtained at a specified interval after medications are taken.
- The nurse is an ideal health professional to assess and make recommendations regarding lifestyle changes that are necessary to prevent symptom recurrence. If symptoms have not begun to diminish over 2 weeks, the nurse should encourage the person to seek medical attention.

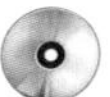

Go to your Companion CD-ROM for Appendices, an Audio Glossary, animations, Drug Dosage Calculators, customizable Patient Self-Assessment forms, and Review Questions for the NCLEX® Examination.

evolve Be sure to visit the companion Evolve site at http://evolve.elsevier.com/Clayton for WebLinks and additional online resources.

MEDICATION SAFETY REVIEW

MATH REVIEW QUESTIONS

1. Order: Ranitidine (Zantac) 50 mg in 100 mL D5W IV over 20 minutes

   Using an infusion pump calibrated in milliliters per hour, at what rate would the infusion pump be set?

   Give at a rate of ____ mL/hr (infusion pump).

2. Order: Famotidine (Pepcid) 35 mg PO stat

   Available: Famotidine (Pepcid) 40 mg/mL oral suspension

   Give ___ mL.

CRITICAL THINKING QUESTIONS

1. A 45-year-old patient has PUD and seems unaware that lifestyle changes are needed to treat the disorder. She has an H_2 antagonist ordered. What teaching approaches would be appropriate for her?
2. A patient complains of intermittent diarrhea. No physical basis for the diarrhea has been identified. She also complains of heartburn. Explore self-treatments available with OTC medicines that could cause the diarrhea.
3. Summarize premedication assessments for each classification of drugs used to treat PUD and GERD.
4. Identify the action of each classification of drugs used in the treatment of PUD and GERD.

CONTENT REVIEW QUESTIONS

1. Antacid therapy requires a premedication assessment of:
   1. renal function studies and/or renal disease present.
   2. mental status data.
   3. serum electrolyte studies.
   4. closed-angle glaucoma.

2. Metoclopramide therapy has possible major reportable side effects of:
   1. irregular heartbeat.
   2. persistent vesicular rash.
   3. extrapyramidal symptoms.
   4. hepatotoxicity.

3. Drugs whose generic names all end in "-dine" belong to a class of drugs known as:
   1. prokinetic agents.
   2. coating agents.
   3. proton pump inhibitors.
   4. histamine (H_2)-receptor antagonists.

4. This classification of drugs has the side effects of blurred vision, constipation, urinary retention, and dryness of mucosa of mouth, nose, and throat.
   1. Anticholinergics
   2. Proton pump inhibitors
   3. Histamine (H_2)-receptor antagonists
   4. Prokinetic agents

5. Ranitidine and famotidine have which of the following benefits over cimetidine?
   1. They must be taken more frequently.
   2. They have fewer drug interactions.
   3. They have an antiandrogenic effect.
   4. They can only be given orally.

6. The mechanism of action of pantoprazole is:
   1. inhibiting the gastric acid pump of the stomach's parietal cells.
   2. coating the lining of the stomach.
   3. increasing gastric emptying.
   4. reducing peristalsis.

7. Gastric acid pump inhibitors and antibiotics are often used in combination to rid which common cause of PUD?
   1. NSAID drugs
   2. Complications of smoking
   3. *H. pylori*
   4. Viruses

CHAPTER

34 Drugs Used to Treat Nausea and Vomiting

evolve http://evolve.elsevier.com/Clayton

Chapter Content

Objectives

1. Compare the purposes of using antiemetic products.
2. State the therapeutic classes of antiemetics.
3. Discuss scheduling of antiemetics for maximum benefit.

Key Terms

nausea
vomiting
emesis
retching
regurgitation
postoperative nausea and vomiting (PONV)
hyperemesis gravidarum
psychogenic vomiting
chemotherapy-induced nausea and vomiting (CINV)
anticipatory nausea and vomiting
delayed emesis
radiation-induced nausea and vomiting (RINV)

NAUSEA AND VOMITING

Nausea is the sensation of abdominal discomfort that is intermittently accompanied by a desire to vomit. Vomiting (also known as emesis) is the forceful expulsion of gastric contents up the esophagus and out the mouth. Nausea may occur without vomiting, and sudden vomiting may occur without prior nausea, but the two symptoms often occur together. Retching is the involuntary labored, spasmodic contractions of the abdominal and respiratory muscles without the expulsion of gastric contents (also known as "dry heaves").

Nausea and vomiting accompany almost any illness and are experienced by virtually everyone at one time or another. They may be due to a wide variety of causes (Box 34-1).

The primary anatomic areas involved in vomiting are shown in Figure 34-1. The vomiting center (VC) located in the medulla of the brain coordinates the vomiting reflex. Nerves from sensory receptors in the pharynx, stomach, intestines, and other tissues connect directly with the VC through the vagus and splanchnic nerves and produce vomiting when stimulated. The vomiting center also responds to stimuli originating in other tissues, such as the cerebral cortex, vestibular apparatus of the inner ear, and blood. These stimuli travel first to the chemoreceptor trigger zone (CTZ), which then activates the VC to induce vomiting. The CTZ is also located in the medulla. An important function of the CTZ is to sample blood and spinal fluid for potentially toxic substances and, when detected, to initiate the vomiting reflex. The CTZ cannot initiate vomiting independently but only by stimulating the VC. Both the VC and the CTZ are much smaller than shown in Figure 34-1.

The cerebral cortex of the brain can be a source of stimulus or suppression of the VC (see Figure 34-1). Vomiting can occur as a conditioned response (e.g., anticipatory nausea and vomiting as described later), or as a reaction to unpleasant sights and smells. Suppression of motion sickness by the person's concentration on some mental activity is an example of cortical control of the vomiting reflex. Psychological factors can play an important role (see psychogenic vomiting, later), although they are usually controlled by physical factors.

When the VC is stimulated, nerve impulses are sent to the salivary, vasomotor, and respiratory centers. The vomiting reflex begins with a sudden deep inspiration

Box 34-1 ***Causes of Nausea and Vomiting***

- Infection
- Gastrointestinal disorders such as gastritis or liver, gallbladder, or pancreatic disease
- Overeating or irritation of the stomach by certain foods or liquids
- Motion sickness
- Drug therapy (nausea and vomiting are the most common side effects of drug therapy)
- Surgical procedures (e.g., abdominal surgery, extraocular and middle ear manipulations, testicular traction)
- Emotional disturbances and mental illness
- Pregnancy
- Pain and unpleasant sights and odors

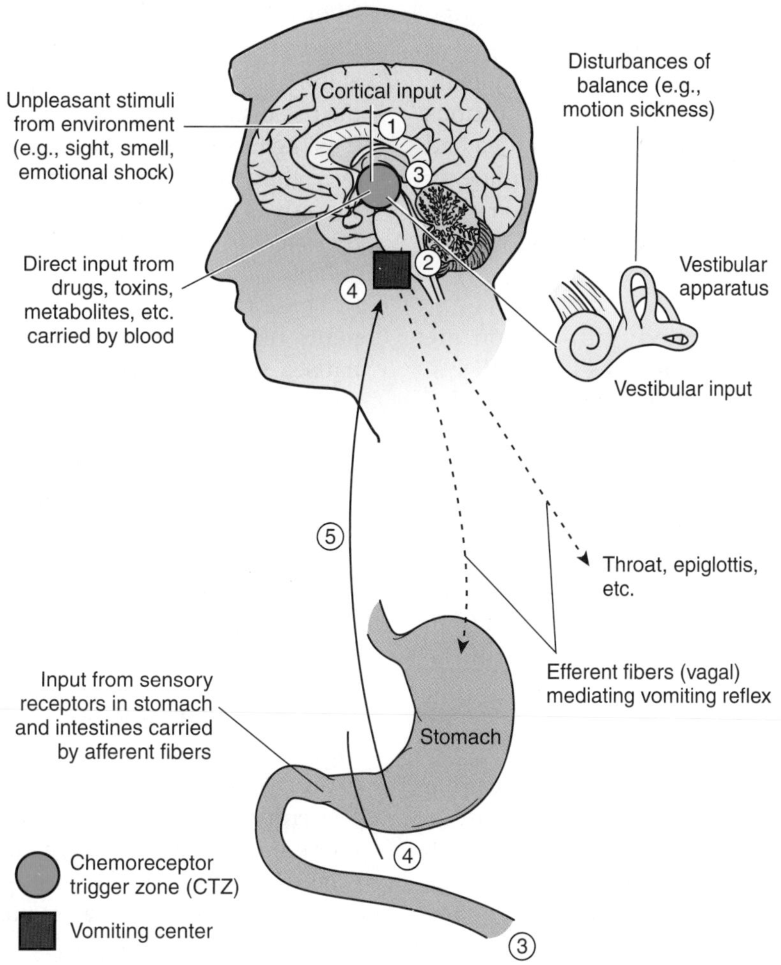

FIGURE **34-1** Sites of action of antiemetic medicines. *(1)* Cerebral cortex—anxiolytic agents; *(2)* vestibular apparatus—antihistamine and anticholinergic agents; *(3)* chemoreceptor trigger zone and gastrointestinal tract—dopamine antagonists; *(4)* serotonin receptors in GI tract and vomiting center—serotonin antagonists; *(5)* neurokinin receptors in vomiting center—neurokinin-1 receptor antagonists.

that increases abdominal pressure, which is further increased by contraction of the abdominal muscles. The soft palate rises and the epiglottis closes, thus preventing the aspiration of vomitus into the lungs. The pyloric sphincter contracts and the cardiac sphincter and esophagus relax, allowing stomach contents to be expelled. The flow of saliva increases to aid the expulsion. Autonomic symptoms of pallor, sweating, and tachycardia cause additional discomfort associated with vomiting. Regurgitation (burping, belching) occurs when the gastric or esophageal contents rise to the pharynx because of greater pressure (gas bubbles, tight clothing, body position) in the stomach and should not be confused with vomiting.

COMMON CAUSES OF NAUSEA AND VOMITING

Postoperative Nausea and Vomiting

Postoperative nausea and vomiting (PONV) constitute a relatively common complication after surgery. The incidence of nausea and vomiting varies with the surgical procedure, gender, age, obesity, anesthetic procedure, and analgesia used. A previous history of motion sickness and PONV also is an indicator of the likelihood of developing this postoperative complication. Factors associated with obesity that may contribute to a higher incidence of nausea and vomiting are a larger residual gastric volume, increased esophageal reflux, and increased gallbladder and gastrointestinal disease. Fat-soluble anesthetics may also accumulate in adipose tissue and continue to be released long after anesthesia is discontinued. Pain not treated with appropriate analgesia also induces nausea and vomiting. Surgical procedures that have a higher incidence of PONV are extraocular muscle and middle-ear manipulations, testicular traction, and abdominal surgery. Women have a higher incidence of PONV, possibly because of hormonal differences. Children ages 11 to 14 years have the highest incidence based on age-group. Patients who have had general anesthesia have a higher incidence of PONV than those who have had regional anesthesia; spinal anesthesia is generally associated with less PONV than general anesthesia; peripheral regional anesthesia is the least emetogenic. Analgesics (e.g., morphine, meperidine, fentanyl, alfentanil) used as premedications or with regional anesthetics frequently induce nausea and vomiting. Patients under nitrous oxide anesthesia have a higher incidence of nausea and vomiting than do those under halothane, enflurane, or isoflurane. Swallowed blood and gas accumulation in the stomach may also induce nausea and vomiting.

Motion Sickness

Nausea and vomiting associated with motion are thought to result from stimulation of the labyrinth system of the ear, with subsequent transmission of this stimulus to the vestibular network located near the vomiting center. When there is strong or frequent stimulation, such as from a rocking ship or airplane, the vestibular network is bombarded with an abnormally high number of impulses that radiate by cholinergic nerve impulses to the adjacent vomiting center. Thus drugs that inhibit the cholinergic nerve impulses from the vestibular network to the vomiting center should be effective in treating motion sickness.

Nausea and Vomiting in Pregnancy

The percentage of women reporting vomiting during the first 16 weeks of gestation is relatively constant at about 40%, decreasing to 20% from 17 to 20 weeks, with only 9% of women complaining of vomiting after 20 weeks of pregnancy. Vomiting is significantly more common among primigravidas, younger women, women with less education, nonsmokers, African Americans, and obese women. Contrary to commonly held beliefs, vomiting is not more common among women who have experienced prior fetal losses or among women with hypertension, proteinuria, or diabetes or those who used diethylstilbestrol. There is also no association between vomiting and cohabitation; unplanned pregnancy; or gallbladder, liver, or thyroid disease.

Although traditionally described as "morning sickness," the majority of women report that symptoms of nausea and vomiting tend to persist to varying degrees throughout the day. The cause of morning sickness is unknown, but its occurrence and severity appear to be related to the levels of free and bound estradiol and sex hormone–globulin binding capacity.

A woman with severe persistent vomiting that interferes with nutrition, fluid, and electrolyte balance may be experiencing **hyperemesis gravidarum,** a condition in which starvation, dehydration, and acidosis are superimposed on the vomiting syndrome. Hospitalization for fluid, electrolyte, and nutritional therapy may be required.

Psychogenic Vomiting

Psychogenic vomiting can be self-induced, or it can occur involuntarily in response to situations that the person considers threatening or distasteful (e.g., eating food whose origin is considered repulsive).

Chemotherapy-Induced Nausea and Vomiting

Chemotherapy-induced nausea and vomiting (CINV) is the most unpleasant adverse effect associated with the use of cancer chemotherapy. Many patients regard it as the most stressful aspect of their disease, more so even than the prospect of dying. Because the object of therapy is to prolong life for a relatively short period, the effect of CINV on the quality of life must be considered.

Three types of emesis have been identified in patients receiving antineoplastic therapy: anticipatory nausea and vomiting, acute CINV, and delayed emesis.

Anticipatory nausea and vomiting is a conditioned response triggered by the sight or smell of the clinic or hospital or by the knowledge that treatment is imminent. The onset of anticipatory nausea and vomiting is usually 2 to 4 hours before treatment and is most severe at the time of chemotherapy administration. Patients who experience anticipatory nausea and vomiting are more likely to be younger and to have received about twice as many courses of chemotherapy with more drugs for about three times as long as patients who do not experience this complication.

Acute CINV may be stimulated directly by chemotherapeutic agents. This type of emesis may begin 1 to 6 hours after chemotherapy is administered and last for up to 24 hours. The emetogenic potential of antineoplastic drugs is highly variable, ranging from an incidence of almost 100% with high-dose cisplatin to less than 10% with chlorambucil. Table 34-1 summarizes chemotherapeutic agents in terms of emetogenicity. Emetogenicity also is influenced by dosage, duration, and frequency of administration.

Patient factors also affect acute CINV. The incidence and severity of CINV are generally greater among younger people, women, those in poor general health, and those with metabolic disorders (e.g., uremia, dehydration, infection, gastrointestinal obstruction). Patients with a history of motion sickness seem to be more sensitive to the emetic effects of cytotoxic agents. The patient's outlook and attitude about cancer and therapy can significantly influence the frequency and severity of nausea and vomiting.

Delayed emesis occurs 24 to 120 hours after the administration of chemotherapy. The mechanisms are not known, but may be induced by metabolic by-products of the chemotherapeutic agent or by destruction of malignant cells. The emesis experienced is usually less severe than that which occurs acutely, but it still can be significant in reducing activity, nutrition, and hydration. Patients who have incomplete control of acute emesis often experience delayed emesis. Events that often trigger delayed nausea and vomiting are brushing teeth, using mouthwash, manipulating dentures, seeing food, and quickly standing up after getting out of bed in the morning.

Table 34-1 Potential of Emesis with Chemotherapeutic Agents

AGENT	FREQUENCY OF EMESIS
VERY HIGH EMETIC POTENTIAL	>90%
carmustine (BNCU) (high dose)	
cisplatin (high dose)	
cyclophosphamide (high dose)	
cytarabine (high dose)	
dacarbazine	
dactinomycin	
lomustine (high dose)	
mechlorethamine	
streptozocin	
HIGH EMETIC POTENTIAL	60%-90%
carboplatin	
carmustine (BNCU)	
cyclophosphamide (dose dependent)	
cytarabine	
dacarbazine	
doxorubicin (Adriamycin) (high dose)	
ifosfamide	
lomustine	
methotrexate (high dose)	
plicamycin (Mithramycin)	
procarbazine (dose dependent)	
MODERATE EMETIC POTENTIAL	30%-60%
doxorubicin (Adriamycin)	
daunorubicin	
epirubicin	
hexamethylmelamine	
idarubicin	
ifosfamide	
irinotecan	
methotrexate	
mitoxantrone	
LOW EMETIC POTENTIAL	10%-30%
capecitabine	
docetaxel	
etoposide	
5-fluorouracil	
gemcitabine	
mitomycin	
methotrexate	
6-mercaptopurine	
paclitaxel	
tamoxifen	
thiotepa	
vinblastine (dose dependent)	
VERY LOW EMETIC POTENTIAL	<10%
bleomycin	
busulfan	
chlorambucil	
corticosteroids	
fludarabine	
hydroxyurea	
thioguanine	
vinblastine	
vincristine	
vinorelbine	

Modified from Borson HL, McCarthy LE: Neuropharmacology of chemotherapy-induced emesis, *Drugs* 25 (Suppl 1):8-17, 1983.

Radiation-Induced Nausea and Vomiting

Another common cause of emesis associated with treatment of cancer is radiation-induced nausea and vomiting (RINV). The use of high-energy radiation (also known as radiotherapy) from x-rays, gamma rays, neutrons, and other sources to kill cancer cells and shrink tumors also induces nausea and vomiting, especially when concurrent chemotherapy is used. Radiation may come from a machine outside the body (external-beam radiation therapy), or it may come from radioactive material placed in the body near cancer cells (internal radiation therapy, implant radiation). Frequency of RINV depends on the treatment site, field exposure, dose of radiation delivered per fraction, and total dose delivered.

DRUG THERAPY FOR SELECTED CAUSES OF NAUSEA AND VOMITING

Control of vomiting is important, not only to relieve the obvious distress associated with it but also to prevent aspiration of gastric contents into the lungs, dehydration, and electrolyte imbalance. Primary treatment of nausea and vomiting should be directed at the underlying cause. Because this is not always possible, treatment with nondrug as well as drug measures is appropriate. Most medicines (antiemetics) used to treat nausea and vomiting act either by suppressing the action of the vomiting center or inhibiting the impulses going to or coming from the center. These agents are generally more effective if administered before the onset of nausea, rather than after it has started. The seven classes of agents used as antiemetics are dopamine antagonists, serotonin antagonists, anticholinergic agents, corticosteroids, benzodiazepines, neurokinin-1 receptor antagonists, and cannabinoids.

Postoperative Nausea and Vomiting

As mentioned, there is no single cause of PONV, and therefore treatment with a single pharmacologic agent for all cases is unlikely. Measures such as limiting patient movement and preventing gastric distention can reduce PONV. Adequate analgesia can also forestall this complication. Nonsteroidal antiinflammatory analgesics are not emetogenic (opioids are emetogenic) and should be given consideration if appropriate to the type of surgical procedure. Antiemetics used include dopamine antagonists, anticholinergic agents, and serotonin antagonists. The H_2 antagonists (e.g., cimetidine, ranitidine) also are occasionally used to reduce gastric secretions to minimize nausea and vomiting.

PONV is usually managed with an as-needed (PRN) order, but patients who are considered to be at moderate to high risk for PONV should be considered for prophylactic antiemetic therapy. In addition to minimizing the risk factors listed, a "multimodal treatment approach" is recommended because of the variety of receptor types associated with PONV. Therapy may include hydration, supplemental oxygen, a benzodiazepine for anxiolysis, a combination of antiemetics that work by different mechanisms (e.g., droperidol, dexamethasone, serotonin antagonist), total intravenous (IV) anesthesia (e.g., propofol and remifentanil), and analgesia with a nonsteroidal antiinflammatory drug (NSAID) (e.g., ketorolac) rather than an opioid. Nonpharmacologic techniques prior to surgery using acupuncture, transcutaneous electrical nerve stimulation (TENS), and acupressure stimulation have also been shown to reduce PONV.

The first step in treating PONV is to identify the cause. If a nasogastric (NG) tube is in place, check its patency and placement in preventing abdominal distention. Do not move an NG tube that was inserted during surgery (e.g., gastric resection); in such cases there is a danger of penetrating the suture line. Irrigation of a blocked NG tube may alleviate the nausea and vomiting. (A health care provider's order to irrigate the NG tube is required.) Administration of PRN antiemetics when the patient first complains of nausea will often prevent vomiting.

Motion Sickness

Most agents used to reduce nausea and vomiting from motion sickness are chemically related to antihistamines. The effectiveness of antihistamines in motion sickness probably results from their anticholinergic properties, not from their ability to block histamine.

Nausea and Vomiting in Pregnancy

In most cases, morning sickness can be controlled by dietary measures alone. The woman should be advised to eat small, frequent dry meals and to avoid fatty foods and other foods found to cause problems. Sometimes it may be difficult or impossible to work in the kitchen around food, and assistance may be required.

In approximately 15% of cases, dietary measures alone will be insufficient, and drug therapy should be considered. Drugs that have been extensively used for treating morning sickness are phenothiazines such as promethazine and prochlorperazine, and antihistamines such as diphenhydramine, dimenhydrinate, meclizine, and cyclizine. Ginger, an herb (see Chapter 48) is used in many cultures to treat pregnancy-induced nausea and vomiting. From a safety standpoint, meclizine, cyclizine, or dimenhydrinate is generally recommended first. If persistent vomiting threatens maternal nutrition, promethazine may be considered. If antidopaminergic antiemetic therapy is required, prochlorperazine is the safest time-tested medicine. Metoclopramide has been shown to be an effective antiemetic in treating hyperemesis gravidarum, and no teratogenic effects have been reported to date.

Psychogenic Vomiting

When a person has chronic or recurrent vomiting, a diagnosis of psychogenic vomiting is made after elimination of all other possible causes. The person with psychogenic vomiting usually does not lose weight and is able to control vomiting in certain situations (e.g., in public). Identification of the causes of psychogenic vomiting and successful resolution of the problem may not be possible. After an extensive workup eliminates other potential causes, a short course of an antiemetic drug, such as metoclopramide, or an antianxiety drug may be prescribed, along with counseling.

Anticipatory Nausea and Vomiting

People with a negative attitude toward therapy, such as the belief that it will be of no benefit, are more likely to develop anticipatory nausea and vomiting. It tends to become more severe as treatments progress unless behavior therapy modifies the conditioned response. Such treatments include progressive muscle relaxation, mind diversion, hypnosis, self-hypnosis, systematic desensitization, and benzodiazepines. Nurses can play a significant role by maintaining a positive, supportive attitude with the patient and making sure the patient receives antiemetic therapy before each course of chemotherapy.

Chemotherapy-Induced Nausea and Vomiting

Antiemetic therapy to minimize acute CINV is based on the emetogenic potential of the antineoplastic agents used. Combinations of antiemetics are often used, based on the assumption that antineoplastic agents produce emesis by more than one mechanism. In general, all patients being treated with chemotherapeutic agents of moderate to very high emetogenic potential should receive prophylactic antiemetic therapy before chemotherapy is started. Combinations of ondansetron, dolasetron, granisetron, or palonosetron; dexamethasone; aprepitant; and possibly metoclopramide are often used. Haloperidol may be substituted for metoclopramide if the latter is not tolerated by the patient. Antiemetic therapy should be continued for 2 to 4 days to prevent delayed vomiting. Emesis induced by moderately emetogenic agents may be treated prophylactically with a similar regimen and therapy should be continued for 24 hours. Dexamethasone with or without a phenothiazine (prochlorperazine) is recommended if the chemotherapy is of low emetic potential. Antiemetic therapy is not recommended with medicines of minimum emetic risk, although prochlorperazine may be used to prevent delayed emesis. All antiemetics should be administered an adequate time before chemotherapy is initiated and should be continued for an appropriate time after the antineoplastic agent has been discontinued.

Delayed Emesis

In general, patients who have complete control of acute emesis have a much lower incidence of delayed-onset emesis. A combination of prochlorperazine, lorazepam, and diphenhydramine given orally 1 hour before meals has been successful in controlling delayed emesis. Recent studies indicate that adding aprepitant, the NK_1

antagonist, in combination with a serotonin antagonist plus dexamethasone, significantly reduces the incidence of delayed emesis.

Radiation-Induced Nausea and Vomiting

Clinical guidelines recommend that patients who will be receiving radiation over a large portion of the body or those receiving a single-exposure, high-dose radiation therapy to the upper abdomen should receive preventive antiemetic therapy. Granisetron, a serotonin antagonist, is approved to treat RINV. Patients at low to intermediate risk for RINV should receive granisetron or prochlorperazine before each dose of radiation. Rescue medicines used to treat RINV include prochlorperazine, metoclopramide, and thiethylperazine. Patients who require rescue antiemetic therapy should be pretreated with a serotonin antagonist before the next dose of rational therapy.

NURSING PROCESS *for Nausea and Vomiting*

Nausea and vomiting are associated with illnesses of the gastrointestinal tract and other body systems and with side effects of medications and food intolerance. Nursing care must be individualized to the patient's diagnosis and needs at all times.

Assessment

History

- Obtain a history of the patient's symptoms—onset, duration, frequency, volume, and description of the vomitus (e.g., color: "coffee ground," greenish yellow, red tinged; consistency, undigested food particles).
- Ask the patient's perception of the precipitating factors, such as foods, odors, medications, stress, or treatment (e.g., chemotherapy, radiation therapy, surgery). Is there actual emesis or is it primarily retching?

Medications. Ask the patient to list all current over-the-counter (OTC) medications being taken (including herbal supplements) or those prescribed by a health care provider. Are any used to treat nausea and vomiting?

Basic Assessment

- Individualize the assessment procedure to the underlying cause of the symptoms if known.
- *Vital signs:* Obtain baseline vital signs, height, and weight.
- *Abdomen:* Assess bowel sounds in all four quadrants of the abdomen. Observe the size and shape of the abdomen. Note any signs of distention, ascites, or masses.
- *Hydration:* Assess and record signs of hydration. Examine for poor skin turgor, sticky oral mucous membranes, excessive thirst, shrunken and deeply furrowed tongue, crusted lips, weight loss, deteriorating vital signs, soft or sunken eyeballs, delayed capillary filling, high urine specific gravity or no urine output, and possible mental confusion.

Laboratory Studies. Review laboratory reports for indications of malabsorption; protein depletion; dehydration; fluid, electrolyte, and acid–base imbalances; and so on (e.g., K^+, Cl^-, pH, Pco_2, bicarbonate, hemoglobin [Hgb] hematocrit [Hct], urinalysis [specific gravity], serum albumin, total protein). The scope of laboratory data gathered will depend on the underlying cause of the nausea and vomiting and severity of the symptoms.

Nursing Diagnoses

- Fluid volume, deficient (indication)
- Nutrition, imbalanced: less than body requirements (indication)

Planning

History. Plan to perform a focused assessment consistent with the symptoms and underlying pathologic condition.

Medications

- Schedule prescribed medications on the medication administration record (MAR), and requisition the medicines from the pharmacy.
- Ensure that prechemotherapy or preradiation therapy antiemetics are marked precisely as ordered on the MAR along with around-the-clock or PRN orders.

Nursing Interventions

- Mark the Kardex or enter data in computer with specific parameters to be recorded: intake and output, vital signs every shift or more frequently depending on patient's status and daily weights.
- Mark the Kardex or enter data in computer with any requested testing of the vomitus (e.g., presence of blood, pH).
- Schedule oral hygiene measures.

Nutrition

- Obtain specific orders relating to nutrition. Diet orders will depend on the underlying cause and severity of the nausea and vomiting.
- Mark the Kardex or enter data in computer regarding nutrition status (e.g., nothing by mouth [NPO], NG suction, IV fluids, enteral or parenteral nutrition).
- As the patient's condition improves, obtain diet orders for a gradual progression of diet.

Laboratory Studies. Order baseline laboratory studies requested by the health care provider, such as electrolytes, white blood cell count with differential, hemoglobin, hematocrit, and albumin. The extent of laboratory studies will depend on the underlying cause and patient's clinical condition.

Implementation

Maintain hydration via oral or parenteral forms as prescribed by the health care provider.

Adults: The usual treatment includes discontinuation of solid foods and the ingestion of oral rehydration solutions or clear juices. Depending on the severity of the condition or underlying cause, the patient may be NPO with an NG tube in place for hydration.

As the patient's condition improves, the diet is advanced from clear liquids to small, frequent low-fat feedings to bland or normal diet. Generally high-fat foods, milk products, whole grains, and raw fruits and vegetables are initially avoided.

Infants: Formula, milk products, and solid foods usually are discontinued. Fluids are offered every 30 to 60 minutes in small amounts (30 to 60 mL). The volume is gradually increased as tolerance improves. Oral rehydration solutions (e.g., Pedialyte, diluted Jell-O water, decarbonated colas, ginger ale) may be offered.

- Monitor for lactose intolerance when formula is reintroduced. Formula is generally given in a diluted form when reinitiated and gradually increased to full strength.
- Monitor hydration status using vital signs, skin turgor, daily weights, and moisture of mucous membranes.
- Perform a physical assessment every shift and a focused assessment at intervals consistent with the patient's status and underlying pathologic condition.
- Initiate hygiene measures to provide patient comfort during and after emesis. Oral hygiene should be scheduled at intervals whenever an NG tube is in place, the patient has stomatitis, or the condition warrants it.
- Patients with significant central nervous system (CNS) depression may have lost the gag reflex; therefore institute aspiration precautions as appropriate.
- Initiate measures to eliminate factors that contribute to nausea and vomiting (e.g., irritating foods, odors, or medications).
- Give antiemetics as prescribed or recommended. With postsurgical patients, administer when symptoms of nausea first occur. Administer before chemotherapy or radiation therapy; depending on treatment, schedule on an around-the-clock basis following chemotherapy or radiation therapy. Administer 30 to 60 minutes before undertaking an activity known to precipitate motion sickness. If the transdermal patch is to be worn during travel, it can be applied behind the ear 4 hours before.
- If young children experience motion sickness while riding in a car, position them so that they are facing forward and can see the horizon; try covering the side windows with screens so that they do not have to suddenly turn their heads to watch rapidly passing objects.
- Provide diversional activities.
- Monitor nutritional needs and status on a continuum.

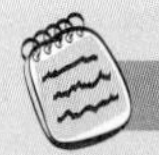

Patient Education and Health Promotion

Nutritional Status

- Ensure that the patient, individual, parent, or significant other understands all aspects of the diet, fluid, and nutritional regimen during hospitalization as well as at discharge for home management.
- Stress the importance of maintaining hydration and following the parameters that must be reported to the health care provider (e.g., weight loss of 2 pounds in a specified period, recurrence of nausea and vomiting).
- For patients receiving cancer treatments, the American Cancer Society has pamphlets with suggestions for supplementing dietary needs. These include, but are not limited to, giving small, frequent low-fat meals; food temperature; and increasing protein content of meals with the use of powdered milk added to puddings, shakes made with nutritional supplements, and frozen yogurt.
- For patients with cardiac disease, help prevent straining and the Valsalva (vasovagal) reflex by giving stool softeners as needed.
- In patients with degenerative neurologic disorders, a bowel program may be necessary, usually performed on an every-other-day basis. Glycerin or bisacodyl suppositories or digital stimulation may be required as part of the regimen.
- Discuss ways to decrease environmental stimuli to vomit, such as removing the emesis basin.
- Antiemetics cause some degree of sedation, and patients are often fatigued after receiving chemotherapy or radiation therapy; therefore caution patients not to drive or operate power equipment until these effects have subsided.

Medications. Verify the patient's and significant others' understanding of all prescribed medications to be given on a scheduled or PRN basis.

Fostering Health Maintenance

- Provide the patient and significant others with important information described in the monograph for drugs prescribed. Additional health teaching and nursing interventions for side effects to expect and report are described in each monograph.
- Seek cooperation and understanding of the following points so that medication adherence is increased: name of medication, dosage, route and times of administration, side effects to expect, and side effects to report.

Written Record. Enlist the patient's aid in developing and maintaining a written record of monitoring parameters (e.g., weight, details of when nausea occurs and amount and appearance of vomitus, food diary of what is being eaten, which foods initiate or aggravate the symptoms) (see Patient Self-Monitoring Form, Appendix I). Complete the Premedication Data column for use as a baseline to track response to drug therapy. Ensure that the patient understands how to use the form and instruct the patient to bring the completed form to follow-up visits. During follow-up visits, focus on issues that will foster adherence with the therapeutic interventions prescribed.

DRUG CLASS: Dopamine Antagonists

Actions

The dopamine antagonists are the phenothiazines, the butyrophenones, and metoclopramide. These medicines inhibit dopamine receptors that are part of the pathway to the vomiting center. Unfortunately dopamine receptors in other parts of the brain are also blocked, potentially producing extrapyramidal symptoms of dystonia, parkinsonism, and tardive dyskinesia (see Chapters 15, 18, and 33) in some patients, especially when higher dosages are required.

Uses

The phenothiazines are primarily used as antiemetics for the treatment of mild to moderate nausea and vomiting associated with anesthesia and surgery, radiation therapy, and cancer chemotherapy. Prochlorperazine is the phenothiazine most widely used as an antiemetic.

The butyrophenones also are used as antiemetics in surgery and cancer chemotherapy. These agents tend to cause less hypotension than the phenothiazines, but they produce more sedation. The most widely used butyrophenone is haloperidol. Droperidol must be administered parenterally.

Metoclopramide is an antagonist of both dopamine and serotonin receptors. In addition to acting on receptors in the brain, it also acts on similar receptors in the gastrointestinal (GI) tract, thus making it particularly useful in treating nausea and vomiting associated with GI cancers, gastritis, peptic ulcer, radiation sickness, and migraine. High-dose metoclopramide is now routinely used to treat nausea and vomiting associated with certain cancer chemotherapies. In higher doses, extrapyramidal symptoms are more common; therefore many cancer chemotherapy protocols now include both high-dose metoclopramide and routine doses of diphenhydramine when highly emetogenic anticancer agents are used. Metoclopramide appears to be of little value in treating motion sickness.

Therapeutic Outcomes

The primary therapeutic outcome expected from the dopamine antagonist antiemetics is relief of nausea and vomiting.

Nursing Process for Dopamine Antagonists

Premedication Assessment

1. Collect data regarding emesis (type, amount, and frequency, on a continuum).
2. Assess data relative to the underlying cause of nausea and vomiting (e.g., pregnancy, postsurgical state, chemotherapy, radiation, bowel obstruction).
3. Obtain baseline data about the patient's degree of alertness before starting therapy because these medications tend to produce some degree of sedation.

Planning

Availability. See Table 34-2.

Implementation

Dosage and Administration. See Table 34-2.

Evaluation

Phenothiazines. See Chapter 18.
Haloperidol. See Chapter 18.
Metoclopramide. See Chapter 33.

DRUG CLASS: Serotonin Antagonists

Actions

The serotonin (5-HT_3) receptor antagonists have made major inroads in the treatment of emesis associated with cancer chemotherapy, radiation therapy, and postoperative nausea and vomiting over the past few years. Serotonin receptors of the 5-HT_3 type are located centrally in the chemoreceptor trigger zone of the medulla and in specialized cells of the GI tract and play a significant role in inducing nausea and vomiting. The serotonin antagonists block these receptors and have been shown to actively control nausea and vomiting associated with cisplatin and several other emetogenic chemotherapeutic agents.

Uses

Studies of ondansetron and metoclopramide demonstrate that ondansetron is more effective than metoclopramide in the control of high-dose cisplatin-induced nausea and vomiting. Studies comparing the efficacy and safety of ondansetron, dolasetron, and granisetron in the control of cisplatin-induced acute emesis and PONV conclude that there are no significant differences among the treatment groups with respect to emetic control, nausea, or adverse reactions. Granisetron is approved to treat nausea and vomiting associated with radiation therapy. Palonosetron has been approved to treat both acute and delayed nausea and vomiting associated with chemotherapy. A particular advantage to this group of compounds is that there is minimal to no dopaminergic blockade, and thus extrapyramidal adverse effects are rare.

Text continued on p. 554

Drug Table 34-2 ANTIEMETIC AGENTS

GENERIC NAME	BRAND NAME	AVAILABILITY	ANTIEMETIC DOSAGE ADULTS	ANTIEMETIC DOSAGE CHILDREN	COMMENTS
DOPAMINE ANTAGONISTS					
Phenothiazines					**Comments for All Phenothiazines**
chlorpromazine	Thorazine, ✱ Largactil	Tablets: 10, 25, 50, 100, 200 mg Syrup: 10 mg/5 mL Concentrate: 100 mg/mL Suppositories: 100 mg Injection: 25 mg/mL	PO: 10-25 mg q4-6h Rectal: 50-100 mg q6-8h IM: 25 mg	PO: 0.25 mg/lb q4-6h Rectal: 0.5 mg/lb q6-8h IM: 0.25 mg/lb q6-8h (maximum IM dose: up to 5 yr: 40 mg/day; 5-12 yr: 75 mg/day)	Phenothiazines may suppress the cough reflex. Ensure that the patient does not aspirate vomitus. Use with caution in patients, especially children, with undiagnosed vomiting.
perphenazine	Perphenazine, ✱ Apo-Perphenazine	Tablets: 2, 4, 8, 16 mg Concentrate: 16 mg/5 mL	PO: 4 mg q4-6h IM: 5 mg	Not recommended	Phenothiazines can mask signs of toxicity of other drugs or mask symptoms of other diseases, such as brain tumor, Reye syndrome, or intestinal obstruction.
prochlorperazine	Compazine, ✱ Stemetil	Tablets: 5, 10 mg Capsules: 10, 15 mg Syrup: 5 mg/mL Suppositories: 2.5, 5, 25 mg Injection: 5 mg/mL	PO: 5-10 mg q6-8h Rectal: 25 mg twice daily IM: 5-10 mg	PO or rectal: 20-29 lb—2.5 mg once or twice daily 30-39 lb—2.5 mg two or three times daily 40-85 lb—2.5 mg three times daily IM: 0.06 mg/lb	Use with extreme caution in patients with seizure disorders.
thiethylperazine	Torecan	Injection: 5 mg/mL	IM: 10 mg 1 to 3 times daily	Not recommended	Discontinue if rashes develop. May cause orthostatic hypotension. See Chapter 18 for a complete list of adverse effects, drug interactions, and nursing interventions.
Butyrophenones					
haloperidol (see Chapter 18, p. 292)					See comment for phenothiazines above.
metoclopramide (see Chapter 33, p. 537)					

✱ Available in Canada.

Drug Table 34-2 ANTIEMETIC AGENTS—cont'd

GENERIC NAME	BRAND NAME	AVAILABILITY	ANTIEMETIC DOSAGE ADULTS	ANTIEMETIC DOSAGE CHILDREN	COMMENTS
DOPAMINE ANTAGONISTS—cont'd					
Butyrophenones—cont'd					
trimethobenzamide	Tigan	Capsules: 300 mg Suppositories: 100, 200 mg Injection: 100 mg/mL	PO: 300 mg three or four times daily Rectal: 200 mg three or four times daily IM: 200 mg three or four times daily	PO: 30-90 lb: 100-200 mg three or four times daily Rectal: <30 lb: 100 mg three or four times daily 30-90 lb: 100-200 mg three or four times daily	Injectable form contains benzocaine. Do not use in patients allergic to benzocaine or local anesthetics. Inject in upper, outer quadrant of gluteal region. Avoid escape of solution along the route. May cause burning, stinging, pain on injection.
SEROTONIN ANTAGONISTS					
dolasetron	Anzemet	Tablets: 50, 100 mg Injection: 20 mg/mL	PO: 100 mg within 1 hr before chemotherapy; 100 mg 2 hr before surgery IV: 100 mg 30 min before chemotherapy; 12.5 mg 15 min before cessation of anesthesia	PO: 1.8 mg/kg 60 min before chemotherapy IV: 1.8 mg/kg 30 min before chemotherapy	Recommended for prevention of nausea and vomiting associated with cancer chemotherapy and postoperative nausea and vomiting.
granisetron	Kytril	Tablets: 1 mg Liquid: 1 mg/5 mL Injection: 1 mg/mL	PO: 1 mg up to 1 hr before chemotherapy, followed by a second dose 12 hr later; or 2 mg once daily IV: 10 mcg/kg infused over 5 min beginning 30 min before chemotherapy	As for adults	Recommended for prevention of nausea and vomiting associated with cancer chemotherapy, postoperative nausea and vomiting, and nausea and vomiting associated with radiation therapy.

Continued

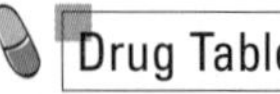Drug Table 34-2 **ANTIEMETIC AGENTS—cont'd**

GENERIC NAME	BRAND NAME	AVAILABILITY	ANTIEMETIC DOSAGE ADULTS	ANTIEMETIC DOSAGE CHILDREN	COMMENTS
SEROTONIN ANTAGONISTS—cont'd					
ondansetron	Zofran	Tablets: 4, 8, 24 mg Tablets, orally disintegrating: 4, 8 mg Injection: 2 mg/mL; 32 mg/50 mL Liquid: 4 mg/5 mL	PO: 8 mg 30 min before chemotherapy, followed by 8 mg 8 hr later IV: 3-0.15 mg/kg doses: (1) 30 min before chemotherapy, (2) 4 hr later, (3) 4 more hr later Or A single dose of 32 mg infused over 15 minutes, 30 minutes before starting chemotherapy	As for adults	Recommended for prevention of nausea and vomiting associated with cancer chemotherapy and postoperative nausea and vomiting.
palonosetron	Aloxi	Injection: 0.25 mg/5 mL	IV: 0.25 mg 30 min before start of chemotherapy. DO NOT repeat within 2 days		Recommended for prevention of nausea and vomiting associated with cancer chemotherapy; prevention of delayed nausea and vomiting from chemotherapy.
ANTICHOLINERGIC AGENTS USED FOR MOTION SICKNESS					
cyclizine	Marezine	Tablets: 50 mg	PO: 50 mg, repeated in 4-6 hr; do not exceed 200 mg daily IM: 50 mg q4-6h	PO: 6-12 yr: 25 mg up to three times daily	May suppress cough reflex. Ensure that patient does not aspirate vomitus. Must be administered 30-45 min before travel.
dimenhydrinate	Dramamine	Tablets: 50 mg Injection: 50 mg/mL Liquid: 12.5 mg/4 mL, 15.6 mg/5 mL	PO: 50-100 mg q4-6h; do not exceed 400 mg in 24 hr IM: 50 mg as needed	PO: 6-12 yr: 25-50 mg q6-8h; do not exceed 150 mg in 24 hr 2-6 yr: up to 25 mg q6-8h; do not exceed 75 mg in 24 hr	Will cause sedation. Beware of operating machinery.

 Drug Table 34-2 **ANTIEMETIC AGENTS—cont'd**

GENERIC NAME	BRAND NAME	AVAILABILITY	ANTIEMETIC DOSAGE ADULTS	ANTIEMETIC DOSAGE CHILDREN	COMMENTS
ANTICHOLINERGIC AGENTS USED FOR MOTION SICKNESS—cont'd					
diphenhydramine	Benadryl, Diphenhist	Tablets: 25, 50 mg Capsules: 25, 50 mg Elixir: 12.5 mg/5 mL Injection: 50 mg/mL Liquid: 6.25, 12.5 mg/5 mL	PO: 25-50 mg three or four times daily IM: 10-50 mg; do not exceed 400 mg/24 hr	PO: over 20 lb: 12.5-25 mg three or four times daily (5 mg/kg/ 24 hr; do not exceed 300 mg/24 hr) IM: 5 mg/kg/ 24 hr, in four divided doses; do not exceed 300 mg in 24 hr	
hydroxyzine	Atarax, Vistaril, ✱ Multipax	Tablets: 10, 25, 50, 100 mg Capsules: 25, 50, 100 mg Syrup: 10 mg/5 mL Suspension: 25 mg/5 mL Injection: 25, 50 mg/mL Liquid: 10 mg/5 mL	PO: 25-100 mg three or four times daily IM: as for PO	PO: Over 6 yr: 10-25 mg q4-6h; under 6 yr: 10 mg q4-6h IM: as for PO	
meclizine	Antivert, ✱ Bonamine	Tablets: 12.5, 25, 50 mg Capsules: 25 mg	PO: 25-50 mg; may be repeated every 24 hr	Not approved for use by children	
scopolamine, transdermal	Transderm-Scop	Transdermal patch: delivers 1.5 mg over 3 days	Patch: apply to skin behind the ear at least 4 hr before antiemetic effect is required. Replace in 3 days if continued therapy is required. Do not cut patches!	Not approved for use by children	
CORTICOSTEROIDS					
dexamethasone	Decadron	Tablets: 0.25, 0.5, 0.75, 1, 1.5, 2, 4, 6 mg Elixir: 0.5 mg/5 mL Injection: 4, 10, 20, 24 mg/mL Liquid: 1 mg/mL, 0.5 mg/5 mL	PO: 4-25 mg q4-6h for 1-2 days IV: as for PO	As for adults	Recommended for prevention of nausea and vomiting associated with chemotherapy.

✱ Available in Canada.

Continued

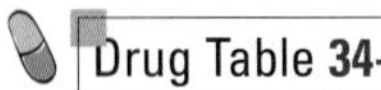

Drug Table 34-2 ANTIEMETIC AGENTS—cont'd

GENERIC NAME	BRAND NAME	AVAILABILITY	ANTIEMETIC DOSAGE: ADULTS	ANTIEMETIC DOSAGE: CHILDREN	COMMENTS
BENZODIAZEPINES					
lorazepam	Ativan	Tablets: 0.5, 1, 2 mg Injection: 2, 4 mg/mL Liquid: 2 mg/mL	PO: 1-4 mg q4-6h IV: as for PO	Not recommended	Recommended for prevention of nausea and vomiting associated with chemotherapy.
midazolam	Versed	Injection: 1, 5 mg/mL in 1-, 2-, 5-, 10-mL vials	IM: 0.07 mg/kg up to 1 hr before chemotherapy	Not recommended	
CANNABINOIDS					
dronabinol (THC)	Marinol	Capsules: 2.5, 5, 10 mg	PO: initial 5-10 mg/m^2 1-3 hr before chemotherapy, then q2-4h for a total of 4-6 doses/day Maximum—15 mg/m^2/dose	Not recommended	Schedule III controlled substance. Common adverse effects include drowsiness, dizziness, muddled thinking, and possible impairment of coordination, sensory, and perceptual functions. Use with caution in hypertension or heart disease.
NEUROKININ-1 RECEPTOR INHIBITOR					
aprepitant	Emend	Capsules: 80, 125 mg	PO: 125 mg 1 hr before chemotherapy on day 1; 80 mg daily in the morning of days 2 and 3	Not recommended	Recommended for prevention of acute and delayed nausea and vomiting associated with initial and repeat courses of highly emetogenic chemotherapy.

Therapeutic Outcomes

The primary therapeutic outcome expected from the serotonin antagonist antiemetics is relief of nausea and vomiting.

Nursing Process for Serotonin Antagonists

Premedication Assessment

1. Collect data regarding emesis (type, amount, and frequency, on a continuum).
2. Assess data relative to the underlying cause of nausea and vomiting (e.g., pregnancy, postsurgical state, chemotherapy, radiation, bowel obstruction).
3. Obtain baseline data about the patient's degree of alertness before initiation of therapy because these medications tend to produce some degree of sedation.

Planning

Availability. See Table 34-2.

Implementation

Dosage and Administration. See Table 34-2.

Evaluation

Side Effects to Expect

Headache, Diarrhea, Constipation, Sedation. These side effects are fairly mild, especially in relation to the prevention of nausea and vomiting. Because only a few doses are administered, frequency and duration of adverse effects are minimal.

Drug Interactions. No clinically significant drug interactions have been reported.

DRUG CLASS: Anticholinergic Agents

Actions

Motion sickness is thought to be caused by an excess of acetylcholine at the chemoreceptor trigger zone and the vomiting center by cholinergic nerves receiving impulses from the vestibular network of the inner ear. Anticholinergic agents are used to counterbalance the excessive amounts of acetylcholine present.

Uses

Anticholinergic agents such as scopolamine and antihistamines (e.g., diphenhydramine, dimenhydrinate, cyclizine, meclizine, promethazine) are used to treat motion sickness and, in the case of the antihistamines, nausea and vomiting associated with pregnancy. The choice of drug depends on the period for which antinausea protection is required and the side effects. Scopolamine is the drug of choice for short periods of motion, and an antihistamine is preferred for longer periods. Of the antihistamines, promethazine is the drug of choice. Higher doses act longer, but sedation is usually a problem. Cyclizine and meclizine have fewer side effects than promethazine but have a shorter duration of action and are less effective for severe conditions. Diphenhydramine has a long duration, but excessive sedation is often a problem, especially after the boat, plane, or car ride is over. For very severe conditions, sympathomimetic drugs such as ephedrine are used in combination with scopolamine or an antihistamine. Anticholinergic agents are usually not effective in chemotherapy-induced nausea and vomiting.

Therapeutic Outcomes

The primary therapeutic outcome expected from the anticholinergic antiemetics is relief of nausea and vomiting.

Nursing Process for Anticholinergic Agents

Premedication Assessment

1. Collect data regarding emesis (type, amount, and frequency, on a continuum).
2. Assess data relative to the underlying cause of nausea and vomiting (e.g., pregnancy, postsurgical state, chemotherapy, radiation, bowel obstruction).
3. Obtain baseline data about the patient's degree of alertness before initiation of therapy because these medications tend to produce some degree of sedation.

Planning

Availability. See Table 34-2.

Implementation

Dosage and Administration. See Table 34-2.

Evaluation

Side Effects to Expect

Sedative Effects. Tolerance may develop over a period, thus diminishing the effect.

Caution patients about operating power equipment or motor vehicles.

Fluid Intake. Maintain fluid intake at eight to ten 8-ounce glasses daily.

Blurred Vision, Constipation, Urinary Retention, Dry Mucosa of the Mouth, Throat, and Nose. These symptoms are the anticholinergic effects produced by these agents. Patients should be monitored for these side effects.

Dryness of the mucosa may be relieved by sucking hard candy or ice chips or by chewing gum.

Stool softeners, such as docusate, or the occasional use of a stimulant laxative, such as bisacodyl, may be required for constipation.

Caution the patient that blurred vision may occur and make appropriate suggestions for personal safety of the individual.

Patients who develop urinary hesitancy should discontinue the medication and contact their health care provider for further evaluation.

Drug Interactions

Enhanced Sedation. CNS depressants, including sleeping aids, analgesics, tranquilizers, and alcohol, will enhance the sedative effects of antihistamines. People who work around machinery, drive a car, or perform other duties in which they must remain mentally alert should not take these medications while working.

DRUG CLASS: Corticosteroids

Actions

Several studies have shown that dexamethasone and methylprednisolone can be effective antiemetics either as single agents or in combination with other antiemetics. The mechanism of action is unknown. Other actions of the corticosteroids, such as mood elevation, increased appetite, and a sense of well-being, may also help in patient acceptance and control of emesis.

Uses

A particular advantage of the steroids, apart from their efficacy, is their relative lack of side effects. Because only a few doses are administered, the usual complications associated with long-term therapy do not arise.

Therapeutic Outcomes

The primary therapeutic outcome expected from the corticosteroids as antiemetics is relief of nausea and vomiting.

Nursing Process for Corticosteroids

Premedication Assessment

1. Collect data regarding emesis (type, amount, and frequency, on a continuum).
2. Assess data relative to the underlying cause of nausea and vomiting (e.g., pregnancy, postsurgical state, chemotherapy, radiation, bowel obstruction).
3. Obtain baseline data about the patient's degree of alertness before initiation of therapy because these medications tend to produce some degree of sedation.

Planning

Availability. See Table 34-2.

Implementation

Dosage and Administration. See Table 34-2.

Evaluation

Side Effects to Expect and Report. Side effects are infrequent because few dosages are administered for nausea and vomiting. See also Chapter 38.

Drug Interactions. See Chapter 38.

DRUG CLASS: Benzodiazepines

Actions

Benzodiazepines act as antiemetics through a combination of effects, including sedation, reduction in anxiety, possible depression of the vomiting center, and an amnesic effect. Of these, the amnesic effect appears to be most important in treating cancer patients, and in this respect lorazepam and midazolam are superior to diazepam.

Uses

Benzodiazepines (e.g., lorazepam, midazolam, diazepam) are effective in reducing not only the frequency of nausea and vomiting but also the anxiety often associated with chemotherapy. Clinically, benzodiazepines are most useful in combination with other antiemetics, such as metoclopramide, dexamethasone, and serotonin antagonists.

Therapeutic Outcomes

The primary therapeutic outcome expected from benzodiazepine antiemetics is relief of nausea and vomiting.

Nursing Process for Benzodiazepines

Premedication Assessment

1. Collect data regarding emesis (type, amount, and frequency, on a continuum).
2. Assess data relative to the underlying cause of nausea and vomiting (e.g., pregnancy, postsurgical state, chemotherapy, radiation, bowel obstruction).
3. Obtain baseline data about the patient's degree of alertness before initiation of therapy because these medications tend to produce some degree of sedation.

Planning

Availability. See Table 34-2.

Implementation

Dosage and Administration. See Table 34-2.

Evaluation

Side Effects to Expect and Report. See Chapter 16.

Drug Interactions. See Chapter 16.

DRUG CLASS: Cannabinoids

Actions

After numerous reports that smoking marijuana reduces the frequency of nausea, the antiemetic properties of the active ingredients tetrahydrocannabinol (THC) and synthetic analogs such as dronabinol, nabilone, and levonantradol have been studied. The cannabinoids act through several mechanisms to inhibit pathways to the vomiting center, however there is no dopamine antagonist activity.

Uses

Cannabinoids have been shown to be more effective than placebo and equally as effective as prochlorperazine in patients receiving moderately emetogenic chemotherapy. They are less effective than metoclopramide. Because of the mind-altering effects and the potential for abuse, the cannabinoids serve as antiemetics only in patients receiving chemotherapy. The cannabinoids are of more use in those younger patients who are refractory to other antiemetic regimens and in whom combination therapy may be more effective.

Therapeutic Outcomes

The primary therapeutic outcome expected from the cannabinoids is relief of nausea and vomiting.

Nursing Process for Cannabinoids

Premedication Assessment

1. Collect data regarding emesis (type, amount, and frequency, on a continuum).
2. Assess data relative to the underlying cause of nausea and vomiting (e.g., pregnancy, postsurgical state, chemotherapy, radiation, bowel obstruction).
3. Obtain baseline data about the patient's degree of alertness before initiation of therapy because these medications tend to produce some degree of sedation.

Planning

Availability. See Table 34-2.

Implementation

Dosage and Administration. See Table 34-2.

Evaluation

Side Effects to Expect and Report

Dysphoric Effects. Depressed mood, hallucinations, dreaming or fantasizing, distortion of perception, paranoid reactions, and elation are more frequent with moderate to high doses. Younger patients appear to tolerate these side effects better than older patients or patients who have not used marijuana.

Patients should be specifically warned not to drive, operate machinery, or engage in any hazardous activity until it is determined that they are able to tolerate the drug and to perform such tasks safely.

Patients should remain under the supervision of a responsible adult during initial use of dronabinol and after dosage adjustments.

Drug Interactions

Drugs That Increase Toxic Effects. Antihistamines, alcohol, analgesics, benzodiazepines, barbiturates, antidepressants, muscle relaxants, and sedative-hypnotics increase toxic effects. Monitor the patient for excessive sedation and reduce the dosage of the other sedative agents, if necessary.

DRUG CLASS: Neurokinin-1 Receptor Antagonists

aprepitant (a prep′ eh tant)

EMEND (e mend′)

Actions

Another neurotransmitter thought to play a role in the vomiting process is substance P. Substance P is a neuropeptide found in high concentrations in the area of the CNS responsible for vomiting, and coexists with serotonin in the enterochromaffin cells and vagal afferent nerves of the GI tract. The actions of substance P are mediated through the neurokinin-1 (NK_1) receptor. Aprepitant is a potent, selective NK_1 antagonist that blocks the effects of substance P in the CNS. It has no affinity for serotonin, dopamine, or corticosteroid receptors.

Uses

Aprepitant is the first oral NK_1 receptor antagonist available in the United States. It is used for the prevention of acute and delayed chemotherapy-induced nausea and vomiting caused by highly emetogenic antineoplastic agents. It is used in combination with a corticosteroid and a 5-HT_3 receptor antagonist. It appears to have its greatest effect on reducing the frequency of delayed emesis. It does not treat CINV once it has started.

Therapeutic Outcomes

The primary therapeutic outcome expected from aprepitant is relief of nausea and vomiting.

Nursing Process for Neurokinin-1 Receptor Antagonists

Premedication Assessment

1. Collect data regarding emesis (type, amount, and frequency, on a continuum).
2. Assess data relative to the underlying cause of nausea and vomiting (e.g., pregnancy, postsurgical state, chemotherapy, radiation, bowel obstruction).

Planning

Availability. 80 and 125 mg capsules

Implementation

Dosage and Administration. *Adult*: PO: Day 1: One 125 mg capsule 1 hour before initiating chemotherapy treatment. Days 2 and 3: One 80 mg capsule each morning for the 2 days following chemotherapy treatment.

Evaluation

Side Effects to Expect and Report. The most common side effects with aprepitant are tiredness, nausea, hiccups, constipation, diarrhea, loss of appetite, headache, and hair loss. Because aprepitant is taken only for up to 3 days at a time, side effects are short lived and rarely troublesome.

Drug Interactions

Drugs That Increase Toxic Effects. Ketoconazole, itraconazole, nefazodone, troleandomycin, clarithromycin, ritonavir, nelfinavir, cisapride, and diltiazem may inhibit the metabolism of aprepitant. Monitor the patient for signs of aprepitant toxicity.

Drugs That Reduce Therapeutic Effects. Rifampin, carbamazepine, paroxetine, and phenytoin induce the metabolism of aprepitant, reducing its therapeutic effect.

Oral Contraceptives. Female patients receiving aprepitant who take oral contraceptives should be advised to use an alternate or additional method of birth control for the next month because aprepitant may enhance the metabolism of estrogens.

Dexamethasone and Methylprednisolone. Aprepitant inhibits the metabolism of these corticosteroids. Oral doses of dexamethasone and methylprednisolone should be reduced by approximately 50% when prescribed concurrently with aprepitant. Intravenous methylprednisolone dosages should be reduced by 25%.

Warfarin. Patients receiving warfarin therapy should be instructed to have an International Normalized Ratio (INR) checked approximately 7 to 10 days after aprepitant therapy because coadministration with aprepitant may result in increased metabolism of warfarin and a reduced INR.

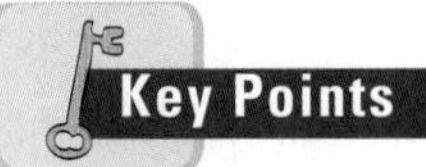

Key Points

- Nausea and vomiting vary from a minor inconvenience to severe debilitation.
- Nonpharmacologic treatments, such as eliminating noxious substances, avoiding fatty or spicy foods, and restricting activity to bed and chair rest to avoid vestibular irritation, are equally important in reducing the frequency of nausea and vomiting.
- The causes of nausea and vomiting should be assessed before treatment is begun, and specific therapy should be selected for each of the causes.

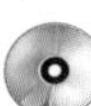

Go to your Companion CD-ROM for Appendices, an Audio Glossary, animations, Drug Dosage Calculators, customizable Patient Self-Assessment forms, and Review Questions for the NCLEX® Examination.

evolve Be sure to visit the companion Evolve site at http://evolve.elsevier.com/Clayton for WebLinks and additional online resources.

MEDICATION SAFETY REVIEW

MATH REVIEW QUESTIONS

1. Order: Ondansetron (Zofran) 3 mg/kg IV in 50 mL D5W at least 20 minutes before chemotherapy. The patient's weight today is 135 pounds.

   Weight is ___ kg.

   The total amount of ondansetron to administer is _____.

   When administering this order, using an infusion pump calibrated in milliliters per hour, set the pump at ___ mL/hr.

2. Order: Dexamethasone 6 mg intramuscular (IM) stat

   Available: Dexamethasone 4 mg/mL

   Give ____ mL.

CRITICAL THINKING QUESTIONS

1. A 65-year-old patient "with the flu" has been vomiting intermittently for 3 days. He is a resident on your unit in the nursing home. What data should be collected and reported to the health care provider for further evaluation and actions?
2. A patient has been vomiting repeatedly after administration of chemotherapy and received metoclopramide 1 hour ago. What is the action of this drug, and what further actions by the nurse are appropriate?
3. Ondansetron (Zofran) is ordered 30 minutes before chemotherapy and again 4 and 8 hours after chemotherapy. However, the prescribed dosage of the chemotherapy agent is not on the nursing unit 30 minutes before the scheduled time. Identify the appropriate nursing actions.
4. Review drugs used for motion sickness and identify those specifically not recommended for use for children.

CONTENT REVIEW QUESTIONS

1. A neighbor is going on a deep-sea fishing trip and tells you she plans on using transdermal patches of scopolamine. How far in advance should the patches be applied?
   1. 30 minutes
   2. 60 minutes
   3. 2 hours
   4. 4 hours

2. You are told that two children, ages 6 and 8, will accompany your neighbor on the deep-sea fishing trip. You should:
   1. ask what specific medication she plans to give the children, if any.
   2. encourage her not to premedicate the children.
   3. have her consult the family health care provider for specific orders.
   4. tell her to wait and see if the children develop seasickness before medicating them.

3. People using dronabinol (THC) (Marinol) for nausea and vomiting should be taught to report:
   1. headache, diarrhea, constipation, and sedation.
   2. sedative effects.
   3. depression, paranoia, or hallucinations.
   4. blurred vision, constipation, or urinary retention.

4. Nausea and vomiting experienced during the first 24 hours after chemotherapy are best described as:
   1. rebound nausea and vomiting.
   2. acute nausea and vomiting.
   3. chronic nausea and vomiting.
   4. anticipatory nausea and vomiting.

5. Which of the following statements about anticipatory nausea and vomiting are true? *(Select all that apply.)*
   1. Antiemetic drugs effectively control anticipatory nausea and vomiting once it has developed.
   2. Anticipatory nausea occurs more frequently than anticipatory vomiting.
   3. Patients are more likely to develop anticipatory nausea and vomiting if they are less than 50 years old.
   4. The earlier it is identified, the greater the likelihood that treatment will be effective.

6. Aprepitant is a selective antagonist of which of the following receptors?
   1. cetylcholine
   2. beta-adrenergic
   3. neurokinin
   4. serotonin

7. Which of the following interventions will help postoperative nausea and vomiting? *(Select all that apply.)*
   1. Check patency of nasogastric tube if one is present
   2. Limit patient movement
   3. Adequate analgesia
   4. Advancing NG tube if one is present

CHAPTER

35 Drugs Used to Treat Constipation and Diarrhea

evolve http://evolve.elsevier.com/Clayton

Chapter Content

Objectives

1. State the underlying causes of constipation.
2. Explain the meaning of "normal" bowel habits.
3. Identify the indications for use, method of action, and onset of action for stimulant laxatives, saline laxatives, lubricant or emollient laxatives, bulk-forming laxatives, and fecal softeners.
4. Describe medical conditions in which laxatives should *not* be used.
5. Cite nine causes of diarrhea.
6. State the differences between locally acting and systemically acting antidiarrheal agents.
7. Identify electrolytes that should be monitored whenever prolonged or severe diarrhea is present.
8. Describe nursing assessments needed to evaluate the patient's state of hydration when suffering from either constipation or dehydration.
9. Cite conditions that generally respond favorably to antidiarrheal agents.
10. Review medications studied to date and prepare a list of those that may cause diarrhea.

Key Terms

constipation
diarrhea
laxatives

CONSTIPATION

Constipation is the infrequent, incomplete, or painful elimination of feces. It may result from decreased motility of the colon or from retention of feces in the lower colon or rectum. In either case, the longer the feces remain in the colon, the greater the reabsorption of water and the drier the stool becomes. The stool is then more difficult to expel from the anus. Causes of constipation are improper diet—too little residue or too little fluid (e.g., lacking fruits and vegetables or high in constipating food such as cheese and yogurt); too little fluid intake, especially considering the climate; lack of exercise and sedentary habits (e.g., "couch potato" with remote control); failure to respond to the normal defecation impulses; muscular weakness of the colon; diseases such as anemia and hypothyroidism; frequent use of constipating medicines (e.g., morphine, codeine, anticholinergic agents); tumors of the bowel or pressure on the bowel from tumors; diseases of the rectum.

Occasional constipation is not detrimental to a person's health, although it can cause a feeling of general discomfort or abdominal fullness, anorexia, and anxiety in some people. Habitual constipation leads to decreased intestinal muscle tone, increased straining at the stool as the person bears down in the attempt to pass the hardened stool, and an increased incidence of hemorrhoids. Using laxatives or enemas daily should be avoided because they decrease the muscular tone and mucus production of the rectum and may result in water and electrolyte imbalance. They also become habit forming: the weakened muscle tone adds to the inability to expel the fecal contents, which leads to the continued use of enemas or laxatives.

Today many people believe that even occasional failure of the bowel to move daily is abnormal and should be treated. Daily bowel movements are frequently not necessary. Many people have "normal" bowel habits even though they have only two or three bowel movements per week. As long as the patient's health is good and the stool is not hardened or impacted, this schedule is acceptable.

DIARRHEA

Diarrhea is an increase in the frequency or fluid content of bowel movements. Because normal patterns of defecation and the patient's perception of bowel function vary, a careful history must be obtained to determine the change in a particular patient's bowel elimination pattern. An important fact to remember about diarrhea is that diarrhea is a symptom rather than a disease. It may be caused by any of the following:

- Intestinal infections
- Spicy or fatty foods
- Enzyme deficiencies
- Excessive use of laxatives
- Drug therapy

- Emotional stress
- Hyperthyroidism
- Inflammatory bowel disease
- Surgical bypass of the intestine

Intestinal Infections

These are most frequently associated with ingestion of food contaminated with bacteria or protozoa (food poisoning) or eating or drinking water that contains bacteria that are foreign to the patient's gastrointestinal (GI) tract. People traveling, especially to other countries, develop what is known as traveler's diarrhea from ingestion of microorganisms that are pathogenic to their GI tracts but not to those of the local residents.

Spicy or Fatty Foods

Spicy or fatty foods may produce diarrhea by irritating the lining of the GI tract. Diarrhea occurs particularly when the patient does not routinely eat these types of foods. This type of diarrhea is not uncommon on vacation (e.g., eating fresh oysters daily while visiting coastal regions).

Enzyme Deficiencies

Patients with deficiencies of digestive enzymes such as lactase or amylase have difficulty digesting certain foods. Diarrhea usually develops because of irritation from undigested food.

Excessive Use of Laxatives

People who use laxatives on a routine, chronic basis but are not under the care of a health care provider for a specific GI problem are laxative abusers. Some do it for weight control, and others use laxatives under the misconception that a person is not normal if the bowels do not move daily.

Drug Therapy

Diarrhea is a common side effect caused by the irritation of the GI lining by ingested medication. Diarrhea may also result from the use of antibiotics that may kill certain bacteria that live in the GI tract and help digest food.

Emotional Stress

Diarrhea is a common symptom of emotional stress and anxiety.

Hyperthyroidism

Hyperthyroidism induces increased GI motility, resulting in diarrhea.

Inflammatory Bowel Disease

Inflammatory bowel diseases such as diverticulitis, ulcerative colitis, gastroenteritis, and Crohn's disease cause inflammation of the GI lining, resulting in muscle spasm and diarrhea.

Surgical Bypass

Surgical bypass procedures of the intestine often result in chronic diarrhea because of the decreased absorptive area remaining after surgery. Incompletely digested food and water rapidly pass through the GI tract.

TREATMENT OF ALTERED ELIMINATION

Constipation

Constipation that does not have a specific cause can often be treated without the use of laxatives. A high-fiber diet (e.g., fruits, grains, nuts, vegetables), adequate hydration (e.g., eight to ten 8-ounce glasses of water daily), and daily exercise (e.g., for physical activity, stress relief) can eliminate most cases of constipation. Laxatives, other than treating acute constipation from a specific cause (e.g., a change in routine such as traveling for long hours in a car or plane), should be avoided. The ingredients of laxative products frequently cause side effects and may be contraindicated in certain patients. The following patients should not take laxatives and should be referred to a health care provider: those with severe pain or discomfort; those who have nausea, vomiting, or fever; patients with a preexisting condition (e.g., diabetes mellitus, abdominal surgery); those taking medicines that cause constipation (e.g., iron, aluminum antacids, antispasmodics, muscle relaxants); patients who have used other laxatives without success; and laxative abusers.

Diarrhea

Diarrhea may be acute or chronic, mild or severe. Because it may be a defense mechanism to rid the body of infecting organisms or irritants, it is usually self-limiting. Chronic diarrhea may indicate a disease of the stomach or small or large intestine, may be psychogenic, or may be one of the first symptoms of cancer of the colon or rectum. If diarrhea is severe or prolonged, it may cause dehydration, electrolyte depletion, and physical exhaustion. Specific antidiarrheal therapy depends on the cause of the diarrhea.

NURSING PROCESS *for Altered Elimination: Constipation and Diarrhea*

Assessment

History

- Obtain a history of the patient's usual bowel pattern and changes that have taken place in the frequency, consistency, odor, color, and number of stools per day. Ask whether the patient has a usual time of defecation daily. Does the individual respond immediately to the urge to defecate or delay toileting until a more convenient time?
- Ask whether the onset of diarrhea or constipation is recent and if it can be associated with travel or stress. Has there been a change in water source or

foods lately? Ask what measures the patient has already initiated, whether prescribed by a health care provider or by self-treatment, to correct the problem and the degree of success achieved.

- Obtain a detailed history of the individual's health. Are any acute or chronic conditions being treated, for example, cancer, GI disorders, neurologic conditions, or intestinal obstruction?

Medications. Ask the patient to give a listing of all current over-the-counter (OTC) medications being taken or prescribed by a health care provider. Are any used to treat diarrhea or constipation? Are any of these medications known to slow intestinal transit time (e.g., narcotic analgesics, aluminum-containing antacids, or anticholinergic agents)? Are any known to cause diarrhea (e.g., magnesium-containing antacids)?

Activity and Exercise. Ask the patient about daily activity level and exercise. Does the patient play vigorous sports, take walks and jog, or have a sedentary job and hobby?

Elimination Pattern. What is the individual's usual pattern of stool elimination (i.e., frequency of the urge to defecate, usual stool consistency, presence of bloating or flatus, fecal incontinence)? Does the individual have a history of, or currently have, anal fissures, hemorrhoids, or abscesses?

Nutritional History

- Ask questions to determine the patient's usual dietary practices: How much coffee, tea, soft drinks (caffeinated or decaffeinated), water, fruit juice, and alcoholic beverages are consumed daily?
- Ask for a description of what the patient has eaten over the past 24 hours. Evaluate the data to identify whether foods from all levels of the food pyramid are being eaten. Are there good sources of dietary fiber? Has the patient introduced new foods not usually eaten into the diet?

Basic Assessment

- Obtain baseline vital signs, height, and weight.
- Assess bowel sounds in all four quadrants. Observe the size and shape of the abdomen. Note any signs of distention, ascites, or masses.
- Assess and record signs of hydration. Examine for poor skin turgor, sticky oral mucous membranes, excessive thirst, a shrunken and deeply furrowed tongue, crusted lips, weight loss, deteriorating vital signs, soft or sunken eyeballs, delayed capillary filling, high urine specific gravity or no urine output, and possible mental confusion.

Laboratory Studies

- Review laboratory reports for indications of malabsorption, dehydration, fluid, electrolyte and acid-base imbalances, and so on (e.g., K^+, Cl^-, pH, Pco_2, bicarbonate, hemoglobin [Hgb], hematocrit [Hct], urinalysis [specific gravity], serum albumin, total protein).
- Check reports of stool specimen sent for laboratory examination.

Nursing Diagnoses

Constipation

- Constipation, risk for (side effects)
- Constipation (indication)
- Constipation, perceived (indication)
- Fluid volume, deficient (indication)
- Diarrhea
- Nutrition, imbalanced: less than body requirements (indication)

Planning

History. Plan to perform a focused assessment consistent with the symptoms and underlying pathology.

Medications, Treatments, and Diagnostics

- Order baseline laboratory studies requested by the health care provider. Schedule prescribed treatments (e.g., enema administration) and diagnostic procedures (e.g., abdominal radiographs, colonoscopy, anorectal manometry).
- Schedule prescribed medications on the medication administration record (MAR), and requisition medicines from the pharmacy.

Assessment

- Mark the Kardex or enter data in the computer with specific parameters to be recorded (e.g., intake and output, frequency and consistency of stools, presence of blood).
- Mark the Kardex or enter data in the computer if stool specimens are to be obtained.

Nutrition. Obtain specific orders relating to nutrition. Diet orders depend on the cause of constipation or diarrhea. A dietary consult may be indicated. Schedule fluid intake of at least 3000 mL/day, unless contraindicated by coexisting conditions (e.g., heart failure, renal disease). Rehydration solutions may be required with severe diarrhea.

Does the patient have any food intolerances or foods known to produce either diarrhea or constipation?

Activity and Exercise. Mark the Kardex or enter data in computer with specific orders regarding ambulation. Whenever possible, encourage frequent ambulation.

Implementation

- Maintain hydration with oral or parenteral solutions as prescribed by the health care provider. Monitor the hydration status with volume of intake, urine output, skin turgor, moisturization of mucous membranes, and daily weights.
- Assess for bowel sounds in all four quadrants. Report absence of bowel sounds immediately to the health care provider. Assess abdomen for distention; measure abdominal girth if necessary.
- Give enemas prescribed according to hospital procedures. (These are not used for long-term treatment of constipation.) Oil-retention enemas may be required to soften the fecal material.

- Initiate nutritional interventions such as high-fiber foods and adequate fluid intake.
- Give prescribed laxatives or stool softeners. Monitor for effectiveness and side effects.
- Give prescribed antidiarrheal agents, antiperistaltic agents (except to patients known to have infectious diarrhea), and antibiotics for infection-based diarrhea.
- Initiate hygiene measures to prevent perianal skin breakdown. Cleanse the perianal area thoroughly after each stool. Apply protective ointment (e.g., zinc oxide) as prescribed; with severe diarrhea, a fecal collection apparatus may be helpful.
- Monitor vital signs and daily weights and perform a focused assessment appropriate to the underlying etiology of the constipation or diarrhea.

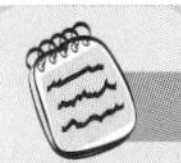

Patient Education and Health Promotion

Nutritional Status

- Be certain the individual, parent, or significant other understands all aspects of the diet and fluid orders prescribed.
- Stress the inclusion of high-fiber foods and adequate fluids to maintain hydration and alleviate constipation.
- Depending on the underlying cause of the symptoms, health teaching is appropriate regarding proper food preparation, storage, and prevention of contamination.
- During travel, use bottled water, when appropriate.

Activity and Exercise. Encourage regular exercise.

Medications

- Explain the consequences of regular use of laxatives and the benefits of handling constipation with diet, exercise, and adequate fluid intake first.
- When codeine or morphine is used regularly for pain control in cancer patients, it is imperative that the individual know that stool softeners should be initiated and continued as long as constipating medicines are being taken.
- If laxatives or enemas are prescribed to cleanse the intestines before diagnostic examination, be certain the individual has written instructions, the time and amount to be administered, and where the laxative or enema can be purchased. Review the correct procedure for self-administering an enema with the patient, or instruct a family member.
- Emphasize the need to be in proximity to a bathroom once laxatives such as GoLYTELY are taken.

Fostering Health Maintenance

- Fecal-oral contamination may cause diarrhea. Teaching proper handwashing and cleansing or disinfection of the toilet, bedpan, or commode.
- For diarrhea associated with chronic GI diseases, it is imperative to reinforce all aspects of health teaching relating to the specific disease underlying the symptomatology.
- Provide the patient and significant others with important information contained in individual drug monographs to identify drugs that cause constipation or diarrhea. Additional health teaching and nursing interventions for side effects to expect and report are described in each monograph.
- Seek cooperation and understanding of the following points for judicious use of laxatives or antidiarrheals: name of medication, dosage, route and times of administration, side effects to expect, and side effects to report. For infectious diarrhea, teach the patient precautions to prevent its spread to others. For all patients with diarrhea, teach the need for adequate fluid intake and any dietary restrictions.

DRUG CLASS: Laxatives

Actions

Laxatives are chemicals that act to promote the evacuation of the bowel. They are usually subclassified based on the mechanism of action.

Stimulant Laxatives

Stimulant laxatives act directly on the intestine, causing an irritation that promotes peristalsis and evacuation. If given orally, these agents act within 6 to 10 hours. If administered rectally, they act within 60 to 90 minutes.

Saline Laxatives

Saline laxatives are hypertonic compounds that draw water into the intestine from surrounding tissues. The accumulated water affects stool consistency and distends the bowel, causing peristalsis. These agents usually act within 1 to 3 hours. Continued use of these products significantly alters electrolyte balance and may cause dehydration.

Polyethylene glycol–electrolyte solution is a relatively new approach to saline laxative therapy. It is a mixture of a nonabsorbable ion-exchange solution and electrolytes that acts as an osmotic agent. When taken orally, it pulls electrolytes and water into the solution in the lumen of the bowel and exchanges sodium ions to replace those removed from the body. The result is a diarrhea that cleanses the bowel for colonoscopy and barium enema x-ray examination with no significant dehydration or loss of electrolytes.

Lubricant Laxatives

Lubricant laxatives lubricate the intestinal wall and soften the stool, allowing a smooth passage of fecal contents. Onset of action is often 6 to 8 hours but may be up to 48 hours because the action is highly dependent on the individual patient's normal GI transit time. Peristaltic activity does not appear to be increased. If used frequently, these oils may inhibit the absorption of fat-soluble vitamins.

Bulk-Producing Laxatives

Bulk-producing laxatives must be administered with a full glass of water. The laxative causes water to be retained within the stool. This increases bulk, which stimulates peristalsis. Onset of action is usually 12 to 24 hours but may be as long as 72 hours depending on the patient's GI transit time. Bulk-forming agents are usually considered to be the safest laxative, even when taken routinely. Fresh fruits, vegetables, and cereals such as bran are natural bulk-forming products.

Fecal Softeners

Fecal softeners, known as wetting agents, draw water into the stool, causing it to soften. They do not stimulate peristalsis and may require up to 72 hours to aid in a soft bowel movement. Action from these agents depends on the patient's state of hydration and the GI transit time.

Uses

Lubricants and bulk-forming laxatives may be used in the geriatric and pregnant patient because there is little cramping accompanying their use. Pediatric patients should also be treated with a change in diet to include cereals, fruits, and grains. Constipation in infants can be treated with malt soup extract, a bulk-forming laxative, or dark corn syrup added to a feeding bottle.

Do not administer laxatives to patients with undiagnosed abdominal pain or inflammation of the GI tract such as gastritis, appendicitis, or colitis.

Bulk-Forming Laxatives

Bulk-forming laxatives are generally considered to be the drug of choice for a person who is incapacitated and needs a laxative regularly. These agents may also be used in patients with irritable bowel syndrome to provide a softer consistency to the stools if a high-fiber diet is not adequate. Bulk-forming laxatives are also used to control certain types of diarrhea by absorbance of the irritating substance, thus allowing its removal from the bowel during defecation.

It is important that bulk-forming laxatives be dispersed in a glass of water or juice before administration. If adequate volumes of water are not taken, obstruction within the GI tract may result from a bulk laxative that forms a sticky mass.

Stimulant and Saline Laxatives

Stimulant and saline laxatives may be used to relieve acute constipation. They are also routinely used as bowel preparations to remove gas and feces before radiologic examination of the kidneys, colon, intestine, or gallbladder. These products should be used only intermittently, because chronic use may cause loss of normal bowel function and dependency on the agent for bowel evacuation.

Stool Softeners

Stool softeners are routinely used for prophylactic purposes to prevent constipation or straining at stool (e.g., in patients recovering from myocardial infarction or abdominal surgery).

Lubricant Laxatives

Lubricant laxatives are quite helpful in producing a soft stool without causing significant bowel spasm. Lubricants are also used prophylactically in patients who should not strain during defecation. Lubricants should not be administered to debilitated patients who are constantly in a recumbent position. The oil can be aspirated into the lungs, causing lipid pneumonia.

Therapeutic Outcomes

The primary therapeutic outcomes expected from laxative therapy are as follows:

- Relief from abdominal discomfort.
- Passage of bowel contents within a few hours of administration.

Nursing Process for Altered Elimination: Constipation

Premedication Assessment

1. Determine usual pattern of elimination.
2. Ask specifically about symptoms that may indicate undiagnosed abdominal pain such as those associated with intestinal obstruction or appendicitis.

Planning

Availability. See Table 35-1.

Implementation

Dosage and Administration. PO: Follow directions on the container. Be sure to give adequate water with bulk-forming agents to prevent esophageal, gastric, intestinal, or rectal obstruction.

Evaluation

Side Effects to Expect

Griping, Minor Abdominal Discomfort. The most common adverse effects are excessive bowel stimulation resulting in griping and diarrhea. Patients who are severely constipated may develop abdominal cramps. The patient should first experience the urge to defecate, then defecate and feel a sense of relief.

Side Effects to Report

Abdominal Tenderness, Pain, Bleeding, Vomiting, Diarrhea, Increasing Abdominal Girth. Failure to defecate or defecation of only a small amount may indicate an impaction. These also are symptoms of an acute abdomen.

Drug Table 35-1 LAXATIVES

PRODUCT	STIMULANT	SALINE	BULK-FORMING	LUBRICANT	FECAL SOFTENER	OTHER
Citrate of Magnesia		Magnesium citrate				
Colace					Docusate sodium	
Colyte						Polyethylene glycol, electrolyte solution
Correctol	Bisacodyl					
Dulcolax	Bisacodyl					
Ex-Lax	Sennosides A&B					
Fiber Con			Polycarbophil			
Go-LYTELY						Polyethylene glycol, electrolyte solution
Haley's M-O		Magnesium hydroxide		Mineral oil		
Metamucil			Psyllium hydrophilic mucilloid			
Modane	Bisacodyl					
Peri-Colace	Sennosides A & B				Docusate sodium	
Phillip's Milk of Magnesia		Magnesium hydroxide				
Phospho-Soda			Sodium phosphates			
Surfak					Docusate calcium	
X-Prep	Senna concentrate					

Drug Interactions

Bisacodyl. Do not administer with milk, antacids, cimetidine, famotidine, nizatidine, or ranitidine. These products may allow the enteric coating to dissolve prematurely, causing nausea, vomiting, and cramping.

Psyllium. Do not administer products containing psyllium (e.g., Metamucil) at the same time as salicylates, nitrofurantoin, or digoxin. The psyllium may inhibit absorption. Administer these medications at least 1 hour before or 2 hours after psyllium.

Mineral Oil. Daily administration of mineral oil for more than 1 to 2 weeks may cause a deficiency of the fat-soluble vitamins.

Docusate. Docusate enhances the absorption of mineral oil. Concurrent use is not recommended to prevent granuloma formation in the liver, lymph nodes, and intestinal lining.

DRUG CLASS: Antidiarrheal Agents

Actions

Antidiarrheal agents include a wide variety of drugs, but they can be divided into two broad categories: locally acting agents and systemic agents. Locally acting agents such as activated charcoal, pectin, psyllium, and activated attapulgite absorb excess water to cause a formed stool and to adsorb irritants or bacteria that are causing the diarrhea.

The systemic agents act through the autonomic nervous system to reduce peristalsis and motility of the GI tract, allowing the mucosal lining to absorb nutrients, water, and electrolytes, leaving a formed stool in the colon. Representatives of the systemically acting agents are diphenoxylate, loperamide, and certain anticholinergic agents (Table 35-2).

The systemically acting agents are associated with more adverse effects (see Table 35-2), which should not be used to treat diarrhea caused by substances toxic to the GI tract, such as bacterial contaminants or other irritants. Because these agents act by reducing GI motility, the systemically acting antidiarrheals tend to allow the toxin to remain in the GI tract longer, causing further irritation.

Uses

Although the ingredients of the antidiarrheal products are in general benign and the majority are available OTC, the decision as to recommend treatment versus when to refer the patient to a health care provider is not to be taken lightly.

Antidiarrheal products are usually indicated under the following conditions:

- The diarrhea is of sudden onset, has lasted more than 2 or 3 days, and is causing significant fluid and water loss. Young children and elderly patients are more susceptible to rapid dehydration

Drug Table 35-2 ANTIDIARRHEAL AGENTS

GENERIC NAME	BRAND NAME	AVAILABILITY	ADULT DOSAGE	COMMENTS
SYSTEMIC ACTION				
difenoxin with atropine	Motofen	Tablets: 1 mg diphenoxin with 0.025 mg atropine	PO: two tablets, then one tablet each loose stool. Do not exceed eight tablets in 24 hr	Inhibits peristalsis Atropine added to minimize potential overdose or abuse May cause drowsiness or dizziness; use caution in performing tasks requiring alertness Do not use in children younger than 2 yr of age
diphenoxylate with atropine	Lomotil, Lomanate	Tablets: 2.5 mg diphenoxylate with 0.025 mg atropine Liquid: 2.5 mg diphenoxylate, with 0.025 mg atropine per 5 mL	PO: 5 mg four times daily	Inhibits peristalsis Atropine added to minimize potential overdose or abuse May cause drowsiness or dizziness; use caution in performing tasks requiring alertness Do not use in children younger than 2 yr of age
loperamide	Imodium, Imodium A-D, Pepto Diarrhea Control	Tablets: 2 mg Capsules: 2 mg Liquid: 1 mg/5 mL; 1 mg/mL	PO: 4 mg initially, followed by 2 mg after each unformed movement. Do not exceed 16 mg/day	Inhibits peristalsis Used in acute, nonspecific diarrhea and to reduce the volume of discharge from ileostomy
opium	Paregoric	Liquid	PO: 5-10 mL four times daily	Inhibits peristalsis and pain of diarrhea; 5 mL of liquid = 2 mg morphine
LOCAL ACTION				
Lactobacillus acidophilus	Lactinex	Capsules, granules, tablets	PO: two to four tablets or capsules, two to four times daily, with milk Granules: one packet added to cereal, fruit juice, milk three or four times daily	Bacteria used to recolonize the gastrointestinal tract in an attempt to treat chronic diarrhea Do not use in acute diarrhea
bismuth subsalicylate	Pepto-Bismol Kaopectate	Tablets, suspension	PO: 30 mL or two tablets chewed every 30-60 min up to eight doses	Used as adsorbent

and electrolyte imbalance and therefore should start antidiarrheal therapy earlier.
- Patients with inflammatory bowel disease develop diarrhea. Rapid treatment shortens the course of the incapacitating diarrhea and allows the patient to live a more normal lifestyle. Other agents such as adrenocorticosteroids or sulfonamides may also be used to control the underlying bowel disease.
- Postgastrointestinal surgery patients develop diarrhea. These patients may require chronic antidiarrheal therapy to allow adequate absorption of fluids and electrolytes.
- The cause of the diarrhea has been diagnosed and the health care provider determines that an antidiarrheal product is appropriate for therapy. Because many cases of diarrhea are self-limiting, therapy may not be necessary.

Therapeutic Outcomes

The primary therapeutic outcome expected from antidiarrheal therapy is relief from the incapacitation and discomfort of diarrhea.

Nursing Process for Altered Elimination: Diarrhea

Premedication Assessment

1. Confer with patient regarding medications that may be contributing to diarrhea, including antacids containing magnesium or laxative products, antibiotics, or products containing large quantities of sorbitol.
2. Review history of onset of diarrhea and precipitating factors. Refer to health care provider if there's a question about administering antidiarrheal agents.

Planning

Availability. See Table 35-2.

Implementation

Dosage and Administration. See Table 35-2. PO: Follow directions on the container. Be sure to give adequate water with bulk-forming agents to prevent esophageal, gastric, intestinal, or rectal obstruction.

Evaluation

Side Effects to Expect

Abdominal Distention, Nausea, Constipation. Locally acting agents have essentially no adverse effects, but if used excessively, they may cause abdominal distention, nausea, and constipation.

Side Effects to Report

Prolonged or Worsened Diarrhea. This may be an indication that toxins are present in the gut and that the systemically acting antidiarrheal is causing retention of these toxins. Refer the patient for medical attention.

Drug Interactions

Diphenoxylate, Difenoxin. The chemical structure of these two antidiarrheal agents is similar to meperidine. These agents should not be used in a patient receiving monoamine oxidase inhibitors (e.g., phenelzine, isocarboxazid, tranylcypromine). There is potential for a hypertensive crisis.

Sedatives, Alcohol, Tranquilizers. Sedation caused by diphenoxylate and difenoxin is potentiated by other medicines with CNS depressant properties.

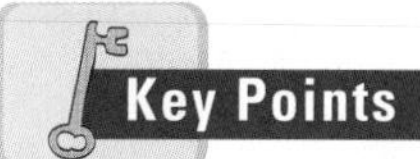

- Constipation and diarrhea are common disorders of the GI tract that most people experience occasionally throughout their lives. Most cases are self-limiting and do not require pharmacologic treatment.
- Constipation is most frequently treated by adding bulk and water to the diet and regular exercise. If drug treatment is required, laxatives that act by a variety of mechanisms are available: bulk formers, stimulants, saline, lubricants, and surfactants.
- Acute diarrhea is usually a symptom of an underlying problem, such as a GI infection. A detailed history of recent events must be taken to assess whether to recommend treatment with antidiarrheal agents.

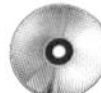

Go to your Companion CD-ROM for Appendices, an Audio Glossary, animations, Drug Dosage Calculators, customizable Patient Self-Assessment forms, and Review Questions for the NCLEX® Examination.

evolve Be sure to visit the companion Evolve site at http://evolve.elsevier.com/Clayton for WebLinks and additional online resources.

MEDICATION SAFETY REVIEW

CRITICAL THINKING QUESTIONS

1. The health care provider tells the office nurse to instruct the mother of a 6-month-old infant on the procedure to insert a glycerin suppository. What information would you give?
2. An 80-year-old patient asks for a laxative on a daily basis. What health teaching should be done? Would you give the PRN laxative daily?
3. Summarize the types of laxatives available and the onset of action for each type.
4. Summarize the types of antidiarrheal products available and identify the action of each.

Continued

CONTENT REVIEW QUESTIONS

1. All systemic antidiarrheal agents act by:
   1. softening the stool.
   2. inhibiting peristalsis.
   3. adsorbent action.
   4. increasing bulk.
2. Kaopectate, a common OTC medication for diarrhea, acts by:
   1. softening the stool.
   2. inhibiting peristalsis.
   3. adsorbent action.
   4. increasing bulk.
3. Stimulant laxatives increase peristalsis within _____ hour(s) when given orally.
   1. 0.5
   2. 1 to 3
   3. 6 to 10
   4. 12 to 24
4. Bulk-forming laxatives have an onset of action of _____ hour(s).
   1. 0.5
   2. 1 to 3
   3. 6 to 8
   4. 12 to 24
5. Which antidiarrheal agent should not be used in children younger than the age of 2?
   1. diphenoxylate
   2. loperamide
   3. bismuth subsalicylate
   4. Kaopectate
6. Which type of laxative should not be administered to debilitated patients who are constantly in a recumbent position?
   1. Saline
   2. Stimulant
   3. Lubricant
   4. Bulk-forming
7. Which type of laxative may cause electrolyte imbalance and dehydration?
   1. Saline
   2. Stimulant
   3. Lubricant
   4. Bulk-forming

36 Drugs Used to Treat Diabetes Mellitus

evolve http://evolve.elsevier.com/Clayton

Chapter Content

Objectives

1. State the current definition of diabetes mellitus.
2. Identify the extent of the disease within the United States.
3. Describe the current classification system for diabetes mellitus.
4. Identify normal fasting glucose levels.
5. Differentiate between the symptoms of type 1 and type 2 diabetes mellitus.
6. Identify the objectives of dietary control of diabetes mellitus.
7. Discuss the action and use of insulin as opposed to oral hypoglycemic and antihyperglycemic agents to control diabetes mellitus.
8. Identify the mechanism of action of the different oral antidiabetic agents.
9. Identify the major nursing considerations associated with the management of the patient with diabetes (e.g., nutritional evaluation, dietary prescription, activity and exercise, and psychological considerations).
10. Differentiate among the signs, symptoms, and management of hypoglycemia and hyperglycemia.
11. Discuss the difference between microvascular and macrovascular complications.
12. Define "intensive therapy."
13. Identify the symptoms of the major complications of diabetes.
14. Discuss the contributing factors, nursing assessments, and nursing interventions needed for patients exhibiting complications associated with diabetes mellitus.
15. Develop a health teaching plan for people taking any type of insulin or oral hypoglycemic agent.

Key Terms

diabetes mellitus
hyperglycemia
type 1 diabetes mellitus
type 2 diabetes mellitus
gestational diabetes mellitus
impaired glucose tolerance (IGT)
impaired fasting glucose (IFG)
prediabetes
microvascular complications
macrovascular complications
neuropathies
paresthesia
hypoglycemia
intensive therapy

DIABETES MELLITUS

Diabetes mellitus is a group of diseases characterized by **hyperglycemia** (fasting plasma glucose >100 mg/dL) and abnormalities in fat, carbohydrate, and protein metabolism that lead to microvascular, macrovascular, and neuropathic complications. Several pathologic processes are associated with the development of diabetes, and patients often have impairment of insulin secretion as well as defects in insulin action, resulting in hyperglycemia. It is now recognized that different pathologic mechanisms are involved for different diseases.

Diabetes mellitus is occurring with increasing frequency in the United States as the population increases both in weight and age. In the United States, the Centers for Disease Control and Prevention (CDC) estimate that the prevalence of diabetes in the general population is approximately 6% (18.3 million people, 5 million of whom are undiagnosed). Direct expenditures of medical care totaled $92 billion in 2002. An additional $40 billion was attributed to lost productivity at work, disability, and premature death. Diabetes is listed as the sixth leading cause of death in the United States. Most diabetes-related deaths are due to cardiovascular disease as the risk of heart disease and stroke is two to four times greater in patients with diabetes compared with those without the disease.

Undiagnosed diabetic adults, with few or no symptoms, present a major challenge to the health profession. Because early symptoms of diabetes are minimal, the patient does not seek medical advice. Indications of the disease are discovered only at the time of routine physical examination. Those with a predisposition to developing diabetes include people who have relatives with diabetes (they have 2.5 times greater incidence of developing the disease), obese people (85% of all diabetic patients are overweight), and older people (four out of five diabetic patients are more than 45 years of age). The incidence of diabetes is higher in African Americans, Hispanics, American Indians, Native Alaskans, and women.

The National Diabetes Data Group of the National Institutes of Health and the World Health Organization Expert Committee on Diabetes (NDDG/WHO) classifies diabetes by the underlying pathology causing hyperglycemia (Box 36-1).

Type 1 diabetes mellitus, formerly known as insulin-dependent diabetes mellitus (IDDM), is present in 5% to 10% of the diabetic population. It is caused by an autoimmune destruction of the beta cells in the pancreas. It occurs more frequently in juveniles, but patients can become symptomatic for the first time at any age. The onset of this form of diabetes usually has a rapid progression of symptoms (a few days to a few weeks) characterized by polydipsia (increased thirst), polyphagia (increased appetite), polyuria (increased urination), increased frequency of infections, loss of weight and strength, irritability, and often ketoacidosis. Because there is no insulin secretion from the pancreas, patients require administration of exogenous insulin. Insulin dosage adjustment is easily influenced by inconsistent patterns of physical activity and dietary irregularities. It is common for patients with type 1 diabetes mellitus to go into remission in the early stages of the disease, requiring little or no exogenous insulin. This condition may last for a few months, and is referred to as the "honeymoon" period.

Type 2 diabetes mellitus, formerly known as non–insulin-dependent diabetes mellitus (NIDDM), represents about 90% of the diabetic population. In contrast to type 1 diabetes mellitus, type 2 diabetes is characterized by a decrease in beta cell activity (insulin deficiency), insulin resistance (reduced uptake of insulin by peripheral muscle cells), or an increase in glucose production by the liver. Over time, the beta cells of the pancreas fail and exogenous insulin may be required. Most people with type 2 diabetes mellitus also have metabolic syndrome, also known as insulin resistance syndrome and syndrome X (see Chapter 21). Type 2 diabetes onset is usually more insidious than that of type 1 diabetes. The pancreas still maintains some capability to produce and secrete insulin. Consequently, symptoms (polyphagia, polydipsia, polyuria) are minimal or absent for a prolonged period of time. The patient may seek medical attention several years later only after symptoms of the disease are apparent (see Complications of Diabetes Mellitus, later). Fasting hyperglycemia can be controlled by diet in some patients, but most patients require the use of supplemental insulin or oral antidiabetic agents, such as metformin or glyburide. Although the onset is usually after the fourth decade of life, type 2 diabetes can occur in younger patients who do not require insulin for control. See Table 36-1 for a comparison of the characteristics of type 1 and type 2 diabetes mellitus.

A third subclass of diabetes mellitus (Box 36-1) includes additional types of diabetes that are a part of other diseases having features not generally associated with the diabetic state. Diseases that may have a diabetic component include pheochromocytoma, acromegaly, and Cushing's syndrome. Other disorders included in this category are malnutrition, infection, drugs and chemicals that induce hyperglycemia, defects in insulin receptors, and certain genetic syndromes.

The fourth category of classification, known as **gestational diabetes mellitus** (GDM), is reserved for women who show abnormal glucose tolerance during pregnancy. Gestational diabetes is diagnosed in about 4% of all pregnancies in the United States, resulting in about 135,000 cases per year. It does not include diabetic women who become pregnant. The majority of gestational diabetic people have a normal glucose tolerance postpartum. Gestational diabetic patients must be reclassified 6 weeks after delivery into one of the following categories: diabetes mellitus, impaired fasting glucose, impaired glucose tolerance, or normoglycemia. Gestational diabetic patients have been put into

Box 36-1 ***Etiologic Classification of Diabetes Mellitus***

I. Type 1 diabetes* (beta cell destruction, usually leading to absolute insulin deficiency)
   Immune mediated
   Idiopathic
II. Type 2 diabetes* (may range from predominantly insulin resistance with relative insulin deficiency to a predominantly secretory defect with insulin resistance)
III. Other specific types
   Genetic defects of beta-cell function
   Genetic defects in insulin action
   Disease of the exocrine pancreas
   Endocrinopathies
   Drug- or chemical-induced
   Infections
   Uncommon forms of immune-mediated diabetes
   Other genetic syndromes sometimes associated with diabetes
IV. Gestational diabetes mellitus (GDM)

Modified from The Expert Committee on the Diagnosis and Classification of Diabetes Mellitus: Report of the Expert Committee on the Diagnosis and Classification of Diabetes Mellitus, *Diabetes Care,* 26(Suppl 1): S7, 2003.

*Patients with any form of diabetes may require insulin treatment at some stage of their disease. Such use of insulin does not, of course, classify the patient.

Table 36-1 Characteristics of Type 1 and Type 2 Diabetes Mellitus*

CHARACTERISTIC	TYPE 1 DIABETES	TYPE 2 DIABETES
Age	<20 years†	>40 years†
Onset	Over a few days to weeks	Gradual
Insulin secretion	Falling to none	Oversecretion for years
Body image	Lean	Obese
Early symptoms	Polyuria, polydipsia, polyphasia	Often absent until complications arise
Ketones at diagnosis	Yes	No
Insulin required for treatment	Yes	No‡
Acute complications	Diabetic ketoacidosis	Hyperosmolar hyperglycemia
Microvascular complications at diagnosis	No	Common
Macrovascular complications at diagnosis	Uncommon	Common

*Clinical presentation is highly variable.
†Age of onset is most commonly less than 20 years of age, but may occur at any age. As the rates of obesity increase, type 2 diabetes is becoming much more prevalent in children, adolescents, and young adults in all ethnic groups.
‡May eventually require insulin therapy over time.

Table 36-2 Criteria for the Diagnosis of Diabetes Mellitus*

DIABETES MELLITUS	PREDIABETES
1. Symptoms of diabetes and a casual† plasma glucose ≥200 mg/dL	N/A
OR	
2. Fasting plasma glucose ≥126 mg/dL‡	100-125 mg/dL (IFG)
OR	
3. 2-hour plasma glucose ≥200 mg/dL during an oral glucose tolerance test (OGTT)	140-199 mg/dL (IGT)

From American Diabetes Association: Standards of medical care in diabetes 2006, *Diabetes Care* 29 (Suppl 1), 2006.
IFG, Impaired fasting glucose; *IGT,* impaired glucose tolerance; *FPG,* fasting plasma glucose.
*In the absence of unequivocal hyperglycemia, these criteria should be confirmed by repeat testing on a different day. The OGTT is not recommended for routine clinical use, but may be required in the evaluation of patients with IFG or when diabetes is still suspected despite a normal FPG as with the postpartum evaluation of women with gestational diabetes mellitus.
†"Casual" is defined as any time of day without regard to time since last meal. The classic symptoms of diabetes include polyuria, polydipsia, and unexplained weight loss.
‡Fasting is defined as no caloric intake for at least 8 hours.

a separate category because of the special clinical features of diabetes that develop during pregnancy and the complications associated with fetal involvement. These women are also at a greater risk of developing diabetes 5 to 10 years after pregnancy.

There is a group of patients who are found to have an **impaired glucose tolerance (IGT)** or **impaired fasting glucose (IFG)**. These patients are often euglycemic in their daily living, but develop hyperglycemia when challenged with an oral glucose tolerance test. In many of these patients, the glucose tolerance returns to normal or persists in the intermediate range for years. This intermediate stage between normal glucose homeostasis and diabetes is now known as **prediabetes**. It is now thought that patients with IGT or IFG are at a higher risk for developing type 1 or type 2 diabetes and cardiovascular disease in the future. Categories of fasting plasma glucose (FPG) levels are:

- FPG less than 100 mg/dL = normal fasting glucose
- FPG at 100 mg/dL or greater but less than 126 mg/dL = IFG
- 2-hour plasma glucose at 140 or greater but less than 199 mg/dL = IGT

See Table 36-2 for criteria for the diagnosis of types 1 and 2 diabetes mellitus.

COMPLICATIONS OF DIABETES MELLITUS

Long-standing hyperglycemia and abnormalities in fat, carbohydrate, and protein metabolism lead to microvascular, macrovascular, and neuropathic complications. **Microvascular complications** are those that arise from destruction of capillaries in eyes, kidneys, and peripheral tissues. **Macrovascular complications** are those associated with atherosclerosis of middle to large arteries such as those in the heart and brain. Comorbid diseases that often arise include (Figure 36-1):

- Hypertension
- Cardiovascular disease (atherosclerosis) leading to myocardial infarction and stroke
- Retinopathy leading to blindness
- Renal disease leading to end-stage renal disease (ESRD) and the need for dialysis
- Peripheral arterial disease leading to nonhealing ulcers, infections, and lower extremity amputations
- Neuropathies with sexual dysfunction, bladder incontinence, paresthesias, and gastroparesis
- Periodontal disease with loss of teeth

Symptoms associated with complications of diabetes may be the first indication of the presence of diabetes. Patients may complain of weight gain or loss. Blurred vision may indicate diabetic retinopathy. **Neuropathies** may be first observed as numbness or

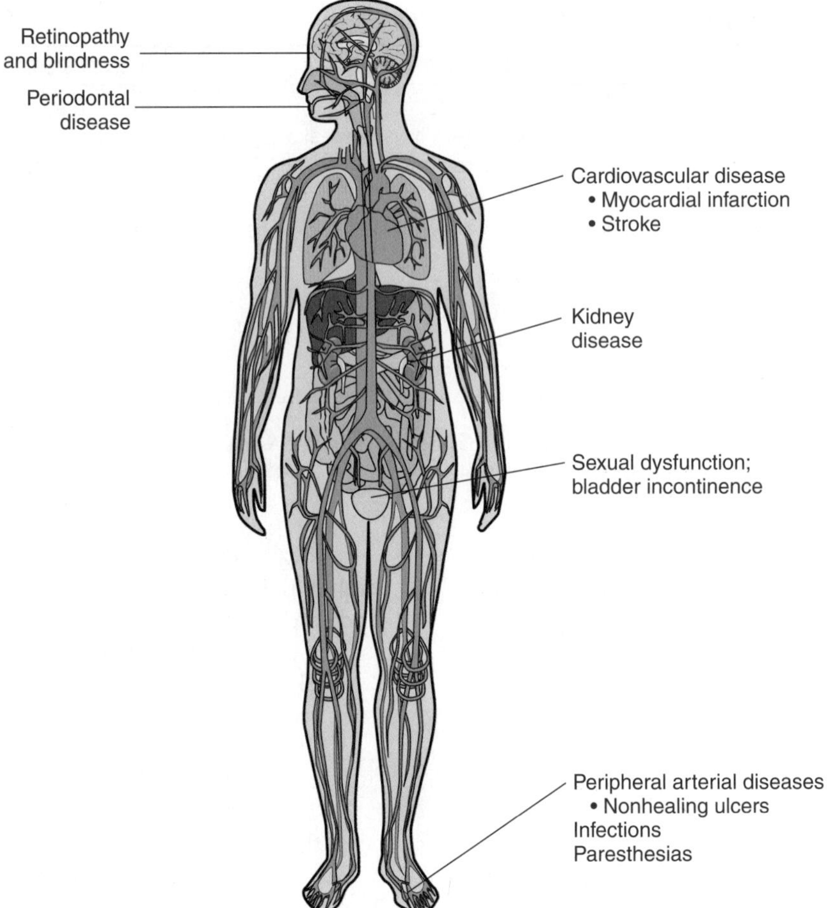

FIGURE **36-1** Complications of diabetes mellitus.

tingling of the extremities (paresthesia), loss of sensation, orthostatic hypotension, impotence, and difficulty in controlling urination (neurogenic bladder). Nonhealing ulcers of the lower extremities may indicate chronic vascular disease. Diabetic complications can be delayed or prevented with continuous normoglycemia accomplished by monitoring blood glucose, drug therapy, and treatment of comorbid conditions as they arise.

TREATMENT OF DIABETES MELLITUS

Although the classification system of the NDDG/WHO was developed to facilitate clinical and epidemiologic investigation, the categorization of patients can also be helpful in determining general principles for therapy. Because a cure for diabetes mellitus is unknown at present, the minimal purpose of treatment is to prevent ketoacidosis and symptoms resulting from hyperglycemia. The long-term objective of control of the disease must involve mechanisms to stop the progression of the complications of the disease. Major determinants to success are a balanced diet, insulin or oral antidiabetic therapy, routine exercise, and good hygiene.

Patients with diabetes can lead full and satisfying lives. However, unrestricted diets and activities are not possible. Dietary treatment of diabetes constitutes the basis for management of most patients, especially those with the type 2 form of the disease. With adequate weight reduction and dietary control, patients may not require the use of exogenous insulin or oral antidiabetic drug therapy. People with type 1 diabetes will always require exogenous insulin as well as dietary control because the pancreas has lost the capacity to produce and secrete insulin. The aims of dietary control are the prevention of excessive postprandial hyperglycemia, the prevention of hypoglycemia (blood glucose <60 mg/dL) in those patients being treated with antidiabetic agents or insulin, the achievement and maintenance of an ideal body weight, and a reduction of lipids and cholesterol. A return to normal weight is often accompanied by a reduction in hyperglycemia. The diet should also be adjusted to reduce elevated cholesterol and triglyceride levels in an attempt to retard the progression of atherosclerosis.

To help maintain adherence to dietary restrictions, the diet should be planned using the American Diabetes Association (ADA) recommendations in relation to the patient's food preferences, economic status, occupation, and physical activity. Emphasis should be placed on what food the patient may have and what exchanges are acceptable. Food should be measured for balanced portions, and the patient

Table 36-3 Treatment Goals for Diabetes and Comorbid Diseases by the American Diabetes Association and the American College of Clinical Endocrinologists

DISEASE	MONITORING PARAMETER	ADA THERAPEUTIC GOALS	ACCE THERAPEUTIC GOALS
Diabetes	Hemoglobin A_{1C}	<7%*	≥6.5%
	Preprandial plasma glucose	90-130 mg/dL	≥110 mg/dL
	Postprandial plasma glucose	<180 mg/dL	≥140 mg/dL
Hypertension	Blood pressure	<130/80 mm Hg	<130/80 mm Hg
Dyslipidemia	LDL cholesterol	<100 mg/dL	<100 mg/dL
	HDL cholesterol	>40 mg/dL	>40 mg/dL
	Triglycerides	<150 mg/dL	<150 mg/dL
Weight		BMI <25 kg/m^2 (see p. 348)	BMI <25 kg/m^2 (see p. 348)

BMI, Body mass index; *HDL,* high-density lipoprotein; *LDL,* low-density lipoprotein.
*The goal A1C level for patients in general is less than 7%, but the ideal goal for individual patients is as close to normal (<6%) as possible without significant hypoglycemia.

should be cautioned not to omit meals or between-meal and bedtime snacks.

Patient education and reinforcement are extremely important to successful therapy. The intelligence and motivation of the diabetic patient and his or her awareness of the potential complications contribute significantly to the ultimate outcome of the disease and the quality of life the patient may lead.

All diabetic patients must receive adequate instruction on personal hygiene, especially regarding care of the feet, skin, and teeth. Infection is a common precipitating cause of ketosis and acidosis and must be treated promptly.

Patients with diabetes must also be aggressively treated for comorbid diseases (smoking cessation, treatment of dyslipidemia, blood pressure control, antiplatelet therapy, influenza, and pneumococcal vaccinations) to help prevent microvascular and macrovascular complications. The American Association of Clinical Endocrinologists (ACCE) has developed the System of Intensive Diabetes Self-Management that applies to type 1 and type 2 diabetes mellitus. The program includes the concepts of care, the responsibilities of the patient and the physician, and the appropriate intervals for laboratory testing and follow-up. Patient education, understanding, and direct participation by the patient in his or her treatment are key components of the long-term success in disease management. The term ***intensive therapy*** describes a comprehensive program of diabetes care that includes self-monitoring of blood glucose four or more times daily, and, for those patients with type 1 diabetes, three or more insulin injections daily or use of an insulin pump for continuous insulin infusion. See Table 36-3 for the treatment goals recommended by the ADA and the ACCE.

DRUG THERAPY FOR DIABETES MELLITUS

The primary treatment goal of type 1 and type 2 diabetes is normalization of blood glucose levels. Insulin is required to control type 1 diabetes and for those patients with other types of diabetes whose blood glucose cannot be controlled by diet, weight reduction, or oral antidiabetic agents. Patients normally controlled with oral antidiabetic agents require insulin during situations of increased physiologic and psychological stress, such as pregnancy, surgery, and infections. The dosage of insulin is usually adjusted according to the blood glucose levels. The patient should test blood glucose before each meal and at bedtime while the insulin and food intake is being regulated.

Oral antidiabetic agents are used in the therapy of type 2 diabetes. They are recommended only for those patients whose diabetes cannot be controlled by diet alone and who are not prone to develop ketosis, acidosis, or infections. Patients most likely to benefit from treatment are those who have developed diabetes after 40 years of age and who require less than 40 units of insulin per day.

A combination of oral antidiabetic agents working by different mechanisms is often required to successfully control hyperglycemia (Figure 36-2).

- *Secretogogues:* The sulfonylureas (e.g., glyburide, glipizide) and the meglitinides (repaglinide, nateglinide) stimulate the pancreas to secrete more insulin. The sulfonylureas also diminish glucose production and metabolism of insulin by the liver. The net effect is a normalization of insulin and glucose levels.
- *Biguanide:* The only biguanide available in the United States is metformin. Metformin decreases hepatic glucose production by inhibiting glycogenolysis and gluconeogenesis, reduces absorption of glucose from the small intestine, and increases insulin sensitivity improving glucose uptake in peripheral muscle and adipose cells. The net result is a significant decrease in fasting and postprandial blood glucose and hemoglobin A1C concentrations.
- *Thiazolidinediones (TZDs):* The TZDs (pioglitazone, rosiglitazone) increase tissue sensitivity to insulin causing greater glucose uptake in

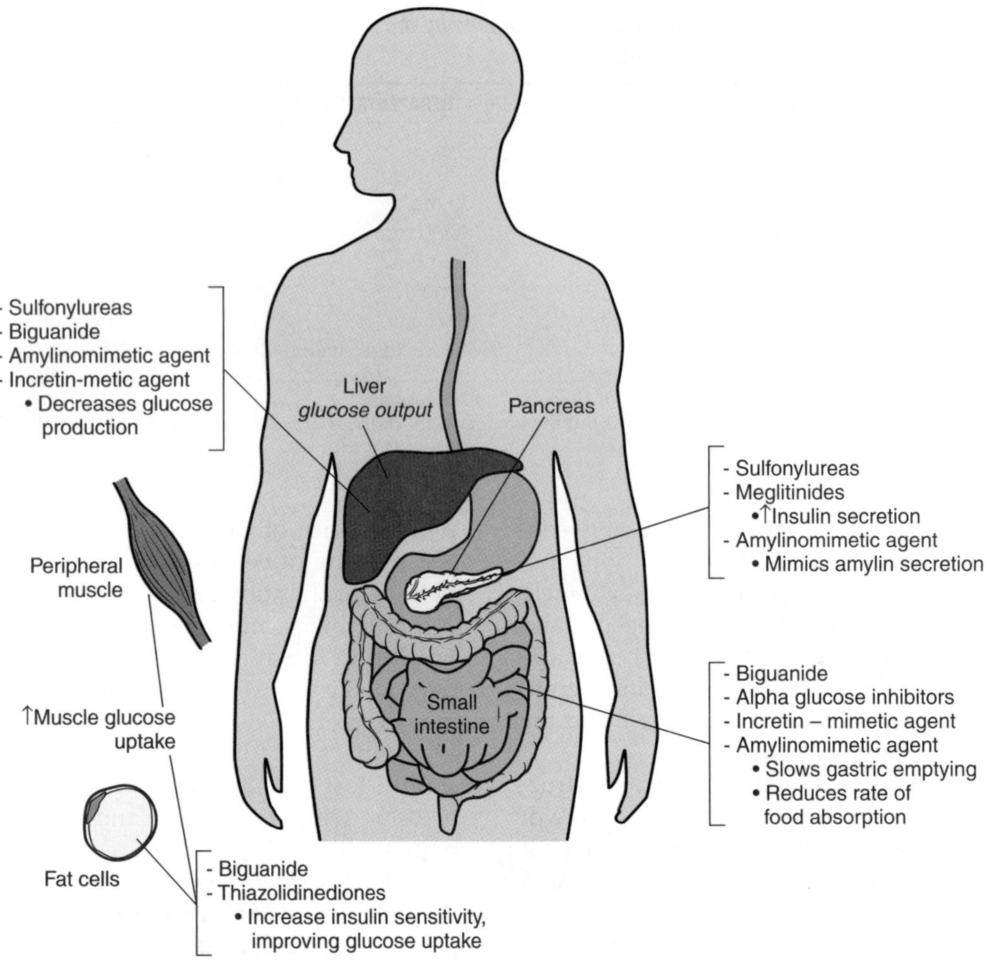

FIGURE **36-2** Mechanisms of action of antidiabetic agents.

Table 36-4 ***Summary of Physiological Effects of Antidiabetic Agents***

DRUG	INSULIN SECRETION	DECREASE IN FASTING BLOOD GLUCOSE	EFFECT ON HEMOGLOBIN A_{1C}	WEIGHT GAIN
Insulin	Decrease	Significant	Significant	Yes
Sulfonylureas	Increase	40-60 mg/dL	1%-2%	Yes
Meglitinides	Increase	30 mg/dL	1.1%	Yes
Biguanide	No change	53 mg/dL	1.4%	No—mild
Thiazolidinediones	No change	25-55 mg/dL	0.1%-0.7%	Yes
Alpha-glucosidase inhibitors	No change	20-30 mg/dL	0.5%-1%	No

Adapted from The American Association of Clinical Endocrinologists Medical Guideline for the Management of Diabetes Mellitus: The ACCE system of intensive diabetes self-management, 2002 Update, *Endocrine Practice* 8 (Suppl 1), 2002.

muscle, adipose, and liver tissue. It also diminishes glucose production by the liver.

- *Alpha-glucosidase inhibitors:* Acarbose and miglitol inhibit enzymes in the small intestine that metabolize complex carbohydrates. This slows the absorption of carbohydrates, reducing postprandial hyperglycemia.

Initial oral antidiabetic therapy for type 2 diabetes is highly dependent on the patient's success with lifestyle modification and diet control. Patients who are near normal in weight are often started on a sulfonylurea to stimulate insulin production. Obese patients are often started on metformin, assuming that there is no contraindication to therapy (e.g., renal insufficiency, heart failure). If initial therapy does not control glucose levels, medicine from a different class should be added to therapy. The most frequently used combination is a sulfonylurea and metformin. A TZD or insulin could be added if a third agent is necessary. An alpha-glucosidase inhibitor could be added if postprandial hyperglycemia is a problem. See Table 36-4 for a comparison of oral antidiabetic agents and their effect on lowering blood glucose levels and hemoglobin A1C concentrations.

NURSING PROCESS *for Patients with Diabetes Mellitus*

A major challenge in nursing is to teach the recently diagnosed diabetic patient all the necessary information to manage self-care and the disease process and to prevent complications. The patient must be taught the entire therapeutic regimen: diet, activity level, blood or urine testing, medication, self-injection techniques, prevention of complications, and effective management of hypoglycemia or hyperglycemia. Many diabetic patients have difficulty understanding the critical balance among the dietary prescription, the prescribed medication, and the maintenance of general health. All are important to the control and effective management of the disease process.

Assessment

The order of performing the assessment depends on the setting and the severity of the patient's symptoms.

Description of Current Symptoms

- Ask the reasons for seeking the current appointment or admission.
- Review symptoms and procedures used to diagnose diabetes mellitus in a general medical-surgical textbook.

Patient's Understanding of Diabetes Mellitus

- Assess the individual's current knowledge of the treatment of diabetes mellitus. Gather additional data about the person's current educational needs with regard to self-management of the disease process.
- Will other family members or significant others be providing part of the care or participating in the health education portion of the individual's care?
- Is there a need to communicate with a child's school regarding the disease process?
- Patients who are readmitted must be assessed for the understanding of the treatment regimen and for adherence with the prescribed diet, medications, and exercise.
- For pregnant women, risk assessment for gestational diabetes mellitus (GDM) should be performed at the first prenatal visit. High-risk women who have an initial negative testing for diabetes should be retested between 24 to 28 weeks of gestation.

The FPG is the preferred test used to screen for diabetes in children and nonpregnant adults.

Psychosocial Assessment

- *Mental status:* Ask specific information to evaluate the patient's current level of consciousness, alertness, comprehension, and appropriateness of responses. Evaluate the person's judgment capabilities and ability to solve problems about the management of the diabetes.
- *Adaptation to disease:* Ask specifically about the person's adjustment to the diagnosis of diabetes mellitus; or, in a recently diagnosed individual, identify prior coping mechanisms used successfully to deal with life events.
- *Feelings:* Assess for fears and the person's perspective of the impact of the disease on his or her life.
- *Support system:* Obtain information regarding who can provide support for the patient. Does the individual live alone? What effect does the disease have on other members of the family structure (e.g., children who are diabetic, people with renal or visual complications)? Does the patient participate in a support group for patients with diabetes?

Nutrition

- Is the patient on a prescribed diet? The recently diagnosed diabetic patient requires a thorough nutritional assessment. Information collected by the nurse or dietitian should include identification of the patient's average daily diet, the ability and willingness to prepare foods, food budget, and level of daily activity and exercise.
- Ask about diet prescription—total daily calories, and distribution pattern of carbohydrates, fats, and proteins.
- Have there been any problems encountered in purchasing or preparing the foods? Has it been difficult to comply with the diet? If so, what problems are being encountered?
- How much alcohol is consumed and how often?
- Has the individual experienced any weight loss or gain recently?
- If the patient is a child, obtain data relating to the individual's growth and development patterns.

Activity and Exercise

- Does the individual experience weakness or fatigue with daily activities? Does the patient get regular exercise? What type, intensity, and duration is it? Has there been any significant variation in the degree of exercise recently?
- Has the patient made any adjustments in the insulin, oral antidiabetic agents, or diet to offset an increase or decrease in exercise?
- Has there been a change in occupation that has affected the level of exercise?

Medications. What medications have been prescribed and what is the degree of adherence with the regimen? What over-the-counter medicines (including herbal medications) does the patient take, and how often? Does the patient consume alcohol? How much and how often? Ask specifically about the type and amount of insulin being taken and the times of administration.

Monitoring. Ask the patient to bring a record of self-monitoring of insulin or antidiabetic agents taken, as well as any blood glucose testing or glycosylated hemoglobin A1C testing that was done. Has the patient done any testing for ketones? If so, what were the results? Other tests to be completed periodically include the fasting lipid profile including cholesterol, high-density lipoprotein (HDL) and low-density lipoprotein (LDL) cholesterol and triglycerides, serum creatinine, and microalbuminuria.

Physical Assessment. Generally, data are collected about all body systems to serve as a baseline for subsequent evaluations throughout the course of treatment. Periodic focused assessments are completed to detect signs and symptoms of complications commonly associated with diabetes mellitus.

- *Hyperglycemia and hypoglycemia:* Have there been any episodes of hypoglycemia or hyperglycemia? If so, obtain details of the occurrences (e.g., has the patient eaten the prescribed diet, taken the prescribed medications, or altered the exercise level?). Record all prescription and over-the-counter medications being taken to assess whether any drug interactions may be causing the hyperglycemia or hypoglycemia.
- *Illnesses/stress:* Have there been any recent illnesses, infections, or stressful events? If so, what treatments have been initiated? Ask specifically about any sores with the skin, feet, or teeth, and for the occurrence of urinary tract infections.
- *Vascular changes:* Obtain baseline vital signs. Does the person have any symptoms of, or is the patient being treated for cerebrovascular, peripheral vascular, or cardiovascular disease (including hypertension), or diabetic retinopathy or nephropathy?

Obtain a current history of the patient's blood pressure and details of any medications being taken to treat hypertension. When hypertension is present, perform a urinalysis and check for protein. If protein is negative, microalbumin testing should be performed to determine the presence of protein in the urine.

- *Neuropathy:* Ask about specific symptoms of *paresthesias* (numbness or tingling sensations), foot injuries and ulcerations, diarrhea, postural hypotension, impotence, or neurogenic bladder.
- *Smoking:* Obtain history of smoking and tobacco use in everyone with diabetes mellitus.

Nursing Diagnoses

- Knowledge, deficient (indication, side effects)
- Infection, risk for (indication)
- Fluid volume, risk for deficient (side effects)
- Nutrition, imbalanced: less or more than body requirements (indication)

Planning

Description of Current Symptoms. Individualize the care plan to address the patient's symptoms (e.g., hypoglycemia, hyperglycemia, diabetic ketoacidosis coma, renal failure). A specific diabetic care plan for children attending school should be developed with the parents and the diabetic care team. The ADA publishes an outline of a care plan that can be used to formulate the plan for the child.

Medications

- Order medications prescribed and schedule these on the medication administration record (MAR).
- Perform focused assessments at regularly scheduled intervals consistent with the patient's status to determine the effectiveness and the side effects to expect or report.
- Initiate a diabetic flow sheet or record in computer where indicated.

Diet

- Schedule a consultation with a dietitian or nutritional educator, as appropriate to the patient's needs. Standardized calorie-level meal patterns based on exchange lists have traditionally been used to plan meals for hospitalized patients. Other meal planning systems include menus based on *Nutrition and Your Health: Dietary Guidelines for Americans,** regular hospital menus, individualized meal plans, or menus using carbohydrate counting. A new system, termed the "consistent-carbohydrate diabetes meal plan," is being developed that uses meal plans without a specific calorie level; instead, it incorporates a consistent carbohydrate content for each meal and snack. The meal plan also includes appropriate fat and protein modifications and emphasizes consistent timing of meals and snacks. A typical day's meals and snacks provide 1500 to 2000 calories with 45% to 65% of the calories from carbohydrate, 15% to 20% from protein, and no more than 30% from fat. If a patient's nutritional needs are more or less than provided by these meal plans, individualized adjustments may be required. Patients who often require adjustments include children, adolescents, metabolically stressed patients, pregnant women, and older adult patients.
- Weight loss is recommended for all overweight (body mass index [BMI] 25 to 29.9 kg/m^2) or obese (BMI ≥30 kg/m^2) adults, who have or are at risk for developing type 2 diabetes. The primary approach for achieving weight loss is therapeutic lifestyle change, which includes a reduction in energy intake and/or an increase in physical activity. A moderate decrease in caloric balance (500 to 1000 kcal/day) will result in slow but progressive weight loss (1 to 2 lb/week). For most patients, weight loss diets should supply at least 1000 to 12000 kcal per day for women and 1200 to 1600 kcal per day for men.
- Order the prescribed diet and clearly mark the Kardex or enter data in the computer regarding fluid intake parameters between meals.

*Departments of Health and Human Services and Agriculture: *Nutrition and your health: dietary guidelines for Americans*, 2005, www.health.gov/dietaryguidelines. Accessed February 2, 2006.

Weight. Mark the Kardex or enter data in the computer with specific intervals for measurement of weight (e.g., daily weights, weight every other day on even days).

Laboratory Studies

- Schedule the laboratory blood draws for fasting blood glucose, glucose tolerance testing, A1C, serum lipid studies, and so on as ordered by the physician.
- Mark the Kardex or enter data in the computer with specific intervals for the performance of fingerstick blood glucose monitoring.
- Indicate clearly if the person is receiving insulin by sliding scale and where orders are written for the amount of insulin to be administered based on the sliding scale (e.g., see MAR for sliding scale parameters).

Referrals. Schedule eye examinations, appointments with diabetes educator, family planning (for women of reproductive age), foot specialists, and other services as indicated.

Health Teaching. Individualize and initiate health teaching forms used by the clinical site to educate the patient and significant others.

Implementation

- Answer questions the patient has regarding any aspect of the care being provided, including the rationale.
- Encourage expression of feelings and concerns the patient has, and address the patient's concerns first. Involve support personnel, as appropriate, in the delivery of care or planning for home management of the diabetes.
- Encourage adequate nutrition by implementing the dietary regimen prescribed. Promote adequate fluid intake to maintain hydration. Support dietary teaching by the health team, and be constantly alert for misperceptions or misunderstanding of the diet.
- Encourage activity and exercise at the prescribed level. Discuss the benefits while providing care.
- Administer prescribed medications (e.g., insulin, oral antidiabetic agents). Monitor for side effects to expect and report, and document associated monitoring parameters on the records (e.g., blood glucose, ketone testing). If the patient is taking insulin, assess the ability and accuracy to self-administer injections. If a family member gives the insulin, assess the ability and accuracy in giving injections.
- If a hypoglycemic reaction occurs, notify the team leader or primary nurse, who will then contact the physician. The underlying cause of the hypoglycemia must be identified to prevent further occurrences. If in doubt about whether the patient is hypoglycemic or hyperglycemic, the nurse should always proceed to treat the individual for hypoglycemia to prevent neurologic damage from prolonged reduction in glucose to the nerve cells (e.g., brain cells).
- With any hyperglycemic reaction, notify the team leader or primary nurse, who will then contact the physician. The goals of treatment include maintaining normal fluid and electrolyte balance and restoration of a normal serum glucose level.
- Perform routine physical assessments every shift as required by the clinical site. Perform focused assessments of areas where complications are anticipated, based on the admission data and subsequent data collected.

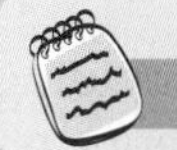

Patient Education and Health Promotion

Knowledge. Teach the individual specifics regarding the type of diabetes that has been diagnosed:

- Type 1 diabetes mellitus results from damage to the beta cells of the pancreas, where insulin is normally produced. Insulin is needed to transport the glucose required by the body cells from the bloodstream to the individual cells to be used as an energy source. Without beta cells, no insulin is produced and the glucose accumulates in the blood (hyperglycemia).
- Type 1 diabetes mellitus requires the administration of insulin injections to replace the insulin the body is no longer able to make. The patient must follow a prescribed diet and exercise program, perform glucose testing, and, during times when hyperglycemia is present, test for ketones in the urine.
- Type 2 diabetes mellitus is an illness characterized by abnormal beta cell function, resistance to insulin action and increased hepatic glucose production. Type 2 diabetes mellitus requires a prescribed diet and exercise program, weight loss to a near-ideal body level, glucose testing, and an oral antidiabetic agent or antihyperglycemic agent if unable to manage the diabetes with diet and exercise alone. During times of illness, or if the oral treatment stops being effective, insulin may be required. Special needs may be required for patients who are pregnant or nursing.

Psychological Adjustment

- When first diagnosed, the patient may experience varying degrees of grief, anger, denial, or acceptance. Let the patient express these concerns, and address those items that are considered to be of greatest importance first.
- Encourage the idea that the patient can control most aspects of diabetes by careful management of diet, medications, and activities. Having a sense of control is important to all people. Stress

that learning to manage the disease process is the best long-term approach.

- Discuss the individual's lifestyle, travel, work, school schedules, and activities, and individualize the care needs.
- Discuss the need for continued, regular monitoring of the diabetes to minimize the effect the disease may have on the patient and family.

Smoking. Health care providers should emphasize the need for smoking cessation as a priority of care for all patients with diabetes.

Nutrition

- Diet is used alone or in combination with insulin or oral antidiabetic agents to control diabetes mellitus. The diabetic patient, whether type 1 or type 2, must follow a prescribed diet to achieve optimal control of the disease.
- The dietary prescription is based on providing the patient with the nutritional and energy requirements necessary to maintain an appropriate weight, lifestyle, and normal growth and development. Diabetic patients are encouraged to maintain a reasonable body weight based on height, gender, and frame size.
- Additional goals for medical nutrition therapy include maintaining a blood glucose level in the normal range to reduce the risk of complications of diabetes; a normal lipid profile to reduce the risk for microvascular disease; and normal blood pressure levels to reduce the risk for vascular disease.
- The ADA no longer endorses any single meal plan or specified percentages of macronutrients as it has in the past. The Institute of Medicine and the ADA recommends, in general, that the diet be composed of 45% to 65% carbohydrates, 15% to 20% protein (0.8 to 1 g protein per kilogram of body weight), and no more than 30% of fat. Monounsaturated and polyunsaturated fat should be the primary fat sources; saturated fats should be limited to no more than 10% of the diet and cholesterol intake to 300 mg or less per day. Trans fatty acids should be avoided when possible. Including high-fiber foods (e.g., legumes, oats, barley) assists in lowering both blood glucose levels and blood cholesterol. Reduced sodium, alcohol, and caffeine consumption is also advisable (see also Chapter 47).
- Diabetic patients, as well as all individuals, need to be encouraged to consume an adequate intake of vitamin and minerals from natural food sources.
- Inclusion of sucrose is now permitted in limited amounts in the diabetic diet; however, the amount eaten must be calculated as part of the carbohydrate intake for the day. Meal plans such as "no concentrated sweets," "no added sugar," "low sugar," and "liberal diabetic diets" are no longer appropriate. These diets do not reflect the diabetes nutrition recommendations and unnecessarily restrict sucrose. Such meal plans may perpetuate the false notion that simply restricting sucrose-sweetened foods will improve blood glucose control.
- The U.S. Food and Drug Administration (FDA) has approved the use of four artificial sweeteners as sugar substitutes: saccharin, aspartame (NutraSweet), sucralose (Splenda), and acesulfame potassium.
- Patients with diabetes should adhere to the same guidelines for ingestion of alcohol as for all Americans: no more than two drinks per day for men and one drink per day for women. People with good control of their diabetes may ingest alcohol in moderation. However, drinking can result in either hypoglycemia or hyperglycemia in diabetic people. The effects of alcohol are influenced by the amount ingested, if ingested on an empty stomach, or if used chronically or excessively. Many alcoholic beverages are high in sugar and should be used with caution; light beer or dry wines are alternatives. One drink is defined as 12 ounces of beer, 5 ounces of wine, or 1.5 ounces of distilled spirits, each of which contains 15 g of alcohol. Because alcohol does affect the blood sugar, it may be wise to test the blood glucose level before and after drinking to identify how the alcohol reacts in a particular patient. Abstinence is recommended for pregnant patients, those with known medical problems aggravated by its use, and by those with a history of abuse.
- Dietary considerations for children and adolescents with type 1 and type 2 diabetes are similar to the needs of all other children. They need to maintain a steady intake of a balanced diet aimed at maintaining normal growth and development. It is important to obtain height and weight values and to compare these to the normal growth curve found on charts to ascertain whether the dietary intake is adequate, deficient, or excessive. The individual's meal planning must be done in such a way as to accommodate irregular meal times and schedules, and the varying activity levels of the child or adolescent.
- All women have similar nutritional needs during pregnancy and lactation whether they have diabetes or not. An individual with gestational diabetes is given education on food choices that are appropriate for normal weight gain, normoglycemia, and absence of ketones. Some individuals with gestational diabetes may require a modest restriction in carbohydrates.
- In older adults, a change in body weight of greater than 10 pounds or 10% of the body weight in less than 6 months is considered sufficient reason to investigate for nutrition-related

causes. In general, older people with diabetes in long-term care settings tend to be underweight rather than overweight. Administering a daily vitamin supplement to older adults, especially those with decreased energy intake may be advisable. It should be noted that specialized diets do not appear to be beneficial to the older adult in long-term care settings where food choices are decidedly limited. It is preferable to make medication adjustments to control blood glucose rather than to implement food restrictions in the long-term care setting. As with everyone, physical activity should be encouraged.

The ADA has several cookbooks and a number of pamphlets available on nutrition for the diabetic person.

Activity and Exercise

- Maintenance of a normal lifestyle is to be encouraged. This includes exercise and activities enjoyed by the individual. The normal daily energy level is used in determining the dietary and medication requirements for the patient. The ADA recommends that initial therapy should be modest, based on the patient's willingness and ability, gradually increasing the duration and frequency to 30 to 45 minutes of moderate aerobic activity 3 to 5 days per week, when possible. Greater activity levels of at least 1 hour per day of moderate (walking) or 30 minutes per day of vigorous (jogging) activity may be needed to achieve successful long-term weight loss.
- As with all individuals who are about to undertake exercise, a proper period of warm-up and cool-down consisting of 5 to 10 minutes of aerobic activity at a low intensity should be done. It is very important to maintain proper foot care in a diabetic patient who is to undertake exercise. Use silica gel or air midsoles as well as polyester or blend socks to prevent blisters and keep the feet as dry as possible. Visible inspection of the feet surfaces before and after exercise is an important component of an exercise regimen and is especially important in diabetic patients who already have peripheral neuropathy. Persons with loss of protective sensation should not use step exercises, jogging, prolonged walking, or treadmills as an exercise regimen. Rather, they should substitute swimming, bicycling, rowing, chair exercises, arm exercises, or other non–weight-bearing exercise.
- Just as it is important for the patient to maintain a certain diet, it is equally important to maintain a certain activity level. Patients who suddenly increase or decrease activity levels are susceptible to developing episodes of hyperglycemia or hypoglycemia. Both dietary and medication prescriptions may require adjustment if the patient does not plan to resume the previous exercise level. The patient should consult with the physician before initiating an exercise program.
- Additional self-monitoring of the blood glucose level may be advisable before, during, and approximately 30 minutes after exercise to provide the physician with data to analyze regarding the effects of exercise on the individual's blood glucose level. The ADA recommends that you not exercise if your glucose level is above 250 mg/dL. Conversely, exercising with hypoglycemia is not advisable. A snack high in carbohydrate (10 to 20 g) should be taken before exercising if the blood sugar is less than 100 mg/dL.
- Exercise helps the cells use glucose; therefore, exercise lowers the glucose level.
- Drink sufficient fluids without caffeine when exercising to prevent dehydration.
- Stop exercising if feeling weak, sick, dizzy, or if experiencing any type of pain.

Medication

- Insulin or oral antidiabetic agent therapy may be required to control diabetes mellitus. No changes in therapy should be made without medical supervision.
- A variety of combinations of insulin or insulin and oral antidiabetic agents may be used to provide control of the blood glucose level. The goal of therapy is to consistently maintain the blood glucose level within the normal range. A variety of administration schedules have evolved over the years to accomplish this goal. The schedules commonly used are as follows:
  1. Divided doses of intermediate-acting insulin (two thirds in the morning, one third in the evening before dinner).
  2. A combination of rapid-acting or short-acting and intermediate-acting insulin in the morning, followed by rapid- or short-acting insulin at dinner and intermediate-acting insulin before bedtime.
  3. Rapid- or short-acting insulin before each meal and intermediate-acting insulin at bedtime.
  4. Rapid-acting or short-acting and long-acting insulin before breakfast, rapid-acting or short-acting insulin before lunch, and rapid-acting or short-acting and long-acting insulin again before dinner.
  5. Continuous infusion of rapid-acting or short-acting insulin using a small, portable insulin infusion pump.
- The regimen chosen depends on each person's response to medications, schedule of daily activities, and compliance with blood glucose monitoring, insulin injections, and diet.
- Medication preparation, dosage, frequency, storage, and refilling should be discussed and taught in detail. See p. 165 for administration of subcutaneous injections, and p. 160 for mixing of

insulins. Also discuss proper disposal of used syringes and needles in the home setting.

- Be certain that the patient understands how to refill prescriptions for insulin or oral antidiabetic agents. When purchasing insulin, ask the patient to double-check the type, concentration (usually U-100), and the expiration date. Insulin types should not be changed without the approval of the prescribing health care provider. The insulin should be stored in the refrigerator (not the freezer) before use. Once it is opened and being used, it can be stored at room temperature for up to 1 month. The patient or nurse should date the bottle when first opened and used. The patient should always have a spare bottle of each type of insulin prescribed available for use.
- When a patient is experiencing an acute illness, injury, or surgery, hyperglycemia may result. When ill, the patient should continue with the regular diet plan and increase noncaloric fluids such as broth, water, and other decaffeinated drinks. The patient should continue to take the oral agents and/or insulin as prescribed, and monitor the blood glucose level at least every 4 hours. If the glucose is greater than 240 mg/dL, urine should be tested for ketones (see later). If the patient is unable to eat the normal caloric intake, he or she should continue to take the same dose of oral agents and/or insulin prescribed, but supplement food intake with carbohydrate-containing fluids such as soups, regular juices, and decaffeinated soft drinks. The health care provider should be notified immediately if the patient is unable to "keep anything down." Patients should understand that medication for diabetes, including insulin, should not be withheld during times of illness because counterregulatory mechanisms in the body often increase the blood glucose level dramatically. Food intake is also necessary because the body requires extra energy to deal with the stress of illness. Extra insulin may also be necessary to meet the demand of illness.
- If pregnancy is suspected, consult an obstetrician as soon as possible about continuing and adjusting medication therapy during pregnancy.

Hypoglycemia. Hypoglycemia, or low blood sugar, can occur from too much insulin, sulfonylureas, insufficient food intake to cover the insulin given, imbalances caused by vomiting and diarrhea, and excessive exercise without additional carbohydrate intake.

Symptoms. Recognize and assess early symptoms of hypoglycemia: nervousness, tremors, headache, apprehension, sweating, cold and clammy skin, and hunger. If uncorrected, hypoglycemia progresses to blurring of vision, lack of coordination, incoherence, coma, and death. Children younger than the age of 6 to 7 years of age may not have the cognitive abilities to recognize and initiate self-treatment of hypoglycemia.

Treatment. If the patient is conscious and able to swallow, give 2 to 4 ounces of fruit juice, or 1 cup of skim milk, or 4 ounces of a nondiet soft drink, or give a piece of candy such as a gumdrop. An alternative is to carry a glucose-containing product (e.g., Glutose gel, Dex4 Glucose tablets) and take as recommended when hypoglycemic. Repeat in 10 to 15 minutes if relief of symptoms is not evident. Do not use hard candy if there is a danger of aspiration. If the patient is unconscious, having a seizure, or unable to swallow, administer glucagon or 20 to 50 mL of glucose 50% intravenously (IV) (only by a qualified individual). People taking insulin should have a family member, significant other, or coworker who is able to administer glucagon. Obtain a blood glucose level at the time of hypoglycemia, if possible.

Hyperglycemia. Hyperglycemia (elevated blood sugar) occurs when the glucose available in the body cannot be transported into the cells for use because of a lack of insulin necessary for the transport mechanism.

Symptoms. Symptoms of hyperglycemia are headache, nausea and vomiting, abdominal pain, dizziness, rapid pulse, rapid shallow respirations, and a fruity odor to the breath from acetone. If untreated, hyperglycemia may also cause coma and death. Glucose levels greater than 240 mg/dL, and ketones present in the urine is an early indication of diabetic ketoacidosis.

Treatment. Treatment of hyperglycemia often requires hospitalization with close monitoring of hydration status, administration of IV fluids, insulin, and blood glucose levels, urine ketones, and potassium levels. Hyperglycemia usually occurs because of another cause; therefore the problem, often an infection, must also be identified and treated to control the hyperglycemia.

Prevention. The risk of hyperglycemia can be minimized by taking the prescribed dose of insulin or oral antidiabetic agent; adhering to the prescribed diet and exercise; reporting fevers, infection, or prolonged vomiting or diarrhea to the physician; and maintaining an accurate written record for the physician to analyze to determine the individual patient's needs. Self-monitoring of blood glucose results and evaluation of urine ketones can provide the physician with valuable data to effectively manage the treatment of the individual.

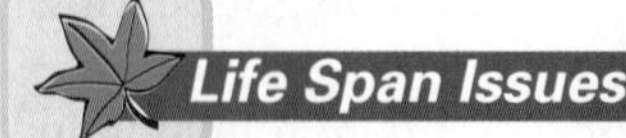

Life Span Issues

Insulin

Virtually all patients receiving insulin will experience a hypoglycemic reaction at one time or another. Symptoms of hypoglycemic reaction vary from patient to patient. Be aware that confusion and lethargy are signs of hypoglycemia but are sometimes overlooked in older adult patients with the thought that slowness and confusion are just symptoms of "age."

Self-Monitoring of Blood Glucose

- Home blood glucose monitoring (self-monitoring) is an accepted practice for managing diabetes mellitus. It is used to evaluate the degree of control of the blood glucose. It can also be used to evaluate when additional insulin must be taken or to determine the effect of exercise on insulin needs.
- Educate the individual using the equipment for self-monitoring that will be used at home. Teach the individual all details of the operation, including calibration, care, handling, and cleansing of the glucose monitor.
- The best time to check blood glucose levels is just before meals, 1 to 2 hours after meals, before bed, and between 2:00 and 3:00 AM. The physician will give specific instructions regarding how often and when glucose testing should be done. When ill, it is important to increase the frequency of glucose monitoring.
- A small sample of capillary blood is obtained, generally using an automatic finger-sticking lancet. The blood sample is applied to a reagent strip, which is then placed in an electronic device that reads the amount of color change and converts this into a numeric value representing the blood glucose level. There also are meters and sensors (that do not use reagent strips) for delivering the glucose results. "Talking" glucometers are on the market for people who are visually impaired. Written records of the blood glucose results should be maintained and taken to all follow-up visits with the physician for analysis.

Urine Testing for Ketones

- Teach the patient to perform urine testing for ketones at least four times daily during times of stress, infection, or when signs or symptoms of hyperglycemia are suspected or present. (Ketone testing should be done when the blood glucose level is consistently greater than 300 mg/dL, during pregnancy, or when symptoms of ketoacidosis, such as nausea, vomiting, or abdominal pain, are present.) The physician may suggest additional times when ketones should be monitored depending on the type of regimen prescribed for controlling blood glucose. An accurate written record of the results should be maintained. Guidelines for reporting abnormal results to the physician should be discussed at the time of discharge. First morning urine tests from pregnant women and up to 30% of first morning specimens in individuals who are fasting may have positive readings. Several drugs also may interfere with the results of ketone urine testing, giving false-positive values. Blood ketone testing methods that quantify beta-hydroxybutyric acid are available for home testing and are preferred over urine ketone testing for monitoring and diagnosing ketoacidosis.
- Suggest ketone testing be initiated when an illness occurs and the serum glucose is elevated above the individual's usual range. Explain when to call the physician. Suggest increasing fluid intake whenever the ketones are positive.

Other Laboratory Glucose Testing

- The A1C test measures the percent of hemoglobin that has been irreversibly glycosylated because of high blood sugar levels. This provides a reflection of the average blood sugar level attained over the past 8 to 10 weeks. This test is used in conjunction with home self-glucose monitoring to assess overall glycemic control.
- The fructosamine test measures the amount of glucose bonded to a protein, fructosamine. This reflects the average blood level attained over the past 1 to 3 weeks.

Complications Associated with Diabetes Mellitus

Cardiovascular Disease. Men and women with diabetes are at an increased risk of dying from complications of cardiovascular disease. Aspirin therapy is a primary prevention strategy for both diabetic men and women. Enteric-coated aspirin in doses of 81 to 325 mg per day is taken by individuals who are older than 21 years of age and by people who do NOT have an aspirin sensitivity.

Peripheral Vascular Disease. The person with diabetes mellitus is more likely to suffer from peripheral vascular disease than is the general population. Reduced blood supply to the extremities may result in intermittent claudication, numbness and tingling, and a greater likelihood of foot infection. The following are symptoms the patient should look for in caring for the extremities:

- *Color:* Observe the color of each hand, finger, leg, and foot; report cyanosis or reddish blue discolorations. Inspect the skin of the extremities for any signs of ulceration.
- *Temperature:* Feel the temperature in each hand, finger, leg, and foot. Report paleness and coldness. Note that these symptoms will be increased if the limbs are elevated above the level of the heart.
- *Edema:* Report edema, its extent, and whether relieved or unchanged when in a dependent position.
- *Limb pain:* Pain with exercise that is relieved by rest may be from claudication and should be reported to the physician.
- *Care:* Prevent ulcers, injury, and infection in the lower extremities with meticulous, regular care. Use lotion to prevent dryness. Inspect the feet daily for any signs of skin breakdown or loss of sensation; report to physician and do not attempt to self-treat. The presence of redness, warmth, or calluses may signal an impending breakdown. Always cut toenails straight across and seek foot care from a podiatrist if problems exist.

Visual Alterations. Visual changes are common in the patient with diabetes mellitus. These individuals frequently suffer from blurred vision associated with an elevated blood sugar. Any diabetic person with intermittently blurred vision should contact the physician for a check of the blood sugar level. Once the hyperglycemia is controlled, the blurred vision usually resolves.

Blindness. In advanced stages of diabetes mellitus, the patient may suffer from changes (microangiopathies) in the small blood vessels of the eyes. Retinal hemorrhages, degeneration of retinal vascular tissue, cataracts, and eventual blindness may occur. The diabetic patient should have regular eye exams to allow early treatment of any apparent alterations.

Renal Disease. People with diabetes mellitus are more susceptible to urinary tract infections; therefore symptoms such as burning on urination or low back pain should be evaluated promptly. Patients are also more susceptible to renal disease. Routine periodic monitoring of protein in the urine determines the presence of renal disease. In patients with type 1 or type 2 diabetes who have microalbuminuria, even a small reduction in protein intake has been shown to improve the glomerular filtration rate and reduce urinary albumin excretion rates.

Infection. Any type of infection can cause a significant loss of control of diabetes mellitus. Patients should check themselves carefully for any signs of redness, tenderness, swelling, or drainage that may occur when there is any break in the skin. Patients should be taught to report immediately early signs of infection, such as fever or sore throat. During an infection, the dosage of insulin may require an adjustment to compensate for a change in metabolic rate, diet, and exercise. Contact the physician for specific directions.

Neuropathies. Explain to appropriate individuals the complication of degeneration of nerves when it exists. Ask the patient to describe sensations (e.g., numbness, tingling) in the extremities. Inspect the feet for blisters, ulcerations, ingrown toenails, or sores. Occasionally the patient will not be aware of these lesions because of the degeneration of nerves in the area. When numbness and lack of sensation are present, always test the water temperature before immersing a limb. Because of impaired sensation, it is easy to be burned and be unaware of it until later.

Impotence. Impotence may occur from a number of causes and should be discussed on an individual basis with the physician.

Hypertension. All patients with diabetes should have a blood pressure measurement, including orthostatic measurements, completed on every routine office visit. The ADA has developed a complete set of guidelines for treatment of hypertension.*

*American Diabetes Association: Standards of medical care in diabetes, *Diabetes Care* 29(Suppl 1):476, 2006.

Fostering Health Maintenance

- Throughout the course of treatment, discuss medication, diet, exercise, and the need to achieve and maintain good glucose control to prevent the complications associated with diabetes mellitus. The patient must achieve a high degree of understanding of diabetes mellitus and its management. The patient and family members must be included in the total educational program.
- With the advent of shorter hospitalizations, it may be necessary to incorporate follow-up care by a visiting nurse association or a home health agency in the discharge planning.
- Seek cooperation and understanding of the following points so that medication compliance is increased: name of medication, dosage, route and time of administration, side effects to expect, and side effects to report.

At Discharge. Develop a list of specific equipment and supplies the patient will need when discharged. Keep in mind the cost of these supplies. Consider the following:

1. Syringes: Disposable syringes are convenient and presterilized but are more expensive. Be sure to tell the patient that disposable syringes are designed to be used once and then discarded. However, recent literature refers to the repeated use of the same syringe by an individual patient as long as the needle remains sharp and is kept clean and covered. CHECK with the individual physician BEFORE instituting this practice. Diabetic people are susceptible to infection, and healing may be a problem. The newer, smaller 30- and 31-gauge needles can become bent with even one use, forming a hook at the end of the needle. If the needle is reused, the hook may result in a laceration to the tissue and lead to adverse effects. Syringes being reused should be stored at room temperature. The potential benefits of storing a syringe and needle for reuse in the refrigerator or of wiping the needle with alcohol are unknown. Cleansing the needle with alcohol may disrupt the silicone coating on the needle, resulting in increased pain at the injection site. Syringes are available in 0.3-, 0.5-, 1-, and 2-mL capacities. In some instances, a pen device may also be prescribed for use by appropriate individuals. Several medical devices have been developed to reduce the incidence of needlesticks and other sharp injuries. When performing patient education in self-administration of insulin, it is important to use the type of syringe and needle device that will be used at home to ensure that the patient knows how to manipulate the device correctly. Insulin can also be administered using a jet injector for people with a phobia of needles or unable to use a syringe. They are not, however, a routine option for use in all patients with diabetes.

2. Insulin pumps: An insulin pump uses regular insulin or the rapid-acting insulin analogs such as lispro, aspart, or glulisine. The use of mixtures of insulins in insulin pumps is not recommended because this approach has not been evaluated.
3. Needles: Disposable needles are more convenient but also more expensive. Patients usually use a 27-, 28-, 29-, 30-, or 31-gauge ½- or ⅝-inch needle, but needles should be adjusted to the individual. An obese patient may require a 1- to 1½-inch-long needle to properly inject the insulin. Several lengths of needles are available, and blood glucose should be monitored when changing from one needle length to another. Always dispose of insulin syringes, needles, and lancets in sharps containers. (See Chapter 10 for further discussion of syringes, needles, and safety during use.)
4. Specialized equipment: Magni-Guides are available for the visually impaired patient. This aid holds the vial of insulin, acts as a guide in withdrawing insulin, and has a magnifying glass to make reading the syringe scale easier. Special automatic insulin syringes (insulin "pens") are available for blind or neurologically impaired patients. A talking glucose measuring device is also available for the visually impaired individual to perform self-monitoring of the capillary blood glucose levels. Persons with diabetes desiring more information on insulin delivery aids can contact the ADA.
5. Self-monitoring equipment for blood glucose: Be certain the individual has or understands where to purchase the supplies used with the specific brand of self-monitoring glucose machine to be used at home. Because numerous models of self-monitoring equipment are available, it is important that the individual be trained on the specific equipment that will be used at home.

Written Record. Enlist the patient's aid in developing and maintaining a written record of monitoring parameters (e.g., blood glucose or urine ketones, insulin dosage, pertinent stress factors, exercise level, illnesses, or major changes in diet or other routine) (see the Patient Self-Monitoring form on p. 584). Complete the Premedication Data column for use as a baseline to track response to drug therapy. Ensure that the patient understands how to use the form and instruct the patient to bring the completed form to follow-up visits. During follow-up visits, focus on issues that will foster adherence with the therapeutic interventions prescribed.

Education. The ADA has developed areas of diabetic education. All aspects of the care outlined in these recommendations are not presented in the sample teaching plan for diabetic people located in Chapter 5, p. 65. The recommendations must be adapted to the individual's needs and it may not be possible to teach the entire program during the hospitalization period.

For children who have diabetes it is essential that the school setting, whether a daycare, preschool, or regular school environment, be familiar with the child's health needs. Figure 36-3 is a Diabetic Health Care Plan for use in school and daycare.

DRUG CLASS: Insulins

Actions

Insulin is a hormone produced in the beta cells of the pancreas and is a key regulator of metabolism. Insulin is required for the entry of glucose into skeletal and heart muscle and fat. It also plays a significant role in protein and lipid metabolism. It is not required for glucose transport into the brain, kidney, gastrointestinal, or liver tissue.

The pancreas secretes insulin at a steady rate of 0.5 to 1 unit per hour. It is released in greater quantities when the blood glucose rises above 100 mg/dL, such as after a meal. The average rate of insulin secretion in an adult is 30 to 50 units per day.

Insulin deficiency reduces the rate of transport of glucose into cells, producing hyperglycemia. Other metabolic reactions are also inhibited by the lack of insulin, resulting in the conversion of protein to glucose (gluconeogenesis), hyperlipidemia, ketosis, and acidosis.

Insulins from the pancreases of different animals have similar activity and were used in human beings for many years. Biosynthetic human insulin is now used by most patients, especially people newly diagnosed with diabetes. It has fewer allergic reactions associated with it than beef and pork insulins.

Uses

The following three factors—onset, peak, and duration—are important in the use of insulin therapy. *Onset* is the time required for the medication to have an initial effect or action; *peak* is when the agent will have the maximum effect; and *duration* is the length of time that the agent remains active in the body. When monitoring insulin therapy, it is important to understand these terms and to associate them with the type of insulin being administered to ascertain when a patient is most susceptible to hyperglycemia or hypoglycemia (Table 36-5).

Four types of insulin, based on onset, peak, and duration, are in use today: rapid-acting, short-acting, intermediate-acting, and long-acting insulins (see Table 36-5).

The most rapid-acting insulins are the insulin analogs, new synthetic forms called lispro, aspart, and glulisine. They are clear solutions that may be injected separately or mixed in the same syringe with an intermediate-acting insulin. Aspart and lispro are equally potent to human regular insulin, but have a more rapid onset and shorter duration of activity. Glulisine has a similar onset of action to lispro and

Text continued on p. 587

PATIENT SELF-ASSESSMENT FORM Antidiabetic Agents

MEDICATIONS	COLOR	TO BE TAKEN

Patient ______________________

Health Care Provider ______________________

Health Care Provider's phone ______________________

Next appt.* ______________________

What I Should Monitor		Premedication Data	Date	Date	Date	Date	Date	Date	Comments
Insulin/oral agent Types AM PM	Temperature / Weight								
	Site AM PM								
	Units AM PM								
Blood glucose levels	Before breakfast After breakfast								
Insert time (e.g., 1 PM)	Before lunch After lunch								
	Before supper After supper								
	Bedtime								
	Other								
Urine (use 2nd voided specimen)	Before breakfast								
	Before lunch								
Sugar / Ketones	Before supper								
	Bedtime								
Diet	Eat all foods allowed								
	Unable to eat								
	Overate or indulged								
Lifestyle	Usual daily activities/exercise								
	Increased amount of exercise								
	Increased stress								
	Normal day-to-day stress								
Injuries or skin integrity	No visible changes in skin of feet								
	Cuts, bruises, open sores								
Hypoglycemia	Symptoms: Sweating, weak, shaky, hungry								
	Blood glucose level (time)								
Hyperglycemia	Symptoms: Urinating frequency, poor appetite, ↑ thirst, weak, dizzy								
	Blood glucose level (time)								
Other									

*Please bring this record with you to your next appointment.
Use the back of this sheet for additional information.

Diabetes Care Plan for ______(name of student)______ School ______ Effective Dates: ______

To be completed by parents/health care team and reviewed with necessary school staff. Copies should be kept in student's classrooms and school records.

Date of Birth: ______ **Grade:** ______ **Homeroom Teacher:** ______

Contact information:

Parent/guardian #1: ______ Address: ______

Telephone - Home: ______ Work: ______ Cell Phone: ______

Parent/guardian #2: ______ Address: ______

Telephone - Home: ______ Work: ______ Cell Phone: ______

Student's Doctor/Health Care Provider: ______ Telephone: ______

Nurse Educator: ______ Telephone: ______

Other emergency contact: ______ Relationship: ______

Telephone - Home: ______ Work: ______ Cell Phone: ______

Notify parent/guardian in the following situations: ______

Blood Glucose Monitoring

Target range for blood glucose: ______ mg/dL to ______ mg/dL Type of blood glucose meter student uses: ______

Usual times to test blood glucose: ______

Times to do extra tests (check all that apply):

______ Before exercise

______ After exercise

______ Other (explain): ______

______ When student exhibits symptoms of hyperglycemia

______ When student exhibits symptoms of hypoglycemia

Can student perform own blood glucose tests? Yes No Exceptions: ______

School personnel trained to monitor blood glucose level and dates of training: ______

Insulin

Times, types, and dosages of insulin injections to be given during school:

Time	Type(s)	Dosage
______	______	______
______	______	______
______	______	______

School personnel trained to assist with insulin injection and dates of training: ______

Can student give own injections?	Yes	No
Can student determine correct amount of insulin?	Yes	No
Can student draw correct dose of insulin?	Yes	No

For Students with Insulin Pumps:

Type of pump: ______

Insulin/carbohydrate ratio: ______

Correction factor: ______

Is student competent regarding pump?	Yes	No
Can student effectively troubleshoot problems (e.g., ketosis, pump malfunction)?	Yes	No

Comments: ______

Meals and Snacks Eaten at School (The carbohydrate content of the food is important in maintaining a stable blood glucose level.)

	Time	Food content/amount
Breakfast	______	______
AM snack	______	______
Lunch	______	______
PM snack	______	______
Dinner	______	______
Snack before exercise? Yes No		______
Snack after exercise? Yes No		______

Other times to give snacks (content/amount): ______

A source of glucose such as ______ should be readily available at all times.

Perferred snack foods: ______

Foods to avoid, if any: ______

Instructions for when food is provided to the class, e.g., as part of a class party or food sampling: ______

Hypoglycemia (Low Blood Sugar)

Usual symptoms of hypoglycemia: ______

Treatment of hypoglycemia: ______

School personnel trained to administer glucagon and dates of training: ______

Glucagon should be given if the student is unconscious, having a seizure (convulsion), or unable to swallow. If required, glucagon should be administered promptly and then 911 (or other emergency assistance) and parents should be called.

Hyperglycemia (High Blood Sugar)

Usual symptoms of hyperglycemia: ______

Treatment of hyperglycemia: ______

Circumstances when urine or blood ketones should be tested: ______

Treatment for ketones: ______

Exercise and Sports

A snack such as ______ should be readily available at the site of exercise or sports.

Restrictions on activity, if any: ______

Student should not exercise if blood glucose is below ______ mg/dL.

Supplies and Personnel

Location of supplies: Blood glucose monitoring equipment: ______ Insulin administration supplies: ______

Glucagon emergency kit: ______ Ketone testing supplies: ______

Snack foods: ______

Personnel trained in the symptoms and treatment of low and high blood sugar and dates of training: ______

Signatures

Reviewed by: [student's health provider/date] Acknowledged/received by: [guardian/date] Acknowledged/received by: [school representative/date]

FIGURE **36-3** Diabetes health care plan.

Drug Table 36-5 COMMERCIALLY AVAILABLE FORMS OF INSULIN

TYPE OF INSULIN	MANUFACTURER	STRENGTH (UNITS/mL)	SOURCE	ONSET (hr)	PEAK (hr)	DURATION* (hr)	HYPERGLYCEMIA†	HYPOGLYCEMIA†
RAPID-ACTING INSULIN								
Insulin Analog Injection								
Novolog (aspart)	Novo Nordisk	100	Semisynthetic	0.2-0.33	1-3	3-5	After lunch (3)	Within 1-3 hr
Humalog (lispro)	Lilly	100	Semisynthetic	0.2-0.33	0.5-2.5	3-6.5	After lunch (3)	Within 1-3 hr
Apidra (glulisine)	Aventis	100	Semisynthetic	0.2-0.33	0.5-1.5	1-2.5	After lunch (3)	Within 1-3 hr
SHORT-ACTING INSULIN								
Insulin Injection								
Humulin R (human)	Lilly	100, 500	Semisynthetic	0.5-4	2.5-5	5-10	Early AM (1)	Before lunch (3)
Novolin R (human)	Novo Nordisk	100	Semisynthetic	0.5	2.5-5	8	Early AM	Before lunch
INTERMEDIATE-ACTING INSULIN								
Isophane Insulin Suspension (NPH)								
Humulin N (human)	Lilly	100	Semisynthetic	1-4	4-12	16-28	Before lunch (2)	3 PM to supper (3)
Novolin N (human)	Novo Nordisk	100	Semisynthetic	1.5	4-12	24	Before lunch	3 PM to supper
Isophane Insulin Suspension and Insulin Injection								
Humulin 50/50 (human)	Lilly	100	Semisynthetic	0.5	4-8	24	Before lunch	3 PM to supper
Humulin 70/30 (human)	Lilly	100	Semisynthetic	0.5	4-12	24	Before lunch	3 PM to supper
Novolin 70/30 (human)	Novo Nordisk	100	Semisynthetic	0.5	2-12	24	Before lunch	3 PM to supper
Lispro Protamine Suspension and Lispro Injection								
Humalog Mix 75/25	Lilly	100	Semisynthetic	0.25-0.5	0.5-1.5	12-24		3 PM to supper
Novolog Mix 70/30	Novo Nordisk	100	Semisynthetic	0.2-0.33	2.4	24		3 PM to supper
Insulin Zinc Suspension								
Lente Iletin II	Lilly	100	Pork	1-1.5	8-12	24	Before lunch	3 PM to supper
Novolin L (human)	Novo Nordisk	100	Semisynthetic	1-4	7-15	20-28	Before lunch	3 PM to supper
LONG-ACTING INSULIN								
Lantus (glargine)	Aventis	100	Semisynthetic	1.1	—‡	241	Mid-am to Mid-pm (1)	—‡
Levemir (detemir)	Novo Nordisk	100	Semisynthetic	1	—‡	Up to 24	Mid-am to Mid-pm (1)	—‡

*The times listed are averages based on a newly diagnosed diabetic patient. Factors modifying these times include patient variation, site and route of administration, and dosage.
†Most often occurs when insulin is administered (1) at bedtime the previous night; (2) before breakfast the previous day; (3) before breakfast the same day.
‡No pronounced peak activity.

aspart, but has a shorter duration of action. Their rapid onset of action is related to a more rapid absorption rate from subcutaneous tissue than regular insulin. Aspart appears to have a slightly more rapid onset than lispro. Aspart, lispro, and glulisine are usually administered within 10 to 15 minutes of a meal. The rationale for the development and use of these newer insulins is that when a meal is ingested, the blood glucose rises for about 2 to 3 hours. After injection, regular insulin takes 30 minutes to start acting, peaks at 2½ to 5 hours, and may have a duration of 5 to 10 hours. Lispro and aspart start to act within 10 minutes of injection, peak within 1 to 2 hours, and are gone by 3 to 5 hours. Glulisine has a similar onset of action, but peaks in 30 to 90 minutes with a duration of action up to 2½ hours. Consequently, the newer, shorter-acting insulins are used to control hyperglycemia associated with meals without having longer-lasting effects with the potential for hypoglycemia. These insulins may also be used alone without any other insulin in patients with type 2 diabetes who only have hyperglycemia associated with ingestion of meals (postprandial hyperglycemia).

Regular insulin has long been used for its rapid onset of activity and relatively short duration of action. Regular insulin is the only dosage form of insulin that is approved to be injected by both intravenous and subcutaneous routes of administration. Human regular insulin is usually administered 30 to 60 minutes before meals.

Neutral protamine Hagedorn (NPH) insulin is an intermediate-acting insulin containing specific amounts of regular insulin and protamine. The protamine binds to the insulin. When administered subcutaneously, the insulin is slowly released from the protamine and becomes active, giving it the intermediate-acting classification.

Lispro and aspart insulin may also be mixed with protamine to prolong its duration of action. Two products are available: 75% lispro protamine suspension and 25% lispro solution (Humalog Mix 75/25) and 70% aspart protamine suspension and 30% aspart solution (Novolog Mix 70/30). The combined effect is a rapid-acting onset with an intermediate duration of action of 12 to 24 hours.

Insulin glargine and insulin detemir are biosynthetic long-acting insulins. They are absorbed from the subcutaneous tissue in a uniform manner without large fluctuations in insulin levels, reducing the possibility of hypoglycemic reactions. Either product is most commonly injected in the evening to serve as a 24-hour basal source of insulin for the body. Rapid-acting insulin is then injected just before meals to control hyperglycemia secondary to the meal, or intermediate-acting NPH can be injected in the morning and late afternoon to treat hyperglycemia from meals. Neither insulin glargine nor detemir should be mixed with other insulins.

Insulin is also available in a dosage form for inhalation (see p. 589).

Storage of Insulin

It is recommended that insulin neither be allowed to freeze nor be heated above a temperature of 98° F. A general rule of thumb is that the bottle of insulin should be stored in the refrigerator (not the freezer) until opened. Because patients find it uncomfortable to inject cold insulin, the bottle (and insulin cartridges for insulin pens) may then be kept at room temperature (68° to 75° F) until gone. For all insulins other than regular, lispro, aspart, or glulisine insulin, the vial should be gently rolled in the palms of the hands (not shaken) to warm and resuspend the insulin. It is recommended that once an insulin vial is opened, it should be discarded in 30 days. Even though the insulin has not "gone bad," there is concern that the contents are no longer sterile and the vial may become a reservoir for infection, especially with patients who reuse needles.

At sustained temperatures above room temperature, insulins lose potency rapidly. Do not leave in a hot car throughout the day.

Excess agitation should be avoided to prevent loss of potency, clumping, or precipitation. When insulins are prefilled in syringes, the syringes should be stored in a refrigerator for up to 30 days in a vertical position with the needle up. The syringe should be rolled between the hands to warm and remix the insulin before administration.

Therapeutic Outcomes

The primary therapeutic outcomes expected from insulin therapy are as follows:

- A decrease in both fasting blood glucose levels and A1C concentrations in the range defined as acceptable for the individual patient.
- Fewer long-term complications associated with poorly controlled diabetes mellitus.

Nursing Process for Insulin

Premedication Assessment

1. Confirm that a blood glucose level was recently measured and was acceptable for the individual patient.
2. Confirm that the patient has had a level of activity reasonable for the individual patient, and the anticipated level of activity planned for the next several hours is balanced with the insulin dose.
3. Confirm that the prescribed diet is being consumed as planned and that no changes in diet are anticipated in relation to insulin dosage over the next several hours.

Planning

Availability. See Table 36-5.

Implementation

Administration Techniques. See Figure 10-26 and Chapter 11 for administration.

Dosage and Administration. Maintenance therapy for newly diagnosed diabetic patients should include the following recommendations.

It is important to understand that effective control of diabetes mellitus requires a balanced food intake, exercise, blood glucose levels measured several times daily, and insulin dosage adjustments based on the blood glucose levels.

Several methods have been developed to initiate insulin therapy. The method chosen depends on such issues as fluctuation of the patient's blood glucose; ability of the patient to measure, mix, and administer the insulin; and adherence with planned exercise and diet.

Before starting a standardized regimen, the diet and physical exercise level must be stabilized. A standard approach is to calculate the initial total daily dose of insulin based on 0.5 to 0.8 unit/kg of whole body (not lean body) weight. Neutral protamine Hagedorn (NPH, human) insulin is often used to initiate therapy. This total daily dose is then split into two doses so that two thirds are administered in the morning before breakfast and one third is administered 30 minutes before the evening meal. The insulin dosage is then adjusted over the next several weeks based on blood glucose measurements taken (usually) four times daily and A1C levels. Diet and exercise may also require adjustment.

Mixing Insulins. Many patients with diabetes mix rapid-acting insulin with either intermediate-acting or long-acting insulins to manage the hyperglycemia that follows a meal or snack. See Table 36-6, and Chapter 10, p. 160 for technique in mixing insulins. When regular insulin, insulin Lispro, or insulin Aspart is combined with another insulin in the same syringe, it should be drawn into the syringe first to avoid contaminating the vial with the other insulin.

Evaluation

Side Effects to Expect and Report

Hyperglycemia. Diabetic or prediabetic patients must be monitored for the development of hyperglycemia, particularly during the early weeks of therapy.

Table 36-6 *Compatibility of Insulin Combinations*

COMBINATION	RATIO	MIX BEFORE ADMINISTRATION
Regular + NPH	Any combination	2 to 3 months
Regular + lente	Any combination	Immediately*
aspart + NPH	Any combination	Immediately
lispro + NPH	Any combination	Immediately
glulisine + NPH	Any combination	Immediately
lentes	Any combination	Stable indefinitely
glargine	Do not mix with other insulin	
detemir	Do not mix with other insulin	

*Must be used immediately to retain properties of regular insulin.

Assess regularly for abnormal blood glucose and in certain patients, as requested by the health care provider, for glycosuria and ketones. If symptoms occur frequently, the health care provider should be notified, and the patient's written records that reflect the results of self-testing should be supplied to the health care provider for analysis. Patients receiving insulin may require an adjustment in dosage.

Hypoglycemia. Insulin overdose or decreased carbohydrate intake may result in hypoglycemia. If untreated, irreversible brain damage may occur. Hypoglycemia occurs most frequently when the administered insulin reaches its peak action (see Table 36-5). Hypoglycemia must be treated immediately. The following conditions may predispose a diabetic patient to a hypoglycemic (insulin) reaction: improper measurement of insulin dosage, excessive exercise, insufficient food intake, concurrent ingestion of hypoglycemic drugs and discontinuation of drugs (see Drug Interactions), or conditions (such as infection or stress) causing hyperglycemia.

Monitor for the following signs of hypoglycemia: headache, nausea, weakness, hunger, lethargy, decreased coordination, general apprehension, sweating, or blurred or double vision.

Allergic Reactions. Allergic reactions, manifested by itching, redness, and swelling at the site of injection, have been common in patients receiving insulin therapy. These reactions may be caused by modifying proteins in NPH insulin, the insulin itself, the alcohol used to cleanse the injection site or sterilize the syringe, the patient's injection technique, or the intermittent use of insulin.

Spontaneous desensitization frequently occurs within a few weeks. Local irritation may be reduced by changing to insulin without protein modifiers (e.g., go to the Lente series) or to insulins derived from biosynthetic sources (e.g., "human" insulin); by using unscented alcohol swabs and disposable syringes and needles; and by checking the patient's injection technique. Acute rashes covering the whole body and anaphylactic symptoms are rare, but must be treated with antihistamines, epinephrine, and steroids.

Lipodystrophies. Rotation of injection sites is important to avoid atrophy or hypertrophy of subcutaneous fat tissue. This dermatologic condition may occur at the site of frequent insulin injections. The hypertrophic areas tend to be used more frequently by diabetic patients because the fat pad becomes anesthetized. In addition to the adverse cosmetic effects, the absorption rate of insulin from these sites becomes significantly prolonged and erratic. Loss of diabetic control may result, particularly in unstable type 1 diabetes patients.

Drug Interactions

Hyperglycemia. The following drugs may cause hyperglycemia, especially in prediabetic and diabetic patients (insulin dosages may require adjustment): albuterol, asparaginase, calcitonin, clozapine, olanzapine, corticosteroids, cyclophosphamide, diazoxide, diltiazem, diuretics (e.g., thiazides, furosemide, bumetanide), dobutamine, epinephrine, glucagon, isoniazid, lithium, morphine, niacin, nicotine, oral contraceptives, pentamidine, phenothiazines, phenytoin, protease inhibitors, terbutaline, somatropin, thyroid hormones.

Diabetic or prediabetic patients must be monitored for the development of hyperglycemia, particularly during the early weeks of therapy.

Assess regularly for elevated blood glucose or glycosuria and report if it occurs with any frequency.

Hypoglycemia. The following drugs may cause hypoglycemia, thereby decreasing insulin requirements, in diabetic patients: anabolic steroids (Durabolin), angiotensin-converting enzyme (ACE) inhibitors, alcohol, nonselective beta adrenergic–blocking agents, calcium, clonidine, disopyramide, fluoxetine, ethanol, fenfluramine, fibrates, guanethidine, lithium, insulin, monoamine oxidase inhibitors (MAOIs), pentamidine, pentoxifylline, pyridoxine, salicylates, sulfonamides, and sulfonylureas.

Monitor for the following signs of hypoglycemia: headache, nausea, weakness, hunger, lethargy, decreased coordination, general apprehension, sweating, or blurred or double vision.

Notify the health care provider if any of the aforementioned symptoms appear.

Beta-Adrenergic Blocking Agents. Beta-adrenergic blocking agents (e.g., propranolol, timolol, nadolol, pindolol) may mask many of the symptoms of hypoglycemia. Notify the health care provider if you suspect that any of these symptoms appear intermittently.

Insulin Inhalation Powder

EXUBERA (ex uh bear' ah)

Actions

Insulin inhalation powder is human insulin produced synthetically by recombinant DNA technology. Insulin regulates glucose metabolism. It lowers blood glucose concentrations by (1) stimulating glucose uptake by skeletal muscle and fat cells and (2) inhibiting glucose production by the liver. Insulin also inhibits fat breakdown (lipolysis) in fat cells, inhibits protein breakdown (proteolysis), and enhances protein synthesis.

Uses

Insulin inhalation powder is used to control hyperglycemia in adult patients with type 1 and type 2 diabetes mellitus. It has an onset of action similar to subcutaneously administered short-acting insulins (e.g., aspart, lispro) and has a duration of glucose-lowering activity similar to subcutaneously administered regular human insulin. The onset of action of glucose-lowering activity occurs within 10 to 20 minutes, the maximum effect occurs approximately 2 hours after inhalation, and the duration of glucose-lowering activity is approximately 6 hours.

In patients with type 1 diabetes, inhaled insulin should be used with longer acting (e.g., intermediate-acting or long-acting) insulins. In patients with type 2 diabetes, inhaled insulin powder may be used alone or in combination with oral antidiabetic agents or longer-acting insulins. As with injectable insulin use, response to inhaled insulin depends on other factors such as the patient's current glycemic control, previous response to injected insulin, duration of diabetes, and dietary and exercise habits.

Because of the effect inhaled insulin may have on pulmonary function, all patients should have pulmonary function assessed with spirometry before initiating therapy, again after 6 months of therapy, and annually thereafter, even in the absence of pulmonary symptoms. Inhaled insulin therapy is not recommended for patients with underlying lung disease (e.g., asthma or chronic obstructive pulmonary disease). During an intercurrent respiratory illness (e.g., bronchitis, upper respiratory infection, rhinitis), inhaled insulin therapy may be continued, but close monitoring of blood glucose concentrations and dosage adjustment may be required.

Inhaled insulin is absolutely contraindicated for patients who smoke or who have quit smoking within the last 6 months. Smokers have a two-fold to five-fold higher absorption of insulin doses, a more rapid onset of glucose-lowering action, greater maximum effect, and a greater total glucose-lowering effect compared with nonsmokers, and are at much greater risk for hypoglycemia. Persons who start or resume smoking while on inhaled insulin therapy should discontinue the use of inhaled insulin therapy and use injectable insulin or oral antidiabetic medicine, if appropriate.

Therapeutic Outcomes

The primary therapeutic outcomes expected from insulin therapy are as follows:

- A decrease in both fasting blood glucose levels and A1C concentrations in the range defined as acceptable for the individual patient.
- Fewer long-term complications associated with poorly controlled diabetes mellitus.

Nursing Process for Insulin

Premedication Assessment

1. Confirm that a blood glucose level was recently measured and was acceptable for the individual patient.
2. Confirm that pulmonary spirometry has been completed before initiating therapy, repeat at 6 months, and then perform annually thereafter.

3. Confirm that the patient has had a level of activity reasonable for the individual patient, and the anticipated level of activity planned for the next several hours is balanced with the insulin dose.
4. Confirm that the prescribed diet is going to be consumed within 10 to 20 minutes of insulin inhalation and that no changes in diet are anticipated in relation to insulin dosage over the next several hours.

Planning

Availability. 1 and 3 mg unit dose blisters.

Implementation

Dosage and Administration. Inhaled insulin must be administered through the manufacturer-supplied Exubera Inhaler and the Exubera Release Unit. The patient must become familiar with the care and use of the inhaler and release unit before attempting to administer insulin.

The initial dosage of inhaled insulin should be individualized for each patient. Initial premeal doses may be calculated using the following formula:

$$\text{Actual body weight (kg)} \times 0.05\ \text{mg/kg} = \text{Premeal dose (mg)}$$

Rounded down the dosage to the nearest whole milligram number (e.g., 4.6 mg is rounded down to 4 mg).

One mg of inhaled insulin is approximately equivalent to 3 units of subcutaneously administered regular insulin and 3 mg is approximately equivalent to 8 units of subcutaneously administered regular insulin. Patients should combine 1 mg and 3 mg blisters so that the least number of blisters per dose are taken (e.g., a 4 mg dose should be administered as one 1-mg blister and one 3-mg blister). For a person who has been inhaling 3-mg blisters, if the 3-mg strength becomes unavailable, two 1-mg blisters may be substituted for one 3-mg blister.

As with all insulins, the blood glucose level should be monitored closely. The time course of inhaled insulin may vary in different individuals or at different times in the same individual.

Evaluation

Side Effects to Expect and Report

Hyperglycemia. Patients must be monitored for the development of hyperglycemia, particularly during the early weeks of therapy. Assess regularly for abnormal blood glucose levels, and in certain patients, as requested by the health care provider, for glycosuria and ketones. If symptoms occur frequently, the health care provider should be notified, and the patient's written records that reflect the results of self-testing should be supplied to the health care provider for analysis. Patients receiving insulin may require an adjustment in dosage.

Hypoglycemia. Insulin overdose or decreased carbohydrate intake may result in hypoglycemia. If untreated, irreversible brain damage may occur. Hypoglycemia occurs most frequently when the administered insulin reaches its peak action (approximately 2 hours after administration for inhaled insulin). Hypoglycemia must be treated immediately. The following conditions may predispose a diabetic patient to a hypoglycemic (insulin) reaction: improper measurement of insulin dose, excessive exercise, insufficient food intake, concurrent ingestion of hypoglycemic drugs, and discontinuation of drugs (see Drug Interactions); conditions such as infection or stress cause hyperglycemia.

Monitor for the following signs of hypoglycemia: headache, nausea, weakness, hunger, lethargy, decreased coordination, general apprehension, sweating, and blurred or double vision.

Drug Interactions

Hyperglycemia. The following drugs may cause hyperglycemia, especially in prediabetic and diabetic patients (insulin dosages may require adjustment): albuterol, asparaginase, calcitonin, clozapine, corticosteroids, cyclophosphamide, diazoxide, diltiazem, diuretics (e.g., thiazides, furosemide, bumetanide), dobutamine, epinephrine, glucagon, isoniazid, lithium, morphine, niacin, nicotine, olanzapine, oral contraceptives, pentamidine, phenothiazines, phenytoin, protease inhibitors, terbutaline, somatropin, thyroid hormones.

Diabetic or prediabetic patients must be monitored for the development of hyperglycemia, particularly during the early weeks of therapy.

Assess regularly for elevated blood glucose or glycosuria and report if it occurs with any frequency.

Hypoglycemia. The following drugs may cause hypoglycemia, thereby decreasing insulin requirements, in diabetic patients: anabolic steroids (Durabolin), ACE inhibitors, alcohol, nonselective beta adrenergic blocking agents, calcium, clonidine, disopyramide, fluoxetine, ethanol, fenfluramine, fibrates, guanethidine, lithium, insulin, MAO inhibitors, pentamidine, pentoxifylline, pyridoxine, salicylates, sulfonamides, and sulfonylureas.

Monitor for the following signs of hypoglycemia: headache, nausea, weakness, hunger, lethargy, decreased coordination, general apprehension, sweating, and blurred or double vision.

Notify the health care provider if any of the aforementioned symptoms appear.

Beta-Adrenergic Blocking Agents. Beta-adrenergic blocking agents (e.g., propranolol, timolol, nadolol, pindolol) may mask many of the symptoms of hypoglycemia. Notify the health care provider if you suspect that any of these symptoms appear intermittently.

DRUG CLASS: Biguanide Oral Antidiabetic Agents

metformin (met for' mihn)

▶ GLUCOPHAGE (glue' ko fahg)

Actions

Metformin represents a class of oral antidiabetic agents known as the biguanides. Metformin decreases hepatic glucose production by inhibiting glycogenolysis and gluconeogenesis, reduces absorption of glucose from the small intestine, and increases insulin sensitivity improving glucose uptake in peripheral muscle and adipose cells. It may also stimulate glucose metabolism by anaerobic glycolysis. The net result is a significant decrease in fasting and postprandial blood glucose and hemoglobin A1C concentrations. Insulin must be present for metformin to be active, and therefore is not effective in type 1 diabetes.

Uses

Metformin is used as an adjunct to diet to lower blood glucose in patients with type 2 diabetes mellitus whose hyperglycemia cannot be controlled by diet and exercise alone. It has the particular advantage that it will not cause hypoglycemia, as can occur with insulin and the sulfonylureas. It may also be used in combination with the sulfonylureas to lower blood glucose because the two agents act by different mechanisms.

Metformin has two other beneficial effects: it does not cause weight gain, and indeed may cause weight loss, contrary to the actions of the sulfonylureas, meglitinides, and insulin; and it also has a favorable effect on triglycerides. It produces a modest decrease in concentrations of serum triglycerides and total and low-density lipoprotein (LDL) cholesterol, with modest increases in concentrations of high-density lipoprotein (HDL) cholesterol. See the cautionary note in the Dosage and Administration section below regarding renal function, heart failure and liver impairment.

Therapeutic Outcomes

The primary therapeutic outcomes expected from biguanide oral antidiabetic agent therapy are as follows:

- A decrease in both fasting blood glucose levels and the A1C concentrations in the range defined as "acceptable" for the individual patient.
- Fewer long-term complications associated with poorly controlled type 2 diabetes mellitus.

Nursing Process for Metformin

Premedication Assessment

1. Confirm that a blood glucose and A1C levels were recently measured and were acceptable for the individual patient.
2. Confirm that the prescribed diet is being consumed as planned and that no changes in diet are anticipated in relation to oral hypoglycemic agent dosage over the next several hours.

Planning

Availability. 500, 850, 1000 mg; 500 mg extended release tablets.

Implementation

Dosage and Administration. *Adult:* PO: Initially, 500 mg twice daily with the morning and evening meals. Dosage is increased by adding 500 mg to the daily dose each week up to 2500 mg daily. In general, most patients require at least 1500 mg daily for therapeutic effect. At dosages of 2000 mg and more, metformin should be administered three times daily (e.g., 1000 mg with breakfast, 500 mg with lunch, and 1000 mg with dinner; or 850 mg each with breakfast, lunch, and dinner). If a patient's blood glucose is not controlled with the maximum dosage, a sulfonylurea or a TZD oral hypoglycemic agent may be added to the regimen.

NOTE: Lactic acidosis is a rare but potentially life-threatening complication that can occur during treatment with metformin. It is recommended that metformin therapy NOT be initiated in patients who:

- Have a creatinine clearance of less than 70 to 80 mL per minute or in men with a serum creatinine of 1.5 mg/dL or in women with a serum creatinine of 1.4 mg/dL.
- Have tissue hypoperfusion, such as in heart failure, shock, or septicemia, and are at risk for developing metabolic acidosis.
- Have clinical or laboratory evidence (hyperbilirubinemia, elevated aspartate aminotransferase [AST], alanine aminotransferase [ALT]) of liver disease.
- Are scheduled to receive radiopaque dyes. Radiopaque dyes often induce temporary renal insufficiency, so metformin should be discontinued 24 to 48 hours before procedures in which radiopaque dye will be administered (e.g., kidney studies). Metformin should not be reinitiated for 2 to 3 days and until normal renal function has been proven.

Evaluation

Side Effects to Expect

Nausea, Vomiting, Anorexia, Abdominal Cramps, Flatulence. These side effects are usually mild and tend to resolve with continued therapy. Taking the medicine with meals will help reduce these adverse effects. Encourage the patient not to discontinue therapy without first consulting the physician.

Side Effects to Report

Malaise, Myalgias, Respiratory Distress, Hypotension. A rare adverse effect of metformin is lactic acidosis. A gradual onset of these symptoms may be an early indication of lactic acidosis developing. Patients with reduced renal function, poor circulation, and/or excessive alcohol intake are most susceptible to developing lactic acidosis.

Drug Interactions

Drugs That May Enhance Toxic Effects. Amiloride, cimetidine, digoxin, furosemide, morphine, procainamide, quinidine, quinine, ranitidine, triamterene, trimethoprim, and vancomycin are excreted by the same route through the kidneys that metformin depends on for excretion. There is a possibility that these drugs block the excretion of metformin, potentially causing lactic acidosis. Monitor for signs of lactic acidosis as discussed previously.

Ethanol. Patients should be cautioned against excessive alcohol intake, either acute or chronic, when taking metformin, because alcohol potentiates the effects of metformin on lactate metabolism.

Hyperglycemia. The following drugs when used concurrently with metformin may decrease the therapeutic effects of metformin: corticosteroids, phenothiazines, diuretics, oral contraceptives, thyroid replacement hormones, phenytoin, diazoxide, and lithium carbonate.

Diabetic and prediabetic patients must be monitored for the development of hyperglycemia, particularly during the early weeks of therapy.

Assess regularly for elevated blood glucose or glycosuria and report if it occurs with any frequency.

Nifedipine. Nifedipine appears to increase the absorption of metformin. Reducing the dosage of metformin may minimize adverse effects.

DRUG CLASS: Sulfonylurea Oral Hypoglycemic Agents

Actions

The sulfonylureas lower blood glucose by stimulating the release of insulin from the beta cells of the pancreas. The sulfonylureas also diminish glucose production and metabolism of insulin by the liver.

Uses

The sulfonylureas are effective in type 2 diabetic patients in whom the pancreas still has the capacity to secrete insulin, but are of no value in the patient with type 1 diabetes, who has no beta cell function. Sulfonylureas may be effective in the treatment of type 2 diabetes mellitus that cannot be controlled by diet and exercise if the patient is not susceptible to developing ketosis, acidosis, or infections. Patients most likely to benefit from oral hypoglycemic treatment are those who develop signs of diabetes after age 40 and who require less than 40 units of insulin per day (indicating that some insulin is still being secreted by the beta cells). Sulfonylureas may induce hypoglycemia due to overproduction of insulin.

Therapeutic Outcomes

The primary therapeutic outcomes expected from sulfonylurea oral hypoglycemic therapy are as follows:

- A decrease in both fasting blood glucose levels and the A1C concentrations in the range defined as acceptable for the individual patient.
- Fewer long-term complications associated with poorly controlled diabetes mellitus.

Nursing Process for Sulfonylurea Oral Hypoglycemic Agents

Premedication Assessment

1. Confirm that blood glucose and A1C levels were recently measured and were hyperglycemic for the individual patient.
2. Confirm that the patient has had a level of activity "reasonable" for the individual patient, and the anticipated level of activity planned for the next several hours is balanced with the oral hypoglycemic agent dosage.
3. Confirm that the prescribed diet is being consumed as planned and that no changes in diet are anticipated in relation to the oral hypoglycemic agent dosage over the next several hours.

Planning

Availability. See Table 36-7.

Implementation

NOTE: In general, sulfonylureas should not be administered to patients who are allergic to sulfonamides. These patients may also be allergic to sulfonylureas.

Dosage and Administration. See Table 36-7. Individual dosage adjustment is essential for the successful use of oral hypoglycemic agents. A patient should be given a 1-month trial on maximum dosage of the sulfonylurea being used before the medicine can be considered a primary failure. If a patient represents a secondary failure (a patient initially controlled on oral agents), changing to an alternative sulfonylurea is occasionally successful in controlling blood sugar.

Evaluation

Side Effects to Expect

Nausea, Vomiting, Anorexia, Abdominal Cramps. These side effects are usually mild and tend to resolve with continued therapy. Encourage the patient not to discontinue therapy without first consulting the health care provider.

Side Effects to Report

Hypoglycemia. Patients receiving oral hypoglycemic therapy are as susceptible to hypoglycemia as diabetic patients on insulin therapy. Consequently, blood glucose levels must be monitored closely, especially in the early stages of therapy.

Monitor for the following signs of hypoglycemia: headache, nausea, weakness, hunger, lethargy, decreased coordination, general apprehension, sweating, or blurred, or double vision.

Hypoglycemia must be treated immediately. Mild symptoms may be controlled by the oral administration of a glucose source—for example, a lump of sugar,

 Drug Table 36-7 **ORAL HYPOGLYCEMIC AGENTS**

GENERIC NAME	BRAND NAME	AVAILABILITY	INITIAL DOSAGE	DOSAGE RANGE	DURATION* (hr)
FIRST GENERATION					
acetohexamide		Tablets: 250, 500 mg	0.5 g daily	0.25-1.5 g daily	12-18
chlorpropamide	Diabinese	Tablets: 100, 250 mg	100 mg daily	100-750 mg daily	24-72
tolazamide	Tolinase	Tablets: 100, 250, 500 mg	100 mg daily	0.1-1 g daily	12-16
tolbutamide	Orinase	Tablets: 500 mg	1 g twice daily	0.25-3 g daily	6-12
SECOND GENERATION					
glimepiride	Amaryl	Tablets: 1, 2, 4 mg	1-2 mg daily	1-8 mg daily	24
glipizide	Glucotrol	Tablets: 5, 10 mg	2.5-5 mg daily	15-40 mg daily	10-24
glipizide XL	Glucotrol XL	Extended release 2.5, 5, 10 mg			
glyburide	Glynase	Prestabs: 1.5, 3, 6 mg	1.5-3 mg daily	0.75-12 mg daily	24
	DiaBeta, Micronase	Tablets: 1.25, 2.5, 5 mg	2.5-5 mg daily	1.25-20 mg daily	24

*The times listed are averages based on a newly diagnosed diabetic patient. Factors modifying these times include patient variation and dosage.

orange juice, carbonated cola beverage (not diet), candy (not chocolate)—or ingestion of a commercially prepared substance such as Glutose. Severe symptoms may be relieved by the administration of intravenous glucose, and parenteral glucagon may be prescribed in some instances. If in doubt about whether the patient is hypoglycemic or hyperglycemic, always treat the individual for hypoglycemia to prevent the possible neurologic complications that can occur from untreated hypoglycemia.

Notify the health care provider immediately if any of the above symptoms appear. The dosage of oral hypoglycemic agents may also have to be reduced.

Hepatotoxicity. The symptoms of hepatotoxicity are anorexia, nausea, vomiting, jaundice, hepatomegaly, splenomegaly, and abnormal liver function tests (e.g., elevated bilirubin, AST, ALT, gamma-glutamyltransferase [GGT], alkaline phosphatase, prothrombin time).

Blood Dyscrasias. Routine laboratory studies (e.g., red blood cell [RBC] and white blood cell [WBC] counts, differential counts) should be scheduled. Stress the need to return for this laboratory work.

Monitor for the development of a sore throat, fever, purpura, jaundice, or excessive and progressively increasing weakness.

Dermatologic Reactions. Report a rash or pruritus immediately. Withhold additional doses pending approval by the health care provider.

Drug Interactions

Hypoglycemia. The following drugs may enhance the hypoglycemic effects of the sulfonylureas: ethanol, methandrostenolone, chloramphenicol, warfarin, nonselective beta-adrenergic blocking agents, salicylates, sulfisoxazole, guanethidine, oxytetracycline, and MAOIs.

Monitor for the following signs of hypoglycemia: headache, nausea, weakness, hunger, lethargy, decreased coordination, general apprehension, sweating, or blurred or double vision.

Notify the health care provider if any of these symptoms appear.

Hyperglycemia. The following drugs, when used concurrently with the sulfonylureas, may decrease the therapeutic effects of the sulfonylureas: corticosteroids, phenothiazines, diuretics, oral contraceptives, thyroid replacement hormones, phenytoin, diazoxide, and lithium carbonate.

Diabetic or prediabetic patients must be monitored for the development of hyperglycemia, particularly during the early weeks of therapy.

Assess regularly for elevated blood glucose or glycosuria and report if it occurs with any frequency.

Patients receiving insulin may require an adjustment in dosage.

Beta-Adrenergic Blocking Agents. Beta-adrenergic blocking agents (e.g., propranolol, timolol, nadolol, pindolol) may induce hypoglycemia but may also mask many of the symptoms of hypoglycemia. Notify the health care provider if any of these symptoms appear intermittently.

Alcohol. Ingestion of alcoholic beverages during sulfonylurea therapy may infrequently result in an Antabuse-like reaction, manifested by facial flushing, pounding headache, feeling of breathlessness, and nausea.

In patients who develop an Antabuse-like reaction to alcohol, the use of alcohol and preparations containing alcohol (such as over-the-counter cough medications, mouthwashes) should be avoided during therapy and up to 5 days after discontinuation of sulfonylurea therapy.

DRUG CLASS: Meglitinide Oral Hypoglycemic Agents

Actions

The meglitinides (mehg lit′ in ides) are non-sulfonylurea oral hypoglycemic agents. They lower blood glucose by stimulating the release of insulin from the beta cells of the pancreas.

Uses

The meglitinides are effective in patients with type 2 diabetes mellitus in which the pancreas still has the capacity to secrete insulin, but are of no value in patients with type 1 diabetes mellitus who have no beta cell function. The meglitinides may be effective in the treatment of type 2 diabetes mellitus that cannot be controlled by diet and exercise if the patient is not susceptible to developing ketosis, acidosis, or infections. Patients most likely to benefit from oral hypoglycemic treatment are those who develop signs of diabetes after age 40 and who require less than 40 units of insulin per day (indicating that some insulin is still being secreted by the beta cells). The meglitinides may be used alone or in combination with metformin to control hyperglycemia. The meglitinides have the advantage of having a short duration of action, thus reducing the potential for hypoglycemic reactions. On the other hand, having to take doses up to four times daily may reduce compliance. The meglitinides may be of particular use in patients normally well controlled on diet, but who may have periods of transient loss of control, such as during an infection.

Therapeutic Outcomes

The primary therapeutic outcomes expected from meglitinide oral hypoglycemic therapy are as follows:

- A decrease in both fasting blood glucose levels and the A1C concentrations in the range defined as "acceptable" for the individual patient.
- Fewer long-term complications associated with poorly controlled diabetes mellitus.

Nursing Process for the Meglitinides

Premedication Assessment

1. Confirm that blood glucose and A1C levels were recently measured and were hyperglycemic for the individual patient.
2. Confirm that the patient has had a level of activity "reasonable" for the individual patient, and the anticipated level of activity planned for the next several hours is balanced with the oral hypoglycemic agent dosage.
3. Confirm that the prescribed diet is being consumed as planned and that no changes in diet are anticipated in relation to the oral hypoglycemic agent dosage over the next several hours.

Planning

Availability. See Table 36-8.

Implementation

Dosage and Administration. See Table 36-8. Doses may be administered within 1 to 30 minutes of the meal.

Individual dosage adjustment is essential for the successful use of the meglitinides. Dosages may be adjusted weekly, based on fasting blood glucose.

Doses may be taken preprandially two, three, or four times daily in response to changes in the patient's meal pattern.

NOTE: Patients should skip a scheduled dose if they skip the meal so that the risk of hypoglycemia is reduced.

Evaluation

Side Effects to Expect and Report

Hypoglycemia. Patients receiving oral hypoglycemic therapy are as susceptible to hypoglycemia as diabetic patients on insulin therapy. Consequently, blood glucose levels must be monitored closely, especially in the early stages of therapy.

Monitor for the following signs of hypoglycemia: headache, nausea, weakness, hunger, lethargy, decreased coordination, general apprehension, sweating, or blurred or double vision.

Hypoglycemia must be treated immediately. Mild symptoms may be controlled by the oral administration of a glucose source—for example, a lump of sugar, orange juice, carbonated cola beverage (not diet), candy (not chocolate)—or ingestion of a commercially prepared substance such as Glutose. Severe symptoms may be relieved by administering intravenous glucose, and parenteral glucagon may be prescribed in some instances. If in doubt about whether the patient is hypoglycemic or hyperglycemic, always treat the individual for hypoglycemia to prevent the possible neurologic complications that can occur from untreated hypoglycemia.

Notify the health care provider immediately if any of the above symptoms appear. The dosage of

Drug Table 36-8 MEGLITINIDE ORAL HYPOGLYCEMIC AGENTS

GENERIC NAME	BRAND NAME	AVAILABILITY	DAILY DOSE	MAXIMUM DAILY DOSE
repaglinide	Prandin	Tablets: 0.5, 1, 2 mg	Initially, 0.5 mg before each meal	16 mg daily
nateglinide	Starlix	Tablets: 60, 120 mg	Initially, 60 to 120 mg before each meal	360 mg daily

oral hypoglycemic agents also may have to be reduced.

Drug Interactions

Hypoglycemia. The following drugs may enhance the hypoglycemic effects of repaglinide: ethanol, nonsteroidal antiinflammatory drugs (NSAIDs), sulfonylureas, gemfibrozil, itraconazole, ketoconazole, methandrostenolone, chloramphenicol, warfarin, salicylates, sulfisoxazole, probenecid, and monoamine oxidase inhibitors.

Monitor for the following signs of hypoglycemia: headache, nausea, weakness, hunger, lethargy, decreased coordination, general apprehension, sweating, or blurred or double vision.

Notify the health care provider if any of the above symptoms appear.

Hyperglycemia. The following drugs, when used concurrently with the meglitinides, may decrease the therapeutic effects of the meglitinides: corticosteroids, phenothiazines, diuretics, estrogens, oral contraceptives, thyroid replacement hormones, niacin, sympathomimetics, calcium channel blockers, phenytoin, diazoxide, and lithium carbonate.

Beta-Adrenergic Blocking Agents. Beta-adrenergic blocking agents (e.g., propranolol, timolol, nadolol, pindolol) may induce hypoglycemia, but may also mask many of the symptoms of hypoglycemia. Notify the physician if you suspect that any of the above symptoms appear intermittently.

Carbamazepine, Barbiturates, Rifampin. These agents may increase repaglinide metabolism. Monitor blood glucose levels closely when any of these agents are started or discontinued.

Erythromycin, Clarithromycin, Ketoconazole, Miconazole. These agents may inhibit repaglinide metabolism. Monitor closely for hypoglycemia if any of these agents are started in a patient receiving repaglinide.

DRUG CLASS: Thiazolidinedione Oral Antidiabetic Agents

Actions

The thiazolidinediones (thigh a zoe' lid een die' owns; TZDs) lower blood glucose by increasing the sensitivity of muscle and fat tissue to insulin, allowing more glucose to enter the cells in the presence of insulin for metabolism. TZDs also may inhibit hepatic gluconeogenesis and decrease hepatic glucose output. Unlike sulfonylureas or meglitinides, TZDs do not stimulate the release of insulin from the beta cells of the pancreas, but insulin must be present for these agents to work.

Uses

The TZDs are effective in patients with type 2 diabetes mellitus in which the pancreas still has the capacity to secrete insulin, but are of no value in the person with type 1 diabetes, who has no beta cell function. TZDs may be effective in the treatment of type 2 diabetes mellitus that cannot be controlled by diet and exercise if the patient is not susceptible to developing ketosis, acidosis, or infections. TZDs are not indicated as initial therapy in patients with type 2 diabetes mellitus. Rosiglitazone and pioglitazone may be used as monotherapy (with diet and exercise), or in combination with insulin, sulfonylureas, or metformin to control blood glucose. Therapy often takes 4 to 6 weeks for notable effect and several months for full therapeutic effect.

Therapeutic Outcomes

The primary therapeutic outcomes expected from TZD oral antidiabetic therapy are as follows:

- A decrease in both fasting blood glucose levels and the A1C concentrations in the range defined as "acceptable" for the individual patient.
- Fewer long-term complications associated with poorly controlled diabetes mellitus.

Nursing Process for the Thiazolidinediones

Premedication Assessment

1. Confirm that blood glucose and A1C levels were recently measured and were hyperglycemic for the individual patient.
2. Perform scheduled baseline laboratory tests. Liver function tests, including bilirubin, AST, ALT, GGT, and alkaline phosphatase should be obtained before initiation of therapy, once a month for the first year and quarterly after the first year. A baseline test should also be completed for body weight, hemoglobin and hematocrit, white blood cell count and total cholesterol, HDL-cholesterol, LDL-cholesterol, and triglycerides.
3. Confirm that the prescribed diet is being consumed as planned and that no changes in diet are anticipated in relation to the oral hypoglycemic agent dosage over the next several hours.
4. Premenopausal, anovulatory women should be informed that the TZDs might induce the resumption of ovulation. These women may be at risk for pregnancy if adequate contraception is not used (see Drug Interactions—Oral Contraceptives).

Planning

Availability. See Table 36-9.

Implementation

Dosage and Administration. See Table 36-9. Individual dosage adjustment is essential for the successful use of hypoglycemic agents. A patient should be given a multiweek (12 weeks for rosiglitazone and pioglitazone therapy) trial before adjusting the dosage or adding additional hypoglycemic agents.

Drug Table 36-9 THIAZOLIDINEDIONE ORAL HYPOGLYCEMIC AGENTS

GENERIC NAME	BRAND NAME	AVAILABILITY	DAILY DOSE	MAXIMUM DAILY DOSE
pioglitazone	Actos	Tablets: 15, 30, 45 mg	PO: Initially, 15-30 mg once daily	45 mg
rosiglitazone	Avandia	Tablets: 2, 4, 8 mg	PO: Initially, 2 mg twice daily or 4 mg once daily	8 mg

Evaluation

Side Effects to Expect

Nausea, Vomiting, Anorexia, Abdominal Cramps. These side effects are usually mild and tend to resolve with continued therapy. Encourage the patient not to discontinue therapy without first consulting the physician.

Side Effects to Report

Hypoglycemia. Patients receiving TZDs are not susceptible to hypoglycemia unless they are also receiving other hypoglycemic therapy such as insulin or sulfonylureas. If patients are receiving multiple hypoglycemic therapies, blood glucose levels must be monitored closely, especially in the early stages of therapy.

Monitor for the following signs of hypoglycemia: headache, nausea, weakness, hunger, lethargy, decreased coordination, general apprehension, sweating, or blurred or double vision.

Hypoglycemia must be treated immediately. Mild symptoms may be controlled by the oral administration of a glucose source—for example, a lump of sugar, orange juice, carbonated cola beverage (not diet), candy (not chocolate)—or ingestion of a commercially prepared substance such as Glutose. Severe symptoms may be relieved by IV administration of glucose, and parenteral glucagon may be prescribed in some instances. If in doubt about whether the patient is hypoglycemic or hyperglycemic, always treat the individual for hypoglycemia to prevent the possible neurologic complications that can occur from untreated hypoglycemia.

Notify the health care provider immediately if any of the above symptoms appear. The dosage of oral hypoglycemic agents also may have to be reduced.

Hepatotoxicity. The symptoms of hepatotoxicity are anorexia, nausea, vomiting, jaundice, hepatomegaly, splenomegaly, and abnormal liver function tests (elevated bilirubin, AST, ALT, GGT, alkaline phosphatase, prothrombin time).

Weight Gain. Weight gain of a few pounds is a common adverse effect of TZD therapy. It also may be a sign of fluid accumulation and increased plasma volume. Monitor patients for signs of edema and report to the health care provider if present.

Drug Interactions

Hypoglycemia. The following drugs may enhance the hypoglycemic effects of the TZDs: sulfonylureas, ethanol, methandrostenolone, chloramphenicol, warfarin, propranolol, salicylates, sulfisoxazole, guanethidine, oxytetracycline, MAOIs, and phenylbutazone.

Monitor for the following signs of hypoglycemia: headache, nausea, weakness, hunger, lethargy, decreased coordination, general apprehension, sweating, or blurred or double vision. Notify the health care provider if any of the above symptoms appear.

Hyperglycemia. The following drugs, when used concurrently with the TZDs, may decrease the therapeutic effects of the TZDs: corticosteroids, phenothiazines, diuretics, oral contraceptives, thyroid replacement hormones, phenytoin, diazoxide, and lithium carbonate.

Diabetic or prediabetic patients need to be monitored for the development of hyperglycemia, particularly during the early weeks of therapy.

Assess regularly for elevated blood glucose or glycosuria and report if it occurs with any frequency.

Patients receiving insulin may require an adjustment in dosage.

Beta-Adrenergic Blocking Agents. Beta-adrenergic blocking agents (e.g., propranolol, timolol, nadolol, pindolol) may induce hypoglycemia, but may also mask many of the symptoms of hypoglycemia. Notify the health care provider if you suspect that any of the above symptoms appear intermittently.

Oral Contraceptives. Pioglitazone may enhance the metabolism of ethinyl estradiol and norethindrone, which may cause a resumption of ovulation in patients taking oral contraceptives. Counseling regarding alternative methods of birth control (e.g., contraceptive foam, condoms) should be planned. This interaction has not been reported with rosiglitazone.

Erythromycin, Ketoconazole, Itraconazole, Calcium Channel Blockers, Cisapride, Corticosteroids, Cyclosporine, Triazolam, Hydroxymethylglutaryl (HMG)-CoA Reductase Inhibitors (Statins). These agents may inhibit the metabolism of pioglitazone. If a TZD hypoglycemic agent is indicated for a patient already receiving one of these agents, rosiglitazone should be considered over pioglitazone because these agents do not inhibit its metabolism.

DRUG CLASS: Alpha-Glucosidase Inhibitor Agents

acarbose (a' kar bohs)

PRECOSE (pre' kohs)

Actions

Acarbose is a type of agent called antihyperglycemic agents. It is an enzyme inhibitor that inhibits pancreatic alpha amylase and gastrointestinal alpha glucoside hydrolase enzymes used in the digestion of sugars. In patients with diabetes, this enzyme inhibition results in delayed glucose absorption and a lowering of postprandial hyperglycemia.

Uses

Acarbose is used as an adjunct to diet to lower blood glucose in patients with type 2 diabetes mellitus whose hyperglycemia cannot be controlled by diet and exercise alone. It has the particular advantage that it will not cause hypoglycemia, as can occur with insulin and the sulfonylureas. It also may be used in combination with the sulfonylureas or metformin to lower blood glucose because the agents act by different mechanisms.

Therapeutic Outcomes

The primary therapeutic outcomes expected from acarbose therapy are as follows:

- A decrease in both postprandial blood glucose levels and the A1C concentrations in the range defined as "acceptable" for the individual patient.
- Fewer long-term complications associated with poorly controlled type 2 diabetes mellitus.

Nursing Process for Acarbose

Premedication Assessment

1. If the patient is also receiving oral hypoglycemic agent or insulin therapy, ensure that the dosages of these medicines are well adjusted before starting acarbose therapy.
2. Review the patient's history to ensure that there is no gastrointestinal malabsorption syndrome or obstruction present.
3. Review the patient's medical history to ensure that no liver abnormalities are present.

Planning

Availability. 50 and 100 mg tablets.

Implementation

Dosage and Administration. *Adult:* PO: Initially, 25 mg three times daily at the start of each main meal. The dosage is adjusted at 4- to 8-week intervals based on 1-hour postprandial blood glucose concentrations and on the severity of adverse effects. The maintenance dosage is 50 to 100 mg three times daily.

The maximum recommended dosage for patients weighing less than 60 kg (132 lb) is 50 mg three times daily. The maximum dosage for patients weighing more than 60 kg is 100 mg three times daily.

Evaluation

Side Effects to Expect

Abdominal Cramps, Diarrhea, Flatulence. These adverse effects are caused by the metabolism of carbohydrates in the large intestine that were blocked from metabolism in the small intestine by acarbose. These side effects are usually mild and tend to resolve with continued therapy. Encourage the patient not to discontinue therapy without first consulting the health care provider.

Side Effects to Report

Hypoglycemia. Although acarbose does not cause hypoglycemia by itself, it can enhance the hypoglycemia caused by a sulfonylurea or insulin. Consequently, blood glucose levels must be monitored closely, especially in the early stages of therapy.

Monitor for the following signs of hypoglycemia: headache, nausea, weakness, hunger, lethargy, decreased coordination, general apprehension, sweating, or blurred or double vision.

Hypoglycemia must be treated immediately. Treatment should be initiated with oral dextrose (Glutose) because its metabolism is not blocked by acarbose. Do not use sucrose (table sugar) because its metabolism is blocked by acarbose. Severe symptoms may be relieved by IV administration of glucose, and parenteral glucagon may be prescribed in some instances.

If in doubt about whether the patient is hypoglycemic or hyperglycemic, always treat the individual for hypoglycemia to prevent the possible neurologic complications that can occur from untreated hypoglycemia.

Notify the health care provider immediately if any of these symptoms appear. The dosage of oral hypoglycemic agents may also have to be reduced.

Hepatotoxicity. Acarbose has been reported to cause elevations of serum aminotransferases (AST and ALT). In rare cases it causes hyperbilirubinemia. It is recommended that serum aminotransferase concentrations be checked every 3 months during the first year of treatment and periodically thereafter.

Drug Interactions

Hyperglycemia. The following drugs, when used concurrently with acarbose, may decrease the therapeutic effects of acarbose: corticosteroids, phenothiazines, diuretics, oral contraceptives, thyroid replacement hormones, phenytoin, diazoxide, and lithium carbonate.

Digestive Enzymes, Intestinal Adsorbents. Digestive enzymes (e.g., amylase, pancreatin) and intestinal adsorbents (e.g., charcoal) may reduce the effect of acarbose. Concurrent therapy is not recommended.

Digoxin. Acarbose may inhibit the absorption of digoxin. Monitor serum digoxin levels and therapeutic effects to assess whether the dosage of digoxin needs to be adjusted. Monitor closely when the dosage of acarbose is increased or discontinued.

miglitol (mig′ lih tohl)
GLYSET (gly′ set)

Actions

Miglitol is an enzyme inhibitor that inhibits pancreatic alpha-amylase and gastrointestinal alpha-glucoside hydrolase enzymes used in the digestion of sugars. In patients with diabetes, this enzyme inhibition results in delayed glucose absorption and a lowering of postprandial hyperglycemia.

Uses

Miglitol is used as an adjunct to diet and exercise to lower blood glucose in patients with type 2 diabetes mellitus whose hyperglycemia cannot be controlled by diet and exercise alone. It has the particular advantage that it will not cause hypoglycemia, as can occur with insulin and the sulfonylureas. It also may be used in combination with the sulfonylureas to lower blood glucose because the agents act by different mechanisms.

Therapeutic Outcomes

The primary therapeutic outcomes expected from miglitol therapy are as follows:

- A decrease in both postprandial blood glucose levels and the A1C concentrations in the range defined as "acceptable" for the individual patient.
- Fewer long-term complications associated with poorly controlled type 2 diabetes mellitus.

Nursing Process for Miglitol

Premedication Assessment

1. If the patient is also receiving a sulfonylurea hypoglycemic agent or insulin therapy, ensure that the dosages of these medicines are well adjusted before starting miglitol therapy.
2. Review the patient's history to ensure that there is no GI malabsorption syndrome or obstruction present.
3. Review the patient's medical history to ensure that no liver abnormalities are present.

Planning

Availability. 25, 50, and 100 mg tablets.

Implementation

Dosage and Administration. *Adult:* PO: Initially, 25 mg three times daily at the start (the first bite) of each main meal. Some patients may start with 25 mg daily to avoid GI adverse effects. The dosage is adjusted at 4- to 8-week intervals based on 1-hour postprandial plasma glucose levels and A1C concentrations and on the severity of adverse effects. The maintenance dosage is 50 to 100 mg three times daily. The maximum recommended dosage is 100 mg three times daily.

Evaluation

Side Effects to Expect

Abdominal Cramps, Diarrhea, Flatulence. These adverse effects are caused by the metabolism of carbohydrates in the large intestine that were blocked from metabolism in the small intestine by miglitol. These side effects are usually mild especially with low initial dosages and tend to resolve with continued therapy. Encourage the patient not to discontinue therapy without first consulting the physician.

Side Effects to Report

Hypoglycemia. Whereas miglitol does not cause hypoglycemia by itself, it can enhance the hypoglycemia caused by a sulfonylurea or insulin. Consequently, blood glucose levels must be monitored closely, especially in the early stages of therapy.

Monitor for the following signs of hypoglycemia: headache, nausea, weakness, hunger, lethargy, decreased coordination, general apprehension, sweating, or blurred or double vision.

Hypoglycemia must be treated immediately. Treatment should be initiated with oral dextrose (Glutose), because its metabolism is not blocked by miglitol. Do not use sucrose (table sugar), because its metabolism is blocked by miglitol. Severe symptoms may be relieved by IV administration of glucose, and parenteral glucagon may be prescribed in some instances.

If in doubt about whether the patient is hypoglycemic or hyperglycemic, always treat the individual for hypoglycemia to prevent the possible neurologic complications that can occur from untreated hypoglycemia.

Notify the physician immediately if any of the above symptoms appear. The dosage of oral hypoglycemic agents may also have to be reduced.

Drug Interactions

Hyperglycemia. The following drugs, when used concurrently with miglitol, may decrease the therapeutic effects of miglitol: corticosteroids, phenothiazines, diuretics, oral contraceptives, thyroid replacement hormones, phenytoin, diazoxide, and lithium carbonate.

Propranolol, Ranitidine. Miglitol may interfere with the absorption of these agents. Concurrent therapy is not recommended.

Digestive Enzymes, Intestinal Adsorbents. Digestive enzymes (e.g., amylase, pancreatin) and intestinal adsorbents (e.g., charcoal) may reduce the effect of miglitol. Concurrent therapy is not recommended.

DRUG CLASS: Incretin-Mimetic Agent

exenatide (ex en' ah tide)

▶ BYETTA (bi et' ah)

Actions

Exenatide is the first of a new type of agent called incretin-mimetic agents. In normal physiology, proteins known as incretin peptides are released from L-cells located in the distal ileum and colon in response to ingestion of carbohydrates and fats. The incretins help control blood glucose levels by:

- Enhancing insulin secretion
- Suppressing glucagon secretion from the liver, suppressing glucose output from the liver

- Delaying gastric emptying, thus slowing carbohydrate and lipid absorption, reducing postprandial hyperglycemia
- Reducing appetite
- Maintaining beta cell function

These actions result in the reduction in basal glucose concentrations and in elevations of postprandial glucose concentrations. There is also a reduced appetite with subsequent body weight reduction. Ultimately, the A1C levels are reduced. Exenatide is a synthetic version of exendin-4, a naturally occurring hormone. Exenatide mimics the actions of incretins for self-regulating glycemic control, resulting in an increase in serum insulin and a reduction in glucose concentrations.

Uses

Exenatide is used as additional therapy to reduce elevated fasting and postprandial hyperglycemia in patients with type 2 diabetes mellitus who are taking metformin, a sulfonylurea, or a combination of metformin and a sulfonylurea, but who have not achieved adequate glycemic control. Particular benefits of exenatide are that it enhances insulin secretion only in the presence of hyperglycemia, and insulin secretion decreases as blood glucose approaches normal levels.

Therapeutic Outcomes

The primary therapeutic outcomes expected from exenatide therapy are as follows:

- A decrease in fasting and postprandial blood glucose levels and the A1C concentrations in the range defined as "acceptable" for the individual patient.
- Fewer long-term complications associated with poorly controlled type 2 diabetes mellitus.

Nursing Process for Exenatide

Premedication Assessment

1. Ensure that the dosages of concurrent oral antidiabetic therapy are well adjusted before starting exenatide therapy.
2. Assess patient's or family member's ability to self-administer injections.

Planning

Availability. Available in 250 mcg/mL prefilled cartridges in a pen injector. Prefilled pens, containing 1.2 or 2.4 mL of solution, are available to deliver 5 mcg or 10 mcg. Each prefilled pen will deliver 60 doses to provide a 30-day supply of the twice-daily medication.

Implementation

Dosage and Administration. *Adult:* Subcutaneous: Initial: 5 mcg per dose administered twice daily at any time within the 60-minute period before the morning and evening meals. Administer as a subcutaneous injection in the thigh, abdomen, or upper arm. Do NOT administer after a meal. Based on clinical response, the dose may be increased to 10 mcg twice daily after 1 month of therapy.

Exenatide is used in conjunction with metformin and/or a sulfonylurea. Dosage adjustment of the metformin is not necessary, but a dosage reduction of the sulfonylurea might be necessary to reduce the risk of hypoglycemia.

Exenatide pens should be stored refrigerated at 36° to 46° F. Do not freeze or use if it has been frozen. Warm to room temperature before use. The pen should be discarded 30 days after first use, even if some of the drug remains in the pen.

Evaluation

Side Effects to Expect

Nausea, Vomiting, Diarrhea. These adverse effects are usually mild to moderate and tend to resolve with continued therapy. Encourage the patient not to discontinue therapy without first consulting the health care provider.

Side Effects to Report

Hypoglycemia. Although exenatide does not cause hypoglycemia by itself, it can enhance the hypoglycemia that may be caused by a sulfonylurea. Consequently, blood glucose levels must be monitored closely, especially in the early stages of therapy.

Monitor for the following signs of hypoglycemia: headache, nausea, weakness, hunger, lethargy, decreased coordination, general apprehension, sweating, or blurred or double vision.

Hypoglycemia must be treated immediately. Mild symptoms may be controlled by the oral administration of a glucose source—for example, a lump of sugar, orange juice, carbonated cola beverage (not diet), candy (not chocolate)—or ingestion of a commercially prepared substance such as Glutose. Severe symptoms may be relieved by IV administration of glucose, and parenteral glucagon may be prescribed in some instances. If in doubt about whether the patient is hypoglycemic or hyperglycemic, always treat the individual for hypoglycemia to prevent the possible neurologic complications that can occur from untreated hypoglycemia.

Notify the health care provider immediately if any of the above symptoms appear. The dosage of oral antidiabetic agents may also have to be reduced.

Drug Interactions

Hypoglycemia. The following drugs may enhance the hypoglycemic effects of the sulfonylureas and exenatide: ethanol, methandrostenolone, chloramphenicol, warfarin, nonselective beta-adrenergic blocking agents, salicylates, sulfisoxazole, guanethidine, oxytetracycline, and MAOIs.

Monitor for the following signs of hypoglycemia: headache, nausea, weakness, hunger, lethargy, decreased coordination, general apprehension, sweating, blurred or double vision.

Notify the health care provider if any of these symptoms appear.

Hyperglycemia. The following drugs, when used concurrently with exenatide, may decrease the therapeutic effects of exenatide: corticosteroids, phenothiazines, diuretics, oral contraceptives, thyroid replacement hormones, phenytoin, diazoxide, and lithium carbonate.

DRUG CLASS: Amylinomimetic Agent

pramlintide (pram′ lin tide)
SYMLIN (sim′ lin)

Actions

Pramlintide is a synthetic analog of amylin. Amylin is a protein secreted from pancreatic beta cells with insulin in response to food intake. Patients with a deficiency of insulin also have a deficiency of amylin. Amylin and pramlintide reduce postprandial glucose levels by:

- Suppressing glucagon secretion from the liver, suppressing glucose output from the liver.
- Delaying gastric emptying, thus slowing carbohydrate and lipid absorption, reducing postprandial hyperglycemia.
- Suppressing the appetite with subsequent potential weight reduction.

Uses

Pramlintide is used as additional therapy to reduce elevated postprandial hyperglycemia in patients with type 1 or type 2 diabetes mellitus who are taking mealtime insulin, or metformin, a sulfonylurea, or a combination of metformin and a sulfonylurea but who have not achieved adequate glycemic control.

Therapeutic Outcomes

The primary therapeutic outcomes expected from pramlintide therapy are as follows:

- A decrease in postprandial blood glucose levels and the A1C concentrations in the range defined as "acceptable" for the individual patient.
- Fewer long-term complications associated with poorly controlled type 1 or type 2 diabetes mellitus.

Nursing Process for Pramlintide

Premedication Assessment

1. Ensure that the dosages of concurrent oral antidiabetic therapy are well adjusted before starting pramlintide therapy.
2. Assess the patient's ability to self-administer injections.
3. Discuss with patients their compliance with current insulin therapy and ability to do self-blood glucose monitoring.
4. Make sure the patient and family understand the signs and symptoms of hypoglycemia and its causes.
5. Identify whether the patient is pregnant or breastfeeding.

Planning

Availability. 0.6 mg/mL in 5-mL vials.

Implementation

Pramlintide should NOT be used in patients with any of the following:

- Poor compliance with a current insulin therapy
- Poor compliance with self-blood glucose monitoring
- An A1C level greater than 9%
- Recurrent severe hypoglycemia requiring assistance during the previous 6 months
- Unawareness of oncoming hypoglycemic episodes
- Need for medicines to stimulate gastric motility

Dosage and Administration. *Adult:* Subcutaneous: pramlintide is administered subcutaneously into the abdomen or thigh. Do not use the upper arm due to variable absorption.

- Do not mix insulin and pramlintide in the same syringe.
- Administer pramlintide and insulin as separate injections at separate sites at least 2 inches apart. Rotate sites.
- If a dose of pramlintide is missed, do not give an additional injection. Wait until the next major meal.

NOTE: Pramlintide dosage differs depending on whether the patient has type 1 or type 2 diabetes.

- *Type 1 diabetes.* Subcutaneous: Initial: 15 mcg immediately before major (≥250 kcal or ≥ 30 g carbohydrate) meals.
  - Reduce preprandial, rapid-acting, or short-acting insulin doses, including fixed-mix insulins (e.g., 75/25) by 50%.
  - Monitor blood glucose levels frequently, including before and after meals and at bedtime.
  - Increase pramlintide dosage by 15 mcg when no significant nausea has occurred for at least 3 days. Maximum dose is 60 mcg.
  - Adjust insulin doses to optimize blood glucose control once the target dose of pramlintide is achieved and nausea (if experienced) has subsided.
- *Type 2 diabetes.* Subcutaneous: Initial: 60 mcg immediately before major (≥250 kcal or ≥30 g carbohydrate) meals.
  - Reduce preprandial, rapid-acting, or short-acting insulin doses, including fixed-mix insulins (e.g., 75/25) by 50%.
  - Monitor blood glucose levels frequently, including before and after meals and at bedtime

- Increase pramlintide dosage to 120 mcg when no significant nausea has occurred for 3 to 7 days. Maximum dose is 120 mcg.
- Adjust insulin doses to optimize blood glucose control once the target dose of pramlintide is achieved and nausea (if experienced) has subsided.

Patients should be cautioned to NOT take their dose of pramlintide if:

- Their blood glucose is low.
- They plan to skip a meal.
- They plan to eat a meal with fewer than 250 calories or 30 g of carbohydrate.
- They are sick and cannot eat a usual meal.
- They are having surgery or a medical test in which they must fast before the test.
- They are pregnant or breastfeeding and have not talked to their health care provider.

Measurement of dosage. Pramlintide is measured using a U-100 insulin syringe, preferably the 0.3-mL size, for more accurate measurement. Use the chart below to measure the microgram dosage in unit increments.

DOSAGE PRESCRIBED (mcg)	INCREMENT USING A U-100 SYRINGE (Units)	VOLUME (mL)
15	2.5	0.025
30	5	0.050
45	7.5	0.075
60	10	0.1
120	20	0.2

Unopened vials of pramlintide should be stored refrigerated at 36° to 46° F. Do not freeze or use if it has been frozen.

Opened (in use) vials may be kept either refrigerated or at room temperature for up to 28 days as long as the temperature is not greater than 77° F. Opened vials, whether or not refrigerated, should be discarded after 28 days.

Evaluation

Side Effects to Expect

Nausea, Vomiting, Indigestion. Nausea is the most common side effect with pramlintide. Mild nausea is more likely during the first weeks after starting therapy and usually does not last long. Starting with a low dose and building up slowly is important. These adverse effects are usually mild to moderate and tend to resolve with continued therapy. Encourage the patient not to discontinue therapy without first consulting the health care provider.

Side Effects to Report

Hypoglycemia. Although pramlintide does not cause hypoglycemia by itself, it can enhance the hypoglycemia that may be caused by a sulfonylurea or insulin. Consequently, blood glucose levels must be monitored closely, especially in the early stages of therapy.

Monitor for the following signs of hypoglycemia: headache, nausea, weakness, hunger, lethargy, decreased coordination, general apprehension, sweating, or blurred or double vision.

Hypoglycemia must be treated immediately. Mild symptoms may be controlled by the oral administration of a glucose source—for example, a lump of sugar, orange juice, carbonated cola beverage (not diet), candy (not chocolate)—or ingestion of a commercially prepared substance such as Glutose. Severe symptoms may be relieved by IV administration of glucose, and parenteral glucagon may be prescribed in some instances. If in doubt about whether the patient is hypoglycemic or hyperglycemic, always treat the individual for hypoglycemia to prevent the possible neurologic complications that can occur from untreated hypoglycemia.

Notify the health care provider immediately if any of the above symptoms appear. The dosage of oral antidiabetic agents may also have to be reduced.

Drug Interactions

Hypoglycemia. The following drugs may enhance the hypoglycemic effects of pramlintide and insulin: sulfonylureas, meglitinides, ACE inhibitors (e.g., captopril, ramipril, lisinopril), disopyramide, fibrates (e.g., gemfibrozil), fluoxetine, MAOIs (e.g., tranylcypromine, isocarboxazid), pentoxifylline, propoxyphene, salicylates, and sulfonamide antibiotics. Monitor for the following signs of hypoglycemia: headache, nausea, weakness, hunger, lethargy, decreased coordination, general apprehension, sweating, blurred or double vision. Notify the health care provider if any of these symptoms appear.

Hyperglycemia. The following drugs, when used concurrently with pramlintide, may decrease the therapeutic effects of pramlintide: corticosteroids, phenothiazines, diuretics, oral contraceptives, thyroid replacement hormones, phenytoin, diazoxide, and lithium carbonate.

DRUG CLASS: Antihypoglycemic Agents

glucagon (glue' kah gohn)

Actions

Glucagon is a hormone secreted by the alpha cells of the pancreas that breaks down stored glycogen to glucose, resulting in elevated blood glucose levels. Glucagon also aids in converting amino acids to glucose (gluconeogenesis). Glucagon is dependent on the presence of glycogen for its action. It has essentially no action in cases of starvation, adrenal insufficiency, or chronic hypoglycemia.

Uses

Glucagon is used to treat hypoglycemic reactions in patients with diabetes mellitus.

Therapeutic Outcomes

The primary therapeutic outcome expected from glucagon therapy is elimination of symptoms associated with hypoglycemia.

Nursing Process for Glucagon

Premedication Assessment

1. Confirm patient unresponsiveness before administration. If conscious, oral antihypoglycemic therapy is usually more appropriate.
2. Hypoglycemia is a medical emergency. If suspected, it should be treated by authorized personnel as soon as possible.

Planning

Availability. Subcutaneous, IM, IV: 1-mg vials.

Implementation

Dosage and Administration. *Adult:* Subcutaneous, IM, IV: Administer 1 mg. Response should be observed within 5 to 20 minutes. If response is minimal, one or two additional doses may be administered. If the patient is slow to arouse, consider glucose to be administered IV.

Evaluation

Side Effects to Expect and Report

Nausea, Vomiting. These side effects may also occur with hypoglycemia. Take precautions to prevent aspiration of vomitus.

Drug Interactions

Warfarin. Glucagon may potentiate the anticoagulant effects of warfarin if used for several days. Monitor the patient's International Normalized Ratio (INR) and reduce the dosage of warfarin accordingly.

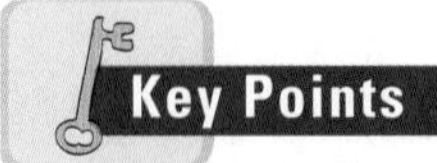

- Diabetes mellitus is a complex group of chronic diseases that has both short- and long-term complications associated with it. The long-term objective of control of the disease must involve mechanisms to stop the progression of the complications of the disease.
- Patient education and reinforcement are extremely important to successful therapy. Major determinants to success are the patient's taking responsibility for a balanced diet, insulin or oral hypoglycemic therapy, routine exercise, and good hygiene.
- The nurse plays a critical role as a health educator in discussion of treatment options, planning for lifestyle changes, counseling before discharge, and reinforcement of key points during office visits. Best results are attained when the patient, family, and nurse work together in developing the care plan.

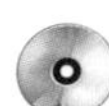

Go to your Companion CD-ROM for Appendices, an Audio Glossary, animations, Drug Dosage Calculators, customizable Patient Self-Assessment forms, and Review Questions for the NCLEX® Examination.

evolve Be sure to visit the companion Evolve site at http://evolve.elsevier.com/Clayton for WebLinks and additional online resources.

MEDICATION SAFETY REVIEW

MATH REVIEW QUESTIONS

1. Order: 22 units NPH (human) insulin to be administered 30 minutes before breakfast

   Available: U-100 NPH (human) insulin

   Give ____ mL.

2. Order: 27 units NPH (human) insulin plus 7 units regular (human) insulin to be administered before breakfast.

   Available: U-100 NPH (human) insulin
   U-100 regular (human) insulin

   What volume of NPH insulin is to be drawn up?

   ____ mL

   What volume of regular insulin is to be drawn up?

   ____ mL

   What total volume is to be injected? ____ mL

CRITICAL THINKING QUESTIONS

An 18-year-old patient was recently diagnosed with type 1 diabetes mellitus. After several days of treatment with adjustment of diet, exercise, and regular insulin, he was placed on U-100 NPH (human) insulin, 20 units 30 minutes before breakfast and 10 units before the evening meal.

1. What are the nursing interventions to be considered when administering the NPH insulin?
2. The patient is having trouble injecting himself. In a moment of frustration, he asks, "Why can't I take insulin pills like my grandfather?" What is your response?

Five days later, the health care provider adds 5 units of regular (human) insulin to the morning dose to be administered with the NPH insulin.

3. Describe how you would teach the patient to mix the morning insulin dose for a single administration.
4. While continuing with the patient's education, he asks again for the difference between the symptoms of hypoglycemia and hyperglycemia. What is your response?

CONTENT REVIEW QUESTIONS

1. The most rapid-acting type of insulins available are:
   1. Lispro and Aspart.
   2. Humulin R.
   3. glargine
   4. Humulin N.
2. After injection, regular insulin takes _____ minutes to start acting and its peak action is in _____ hours.
   1. 10 minutes; 1 to 2 hours
   2. 20 minutes; 2 to 4 hours
   3. 30 minutes; 2.5 to 5 hours
   4. 50 minutes; 4 to 6 hours
3. Hypoglycemia can occur as a result of:
   1. increased carbohydrate intake; usual daily insulin dose.
   2. increased protein intake with decreased physical activity.
   3. intake of diuretic agents with insulin.
   4. insulin overdose; decreased carbohydrate intake.
4. This classification of commonly prescribed drugs may mask the symptoms of hypoglycemia when taken concurrently with insulin.
   1. Glucagon
   2. Oral contraceptives
   3. Corticosteroids
   4. Beta-adrenergic blocking agents
5. The action of TZDs lower blood glucose by:
   1. stimulating release of insulin from beta cells in pancreas.
   2. an unknown mechanism of action.
   3. increasing muscle and fat tissue sensitivity to allow more glucose to enter the cell in the presence of insulin.
   4. affecting certain enzymes used in digestion of sugars that results in delayed glucose absorption.
6. A patient screened for diabetes at a clinic has a fasting plasma glucose of 130 mg/dL (6.7 mmol/L). The nurse knows that this result may indicate:
   1. a normal finding.
   2. impaired fasting glucose.
   3. impaired glucose tolerance.
7. During a clinic visit 3 months following a diagnosis of type 2 diabetes, the patient reports that she has been following her reduced-calorie diet, but she has not lost any weight. She has also neglected to bring her record of glucose monitoring results. The nurse recognizes that the best indicator of the patient's control of her diabetes since her initial diagnosis and instruction is:
   1. a fasting glucose level.
   2. analysis for microalbuminuria.
   3. A1C level.
   4. the patient's verbal report of her symptoms.
8. A patient receives a daily injection of 25 units NPH insulin at 7:00 AM. The nurse expects that a hypoglycemic reaction is most likely to occur between:
   1. 0800 and 1000.
   2. 1500 and 1800.
   3. 1900 and 2100.
   4. 2200 and 2400.
9. A rare but life-threatening complication that can occur with metformin is:
   1. lactic acidosis.
   2. kidney failure.
   3. status epilepticus.
   4. hypoglycemia.

CHAPTER

37 Drugs Used to Treat Thyroid Disease

evolve http://evolve.elsevier.com/Clayton

Chapter Content

Objectives

1. Describe the signs, symptoms, treatment, and nursing interventions associated with hypothyroidism and hyperthyroidism.
2. Identify the two classes of drugs used to treat thyroid disease.
3. State the drug of choice for hypothyroidism.
4. Explain the effects of hyperthyroidism on doses of warfarin and digoxin and on people taking oral hypoglycemic agents.
5. Cite the actions of antithyroid medications on the formation and release of the hormones produced by the thyroid gland.
6. State the three types of treatment for hyperthyroidism.
7. Explain the nutritional requirements and activity restrictions needed for an individual with hyperthyroidism.
8. Identify the types of conditions that respond favorably to the use of radioactive iodine-131.
9. Cite the action of propylthiouracil on the synthesis of T_3 and T_4.

Key Terms

thyroid-stimulating hormone	myxedema
triiodothyronine (T_3)	cretinism
thyroxine (T_4)	hyperthyroidism
hypothyroidism	thyrotoxicosis
	iodine-131

THYROID GLAND

The thyroid gland is a large, reddish, ductless gland in front of and on either side of the trachea. It consists of two lateral lobes and a connecting isthmus and is roughly butterfly shaped. It is enclosed in a covering of areolar tissue. The thyroid is made up of numerous closed follicles containing colloid matter and is surrounded by a vascular network. This gland is one of the most richly vascularized tissues in the body.

As with other endocrine glands, thyroid gland function is regulated by the hypothalamus and the anterior pituitary gland. The hypothalamus secretes thyrotropin-releasing hormone (TRH), which stimulates the anterior pituitary gland to release **thyroid-stimulating hormone** (TSH). Thyroid-stimulating hormone stimulates the thyroid gland to release its hormones **triiodothyronine (T_3)** and **thyroxine (T_4)**.

The thyroid hormones regulate general body metabolism. Imbalance in thyroid hormone production may also interfere with the following body functions: growth and maturation; carbohydrate, protein, and lipid metabolism; thermal regulation; cardiovascular function; lactation; and reproduction.

THYROID DISEASES

Hypothyroidism is the result of inadequate thyroid hormone production.

Myxedema is hypothyroidism that occurs during adult life. The onset of symptoms is usually mild and vague. Patients develop a slowness in motion, speech, and mental processes. They often develop more lethargic, sedentary habits; have decreased appetites; gain weight; are constipated; cannot tolerate cold; become weak; and fatigue easily. The body temperature may be subnormal; the skin becomes dry, coarse, and thickened; and the face appears puffy. Patients often have decreased blood pressure and heart rate and develop anemia and high cholesterol levels. These patients have an increased susceptibility to infection and are sensitive to small doses of sedative-hypnotics, anesthetics, and narcotics. Myxedema may be caused by excessive use of antithyroid drugs used to treat hyperthyroidism, radiation exposure, thyroid surgery, acute viral thyroiditis, or chronic thyroiditis.

Congenital hypothyroidism occurs when a child is born without a thyroid gland or one that is hypoactive. The historical name of this disease is **cretinism.** Fortunately, this disorder is becoming rare because most states require diagnostic testing of the newborn for hypothyroidism.

Although the symptoms of hypothyroidism in both infants and adults are for the most part classical, the final diagnosis is usually not made until diagnostic tests have been completed. These tests include drawing serum levels of circulating T_3 and T_4 hormones. If the levels are low, the patient is considered to be hypothyroid. Further diagnostic testing is required to determine the cause of thyroid hypofunction.

Hyperthyroidism is caused by excess production of thyroid hormones. Disorders that may cause hyperactivity of the thyroid gland are Graves' disease, nodular goiter, thyroiditis, thyroid carcinoma, overdoses of thyroid hormones, and tumors of the pituitary gland.

The clinical manifestations of hyperthyroidism are rapid, bounding pulse (even during sleep); cardiac enlargement; palpitations; and dysrhythmias. Patients are nervous and easily agitated. They develop tremors, a low-grade fever, and weight loss, despite an increased appetite. Hyperactive reflexes and insomnia are also usually present. Patients are intolerant of heat; the skin is warm, flushed, and moist, with increased sweating; edema of the tissues around the eyeballs produces characteristic eye changes, including exophthalmos. Patients develop amenorrhea; dyspnea with minor exertion; hoarse, rapid speech; and an increased susceptibility to infection. Elevated circulating thyroid hormone tests easily diagnose hyperthyroidism. Further diagnostic studies are required to determine the cause of hyperthyroidism.

Excessive formation of thyroid hormones and their secretion into the circulatory system causes hyperthyroidism, also known as **thyrotoxicosis.** Symptoms include increased metabolic rate, increased pulse rate (to perhaps 140 beats/minute), increased body temperature, restlessness, nervousness, anxiety, sweating, muscle weakness and tremors, and a sensation of feeling too warm. This condition is treated with antithyroid drugs or surgical removal of the thyroid gland.

TREATMENT OF THYROID DISEASES

The primary goal of therapy for both hyperthyroidism and hypothyroidism is to return the patient to a normal thyroid (euthyroid) state. Hypothyroidism can be treated successfully by replacement of thyroid hormones (see individual agents). After therapy is initiated, the dosage of thyroid hormone is adjusted until serum levels of the thyroid hormones are within the normal range.

Three types of treatment can be used to reduce the hyperthyroid state: subtotal thyroidectomy, radioactive iodine, and antithyroid medications. Until treatment is under way, the patient requires nutritional and psychological support.

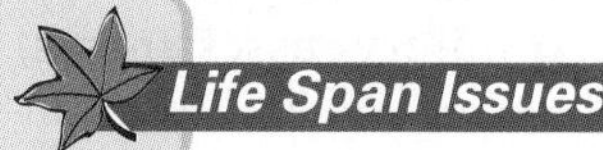

Life Span Issues

Treatment of Hypothyroid State

During initial treatment of the hypothyroid state in the older adult client, be alert for and report increased frequency of angina or symptoms of heart failure.

DRUG THERAPY FOR THYROID DISEASES

Two general classes of drugs used to treat thyroid disorders are (1) those used to replace thyroid hormones in patients whose thyroid glandular function is inadequate to meet metabolic requirements (hypothyroidism) and (2) antithyroid agents used to suppress synthesis of thyroid hormones (hyperthyroidism). Thyroid hormone replacements available are levothyroxine (T_4), liothyronine (T_3), liotrix, and thyroid, USP. Antithyroid drugs interfere with the formation or release of the hormones produced by the thyroid gland. Antithyroid agents to be discussed include radioactive iodides, propylthiouracil, and methimazole.

NURSING PROCESS *for Thyroid Disorders*

Hypothyroidism and hyperthyroidism are primarily treated on an outpatient basis unless surgery is indicated or complications occur. Nurses must be able to offer guidance to the patients requiring treatment on an inpatient or ambulatory basis.

In general, body processes are slowed with hypothyroidism and accelerated with hyperthyroidism.

Assessment

History. Take a history of treatment prescribed for hypothyroidism or hyperthyroidism (e.g., surgery, iodine-131, or hormone replacement). Ask for specific information regarding treatment for any cardiac disease or adrenal insufficiency.

Medications. Request a list of all prescribed and over-the-counter (OTC) medications being taken. Ask if any of the prescribed medications are taken on a regular basis. If not taken regularly, what factors have caused the patient to decrease administration?

Description of Current Symptoms. Ask the patient to explain symptoms experienced and what changes in functioning have occurred over the past 2 to 3 months.

Focused Assessment. Perform a focused assessment of the body systems generally affected by hypothyroid or hyperthyroid states:

- *Cardiovascular:* Take current vital signs, including an apical pulse. Note bradycardia or tachycardia and any alterations in rhythm, subnormal or elevated temperature, and hypertension. Ask whether the pulse rate is decreased or elevated on awakening, before any stimulus. Does the patient experience any palpitations or a feeling that the pulse is rapid and bounding? Record heart sounds and any abnormal characteristics heard (or have a qualified nurse perform this).
- *Respiratory:* Does the patient experience dyspnea? Is it made worse by mild exertion?
- *Gastrointestinal:* Measure the person's height and weight. Ask for a history of increase or decrease in weight over the past 3 months. Has there been

a change in appetite? Does the individual experience nausea and vomiting? What have the characteristics of the stools been over the past several months—constipation or diarrhea? Check and record bowel sounds.
- *Integumentary:* Note the temperature, texture, and condition of the skin and the characteristics of the hair and nails. Does the patient complain of intolerance to heat or cold?
- *Musculoskeletal:* What activity level is maintained? Does the person feel or act sluggish or hyperactive? Is the pattern of activity a change from the recent past? If so, when did this become apparent? Is there muscle weakness, wasting, or discomfort? Is dependent edema present?
- *Neurologic:* What is the patient's mental status—oriented to time, date, and place? What is the degree of alertness and pace of responsiveness (e.g., sluggish and slow in contrast with quickness or fast paced). Is the individual depressed, stuporous, or hyperactive? Has the individual or family and significant others noticed any change in personality in the recent past? Has the individual had tremors of hands, eyelids, or tongue? Has the individual experienced insomnia?
- *Sensory:* What is the condition of the eyes? Do the eyelids retract or is exophthalmos present?
- *Reproductive:* Obtain a history of changes in the pattern of menses and libido.
- *Immunologic:* Has the individual had any recent infections?

Laboratory/Diagnostic Studies. Review laboratory and diagnostic studies available on the chart associated with thyroid disorders such as total thyroxine (TT_4) and total triiodothyronine (TT_3), free thyroxine (FT_4) and free triiodothyronine (FT_3) tests, TSH levels, TRH stimulation test, thyroid autoantibodies, thyroglobulin, calcitonin assay, ultrasound, fine-needle biopsy, radioactive iodine uptake, electrocardiogram (ECG), and thyroid scan.

Nursing Diagnoses

Hyperthyroidism
- Nutrition, imbalanced: less than body requirements (indication)
- Diarrhea (indication)
- Sleep pattern, disturbed (indication)
- Fatigue (indication)
- Hypothyroidism
- Nutrition, imbalanced: more than body requirements (indication)
- Constipation (indication)

Note that an excessive dosage of thyroid medication for a person with hypothyroid disease may produce the nursing diagnoses for hyperthyroidism, which would be appropriate nursing diagnoses associated with adverse drug effects.

Planning

Environment
- For the hyperthyroid individual, plan to provide a cool, quiet, structured environment because the patient lacks the ability to respond to change and anxiety-producing situations and has an intolerance to heat.
- For the hypothyroid individual, plan to provide a warm, quiet, structured environment that supports the patient's needs.

Nutrition
- *Hyperthyroid:* Order the prescribed diet, usually a high-calorie diet of 4000 to 5000 calories per day with balanced nutrients. Mark the Kardex or enter data in the computer for no caffeine products (e.g., coffee, tea, colas) or tobacco. If diarrhea is present, mark the Kardex or enter data in the computer to check trays for any foods with a laxative or stimulating effect such as bran products, fruits, and fresh vegetables.
- *Hypothyroid:* Order the prescribed diet, usually a low-calorie diet with increased bulk to alleviate constipation. Encourage adequate fluid intake, unless coexisting conditions prohibit.

Psychosocial
- Mark the Kardex or enter data in the computer to monitor the mental status at least every shift.
- Plan to incorporate family into the health teaching plan because the patient may be unable to understand or implement all facets of the therapeutic regimen.

Activity and Exercise. Mark the Kardex or enter data in the computer with the prescribed level of activity ordered by the health care provider. Institute safety precautions for individuals with muscle weakness, wasting, or pain that would place them at risk for injury.

Medications. Order the prescribed medications and transcribe orders to the medication administration record (MAR) or enter data in the computer. Thyroid medications are usually scheduled early in the day to prevent insomnia.

Assessment

- Schedule regular assessment of intake and output, vital signs, mental status, and daily weights on the Kardex or computer.
- If surgery is scheduled for hyperthyroidism, schedule routine postoperation vital signs, and order a tracheostomy set for the bedside. Mark the Kardex/care plan/computer to check dressings for bleeding, perform respiratory assessments, perform voice checks for hoarseness, and monitor for development of tetany for first 24 to 48 hours, as ordered by the health care provider. Have calcium gluconate and supplies needed for intravenous (IV) administration ready in the immediate environment.

Implementation

- Implement monitoring parameters for vital signs, intake and output, daily weights, and mental status checks.
- Encourage the patient to comply with dietary orders.
- Give prescribed medications and monitor for response to therapy.
- Provide support and give directions slowly and with patience because the individual may have difficulty processing the information. Incorporate the family into the provision of care, as appropriate.
- Monitor the pattern of bowel elimination and give as-needed (PRN) medications prescribed for diarrhea or constipation.
- Monitor for cardiac symptoms (e.g., heart failure) and for increased susceptibility to infection.

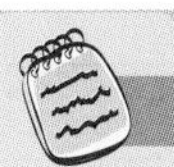

Patient Education and Health Promotion

Medications

- Stress the need for lifelong administration of medications for the treatment of hypothyroidism and the need for periodic laboratory studies and evaluation by the health care provider.
- Stress that several medications interact with thyroid drugs so it is important to inform any prescribing health care provider of the thyroid disease and the medications being taken.
- People scheduled for outpatient diagnostics must receive detailed, written instructions regarding the prescribed medications to be taken in preparation for testing.
- The patient and, as appropriate, family or significant others must understand the anticipated therapeutic response sought from prescribed medications. Teach specific indications of a satisfactory response to pharmacologic therapy. Stress the need to contact the health care provider if signs of an excess or deficit in dosage occur. Ensure that the individual can monitor the resting pulse.

Environment

- Explain the need for a cool environment for a patient with hyperthyroidism; for a warm environment for the person with hypothyroidism.
- Involve the family and significant others in identifying an appropriate home environment that will support the individual's needs until a preillness status is reached.

Nutrition

- In patients with diarrhea secondary to hyperthyroidism, explain the need for a high-calorie diet with reduced roughage.
- Explain the need for a low-calorie diet with increased roughage to the individual with hypothyroidism. Encourage patients with constipation to drink eight to ten 8-ounce glasses of water each day.
- As the patient returns to a more normal thyroid function through medication, the caloric requirements of the diet will also change.

Psychosocial. The patient may have had a major personality change, may be depressed, or (at the other end of the spectrum) may be hyperactive. Explain these symptoms to the family and involve them in examining potential interventions that can be used in the home environment until the individual returns to the pre-illness level of functioning.

Activity and Exercise

- Provide for patient safety during ambulation if muscle weakness, wasting, or discomfort is present. Discuss measures needed to provide for patient safety with family and significant others.
- As the patient returns to a more normal thyroid function through medication, the activity level should change. Encourage moderate exercise.

Fostering Health Maintenance

- Throughout the course of treatment, discuss medication information and how it will benefit the patient. Recognize that nonadherence with lifelong treatment, when prescribed, may occur, and stress positive outcomes that occur with regular medication adherence.
- Provide the patient and significant others with important information contained in the specific drug monograph for the medicines prescribed. Additional health teaching and nursing interventions for the side effects to expect and report are described in the drug monographs.
- Seek cooperation and understanding of the following points so that medication adherence is increased: name of medication, dosage, route and times of administration, side effects to expect, and side effects to report.
- When laboratory studies for thyroid function are scheduled, thyroid preparations may be discontinued for one or more days in advance of the tests. Always consult the physician for detailed instructions.

Written Record. Enlist the patient's aid in developing and maintaining a written record (see Patient Self-Monitoring forms for Thyroid Medications on p. 608 and Antithyroid Medications on p. 609). Complete the Premedication Data for use as a baseline to track response to drug therapy. Ensure that the patient understands how to use the form and instruct the patient to bring the completed form to follow-up visits. During follow-up visits, focus on issues that will foster adherence with the therapeutic interventions prescribed.

DRUG CLASS: Thyroid Replacement Hormones

Actions

Hypothyroidism is treated by replacing the deficient T_3 and T_4 hormones.

PATIENT SELF-ASSESSMENT FORM Thyroid Medications

MEDICATIONS	COLOR	TO BE TAKEN

Patient ____________________

Health Care Provider ____________________

Health Care Provider's phone ____________________

Next appt.* ____________________

What I Should Monitor		Premedication Data	Date	Date	Date	Date	Date	Date	Comments
Pulse									
Temperature									
Weight									
Desire to eat Eat all the time (10) — Normal (5) — None (1)									
Use this scale to rate tolerance of:	Heat								
	Cold								
Cannot tolerate (10) — Moderate toleration (5) — Normal (1)									
Fatigue level Tired all the time (10) — Normal (5) — Not tired: cannot stop (1)									
Skin condition: Dry, leathery; oily; normal									
How I feel about life Feel awful (10) — Getting better (5) — Feel good (1)									
Tolerance for exercise Difficulty breathing with exercise (10) — Normal (5) — Endless energy, no problem (1)									
Sleep pattern Poor (10) — Normal (5) — Excessive (1)									
Menses Excessive (10) — Normal (5) — Scant/absent (1)									
Other									

*Please bring this record with you to your next appointment.
Use the back of this sheet for additional information.

PATIENT SELF-ASSESSMENT FORM Antithyroid Medications

MEDICATIONS	COLOR	TO BE TAKEN

Patient ______

Health Care Provider ______

Health Care Provider's phone ______

Next appt.* ______

What I Should Monitor		Premedication Data	Date	Date	Date	Date	Date	Date	Comments
Pulse									
Temperature									
Weight									
Desire to eat Eat all the time (10) — Normal (5) — None (1)									
Use this scale to rate tolerance of:	Heat								
	Cold								
Cannot tolerate (10) — Moderate toleration (5) — Normal (1)									
Fatigue level Tired all the time (10) — Normal (5) — Not tired: cannot stop (1)									
Skin condition: Dry, leathery; oily; normal									
How I feel about life Feel awful (10) — Getting better (5) — Feel good (1)									
Tolerance for exercise Difficulty breathing with exercise (10) — Normal (5) — Endless energy, no problem (1)									
Sleep pattern Poor (10) — Normal (5) — Excessive (1)									
Menses Excessive (10) — Normal (5) — Scant/absent (1)									
Other									

*Please bring this record with you to your next appointment.
Use the back of this sheet for additional information.

Uses

The primary goal of therapy is to return the patient to a normal thyroid (euthyroid) state. Several forms of thyroid hormone replacement are available from natural and synthetic sources.

Thyroxine (T_4) is one of the two primary hormones secreted by the thyroid gland. It is partially metabolized to triiodothyronine (T_3), so therapy with thyroxine provides physiologic replacement of both hormones. Synthetic levothyroxine (T_4) is now considered to be the drug of choice for hormone replacement in hypothyroidism.

Liothyronine is a synthetic form of the natural thyroid hormone, triiodothyronine, T_3. Its onset of action is more rapid than that of levothyroxine, and it is occasionally used as a thyroid hormone replacement when prompt action is necessary. It is not recommended for patients with cardiovascular disease unless a rapid onset of activity is deemed essential.

Liotrix is a synthetic mixture of levothyroxine and liothyronine in a ratio of 4:1, respectively. A few endocrinologists prefer this combination because of the standardized content of the two hormones that results in consistent laboratory test results, more in agreement with the patient's clinical response.

Thyroid, USP (desiccated thyroid) is derived from pig, beef, and sheep thyroid glands. Thyroid is the oldest thyroid hormone replacement available and the least expensive. Because of its lack of purity, uniformity, and stability, however, it is generally not the drug of choice for the initiation of thyroid replacement therapy.

Therapeutic Outcomes

The primary therapeutic outcome expected from thyroid hormone replacement therapy is return of the patient to a euthyroid metabolic state.

Nursing Process for Thyroid Hormone Replacement Therapy

Premedication Assessment

1. Record baseline vital signs including apical pulse, weight, and bowel elimination patterns before initiating therapy. Establish a once-daily schedule in which these assessments are retaken. Assess for patterns that may indicate early signs of hyperthyroidism (e.g., weight loss, nervousness, diaphoresis, muscle cramps, palpitations, angina pectoris).
2. Ensure that laboratory studies (e.g., thyroid hormone levels) have been completed before administration of the medicine.

Planning

Availability. See Table 37-1.

Implementation

NOTE: The age of the patient, severity of hypothyroidism, and other concurrent medical conditions determine the initial dosage and the interval of time necessary before increasing the dosage. Hypothyroid patients are sensitive to replacement of thyroid hormones. Monitor patients closely for adverse effects.

Dosage and Administration. *Adult:* PO: Therapy may be initiated in low doses of levothyroxine, such as 0.05 to 0.1 mg daily. Dosages are gradually increased over the next few weeks to an average daily maintenance dose of 0.1 to 0.2 mg.

Evaluation

Side Effects to Expect and Report

Signs of Hyperthyroidism. Adverse effects of thyroid replacement preparations are dose related and may occur 1 to 3 weeks after changes in therapy have

Drug Table 37-1 THYROID HORMONES

GENERIC NAME	BRAND NAME	AVAILABILITY	COMPOSITION	DOSAGE RANGE
levothyroxine	Synthroid Levoxyl	Tablets: 0.025, 0.05, 0.075, 0.088, 0.1, 0.112, 0.125, 0.137, 0.15, 0.175, 0.2, 0.3 mg Injection: 200 and 500 mcg/vial in 6 and 10 mL vials	Thyroxine (T_4)	PO: Initial—0.025 mg daily Maintenance—0.1 to 0.2 mg daily
liothyronine	Cytomel	Tablets: 5, 25, 50 mcg Injection: 10 mcg/mL in 1 mL vials	Liothyronine (T_3)	PO: Initial—25 mcg daily; Maintenance—25 to 75 mcg daily
liotrix	Thyrolar	Tablets: 15, 30, 60, 120, 180 mg thyroid equivalents	T_4:T_3 = 4:1	PO: Maintenance—60-180 mg thyroid equivalents daily
thyroid, USP	—	Tablets and capsules: 15, 30, 60, 90, 120, 180, 240, 300 mg	Unpredictable T_4;T_3 ratio	PO: Maintenance—60-180 mg daily

been initiated. Symptoms of adverse effects are tachycardia, anxiety, weight loss, abdominal cramping and diarrhea, cardiac palpitations, dysrhythmias, angina pectoris, fever, and intolerance to heat.

Symptoms may require a reduction or discontinuation of therapy. Patients may require up to a month without medication for toxic effects to fully dissipate.

Therapy must be restarted at lower dosages after symptoms have stopped.

Drug Interactions

Warfarin. Patients with hypothyroidism require increased dosage of anticoagulants. If thyroid replacement therapy is initiated while the patient is receiving warfarin therapy, the patient should have frequent prothrombin time (INR) determinations and should be counseled to observe closely for development of petechiae, ecchymoses, nosebleeds, bleeding gums, dark tarry stools, and bright red or "coffee ground" emesis.

The dosage of warfarin may have to be reduced by one third to one half over the next 1 to 4 weeks.

Digoxin. Patients with hypothyroidism require a decreased dosage of digoxin. If thyroid replacement therapy is started while receiving digoxin, a gradual increase in the glycoside will also be necessary to maintain adequate therapeutic activity.

Estrogens. Patients who have no thyroid function and who start estrogen therapy may require an increase in dosage of the thyroid hormone. Estrogens increase thyroid binding globulin levels, which reduce the level of circulating free T_4. The total level of T_4 is either normal or increased. Do not adjust the thyroid hormone dosage until the patient shows clinical signs of hypothyroidism.

Cholestyramine. To prevent binding of thyroid hormones by cholestyramine, administer doses at least 4 hours apart.

Hyperglycemia. Diabetic or prediabetic patients should be monitored for the development of hyperglycemia, particularly during the early weeks of therapy.

Assess regularly for hyperglycemia or glycosuria and report if it occurs with any frequency.

Patients receiving oral hypoglycemic agents or insulin may require an adjustment in dosage.

DRUG CLASS: Antithyroid Medicines

Iodine-131 (^{131}I)

Actions

The synthesis of thyroid hormones and their maintenance in the bloodstream in adequate amounts depend on sufficient iodine intake through food and water. Iodine is converted to iodide and stored in the thyroid gland before reaching the circulation.

Iodine-131 (^{131}I) is a radioactive isotope of iodine. When administered, it is absorbed into the thyroid gland in high concentrations. The liberated radioactivity destroys the hyperactive thyroid tissue, with essentially no damage to other tissues in the body.

Uses

Radioactive iodine is most commonly used for treating hyperthyroidism in the following individuals: older patients who are beyond the childbearing years, those with severe complicating diseases (e.g., heart disease), those with recurrent hyperthyroidism after previous thyroid surgery, those who are poor surgical risks, and those who have unusually small thyroid glands.

It often takes 3 to 6 months after a dose of radioactive iodine to fully assess benefits gained. Normal thyroid function occurs in about 60% of patients after one dose; the remaining patients require two or more doses. If more than one dose is required, an interval of at least 3 months between doses is required.

Therapeutic Outcomes

The primary therapeutic outcome expected from radioactive iodine is return to a normal thyroid state.

Nursing Process for Radioactive Iodine

Premedication Assessment

1. Review policy for both hospital personnel and the patient regarding precautions, storage, handling, administration, and disposal of radioactive substances.
2. Have all supplies immediately available in case of a spill.
3. Have all supplies needed according to hospital procedure to dispose of patient's excreta.

Planning

Availability. Each dose is prepared for an individual patient from a nuclear pharmacy.

Implementation

Administration of Radioactive Iodine. Administration of radioactive iodine preparations seems simple: it is added to water and swallowed. It has no color or taste. The radiation, however, is extremely dangerous.

- Minimize exposure as much as possible. Wear latex gloves whenever administering radioactive iodine or disposing of the patient's excreta.
- If the radioactive iodine or the patient's excreta should spill, follow hospital policy. In general, collect the clothing, bedding, bedpan, urinal, and any other contaminated materials and place them in special containers for radioactive waste disposal.
- *Avoid spills! Report any accidental contamination at once to your supervisor, and follow directions for hospital contamination cleanup technique.*
- In the event of a spill, complete an incident report.

Evaluation

Side Effects to Expect and Report

Tenderness in the Thyroid Gland. Side effects include radioactive thyroiditis, which causes tenderness over the thyroid area and occurs during the first few days or few weeks after radioactive iodine therapy.

Hyperthyroidism. A return of symptoms of hyperthyroidism occurs in about 40% of patients who received one dose of radioactive iodine. Additional doses may be required.

Hypothyroidism. Some patients who receive radioactive iodine develop hypothyroidism, which requires thyroid hormone replacement therapy.

Drug Interactions

Lithium Carbonate. Lithium and iodine may cause synergistic hypothyroid activity. Concurrent use may result in hypothyroidism. Monitor patients for both hypothyroidism and bipolar disorder.

propylthiouracil (pro pil thy o you' rah sil)
PTU, PROPACIL
methimazole (meth im' ah zohl)
TAPAZOLE (tap' ah zoal)

Actions

Propylthiouracil and methimazole are antithyroid agents that act by blocking synthesis of T_3 and T_4 in the thyroid gland. They do not destroy any T_3 or T_4 already produced, so there is usually a latent period of a few days to 3 weeks before symptoms improve once therapy is started.

Uses

Propylthiouracil and methimazole may be used for long-term treatment of hyperthyroidism or for short-term treatment before subtotal thyroidectomy. Therapy for long-term use is often continued for 1 to 2 years to control symptoms. After discontinuation, some patients gradually return to the hyperthyroid state, and antithyroid therapy must be reinitiated.

Therapeutic Outcomes

The primary therapeutic outcome expected from propylthiouracil or methimazole is gradual return to normal thyroid metabolic function.

Nursing Process for Propylthiouracil and Methimazole

Premedication Assessment

1. Record baseline vital signs, weight, and bowel elimination patterns before initiating therapy. Establish an every-other-day schedule in which these assessments are retaken. Assess for patterns that may indicate early signs of hypothyroidism.
2. Ensure that laboratory studies (e.g., thyroid hormone levels, TSH, complete blood count with differential, blood urea nitrogen [BUN], serum creatinine, liver enzymes) have been completed before administering the medicine.

Planning

Availability. PO: Propylthiouracil: 50 mg tablets. PO: Methimazole: 5 and 10 mg tablets.

Implementation

Dosage and Administration. Adult: Propylthiouracil, PO: initially 100 to 150 mg every 6 to 8 hours. Dosage ranges up to 900 mg daily. The maintenance dosage is 50 mg two or three times daily. Methimazole, PO: initially 5 to 20 mg every 8 hours. Daily maintenance dosage is 5 to 15 mg.

Evaluation

Side Effects to Expect and Report

Purpuric, Maculopapular Rash. The most common reaction (in 5% of all patients) that occurs with propylthiouracil is a purpuric, maculopapular skin eruption. This skin eruption often occurs during the first 2 weeks of therapy and usually resolves spontaneously, without treatment. If pruritus becomes severe, a change to methimazole may be necessary. Cross-sensitivity is uncommon.

Headaches, Salivary Gland and Lymph Node Enlargement, Loss of Taste. These side effects are usually mild and tend to resolve with continued therapy. Encourage the patient not to discontinue therapy without first consulting the health care provider.

Bone Marrow Suppression. Routine laboratory studies (e.g., red blood cell [RBC], white blood cell [WBC], differential counts) should be scheduled. Stress the importance of returning for this laboratory work.

Monitor the patient for the development of a sore throat; fever; purpura; jaundice; or excessive, progressive weakness.

Hepatotoxicity. The symptoms of hepatotoxicity are anorexia, nausea, vomiting, jaundice, hepatomegaly, splenomegaly, and abnormal liver function tests (e.g., elevated bilirubin, aspartate aminotransferase [AST], alanine aminotransferase [ALT], gamma-glutamyltransferase [GGT], alkaline phosphatase, prothrombin time).

Nephrotoxicity. Monitor urinalyses and kidney function tests for abnormal results. Report increased BUN and creatinine, decreased urine output or decreased specific gravity (despite amount of fluid intake), casts or protein in the urine, frank blood or smoky-colored urine, or RBCs in excess of 0 to 3 on the urinalysis report.

Drug Interactions

Warfarin. Patients with hyperthyroidism require reduced dosage of anticoagulants. If antithyroid therapy is initiated while the patient is receiving warfarin therapy, the patient should have frequent prothrombin time determinations and should be counseled to observe closely for development of petechiae, ecchymoses, nosebleeds, bleeding gums, dark tarry stools, and bright red or "coffee ground" emesis.

The dosage of warfarin may have to be increased over the next 1 to 4 weeks.

Digoxin. Patients with hyperthyroidism require an increased dosage of digoxin. If antithyroid replacement therapy is started while receiving digoxin, a gradual reduction in the digoxin will be necessary to prevent signs of toxicity. Monitor for the development of dysrhythmias, bradycardia, increased fatigue, nausea, and vomiting.

Key Points

- Thyroid disease is a relatively common disorder that is easily treated.
- Most therapies require long-term treatment to maintain normal thyroid function.
- Nurses can play a significant role in education and reinforcement of the treatment plan. Best results are attained when the patient, family, and nurse work together in reinforcing the care plan.

Go to your Companion CD-ROM for Appendices, an Audio Glossary, animations, Drug Dosage Calculators, customizable Patient Self-Assessment forms, and Review Questions for the NCLEX® Examination.

evolve Be sure to visit the companion Evolve site at http://evolve.elsevier.com/Clayton for WebLinks and additional online resources.

MEDICATION SAFETY REVIEW

MATH REVIEW QUESTIONS

1. Order: levothyroxine (Synthroid) 0.1 mg, PO, daily
   Available: levothyroxine (Synthroid) 0.05 mg tablets

   Give: _____ tablets.

2. Order: levothyroxine (Synthroid) 200 mcg
   Convert 200 mcg to mg

   ______ mg

CRITICAL THINKING QUESTIONS

1. A patient's baseline vital signs are: BP 140/60 mm Hg, pulse 104, respirations 24. The patient has been receiving levothyroxine (Synthroid) 0.1 mg PO daily for the past 6 weeks for treatment of hypothyroidism, and reports resting pulse, on awakening, has been between 90 and 112 over the past week.

Should these findings be reported to the health care provider and, if so, what additional data should be assembled before initiating physician contact?

2. A patient is taking propylthiouracil 50 mg, PO, tid. What patient education should be provided to her regarding side effects to expect and side effects to report?
3. Research appropriate patient education for a patient having cardiac symptoms who is receiving antithyroid medications.
4. List premedication assessments for thyroid replacement and antithyroid medications.

CONTENT REVIEW QUESTIONS

1. A patient receiving levothyroxine should be monitored for which of these signs and symptoms of overdose?
   1. Bradycardia, weight gain
   2. Cold intolerance, bradycardia
   3. Palpitations, tachycardia, heat intolerance
   4. Sluggish, slow speech; increasing confusion
2. Patients with hyperthyroidism would require a _____ dose of digoxin.
   1. normal
   2. decreased
   3. increased
   4. staggered
3. Propylthiouracil acts by:
   1. converting iodine to active iodine.
   2. blocking synthesis of T_3 and T_4 in the thyroid gland.
   3. destroying T_3 and T_4.
   4. being a synthetic form of thyroid.
4. Special equipment that the nurse places in the patient's room before the patient returns to the surgical unit following a thyroidectomy includes:
   1. a tracheostomy tray.
   2. padded tongue blades.
   3. a closed chest drainage system.
   4. a prefilled syringe of 50% glucose.

Continued

CONTENT REVIEW QUESTIONS—cont'd

5. Congenital hypothyroidism is referred to as:
   1. cretinism.
   2. myxedema.
   3. Graves' disease.
   4. thyrotoxicosis.

6. When administering radioactive iodine, which precautions must the nurse take? *(Select all that apply.)*
   1. Wear gloves.
   2. Place contaminated items with excreta in regular laundry bags.
   3. Report spills to supervisor immediately.
   4. Wear a radioactive suit when administering medication.

7. The action of radioactive iodine is to:
   1. destroy the hyperactive thyroid tissue.
   2. block synthesis of T_3 and T_4.
   3. replace deficient hormones.
   4. destroy the thyroid gland.

8. Patients with hyperthyroidism require _____ dosages of anticoagulants.
   1. increased
   2. reduced
   3. normal
   4. staggered

CHAPTER

38 Corticosteroids

evolve http://evolve.elsevier.com/Clayton

Chapter Content

Objectives

1. Review the functions of the adrenal gland.
2. State the normal actions of mineralocorticoids and glucocorticoids in the body.
3. Cite the disease states caused by hypersecretion or hyposecretion of the adrenal gland.
4. Identify the baseline assessments needed for a patient receiving corticosteroids.
5. Prepare a list of the clinical uses of mineralocorticoids and glucocorticoids.
6. Discuss the potential side effects associated with the use of corticosteroids, and give examples of specific patient education needed for the patient who will be taking these agents.
7. Develop measurable objectives for patient education for people taking corticosteroids.

Key Terms

corticosteroids
mineralocorticoids
glucocorticoids
cortisol

CORTICOSTEROIDS

Corticosteroids are hormones secreted by the adrenal cortex of the adrenal gland. Corticosteroids are divided into two categories based on structure and biologic activity. The **mineralocorticoids** (fludrocortisone and aldosterone) maintain fluid and electrolyte balance and are used to treat adrenal insufficiency caused by hypopituitarism or Addison's disease. The **glucocorticoids** (cortisone, hydrocortisone, prednisone, and others) regulate carbohydrate, protein, and fat metabolism. Glucocorticoids have antiinflammatory, antiallergenic, and immunosuppressant activity. (See p. 620 for clinical uses of glucocorticoids.)

NURSING PROCESS *for Corticosteroid Therapy*

Assessment

The minimum assessment data for a patient receiving corticosteroids include baseline weight, blood pressure, and results of electrolyte and glucose studies. Monitoring of all aspects of intake, output, diet, electrolyte balance, and state of hydration is important to the long-term success of corticosteroid therapy.

Although many of the parameters used for assessment may initially be normal, it is important that a baseline for these parameters be established so that they may be used to monitor steroid therapy.

History

- Ask the patient to describe the current problems that initiated this visit or admission.
- How long have the symptoms been present?
- Is this a recurrent problem? If so, how has it been treated?
- If an infectious process is suspected, determine when the patient was last tested for tuberculosis.

History of Pain Experience. See the nursing process for pain management, Chapter 20, p. 319.

Medication History. Obtain a detailed history of all prescribed and over-the-counter medications (including herbal medicines). Ask if the patient understands why each is being taken. Ask specifically whether corticosteroids have been taken within the past year, and for what purpose. Tactfully determine if the prescribed medications are being taken regularly and if not, why not?

Central Nervous System

- *Mental status:* A patient receiving a higher dosage of corticosteroids is susceptible to psychotic behavioral changes. The most susceptible patient is one with previous histories of mental dysfunction. Perform a baseline assessment of the patient's ability to respond rationally to the environment and the diagnosis of the underlying disease. Check for orientation to date, time, and place and assess for level of confusion, restlessness, or irritability. Make regularly scheduled mental status evaluations and compare the findings.
- *Anxiety:* What degree of apprehension is present? Did stressful events precipitate the anxiety?

History of Ulcers. Patients receiving corticosteroid therapy have higher incidences of peptic ulcer disease.

Ask the patient about any previous treatment for an ulcer, heartburn, or stomach pain. Periodic testing of stools for occult blood may be ordered.

Physical Assessment

- *Blood pressure:* Take a baseline blood pressure reading in the sitting, lying, and standing positions. Because patients receiving corticosteroids accumulate fluid and gain weight, hypertension may develop.
- *Temperature:* Record temperature daily, and monitor more frequently if elevated. Patients receiving corticosteroids are more susceptible to infection, and fever is often an early indicator of infection. Glucocorticoids, however, sometimes suppress a febrile response to infection.
- *Weight and fat distribution:* Obtain the patient's weight on admission and use as a baseline in assessing therapy. Because patients receiving corticosteroids have a tendency to accumulate fluid and gain weight, the daily weight is an important tool in assessing ongoing therapy. Observe for any changes in the distribution of fat and for any muscle weakness or muscle wasting.
- *Pulse:* Record the rate, quality, and rhythm of the pulse.
- *Heart and lung sounds:* Nurses with advanced skills can perform auscultation and percussion to note changes in heart size and heart and lung sounds. (Consult a medical-surgical nursing textbook for details in performing these assessments.) Lung fields are assessed in a sitting position to detect abnormal lung sounds (e.g., wheezes, rales, crackles, and accumulation of fluid).
- *Skin color:* Note the color of the skin, mucous membranes, tongue, earlobes, and nailbeds. Note in particular the development of a rash or the development of ecchymoses (bruises).
- *Neck veins:* Record any jugular vein distention. This may be an indication of fluid overload.

Status of Hydration

- *Dehydration:* Assess and record significant signs of dehydration in the patient. Observe for the following signs: poor skin turgor, sticky oral mucous membranes, a shrunken or deeply furrowed tongue, crusted lips, weight loss, deteriorating vital signs, soft or sunken eyeballs, weak pedal pulses, delayed capillary filling, excessive thirst, high urine specific gravity (or no urine output), and possible mental confusion.
- *Skin turgor:* Check skin turgor by gently pinching the skin together over the sternum, forehead, or on the forearm. In the well-hydrated patient elasticity is present and the skin rapidly returns to a flat position. With dehydrated patients, the skin remains pinched or peaked and returns very slowly to the flat, normal position.
- *Oral mucous membranes:* When adequately hydrated, the membranes of the mouth feel smooth and glisten. In dehydrated patients, they are sticky and appear dull.
- *Laboratory changes:* The values of the hematocrit, hemoglobin, blood urea nitrogen (BUN), and electrolytes will appear to fluctuate, based on the state of hydration. A dehydrated patient will show higher values as a result of hemoconcentration. When a patient is overhydrated, the values appear to drop because of hemodilution.
- *Overhydration:* Increased abdominal girth and circumference of the medial malleolus, weight gain, and neck vein engorgement are indications of overhydration. Measure the abdominal girth daily at the umbilical level. Measure the extremities bilaterally every day, approximately 5 cm above the medial malleolus.
- *Edema:* Is edema present? Where is it located? Is it pitting or nonpitting? It may be an indicator of fluid and electrolyte imbalance.

Laboratory Tests

- Patients taking corticosteroids are particularly susceptible to the development of electrolyte imbalance. Physiologically, corticosteroids cause sodium retention (hypernatremia) and potassium excretion (hypokalemia).
- Patients most likely to develop electrolyte disturbances are those who, in addition to receiving corticosteroids, have histories of renal or cardiac disease, hormonal disorders, massive trauma or burns, or are on diuretic therapy.
- Review laboratory tests and report abnormal results to the health care provider promptly. Tests may include serum electrolytes, especially sodium, potassium, calcium, and magnesium; arterial blood gases; electrocardiogram (ECG); chest x-ray; urinalysis and kidney function, and hemodynamic assessments.
- Because the symptoms of most electrolyte imbalances are similar, the nurse should assess changes in the patient's mental status (alertness, orientation, and confusion), muscle strength, muscle cramps, tremors, nausea, and general appearance.

Nutrition. Obtain a history of the patient's diet. Ask questions regarding appetite and the presence of nausea and vomiting. Anorexia, nausea, and vomiting are early indications of corticosteroid insufficiency.

Hyperglycemia. Corticosteroid therapy may induce hyperglycemia, particularly in prediabetic or diabetic patients. All patients must be monitored for the development of hyperglycemia, especially during the early weeks of therapy. Assess regularly for glycosuria and blood glucose, and report frequent occurrences.

Activity and Exercise

- Ask questions to obtain information about the effect of exercise on the patient's functioning.

- Is the person normally sedentary, moderately active, or very active?
- Has there been a reduction in activity level to cope with associated fatigue or dyspnea?
- Are the activities of daily living being performed by the person?

Nursing Diagnoses

- Activity intolerance (indication)
- Fluid volume, excess (indication)
- Pain, acute or chronic (indication)
- Tissue perfusion, ineffective (indication)
- Injury, risk for (side effects)

Planning

History of Illness. If an infectious disease process is suspected and tuberculosis testing is planned, it should be performed before initiating corticosteroid therapy.

Medication History. Review prescription medications as well as over-the-counter medicines (including herbal medications) being taken, and establish whether they are being taken correctly. Analyze nonadherence issues and plan interventions with the patient. Plan to review drug administration as needed.

Medication Administration

- Glucocorticoids may cause hyperglycemia, necessitating the monitoring of blood glucose levels at appropriate intervals. If elevated, insulin therapy may be required. Initiate a diabetic flow sheet, and mark the medication administration record (MAR) or computer to clearly identify the insulin orders.
- During steroid replacement therapy, the administration schedule for the replacement drugs should mimic the body's normal circadian rhythm. Therefore glucocorticoids ordered twice daily are usually scheduled with two thirds of the dose administered before 9:00 AM (usually with breakfast) and one third of the dose in the late afternoon (usually with dinner). Alternate-day therapy is also used in some instances to maintain a more normal body rhythm. Mineralocorticoids are usually given once daily in the evening.
- Steroid replacement therapy is gradually discontinued in small increments (tapered) to ensure that the patient's adrenal glands are able to start secreting steroids appropriately as the drug dosage is reduced.

Central Nervous System. Plan for stress reduction education and discussion of effective means of coping with stressful events. Note on the Kardex or computer file to monitor patient's mental status every shift.

Fluid Volume Status. Plan to monitor intake and output at intervals appropriate to the patient's condition. Report intake that exceeds output.

Nutritional History. Examine the dietary history to determine if referral to a nutritionist would help the patient understand the diet regimen. Plan interventions needed to deal with dietary nonadherence.

Laboratory Tests. Order stat and subsequent laboratory studies.

Implementation

Medications. Order medications prescribed, and schedule these on the MAR. Corticosteroids should be scheduled to be taken with food. Perform focused assessments to determine effectiveness and side effects of pharmacologic interventions. Monitor for hyperglycemia.

Pain Management. When pain is present, comfort measures must be implemented to allow the patient to decrease the pain. Fatigue may increase pain perception; spacing activities so that fatigue does not occur is recommended. Maintain a flow sheet of pain ratings and evaluate for the effectiveness of medications in the management of pain.

Central Nervous System

- Perform neurologic assessment to determine changes in mental status.
- Deal calmly with an anxious patient; offer explanations of procedures being performed; listen to concerns and intervene appropriately.

Vital Signs and Status of Hydration

- Monitor vital signs and perform focused assessment of heart, respiratory, and hydration status at specified intervals.
- Perform daily weights using the same scale, in clothing of approximately the same weight, and at the same time, usually before breakfast. Record and report significant weight changes. (Weight gains and losses are the best indicators of fluid gain or loss.) As appropriate to patient's condition, obtain and record abdominal girth measurements.
- When fluid restrictions are prescribed, one half of fluids is generally given with meals. The other half is given on a per-shift basis.
- Monitor the rate of intravenous (IV) infusions carefully; contact the health care provider regarding concentration of admixtures of drugs to IV infusion solution when limited fluids are indicated.

Nutrition. Schedule meetings with the nutritionist to learn how to manage specific dietary modifications prescribed (e.g., a low-sodium, high-potassium diet with weight reduction parameters for obese patients). If possible, instruct the patient to practice food selections from the daily menus while still in the hospital. The nurse can then offer guidance. Teach the patient which foods are low in sodium and high in potassium. Potassium restrictions may be indicated if the patient is taking a potassium-sparing diuretic. Salt substitutes are high in potassium; therefore use must be limited.

Laboratory Studies. Check for and report abnormal laboratory values (e.g., hypokalemia, hyperkalemia, hypoglycemia, hyperglycemia, hyponatremia, hypernatremia), depending on the underlying disease pathology.

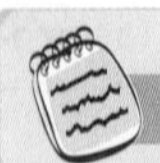

Patient Education and Health Promotion

Contact with Health Care Provider's Office

- Assess the patient's understanding of symptoms that should be reported to the health care provider: dyspnea; productive cough; worsening fatigue; edema in the feet, ankles, or legs; weight gain; or development of angina (chest pain), palpitations, or confusion.
- Instruct the patient to perform daily weights using the same scale, in clothing approximately the same weight, and at the same time, usually before breakfast. Record and report significant weight changes; weight gains and losses are the best indicators of fluid gain or loss. Usually a gain of 2 pounds in 2 days should be reported.

Skin Care. Teach appropriate skin care and the need to change positions at least every 2 hours, especially when edema is present. Have the patient inspect the ankles, feet, and abdomen for edema daily. If the patient is using a recliner or bed, the sacral area should also be checked regularly for edema.

Coping with Stress

- Patients receiving high doses of corticosteroids do not tolerate stress well. Patients should be instructed to notify the health care provider before exposure to additional stress, such as dental procedures. If a patient sustains an accidental injury or sudden emotional stress, the attending health care provider should be notified that the patient is receiving steroid therapy. An additional steroid dose may be needed to support the patient through a stressful situation.
- Explore the mechanisms the person uses to cope with stress. Discuss how the patient is adapting to the needed lifestyle changes to manage the disease process. Address depression issues, if present.

Avoid Infections. Advise the patient to avoid crowds or people known to have infections. Report even minor signs of an infection (e.g., general malaise, sore throat, low-grade fever) to the physician.

Nutritional Status

- Assist the patient in developing a specific schedule for spacing daily fluid intake and planning sodium restrictions, as prescribed by the physician.
- If weight gain is a specific problem (not related to fluid accumulation), plan for calorie restrictions and spacing of daily intake.
- If a high-potassium diet is prescribed, help the patient become familiar with foods that should be consumed. Teach the signs and symptoms of potassium deficiency or excess, depending on medications prescribed.
- Further dietary needs may include increases in vitamin D and calcium.
- Fluid restrictions may be imposed; discuss specific ways to manage these limitations.

Activity and Exercise

- Participation in regular exercise is essential. The patient may resume activities of daily living within the boundaries set by the health care provider. Encourage such activities as regular and moderate exercise, meal preparation, resumption of usual sexual activity, and social interactions. Help the patient plan for appropriate alterations, depending on the disease process and degree of impairment.
- Encourage weight-bearing measures to prevent calcium loss. Active and passive range-of-motion exercises maintain mobility and joint and muscle integrity.
- Individuals unable to attain the degree of activity anticipated as a result of drug therapy may become frustrated. Allow for verbalization of feelings, and then implement actions appropriate to the circumstances.

Fostering Health Maintenance

- Throughout the course of treatment, discuss medication information and how the medication will benefit the patient.
- Drug therapy is one component of the treatment of illnesses for which steroids are prescribed; it is critical that the medications be taken as prescribed. Ensure that the patient understands the entire medication regimen including the importance of not adjusting the dosage without health care provider approval. If corticosteroid therapy is to be discontinued, a tapering schedule is used. Stress the importance of not suddenly withdrawing the prescribed medication.
- Patients on steroid therapy should carry identification cards or a bracelet with the name of the health care provider to contact in an emergency, as well as the drug name, dosage, and frequency of use. Emphasize situations requiring health care provider consultation for drug dosage adjustments (e.g., stress, dental procedures, infection).
- Provide the patient and significant others with the important information contained in the specific drug monograph for the drugs prescribed. Additional health teaching and nursing interventions for drug side effects to expect and report are in each drug monograph.
- Seek cooperation and understanding of the following points so that medication adherence is increased: name of medication, dosage, route and times of administration, side effects to expect, and side effects to report.

Written Record. Enlist the patient's aid in developing and maintaining a written record of monitoring parameters (e.g., pulse rate, blood pressure, body weight, edema, exercise tolerance, pain relief) (see the Patient Self-Monitoring form on p. 619). Instruct the patient to take this written record to follow-up visits. ■

PATIENT SELF-ASSESSMENT FORM Corticosteroids

MEDICATIONS	COLOR	TO BE TAKEN

Patient ____________________

Health Care Provider ____________________

Health Care Provider's phone ____________________

Next appt.* ____________________

What I Should Monitor		Premedication Data	Date	Date	Date	Date	Date	Date	Comments
Weight									
Blood pressure									
Pulse rate									
Notify doctor of sudden stress in life (e.g., surgery, injury, trauma, death in family or of friend)									
Pain relief No relief — Improved — No pain 10 — 5 — 1									
Assessment of how I feel Good — Improved — Bad 10 — 5 — 1									
Breast tenderness	None								
	Occasionally uncomfortable								
	Increasing								
Hair distribution	No changes seen								
	Hair growth increased: Site ________								
Edema	Swelling noted (where) ________								
	Time of day swelling occurs?								
Other									

*Please bring this record with you to your next appointment.
Use the back of this sheet for additional information.

DRUG THERAPY WITH CORTICOSTEROIDS

DRUG CLASS: Mineralocorticoids

fludrocortisone (flu droh kort′ ih sown)
▶ FLORINEF (flohr′ in ehf)

Actions

Fludrocortisone is an adrenal corticosteroid with potent mineralocorticoid and glucocorticoid effects. It affects fluid and electrolyte balance by acting on the distal renal tubules, causing sodium and water retention and potassium and hydrogen excretion.

Uses

Fludrocortisone is used in combination with glucocorticoids to replace mineralocorticoid activity in patients who suffer from adrenocortical insufficiency (Addison's disease) and to treat salt-losing adrenogenital syndrome.

Therapeutic Outcomes

The primary therapeutic outcomes expected from fludrocortisone therapy are as follows:

- Control of blood pressure.
- Restoration of fluid and electrolyte balance.

Nursing Process for Fludrocortisone

Premedication Assessment

1. Check the electrolyte reports for early indications of electrolyte imbalance.
2. Keep accurate records of intake and output, daily weights, and vital signs.
3. Ask the patient about any signs of infection (e.g., sore throat, fever, malaise, nausea, vomiting). Corticosteroid therapy can mask symptoms of infection.
4. Perform a baseline assessment of the patient's degree of alertness; orientation to name, place, and time; and rationality of responses.
5. Ask the patient about previous treatment for an ulcer, heartburn, or stomach pain. Testing stools for occult blood should be done periodically.

Planning

Availability. PO: 0.1 mg tablets.

Implementation

Dosage and Administration. *Adult:* PO: 0.1 mg daily. Dosage may be adjusted as needed. Cortisone or hydrocortisone also is usually administered to provide additional glucocorticoid effect.

Evaluation

Because fludrocortisone is a natural hormone, side effects reflect fludrocortisone excess, such as sodium accumulation and potassium depletion.

Side Effects to Expect and Report. See Glucocorticoids.

Drug Interactions. See Glucocorticoids.

DRUG CLASS: Glucocorticoids

Actions

The major glucocorticoid of the adrenal cortex is cortisol. The hypothalamic-pituitary axis regulates the secretion of cortisol by increasing or decreasing the output of corticotropin-releasing factor (CRF) from the hypothalamus. CRF stimulates the release of adrenocorticotropic hormone (ACTH) from the pituitary gland; ACTH then stimulates the adrenal cortex to secrete cortisol. As serum levels of cortisol increase, the amount of CRF secreted by the hypothalamus is decreased, resulting in diminished secretion of cortisol from the adrenal cortex.

Uses

Glucocorticoids are usually given because of their anti-inflammatory and antiallergenic properties. They do not cure disease, but relieve the symptoms of tissue inflammation. When used to control rheumatoid arthritis, symptom relief is noted within a few days. Joint and muscle stiffness, muscle tenderness and weakness, joint swelling, and soreness are significantly reduced. However, it is important to assess the patient's predrug activity level because pain relief may lead to overuse of the diseased joints. Appetite, weight, and energy are increased; fever is reduced; and sedimentation rates are reduced or return to normal. Anatomic changes and joint deformities already present remain unchanged. Symptoms usually return shortly after glucocorticoid withdrawal.

Glucocorticoids are also effective for immunosuppression in the treatment of certain cancers, organ transplantation, autoimmune diseases (e.g., lupus erythematosus, dermatomyositis, rheumatoid arthritis), relief of allergic manifestations (e.g., serum sickness, severe hay fever, status asthmaticus), and treatment of shock. They also may be used to treat nausea and vomiting secondary to chemotherapy (see Chapter 34).

Therapeutic Outcomes

The primary therapeutic outcomes expected from glucocorticoid therapy are as follows:

- Reduced pain and inflammation.
- Minimized shock syndrome and faster recovery.
- Reduced nausea and vomiting associated with chemotherapy.

Nursing Process for Glucocorticoids

Premedication Assessment

1. Check the electrolyte and glucose reports for early indications of electrolyte imbalance or hyperglycemia.
2. Keep accurate records of intake and output, daily weights, and vital signs.
3. Ask the patient about any signs of infection (e.g., sore throat, fever, malaise, nausea, vomiting). Corticosteroid therapy can mask symptoms of infection.
4. Perform a baseline assessment of the patient's degree of alertness; orientation to name, place, and time; and rationality of responses.
5. Ask the patient about previous treatment for an ulcer, heartburn, or stomach pain. Testing stools for occult blood should be done periodically.

Planning

Availability. See Table 38-1.

Implementation

NOTE: Glucocorticoids are potent agents that produce many undesirable side effects as well as therapeutic benefits. Unless immediate, life-threatening conditions exist, other therapeutic methods should be exhausted before corticosteroid therapy is initiated. Many of the side effects of the steroids are related to dosage and duration of therapy.

These drugs must be used with caution in patients with diabetes mellitus, heart failure, hypertension, peptic ulcer disease, mental disturbance, and suspected infections.

Dosage and Administration. NOTE: When a therapeutic dosage is administered for 1 week or longer, it must

Drug Table 38-1 CORTICOSTEROID PREPARATIONS*

GENERIC NAME	BRAND NAME	DOSAGE FORMS
alclometasone	Aclovate	Cream, ointment
amcinonide	Cyclocort	Cream, ointment, lotion
betamethasone	Celestone, Valisone, Diprosone, Luxiq, others	Tablets, syrup, injection, cream, ointment, lotion, aerosol, gel, foam, powder
clobetasol	Temovate, Embeline E	Cream, ointment, scalp application, lotion
clocortolone	Cloderm	Cream
cortisone	Cortisone	Tablets
desonide	Tridesilon, DesOwen	Cream, ointment, lotion
desoximetasone	Topicort	Cream, ointment, gel
dexamethasone	Decadron, Dexone, Hexadrol, Decaspray	Cream, aerosol, injection, tablets, elixir
diflorasone	Florone, Maxiflor, Psorcon E	Cream, ointment
fludrocortisone	Florinef	Tablets
fluocinolone	Synalar, Flurosyn	Cream, ointment, solution, shampoo, oil
fluocinonide	Lidex	Cream, ointment, gel, solution
flurandrenolide	Cordran	Cream, ointment, tape, lotion
fluticasone	Cutivate	Cream, ointment
halcinonide	Halog, Halog E	Cream, ointment, solution
halobetasol	Ultravate	Cream, ointment
hydrocortisone	Cortef, Solu-Cortef, Hydrocortone	Cream, ointment, tablets, enema, gel, lotion, suppositories, injection, oral suspension, spray
methylprednisolone	Solu-Medrol, Depo-Medrol, Medrol	Tablets, injection, powder
mometasone	Elocon, Asmanex, Nasonex	Cream, ointment, lotion, spray, inhalant
prednicarbate	Dermatop E	Cream, ointment
prednisolone	Prelone	Injection, tablets, syrup, suspension, solution
prednisone	Deltasone, Orasone, ✤ Apo-Prednisone	Tablets, solution
triamcinolone	Aristocort, Kenalog, Nasacort HFA	Cream, ointment, lotion, injection, tablets, syrup, aerosol, paste, inhalant, spray

*Ophthalmic products, Chapter 41; nasal inhalation products, Chapter 30.
✤ Available in Canada.

be assumed that the internal production of corticosteroids is suppressed. Abrupt discontinuation of glucocorticoids may result in adrenal insufficiency. Therapy should be withdrawn gradually (often called a "steroid taper"). The time required to decrease glucocorticoids depends on the duration of treatment, the dosage amount, the mode of administration, and the glucocorticoid being used.

- *Abrupt discontinuation:* Patients who have received corticosteroids for at least 1 week must not abruptly discontinue therapy. Symptoms of abrupt discontinuation include fever, malaise, fatigue, weakness, anorexia, nausea, orthostatic dizziness, hypotension, fainting, dyspnea, hypoglycemia, muscle and joint pain, and possible exacerbation of the disease process.

- *Application:* Topical corticosteroids are applied as directed by the manufacturer. Specific instructions regarding use of an occlusive dressing should be clarified before application.
- *Alternate-day therapy:* Alternate-day therapy may be used to treat chronic conditions. Corticosteroids are usually given between 6:00 AM and 9:00 AM on alternate days to minimize suppression of normal adrenal function. Administer with meals to minimize gastric irritation.
- *Pediatric patients:* The correct dosage for a child is usually based on the disease being treated rather than the patient's weight. Monitoring of skeletal growth may be required in children if prolonged therapy is required.

Evaluation

Side Effects to Expect and Report

Electrolyte Imbalance, Fluid Accumulation. The electrolytes most commonly altered are potassium (K^+), sodium (Na^+), and chloride (Cl^-). Hypokalemia is most likely to occur.

Many symptoms associated with altered fluid and electrolyte balance are subtle and interspersed with general symptoms of drug toxicity or the disease process itself.

Obtain data about changes in the patient's mental status (alertness, orientation, and confusion), muscle strength, muscle cramps, tremors, nausea, and general appearance (drowsy, anxious, or lethargic).

Always check the electrolyte reports for early indications of electrolyte imbalance.

Keep accurate records of intake and output, daily weights, and vital signs.

Susceptibility to Infection. Always question the patient before initiation of therapy about any signs and symptoms of possible infection. Corticosteroid therapy often masks symptoms of infection.

Monitor the patient for signs of infection such as sore throat, fever, malaise, nausea, and vomiting.

Encourage the patient to avoid exposure to infections.

Behavioral Changes. Psychotic behaviors are more likely to occur in patients with previous histories of mental instability.

Perform a baseline assessment of the patient's degree of alertness; orientation to name, place, and time; and rationality of responses *before* initiating therapy. Make regularly scheduled mental status evaluations, and compare the findings. Report the development of alterations.

Hyperglycemia. Diabetic or prediabetic patients must be monitored for the development of hyperglycemia, particularly during the early weeks of therapy.

Assess regularly for glycosuria and blood glucose and report any frequent occurrences.

Patients receiving oral hypoglycemic agents or insulin may require an adjustment in dosage.

Peptic Ulcer Formation. Before initiating therapy, ask the patient about any previous treatment for an ulcer, heartburn, or stomach pain.

Periodic testing of stools for occult blood may be ordered. Antacids may also be recommended by the physician to minimize gastric symptoms.

Delayed Wound Healing. Surgical sites of patients who have recently had surgery must be monitored closely for signs of dehiscence.

Teach surgical patients to splint the wounds while coughing and breathing deeply.

Inspect surgical sites and report statements such as, "When I coughed, I felt something pop."

Visual Disturbances. Visual disturbances noted by patients on long-term therapy must be reported. Glucocorticoid therapy may produce cataracts.

Drug Interactions

Diuretics (e.g., Furosemide, Bumetanide, Thiazides). Corticosteroids may enhance the loss of potassium. Check potassium levels and monitor the patient more closely for hypokalemia when these agents are used concurrently.

Many symptoms of altered fluid and electrolyte balance are subtle and interspersed with general symptoms of drug toxicity or the disease process itself.

Gather data about changes in the patient's mental status (alertness, orientation, and confusion), muscle strength, muscle cramps, tremors, nausea, and general appearance (drowsy, anxious, and lethargic).

Always check the electrolyte reports for early indications of electrolyte imbalance.

Keep accurate records of intake and output, daily weights, and vital signs.

Warfarin. Steroids may enhance or decrease the anticoagulant effects of warfarin. Observe for the development of petechiae, ecchymoses, nosebleeds, bleeding gums, dark tarry stools, and bright red or "coffee ground" emesis. Monitor the prothrombin time (INR), and adjust the dosage of warfarin if necessary.

Because of the ulcerogenic potential of steroids, close observation of patients taking anticoagulants is necessary to reduce the possibility of hemorrhage.

Hyperglycemia. Diabetic or prediabetic patients must be monitored for the development of hyperglycemia, particularly during the early weeks of therapy.

Assess regularly for hyperglycemia or glycosuria, and report any frequent occurrences.

Patients receiving oral hypoglycemic agents or insulin may require an adjustment in dosage.

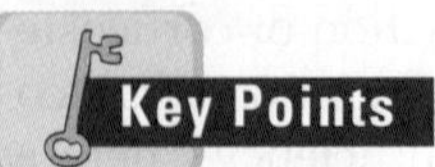

- Corticosteroids are potent agents that produce many therapeutic benefits as well as undesirable side effects.
- Many of the side effects of the steroids are related to dosage and duration of therapy. These drugs must be

used with caution in patients with diabetes mellitus, heart failure, hypertension, peptic ulcer disease, mental disturbance, and suspected infections.
- Nurses can play a significant role in helping patients monitor therapy and can assist them in seeking medical attention at the earliest signs of impending trouble.

Go to your Companion CD-ROM for Appendices, an Audio Glossary, animations, Drug Dosage Calculators, customizable Patient Self-Assessment forms, and Review Questions for the NCLEX® Examination.

evolve Be sure to visit the companion Evolve site at http://evolve.elsevier.com/Clayton for WebLinks and additional online resources.

MEDICATION SAFETY REVIEW

MATH REVIEW QUESTIONS

The package insert accompanying prednisone states that the physiologic replacement dose (pediatric) is 0.1 to 0.15 mg/kg/day PO in equal divided doses q12h. The child's weight is 22 pounds.

1. 22 lb = _____ kg

Using the dosage parameters described, calculate the minimum and maximum dosage per day for this child's weight.

2. _____ mg minimum
3. _____ mg maximum

CRITICAL THINKING QUESTIONS

1. A patient is receiving prednisone for treatment of hypercalcemia associated with cancer. He tells you, with great excitement, that his young grandchildren are coming to stay at his home for the next several months. What precautions should be taught to him and immediate family members regarding exposure to the grandchildren, especially during times when pediatric immunizations may be being received?
2. What data would indicate a positive clinical response after administration of adrenal cortical hormones prescribed for the treatment of Addison's disease?
3. Summarize the premedication assessments needed before administering mineralocorticoids or glucocorticoids.

CONTENT REVIEW QUESTIONS

1. Patients receiving a corticosteroid should be questioned regarding any history of:
   1. ulcers.
   2. blood dyscrasias.
   3. heart disease.
   4. respiratory disease.
2. Fludrocortisone (Florinef) is used for:
   1. inflammatory processes.
   2. allergic reactions.
   3. severe itching and hives.
   4. mineralocorticoid replacement.
3. The use of alternate-day administration of corticosteroids is to:
   1. minimize the suppression of normal adrenal activity.
   2. maximize the effects on the electrolytes.
   3. reduce likelihood of hypokalemia.
   4. reduce potential for cataract development.
4. Symptoms of abrupt discontinuation of glucocorticoids may result in:
   1. adrenal insufficiency.
   2. adrenal oversecretion.
   3. pituitary insufficiency.
   4. pituitary oversecretion.
5. In diabetic or prediabetic patients, corticosteroid therapy may induce:
   1. hypoglycemia.
   2. hyperglycemia.
   3. insulin resistance.
   4. no effects.
6. What two types of electrolyte imbalances are corticosteroids most likely to cause?
   1. Hyperkalemia and hyponatremia
   2. Hypokalemia and hypernatremia
   3. Hypercalcemia and hypermagnesemia
   4. Hypocalcemia and hypomagnesemia
7. Steroid replacement therapy should be gradually discontinued in small increments to:
   1. ensure that the patient's adrenal glands are able to start secreting steroids appropriately.
   2. lessen the risk of side effects.
   3. maintain a more normal body rhythm.
   4. decrease the risk of electrolyte imbalance.

CHAPTER

39 Gonadal Hormones

evolve http://evolve.elsevier.com/Clayton

Chapter Content

Objectives

1. Describe the body changes that can be anticipated with the administration of androgens, estrogens, or progesterone.
2. State the uses of estrogens and progestins.
3. Compare the side effects seen with the use of estrogen hormones with those seen with a combination of estrogen and progesterone.
4. Differentiate between the side effects to expect and those requiring consultation with the physician that occur with the administration of estrogen or progesterone.
5. Identify the rationale for administering androgens to women who have certain types of breast cancer.

Key Terms

gonads	**ovaries**
testosterone	**estrogen**
androgens	**progesterone**

THE GONADS AND GONADAL HORMONES

The **gonads** are the reproductive glands: the testes of the male and the ovaries of the female. In addition to producing sperm, the testes produce **testosterone,** the male sex hormone. Testosterone controls the development of the male sex organs and influences characteristics such as voice, hair distribution, and male body form. **Androgens** are other steroid hormones that produce masculinizing effects.

The **ovaries** produce estrogen and progesterone. These are hormones that stimulate maturation of the female sex organs. They influence breast development, voice quality, and the broader pelvis of the female body form. Menstruation is established because of the hormone production of the ovaries. **Estrogen** is responsible for most of these changes. **Progesterone** is thought to be associated mainly with body changes that favor the implantation of the fertilized ovum, continuation of pregnancy, and preparation of the breasts for lactation.

NURSING PROCESS *for Gonadal Hormones*

Assessment

History. Ask the patient to describe the current problems that initiated this visit. How long have the symptoms been present? Is this a recurrent problem? If so, how was it treated?

Reproductive History. Ask the patient to describe the following, as appropriate: age of menarche; usual pattern of menses (i.e., duration, number of pads used, last menstrual period); number of pregnancies, live births, miscarriages, and abortions; vaginal discharges, itching, infections, and how treated; and breast self-examination routine (if not being performed regularly, explain the correct procedure). Male patients should be asked whether testicular self-examinations are performed (if not being performed regularly, explain the correct procedure). As appropriate, obtain information regarding impotence, sterility, or alterations in libido.

History of Prior Illnesses. Any indication of hypertension, heart or liver disease, thromboembolic disorders, or cancers of the reproductive organs is of particular concern.

Medication History. Obtain a detailed history of all prescribed medicines, including oral contraceptives, over-the-counter medications, including herbal medicines (e.g., dong quai, black cohosh) and any street drugs (e.g., "muscle-building" steroids). Ask patients if they understand why each is being taken. Tactfully determine if the prescribed medications are being taken regularly and if not, why not?

Smoking History. Does the person smoke?

Physical Examination

- A complete physical examination is usually done as part of the preliminary workup before treatment of any disorders using gonadal hormones. With children and adolescent patients, include questions to collect data regarding growth and development (note in particular the development of long bones), changes in hair growth and distribution, and the size of genitalia.
- Record basic patient data: height, weight, and vital signs. Blood pressure readings are of particu-

lar concern so that recordings on future visits can be evaluated for any change.
- Collect urine for urinalysis and blood samples for hemoglobin, hematocrit, measurement of gonadotropic hormones, and other laboratory studies deemed appropriate by the health care provider. Usually, patients with family histories of diabetes mellitus should be tested for hyperglycemia before starting gonadal hormone therapy.
- The physical examination for a female patient should include a breast examination and a pelvic examination including a Papanicolaou test. Observe the distribution of body hair and the presence of scars. Stress the need for periodic physical examinations while receiving gonadal hormones.

Psychosocial. Patients requiring androgen therapy may need to be encouraged to discuss feelings relating to sexuality, sterility, or altered libido.

Nursing Diagnoses
- Fluid volume, excess (side effect)
- Body image, disturbed (side effect)

Planning
- Most gonadal hormones are prescribed to patients for prolonged self-administration. Therefore planning should stress patient education specific to the type of gonadal hormone prescribed and its intended actions, including monitoring of side effects to expect and side effects to report. Ensure that the individual understands the dosage and specific time schedule for administration of the prescribed medication.
- Schedule follow-up health care provider visits and laboratory studies. Always note on laboratory slips that a patient is receiving estrogen.
- Plan to teach the individual to monitor vital signs and to weigh himself/herself daily.

Implementation
- Obtain baseline data for subsequent evaluation of therapeutic response to therapy (e.g., weight, vital signs, and blood pressure in sitting, lying, and standing positions).
- Assist with the physical examination.

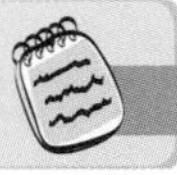

Patient Education and Health Promotion

Expectations of Therapy. Discuss the expectations of therapy with the patient (e.g., degree of pain relief, frequency of use of therapy, relief of menopausal symptoms, sexual maturation, regulation of menstrual cycle, sexual activity, maintenance of mobility, activities of daily living and/or work).

Smoking. Explain the risks of continuing to smoke, especially when the patient is receiving estrogen or progestin therapy. (The incidence of fatal heart attacks is increased for women more than 35 years of age.)

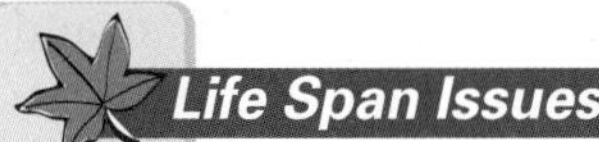

Life Span Issues

Diabetes Mellitus

Patients with diabetes mellitus who receive gonadal hormones may experience alterations in the blood glucose levels. Parameters should be established and a written record for glucose monitoring maintained for reporting to the physician or health care provider.

Physical Examination. Stress the need for regular periodic medical examinations and laboratory studies.

Fostering Health Maintenance
- Discuss medication information and how it will benefit the course of treatment to produce an optimal response.
- Seek cooperation and understanding of the following points so that medication adherence is increased: name of medication, dosage, route and times of administration, side effects to expect, and side effects to report. If taking estrogen for the purpose of delaying the advancement of osteoporosis, it is important to adhere to the regimen to achieve the maximum effect.

Written Record. Enlist the patient's aid in developing and maintaining a written record of monitoring parameters (e.g., blood pressure, pulse, daily weight, degree of pain relief, menstrual cycle information, breakthrough bleeding, nausea, vomiting, cramps, breast tenderness, hirsutism, gynecomastia, masculinization, hoarseness, headaches, sexual stimulation) (see Patient Self-Assessment form in Appendix I). Complete the Premedication Data column for use as a baseline to track response to drug therapy. Ensure that the patient understands how to use the form and instruct the patient to take the completed form to follow-up visits. During follow-up visits, focus on issues that will foster adherence with the therapeutic interventions prescribed.

DRUG THERAPY WITH GONADAL HORMONES

DRUG CLASS: Estrogens

Actions

The natural estrogenic hormone released from the ovaries comprises several closely related chemical compounds: estradiol, estrone, and estriol. The most potent is estradiol. It is metabolized to estrone, which is half as potent. Estrone is further metabolized to estriol, which is considerably less potent. Estrogens are responsible for the development of the sex organs during growth in the uterus and for maturation at puberty. They are also responsible for characteristics such as growth of hair, texture of skin, and distribution of body fat. Estrogens also affect the release of pituitary gonadotropins; cause capillary dilatation, fluid retention, and protein metabolism; and inhibit ovulation and postpartum breast engorgement.

Uses

Estrogen products are used for relieving the hot flash symptoms of menopause; for contraception; for hormone replacement therapy after an oophorectomy; in conjunction with appropriate diet, calcium, and physical therapy in the treatment of osteoporosis; for treatment of severe acne in females; and to slow the disease progress (and minimize discomfort) in patients with advanced prostatic cancer and certain types of breast cancer.

Therapeutic Outcomes

The primary therapeutic outcomes expected from estrogen therapy are as follows:

- Contraception.
- Hormonal balance.
- Prevention of osteoporosis.
- Palliative treatment of prostate and breast cancer.
- Treatment of severe acne in females.

Nursing Process for Estrogen Therapy

Premedication Assessment

1. Determine whether the patient is pregnant before starting estrogen therapy; withhold the medicine and consult the physician if there is a possibility of pregnancy.
2. Obtain baseline weight and vital signs, especially accurate blood pressure readings.
3. Ask whether the individual has a history of thromboembolic disorders or cancer of the reproductive organs; if so, hold medication and contact the health care provider.

Planning

Availability. See Table 39-1.

Implementation

NOTE: The use of estrogens during early pregnancy is contraindicated. Serious birth defects have been reported, and it has been found that the female offspring have an increased risk of developing vaginal or cervical cancer later in life.

Drug Table 39-1 ESTROGENS

GENERIC NAME	BRAND NAME	AVAILABILITY	USES	DOSES
Conjugated estrogen	Premarin	Tablets: 0.3, 0.45, 0.625, 0.9, 1.25 mg	Menopause	PO: 0.625-1.25 mg daily cyclically*
		IV: 25 mg/5-mL vial	Atrophic vaginitis	PO: 0.3-1.25 mg daily cyclically*
	✤ C.E.S.	Cream: 0.625 mg/g	Female hypogonadism	PO: 0.3-0.625 mg daily for 20 days, followed by 10 days off
			Ovarian failure or post-oophorectomy	PO: 1.25 mg daily cyclically*
			Osteoporosis	PO: 0.625 mg daily cyclically*
			Breast carcinoma	PO: 10 mg three times daily
			Prostatic carcinoma	PO: 1.25-2.5 mg three times daily
Esterified estrogen	Menest	Tablets: 0.3, 0.625, 1.25, 2.5 mg	Menopause, atrophic vaginitis	PO: 0.3-1.25 mg daily cyclically*
			Female hypogonadism, postoophorectomy, ovarian failure	PO: 1.25-7.5 mg daily cyclically*
			Breast carcinoma	PO: 10 mg three times daily
			Prostatic carcinoma	PO: 1.25-2.5 mg three times daily
estradiol	Estrace	Tablets: 0.45, 0.5, 1, 1.5, 1.8, 2 mg Injections: Cypionate in oil: 5 mg/mL	Menopause, atrophic vaginitis, hypogonadism, postoophorectomy, ovarian failure	PO: 1-2 mg daily cyclically* IM: Cypionate: 1-5 mg every 3-4 weeks Valerate: 10-20 mg every 4 weeks
		Valerate in oil: 10, 20, 40 mg/mL Cream: vaginal	Prostatic carcinoma	PO: 1-2 mg three times daily IM: Valerate: 30 mg every 1-2 weeks
			Breast carcinoma	PO: 10 mg three times daily

*Cyclically = 3 weeks of daily estrogen followed by 1 week off.
†Alora, Estraderm, Esclim, Vivelle, Vivelle-Dot are applied 2 times weekly. Climara and Menostar are applied once weekly.
✤ Available in Canada.

Drug Table 39-1 ESTROGENS—cont'd

GENERIC NAME	BRAND NAME	AVAILABILITY	USES	DOSES
estradiol—cont'd	Vivelle†	Transdermal patch: 0.014, 0.025, 0.0375, 0.05, 0.06, 0.075, 0.1 mg	Menopause Female hypogonadism Primary ovarian failure Atrophic vaginitis Postoophorectomy Prevention of osteoporosis	Transdermal system†: a patch should be placed on a clean, dry area of the skin on the trunk (usually abdomen or buttock) twice weekly on a cyclic schedule (3 weeks of therapy followed by 1 week without). Rotate application site; interval of 1 week between uses of same site.
	Estrasorb	Topical emulsion: 4.35 mg/pouch	Menopause	Topical: Apply contents of 1 pouch to left leg and 1 pouch to right leg daily. Rub from upper thigh area to ankles. Allow to dry. Wash hands with soap and water. If uterus is intact, progestin should also be taken to prevent endometrial cancer.
	Estrogel	Topical gel: 0.06% in tube or pump	Menopause; vaginal atrophy	Topical: Apply contents of 1 applicator or 1 pump daily to 1 arm, spreading from wrist to upper arm on all sides. Allow to dry. Wash hands with soap and water. If uterus is intact, progestin should also be taken to prevent endometrial cancer. Alcohol gel is flammable until dry; avoid fire, flame, or smoking until dry.
estropipate	Ogen	Tablets: 0.625, 1.25, 2.5, 5 mg	Menopause, atrophic vaginitis	PO: 0.625-6 mg daily cyclically*
		Cream: Vaginal	Female hypogonadism, postoophorectomy, ovarian failure	PO: 1.25-9 mg daily cyclically*
			Osteoporosis prevention	PO: 0.75 mg daily cyclically*
ethinyl estradiol	Estinyl	Tablets: 0.02, 0.05, 0.5 mg	Menopause	PO: 0.625 mg daily cyclically*
			Female hypogonadism	PO: 0.02-0.05 mg daily cyclically* PO: 0.05 one to three times daily for 2 weeks followed by 2 weeks of progesterone
			Breast carcinoma	PO: 1 mg three times daily
			Prostatic carcinoma	PO: 0.15-2 mg daily

Dosage and Administration. See Table 39-1.

Evaluation

Side Effects to Expect

Weight Gain, Edema, Breast Tenderness, Nausea. These symptoms tend to be mild and resolve with continued therapy. If they do not resolve or become particularly bothersome, the patient should consult a physician.

Side Effects to Report

Hypertension, Hyperglycemia, Thrombophlebitis, Breakthrough Bleeding, Any Other Symptoms the Patient Recognizes as Being of Concern. These are all complications associated with estrogen therapy. It is extremely important that the patient is evaluated by the health care provider to consider alternative therapy.

Drug Interactions

Warfarin. This medication may diminish the anticoagulant effects of warfarin. Monitor the prothrombin time (INR) and increase the dosage of warfarin if necessary.

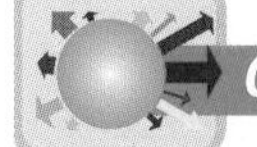

Clinical Landmine

Use of Gonadal Hormones during Pregnancy

The use of estrogens during early pregnancy is contraindicated. Serious birth defects have been reported, and it has been found that the female offspring have an increased risk of developing vaginal or cervical cancer later in life. The use of progestins in early pregnancy has been associated with birth defects. If pregnancy is suspected, the physician should be consulted immediately.

Phenytoin. Estrogens may inhibit the metabolism of phenytoin, resulting in phenytoin toxicity.

Monitor patients with concurrent therapy for signs of phenytoin toxicity (e.g., nystagmus, sedation, lethargy). Serum levels may be ordered, and a reduced dosage of phenytoin may be required.

Thyroid Hormones. Patients who have no thyroid function and who start estrogen therapy may require an increase in thyroid hormone dosage. Estrogens increase thyroid binding globulin levels, which reduce the level of circulating free T_4. The total level of T_4 is either normal or increased. Do not adjust the thyroid dosage until the patient shows clinical signs of hypothyroidism.

DRUG CLASS: Progestins

Actions

Progesterone and its derivatives (the progestins) inhibit the secretion of pituitary gonadotropins, preventing maturation of ovarian follicles and thus inhibiting ovulation.

Uses

Progestins are used primarily to treat secondary amenorrhea, breakthrough uterine bleeding, and endometriosis, but they may also be used in combination with estrogens as contraceptives. (See the section on oral contraceptives in Chapter 41.)

Therapeutic Outcomes

The primary therapeutic outcomes expected from progestin therapy are as follows:

- Contraception.
- Relief of symptoms of endometriosis.
- Hormonal balance to relieve amenorrhea or abnormal uterine bleeding.

Nursing Process for Progestins

Premedication Assessment

1. Determine whether the patient is pregnant before starting progestin therapy; hold the medicine and consult the physician if there is a possibility of pregnancy.
2. Obtain baseline weight and vital signs, especially accurate blood pressure readings.
3. Ask whether the individual has a history of thromboembolic disorders or cancer of the reproductive organs; if so, withhold medication and contact the health care provider.

Planning

Availability. See Table 39-2.

Implementation

NOTE: The use of progestins in early pregnancy has been associated with birth defects. If pregnancy is suspected, the health care provider should be consulted immediately.

Dosage and Administration. See Table 39-2.

Evaluation

Side Effects to Expect

Weight Gain, Edema, Nausea, Vomiting, Diarrhea, Tiredness, Oily Scalp, Acne. These symptoms tend to be mild and resolve with continued therapy. If they do not resolve or become particularly bothersome, instruct the patient to consult the health care provider.

Side Effects to Report

Breakthrough Bleeding, Amenorrhea, Continuing Headache, Cholestatic Jaundice, Mental Depression. These are all complications associated with progestin therapy. It is extremely important that the patient is evaluated by the health care provider to consider alternatives in therapy.

Pregnancy. Because of the possibility of birth defects, a health care provider should be consulted immediately.

Drug Table 39-2 PROGESTINS

GENERIC NAME	BRAND NAME	AVAILABILITY	USES	DOSES
hydroxyprogesterone	Hylutin	Injection: 125, 250 mg/mL	Amenorrhea; abnormal uterine bleeding	IM: 375 mg
medroxyprogesterone	Provera, Amen, Curretab	Tablets: 2.5, 5, 10 mg	Secondary amenorrhea Abnormal uterine bleeding	PO: 5-10 mg daily for 5-10 days PO: 5-10 mg daily for 5-10 days, beginning on the 16th or 21st day of the menstrual cycle
norethindrone	Aygestin	Tablets: 5 mg	Amenorrhea, abnormal uterine bleeding Endometriosis	PO: 2.5-10 mg starting with the 20th and ending on the 25th day of the menstrual cycle PO: 5 mg for 2 weeks; increase in increments of 2.5 mg/day every 2 weeks until 15 mg/day is reached
norgestrel	Ovrette	Tablets: 0.075 mg	Oral contraceptive	PO: 1 tablet daily
progesterone	Progesterone	Injection: 50 mg/mL Vaginal gel 4%, 8%	Amenorrhea, functional uterine bleeding	IM: 5-10 mg for 6-8 consecutive days

Drug Interactions

Rifampin. Rifampin may enhance the metabolism of progestins. The dosage of progestins may need to be increased to provide therapeutic benefit.

DRUG CLASS: Androgens

Actions

The dominant male sex hormone is testosterone. It is the primary natural androgen produced by the testicles. Androgens are responsible for the normal growth and development of male sex organs and for maintenance of secondary sex characteristics. These effects include the growth and maturation of the prostate, seminal vesicles, penis, and scrotum; the development of male hair distribution; laryngeal enlargement (Adam's apple); vocal cord thickening; alterations in body musculature; and fat distribution.

Uses

Androgens are used to treat hypogonadism, eunuchism, androgen deficiency, and palliation of breast cancer in postmenopausal women with certain cell types of cancer. When androgens are used for palliation of cancer in women, they suppress cancer cell growth.

Therapeutic Outcomes

The primary therapeutic outcomes expected from androgen therapy are as follows:

- Restoration of hormonal balance in androgen deficiency.
- Reduced discomfort associated with breast cancer.

Nursing Process for Androgens

Premedication Assessment

1. Obtain baseline vital signs and weight, and assess mental status.
2. Check baseline electrolyte values; report abnormal findings. Be especially alert for hypercalcemia.
3. Identify baseline glucose levels for individuals initiating androgen therapy who are taking insulin or oral hypoglycemic agents since the use of androgens may cause hypoglycemia.

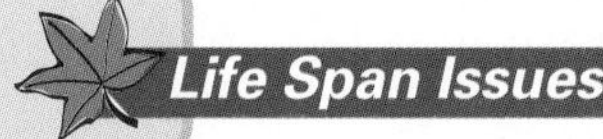

Androgens

Male children receiving androgens must have the effects of the drug on long bones monitored by periodic x-ray of long bones. Usually, x-rays of long bones are performed every 3 to 6 months to check the status of the epiphyseal line. Androgens may prematurely close the epiphyseal line, preventing bone elongation.

Planning

Availability. See Table 39-3.

Implementation

Dosage and Administration. See Table 39-3.

Evaluation

Side Effects to Expect

Gastric Irritation. If gastric irritation occurs, administer drug with food or milk. If symptoms persist or increase in severity, report for physician evaluation.

Side Effects to Report

Electrolyte Imbalance, Edema. The most commonly altered electrolytes are potassium (K^+), sodium (Na^+), and chloride (Cl^-). Hyperkalemia is most likely to occur.

Many symptoms associated with altered fluid and electrolyte balance are subtle and interspersed with general symptoms of drug toxicity or the disease process itself.

Gather data about changes in the patient's mental status (e.g., alertness, orientation, confusion), muscle strength, muscle cramps, tremors, nausea, and general appearance (e.g., drowsy, anxious, lethargic).

Always check the electrolyte reports for early indications of electrolyte imbalance.

Keep accurate records of intake and output, daily weights, and vital signs.

Patients should report weight gains of more than 2 pounds per week. Diuretic therapy, with or without dietary reduction of salt, may be prescribed if edema is significant.

Masculinization. Women receiving high doses of androgens may develop signs of masculinization. Women should be monitored for signs of masculinization (e.g., deepening of the voice, hoarseness, growth of facial hair, clitoral enlargement, and menstrual irregularities) during androgen therapy. The drug should usually be discontinued when mild masculinization is evident because some adverse androgenic effects (e.g., voice changes) may not reverse with discontinuation of therapy. In consultation with the health care provider, the woman may decide that some masculinization is acceptable during treatment for carcinoma of the breast. Help patients adjust to a possible change in self-image or self-esteem caused by the effects of masculinization.

Males should be carefully monitored for the development of gynecomastia, priapism, or excessive sexual stimulation. These are indications of androgen overdose.

Hypercalcemia. In immobilized patients and patients with breast cancer, androgen therapy may cause hypercalcemia. Monitor patients for nausea, vomiting, constipation, poor muscle tone, and lethargy. These are indications of hypercalcemia and are indications for discontinuation of androgen therapy.

Drug Table 39-3 ANDROGENS

GENERIC NAME	BRAND NAME	AVAILABILITY	USES	DOSES
SHORT-ACTING				
testosterone gel	AndroGel 1%, Testim	Topical gel 1%	Hypogonadism	Topical: Open one or more hormone packets (depending on dosage), squeeze entire contents onto palm of hand and apply to clean, dry, intact skin of shoulders, upper arms, and abdomen. Allow to dry prior to dressing. Wash hands with soap and water. Do not apply to genitals.
testosterone USP in gel base	Androderm Transdermal System; Testoderm TTS	Transdermal patch: 12.5, 25 mg	Androgen deficiency	Transdermal system: 1-3 patches applied to skin, on hips, abdomen, thighs, or buttocks nightly for 24 hours; replace every 24 hours; do not apply to scrotum
	Testoderm	Transdermal patch: 4, 6 mg	Androgen deficiency	Transdermal system: Shave scrotal area. Apply a 4 or 6 mg patch to the scrotum once daily at about the same time each day. Apply to clean, dry skin. Do not apply to other skin surfaces. The drug is poorly absorbed from other tissues.
LONG-ACTING				
testosterone pellets	Testopel	Pellets: 75 mg	Hypogonadism; delayed puberty	Subcutaneous: 2 to 6 pellets implanted subcutaneously every 3 to 6 months
testosterone enanthate	Delatestryl	IM: 200 mg/mL	Eunuchism, androgen deficiency Oligospermia	IM: 200-400 mg every 4 weeks IM: 100-200 mg every 4-6 weeks
testosterone cypionate	Depo-Testosterone	IM: 100, 200 mg/mL	As for testosterone enanthate	As for testosterone enanthate
ORAL PRODUCTS				
testosterone	Striant	Buccal system: 30 mg	Hypogonadism	PO: 1 buccal system applied to the gum above the incisor tooth every 12 hours. Alternate with opposite side for each new dose. When applying, hold the rounded surface against the gum for 30 sec to ensure adhesion. Do not chew or swallow.
methyltestosterone	Methitest, Testred, Virilon	Tablets: 10, 25 mg Capsules: 10 mg Buccal tablets: 10 mg	Eunuchism Cryptorchidism Breast carcinoma	PO: 10-40 mg daily PO: 30 mg daily PO: 50-200 mg daily
fluoxymesterone		Tablets: 10 mg	Male hypogonadism Female breast carcinoma	PO: 2-10 mg daily PO: 10-40 mg daily

Force fluids to minimize the possibility of renal calculi. Encourage the patient to drink eight to twelve, 8-ounce glasses of water daily.

Perform weight-bearing and active and passive exercises to the degree tolerated by the patient to minimize loss of calcium from bones.

Hepatotoxicity. The symptoms of hepatotoxicity are anorexia, nausea, vomiting, jaundice, hepatomegaly, splenomegaly, and abnormal liver function test results (e.g., elevated bilirubin, aspartate aminotransferase [AST], alanine aminotransferase [ALT], gamma-glutamyltransferase [GGT], alkaline phosphatase, prothrombin time).

Drug Interactions

Warfarin. Androgens may enhance the anticoagulant effects of warfarin. Observe for the development of petechiae, ecchymoses, nosebleeds, bleeding gums, dark tarry stools, and bright red or "coffee ground" emesis. Monitor the prothrombin time (INR), and reduce the dosage of warfarin if necessary.

Oral Antidiabetic Agents, Insulin. Monitor for hypoglycemia: headache, weakness, decreased coordination, general apprehension, diaphoresis, hunger, and blurred or double vision. The dosage of the hypoglycemic agent or insulin may need to be reduced. Notify the health care provider if any of the aforementioned symptoms appear.

Corticosteroids. Concurrent use may increase the possibility of electrolyte imbalance and fluid retention. See earlier in this chapter for monitoring parameters.

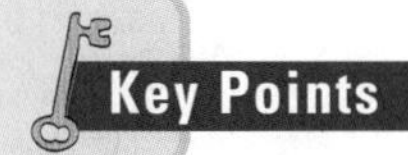

- The gonadal hormones are necessary for the body to grow and mature into the adult form and for reproduction.
- Male and female gonads secrete hormones. The male testes secrete predominantly androgens, and the female ovaries secrete primarily estrogens and progesterone.
- These hormones are responsible for the shape and secondary sex characteristics associated with the male and female body form.

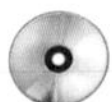

Go to your Companion CD-ROM for Appendices, an Audio Glossary, animations, Drug Dosage Calculators, customizable Patient Self-Assessment forms, and Review Questions for the NCLEX® Examination.

evolve Be sure to visit the companion Evolve site at http://evolve.elsevier.com/Clayton for WebLinks and additional online resources.

MEDICATION SAFETY REVIEW

MATH REVIEW QUESTIONS

1. Order: hydroxyprogesterone 375 mg IM
   Available: hydroxyprogesterone 250 mg/mL
   Give: _____ mL.
2. Order: progesterone 10 mg IM daily for 6 days
   Available: progesterone 50 mg/mL
   Give: _____ mL.

CRITICAL THINKING QUESTIONS

1. A 62-year-old patient is receiving methyltestosterone 200 mg PO daily for palliation of breast cancer. She asks you why she is taking this particular medication and expresses concern that this medication, like other medications she has taken for treatment of the cancer, will make her feel ill. What should you tell her?
2. Identify premedication assessments used with androgens, progestins, and estrogens. Distinguish among the intended actions of androgens, progestins, and estrogens.

CONTENT REVIEW QUESTIONS

1. Androgens, when given to an immobilized patient or a patient with breast cancer, may result in development of:
   1. hypertension.
   2. fluid loss and dehydration.
   3. feminization.
   4. hypercalcemia.
2. Androgens given to male children may result in:
   1. hypercalcemia.
   2. premature closure of epiphyseal line.
   3. delayed closure of epiphyseal line.
   4. developmental delay.

Continued

CONTENT REVIEW QUESTIONS—cont'd

3. Conjugated estrogen (Premarin) is prescribed during menopause for:
   1. amenorrhea.
   2. breast cancer.
   3. hot flashes.
   4. breakthrough uterine bleeding.

4. An action of progestin is to:
   1. inhibit ovulation.
   2. promote ovulation.
   3. promote growth of secondary sex characteristics.
   4. treat prostatic cancer.

5. If symptoms of masculinization occur after taking androgen therapy, the drug should be:
   1. monitored.
   2. decreased.
   3. discontinued.
   4. continued.

6. Which of the following medications may be affected by estrogen therapy? *(Select all that apply.)*
   1. warfarin
   2. phenytoin
   3. digoxin
   4. Thyroid hormones

7. Which of the following medications may be affected by androgen therapy? *(Select all that apply.)*
   1. warfarin
   2. phenytoin
   3. Oral antidiabetic medication
   4. Corticosteroids

40 Drugs Used in Obstetrics

evolve http://evolve.elsevier.com/Clayton

Chapter Content

Objectives

1. Describe nursing assessments and nursing interventions needed for the pregnant patient during the first, second, and third trimesters of pregnancy.
2. Identify appropriate nursing assessments, nursing interventions, and treatment options used for the following obstetric complications: infection, hyperemesis gravidarum, miscarriage, abortion, preterm labor, premature rupture of membranes, gestational diabetes, and pregnancy-induced hypertension.
3. State the methods and time parameters of each approach to the termination of a pregnancy.
4. Summarize the care needs of the pregnant woman during labor and delivery and the immediate postpartum period including the patient education needed before discharge to promote safe self-care and care of the newborn.
5. State the purpose of administering glucocorticoids to certain women in preterm labor.
6. State the actions, primary uses, nursing assessments, and monitoring parameters for uterine stimulants, uterine relaxants, clomiphene citrate, magnesium sulfate, and $Rh_0(D)$ immune globulin.
7. Compare the effects of uterine stimulants and uterine relaxants on a pregnant woman's uterus.
8. Describe specific nursing concerns and appropriate nursing actions when uterine stimulants are administered for induction of labor, augmentation of labor, and postpartum atony and hemorrhage.
9. Cite the effects of adrenergic agents on beta-1 and beta-2 receptors, then identify the relationship of these actions to the side effects to report when adrenergic agents are used to inhibit preterm labor.
10. Describe specific assessments needed before and during the use of terbutaline or magnesium sulfate.
11. Identify emergency supplies that should be available during magnesium sulfate therapy.
12. Identify the action, specific dosage, administration precautions, and proper timing of the administration of $Rh_0(D)$ immune globulin and rubella vaccine.
13. Summarize the immediate nursing care needs of the newborn following delivery.

Key Terms

pregnancy-induced hypertension (PIH)
lochia
precipitous labor and delivery
augmentation
dysfunctional labor

OBSTETRICS

NURSING PROCESS *for Obstetrics*

Assessment

Assessment of the Pregnant Woman

Prenatal Visit. Obtain basic historical information about the woman and family concerning diseases, surgeries, and deaths.

- Has the patient been treated for kidney or bladder problems; high blood pressure; heart disease; rheumatic fever; hypothyroidism or hyperthyroidism; diabetes mellitus; allergies to any foods, drugs, or environmental substances; or sexually transmitted diseases?
- Has the patient been exposed to any communicable diseases since becoming pregnant?
- Has the patient received blood or blood products?
- Does the patient smoke?

If the woman answers yes to any of these questions, find out what health care provider made the diagnosis, when the disorder occurred, and how the disorder was treated. Request the approximate date of the last Papanicolaou (Pap) test and results.

Gather data about menstrual pattern (e.g., age of initial onset, duration and frequency of monthly periods, date of last full menstrual cycle, any bleeding since the last full menstrual period) and contraceptive use (e.g., condoms, foam, diaphragm, sponge, oral contraceptives, intrauterine devices).

Take an obstetric history. Ask the woman if she had any previous live births, stillbirths, miscarriages, or induced abortions. If any of the deliveries were premature, obtain additional information about the infant's age of gestation, survival of the child, suspected causes, and infections. Have any of the births required a cesarean section? If yes, why?

Ask if $Rh_o(D)$ immune globulin (RhoGAM) has been received for Rh factor incompatibility.

Nutritional History

- What is the patient's usual weight? How much weight has she gained or lost in the past 3 months?
- What are the woman's favorite foods? Are there any foods she avoids? How often does she eat? What has she eaten in the past 3 days? Does she normally take a daily vitamin, minerals, or herbal products?
- Are there any cultural food practices to be maintained during the pregnancy?

Elimination Pattern

- What is the patient's elimination pattern?
- How often does she have bowel movements?
- What is the stool consistency and color?
- Is there any bleeding?
- Are laxatives ever needed? If so, how often?

Psychosocial Culture History. Determine how the woman feels about this pregnancy (e.g., excited, nervous, or if the baby is unwanted). Determine cultural patterns regarding prenatal care (e.g., language spoken, activities that she cannot do while pregnant, and whether she prefers a female caregiver). Ask the pregnant woman what specific cultural practices she would like to follow during the pregnancy.

Who makes up her support group: husband, boyfriend, friends, family, tribal healer?

Ask about her employment status and what type of work she performs.

Determine the woman's level of education, economic status, and general interest in learning more about effective management of the pregnancy. Will referral to social services agencies be necessary?

Medication History. Ask the woman if she takes any prescribed, over-the-counter (OTC) medications, or herbal remedies. If she is not currently taking any medications, ask whether any have been taken over the past 6 months. Determine which have been prescribed and for what purpose.

Determine the use of alcohol or street drugs of any kind, including what, how much, and how frequently.

Physical Examination. Assist the woman to undress and prepare for examination, including a pelvic examination and Pap smear.

- *Height and weight:* Record height and weight. (See an obstetric textbook for a detailed guide to all aspects of a prenatal visit and the initial assessments performed.)
- *Hypertension:* Take the blood pressure. Ask if any treatment has been given for high blood pressure. If so, inquire about the onset, treatment, and degree of control achieved.
- *Heart rate:* At prenatal visits, count the pulse for 1 full minute. Report irregularities in rate, rhythm, or volume. On subsequent visits, anticipate an increase in rate of approximately 10 beats per minute during the course of the pregnancy.
- *Respirations:* Record the rate of respirations. As the pregnancy progresses, observe for hyperventilation and thoracic breathing.
- *Temperature:* If the temperature is elevated, ask about any signs of infection or exposure to people with known communicable diseases.
- *Laboratory and diagnostic studies:* Obtain a urine specimen using the clean-catch method.
- Blood samples for complete blood count (CBC), hemoglobin, hematocrit, hemoglobin electrophoresis, rubella titer, Rh factor, and sexually transmitted diseases (STDs) (e.g., syphilis, gonorrhea, chlamydia) may be ordered at this initial visit. Blood tests may include an antibody, sickle cell, and thalassemia screen; folic acid level; and, as appropriate, purified protein derivative (PPD), human immunodeficiency virus (HIV), hepatitis B screen, and toxicology screen. With a history of diabetes mellitus, hypertension, or renal disease, additional laboratory testing may be ordered (e.g., 1-hour glucose tolerance, creatinine clearance, total protein excretion).

Assessment during First, Second, and Third Trimesters. Assessment done at routine visits during the pregnancy includes: weight; measurement of blood pressure, pulse, and respirations; and examination of the abdomen with measurement of fundal height and fetal heart sounds. Any problems or concerns should be discussed. Hemoglobin and hematocrit may be periodically rechecked.

The pregnant woman who does not experience complications is usually examined monthly for the first 6 months, every 2 weeks in the seventh and eighth months, and weekly during the last month. Vaginal examinations are usually performed on the initial visit and are not repeated until 2 to 3 weeks before the estimated date of confinement (EDC), or due date, at which time the cervical status, degree of engagement, and fetal presentation are evaluated. A sonogram may be done in early pregnancy.

Assessment of the Pregnant Patient at Risk

- Assess for signs and symptoms of potential obstetric complications (see an obstetrics text for further details of each complication): infection, hyperemesis gravidarum, miscarriage, abortion, preterm labor, premature rupture of membranes (PROM), gestational diabetes, and pregnancy-induced hypertension, intrauterine fetal death, and HELLP (hemolysis, elevated liver enzymes, and low platelet count) syndrome.
- *Infection:* Record the temperature. Report any elevations to the health care provider immediately for further evaluation. As appropriate obtain urine for urinalysis.

- *Hyperemesis gravidarum:* Obtain details of persistent, severe vomiting.
- *Miscarriage, placental separation, abortion:* Assess for signs of bleeding. Gather specific information about the onset, duration, volume (number of pads used), and color, and report any clots or tissue.
- Ask the patient to describe any pain experienced. Has she had any backache or pelvic cramping, sharp abdominal pain, faintness, or pain in the shoulder area?
- Vital signs should be taken and compared with baseline data whenever bleeding is suspected. Assess for development of shock: restlessness, perspiration, pallor, clammy skin, dyspnea, tachycardia, and blood pressure changes. Record fetal heart tones at regular intervals.
- *Preterm labor:* Preterm labor is defined as:
  - Labor occurring after 20 and before 37 completed weeks of gestation; plus
  - Clinically documented uterine contractions (4/20 minutes or 6/60 minutes); plus
  - Ruptured membranes; or
  - Intact membranes and cervical dilation greater than 2 cm; or
  - Intact membranes and cervical effacement greater than 80%; or
  - Intact membranes and cervical change during observation. These can be measured by changes in dilation or effacement, or by changes in cervical length measured clinically, or by ultrasound.

Assess the status of the fetus (Figure 40-1) by fetal movement counts, contraction stress testing, biophysical profile, and ultrasonography for placental placement and measurement of maturity indicators. An amniocentesis may be performed to assess fetal lung maturity. Home uterine activity monitoring (HUAM) using a tocodynamometer may be used to detect excessive uterine contractions.

A fetal fibronectin test may be ordered to assess the presence of preterm labor in patients whose presenting symptoms are questionable, so that early intervention (e.g., tocolytic therapy, corticosteroids, transport to a tertiary center) can be initiated when indicated or, if negative, avoid unnecessary interventions. This test is for women with intact membranes and cervical dilation of less than 3 cm. This test detects preterm labor from 24 to 34 weeks' gestation. If the test is negative, the patient is highly unlikely to experience preterm delivery in the next 7 to 14 days.

- *Premature rupture of membranes:* Assess for and obtain specifics of any signs of leakage of amniotic fluid from the vagina.
- *Gestational diabetes:* Review urinalysis reports for glycosuria. Review history of symptoms, especially during previous pregnancies. Review 1- and 3-hour glucose tolerance test results.
- *Pregnancy-induced hypertension:* Assess for and report sudden hypertension (an elevation of systolic pressure 30 mm Hg or more above prior readings, systolic blood pressure of 140 mm Hg or more, or diastolic pressure of 90 mm Hg or more). **Pregnancy-induced hypertension (PIH)** includes preeclampsia (elevated blood pressure, proteinuria) and eclampsia (convulsions accompanying preeclampsia).
- Assess for edema of any body parts (e.g., fingers, hands, face, legs, ankles). Assess hydration status, and, in particular, obtain daily weights.

The status of the fetus may be assessed by fetal movement counts, contraction stress testing, biophysical profile, and ultrasonography for placental placement and measurement of maturity indicators. Amniocentesis may be performed to assess fetal lung maturity and detect fetal disorders.

Review laboratory reports for indications of abnormal electrolytes, elevated uric acid or hematocrit levels, thrombocytopenia, and the presence of red blood cells (RBCs) and protein in the urine.

- Assess for signs and symptoms of seizure activity.
- Monitor fetal heart rate and movements.
- Assess for start of labor or signs of other complications such as pulmonary edema, disseminated intravascular coagulation (DIC), heart failure, abruptio placentae, or cerebral hemorrhage.

When giving magnesium sulfate for PIH, assess deep tendon reflexes, respiratory status (report depression), sedation level, intake and output, seizure precautions, and cardiac status. (Always have calcium gluconate, the antidote for magnesium sulfate, available.)

Assessment during Normal Labor and Delivery

History of Pregnancy. On admission to the hospital, obtain the following information:

- Name and age
- Obstetric history: gravida, para, abortions, fetal deaths, birthweight of previous children, and complications during previous deliveries
- Estimated due date, estimated gestational age, and day of last menstrual period (LMP)
- Prenatal care: type and amount, any significant problems
- Prenatal education: type and extent of childbirth preparation
- Plan for infant feeding
- Status of membranes: intact, ruptured, time ruptured, amount, and color of fluid that escaped
- Status of labor: time of onset of contractions, frequency, duration and intensity, how patient is coping with contractions
- Time of last meal

Physical Examination. The physical examination should include the following:

- Height, weight, vital signs (temperature, blood pressure, pulse, and respirations)
- State of hydration, including presence of edema
- Size and contour of abdomen and fundus
- Frequency of contractions

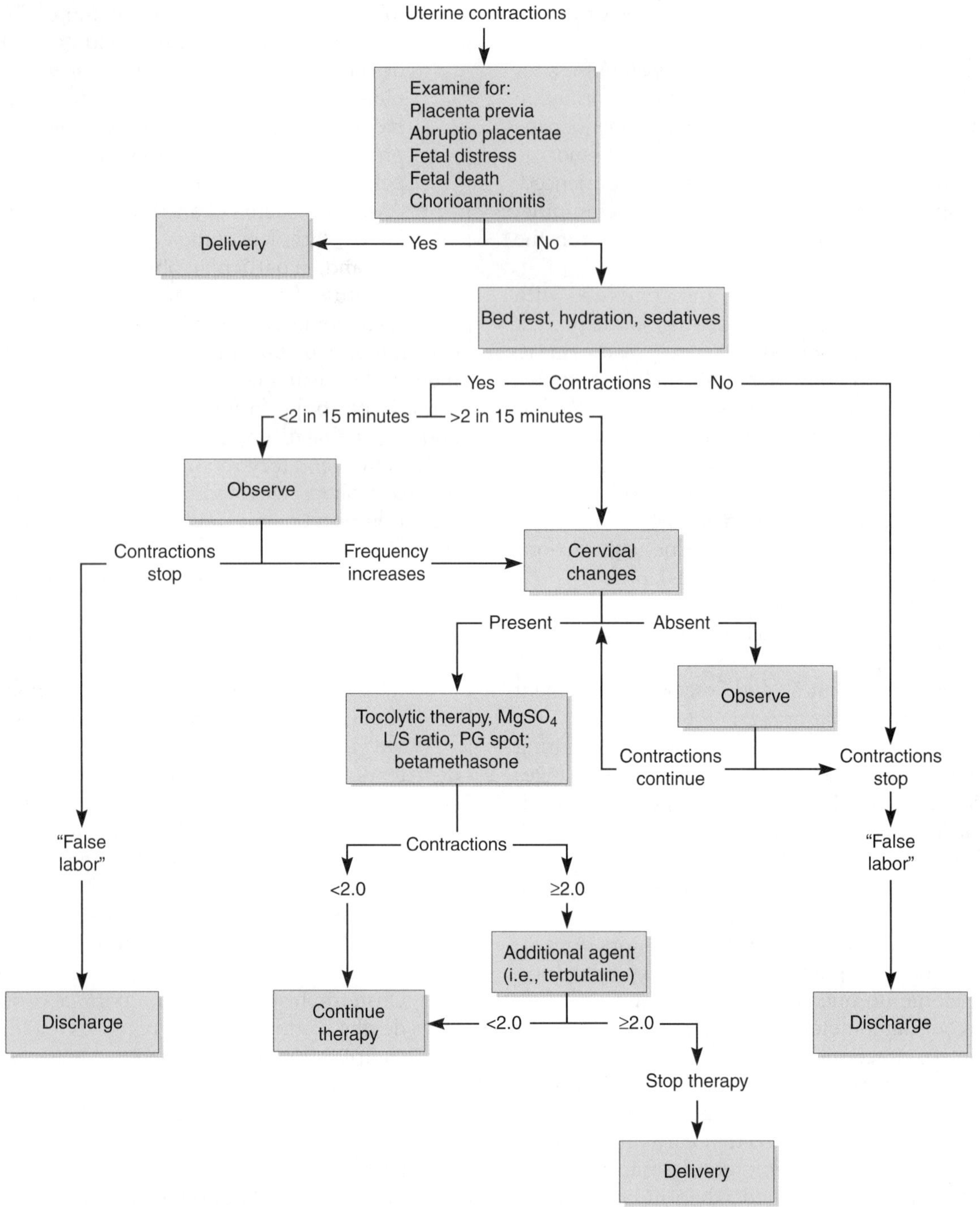

FIGURE 40-1 Alternatives in the treatment of preterm labor.

- Fetal heart rate
- Vaginal examination: cervical dilation and effacement, status of membranes, and presentation and position of fetus

Assessment after Delivery and During Postpartum Care

- The vital signs should be checked every 15 minutes during the first hour or until the woman is stable, then every 30 minutes for the next 2 hours.
- Inspect the perineum and note any abnormal swelling or bruising.
- Assess fundal height and firmness every 15 minutes for 1 hour, then every 30 minutes for the next 4 hours. Continue to assess fundal height and position until the woman is discharged.
- Describe the amount of **lochia** and the color and the presence of clots every 15 minutes for 1 hour, every 30 minutes for 4 hours, and hourly for the next 12 hours.
- Assess breasts for colostrum and breast milk approximately 3 to 4 hours after delivery. Check for breast engorgement and discomfort.

Assessment of the Neonate

- Ensure a patent airway.
- Umbilical cord is observed until pulsations cease, then clamped or ligated.
- Assess neonate's health status at 1 minute and 5 minutes after delivery using the Apgar rating system (Table 40-1).
- Rapid estimation of gestational age is also performed (Table 40-2).

Nursing Diagnoses

- Nutrition, imbalanced: less than body requirements (indication)
- Body image, disturbed (indication)
- Injury, risk for (indication, side effects)
- Anxiety (indication, side effects)
- Sleep pattern, disturbed (indication)
- Tissue perfusion, ineffective (specify type) (indication)

Planning

A large part of maternity care occurs in the clinic setting, so the care plan must be individualized to the patient's needs and available resources. Incorporate cultural aspects of care, education level and capabilities, family structure, economic resources, and access to health care and community resources. To ensure optimal health for the mother to support fetal development, an integral part of the plan must include health teaching to meet the following needs: nutrition; activity and exercise; elimination; sleep requirements; cessation of smoking, alcohol consumption, and recreational drug use; and management of usual discomforts of pregnancy. Provide information in a timely manner regarding self-monitoring for complications and for signs of true or false labor.

During the first trimester, initiate discussion of infant feeding options. Schedule follow-up appointments and appropriate laboratory and diagnostic studies.

Cooperatively plan with the mother (and father) for attendance at childbirth and parenting classes.

The patient with diabetes should have multiple laboratory tests including glycosylated hemoglobin (AIC), serum creatinine, urine microalbumin, and other tests consistent with the history. The woman with diabetes must understand the importance of having a sustained record of preconception glycemic control to prevent maternal and fetal complications.

Implementation

Prenatal

- Collect information relating to the person's health status and the pregnancy. Observe for signs of potential complications of pregnancy.
- Assist with routine prenatal examinations and diagnostic procedures.
- Review laboratory and diagnostic studies performed; report abnormal findings to the health care provider.
- During the first trimester, initiate discussion of infant feeding options available; provide information needed for parents to make a decision.

Complications of Pregnancy

- *Infection*: Monitor for infections and intervene according to the health care provider's orders when an infection is confirmed.
- *Hyperemesis gravidarum* (see Chapter 34): Monitor hydration status, daily weight, and vital signs. Provide for dietary needs through intravenous therapy, nutritional supplements, and gradual progression of diet as tolerated.

Table 40-1 ***The Apgar Scoring System***

SIGN	0	1	2
Heart rate	Absent	Slow (below 100)	Over 100
Respiratory effort	Absent	Slow, irregular	Good, crying
Muscle tone	Flaccid	Some flexion of extremities	Active motion
Reflex irritability	No response	Grimace	Cry
Color	Blue, pale	Body pink, extremities blue	Completely pink

Table 40-2 ***Gestational Age***

SITES	36 WEEKS OR LESS	37-38 WEEKS	39 WEEKS OR MORE
Sole creases	Anterior transverse creases only	Occasional creases anterior two thirds	Sole covered with creases
Breast nodule diameter	2 mm	4 mm	7 mm
Scalp hair	Fine, fuzzy	Fine, fuzzy	Coarse and silky
Earlobes	Pliable, no cartilage	Some cartilage	Stiffened by thick cartilage
Testes and scrotum	Testes in lower canal, scrotum small, few rugae	Intermediate	Testes pendulous, scrotum full, extensive rugae

From Cunningham FG, MacDonald PC, Grant NF: *Williams' obstetrics*, ed 18, Norwalk, Conn, 1989, Appleton & Lange.

- *Bleeding, miscarriage, abortion:* Ensure that the patient adheres to bed rest, and give sedatives as prescribed. Monitor maternal vital signs, fetal heart rate and activity, and the volume (frequency of change and number of pads used) of bleeding present. When bleeding is present, blood studies for hemoglobin, hematocrit, white blood cells (WBCs), human chorionic gonadotropin (hCG) titer, and blood type and crossmatch may be ordered. Other diagnostic procedures such as culdoscopy, sonography, laparoscopy, fetoscopy, and pregnancy tests may be performed.

Preterm Labor

- Monitor uterine contractions, and continue external fetal and uterine monitoring.
- Position the mother on her side, increase fluid intake, start an intravenous (IV) infusion as ordered. Monitor hydration, maintain accurate intake and output records, and take daily weights.
- Assist with obtaining cervical and vaginal cultures, as ordered.
- Perform cervical examination to determine dilation and effacement. Assess for leakage of amniotic fluid.
- Take maternal vital signs. Record fetal heart rate and frequency and intensity of uterine contractions.
- Administer prescribed uterine relaxants, for example, terbutaline, or magnesium sulfate. (See individual drug monographs for administration information and monitoring parameters.) Glucocorticoids, usually betamethasone or dexamethasone, may be administered intramuscularly (IM) to accelerate lung maturation to minimize fetal respiratory distress syndrome. It may be used in cases in which it is anticipated that premature labor should be stopped for only 36 to 48 hours, such as with premature rupture of the membranes. Usual dosage for betamethasone is 12 mg IM, repeated in 24 hours. Dexamethasone is usually administered 6 mg IM every 12 hours for a total dose of 24 mg.
- Review available laboratory studies and report findings to the health care provider (e.g., fetal fibronectin, electrolyte studies, CBC with differential, thrombocytopenia, uric acid level, hematocrit, serum estriol, lecithin/sphingomyelin [L/S] ratio).
- All patients in preterm labor are considered to be at high risk for neonatal group B streptococcal infection and therefore often receive prophylactic antibiotics. Antibiotics frequently used are penicillin G, ampicillin, or clindamycin for patients allergic to penicillins.
- Provide appropriate psychological support. Involve pastoral care appropriately.

Premature Rupture of Membranes

- Check fetal heart tones and fetal activity.
- Describe the color, characteristics, and amount of amniotic fluid leakage.
- Check maternal vital signs; report elevated temperature, chills, or malaise immediately.

Gestational Diabetes Mellitus (GDM)

- Assist with the performance of glucose tolerance testing.
- Perform blood glucose testing four times a day, and assist the patient in administering prescribed insulin. While reviewing the self-monitoring blood glucose (SMBG) levels, ensure that the patient understands her individualized insulin dosage adjustment.
- Encourage adherence to diet and exercise prescribed to achieve tight glucose control to maintain desired weight gain during the pregnancy and to prevent complications (e.g., neonatal hypoglycemia or stillbirth).
- Women with gestational diabetes have twice the risk of developing hypertension than other pregnant women, so the blood pressure should be monitored regularly.
- Monitor for development of hypoglycemia and hyperglycemia. Consult current American Diabetes Association (ADA) guidelines for monitoring GDM.
- During labor, monitor glucose level every 2 hours; maintain adequate hydration.
- During the postpartum period, continue to monitor glucose levels. (Usually with gestational diabetes, the mother's glucose reverts to normal during the postpartum period. Therefore careful monitoring of glucose and adjustment of insulin dosages is required.)

Pregnancy-Induced Hypertension

- Monitor maternal vital signs, fetal heart tones, and fetal movement at appropriate intervals consistent with presenting symptoms. Maintain the patient on bed rest in a lateral position to promote uteroplacental circulation and to reduce compression of the vena cava.
- Maintain hydration by oral or IV routes (usually 1000 mL plus the amount of urine output over the past 24 hours). Maintain accurate intake and output, and obtain daily weights. Salt intake is generally maintained at a normal level, although heavy use should be discouraged.
- Test the urine for protein and specific gravity every hour. Report a steady decrease in hourly output or output of less than 30 mL per hour.
- Review available laboratory studies and report findings to the health care provider (e.g., electrolyte studies, CBC with differential, thrombocytopenia, uric acid level, hematocrit, serum estriol, L/S ratio).

- Monitor for signs of seizure activity (e.g., increased drowsiness, hyperreflexia, visual disturbances, and development of severe pain). If symptoms are present, report immediately.
- If seizures occur, give supportive care, provide a nonstimulating environment, and have oxygen and suction available. Institute seizure precautions.
- Be alert for complications (e.g., start of labor, pulmonary edema, DIC, heart failure, abruptio placentae, cerebral edema).
- Administer prescribed drugs (e.g., diazepam or phenobarbital, antihypertensives). The vasodilator hydralazine is usually administered to control blood pressure. It may be administered orally or IV, depending on the severity of the condition. If given IV, monitor the maternal and fetal heart rates and the mother's blood pressure every 2 to 3 minutes after the initial dose and every 10 to 15 minutes thereafter. The diastolic pressure is usually maintained at 90 to 100 mm Hg. Anticonvulsants such as magnesium sulfate or phenytoin may be given for seizure activity (see drug monograph regarding administration and monitoring of the patient during drug therapy).

Termination of Pregnancy

- If bleeding occurs near the EDC, the infant may be delivered by cesarean birth. If it appears that a miscarriage is occurring, the woman may be hospitalized for observation and bed rest, diagnosis for possible causes (e.g., infection), and fluid replacement.
- If a pregnancy is to be terminated (aborted), the following methods may be used:
  - Before 12 weeks' gestation: suction curettage or dilation and evacuation (D&E)
  - 12 to 20 weeks' gestation: intraamniotic instillation of hypertonic saline (20% solution) or prostaglandin administered intraamniotically, intramuscularly, or by vaginal suppository
  - Intrauterine fetal death after 20 weeks' gestation: prostaglandin suppositories with or without oxytocin augmentation (see the section on uterine stimulants, on p. 642).
- Encourage the persons involved in the loss of an infant to talk about their feelings of grief, sadness, or anger. Have pastoral care involved in supportive processes as appropriate. Listen and allow them to vent feelings. Give answers (if known) regarding future pregnancies. Refer for other counseling as appropriate. Anticipate that depression may develop over the next few weeks and may need treatment.
- Administer Rh_0(D) immune globulin to an Rh-negative mother within 72 hours of the termination of pregnancy (see p. 653). Also check the patient's rubella titer; if low, obtain an order for inoculation immediately after pregnancy.

Normal Labor and Delivery

- Perform routine admission procedures (e.g., vital signs, perineal preparation).
- Follow institutional guidelines regarding activity level of the mother; some permit ambulation during early stages of labor.
- During labor provide pain relief, alternate side-to-side positioning (avoid lying flat on back), intervene with comfort measures (e.g., backrubs, pelvic rocking, effleurage, warm shower, music). Encourage leg extension and dorsiflexion of the foot to relieve spasms and cramping.
- Provide privacy, and support the woman and coach when necessary.
- Check for bladder distention. Have patient void every 2 hours.
- Maintain adequate hydration by giving ice chips or clear liquids. Check hydration status throughout labor—observe mucous membranes, dryness of lips, and skin turgor. Give oral hygiene frequently. Do not give solid foods unless specifically approved by the health care provider.
- As labor progresses, continue to monitor the maternal and fetal vital signs and the frequency, duration, and intensity of uterine contractions.
- Report contractions of 90 seconds or more and those not followed by complete uterine relaxation. Report abnormal patterns on the fetal monitor, such as decreased variability, late decelerations, and variable decelerations.
- Continue to coach when necessary.
- As vaginal discharge increases, wash the perineum with warm water, then dry the area. Change the bed sheets, pad, and gown when necessary.
- Monitor the temperature every 4 hours while membranes are intact and temperature remains within normal range. Monitor every 2 hours if the temperature is elevated or if the membranes have ruptured.
- After delivery, record the time of delivery and position of the infant; the type of episiotomy or tear, and type of suture used in repair, if appropriate; any anesthetic or analgesic used during repair; the time of placental delivery; and any complications (e.g., additional bleeding or neonatal distress).
- Administer and record oxytocic agent, as ordered.

Immediate Neonatal Care. Before delivery the maternal history through the current stage of labor should be reviewed to identify potential complications that may arise for the neonate. Although a complete physical examination of the neonate will be performed later, a preliminary assessment and recording of data must be completed at the time of birth.

The following procedures must be completed by the health care provider or nurse immediately after delivery.

Airway. Ensure that the airway remains open. As soon as the head is delivered, suction the oropharynx and nasal passages with a small bulb syringe. Immediately after delivery, hold the newborn with the head lowered at a 10- to 15-degree angle to help drain amniotic fluid, mucus, and blood. Resuction with the bulb syringe as necessary.

Clamping the Umbilical Cord. Consult with the mother before delivery if she is participating in cord blood banking. If so, special containers must be used for blood storage and registration. When the airway is opened and the respirations have stabilized, the neonate should be held at the same level as the uterus until cord pulsations cease. The cord is then clamped or ligated.

Health Status. The health status of the neonate is estimated at 1 minute and 5 minutes after delivery using the Apgar rating system (see Table 40-1). Rapid estimation of gestational age is also performed (see Table 40-2).

Temperature Maintenance. The neonate should be dried immediately and body temperature maintained with the use of prewarmed blankets, a heated bassinet, or an infrared heat lamp. If the neonate is term and in stable condition as assessed by the Apgar score, temperature may be maintained by skin-to-skin contact with the mother.

Eye Prophylaxis. It is a legal requirement that every newborn baby's eyes be treated prophylactically for *Neisseria gonorrhoeae.* Another rapidly emerging neonatal conjunctival infection is chlamydial ophthalmia neonatorum, which is caused by *Chlamydia trachomatis.* The neonate may have become infected during birth if the mother is infected. Ophthalmic erythromycin or tetracycline is used for prophylactic treatment of neonatal conjunctivitis caused by *N. gonorrhoeae* or *C. trachomatis.* Instillation of the ophthalmic agent may be delayed up to 2 hours to facilitate parent-child bonding.

Other Procedures. While the parents are bonding with the newborn infant, the nurse should prepare an infant identification bracelet and place it on the baby, examine the placenta and cord for anomalies, and verify the presence of one vein and two arteries. Samples of cord blood may be collected for analysis of the Rh factor, blood grouping, and hematocrit. The baby is then taken to the nursery where it is weighed, measured, and given a complete physical examination. Some health care providers also order an IM injection of vitamin K as prophylaxis against hemorrhage. Evaluation of the infant's vital signs and color is performed on a continuum. Alterations from baseline are evaluated and reported.

Postpartum Care. *Postpartum* is defined as the time between delivery and return of the reproductive organs to prepregnancy status.

- An Rh-negative mother may receive $Rh_o(D)$ immune globulin within 72 hours of the completion of the pregnancy.
- If the mother's rubella titer is low, an appropriate time for inoculation is immediately after pregnancy.
- Continue to assess the fundal height, position, and lochia until the woman is discharged. The lochia normally progresses from blood red (bright) to darker red with some small clots (1 to 3 days postpartum), to pinkish thin, watery consistency (4 to 10 days), to a yellowish or creamy color (11 to 21 days). The odor should be similar to that of a normal menstrual flow; a foul-smelling odor should be reported. Pads should be changed at frequent regular intervals rather than waiting for them to become heavily laden.
- On delivery, the breasts secrete a thin yellow fluid called colostrum. Within 3 to 4 days, breast milk becomes available. This may produce some discomfort for the mother as the breasts become congested. Engorgement in the breastfeeding mother can be minimized by having the infant nurse more frequently (every 90 minutes), or massaging and hand-expressing or pumping milk to empty the breasts completely. A warm shower or application of warm, moist heat may also provide relief.
- The quantity of breast milk varies among mothers. Diet, fluid intake, and level of anxiety all affect lactation.
- Monitor the number of infant voidings, usually six to eight in 24 hours, and record stools, usually one in 24 hours.
- Weigh the infant daily. A weight gain of 0.75 to 1 ounce per day indicates that the infant is receiving adequate nutritional intake.
- Help the mother to hold the baby correctly and provide instruction and guidance on the correct technique of breastfeeding, bottle-feeding, and burping the baby.
- Suppression of lactation in the nonnursing mother includes having the woman wear a supportive, well-fitting bra within 6 hours of delivery. The bra is removed only during bathing. Ice packs may be applied to the axillary area of the breast for 15 to 20 minutes four times daily. Teach the mother to avoid any stimulation of her breasts until the feeling of fullness has subsided (usually 5 to 7 days). Do not use a breast pump, and when showering, allow the warm water to run down her back to avoid stimulating lactation.
- Encourage the mother who is breastfeeding or formula feeding to eat a well-balanced diet with adequate protein, vitamins, and fluids to help restore the body to the optimal level.
- Continue to provide emotional support to the new mother and support personnel.

- Afterpains often require a mild analgesic. For the breastfeeding mother who is experiencing afterpains, administering a mild analgesic approximately 40 minutes before nursing may relieve discomfort.
- Check on voiding and return of normal bowel elimination during the postpartum period.
- Check vital signs every shift or more frequently when indicated.
- Monitor laboratory reports during the postpartum period. The hematocrit may rise during the initial period after childbirth; WBCs, mainly neutrophils, may be elevated as well, making it difficult to diagnose an infection.
- Monitor for thromboembolisms during the postpartum period. Clotting factors and fibrinogen are increased during pregnancy and the immediate postpartum period.

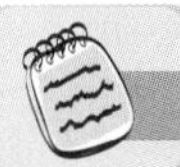

Patient Education and Health Promotion

- Encourage open communication with the expectant family. They must be guided to understand the need for prenatal care. Keep emphasizing those things the family can do to optimize the chances for a healthy baby, including maintaining general health, nutritional needs, adequate rest and appropriate exercise, and continuing prescribed medication therapy.
- The amount of information provided to the expectant mother or parents is individualized. The following health teaching is an overview of information that may be given (see a maternity textbook to cover the areas not addressed).

Adequate Rest and Relaxation. Assist the individual to plan for adequate rest periods throughout the day to prevent fatigue, irritability, and exhaustion. Talk with the individual about planning rest periods during lunch breaks at work, when preschoolers are napping, or when the father is home to care for children. A short period of relaxation in a reclining chair or elevation of the feet may be beneficial when there is no time during the day for sleep. Advise the patient to avoid long periods of standing in one place and to perform some daily activities while sitting.

Activity and Exercise. Usually, the woman can continue to perform common activities of daily living. New attempts at strenuous exercise (such as jogging or aerobics) should not be started during pregnancy. Daily walks in fresh air are encouraged.

Any changes in activity level should be discussed with the health care provider *before* starting.

Encourage good posture and participation in prenatal classes in which exercises are taught to strengthen the abdominal muscles and to relax the pelvic floor muscles.

The woman should avoid lifting heavy objects and anything that might cause physical harm, especially as the pregnancy progresses, and because balance may be affected.

Employment. Advice about continued employment should be based on the type of job; working conditions; amount of lifting, standing, or exposure to toxic substances; and the individual's state of health.

General Personal Hygiene. Encourage maintenance of general hygiene through daily tub baths or showers. Tub baths near the end of pregnancy may be discouraged because of the danger of slipping and falling while getting in and out of the tub. Tub baths should not be taken once the membranes have ruptured.

Encourage the use of plain soap and water to cleanse the genital area and prevent odors. Deodorant sprays should *not* be used because of possible irritation. Tell the pregnant woman that an increase in vaginal discharge is common. Discharge that is yellowish or greenish, is foul smelling, or causes irritation and itching should be reported for further evaluation.

Clothing. Encourage the mother to dress in nonconstricting clothing. As the pregnancy progresses, the mother may be more comfortable with a maternity girdle to support the abdomen. Encourage the mother to wear a well-fitting brassiere to provide proper breast support. The pregnant woman should avoid restrictive circular garters, which may impede lower limb circulation. Encourage low-heeled well-fitting shoes that provide good support. Properly fitting shoes can prevent lower back fatigue as well as tired feet.

Oral Hygiene. Encourage the pregnant patient to have a thorough dental examination at the beginning of the pregnancy. She should tell the dentist she is pregnant at the time of the examination. Encourage thorough daily brushing and flossing.

Sexual Activity. Refer to an obstetrics text for discussion of alterations in sexuality during pregnancy. The wide range of feelings, needs, and intervention deserve more consideration than can be presented in this text.

Smoking and Alcohol. The pregnant woman should be encouraged to abstain from smoking or drinking alcohol during pregnancy. A vast amount of data indicate that smoking and drinking are dangerous to the fetus. An increased incidence of neonatal mortality, low birthweight, and prematurity have been well reported. (See also Chapter 49.)

Nutritional Needs. Balanced nutrition is always to be encouraged, but is especially important throughout the course of the pregnancy. Recommended daily allowances vary based on the individual's age, weight at the time of pregnancy, and daily activity level. At all times allowances must be made to maintain the nutritional needs of the mother and fetus. Refer to a nutrition text for specific recommendations.

Encourage limiting the caffeine content of the diet during pregnancy. Limit the consumption of coffee, tea, cola beverages, and cocoa. Tell the pregnant woman to check labels for specific caffeine content because many soft drinks contain a significant quantity of caffeine.

Tell the woman to avoid highly spiced foods and any foods that she knows have caused heartburn.

Usual weight gain is 3.5 to 5 pounds during the first trimester, followed by an average gain of 1 pound per week during the second and third trimesters. The rate of weekly weight gain may be slightly higher for an underweight woman and slightly lower for overweight women. Stress the need to report a weight gain of 2 or more pounds in any 1 week for further evaluation.

Bowel Habits. Assess the individual's usual pattern of elimination, and anticipate its continuance until later in pregnancy. Pressure on the lower bowel from the presenting part of the fetus may cause constipation and hemorrhoids. Stool softeners or a bulk laxative may be prescribed if problems persist.

Encourage the consumption of fresh fruits and vegetables, whole-grain and bran products, along with an adequate intake of six to eight 8-ounce glasses of fluid daily.

Douching. Discourage any type of douching unless specifically prescribed by the health care provider. Be certain when douching is prescribed that the patient is given simple, explicit instructions.

Discomforts of Pregnancy. Use assessment data as pregnancy progresses to determine individualized teaching needed to deal with discomforts such as backache, leg cramps, hemorrhoids, and edema.

Complications of Pregnancy. Individualize health teaching to deal with complications as they arise. The woman should always immediately report loss of fluid vaginally; dizziness; double or blurred vision; severe headache, abdominal pain or persistent vomiting; fever; edema of the face, fingers, legs, or feet; and weight gain in excess of 2 pounds per week.

Teach signs of true and false labor and when to contact the health care provider.

At Discharge

- Review instructions on self-care (e.g., breast care, fundal height, lochia, incisional or perineal care, bowel and bladder expectations, nutritional and fluid intake, activity). Stress signs of problems that should be reported to the health care provider.
- Contraceptives: Discuss appropriate sexual activity and limitations. Remind the woman that breastfeeding is not a form of contraception. Alternative methods of contraception should be used if the patient does not wish to become pregnant immediately.
- Review infant care needs, bathing, vital signs, fontanel assessment, care of the umbilical cord and circumcision, normal sleep pattern, and feeding.
- Stress the need for follow-up care of the mother and infant. Provide the specific date and time of health care provider appointments. The mother usually returns for a follow-up examination at the health care provider's office 6 to 8 weeks after delivery.

Fostering Health Maintenance

- Discuss any medications prescribed for the mother or infant and how they will benefit the course of treatment to produce optimal response.
- Seek cooperation and understanding of the following points so that medication adherence is increased; name of medication, dosage, route and times of administration, side effects to expect, and side effects to report.

Written Record. Enlist the mother's aid in developing and maintaining a written record of monitoring parameters (e.g., blood pressure, pulse, daily weight, presence and relief of discomfort, exercise tolerance, fetal movement) (see the Patient Self-Assessment forms on pp. 643 and 644). Complete the Premedication Data column for use as a baseline to track response to drug therapy, progression of the pregnancy, and postpartum recovery. Ensure that the patient understands how to use the form and instruct the patient to take the completed form to follow-up visits. During follow-up visits, focus on issues that will foster adherence with the therapeutic interventions prescribed. ■

DRUG THERAPY IN PREGNANCY

DRUG CLASS: Uterine Stimulants

Uses

There are four primary clinical indications for the use of uterine stimulants: (1) induction or augmentation of labor, (2) control of postpartum atony and hemorrhage, (3) control of postsurgical hemorrhage (as in cesarean birth), and (4) induction of therapeutic abortion.

Induction of labor: Uterine stimulants, primarily oxytocin, may be prescribed in cases in which, in the health care provider's judgment, continuation of the pregnancy is considered to be a greater risk to the mother or fetus than the risk associated with drug-induced induction of labor. A history of **precipitous labor and delivery,** postterm pregnancy, prolonged pregnancy with placental insufficiency, prolonged rupture of the membranes, or pregnancy-induced hypertension may indicate the need to induce labor. Vaginal inserts and gels and oral dosage forms of prostaglandins are being tested as adjunctive therapy to help ripen the cervix.

Augmentation of labor: In general, oxytocin should not be used to hasten labor. The type and force of contraction induced by the oxytocin may be harmful to the mother and fetus. In occasional cases of **dysfunctional labor,** there is a prolonged latent phase of cervical dilatation or arrest of descent through the birth canal. Oxytocin infusions starting with low dosages and continuous fetal monitoring may be beneficial in these cases.

Postpartum atony and hemorrhage: After delivery of the fetus and the placenta, the uterus sometimes remains flaccid and "boggy." Continued intravenous infusions of low-dose oxytocin or intramuscular injections of ergonovine or methylergonovine may be used

PATIENT SELF-ASSESSMENT FORM Prenatal Care

MEDICATIONS	COLOR	TO BE TAKEN

Patient ____________

Health Care Provider ____________

Health Care Provider's phone ____________

Next appt.* ____________

What I Should Monitor		Premedication Data	Date	Date	Date	Date	Date	Date	Comments
Weight									
Blood pressure									
Pulse									
Pain	Cramps								
	Backache								
	Abdominal pain								
Bleeding	With cramps								
	# pads/day								
	Describe color: Bright or dark red								
Edema	Morning								
	Evening								
	Other								
	Location: hands, feet, ankles								
Fatigue **All day** (10) — **After exercise** (5) — **Normal** (1)									
Exercise **Poor toleration** (10) — **Moderate exercise** (5) — **Normal** (1)									
Fetal movement	Normal								
	None								
Bowel movements **Constipated** (10) — **Normal** (5) — **Diarrhea** (1)									
Other									

*Please bring this record with you to your next appointment.
Use the back of this sheet for additional information.

PATIENT SELF-ASSESSMENT FORM Postpartum Care

MEDICATIONS	COLOR	TO BE TAKEN

Patient ____________________

Health Care Provider ____________________

Health Care Provider's phone ____________________

Next appt.* ____________________

What I Should Monitor		Premedication Data	Date	Date	Date	Date	Date	Date	Comments
Weight									
Blood pressure	AM / PM								
Pulse	AM / PM								
Lochia	# pads/day								
	Color of vaginal discharge								
Cramps (Frequent 10, Moderate 5, None 1)									
Breast tenderness	↑ Discomfort								
	↓ Discomfort								
	No problem								
Nipple condition	Sore								
	Cracking								
	No problem								
Sexual activity	Persistently painful								
	Uncomfortable								
	Normal								
Bowel movements	Constipation								
	Normal								
Other									

*Please bring this record with you to your next appointment.
Use the back of this sheet for additional information.

to stimulate firm uterine contractions to reduce the risk of postpartum hemorrhage from an atonic uterus. Occasionally oral dosages of ergonovine or methylergonovine are administered for a few days after delivery to assist in uterine involution.

Therapeutic abortion: Pharmacologic agents are usually not effective in evacuating uterine contents until several weeks into the second trimester of pregnancy. Various dosage forms of prostaglandins and hypertonic (20%) sodium chloride may be effective. Uterine smooth muscle is not very responsive to oxytocin stimulation until late in the third trimester, so even large doses of oxytocin are not indicated in therapeutic abortion. Regardless of the stage of pregnancy, stimulants such as ergonovine or methylergonovine may be prescribed after the uterus is emptied to control bleeding and maintain uterine muscle tone.

dinoprostone (die no prahs' tone)
PROSTIN E_2, PREPIDIL, CERVIDIL

Actions

Dinoprostone (prostaglandin E_2) is a natural chemical in the body that causes uterine and gastrointestinal smooth muscle stimulation. It also plays an active role in cervical softening and dilation (cervical ripening) unrelated to uterine muscle stimulation. When used during pregnancy, it produces cervical softening and dilatation and, in higher doses, increases the frequency and strength of uterine contractions.

Uses

Dinoprostone is used to start and continue cervical ripening at term. In larger doses it is also used to expel uterine contents in cases of intrauterine fetal death, benign hydatidiform mole, missed spontaneous miscarriage, and second-trimester abortion. Occasionally oxytocin and dinoprostone are used together to shorten the duration of time required to expel uterine contents.

Therapeutic Outcomes

The primary therapeutic outcomes associated with dinoprostone therapy are as follows:

- Cervical softening and dilation before labor
- Evacuation of uterine contents

Nursing Process for Dinoprostone

Premedication Assessment

1. Obtain baseline vital signs. Temperature and vital signs should be monitored every half hour after initiation of therapy.
2. Assess the state of hydration.
3. Assess uterine activity, including amount and characteristics of any vaginal discharge.
4. Check for antiemetic and antidiarrheal medications ordered at prescribed times or as needed (PRN).

Planning

Availability. Vaginal suppository: 20 mg (Prostin E_2); vaginal insert: 10 mg (Cervidil); cervical gel: 0.5 mg in 2.5-mL prefilled syringe (Prepidil).

Implementation

Dosage and Administration. *Adult:* For cervical ripening:

- *Intravaginal insert administration:* The slab (Cervidil) is placed transversely in the posterior fornix of the vagina after removal from foil wrap. Patients should remain supine for 2 hours after insertion but may be ambulatory thereafter. Cervidil is removed at the onset of labor or 12 hours after insertion. The product does not need to be warmed before insertion.
- *Intracervical gel:* Allow the prefilled syringe of gel (0.5 mg) to warm to room temperature. Do not force the warming process with a water bath or other external source of heat (e.g., microwave oven). A catheter is attached to the syringe (20 mm if the cervix is less than 50% effaced; 10 mm if more than 50% effaced). The patient is placed in a dorsal position and the cervix visualized with a speculum. Using sterile technique, the gel is introduced through the catheter into the cervical canal just below the level of the internal os. The catheter is removed after placement of the gel. After administration the patient should remain supine for 15 to 30 minutes to minimize leakage from the cervical canal. Dosages may be repeated in 6 hours. The maximum recommended cumulative dose for a 24-hour period is 1.5 mg (7.5 mL).

For evacuation of uterine contents:

- Intravaginal suppository: Before removing the foil, allow the suppository (Prostin E_2) to warm to room temperature. Insert one suppository high into the posterior vaginal fornix. Patients should remain supine for at least 10 minutes after each insertion. Suppositories should be inserted every 2 to 5 hours, depending on uterine activity and tolerance to side effects.

Evaluation

Side Effects to Expect

Nausea, Vomiting, Diarrhea. The most frequently observed gastrointestinal side effects are nausea, vomiting, and diarrhea. Premedication with an antiemetic such as prochlorperazine and an antidiarrheal agent (loperamide or diphenoxylate) will reduce, but usually not completely eliminate, these adverse effects.

Fever. Chills and shivering may occur in patients receiving dinoprostone. Temperature elevations to approximately 38° C (100.6° F) occur within 15 to 45 minutes and continue for up to 6 hours. Sponge baths with water and maintaining fluid intake may provide symptomatic relief.

Aspirin does not inhibit dinoprostone-induced fever.

Patients should be observed for clinical indications of intrauterine infection. Monitor temperature and vital signs every half hour.

Side Effects to Report

Orthostatic Hypotension. Transient hypotension with a drop in diastolic pressure of 20 mm Hg, dizziness, flushing, and dysrhythmias have all been reported. Although these effects are infrequent and generally mild, dinoprostone may cause some degree of orthostatic hypotension manifested by dizziness, flushing, and weakness, particularly when therapy is initiated.

Monitor blood pressure in the supine and standing positions.

Anticipate the development of postural hypotension and take measures to prevent it. For ambulatory patients, teach the patient to rise slowly from a supine or sitting position, and encourage her to sit or lie down if feeling faint. Report rapidly falling blood pressure, bradycardia, paleness, and other alterations in vital signs.

Drug Interactions. No clinically significant interactions have been reported.

misoprostol (mis oh pros′ tohl)
CYTOTEC (site′ oh tech)

Actions

Misoprostol is a synthetic prostaglandin E used to prevent nonsteroidal antiinflammatory drug (NSAID)–induced ulcer disease. The prostaglandin E analogs also induce uterine contractions in the pregnant uterus.

Uses

Although not approved by the U.S. Food and Drug Administration (FDA), misoprostol is used as a cervical ripening agent, for induction of labor, and for treatment of serious postpartum hemorrhage in the presence of uterine atony. It is also used in combination with mifepristone as an abortifacient. Misoprostol should not be used to induce labor in women who have had a previous cesarean delivery.

Therapeutic Outcomes

The primary therapeutic outcomes associated with misoprostol therapy in pregnancy are as follows:

- Cervical softening and dilation before labor.
- Induction of active labor.
- Reduction in postpartum hemorrhage in the presence of uterine atony.
- Evacuation of uterine contents.

Nursing Process for Misoprostol

Premedication Assessment

1. Obtain baseline vital signs. Temperature and vital signs should be monitored every half hour after initiation of therapy.
2. Assess the state of hydration.
3. Assess uterine activity, including amount and characteristics of any vaginal discharge.
4. Check for antiemetic and antidiarrheal medications ordered at prescribed times or PRN.

Planning

Availability. 100 and 200 mcg tablets.

Implementation

Dosage and Administration. *Adult:* PO: 50 to 100 mcg every 4 to 6 hours for two or three doses. Intravaginal: 25 to 50 mcg (¼ or ½ of a 100-mcg oral tablet) initially. Additional 25- to 50-mcg doses are administered intravaginally every 3 to 6 hours for two or three doses.

Evaluation

Side Effects to Expect and Report. Misoprostol for short-term obstetric use has not been studied in large well-controlled trials, so the type and frequency of adverse effects is not well documented. Because it is a member of the prostaglandin E family, it may be expected to have side effects similar to dinoprostone. (See the dinoprostone monograph earlier.) Rare adverse effects of uterine hyperstimulation with subsequent fetal hypoxia, uterine rupture, and amniotic fluid embolism have been reported.

Drug Interactions. No significant drug interactions have been reported.

ergonovine maleate (er gon′ oh veen mal′ ee ate)
▸ ERGOTRATE MALEATE (er′ go trayt)
methylergonovine maleate (meth il er gon′ oh veen mal′ ee ate)
▸ METHERGINE (meth′ er jin)

Actions

Ergonovine and methylergonovine are structurally similar ergot derivatives that share similar actions. Both drugs directly stimulate uterine contractions. Small doses produce contractions with normal resting muscle tone; intermediate doses cause more forceful and prolonged contractions with an elevated resting muscle tone; and large doses cause severe, prolonged contractions. Because of this sudden, intense uterine activity, which is dangerous to the fetus, these agents cannot be used for induction of labor.

Uses

Ergonovine and methylergonovine produce more sustained contractions than oxytocin and are used in small doses in postpartum patients to control bleeding and maintain uterine firmness.

Therapeutic Outcomes

The primary therapeutic outcome associated with ergonovine and methylergonovine therapy is reduced postpartum blood loss.

Nursing Process for Ergonovine and Methylergonovine

Premedication Assessment

1. Obtain baseline vital signs, especially blood pressure and pulse.
2. Assess amount and characteristics of vaginal discharge and fundal height and contractility.

Planning

Availability. PO: 0.2 mg tablets. Injection: 0.2 mg/mL in 1-mL ampules.

Implementation

NOTE: Use with extreme caution in patients with hypertension, preeclampsia, heart disease, venoatrial shunts, mitral valve stenosis, sepsis, or hepatic or renal impairment.

Dosage and Administration. *Adult:* PO: 0.2 mg every 6 to 8 hours after delivery for a maximum of 1 week. IM: 0.2 mg every 2 to 4 hours, to a maximum of five doses.

Evaluation

Side Effects to Expect

Nausea, Vomiting. These side effects are usually mild and tend to resolve with continued therapy. Encourage the patient not to discontinue therapy without first consulting the health care provider.

Abdominal Cramping. This is normally an indication of therapeutic activity, but, if severe, reduction or discontinuation of medication may be necessary.

Side Effects to Report

Hypertension. Certain patients, especially those who are eclamptic or previously hypertensive, may be particularly sensitive to the hypertensive effects of these agents. These patients have a higher incidence of developing generalized headaches, severe dysrhythmias, and strokes. Monitor the patient's blood pressure and pulse rate and rhythm. Report immediately if the patient complains of headache or palpitations.

Drug Interactions

Inhibition of Prolactin. Do not use ergonovine in patients who wish to breastfeed. Methylergonovine may be used as an alternative because it will not inhibit stimulation of milk production by prolactin.

Caudal or Spinal Anesthesia. Hypertension and headaches may develop in patients who have received caudal or spinal anesthesia followed by a dosage of either ergonovine or methylergonovine. Monitor the patient's blood pressure and heart rate and rhythm.

oxytocin (ok se to' sin)
PITOCIN (pih to' sin)

Actions

Oxytocin is a hormone produced in the hypothalamus and stored in the pituitary gland. When released, it stimulates the smooth muscle of the uterus, blood vessels, and the mammary glands. When administered during the third trimester of pregnancy, active labor may be initiated.

Uses

Oxytocin is the drug of choice for inducing labor at term and for augmenting uterine contractions during the first and second stages of labor. Oxytocin is routinely administered immediately postpartum to control uterine atony and postpartum hemorrhage.

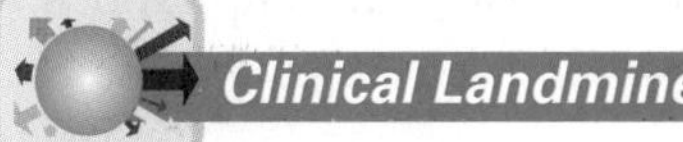

Oxytocin Infusion

Before starting the infusion, establish records of baseline vital signs and intake and output. A constant infusion pump is recommended for controlling the rate of administration. If the infant develops sudden distress, reduce the oxytocin infusion to the slowest possible rate according to hospital policy, turn the mother to the left lateral position, administer oxygen by nasal cannula or face mask, and call the physician immediately.

Therapeutic Outcomes

The primary therapeutic outcomes associated with oxytocin therapy are as follows:

- Initiation of labor.
- Support of uterine contractions during the first and second stages of labor.
- Control of postpartum bleeding.

Nursing Process for Oxytocin

Premedication Assessment

Never leave a patient receiving an oxytocin infusion unattended. Ensure that the IV site is functional before adding oxytocin; use an infusion pump.

1. Monitor maternal vital signs, especially blood pressure and pulse rate.
2. Obtain baseline assessment data of the mother's hydration status. Continue to monitor urine output and intake and output throughout drug therapy.
3. Monitor characteristics of uterine contractions, for example, frequency, rate, duration, and intensity.
4. Monitor fetal heart rate and rhythm. Be alert for signs of fetal distress.
5. Perform reflex testing.
6. Check amount and characteristics of vaginal discharge.

Planning

Availability. IV: 10 units/mL in 1-, 3-, and 10-mL vials and 1-mL disposable syringes.

Implementation

NOTE: Overdosage of oxytocin may cause hyperstimulation of the uterus, resulting in severe contractions with possible abruptio placentae, cervical lacerations, impaired uterine blood flow, and fetal trauma.

Dosage and Administration

- *Starting the infusion:* Establish records of baseline vital signs and intake and output. Oxytocin administered IV should be added to the solution after the IV is shown to be patent and running.
- *Rate:* Careful monitoring of the prescribed rate of infusion is imperative. Should the IV line suddenly open, the resulting severe contractions could be extremely dangerous to the mother.
- *Infusion pump:* A constant infusion pump is recommended to control the rate of administration. Keep in mind that a pump can fail. Continue to monitor the number of drops per minute from the drip chamber.
- *Induction of labor:* IV: Initial rate: 1 to 2 milliunits (mU) per minute. It is strongly recommended that

an infusion pump be used to help control the rate of oxytocin infusion. Most pregnancies close to term will respond well to 2 to 10 mU per minute. Rarely will a patient require more than 20 mU per minute. Those patients at 32 to 36 weeks of gestation often require 20 to 30 mU per minute or more to develop a labor-like contraction pattern. Rates of infusion should not be altered more frequently than every 20 to 30 minutes. It is frequently necessary to reduce or discontinue the infusion as spontaneous uterine activity develops and labor progresses.

- *Augmentation of labor:* IV: Occasionally a labor that started spontaneously may not progress satisfactorily. Labor may be augmented by oxytocin infusions at rates of 0.5 to 2 mU per minute.
- *Postpartum hemorrhage:* IM: 10 units given after delivery of the placenta. IV: 10 to 40 units may be added to 1000 mL of normal saline solution and run at a rate necessary to control uterine atony.

Evaluation

Side Effects to Expect

Uterine Contractions. Oxytocin infusions should be monitored by both a tocometer (an instrument that measures uterine contractions) and a fetal heart monitor.

Maintain an ongoing record of the frequency, duration, and intensity of uterine contractions. Contractions longer than 90 seconds require the flow rate of the oxytocin to be slowed or discontinued.

Nausea, Vomiting. Although uncommon, these side effects may occur. Reduction in dosage may control symptoms.

Side Effects to Report

Fetal Distress. Fetal heart rate should be monitored continuously, but especially closely during uterine contractions. (Normal fetal heart rate is greater than 120 to 160 beats/minute.) Indications of fetal distress may be manifested by tachycardia (>160 beats/minute) followed by bradycardia (<120 beats/minute). As the degree of distress progresses, bradycardia occurs more frequently and lasts longer than 15 seconds after contractions.

If the infant develops sudden distress, reduce the oxytocin infusion to the slowest possible rate according to hospital policy, turn the mother to the left lateral position, administer oxygen by nasal cannula or face mask, and call the health care provider immediately.

Hypertension, Hypotension. Check the mother's blood pressure and pulse rate at least every 30 minutes during oxytocin infusion. Report trends upward or downward, because oxytocin may cause hypertension or hypotension.

Water Intoxication. Oxytocin can alter fluid balance by stimulating antidiuretic hormone, causing the body to accumulate water. This is particularly likely to occur if oxytocin is administered with electrolyte solutions.

Symptoms of water intoxication include drowsiness, listlessness, headache, confusion, anuria, edema, and, in extreme cases, seizures.

Dehydration. Because mothers are routinely placed on nothing by mouth (NPO) status during labor, an occasional patient may develop dehydration even though an IV is running. Monitor urine output, dry crusted lips, and requests for water. Report to the health care provider, and request ice chips and additional IV fluids if appropriate.

Postpartum Hemorrhage. Early postpartum hemorrhage occurs within the first 24 hours after delivery and is usually defined as a blood loss of 500 mL or greater.

The hemorrhage may be caused by uterine atony, retained fragments of placenta, or lacerations of the vaginal tract. Less frequent causes include defective blood clotting mechanisms, uterine eversion, and uterine infections.

Oxytocin is routinely administered after delivery of the placenta to cause the uterus to contract and to decrease blood loss. Always check the height of the fundus of the uterus (usually at umbilical level) every 5 minutes after delivery. Report if the uterus is not firm or the height is rising. (This may be an indication of urinary retention or a uterus filling with blood.) When the uterus becomes boggy, uterine massage is necessary until it becomes firm.

Check the vaginal flow rate on each perineal pad at least every half hour. With uterine atony or retained placental fragments, the uterus becomes boggy and *dark* vaginal bleeding is present; with a laceration of the cervix or vagina, the bleeding is *bright* red and the uterus is firm. Regardless of the cause, the woman must be observed carefully for signs of hypovolemic shock.

Monitor vital signs as ordered by the health care provider or every 15 minutes until stable, every 30 minutes for 2 hours, then every hour until definitely stable. Report an increasing respiratory rate; pulse rate that increases and becomes thready; a pulse deficit; blood pressure that indicates hypotension; skin that is pale, cold, and clammy; or nail beds, lips, and mucous membranes that are pale or cyanotic. Monitor hourly urine output and report an output of 30 mL per hour or less. Observe for restlessness and complaints of thirst and for any decrease in level of consciousness.

Drug Interactions

Anesthetics. Monitor the blood pressure and heart rate and rhythm closely. Report significant changes.

For those patients receiving a local anesthetic containing epinephrine, immediately report any complaints of diaphoresis, fever, chest pain, palpitations, or severe throbbing headache.

DRUG CLASS: Uterine Relaxants

Uterine relaxants, also known as tocolytic agents, are used primarily to delay or prevent preterm labor and delivery in selected patients (p. 638). Tocolytic agents act by inhibiting uterine muscle contractions. They are most commonly used to inhibit labor for 2 to 7 days in order for corticosteroids to be administered to mature fetal lungs, and to transport the mother to a hospital with a neonatal intensive care unit. The FDA has not approved any medicine for use as a tocolytic agent, but agents that are most commonly used are magnesium sulfate and terbutaline. Calcium channel blockers such as nifedipine or prostaglandin inhibitors (e.g., indomethacin, ketorolac, sulindac) may be used in specific circumstances.

magnesium sulfate

Actions

Magnesium is an ion normally found in the blood in concentrations of 1.8 to 3 mEq/L. When administered parenterally in doses sufficient to produce levels greater than 4 mEq/L, the drug may depress the central nervous system and block peripheral nerve transmission, producing anticonvulsant effects and smooth muscle relaxation.

Uses

Magnesium sulfate is used in obstetrics primarily to inhibit premature labor. It may also be used to control seizure activity associated with preeclampsia or eclampsia. When used as an anticonvulsant or to inhibit labor, blood levels should be maintained at 4 to 8 mEq/L.

Patients maintained at a magnesium serum level between 3 and 5 mEq/L rarely show any side effects from hypermagnesemia. At levels approximately 5 to 8 mEq/L, patients begin to show increasing signs of toxicity that correlate fairly well to serum levels. Early signs of maternal toxicity are complaints of "feeling hot all over" and "being thirsty all the time," flushed skin, and diaphoresis. Patients may then become hypotensive and have depressed patellar, radial, and biceps reflexes, and flaccid muscles. Later signs of hypermagnesemia are central nervous system depression shown first by anxiety, then confusion, lethargy, and drowsiness. If serum levels continue to increase, cardiac depression and respiratory paralysis may result. Magnesium sulfate should be administered with extreme caution to patients with impaired renal function and whose urine output is less than 100 mL over the past 4 hours.

Therapeutic Outcomes

The primary therapeutic outcomes associated with magnesium sulfate therapy are as follows:

- Arrest of preterm labor.
- Elimination of seizure activity.

Nursing Process for Magnesium Sulfate

Premedication Assessment

1. Obtain baseline vital signs, especially blood pressure, pulse, and respirations.
2. Perform a mental status examination: level of consciousness, orientation, and anxiety level.
3. Check deep tendon reflexes; report hyporeflexia or absence of reflexes.
4. Review intake and output record; report declining output.
5. Have calcium gluconate or calcium chloride and equipment for IV administration available if needed.
6. Obtain baseline laboratory values (e.g., serum magnesium level).
7. Monitor fetal heart rate and uterine activity; report distress.

Planning

Availability. Injection: 4% (0.325 mEq/mL); 12.5% (1 mEq/mL), and 50% (4 mEq/mL) solutions.

Implementation

Dosage and Administration

- *IM:* Intramuscular injection is extremely painful. Avoid if possible, or administer in conjunction with a local anesthetic.
- *IV:* It is absolutely essential that an infusion pump be used to help control the infusion of the loading dose and continuous drip.

Anticonvulsant

- *IM:* Loading dose: 10 g of 50% solution (20 mL) is divided into two doses of 5 g each (10 mL) and is injected by deep IM injection into each buttock; 1% lidocaine or procaine may be added to each syringe to reduce the pain on injection. The IM loading dose is usually administered at the same time that 4 g is given intravenously. Maintenance dose: 4 to 5 g of 50% solution (10 mL) IM every 4 hours in alternate buttocks.
- *IV:* Loading dose: 4 g of magnesium sulfate is added to 250 mL of D5W and infused slowly at a rate of 10 mL per minute. (The IV loading dose is usually administered at the same time as a 10 g IM loading dose.) Maintenance dose is 1 to 2 g per hour by continuous infusion.

Preterm Labor. *IV:* Loading dose: 4 g of magnesium sulfate intravenously over 15 to 20 minutes. Maintenance dose: 1 to 3 g per hour by continuous infusion.

NOTE: Deep tendon reflexes, intake and output, vital signs, and orientation to the environment must be monitored on a regular, ongoing basis.

Evaluation

Side Effects to Report

Deep Tendon Reflexes. The presence or absence of patellar reflex (knee-jerk reflex), biceps reflex, or radial reflex are primary monitoring parameters for magnesium sulfate therapy.

The patellar reflex should be monitored hourly if the patient is receiving a continuous IV infusion or before every dose if being administered intermittently IM or IV. If the reflex is absent, further doses should be withheld until it returns. If the patellar reflex cannot be used because of epidural anesthesia, the biceps or radial reflex may be used.

Intake and Output. Magnesium toxicity is more likely to occur in patients with reduced renal output. Report urine outputs of less than 30 mL per hour or less than 100 mL over 4 hours. Observe the urine color, and measure the specific gravity.

Note any other fluid and electrolyte loss such as vaginal bleeding, diarrhea, or vomiting.

Vital Signs. Vital signs (blood pressure, heart rate, and rhythm) should be measured every 15 to 30 minutes when a patient is receiving a continuous IV infusion. Take vital signs before and after each administration for patients receiving intermittent therapy.

The respiratory rate should be at least 16 breaths per minute before the administration of further doses of magnesium sulfate.

Do not administer additional doses if there is a reduced respiratory rate, a drop in blood pressure, or fetal heart rate, or other signs of fetal distress.

Confusion. Perform a baseline assessment of the patient's degree of alertness and orientation to name, place, and time *before* initiating therapy. Make regularly scheduled mental status evaluations to ensure that the patient is oriented.

Overdose. The antidote for magnesium intoxication (shown by respiratory depression and heart block) is calcium gluconate. A 10% solution of calcium gluconate should be kept at the patient's bedside ready for use. The dosage is 5 to 10 mEq (10-20 mL) IV over 3 minutes.

Administer cardiopulmonary resuscitation until the patient responds appropriately.

Neonates. Infants born of mothers who receive magnesium sulfate must be monitored for hypotension, hyporeflexia, and respiratory depression.

Drug Interactions

Central Nervous System Depressants. Central nervous system depressants, including barbiturates, analgesics, general anesthetics, tranquilizers, and alcohol, will potentiate the central nervous system depressant effects of magnesium sulfate.

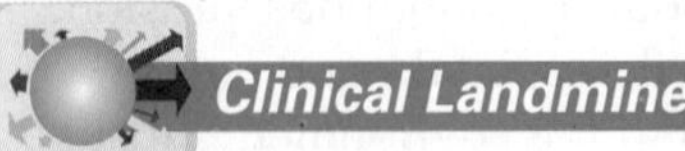

Magnesium Toxicity

Early signs of maternal toxicity are complaints of "feeling hot all over" and "being thirsty all the time," flushed skin color, and diaphoresis. Patients may then become hypotensive; have depressed patellar, radial, and biceps reflexes; and have flaccid muscles. Later signs of hypermagnesemia are central nervous system depression shown first by anxiety, followed by confusion, lethargy, and drowsiness. If serum levels continue to increase, cardiac depression and respiratory paralysis may result. The patellar reflex should be monitored hourly if the patient is receiving a continuous IV infusion or before every dose if administered intermittently IM or IV. If the reflex is absent, further doses should be withheld until it returns. If the patellar reflex cannot be used because of epidural anesthesia, the biceps or radial reflex may be used.

Periodically check orientation to make sure the patient is not suffering from magnesium toxicity.

Neuromuscular Blockade. Concurrent use of neuromuscular blocking agents and magnesium sulfate will further depress muscular activity. Monitor the patient closely for depressed reflexes and respiration.

terbutaline sulfate (ter bew' tal een)
▶ BRETHINE (breh' theen)

Actions

Terbutaline is a beta-adrenergic receptor stimulant, acting predominantly on the beta-2 receptors but, especially in higher dosages, also on the beta-1 receptors. Stimulation of the beta-2 receptors produces relaxation of the uterine, bronchial, and vascular smooth muscle. Beta-1 receptor stimulation causes an increased heart rate.

Unfortunately the receptors that are stimulated by beta-receptor agents are found in muscles of the heart, blood vessels, bronchopulmonary tree, and gastrointestinal, urinary, and central nervous systems, as well as the reproductive system. They also help regulate fat and carbohydrate metabolism. For this reason, many side effects can be expected from this agent, particularly if used too frequently or in higher than recommended doses.

Uses

Because of selective relaxant properties on the uterus, causing a reduction in the intensity and frequency of uterine contractions, terbutaline is used to arrest premature labor in situations in which it has been determined that there is no underlying pathology that would indicate that pregnancy should not be allowed to progress to completion.

Therapeutic Outcomes

The primary therapeutic outcome associated with terbutaline therapy is arrest of preterm labor.

Nursing Process for Terbutaline

Premedication Assessment

1. Obtain baseline vital signs and weight.
2. Monitor maternal and fetal heart rates.
3. Perform baseline mental status examination (e.g., alertness, orientation, anxiety level, muscle strength, tremors).
4. Obtain baseline laboratory studies ordered (e.g., electrolytes, glucose, hematocrit, carbon dioxide).
5. In patients with diabetes, obtain baseline glucose and plan to monitor closely for subsequent hyperglycemia and possible changes in insulin dosage.

Planning

Availability. PO: 2.5 and 5 mg tablets. Injection: 1 mg/mL in 1-mL ampules.

Implementation

Dosage and Administration. See Box 40-1. IV rate: An infusion pump is absolutely essential for the safe delivery of this agent. PO: Administer with food or milk to reduce gastric irritation.

Evaluation

Side Effects to Report

Tachycardia, Palpitations, Hypertension, Hypotension. Because most symptoms are dose related, alterations should be reported to the health care provider. Monitor the maternal and fetal heart rates and rhythms at regular intervals throughout therapy. Report heart rates significantly higher than baseline values. These include maternal and fetal tachycardia averaging 130 and 164 beats per minute, respectively. Maternal systolic blood pressure increases to a range of 96 to 162 mm Hg, and diastolic pressures drop to a range of 0 to 76 mm Hg.

Always report palpitations and suspected dysrhythmias.

Box 40-1 ***Guidelines for Use of Terbutaline with Premature Labor****

1. Initiate a control IV of 5% dextrose, Ringer's lactate, or saline solution and administer 400 to 500 mL 15 to 20 minutes before the initiation of the medication. Then decrease to 100 to 125 mL/hour.
2. Add 20 mg of terbutaline to 1000 mL of D5W.
3. Place the patient in a left lateral, horizontal position with a blood pressure cuff in position.
4. Administer a loading dose of 250 mcg IV over 1 to 2 minutes. Monitor closely for hypotension.
5. Start the infusion at a rate of 10 mcg IV (30 mL/hour).
6. Increase the infusion rate by 3.5 mg/minute (10 mL/hour) every 10 minutes until labor has stopped or a maximum dose of 26 mcg/minute (80 mL/hour) has been attained.
7. Maintain the effective dose for 1 hour or more, then begin decreasing the rate by 2 mcg/minute (6 mL/hour) every 30 minutes until the lowest effective dose is reached. Maintain the total IV fluid intake at 125 mL/hour.
8. When the lowest effective IV dose is reached, begin PO terbutaline, 2.5 mg every 4 hours.
9. If labor has stopped, discontinue the IV infusion 24 hours after PO administration was initiated if the uterus is not irritable.
10. Continue the PO regimen (2.5 mg every 4 hours or 5 mg every 8 hours) until 36 weeks' gestation.
11. If labor begins again, restart the IV infusion as above.

*Note: Terbutaline is not approved by the FDA for use in premature labor. It may be used, however, in emergency situations when the physician judges that it is in the best interests of the patient and infant. When terbutaline is used for premature labor, sometimes a significant drop in blood pressure (due to vasodilatory effects) can be observed at the time of the loading dose and when the infusion is started. Blood pressure and pulse monitoring should be done before and every 5 minutes after the loading dose has been administered and the infusion started, until the patient is stable. Use continuous fetal monitoring. If the maternal pulse exceeds 120 beats/minute and does not decrease with an increase in fluids or when the patient is rolled onto her left side, or if there is any evidence of a decrease in uterine perfusion, discontinue the infusion.

Tremors. Instruct the patient to notify the health care provider if tremors develop after starting any of these medications. A dosage adjustment may be necessary.

Nervousness, Anxiety, Restlessness, Headache. Perform a baseline assessment of the patient's mental status (e.g., degree of anxiety, nervousness, alertness); compare at regular intervals with the findings obtained. Report escalation of tension.

Nausea, Vomiting. Monitor all aspects of the development of these symptoms.

Administer the oral medication with food and a full glass of water or milk. Report if the symptoms are not relieved.

Dizziness. Provide patient safety during episodes of dizziness; report for further evaluation.

Hyperglycemia. Terbutaline routinely increases serum glucose and insulin levels, although these tend to return to normal within 48 to 72 hours with continued infusion. Diabetic or prediabetic patients must be monitored for the development of hyperglycemia, particularly during the early days of therapy.

Assess regularly for hyperglycemia and report if it occurs frequently.

Insulin requirements may double in these patients during terbutaline therapy.

Electrolyte Imbalance. The electrolyte most commonly altered is potassium (K^+). Hypokalemia is most likely to occur. Serum potassium levels may drop during IV administration. Urinary losses generally do not increase; much of the losses are due to intracellular redistribution, which return to the blood after therapy is discontinued.

Many symptoms associated with altered fluid and electrolyte balance are subtle.

Gather data relative to changes in the patient's mental status (e.g., alertness, orientation, confusion), muscle strength, muscle cramps, tremors, nausea, and general appearance (e.g., drowsy, anxious, lethargic).

Always check the electrolyte reports for early indications of electrolyte imbalance.

Keep accurate records of intake and output, daily weights, and vital signs.

The Neonate. Neonatal adverse effects are uncommon, but hyperglycemia, followed by hypoglycemia, hypocalcemia, hypotension, and paralytic ileus have been reported. Monitor these newborns closely over the next several hours. Make sure that the infant's sleep after birth is not masking these conditions.

Drug Interactions

Drugs That Enhance Toxic Effects. Tricyclic antidepressants (e.g., imipramine, amitriptyline, nortriptyline, doxepin), monoamine oxidase inhibitors (e.g., tranylcypromine, isocarboxazid, and phenelzine), and other sympathomimetic agents (e.g., metaproterenol, isoproterenol) enhance toxic effects.

Monitor for increases in severity of drug effects such as nervousness, tachycardia, tremors, and dysrhythmias.

Drugs That Reduce Therapeutic Effects. Beta adrenergic–blocking agents (e.g., propranolol, timolol, nadolol, pindolol). Monitor for lack of therapeutic effect.

Corticosteroids. Concurrent use may rarely result in pulmonary edema. There is a higher incidence in patients with multiple pregnancy, occult cardiac disease, and fluid overload. Persistent tachycardia may be a sign of impending pulmonary edema. Observe patient closely; monitor fluid input and output, breath sounds, and heart rate, as well as the anxiety level and state of well-being.

Antihypertensive Agents. Sympathomimetic agents may reduce the therapeutic effects of antihypertensive agents. Monitor blood pressure for an indication of loss of antihypertensive control.

Anesthetics. Concurrent use with general anesthetics may result in additional hypotensive effects. Monitor blood pressure and heart rate and rhythm regularly.

DRUG CLASS: Other Agents

clomiphene citrate (klom′ ih feen si′ trayt)

▶ CLOMID (klo′ mid)

Actions

Clomiphene is a chemical compound that is structurally similar to natural estrogens. When administered, it binds to estrogen receptor sites, reducing the number of sites available for circulating estrogens. The receptors send back signals to the hypothalamus and pituitary gland, indicating a lack of circulating estrogens. The hypothalamus responds by increasing the secretion of hypothalamic-releasing factor. This stimulates the pituitary gland to release luteinizing hormone (LH) and follicle-stimulating hormone (FSH), which in turn stimulate the ovaries to release ova for potential fertilization.

Uses

Clomiphene is used to induce ovulation in women who are not ovulating because of reduced circulating estrogen levels. Studies indicate that pregnancy occurs in 25% to 30% of patients treated. Ovulation of more than one ovum per cycle with potential fertilization of multiple ova may occur in 5% to 10% of patients treated.

Therapeutic Outcomes

The primary therapeutic outcome associated with clomiphene therapy is ovulation, followed by fertilization and pregnancy.

Nursing Process for Clomiphene

Premedication Assessment

1. Check to ensure that the patient has had a complete physical examination, including pregnancy testing, before initiating therapy.
2. Obtain baseline data regarding any gastrointestinal or visual disturbances present before initiating therapy.

Planning

Availability. PO: 50-mg tablets.

Implementation

NOTE: It is mandatory that patients have a complete physical examination to rule out other pathologic causes for lack of ovulation before initiating clomiphene therapy.

Patients must be informed of the possibility of multiple fetuses with clomiphene treatment.

Possible Pregnancy. Clomiphene should not be administered if pregnancy is suspected. Basal temperatures should be followed for 1 month after therapy. Instruct the patient on how to take and record basal temperatures and how to report a biphasic temperature distribution. If the body temperature follows a biphasic distribution (peaks twice within a few days) and is not followed by menses, the next course of clomiphene therapy should not be scheduled until pregnancy tests have been completed.

Timing of Intercourse. Intercourse timing is important to the therapy's success. Make sure the patient understands the importance of having intercourse during the time of ovulation, usually 6 to 10 days after the last dose of medication.

Dosage and Administration. *Adult:* PO: 50 mg daily for 5 days. Start therapy at any time if there has been no recent bleeding. If spontaneous bleeding occurs before therapy, start on or about the fifth day for 5 days.

If ovulation does not occur after the first course, give a second course of 100 mg per day for 5 days. Start this course no earlier than 30 days after the previous course.

A third course may be administered at 100 mg per day for 5 days. However, most patients who respond will have done so in the first two courses. Reevaluation of the patient is necessary.

Evaluation

Side Effects to Expect

Nausea, Vomiting, Diarrhea, Constipation, "Hot Flashes," Abdominal Cramps. These side effects are usually mild and tend to resolve with continued therapy. Encourage the patient not to discontinue therapy without first consulting the health care provider.

Side Effects to Report

Severe Abdominal Cramps. Patients should be informed to report significant abdominal or pelvic pain and bloating that develop during therapy.

Visual Disturbances. Patients developing visual blurring, spots, or double vision should report for an eye examination. The drug is usually discontinued, and visual disturbances pass within a few days to weeks after discontinuation.

Caution the patient to temporarily avoid tasks that require visual acuity, such as driving or operating power machinery.

Dizziness. Provide patient safety during episodes of dizziness; report for further evaluation.

Drug Interactions. No clinically significant drug interactions have been reported.

Rh_o(D) immune globulin IM [Rh_o(D) IGIM]
HyperRHO S/D Full Dose; RhoGAM
Rh_o(D) immune globulin micro-dose [Rh_o(D) IG micro-dose]
HyperRHO S/D Mini-Dose; MICRhoGAM
Rh_o(D) immune globulin IV (human) [Rh_o(D) IGIV]
WinRho SDF; Rhophylac

Actions

Rh_o(D) immune globulin suppresses the stimulation of active immunity by Rh-positive foreign red blood cells that enter the maternal circulation either at the time of delivery, at the termination of a pregnancy, or during a transfusion of inadequately typed blood.

Rh hemolytic disease of the newborn can be prevented in subsequent pregnancies by administering Rh_o(D) immune globulin [Rh_o(D) antibody] to the Rh-negative mother shortly after delivery of an Rh-positive child.

Uses

Rh_o(D) immune globulin (human) is used to prevent Rh immunization of the Rh-negative patient exposed to Rh-positive blood as the result of a transfusion accident, during termination of a pregnancy, or as the result of a delivery of an Rh-positive infant. Full-dose Rh_o(D) IGIM and Rh_o(D) IGIV are used when there has been a transfusion accident, during termination of a pregnancy greater than 12 weeks' gestation, or as the result of a delivery of an Rh-positive infant. Rh_o(D) IGIM Microdose is used to prevent Rh immunization of the Rh-negative patient exposed to Rh-positive red blood cells at the time of spontaneous or induced abortion of up to 12 weeks' gestation.

In addition to preventing Rh immunization of the Rh-negative patient for the above causes, Rh_o(D) immune globulin IV (human) [Rh_o(D) IGIV] also is used to treat idiopathic thrombocytopenic purpura (ITP), a condition of spontaneous destruction of platelets. The mechanism by which Rh_o(D) immune globulin IV (human) reduces spontaneous rupture of platelets is unknown.

Therapeutic Outcomes

The primary therapeutic outcome associated with Rh_o(D) immune globulin (human) therapy is prevention of Rh hemolytic disease. The primary therapeutic outcome associated with Rh_o(D) immune globulin IV (human) [Rh_o(D) IGIV] therapy is prevention of Rh hemolytic disease and platelet destruction in acute cases of ITP.

Nursing Process for Rh_o(D) Immune Globulin (Human)

Premedication Assessment

1. Check Rh status of mother; she must be Rh negative. Has the mother previously been sensitized to Rh factor through blood transfusion or previous pregnancy?
2. Check the platelet count of those patients being treated for ITP.

Planning

Availability. IM: Rh_o(D) immune globulin micro-dose (HyperRHO S/D Mini Dose, MICRhoGAM): single-dose vial; Rh_o(D) immune globulin (HyperRHO S/D, RhoGAM): single-dose vial or prefilled syringe; IV: WinRho SDF: 600, 1500, 5000 international units in single-dose vials; Rhophylac: 1500 international units in prefilled syringe.

Implementation

Dosage and Administration

Pregnancy and Transfusion Accident

- *Previous immunization:* Although there is no need to administer Rh_o(D) immune globulin to a woman who is already sensitized to the Rh factor, the risk is no more than when given to a woman who is not sensitized. When in doubt, administer Rh_o(D) immune globulin.
- Before administration:
  1. *Never* administer the IGIM full-dose or micro-dose products intravenously. (However, the IVIG full-dose product may be administered intramuscularly or intravenously.)
  2. *Never* administer to a neonate.
  3. *Never* administer to an Rh-negative patient who has been previously sensitized to the Rh antigen.
  4. *Confirm* that the mother is Rh negative.
- *Pregnancy:* Postpartum prophylaxis: 1 standard-dose vial of IGIM intramuscularly or 1 standard-dose vial of IGIV intramuscularly or intravenously. Additional vials may be necessary if there was unusually large fetal-maternal hemorrhage.
- *Antepartum prophylaxis:* One standard-dose vial IM at about 28 weeks' gestation. This must be followed by another vial administered within 72 hours of delivery. After amniocentesis, miscarriage, abortion, or ectopic pregnancy and less than 13 weeks' gestation: one micro-dose vial IM within 72 hours; 13 or more weeks of gestation: one standard dose vial IM within 72 hours.

- *Transfusion accident:* Rh-negative, premenopausal women who receive Rh-positive red cells by transfusion: One standard-dose vial IM for each 15 mL of transfused packed red cells.

Idiopathic Thrombocytopenic Purpura (ITP)

- Before administration:
  1. *Confirm* that the person is Rh positive.
  2. *Follow* manufacturer's instructions on dilution and administration of $Rh_o(D)$ IGIV.
  3. IV: Initial dose: 250 units/kg as a single injection. Additional doses depend on response.

Evaluation

Side Effects to Expect

Localized Tenderness. Inform patients that they may experience stiffness at the site of injection for a few days.

Fever, Arthralgias, Generalized Aches, Pains. Monitor on a regular basis for these symptoms. Follow routine orders of the health care provider or hospital concerning the use of analgesics (usually acetaminophen; do not use aspirin or other antiinflammatory agents) for patient discomfort.

Side Effects to Report

Urticaria, Tachycardia, Hypotension. Allergic reactions require immediate treatment. Monitor patients for 20 to 30 minutes after administration. Have emergency supplies readily available.

Drug Interactions. No significant drug interactions have been reported.

DRUG CLASS: Neonatal Ophthalmic Solutions

erythromycin ophthalmic ointment

ILOTYCIN (eye lo ty' sin)

Actions and Uses

Erythromycin (Ilotycin) is a macrolide antibiotic used prophylactically to prevent ophthalmia neonatorum, which is caused by *N. gonorrhoeae*. It is also effective against *C. trachomatis*.

Therapeutic Outcomes

The primary therapeutic outcome associated with erythromycin ophthalmic ointment therapy is prevention of postpartum gonorrhea or *Chlamydia* eye infection.

Nursing Process for Erythromycin Ophthalmic Ointment

Premedication Assessment

Describe any drainage present in the eye or on the lids; cleanse thoroughly.

Planning

Availability. Ophthalmic ointment: 0.5% in 3.5-g tubes.

Implementation

Dosage and Administration

- *Ointment:* A new tube should be started for each infant.
- *Wash hands:* Wash hands immediately before administration to prevent bacterial contamination. Put on gloves.
- *Cleanse the eyes:* Using a separate sterile absorbent cotton or gauze pledget for each eye, wash the unopened lids from the nose outward until free of blood, mucus, or meconium.
- *Open the eyes and instill medication:* Separate the eyelids and instill a narrow ribbon of erythromycin ointment along the lower conjunctival surface.
- *Instillation:* Instill a ¼-inch ribbon along the lower conjunctival surface of both eyes. Administration should be done within 2 hours of birth.
- *Irrigation:* DO NOT irrigate the eyes after instillation.

Evaluation

Side Effects to Expect

Mild Conjunctivitis. Mild conjunctival inflammation occurs in the neonate and may interfere with the ability to focus. This side effect generally disappears in 1 to 2 days. Assure the family that the redness is temporary.

Drug Interactions. No significant drug interactions have been reported.

phytonadione (fy toe nah di' own)

AQUAMEPHYTON (ak wah mef' i ton)

Actions

Vitamin K is a fat-soluble vitamin necessary for the production of the blood-clotting factors prothrombin (factor II), proconvertin (factor VII), plasma thromboplastin component (factor IX), and Stuart factor (factor X) in the liver. Vitamin K is absorbed from the diet and is normally produced by the bacterial flora in the gastrointestinal tract, from which it is absorbed and transported to the liver for clotting factor production. Newborns have not yet colonized the colon with bacteria and are often deficient in vitamin K. They also may be deficient in these clotting factors and are therefore more susceptible to hemorrhagic disease in the first 5 to 8 days after birth.

Uses

Phytonadione is routinely administered prophylactically to protect against vitamin K deficiency bleeding (VKDB) of the newborn, (formerly known as hemorrhagic disease of the newborn).

Therapeutic Outcomes

The primary therapeutic outcome associated with phytonadione therapy is prevention of VKDB of the newborn.

Nursing Process for Phytonadione

Premedication Assessment

No assessment is required.

Planning

Availability. Injection: 2 mg/mL in 0.5-mL prefilled syringes.

Implementation

IM: DO NOT administer intravenously! Severe reactions, including hypotension, cardiac dysrhythmias, and respiratory arrest, have been reported.

Dosage and Administration. IM: 0.5 to 1 mg in the lateral aspect of the thigh.

Evaluation

Side Effects to Report

Bruising, Hemorrhage. Observe for bleeding (usually occurring on the second or third day). Bleeding may be seen as petechiae, generalized ecchymoses, or bleeding from the umbilical stump, circumcision site, nose, or gastrointestinal tract. Assess results of serial prothrombin times.

Drug Interactions. No significant drug interactions have been reported.

- Today's health care system is placing more emphasis on self-care for the mother and her newborn. Shortened hospital stays have heightened the health care professional's awareness of the need to provide more education to the mother and significant others, not only in the care needs of the mother but also for the newborn.
- Every encounter with the mother is an opportunity to enhance her learning and preparation for parenting. Community resources for prenatal and parenting classes should be encouraged.
- The prenatal examination provides a basis for establishing the future health care needs of the mother and infant. Psychosocial and cultural aspects of care must be incorporated into the assessments and interventions planned for self-care. At subsequent prenatal visits, relevant information must be provided on all aspects of self-care to enhance the normal growth and development of the fetus and to prevent or manage potential complications of pregnancy.
- After delivery, the mother should attend discharge classes and be provided with telephone follow-up, home visitations, and referrals to available community resources to meet the care needs of the mother and newborn at home.

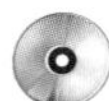

Go to your Companion CD-ROM for Appendices, an Audio Glossary, animations, Drug Dosage Calculators, customizable Patient Self-Assessment forms, and Review Questions for the NCLEX® Examination.

evolve Be sure to visit the companion Evolve site at http://evolve.elsevier.com/Clayton for WebLinks and additional online resources.

MEDICATION SAFETY REVIEW

MATH REVIEW QUESTIONS

1. Order: Methylergonovine maleate (Methergine) 0.2 mg IM immediately after delivery of the placenta

   Available: Use the drug monograph in the textbook to determine the availability of the drug.

   Give: _____ mL.

2. Order: magnesium sulfate 1 g/hour by continuous infusion

   Available: magnesium sulfate 4 g added to 250 mL D5W

   Set the infusion pump at: _____ mL/hour.

Continued

CRITICAL THINKING QUESTIONS

1. After delivery of a newborn, an Rh-negative mother asks you why she must receive RhoGAM. Give an explanation of the rationale that she'll be able to understand.
2. Why is it necessary to prehydrate the mother before administration of terbutaline IV?
3. During administration of terbutaline IV, the woman's pulse elevates to 150 beats per minute and the fetal heart rate is 200 beats per minute. What actions would you take?
4. Identify nursing assessments needed when a uterine relaxant is prescribed.
5. Explain the primary use of uterine stimulants.
6. Develop a detailed listing of premedication assessments needed for oxytocin.

CONTENT REVIEW QUESTIONS

1. Oxytocin (Pitocin) is administered:
   1. subcutaneously.
   2. intramuscularly.
   3. intravenously using an infusion pump.
   4. in fractional doses every hour.
2. During terbutaline (Brethine) administration, the patient's pulse rate is 150 and blood pressure is 170/100 mm Hg. The nurse should:
   1. increase the infusion rate and retake vitals in 20 minutes.
   2. administer an antihypertensive PRN.
   3. check fetal heart rate and report all findings to the health care provider.
   4. report findings to the health care provider.
3. During the administration of magnesium sulfate, the nurse should have _____ available. *(Select all that apply.)*
   1. calcium carbonate
   2. calcium gluconate
   3. calcium citrate
   4. calcium chloride
4. Phytonadione (AquaMEPHYTON) is given to the newborn to:
   1. prevent intestinal flora from developing.
   2. increase water-soluble vitamin supply.
   3. prevent production of prothrombin (factor II).
   4. prevent hemorrhagic disease.
5. Uses for Cytotec include which of the following? *(Select all that apply.)*
   1. Cervical softening and dilation before labor
   2. Induction of active labor
   3. Reduction in postpartum hemorrhage in the presence of uterine atony
   4. Evacuation of uterine contents
6. Which laboratory test may be ordered to assess for the presence of preterm labor in patients whose presenting symptoms are questionable?
   1. Fetal fibronectin
   2. Creatinine clearance
   3. Alpha fetoprotein
   4. Folic acid level
7. All patients in preterm labor are at risk for neonatal group B streptococcal infection. What is the antibiotic most frequently used to treat this if there are no allergies to this medication?
   1. vancomycin
   2. tetracycline
   3. penicillin G
   4. cotrimoxazole

CHAPTER

41 Drugs Used in Men's and Women's Health

evolve http://evolve.elsevier.com/Clayton

Chapter Content

Objectives

1. Identify common organisms known to cause leukorrhea.
2. Cite the generic and brand names of products used to treat *Candida albicans*, *Trichomonas vaginalis*, and *Gardnerella vaginalis*.
3. Review specific techniques for administering vaginal medications.
4. Develop a plan for teaching self-care to women and men with sexually transmitted diseases. Include personal hygiene measures, medication administration, methods of pain relief, and prevention of spread of infection or reinfection.
5. Discuss specific interviewing techniques that can be used to obtain a history of sexual activity.
6. Compare the active ingredients in the two types of oral contraceptive agents.
7. Differentiate between the actions and the benefits of the combination pill and the minipill.
8. Describe the major adverse effects and contraindications to the use of oral contraceptive agents.
9. Develop specific patient education plans to be used to teach a patient to initiate oral contraceptive therapy with the combination pill and the minipill.
10. Identify the patient teaching necessary with the administration of the transdermal contraceptive and the intravaginal hormonal contraceptive.
11. Describe pharmacologic treatments of benign prostatic hyperplasia.
12. Describe the pharmacologic treatment of erectile dysfunction.

Key Terms

leukorrhea
sexually transmitted diseases
dysmenorrhea

VAGINITIS

Secretions from the vagina usually represent a normal physiologic process, but if the discharge becomes excessive, it is known as leukorrhea, an abnormal, usually whitish, vaginal discharge that may occur at any age. It affects almost all females at some time in their lives. Leukorrhea is not a disease but a symptom of an underlying disorder. The most common cause is an infection of the lower reproductive tract, but other physiologic and noninfectious causes of vaginal discharge are well known (Table 41-1).

The most common organisms causing the infectious type of leukorrhea are *Candida albicans*, *Trichomonas vaginalis*, and *Gardnerella vaginalis* (Box 41-1). Occasionally *C. albicans* infections of the mouth, gastrointestinal tract, or vagina may develop as secondary infections during the use of broad-spectrum antibiotics, such as penicillins, tetracyclines, and cephalosporins.

Pathogens that are commonly transmitted by sexual contact are called sexually transmitted diseases (STDs) (see Box 41-1). In some diseases, such as gonorrhea, syphilis, chlamydia, and genital herpes simplex virus infection, sexual transmission is the primary mode of transmission. In others, such as giardiasis, shigellosis, and the hepatitis viruses, other important nonsexual means of transmission also exist. Unfortunately, the true incidence of STDs is not known in the United States because of large numbers of unreported cases.

DRUG THERAPY FOR LEUKORRHEA AND GENITAL INFECTIONS

See Table 41-2.

NURSING PROCESS *for Men's and Women's Health*

Assessment

NOTE: Nurses must be aware of our changing society and the increasing frequency with which young adolescents are sexually active. The following assessment questions apply to all age groups.

Table 41-1 Causes of Vaginal Discharge

PHYSIOLOGIC	INFECTIOUS	NONINFECTIOUS
Ovulation	Vaginal	Atrophic vaginitis
Coitus	*Candida*	Foreign body
Oral contraceptives	*Trichomonas*	Vaginal adenosis
Pregnancy	*Gardnerella*	Allergic vulvovaginitis
Premenstruation	Toxic shock syndrome	Vulvar, vaginal carcinoma
Premenarche	Vulvar	Cervical polyps
Intrauterine device	Herpes	Cervical erosions/ulcers
	Condylomata acuminata	Uterine carcinoma
	Syphilis	Endometrial myoma
	Bartholinitis	Vesicovaginal fistula
	Lymphogranuloma venereum	Enterovaginal fistula
	Chancroid	
	Granuloma inguinale	
	Urethritis	
	Pyoderma	
	Cervical	
	Gonorrhea	
	Chlamydial or bacterial cervicitis	
	Chronic cervicitis	
	Pelvic inflammatory disease	

From Reilly BM: *Practical strategies in outpatient medicine,* Philadelphia, 1984, WB Saunders.

Box 41-1 Sexually Transmitted Diseases

Bacteria
Neisseria gonorrhoeae
Gardnerella vaginalis
Treponema pallidum
Calymmatobacterium granulomatis
Haemophilus ducreyi

Chlamydiae
Chlamydia trachomatis

Ectoparasites
Sarcoptes scabiei
Phthirus pubis

Fungi
Candida albicans

Mycoplasma
Ureaplasma urealyticum
Mycoplasma hominis

Protozoa
Trichomonas vaginalis
Entamoeba histolytica
Giardia lamblia

Viruses
Herpes simplex virus
Hepatitis A, B, C
Cytomegalovirus
Human papillomavirus
Poxvirus
Human immunodeficiency virus

Female Reproductive History. Assess for the following:

- Age of menarche
- Usual pattern of menses: duration, number of pads used, last menstrual period
- Pain, discomfort, spotting between periods, or extended time of menstrual flow
- Number of pregnancies, live births, miscarriages, or abortions
- Vaginal discharges, infections, genital lesions, or warts. Describe color, odor, and amount of discharge; describe lesions or any itching. Is there pain with urination or sexual intercourse?
- Contraceptive methods used (e.g., oral contraceptives, intrauterine device, condoms, or spermicidal products)
- If taking oral contraceptives, what types? How long has therapy been used? Are they taken regularly? What, if any, side effects have been experienced?
- History of multiple sexual partners—male, female, or both. What type of protection is used during sexual intercourse?
- Breast self-examination routine (if not being performed regularly, explain correct procedure)
- Age of menopause
- Postmenopausal women: Is there any vaginal bleeding?
- History and frequency of Papanicolaou (Pap) smears
- Reproductive problems (e.g., endometriosis, ovarian cysts, and uterine fibroids)
- History of STDs (e.g., chlamydia, syphilis, gonorrhea, yeast infections, genital herpes, human immunodeficiency virus [HIV]), genital warts (human papillomavirus [HPV]). If so, when, and what was the treatment?
- If the person is seeking a prescription for oral contraceptive therapy, ask about any indication of hypertension, heart or liver disease, thromboembolic disorders, or cancer of the reproductive organs. Does the individual smoke?

Drug Table 41-2 CAUSATIVE ORGANISMS AND PRODUCTS USED TO TREAT GENITAL INFECTIONS

CAUSATIVE ORGANISM	GENERIC NAME	BRAND NAME	DRUG MONOGRAPH, NURSING IMPLICATIONS
VULVOVAGINITIS			
Candida albicans (fungus)	butoconazole vaginal cream	Gynazolel; Mycelex-3	(p. 778)
	clotrimazole vaginal cream, vaginal tablets	Gyne-Lotrimin, Mycelex-7	(p. 778)
	fluconazole oral tablets	Diflucan	(p. 781)
	miconazole vaginal cream, suppositories	Monistat	(p. 778)
	terconazole vaginal cream, suppositories	Terazol 7, Terazol 3	(p. 779)
	tioconazole vaginal ointment	Vagistat	(p. 779)
Trichomonas vaginalis (protozoa)	metronidazole oral tablets	Flagyl	(p. 773)
	tinidazole oral tablets	Tindamax	(p. 775)
Gardnerella vaginalis (bacteria)	metronidazole oral tablets, vaginal gel	Flagyl; MetroGel-Vaginal	(p. 773)
	clindamycin vaginal cream	Cleocin	(p. 772)
GONORRHEA			
Neisseria gonorrhea (bacteria)	ceftriaxone	Rocephin	(p. 755)
	spectinomycin	Trobicin	(p. 774)
	cefixime	Suprax	(p. 755)
	ciprofloxacin	Cipro	(p. 763)
	ofloxacin	Floxin	(p. 763)
	levofloxacin	Levaquin	(p. 763)
SYPHILIS			
Treponema pallidum (spirochete)	penicillin G, benzathine	Bicillin C-R	(p. 761)
	tetracycline	Tetracycline	(p. 767)
	doxycycline	Vibramycin	(p. 767)
	azithromycin	Zithromax	(p. 759)
GENITAL HERPES			
Herpes simplex genitalis (virus)	acyclovir oral capsules	Zovirax	(p. 786)
	famciclovir oral tablets	Famvir	(p. 794)
	valacyclovir oral tablets	Valtrex	(p. 798)
CHLAMYDIAE			
Chlamydia trachomatis (chlamydia)	doxycycline	Vibramycin	(p. 767)
	erythromycin	Erythromycin	(p. 759)
	azithromycin	Zithromax	(p. 759)
	ofloxacin	Floxin	(p. 763)
	levofloxacin	Levaquin	(p. 763)

From Centers for Disease Control and Prevention: Sexually transmitted diseases treatment guidelines, *MMWR* 2006:55 (No. RR-11), 2006.

Male Reproductive History. Assess for the following:

- Pattern of urination. Has there been a recent change in the pattern of urination (e.g., difficulty initiating urine stream, need to strain to empty the bladder, frequency of nocturia, pain on urination, frequency, urgency, hematuria, incontinence, dribbling, or urinary retention)?
- Presence of a urethral discharge or genital or perianal lesions. Is there any swelling of the penis?
- Is there pain in the lower back, perineum, or pelvis?
- History of prostatitis, benign prostatic hyperplasia, or prostatic cancer
- Testicular self-examination? How frequently? (If not being performed regularly, explain the correct procedure)
- History of STDs (e.g., chlamydia, syphilis, gonorrhea, yeast infections, genital herpes, human immunodeficiency virus [HIV]), genital warts (human papillomavirus [HPV]). If so, when and what was the treatment?
- History of multiple sexual partners—male, female, or both. What type of protection is used during sexual intercourse?
- History of erectile dysfunction and description of pattern of altered erectile functioning

- History of arthralgia, fever, chills, malaise, pharyngitis, or oral lesions
- History of prior illnesses
- If erectile dysfunction has occurred, ask specifically about vascular disorders that may lead to changes in blood flow to the penis (e.g., stroke). Ask about smoking and use of drugs that may affect the vascular system (e.g., antihypertensive agents).
- Has the individual had prostate surgery? If so, was the onset of the erectile dysfunction before or after the surgery?
- Other neurologic disorders (e.g., Parkinson's disease and spinal cord injuries) may cause problems with sexual functioning. Has the individual had any other genitourinary conditions (e.g., testicular injury)?
- Endocrine disorders such as thyroid disease, adrenal disorders, and diabetes mellitus are also associated with sexual dysfunction. Does the patient have any of these illnesses?

History of Current Symptoms. Ask the patient to describe the current problem or problems that initiated this visit. How long have the symptoms existed? Is there a recurrence of symptoms that were treated previously?

Medication History

- Has the individual taken steroids or antibiotics recently? If so, what condition was being treated and for how long? How long ago was therapy discontinued?
- Are over-the-counter (OTC), herbal, prescribed, or recreational drugs being taken? If so, what, why, and for how long?
- Are there any allergies to medications (e.g., antibiotics)?
- If having a recurrence of an STD, what was the previous treatment?
- In the presence of erectile dysfunction, a number of drugs may contribute to the problem (e.g., antihypertensives, antipsychotics, tricyclic antidepressants, monoamine oxidase inhibitors, hormones, sedative-hypnotics, stimulants, hormonal chemotherapeutics, opiates, steroids, and recreational drugs); therefore a medication history is extremely important.

Psychosocial

- Sexually transmitted diseases cause a high degree of anxiety. The intimate nature of the questioning required to obtain a sexual history may be embarrassing. Vaginal or urethral discharge may also be alarming to the patient seeking health care. When an STD diagnosis is suspected, explain the confidentiality policy of the facility before asking about sexual partners. (Many individuals do not return for follow-up appointments; there may be only one chance to obtain relevant information about contacts.)
- Ask about lifestyle orientation (e.g., heterosexual, bisexual, or homosexual and number of partners). Has there been known contact with people with STDs? Are precautions used during sexual contacts?
- Assess the level of anxiety present and adaptive responses and coping mechanisms used.

Laboratory and Diagnostic Studies

- Review reports on Gram stains and cultures from the anus, throat, and urethra for gonorrhea; Venereal Disease Research Laboratory (VDRL) and rapid plasma reagin (RPR), fluorescent treponema antibody absorption (FTA-ABS), for syphilis; tissue cultures for herpes simplex virus (HSV)–2; HIV testing (antibodies against HIV-1 and HIV-2 starting with enzyme immunoassay [EIA]); confirm using the Western blot (WB) or an immunofluorescence assay [IFA]). HIV testing should be offered to everyone evaluated for any type of STD.
- Diagnostic studies are individualized to the suspected etiology of the signs and symptoms (e.g., complete blood count [CBC], prostate specific antigen [PSA], cultures of prostate secretions, urine cultures, blood urea nitrogen [BUN], creatinine) for prostatic disorders.

Physical Examination

- Perform routine physical examination of the woman including pelvic examination, Pap smear, cultures, and breast examination.
- Perform routine physical examination of the man including testicular examination (rectal examination with palpation of prostate after age 40). An anorectal examination and examination of throat, tonsils, and mouth should be completed with men of homosexual or bisexual orientation.

Nursing Diagnoses

- Infection, risk for (indication)
- Health maintenance, ineffective (indication)
- Pain, acute or chronic pain (indication)
- Knowledge, deficient (indication, side effects)
- Sexuality patterns, ineffective (indication, side effects)

Planning

- Most of the conditions discussed in this chapter are treated in the health care provider's office and managed through self-care. Therefore planning is focused on self-care issues, preventing transmission of infectious disorders, and seeking appropriate follow-up care.
- For patients with menstrual irregularities or needing contraceptive therapy, education regarding medications and personal health practices must be given.
- For patients with infections of the reproductive tract, education regarding personal hygiene, proper medi-

cation administration and adherence, and prevention of spread of infection and reinfection are crucial.

- Discuss sex practices, mode of transmission of STDs, prevention measures, and follow-up with people of all age-groups (adolescents, adults). Be aware of possible child abuse as a cause of STDs in infants, children, and adolescents.
- Stress the need for an annual Pap smear to detect cervical cancer that originates from cervical intraepithelial neoplasia (CIN). Men need annual physical examinations after age 40 that include a rectal examination to palpate the prostate. Men and women older than age 50 should have a periodic sigmoidoscopy to assess for colon cancer.

Implementation

- Record basic patient data (e.g., height, weight, vital signs).
- Prepare the patient for and assist with a physical examination.
- Observe distribution of body hair and presence of any scars, lesions, body rashes, pubic lice, or mites.
- Assist with specimen collection (e.g., vaginal smears, cultures of discharge).
- Inspect the penis and scrotum for swelling or abnormalities; observe for urethral discharge.
- Provide psychological support and refer for available counseling, as appropriate.

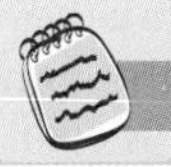

Patient Education and Health Promotion

Instructions for Adolescents. The rate of STDs is high in this age group, so it is important to do a thorough assessment of sexual activity and practices. For those who are sexually active, counseling regarding safe sex practices and voluntary testing and treatment should be offered. Medical care for STDs can be provided without parental consent or knowledge. Check individual state laws for those that allow testing and counseling for HIV. All adolescents should be thoroughly taught about the alternative of abstinence and safe sexual practices.

Instructions for Women

- Refrain from using irritating vaginal substances such as deodorants, scented toilet paper, and perfumed soaps, sprays, and douches.
- Warm sitz baths may help relieve vaginal or perineal irritation.
- Douching is generally avoided unless specifically prescribed by the health care provider. Douching alters the pH of the vagina and may actually encourage the growth of inappropriate organisms.
- Personal hygiene should include wiping from front to back after voiding and defecation, voiding before and after intercourse, thorough cleansing of genitals before and after intercourse, and changing menstrual tampons or pads frequently. Avoid wearing underwear made of synthetic materials; cotton materials help prevent moisture accumulation.
- Contraceptive methods (e.g., oral and other hormonal contraceptives, intrauterine devices) or surgical procedures such as hysterectomy do not provide any protection for HIV or other STDs. It is necessary to use chemical and physical barriers (e.g., condoms, foam spermicides).

Instructions for Men

- Practice good personal hygiene. Keep the penis, scrotum, and perianal area thoroughly cleansed. Wash areas before and after intercourse. Urinate after intercourse. Wash hands well.
- Prostatitis is treated with antibiotics, antiinflammatory agents, and stool softeners. The local application of heat with a sitz bath, drinking plenty of fluids, and adequate rest are also usually used for relief of the symptoms of prostatitis.
- Discuss appropriate interventions for men with altered sexual function that may be treated with medicine such as phosphodiesterase inhibitors or surgical intervention (e.g., penile prosthesis). Remind the patient of the need for consultation with a health care provider before using phosphodiesterase inhibitors. Although the drugs are readily available over the Internet, people with cardiovascular disorders are particularly susceptible to life-threatening consequences with their use.
- Latex condoms can be effective in reducing sexual transmission of HIV and some other STDs (e.g., gonorrhea, trichomonas, chlamydia), but condoms are not as effective against STDs transmitted by skin-to-skin contact such as herpes simplex virus, human papillomavirus [HPV], syphilis, and chancroid).
- Men having homosexual relationships and people who inject drugs should be vaccinated for hepatitis A. The frequent use of nonoxynol-9 spermicide during anal intercourse irritates the epithelial lining of the rectum, providing a portal of entry for HIV and other STDs.

Instructions for Women and Men

- When infections are present, abstain from sexual intercourse. Stress the need to prevent reinfection. When sexual practices are resumed, use latex condoms. Recent research demonstrates that vaginal

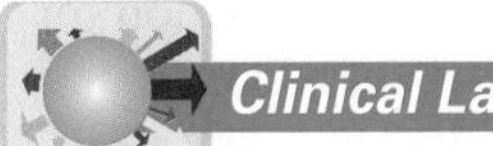

Clinical Landmine

Limitations of Condoms in Preventing STDs

The consistent use of male latex condoms significantly reduces the risk of HIV infection in men and women and of gonorrhea in men, but male condoms may be less effective in protecting against those STDs that are transmitted by skin-to-skin contact (e.g., genital herpes, syphilis), because the infected areas may not be covered by the condom.

spermicides containing nonoxynol-9 may not be effective in preventing cervical gonorrhea, chlamydia, or HIV infection. According to the Centers for Disease Control and Prevention (CDC, 2002), the role of spermicides, sponges, and diaphragms for preventing transmission of HIV has not been evaluated. A recent study indicates that the frequent use of nonoxynol-9 may actually increase the risk of HIV infection during vaginal intercourse due to irritation of vaginal tissues.

- Use sexual abstinence during the communicable phase of any disease. Remember that when having sex with an individual, one is also having sex with all previous sexual partners and should consider the infectious possibilities.
- If having sex with a partner with an unknown status or one infected with HIV or another STD, a new condom should be used for each insertive intercourse.
- It is advised that both partners have tests for STDs, including HIV, before the first sexual encounter.
- Practice safe sex, if not abstinence. Use latex condoms. Discuss proper techniques for applying, using, removing, and discarding condoms.
- Arrange for follow-up appointments with the health care provider and appropriate referrals for counseling or with social service department as needed.
- All sexual partners need to understand the importance of "partner services," the documentation of all sexual partners for the purpose of providing evaluation and treatment to anyone who may have been exposed to an STD before the infected individual became clinically symptomatic. Reporting of syphilis, gonorrhea, chlamydia, and AIDS cases is done in every state.

Medications

For Women. Teach the patient the proper way to apply medications topically or intravaginally using ointments, troches, or suppositories. It is imperative that proper cleansing of the genital area be done regularly using soap and water; rinse and dry well. Hands should be washed before and after the application or insertion of medications and before and after toileting. After every use the vaginal applicator should be thoroughly washed with soap and water, then dried. After inserting a vaginal medication (cream or suppository) the woman should remain in a recumbent position for 30 minutes to allow time for drug absorption. Wear a minipad to catch remaining drainage.

With oral contraceptive therapy, teach not only the medication schedule and dosage but also what to do if a dose is missed, frequency of follow-up care, and side effects to expect and report.

For Men and Women. Teach the medication regimen and who must take the medications—both partners in a sexual relationship.

Fostering Health Maintenance

- Throughout the course of treatment, discuss medication information and how it will benefit the patient. Stress the importance of the nonpharmacologic interventions such as maintaining general health, and proper nutrition and hygiene. Stress the need for adherence with the treatment regimen.
- Provide the patient and significant others with important information contained in the specific drug monographs for the drugs prescribed. Additional health teaching and nursing interventions for drug side effects to expect and report are found in each monograph.
- Seek cooperation and understanding of the following points so that medication adherence is increased: name of medication, dosage, route and times of administration, side effects to expect, and side effects to report.

Written Record. Enlist the patient's aid in developing and maintaining a written record of monitoring parameters (e.g., blood pressure, pulse, weight, degree of relief from menstrual pain, menstrual cycle information for women on oral contraceptives) (see Appendix I: Template for Developing a Written Record for Patients to Monitor Their Own Therapy). For patients with STDs, a listing of the symptoms present and degree of relief obtained may be appropriate. Complete the Premedication Data column for use as a baseline to track response to drug therapy. Ensure that the patient understands how to use the form and instruct the patient to bring the completed form to follow-up visits. During follow-up visits, focus on issues that will foster adherence with the therapeutic interventions prescribed.

DRUG THERAPY FOR CONTRACEPTION

Oral (hormonal) contraceptives (birth control pills) became available in 1960. They now represent one of the most common forms of artificial birth control in the United States. It is estimated that approximately one third of all women between 18 and 44 years of age use oral contraceptives.

DRUG CLASS: Oral Contraceptives

Actions

Estrogens and progestins, to some extent, induce contraception by inhibiting ovulation. The estrogens block pituitary release of follicle-stimulating hormone (FSH), preventing the ovaries from developing a follicle from which the ovum is released. Progestins inhibit pituitary release of luteinizing hormone (LH), the hormone responsible for releasing an ovum from a follicle. Other mechanisms play a contributory role in preventing conception. Estrogens and progestins alter cervical mucus by making it thick and viscous, inhibiting sperm migration. Hormones also change the endometrial wall, impairing implantation of the fertilized ovum.

The progestin-only pills, or minipills, represent a relatively new direction in oral contraceptive therapy. Many of the adverse effects of combination-type contraceptives are caused by the estrogen component of the tablet. For those women particularly susceptible to adverse effects of estrogen therapy, the minipill provides an alternative. Women who might prefer the minipill are those with a history of migraine headaches, hypertension, mental depression, weight gain, and breast tenderness and those who want to breastfeed postpartum. The minipill is not without its disadvantages, however. Between 30% and 40% of women on the minipill continue to ovulate. Birth control is maintained by progestin activity on cervical mucus, uterine and fallopian transport, and implantation. There is a slightly higher incidence of both uterine and tubal pregnancy. **Dysmenorrhea,** manifested by irregular periods, infrequent periods, and spotting between periods, is common among women taking the minipill.

Uses

There are two types of oral contraceptives: the combination pill, which contains both an estrogen and a progestin; and the minipill, which contains only a progestin. The combination pills are subdivided into fixed combination or monophasic (Table 41-3), biphasic (Table 41-4), and triphasic (Table 41-5) products. The monophasic combination pills contain a fixed ratio of estrogen and progestin given daily for 21 days beginning on day 5 of the menstrual cycle. The biphasic product contains a fixed dose of estrogen and a progestin dose on days 1 to 10 that is lower than that on days 11 to 21 of the menstrual cycle. The triphasic combination pills provide three concentrations of estrogen and progestin. The purpose of the variable concentrations of hormones is to provide contraception with the lowest necessary dose of hormones. The combination pills are also packaged in 28-tablet containers. The last 7 tablets are inert but are supplied so that there is no break in the routine of taking 1 tablet daily. The progestin-only products are packaged in units of 28 tablets. All tablets contain active hormone; 1 tablet should be taken daily at approximately the same time each day.

A new form of combination oral contraceptive approved by the U.S. Food and Drug Administration (FDA) was marketed in 2005 under the brand name Seasonale. Seasonale reduces the number of yearly menstrual periods from 13 to 4, so women menstruate only once each season. Seasonale contains a combination of two hormones, an estrogen (ethinyl estradiol) and a progestin (levonorgestrel), but in lower doses than many other combination oral contraceptives. The product package contains 84 active tablets and 7 inert tablets; 1 tablet is taken daily. The active tablets are taken for 84 days (rather than the usual 21 days) before the inert tablets are taken, during which menstruation starts. With sustained hormone use, there is greater suppression of endometrial growth, reducing pregnancy risk, and a lighter period, if any, lasting about 2 days during the 7 days off the active tablets. Another advantage to this product, in addition to fewer periods, is a lower cumulative dose of hormones taken compared with oral contraceptives cycled monthly.

Therapeutic Outcomes

The primary therapeutic outcome associated with oral contraceptive therapy is prevention of pregnancy.

Nursing Process for Oral Contraceptives

Premedication Assessment

1. Review the medical history. If there is a history of obesity, smoking, hypertension, gallbladder disease, diabetes mellitus, severe varicose veins, seizure disorders, oligomenorrhea or amenorrhea, rheumatic heart disease, thromboembolic disease, stroke, malignancy of breast or the reproductive system, renal or liver disease, severe mental depression, suspected pregnancy, or repeated contraceptive failure, consult with a health care provider before dispensing birth control pills.
2. Take a baseline body weight measurement along with blood pressure measurement in the supine and sitting positions.
3. Ensure that a pregnancy test has been given and the patient is not pregnant.

Planning

Availability. See Tables 41-3, 41-4, and 41-5.

Implementation

Before Initiating Therapy. The patient should have a complete physical examination that includes blood pressure, body weight, pelvic and breast examinations, Pap smear, urinalysis, and hemoglobin or hematocrit.

Instructions for Using Combination Oral Contraceptives. Start the first pill on the first Sunday after your period begins. Take one pill daily, at the same time, until the pack is gone. If using a 21-day pack, wait 1 week and restart on the next Sunday. If using a 28-day pack, start a new pack the day after finishing the last pack. Use another form of birth control (condoms, foam) during the first month. You may not be fully protected by the pill during the first month. If the product prescribed also contains an iron supplement, be sure to take the 7 inert tablets monthly. The iron supplement is in the 7 inert tablets, not the 21 tablets containing hormones. (Many women skip the inert tablets each month, thinking they have no benefit.)

- *Missed pills:* If you miss one pill, take it as soon as you remember it; take the next pill at the regularly scheduled time. If you miss two pills, take two pills as soon as you remember and two the next day. Spotting may occur when two pills are missed. Use another form of birth control

Text continued on p. 667

Drug Table 41-3 MONOPHASIC ORAL CONTRACEPTIVES

	PROGESTIN					ESTROGEN		
PRODUCT	NORETHINDRONE (mg)	NORETHINDRONE ACETATE (mg)	ETHYNODIOL DIACETATE (mg)	DESOGESTREL (mg)	LEVONORGESTREL (mg)	ETHINYL ESTRADIOL (mcg)	MESTRANOL (mcg)	OTHER INGREDIENTS
Alesse (28)					0.1	20		
Apri (28)				0.15		30		
Aviane (28)					0.1	20		
Brevicon (28)	0.5					35		
Cryselle (21, 28)						30		Norgestrel 0.3 mg
Demulen 1/35 (21, 28)			1			35		
Demulen 1/50 (21, 28)			1			50		
Desogen (28)				0.15		30		
Junel Fe 1.5/35E (28)		1.5				30		Ferrous fumarate 75 mg
Junel Fe 1/20 (28)		1				20		Ferrous fumarate 75 mg
Lessina (21,28)					0.1	20		
Levlen (28)					0.15	30		
Levlite (21, 28)					0.1	20		
Levora (28)					0.15	30		
Loestrin-21 1/20 (21)		1				20		
Loestrin Fe 1/20 (28)		1				20		Ferrous fumarate 75 mg
Loestrin-21 1.5/30 (21)		1.5				30		
Loestrin Fe 1.5/30 (28)		1.5				30		Ferrous fumarate 75 mg
Low-Ogestrel (28)						30		Norgestrel 0.3 mg
Lo/Ovral (21,28)						30		Norgestrel 0.3 mg
Lutera (28)					0.1	20		
Microgestin Fe 1/20 (28)		1				20		Ferrous fumarate 75 mg

Microgestin Fe 1.5/30 (28)		1.5				30		Ferrous fumarate 75 mg
Modicon (28)	0.5					35		
MonoNessa (28)						35		Norgestimate 0.25 mg
Necon 0.5/35 (21, 28)	0.5					35		
Necon 1/35 (21, 28)	1					35		
Necon 1/50 (21, 28)	1						50	
Nordette (28)					0.15	30		
Norinyl 1 + 35 (28)	1					35		
Norinyl 1 + 50 (28)	1						50	
Nortrel 0.5/35 (21, 28)	0.5					35		
Nortrel 1/35 (21, 28)	1					35		
Ogestrel 0.5/50 (28)						50		Norgestrel 0.5 mg
Ortho-Cept (28)				0.15		30		
Ortho-Cyclen (28)						35		Norgestimate 0.25 mg
Ortho-Novum 1/35 (28)	1					35		
Ortho-Novum 1/50 (28)	1						50	
Ovcon-35 (28)	0.4					35		
Ovcon-50 (21,28)	1					50		
Ovral (28)						50		Norgestrel 0.5 mg
Portia (21, 28)					0.15	30		
Seasonale* (91)					0.15	30		
Solia (21, 28)				0.15		30		
Sprintec (28)						35		Norgestimate 0.25 mg
Yasmin (28)						30		Drospirenone 3 mg
Zovia 1/35 E (21, 28)			1			35		
Zovia 1/50 E (21, 28)			1			50		

*Seasonale is a 90-day-cycle product; 1 pink (active) tablet is taken daily for 84 consecutive days, followed by 7 days of white (inert) tablets.

Drug Table 41-4 BIPHASIC ORAL CONTRACEPTIVES

	PROGESTIN		ESTROGEN
PRODUCT	NORETHINDRONE (mg)	DESOGESTREL (mg)	ETHINYL ESTRADIOL (mcg)
Kariva* (28)		5 white tabs—0.15	21 white tabs—20 5 blue tabs—10
Mircette† (28)		21 white tabs—0.15	21 white tabs—20 5 yellow tabs—10
Necon 10/11 (28)	10 tabs—0.5 11 tabs—1		35 35
Ortho Novum 10/11 (21, 28)	10 tabs—0.5 11 tabs—1		35 35

*1 white tablet is taken daily for 21 days, followed by 1 light green (inert) tablet for 2 days, then 1 light blue (active) tablet daily for 5 days.
†1 white tablet is taken daily for 21 days, followed by 1 green (inert) tablet for 2 days, then 1 yellow (active) tablet daily for 5 days.

Drug Table 41-5 TRIPHASIC AND PROGESTIN-ONLY ORAL CONTRACEPTIVES

	PROGESTIN				ESTROGEN	
PRODUCT	DESOGESTREL	NORETHINDRONE (mg)	NORGESTIMATE (mg)	LEVONORGESTREL (mg)	ETHINYL ESTRADIOL (mcg)	OTHER INGREDIENTS
Aranelle		7 tabs—0.5 9 tabs—1 5 tabs—0.5			35 35 35	
Cesia	7 tabs—0.1 7 tabs—0.125 7 tabs—0.15				25 25 25	
Cyclessa (28)	7 tabs—0.1 7 tabs—0.125 7 tabs—0.15				25 25 25	
Enpresse (28)				6 tabs—0.05 5 tabs—0.075 10 tabs—0.125	30 40 30	
Estrostep 21 (21)		5 tabs—1 7 tabs—1 9 tabs—1			20 30 35	
Estrostep Fe (28)		5 tabs—1 7 tabs—1 9 tabs—1			20 30 35	Ferrous fumarate 75 mg
Leena		7 tabs—0.5 9 tabs—1 5 tabs—0.5			35 35 35	
Necon 7/7/7		7 tabs—0.5 7 tabs—0.75 7 tabs—1			35 35 35	
Ortho-Novum 7/7/7 (21, 28)		7 tabs—0.5 7 tabs—0.75 7 tabs—1			35 35 35	
Ortho Tri-Cyclen (21, 28)			7 tabs—0.180 7 tabs—0.215 7 tabs—0.250		35 35 35	

Drug Table 41-5 TRIPHASIC AND PROGESTIN-ONLY ORAL CONTRACEPTIVES—cont'd

	PROGESTIN				ESTROGEN	
PRODUCT	DESOGESTREL	NORETHINDRONE (mg)	NORGESTIMATE (mg)	LEVONORGESTREL (mg)	ETHINYL ESTRADIOL (mcg)	OTHER INGREDIENTS
Tri-Levlen (21, 28)				6 tabs—0.05 5 tabs—0.075 10 tabs—0.125	30 40 30	
TriNessa			7 tabs—0.180 7 tabs—0.215 7 tabs—0.250		35 35 35	
Tri-Norinyl (21, 28)		7 tabs—0.5 9 tabs—1 5 tabs—0.5			35 35 35	
Triphasil (21, 28)				6 tabs—0.05 5 tabs—0.075 10 tabs—0.125	30 40 30	
Triprevifem			7 tabs—0.180 7 tabs—0.215 7 tabs—0.250		35 35 35	
TriSprintec			7 tabs—0.180 7 tabs—0.215 7 tabs—0.250		35 35 35	
Trivora-28 (28)				6 tabs—0.05 5 tabs—0.075 10 tabs—0.125	30 40 30	
Velivet	7 tabs—0.1 7 tabs—0.125 7 tabs—0.15				25 25 25	
PROGESTIN-ONLY CONTRACEPTIVES						
Camila		0.35				
Errin		0.35				
Jolivet		0.35				
Ortho-Micronor		0.35				
Nora-BE		0.35				
Nor-Q.D.		0.35				
Ovrette						Norgestrel 0.075 mg

(condoms, foam) until you finish this pack of pills. If you miss *three or more,* start using another form of birth control immediately. Start a new pack of pills on the next Sunday even if you are menstruating. Discard your old packs of pills. Use other forms of birth control through the next month after missing three or more pills.

- *Missed pills and skipped periods:* Return to your health care provider for a pregnancy test.
- *Skipping one period but not missing a pill:* It is not uncommon for a woman to occasionally miss a period when on the pill. Start the next pack on the appropriate Sunday.
- *Spotting for two or more cycles:* See your health care provider. A dosage adjustment may be necessary.
- *Periodic examinations:* A yearly examination should include blood pressure tests, pelvic examination, urinalysis, breast examination, and Pap smear.

- *Discontinuing the pill for conception:* Because of a possibility of birth defects, the pill should be discontinued 3 months before attempting pregnancy. Use other methods of contraception for these 3 months.
- *Duration of oral contraceptive therapy:* Many health care providers prefer to have patients discontinue the pill for 3 of every 28 months. This allows the body to return to a normal cycle. Be sure to use other forms of contraception during this time. Long-term use (3 or more years) must be determined on an individual basis.
- *Side effects to be reported as soon as possible:* Severe headaches, dizziness, blurred vision, leg pain, shortness of breath, chest pain, and acute abdominal pain. Although these side effects are usually of minor consequence, a more serious condition must be ruled out.
- NOTE: When being seen by a health care provider or a dentist for other reasons, be sure to mention that you are taking oral contraceptives.

Instructions for Using the Minipill. Start using the minipill on the first day of menstruation. Take 1 tablet daily, every day, regardless of when your next period is. Tablets should be taken at approximately the same time every day.

- *Missed pills:* If you miss one pill, take it as soon as you remember, and take your next pill at the regularly scheduled time. Use another form of birth control until your next period. If you miss two pills, take one of the missed pills immediately and take your regularly scheduled pill for that day on time. The next day, take the regularly scheduled pill as well as the other missed pill. Use another method of birth control until your next period.
- *Missed periods:* Some women note changes in the time as well as duration of their periods while using minipills. This is to be expected. If menses is every 28 to 30 days, ovulation may still be occurring. For maximal safety, use alternative forms of contraception on days 10 through 18. If irregular bleeding occurs every 25 to 45 days, ovulation is probably not regular. You may feel more comfortable if you use other forms of contraception with the minipill or discuss switching to an estrogen-containing (combination) contraceptive. If you have taken all tablets correctly but have not had a period for more than 60 days, speak to your health care provider concerning a pregnancy test.
- NOTE: Report sudden, severe abdominal pain, with or without nausea and vomiting, to your health care provider immediately. There is a higher incidence of ectopic pregnancy with the minipill because it does not inhibit ovulation in all women.
- *Side effects to be reported as soon as possible:* Severe headaches, dizziness, blurred vision, leg pain, shortness of breath, chest pain, and acute abdominal pain. Although these side effects are usually of minor consequence, a more serious condition must be ruled out.
- *Duration of oral contraceptive therapy:* Many health care providers prefer to have their patients discontinue the pill for 3 of every 28 months. This allows the body to return to a normal cycle. Be sure to use other forms of contraception during this time. Long-term use (3 or more years) must be determined on an individual basis.
- *Discontinuing the pill for conception:* Because of a possibility of birth defects, discontinue the pill 3 months before attempting pregnancy. Use other methods of contraception for these 3 months.

Dosage and Administration. The estrogenic component of the combination-type pills is responsible for most of the adverse effects associated with therapy. The FDA has recommended that therapy be initiated with a product containing a low dose of estrogen. Side effects must be reviewed in relation to individual case histories, but many health care providers initiate therapy with Norinyl 1 + 50 or Ortho-Novum $1/50$. Therapy, and therefore products, may be adjusted based on the incidence and type of side effects.

Evaluation

Side Effects to Expect

Nausea, Weight Gain, Spotting, Changed Menstrual Flow, Missed Periods, Depression, Mood Changes, Chloasma, Headaches. These are the most common side effects of hormonal contraceptive therapy. If these symptoms are not resolved after 3 months of therapy, the woman should return to the health care provider for re-evaluation and a possible change in prescription.

Side Effects to Report

Vaginal Discharge, Breakthrough Bleeding, Yeast Infection. These symptoms represent the development of secondary disorders. Examination, a change in oral contraceptive, and possible treatment with other medications may be necessary.

Blurred Vision, Severe Headaches, Dizziness, Leg Pain, Chest Pain, Shortness of Breath, Acute Abdominal Pain. Report as soon as possible. These side effects are usually of minor consequence, but they may be early indications of serious adverse effects.

Drug Interactions

Drugs That Reduce Therapeutic Effects

- Barbiturates, carbamazepine, oxcarbazepine, felbamate, phenytoin, primadone, topiramate, St. John's wort, and the antiviral protease inhibitors (e.g., saquinavir, ritonavir, indinavir, nelfinavir, amprenavir). These agents may increase the rate of metabolism of the oral contraceptive hormones in the liver, possibly decreasing contraceptive effect. An alternate or additional form of birth control is advisable during concurrent use.
- Antibacterial agents (e.g., penicillins, tetracyclines, rifampin, isoniazid, griseofulvin). These agents apparently alter metabolism of hormones

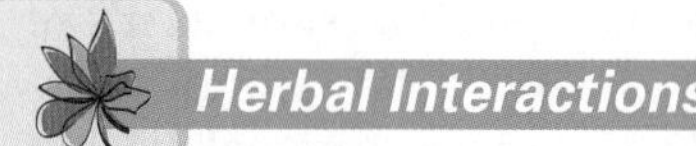

St. John's Wort

St. John's wort may increase the liver's metabolism of oral contraceptive hormones, possibly resulting in decreased contraceptive effect. An alternate or additional form of birth control is advisable during concurrent use.

in the gut, making the contraceptive less effective. An alternate or additional form of birth control is advisable during concurrent use.

Drugs That Enhance Therapeutic and Toxic Effects. Itraconazole and ketoconazole may inhibit the metabolism of oral contraceptives. Menstrual irregularities also may be noted. Adjustment of hormone dosage may be necessary.

Warfarin. Oral contraceptives may diminish the anticoagulant effects of warfarin. Monitor the prothrombin time and the International Normalized Ratio (INR) and increase the dosage of warfarin if necessary.

Phenytoin. Monitor patients with concurrent therapy for signs of phenytoin toxicity: nystagmus, sedation, and lethargy. Serum levels may be ordered, and a reduced dosage of phenytoin may be required.

Thyroid Hormones. Patients who have no thyroid function and who start estrogen therapy may require an increase in thyroid hormone dosage. Estrogens increase thyroid-binding globulin levels, which reduce the level of circulating free thyroxine (T_4). The total level of T_4 is either normal or increased. Do not adjust the thyroid hormone dosage until the patient shows clinical signs of hypothyroidism.

Benzodiazepines. Oral contraceptives appear to have a variable effect on the metabolism of benzodiazepines. Those that have reduced metabolism with an increase in therapeutic response and toxic effect are alprazolam, clorazepate, chlordiazepoxide, diazepam, flurazepam, halazepam, and prazepam. Benzodiazepines that have enhanced metabolism and reduced therapeutic activity when taken with oral contraceptives are lorazepam, oxazepam, and temazepam. Adjust the dosage of benzodiazepine accordingly.

DRUG CLASS: Transdermal Contraceptives

norelgestromin–ethinyl estradiol transdermal system (nor ehl ges′ troh min)

ORTHO EVRA

Actions

Ethinyl estradiol, an estrogen, and norelgestromin, a progestin, work together as a contraceptive by inhibiting ovulation. Estrogens block pituitary release of FSH, preventing the ovaries from developing a follicle that releases an ovum. Progestins inhibit pituitary release of LH, the hormone responsible for releasing an ovum from a follicle. Other mechanisms play a contributory role in preventing conception. Estrogens and progestins alter cervical mucus by making it thick and viscous, inhibiting sperm migration. Hormones also change the endometrial wall, impairing implantation of the fertilized ovum.

Uses

The Ortho Evra transdermal contraceptive system works very much like the combination oral contraceptives, except that the estrogen and progestin hormones are in a transdermal patch dosage form that is applied weekly for 3 weeks. During the fourth week of the menstrual cycle, no patch is worn, and withdrawal bleeding (menses) should begin.

In November 2005, the FDA issued a cautionary note about concern for greater exposure to estrogens from the patch compared with taking a similar oral contraceptive tablet product. In general, increased estrogen exposure may increase the risk of blood clots. However, it is not known whether women using Ortho Evra are at a greater risk of experiencing these serious side effects. The FDA encourages women to discuss the issue with their health care provider, particularly if they are at higher risk for cardiovascular diseases based on the presence of hypertension, obesity, diabetes, smoking, and/or age.

Therapeutic Outcomes

The primary therapeutic outcome associated with transdermal contraceptive therapy is prevention of pregnancy.

Nursing Process for Transdermal Contraceptives

Premedication Assessment

1. Review the medical history. If there is a history of hypertension, gallbladder disease, diabetes mellitus, severe varicose veins, seizure disorders, oligomenorrhea or amenorrhea, rheumatic heart disease, thromboembolic disease, stroke, malignancy of breast or the reproductive system, renal or liver disease, severe mental depression, suspected pregnancy, or repeated contraceptive failure, or if the patient smokes, consult with the health care provider before dispensing birth control patches.
2. Take a baseline blood pressure in the supine and sitting positions.
3. Ensure that a pregnancy test has been given and the patient is not pregnant.

Planning

Availability. Transdermal patch: 6 mg norelgestromin and 0.75 mg ethinyl estradiol per patch. The patch releases 150 mcg of norelgestromin and 20 mcg of ethinyl estradiol per 24 hours.

Implementation

Before Initiating Therapy. The patient should have a complete physical examination that includes blood pressure, pelvic and breast examinations, Pap smear, urinalysis, and hemoglobin or hematocrit. A pregnancy test should be performed on sexually active female patients.

Instructions for Using Transdermal Contraceptives. A new patch should be applied on the same day of the week. This day is known as Patch Change Day. The patch should be applied to clean, dry, intact, healthy skin on the buttock, abdomen, upper outer arm, or upper torso in a place where it will not be rubbed by tight clothing. Patches should not be placed on red irritated skin or on the breasts. Patches should not be cut. Topical products such as makeup, powder, lotions, or creams should not be applied to the skin or to the patch area because the patch may not adhere properly and absorption of the hormones may be impaired.

- Select one of the following methods:
  1. *First day start:* Apply the first patch during the first 24 hours of the menstrual period. Note on a calendar the day of the week as a reminder of Patch Change Day. If the patch is started after the first 24 hours of the menstrual cycle, a nonhormonal backup contraceptive (condoms, spermicidal foam, diaphragm) should be used concurrently for the first 7 consecutive days of the first cycle.
  2. *Sunday start:* Start the first patch on the first Sunday after menses begins. A nonhormonal backup contraceptive (condoms, spermicidal foam, diaphragm) should be used concurrently for the first 7 consecutive days of the first cycle.
- If a patch is partially or completely detached:
  1. *For less than 24 hours:* Try to reapply the patch in the same place or replace it with a new patch immediately. No backup contraception is necessary. Patch Change Day will remain the same. Do not try to reapply the patch if the adhesive will not adhere to the skin. Do not use other adhesives or tape to hold a patch in place. Apply a new patch in a different location.
  2. *For more than 24 hours or if not sure how long since detachment:* Because there may be a lack of protection from pregnancy, stop the current contraceptive cycle and start a new cycle immediately by applying a new patch. This is a "new day 1" and a new Patch Change Day. A nonhormonal backup contraceptive (condoms, spermicidal foam, diaphragm) should be used concurrently for the first 7 consecutive days of the new cycle.
- If a woman forgets to change the patch:
  1. *At the start of any patch cycle (week 1/day 1):* There may be a lack of protection from pregnancy. Apply the new patch as soon as it's remembered. This is a new day 1 and a new Patch Change Day. A nonhormonal backup contraceptive (condoms, spermicidal foam, diaphragm) should be used concurrently for the first 7 consecutive days of the new cycle.
  2. *In the middle of the patch cycle (week 2/day 8 or week 3/day 15):*
     For up to 48 hours: Apply a new patch immediately. The next patch should be applied on the usual Patch Change Day. No backup contraception is needed.
     For more than 48 hours: Because there may be a lack of protection from pregnancy, stop the current contraceptive cycle and start a new 4-week cycle immediately by applying a new patch. This is a new day 1 and a new Patch Change Day. A nonhormonal backup contraceptive (condoms, spermicidal foam, diaphragm) should be used concurrently for the first 7 consecutive days of the new cycle.
     At the end of the patch cycle (week 4/day 22): The patch should be removed as soon as the woman remembers to remove it. The new cycle should be started on the usual Patch Change Day, which is the day after day 28. No backup contraception is needed.
- *Switching from oral contraceptives to the patches:* Apply a patch on the first day of the menses. If there is no withdrawal bleeding within 5 days of the last active hormone tablet (after day 21), a pregnancy test should be completed to ensure that there is no pregnancy before the patch is started.
- Missed patches and skipped periods:
  1. Return to your health care provider for a pregnancy test.
  2. *Skipping one period but not missing a patch:* It is not uncommon for a woman to occasionally miss a period when receiving hormone therapy. Start the next cycle on the same Patch Change Day. If two consecutive periods are missed, a pregnancy test is in order. Contraceptive therapy should be discontinued if pregnancy is confirmed.
  3. *Spotting for two or more cycles:* See your health care provider to have other causes of bleeding assessed.
- *Periodic examinations:* A yearly examination should include blood pressure tests, pelvic examination, urinalysis, breast examination, and Pap smear.
- *Side effects to be reported as soon as possible:* Severe headaches, dizziness, blurred vision, leg pain, shortness of breath, chest pain, and acute abdominal pain. Although these side effects are usually of minor consequence, absence of serious adverse effects such as thromboembolism or ectopic pregnancy must be confirmed.

- NOTE: When being seen by a health care provider or a dentist for other reasons, be sure to mention that oral contraceptives are being taken.

Evaluation

Side Effects to Expect

Nausea, Weight Gain, Spotting, Changed Menstrual Flow, Missed Periods, Depression, Mood Changes, Chloasma, Headaches. These are the most common side effects of hormonal contraceptive therapy. If these symptoms are not resolved after 3 months of therapy, the woman should return to the health care provider for reevaluation and a possible change in prescription.

Side Effects to Report

Vaginal Discharge, Breakthrough Bleeding, Yeast Infection. These symptoms represent the development of secondary disorders. Examination, a change in contraceptive, and possible treatment with other medications may be necessary.

Blurred Vision, Severe Headaches, Dizziness, Leg Pain, Chest Pain, Shortness of Breath, Acute Abdominal Pain. Report as soon as possible. These side effects are usually of minor consequence, but they may be early indications of serious adverse effects.

Drug Interactions. See Drug Interactions for Oral Contraceptives.

DRUG CLASS: Intravaginal Hormonal Contraceptive

etonogestrel–ethinyl estradiol vaginal ring

NuvaRing

Actions

Ethinyl estradiol, an estrogen, and norelgestromin, a progestin, work together as a contraceptive by inhibiting ovulation. Estrogens block pituitary release of FSH, preventing the ovaries from developing a follicle that releases an ovum. Progestins inhibit pituitary release of LH, the hormone responsible for releasing an ovum from a follicle. Other mechanisms play a contributory role in preventing conception. Estrogens and progestins alter cervical mucus by making it thick and viscous, inhibiting sperm migration. Hormones also change the endometrial wall, impairing implantation of the fertilized ovum.

Uses

The NuvaRing vaginal ring works very much like the combination oral contraceptives, except that the estrogen and progestin hormones are in a plastic ring dosage form that the woman inserts in her vagina for 3 weeks. The ring is removed for a 1-week break, during which withdrawal bleeding (menses) should begin.

Therapeutic Outcomes

The primary therapeutic outcome associated with intravaginal hormone contraceptive therapy is prevention of pregnancy.

Nursing Process for Intravaginal Hormone Contraceptive

Premedication Assessment

1. Review the medical history. If there is a history of hypertension, gallbladder disease, diabetes mellitus, severe varicose veins, seizure disorders, oligomenorrhea or amenorrhea, rheumatic heart disease, thromboembolic disease, stroke, malignancy of breast or the reproductive system, renal or liver disease, severe mental depression, suspected pregnancy, or repeated contraceptive failure, or if the patient smokes, consult with the health care provider before dispensing the birth control ring.
2. Take a baseline blood pressure in the supine and sitting positions.
3. Ensure that a pregnancy test has been given and the patient is not pregnant.

Planning

Availability. NuvaRing that releases 0.12 mg etonogestrel and 0.015 mg ethinyl estradiol per day.

Implementation

Before Initiating Therapy. The patient should have a complete physical examination that includes blood pressure, pelvic and breast examinations, Pap smear, urinalysis, and hemoglobin or hematocrit.

Instructions for Using the Intravaginal Hormonal Contraceptive

- *Insertion:* Selecting a comfortable position, compress the ring and insert into the vagina. The exact position inside the vagina is not critical for its function. Insert on the appropriate day as described below, and leave in place for 3 consecutive weeks.
- *Removal:* Remove the ring 3 weeks later on the same day of the week as it was inserted and at about the same time. Remove by hooking the index finger under the forward rim or by grasping the rim between the index and middle fingers and pulling it out. Place the used ring in the foil pouch and discard in a waste receptacle out of reach of children and pets. Do not flush down the toilet.

Select one of the following methods to start contraception:

- *If no hormonal contraceptive was in use in the past month:* Counting the first day of menstruation as day 1, insert the contraceptive ring on or prior to day 5 of the cycle, even if menses is continuing. Note on a calendar the day of the week as a reminder of the removal day 3 weeks later. A nonhormonal backup contraceptive (e.g., condoms, spermicidal foam, diaphragm) should be used concurrently for the first 7 consecutive days of continuous ring use.
- *Switching from a combination oral contraceptive:* Insert the ring anytime within 7 days after the last

active combined oral contraceptive tablet, and no later than the day that a new cycle of pills would have been started. No backup contraception is necessary.

- *Switching from a progestin-only minipill:* Insert the ring the following day after discontinuing the minipill. A nonhormonal backup contraceptive (e.g., condoms, spermicidal foam, diaphragm) should be used concurrently for the first 7 consecutive days of continuous ring use.

If the ring is expelled, removed, or there is a prolonged ring-free interval during the active 3 weeks:

- *For less than 3 hours:* Rinse the ring in cool or lukewarm (not hot) water and reinsert as soon as possible.
- *For greater than 3 hours or if not sure how long since expelled:* If the ring has been out for longer than 3 hours, there may be a lack of protection from pregnancy. Reinsert the ring, but use a nonhormonal backup contraceptive (e.g., condoms, spermicidal foam, diaphragm) for the next 7 consecutive days of continuous ring use.
- If a woman forgets to change the ring:
    1. *If left in place for up to 1 extra week (4 weeks total):* Remove it and insert a new ring after a 1-week ring-free interval. Use a nonhormonal backup contraceptive (e.g., condoms, spermicidal foam, diaphragm) for the next 7 consecutive days of continuous ring use.
    2. *If left in place for more than 4 weeks:* Remove the ring. Rule out pregnancy. Insert a new ring after a 1-week ring-free interval if not pregnant. Use a nonhormonal backup contraceptive (e.g., condoms, spermicidal foam, diaphragm) for the next 7 consecutive days of continuous ring use.
- *Missing one period but being adherent to the program:* It is not uncommon for a woman to occasionally miss a period when receiving hormone therapy. Start the next cycle on the same insertion day (i.e., on the 29th day). If two consecutive periods are missed, a pregnancy test is in order. Contraceptive therapy should be discontinued if pregnancy is confirmed.
- *Missed one period and the ring was out for more than 3 hours, or was left in for more than 4 weeks:* Return to the health care provider for a pregnancy test.
- *Spotting for two or more cycles:* See your health care provider to have other causes of bleeding assessed.
- *Periodic examinations*: A yearly examination should include blood pressure tests, pelvic examination, urinalysis, breast examination, and Pap smear.
- *Side effects to be reported as soon as possible:* Severe headaches, dizziness, blurred vision, leg pain, shortness of breath, chest pain, and acute abdominal pain. Although these side effects are usually of minor consequence, absence of serious adverse effects such as thromboembolism or ectopic pregnancy must be confirmed.
- NOTE: When being seen by a health care provider or a dentist for other reasons, be sure to mention that oral contraceptives are being taken.

Evaluation

Side Effects to Expect

Nausea, Weight Gain, Spotting, Changed Menstrual Flow, Missed Periods, Depression, Mood Changes, Chloasma, Headaches. These are the most common side effects of hormonal contraceptive therapy. If these symptoms are not resolved after 3 months of therapy, the woman should return to the health care provider for reevaluation and a possible change in prescription.

Side Effects to Report

Vaginal Discharge, Breakthrough Bleeding, Yeast Infection. These symptoms represent the development of secondary disorders. Examination, a change in contraceptive, and possible treatment with other medications may be necessary.

Blurred Vision, Severe Headaches, Dizziness, Leg Pain, Chest Pain, Shortness of Breath, Acute Abdominal Pain. Report as soon as possible. These side effects are usually of minor consequence, but they may be early indications of serious adverse effects.

Drug Interactions. See Drug Interactions for Oral Contraceptives.

DRUG THERAPY FOR BENIGN PROSTATIC HYPERPLASIA (BPH)

The prostate gland functions as part of the male reproductive system. It is a firm organ, weighing about 20 g, the size of a walnut. It is located at the base of the urinary bladder and completely surrounds the proximal urethra. As part of the reproductive system, it produces a fluid during ejaculation that mixes with sperm from the testes and fluid from the seminal vesicles to form semen. The gland may also protect against urinary tract infections through secretion of prostatic antibacterial factor (PAF). Two other chemicals secreted by the prostate gland are acid phosphatase and prostate-specific antigen (PSA).

Enlargement of the prostate gland as men age is an almost universal phenomenon. A condition called enlarged prostate, prostatism, or BPH is common later in life, affecting more than half of men in their 60s and as much as 90% in their 70s and 80s. Many men with BPH will need some type of treatment. Although an enlarged prostate is an apparently normal part of aging, problems with urination that often accompany this enlargement are not normal.

BPH is much more common than prostate cancer; however, an enlarged prostate gland can be caused by prostate cancer. Because the signs of enlarged prostate are often the same as the signs and symptoms of prostate cancer, it is important to get a health care provider's opinion so the proper diagnosis can be made. The health care provider may also need to rule out prostate infection and other possible causes of the patient's symptoms.

Table 41-6 ***Symptoms of Benign Prostatic Hyperplasia***

OBSTRUCTIVE	IRRITATIVE
Reduced force of urinary stream	Increased frequency
Resistance to initiate voiding	Nocturia
Prolonged dribbling after urination	Difficult or painful urination (dysuria)
Sensation of incomplete bladder emptying	Sudden urgency
Decreased or interrupted stream	Urge incontinence
Double voiding	
Strain or push to urinate	

The pathogenesis of BPH is not well understood, but appears to involve the presence of increasing levels of dihydrotestosterone (DHT), either due to a slow increase in production or reduced clearance, or both, which stimulates the growth of new prostate cells. DHT is formed in the prostate gland from testosterone from the testes. The conversion of testosterone to DHT is catalyzed by 5-alpha reductase.

The symptoms of BPH are highly variable and patient specific, and are divided into two categories: obstructive and irritative (Table 41-6). Obstructive symptoms result directly from narrowing of the bladder neck and urethra. Irritative symptoms result from incomplete bladder emptying or urinary tract infection secondary to prostatic obstruction. As the prostate gland enlarges, it compresses the urethra, partially or completely obstructing urine flow from the bladder. Over time, symptoms become progressively worse, requiring medical attention. When necessary, the hyperplastic tissue may be removed surgically to reduce the urinary obstruction. Transurethral resection or laser therapy may be used to treat glands smaller than 60 g, whereas larger glands are removed surgically (prostatectomy). Intermittent catheterization several times daily or placement of a permanent indwelling catheter may be used if the patient is not a candidate for surgery.

BPH may also be treated successfully with medicines. Alpha-1 adrenergic blocking agents (e.g., doxazosin, terazosin) (p. 380) and alfuzosin or tamsulosin are used to relax the smooth muscle of the bladder and prostate. Antiandrogen agents, such as finasteride and dutasteride, selectively block androgens at the prostate cellular level and cause the prostate gland to shrink. Recent studies indicate that a combination of an alpha-blocker with a 5-alpha reductase inhibitor is more effective in slowing the progression of BPH than either agent alone.

DRUG CLASS: Alpha-1 Adrenergic Blocking Agents

alfuzosin (al fuse oh' sin)

UROXATRAL (uhr ox' ah tral)

Actions

Alfuzosin is an alpha-1 blocking agent that has selectivity for the alpha-1A receptor subtype found on the prostate gland. Approximately 70% of the alpha-1 receptors in the human prostate are of the alpha-1A subtype. Alfuzosin blocks alpha-1 receptors on the prostate gland and certain areas of the bladder neck, causing muscle relaxation, allowing greater urinary outflow in men with an enlarged prostate gland. The alpha-1 blocking agents do not reduce prostate size or inhibit testosterone synthesis like the 5-alpha-reductase inhibitors do, nor do they affect PSA levels.

Uses

Alfuzosin is used to reduce mild to moderate urinary obstruction manifestations (e.g., hesitancy, terminal urine dribbling, interrupted stream, impaired size and force of stream, and sensation of incomplete bladder emptying) in men with BPH. A1fuzosin produces a 20% to 30% increase in urine flow rate in up to 50% of men with urinary symptoms. Symptoms show improvement after 1 week of therapy, but 2 to 3 months of continued therapy are required to assess full effect. Alfuzosin is not used to treat hypertension.

Therapeutic Outcomes

The primary therapeutic outcomes expected from alfuzosin therapy are reduced symptoms and improvement in urine flow associated with prostate gland enlargement.

Nursing Process for Alfuzosin

Premedication Assessment

1. Obtain baseline blood pressure readings in supine and standing positions.
2. Check if the patient has a history of severe cerebral or coronary arteriosclerosis, gastritis, or peptic ulcer disease. (Reduction of blood pressure may diminish blood flow to these regions, causing therapy to worsen the condition.)

Planning

Availability. 10-mg extended release tablets.

Implementation

Dosage and Administration. PO: 10 mg daily to be taken immediately after the same meal each day. The tablets should not be chewed or crushed.

NOTE: The initial doses of alfuzosin may cause dizziness (<6%) and hypotension with tachycardia, and fainting (<0.5%) in patients starting therapy. This effect may be minimized by giving the first doses with food. Patients should be warned that this side effect might occur, that it is transient and they should lie down immediately if symptoms develop.

Evaluation

Side Effects to Expect

Drowsiness, Headache, Dizziness, Weakness, Lethargy. Tell the patient that these side effects may occur but that they tend to be self-limiting. The patient should not stop taking the medication and should consult the health care provider if the problem becomes unacceptable.

Dizziness, Tachycardia, Fainting. These side effects occur in less than 0.5% of patients when therapy is initiated. They develop 15 to 90 minutes after the first dose is taken. To decrease the incidence, administer the first dose with food.

Instruct the patient to lie down immediately if these symptoms occur.

Provide for the patient's safety.

Drug Interactions

Drugs That Enhance Toxic Effects. Ketoconazole, itraconazole, ritonavir, and diltiazem inhibit the metabolism of alfuzosin and should not be used concurrently with alfuzosin.

Diuretics, tranquilizers, alcohol, barbiturates, antihistamines, beta-adrenergic blocking agents (e.g., propranolol, atenolol, pindolol), and other antihypertensive agents. Monitor the blood pressure response to the cumulative effects of antihypertensive agents. Take the blood pressure in supine and erect positions.

Monitor for an increase in severity of side effects such as sedation, hypotension, and bradycardia or tachycardia.

tamsulosin (tam suhl oh' sin)

FLOMAX (floh' max)

Actions

Tamsulosin is an alpha-1 blocking agent that has selectivity for the alpha-1A receptor subtype similar to alfuzosin.

Uses

Tamsulosin is used to reduce mild to moderate urinary obstruction manifestations (e.g., hesitancy, terminal urine dribbling, interrupted stream, impaired size and force of stream, and sensation of incomplete bladder emptying) in men with BPH. Tamsulosin is not used to treat hypertension.

Therapeutic Outcomes

The primary therapeutic outcomes expected from tamsulosin therapy are reduced symptoms and improvement in urine flow associated with prostate gland enlargement.

Nursing Process for Tamsulosin

Premedication Assessment

1. Obtain baseline blood pressure readings in supine and standing positions.
2. Check if the patient has a history of severe cerebral or coronary arteriosclerosis, gastritis, or peptic ulcer disease. (Reduction of blood pressure may diminish blood flow to these regions, causing therapy to worsen the condition.)

Planning

Availability. Capsules 0.4 mg.

Implementation

Dosage and Administration. PO: 0.4 mg daily, administered approximately 30 minutes following the same meal each day. If symptoms are not adequately controlled after 2 to 4 weeks of therapy, the dose may be increased to 0.8 mg once daily. If administration is discontinued or interrupted for several days at either the 0.4- or 0.8-mg dose, start therapy again with the 0.4-mg once-daily dose.

NOTE: The initial doses of tamsulosin may cause hypotension with dizziness, tachycardia, and fainting; these adverse effects occurred in 7% of patients starting therapy. This effect may be minimized by giving the first doses with food and limiting the initial dose to 0.4 mg. Patients should be warned that this side effect might occur, that it is transient, and they should lie down immediately if symptoms develop.

Evaluation

Side Effects to Expect

Drowsiness, Headache, Dizziness, Weakness, Lethargy. Tell the patient that these side effects may occur but that they tend to be self-limiting. The patient should not stop taking the medication and should consult the health care provider if the problem becomes unacceptable.

Dizziness, Tachycardia, Fainting. These side effects occur in about 7% of patients when therapy is initiated. They develop 15 to 90 minutes after the first dose is taken. To decrease the incidence, administer the first dose with food and limit the initial dose to 0.4 mg.

Instruct the patient to lie down immediately if these symptoms occur.

Provide for the patient's safety.

Drug Interactions

Drugs That Enhance Therapeutic and Toxic Effects. Cimetidine, diuretics, tranquilizers, alcohol, barbiturates, antihistamines, beta-adrenergic blocking

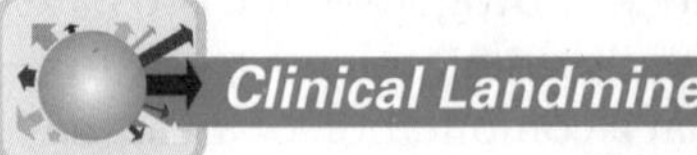

Tamsulosin

The initial doses of tamsulosin may cause hypotension with dizziness, tachycardia, and fainting; these adverse effects occurred in 7% of patients starting therapy. This effect may be minimized by giving the first doses with food and limiting the initial dose to 0.4 mg. Patients should be warned that this side effect might occur, that it is transient and they should lie down immediately if symptoms develop.

agents (e.g., propranolol, atenolol, pindolol), and other antihypertensive agents. Monitor the blood pressure response to the cumulative effects of antihypertensive agents. Take the blood pressure in supine and erect positions.

Monitor for an increase in severity of side effects such as sedation, hypotension, and bradycardia or tachycardia.

DRUG CLASS: Antiandrogen Agents

dutasteride (du tas′ ter ide)
▶ AVODART (av′ oh dart)

Actions

Dutasteride is an androgen hormone inhibitor that acts by inhibiting the enzyme 5-alpha reductase. The conversion of testosterone to DHT is catalyzed by type 1 and type 2, 5-alpha reductase. Reduction in DHT levels reduces the hyperplastic cell growth associated with prostatic hyperplasia.

Uses

Dutasteride inhibits both type 1 and type 2, 5-alpha reductase. Dutasteride is used to treat the symptoms associated with benign prostatic hyperplasia, to reduce the risks associated with urinary retention, and minimize the need for surgery associated with BPH. More than 6 to 12 months of treatment may be necessary to assess whether a therapeutic response has been achieved. Patients who respond to therapy have fewer symptoms associated with partial obstruction, improved urinary flow rates, and a smaller prostate gland. Dutasteride is not approved by the FDA to treat male pattern baldness.

Therapeutic Outcomes

The primary therapeutic outcomes expected from dutasteride therapy are as follows:

- Reduced symptoms and improvement in urine flow associated with prostatic enlargement.
- Reduced need for surgery for prostatic hyperplasia.

Nursing Process for Dutasteride

Premedication Assessment

Obtain a baseline PSA blood level. Dutasteride causes a decrease in serum PSA levels by about 50% in patients with BPH, even in the presence of prostate cancer. Any sustained increase in PSA levels while receiving dutasteride should be investigated, including consideration of prostate cancer and noncompliance with therapy.

Planning

Availability. Capsules: 0.5 mg.

Implementation

Dosage and Administration. PO: 0.5 mg once daily, with or without food.

NOTE: Dutasteride is contraindicated in women who are or may become pregnant. Dutasteride may cause abnormalities of the external genitalia of a male fetus of a pregnant woman who received dutasteride. A woman who is pregnant or who may become pregnant should not handle crushed or broken dutasteride capsules.

Men treated with dutasteride should not donate blood until at least 6 months after stopping therapy to avoid introducing the drug to a pregnant woman.

Evaluation

Side Effects to Expect

Impotence, Decreased Libido, Decreased Volume of Ejaculate. These side effects appear in small numbers of men receiving higher doses of dutasteride. Tell the patient that these side effects may occur but that they tend to be self-limiting. The incidence of impotence, decreased libido, and ejaculation disorder decreases with increasing duration of treatment. Decreased volume of ejaculate does not appear to interfere with normal sexual function. The patient should not stop taking the medication and should consult the health care provider if the problem becomes unacceptable.

Drug Interactions

Drugs That Enhance Toxic Effects. Ketoconazole, itraconazole, ritonavir, diltiazem, verapamil, cimetidine, ciprofloxacin, troleandomycin. These drugs inhibit the metabolism of dutasteride. Dutasteride should be used with extreme caution in men taking any of these medicines.

finasteride (fin as′ ter ide)
▶ PROSCAR (pro′ scar), PROPECIA (pro peesh′ ee ah)

Actions

Finasteride is an androgen hormone inhibitor that acts by inhibiting the enzyme 5-alpha reductase. The conversion of testosterone to DHT is catalyzed by 5-alpha reductase. Reduction in DHT levels reduces the hyperplastic cell growth associated with prostatic hyperplasia. Elevated DHT levels also induce androgenetic alopecia, more commonly known as male pattern baldness (vertex and anterior midscalp).

Uses

Finasteride inhibits type 2, 5-alpha reductase. Finasteride (Proscar, 5 mg) is used to treat the symptoms associated with benign prostatic hyperplasia, to reduce the risks associated with urinary retention, and minimize the need for surgery associated with BPH. More than 6 to 12 months of treatment may be necessary to assess whether a therapeutic response has been achieved. Patients who respond to therapy have fewer symptoms associated with partial obstruction, improved urinary flow rates, and a smaller prostate gland.

Finasteride (Propecia, 1 mg) is used to treat androgenetic alopecia. After at least 3 months of daily use, finasteride maintains hair count and stimulates new hair growth in those who respond. Continued use is necessary to sustain the results. With discontinuation of treatment, the effects are reversed within 1 year. Finasteride does not appear to affect nonscalp body hair.

Therapeutic Outcomes

The primary therapeutic outcomes expected from finasteride therapy are as follows.

- Reduced symptoms and improvement in urine flow associated with prostatic enlargement.
- Reversal of male pattern hair loss.

Nursing Process for Finasteride

Premedication Assessment

Obtain a baseline PSA blood level. Finasteride causes a decrease in serum PSA levels by about 50% in patients with BPH, even in the presence of prostate cancer. Any sustained increase in PSA levels while receiving finasteride should be investigated, including consideration of prostate cancer and noncompliance with therapy.

Planning

Availability. Proscar tablets: 5 mg; Propecia tablets: 1 mg.

Implementation

Dosage and Administration. *BPH:* PO: 5 mg once daily, with or without food. Androgenetic alopecia: PO: 1 mg once daily, with or without food.

NOTE: Finasteride is contraindicated in women who are or may become pregnant. Finasteride may cause abnormalities of the external genitalia of a male fetus of a pregnant woman who received finasteride. A woman who is pregnant or who may become pregnant should not handle crushed or broken finasteride tablets. Tablets are coated and will prevent contact with the active ingredient during normal handling.

Evaluation

Side Effects to Expect

Impotence, Decreased Libido, Decreased Volume of Ejaculate. These side effects appear in small numbers of men receiving higher doses of finasteride. Tell the patient that these side effects may occur but that they tend to be self-limiting. The decreased volume of ejaculate does not appear to interfere with normal sexual function. The patient should not stop taking the medication and should consult the health care provider if the problem becomes unacceptable.

Drug Interactions. No clinically significant drug interactions have been reported to date.

DRUG THERAPY FOR ERECTILE DYSFUNCTION

There has been a significant increase in discussion about erectile dysfunction (ED), sometimes called impotency, because of the availability and high efficacy of an oral dosage form of medicine used to treat certain cases of ED. ED is the consistent inability to achieve or maintain an erection sufficient for satisfactory sexual activity. The prevalence of ED increases with age, although it is not an inevitable outcome of aging. Approximately 5% of men experience the problem at the age of 40, and 15% to 25% 65 years of age or older are affected.

ED usually is the result of a combination of vascular, neurologic, and psychological factors. Vascular and neurogenic causes of ED increase with age. Risk factors include cigarette smoking, hyperlipidemia, hypertension, diabetes mellitus, coronary artery disease, and peripheral vascular disease. Other causes of ED are psychological (e.g., stress, depression, interpersonal relationships), damage to neurologic pathways (e.g., trauma from bicycle seats, prostatectomy, transurethral resection of the prostate, diabetes mellitus, and alcohol abuse). A common cause of ED is the use of medicines for other medical conditions (Table 41-7). It is often difficult to determine whether ED is caused by medicines, the condition for which the medicine is used, or both.

The diagnosis of ED is based on a medical and sexual history, physical examination, and laboratory studies. An abrupt onset and intermittent pattern of difficulty achieving or maintaining an erection may suggest a psychological etiology, whereas a gradual onset in ED is more likely due to a vascular or neurologic cause. The etiology of ED is usually multifactorial. A variety of treatments have been developed for ED, each with advantages and disadvantages: psychotherapy, intracavernosal injection with prostaglandins, intraurethral prostaglandin, vacuum constriction devices, vascular surgery, hormonal therapy, penile prostheses, and oral phosphodiesterase inhibitor therapy.

DRUG CLASS: Phosphodiesterase Inhibitors

Actions

Phosphodiesterase inhibitors are selective inhibitors of phosphodiesterase type 5 (PDE5) enzyme. Recent research indicates that a previously unknown metabolic pathway mediates penile erection. Nitric oxide, a naturally occurring neurotransmitter found in nerve endings and endothelial cells, activates the enzyme guanylate cyclase, which converts guanosine triphosphate to cyclic guanosine monophosphate (cGMP) in smooth muscle cells. The increase in cGMP causes smooth muscle relaxation. In the corpus cavernosum of the penis, smooth muscle relaxation allows blood inflow to fill the many small sinusoidal spaces, resulting in an erection.

Table 41-7 ***Drugs That May Cause Erectile Dysfunction***

ANTIHYPERTENSIVE AGENTS	CENTRAL NERVOUS SYSTEM DEPRESSANTS	CARDIOVASCULAR AGENTS	MISCELLANEOUS AGENTS
Thiazide diuretics (most common) Beta-adrenergic blocking agents (especially propranolol and nonselective agents; less so with beta-1 selective agents) Alpha-adrenergic blocking agents (e.g., prazosin, terazosin) Sympatholytic agents (e.g., clonidine, methyldopa, reserpine, guanethidine) Spironolactone (antiandrogen effect)	Phenothiazine antipsychotic agents (e.g., fluphenazine, thioridazine) Monoamine oxidase inhibitors Tricyclic antidepressants Serotonin reuptake inhibitors (e.g., sertraline, paroxetine)	digoxin (estrogen effect) clofibrate gemfibrozil	Substances of abuse (e.g., smoking, alcohol, cocaine, marijuana) Alkylating agents (e.g., chlorambucil, cyclophosphamide) Anabolic steroids Estrogens Corticosteroids cimetidine (antiandrogen effect) 5-alpha reductase inhibitors (finasteride, dutasteride)

From Koeneman KS, Mulhall JP, Goldstein I: Sexual health for the man at midlife: in-office workup, *Geriatrics* 52:76-86, 1997; and Brock GB, Lue TF: Drug-induced male sexual dysfunction, an update, *Drug Safety* 8(6):414-426, 1993.

In the corpus cavernosum, the enzyme PDE5 inactivates cGMP. The phosphodiesterase inhibitors enhance the relaxant effect of nitric oxide released in response to sexual stimulation by increasing cGMP concentrations in the corpus cavernosum, resulting in smooth muscle relaxation and greater blood flow into the corpus cavernosum, which produces an erection.

Uses

Sildenafil was approved in 1998 as the first oral therapy to treat male erectile dysfunction. Two other products, vardenafil and tadalafil, have since been approved. Sexual stimulation is required for an erection because the phosphodiesterase inhibitors do not have a direct relaxant effect on the smooth muscle of the corpus cavernosum. In the absence of sexual stimulation, these agents have no pharmacologic effect. They are not an aphrodisiac; they do not increase sexual desire or sexual stimulation or affect the frequency of sexual intercourse. Sildenafil and vardenafil are taken anywhere from 30 minutes to 4 hours before sexual activity. Tadalafil also starts to work within 30 minutes, but may last for up to 36 hours. Sexual stimulation is required with all three agents for erection. The erection lasts for an hour or so, although it is highly variable based on continued sexual stimulation, attainment of orgasm, and the individual patient. The phosphodiesterase inhibitors should not be taken more often than once every 24 hours. The phosphodiesterase inhibitors have been tested in women to treatment of sexual dysfunction, but the results to date have been inconclusive, so phosphodiesterase inhibitors are not recommended for women.

Phosphodiesterase inhibitors are also finding a new therapeutic use in a rare lung condition known as pulmonary arterial hypertension. By similar mechanisms in lung tissue as described above in penile tissue, phosphodiesterase inhibitors cause an increase in cGMP in pulmonary tissue, leading to relaxation of smooth muscle and vasodilation of the pulmonary arterial bed, reducing hypertension. Silfenafil has been approved for use in pulmonary arterial hypertension under the brand name of Revatio.

Therapeutic Outcomes

The primary therapeutic outcome expected from phosphodiesterase inhibitor therapy is improved erectile function and overall sexual satisfaction in men with ED.

Nursing Process for Phosphodiesterase Inhibitors

Premedication Assessment

Obtain baseline vital signs and a history of recent use of medicines, including recreational drugs. Patients with cardiovascular disease should seek their health care provider's approval before starting phosphodiesterase inhibitor therapy.

Planning

Availability. See Table 41-8.

Implementation

Dosage and Administration. See Table 41-8.

NOTE: Phosphodiesterase inhibitors do not protect against sexually transmitted diseases or pregnancy. Use of a condom and a spermicide containing nonoxynol-9 will help protect against some sexually transmitted diseases and unwanted pregnancy. Phosphodiesterase inhibitors do not affect sperm count or motility and do not reduce fertility.

Evaluation

Side Effects to Expect

Headache, Flushing of the Face and Neck. These side effects appear in small numbers of men receiving higher doses of phosphodiesterase inhibitors. Tell the patient that these side effects may occur but they tend

Drug Table 41-8 PHOSPHODIESTERASE INHIBITORS USED FOR ERECTILE DYSFUNCTION

GENERIC NAME	BRAND NAME	AVAILABILITY	DOSAGE RANGE
sildenafil	Viagra	Tablets: 25, 50, 100 mg	Initial: 50 mg Maximum: 100 mg/24 hr
tadalafil	Cialis	Tablets: 5, 10, 20 mg	Initial: 10 mg Maximum: 20 mg/24 hr
vardenafil	Levitra	Tablets: 2.5, 5, 10, 20 mg	Initial: 10 mg Maximum: 20 mg/24 hr

to be self-limiting. If they continue to be a problem, a reduced dosage may eliminate the adverse effects. The patient should consult a health care provider if the problem becomes unacceptable.

Color Vision Impairment. Mild, transient reversible impairment of blue or green color interpretation may occur. This is thought to be due to inhibition of the PDE6 enzyme that plays a role in phototransduction in the retina. If this continues to be problem, a reduced dosage may eliminate the adverse effect. Tell the patient to consult a health care provider if the problem becomes unacceptable.

Side Effects to Report

Hypotension, Dizziness, Angina. Patients with heart disease, angina, diabetes mellitus, and hypertension should seek their health care provider's approval before using phosphodiesterase inhibitors. Patients receiving nitroglycerin or isosorbide should not take phosphodiesterase inhibitors due to a potentially fatal interaction. If hypotension, dizziness, or angina develops, the patient should lie down, discontinuing sexual activity. DO NOT TAKE NITROGLYCERIN FOR ANGINA. It may worsen the symptoms. Seek medical attention, as needed.

Sustained Erection. Priapism is an erection that won't go away. If an erection lasts more than 4 hours, medical attention should be sought quickly. Priapism must be treated as soon as possible or lasting damage can happen to the penis, including the inability to have erections.

Drug Interactions

Nitroglycerin Patches, Nitroglycerin Ointment, Nitroglycerin Spray, Amyl Nitrate. Nitrates increase the production of nitric oxide, potentially causing hypotension and arrhythmias. It is thought that nitrates that are inhaled for recreational use during sexual activity (including butyl nitrate and amyl nitrate/nitrite, or "poppers") will have the same effect when combined with phosphodiesterase inhibitors. Nitrates from food sources do not react with phosphodiesterase inhibitors.

Cimetidine, Erythromycin, Ketoconazole, Itraconazole, Ritonavir, Indinavir, Saquinavir. These medicines inhibit the metabolism of phosphodiesterase inhibitors, potentially causing an increased incidence of side effects such as flushing, hypotension, and dizziness. A lower dosage of the phosphodiesterase inhibitor may be necessary.

Alcohol. Alcohol and phosphodiesterase inhibitors are mild vasodilators. Excessive consumption of alcohol in combination with phosphodiesterase inhibitors may cause decreased blood pressure, dizziness, and orthostatic hypotension. Use caution when combining phosphodiesterase inhibitors and alcohol.

Alpha-Adrenergic Blocking Agents. Use of alpha-adrenergic blocking agents (e.g., terazosin, doxazosin, prazosin, tamsulosin, alfuzosin) and vardenafil or tadalafil is CONTRAINDICATED. Significant hypotension may result. Use with sildenafil is not contraindicated, but a lower dose of sildenafil may be required to prevent hypotension.

Rifampin. This drug may enhance the metabolism of sildenafil and tadalafil, reducing its duration of action. An increase in dosage or earlier sexual activity may resolve the problem.

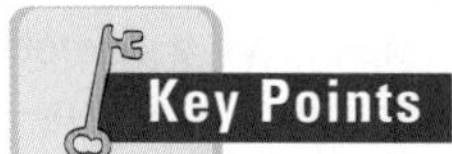

Key Points

- There is a great need for counseling about contraception and about modes of transmission of STDs for all sexually active people. One age group that is frequently not receiving adequate counseling on safe sex practices is the adolescent, many of whom are sexually active.
- Nurses must be leaders in encouraging people to report STDs and seek health care as soon as an STD is suspected.
- Nurses must be leaders in promoting health and wellness, encouraging men and women to complete annual physical examinations that could detect the early onset of disease.
- It is important for the consumer to be aware that hormonal contraceptives have reduced effectiveness when taken in combination with many other medications, thus requiring an alternate form of contraception.

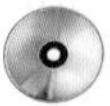

Go to your Companion CD-ROM for Appendices, an Audio Glossary, animations, Drug Dosage Calculators, customizable Patient Self-Assessment forms, and Review Questions for the NCLEX® Examination.

evolve Be sure to visit the companion Evolve site at http://evolve.elsevier.com/Clayton for WebLinks and additional online resources.

MEDICATION SAFETY REVIEW

MATH REVIEW QUESTIONS

1. Order: Acyclovir (Zovirax) 200 mg, PO, q4h while awake for a total of five capsules per day.

   The total daily dose would be _____ mg.

   A prescription that is to last for 2 weeks, until the patient is seen in the clinic again, would need to contain a total of ____ capsules.

2. Order: Doxycycline (Doryx) 100 mg, q12h, PO for the first day followed by 100 mg/day, PO for 10 days.

   When the prescription comes from the pharmacy, how many capsules should be in the bottle (the product is available in 100-mg capsules)?

   _____ capsules

CRITICAL THINKING QUESTIONS

1. A patient is being started on a combination oral contraceptive. You are to provide her the initial health teaching regarding the prescription. What would you explain?
2. A 22-year-old patient comes to the clinic for an annual physical examination and renewal of her oral contraceptive prescription. She tests positive for *Chlamydia* and becomes very upset when informed of this. How would you handle this situation?
3. When a client is being initiated on phosphodiesterase inhibitors, what preassessment screening should be performed? Identify specific drug classifications that should be asked about when performing a medication history for a male client with sexual dysfunction.
4. Discuss important premedication assessments to be used with all types of contraceptives.

CONTENT REVIEW QUESTIONS

1. When combination oral contraceptive products are administered, the action of the _____ is on the release of FSH (follicle stimulating hormone) and the action of _____ is on LH (luteinizing hormone).
   1. enzyme 5-alpha reductase; alpha-1 blocking agent
   2. progestins; estrogens
   3. estrogens; progestins
   4. sympathetic agents; alpha-adrenergic blocking agents
2. Sildenafil (Viagra) requires a premedication assessment for:
   1. STDs.
   2. diabetes mellitus.
   3. gastritis or peptic ulcer disease.
   4. cardiovascular disease.
3. A transdermal contraceptive is applied:
   1. for 28 consecutive days.
   2. for 1 week on, 1 week off.
   3. for 21 days on, 7 days off.
   4. for 14 days on, 14 days off.
4. If the NuvaRing has been out of the vagina longer than 3 hours, the patient should be instructed:
   1. that no backup contraceptive is necessary.
   2. to reinsert the ring and use a nonhormonal contraceptive for 7 consecutive days.
   3. to reinsert the ring and use the minipill for 7 consecutive days.
   4. to reinsert the ring and use a combination contraceptive for 7 consecutive days.
5. Increased estrogen exposure may increase the risk of:
   1. blood clots.
   2. diabetes.
   3. hypertension.
   4. STDs.
6. The name of the oral contraceptive that reduces the number of yearly menstrual periods from 13 to 4 is:
   1. Ortho-Novum.
   2. Ovrette.
   3. Ortho Evra.
   4. Seasonale.
7. Which classification of drugs helps reduce the symptoms of benign prostatic hyperplasia? *(Select all that apply.)*
   1. alpha-1 adrenergic blocking agents
   2. antiandrogen agents
   3. phosphodiesterase inhibitors
   4. antiinflammatory agents

UNIT **NINE** DRUGS AFFECTING OTHER BODY SYSTEMS

CHAPTER 42 Drugs Used to Treat Disorders of the Urinary System

evolve http://evolve.elsevier.com/Clayton

Chapter Content

Objectives

1. Explain the major action and effects of drugs used to treat disorders of the urinary tract.
2. Identify baseline data the nurse should collect on a continuous basis for comparison and evaluation of drug effectiveness.
3. Identify important nursing assessments and interventions associated with the drug therapy and treatment of diseases of the urinary system.
4. Identify essential components involved in planning patient education that will enhance compliance with the treatment regimen.
5. Analyze Table 42-1 and identify specific portions of a urinalysis report that would indicate proteinuria, dehydration, infection, or renal disease.
6. Prepare a chart of antimicrobial agents used to treat urinary tract infections. Give the drug names, the organisms treated, and special considerations (such as the need for acidic urine, changes in urine color, and effect on urine tests).
7. Identify the symptoms, treatment, and medication used for overactive bladder syndrome.
8. Develop a health teaching plan for an individual who has repeated urinary tract infections.

Key Terms

pyelonephritis
cystitis
prostatitis
urethritis
acidification
frequency
urgency
incontinence
urge incontinence
nocturia
overactive bladder (OAB) syndrome
urinary antispasmodic agents

URINARY TRACT INFECTIONS

Urinary tract infections (UTIs) are among the most common infectious diseases in humans, accounting for more than 11 million physicians' office visits yearly. Urinary tract infections are second only to upper respiratory tract infections as a cause of morbidity from infection. Urinary tract infections encompass several different types of infection of local tissue: **pyelonephritis** (the kidney), **cystitis** (the bladder), **prostatitis** (the prostate gland), and **urethritis** (the urethra).

The incidence of urinary tract infections in women is approximately 10 times higher than in men. The incidence increases in women with age, so that by 60 years of age, up to 20% of women will have suffered from at least one urinary tract infection in their lives.

Gram-negative aerobic bacilli from the gastrointestinal tract cause most urinary tract infections. *Escherichia coli* accounts for about 80% of noninstitutionally acquired uncomplicated urinary tract infections. Other common infecting organisms are *Staphylococcus saprophyticus, Klebsiella pneumoniae, Enterobacter, Proteus mirabilis,* and *Pseudomonas aeruginosa.* Nosocomial urinary tract infections and those associated with urinary tract pathologic abnormalities are considered to be complicated urinary tract infections. The pathogens tend to be the same types of bacteria, but they are frequently more resistant to the antibiotics commonly used. This requires the use of more potent antibiotics for longer courses of therapy, placing the patient at a greater risk for complications secondary to drug therapy.

The use of an indwelling urinary catheter should be avoided if possible. When used, adherence to strict aseptic technique and attachment to a closed drainage system is necessary to reduce the rate of infection.

NURSING PROCESS *for Urinary System Disease*

The information the nurse gains through assessment of the patient's clinical signs and symptoms is important to the health care provider when analyzing data for diagnosis and for evaluation of the patient's response to prescribed treatment.

Assessment

History of Urinary Tract Symptoms

- Does the individual have a history of a congenital disorder of the urinary tract, sexually transmitted disease, recent delivery of a baby, prostatic disease, recent catheterization, urologic instrumentation or surgical procedure, renal calculi, gout, urinary tract infection, or bladder dysfunction of neurologic origin? Obtain details applicable to the patient's responses.
- Is there a problem with defecation? When was the last bowel movement?

History of Current Symptoms. Has the individual had any chills, fever, general malaise, or a change in mental status? New confusion in an elderly patient may be the only sign of a urinary tract infection. Ask questions relating to personal hygiene practices and sexual intercourse to evaluate for the possibility of bacterial contamination as an underlying cause of cystitis. Has the person been on prolonged bed rest for any reason?

- *Pattern of urination:* Ask the individual to describe the symptoms that affect the ability to void. What is current urination pattern, and have there been recent changes? Such details as frequency, dysuria, incontinence, changes in the stream, hesitancy in starting to void, hematuria, nocturia (does he or she awaken at night with the desire to urinate, and if so, how many times does this occur during an average night?), and urgency are all of significance. Ask if he or she is able to sit through a 2-hour meeting or ride in a car for 2 hours without urinating. State the onset, course of progression of the symptoms, and any self-treatment that has been attempted and response achieved. Is there blood or pus in the urine? Is it difficult to postpone urination when the urge to urinate is felt? Are there urine leaks? If so, when does this happen and what causes it? Is there leaking when coughing, walking, running, or lifting a heavy object? Is there a leak if unable to reach a toilet immediately?
- *Pattern of pain:* Record the details of any pain the patient describes: frequency, intensity, duration, and location. Pain associated with renal pathology usually occurs at the groin, back, flank, and suprapubic area and on urination (dysuria). Does the pain radiate? If so, obtain details.
- *Intake and output:* Ask specifically about the individual's usual daily fluid intake. How frequently does the patient usually void? What is the amount of each voiding?

Medication History. Ask for a list of all prescribed, over-the-counter (OTC) medicines and herbal products being taken. Many pharmacologic agents (e.g., anticholinergic agents, cholinergic agents, antihistamines, antihypertensives, chemotherapeutic agents, and immunosuppressants) can induce urinary retention or an altered urinary elimination pattern or urologic symptoms. Has the person recently been on medications to prevent or treat a UTI?

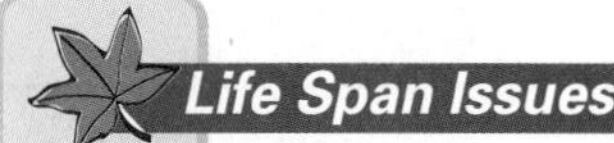

Life Span Issues

Urinary Tract Infections

In children and adult males, urinary tract infections may have a more serious etiology than that of a case of cystitis. Therefore all urinary tract infections must be thoroughly investigated to identify the underlying etiology.

Nutritional History. Has the individual been fasting for any prolonged period? How much alcoholic beverage has been consumed? Are vitamins, minerals, or other dietary supplements taken regularly? What kinds of fluids are taken daily? How many dairy or meat products are consumed daily? Do you drink coffee or colas, eat chocolate, or spice your foods heavily?

Laboratory and Diagnostic Studies. Review diagnostic and laboratory reports (e.g., urinalysis, renal function tests, voiding evaluatory procedures, cystoscopy, and complete blood count [CBC] with differential).

Urinalysis is a physical, chemical, and microscopic examination of the urine, and it is the most routine test the nurse encounters. The color, appearance (e.g., clear, foamy, turbid), and odor of the urine are noted, and the pH, protein, glucose, and ketones are determined with reagent dipsticks. Specific gravity is measured with a refractometer, and a microscopic examination of the urinary sediment is performed to detect the presence of red and white blood cells, bacteria, casts, and crystals. An understanding of the significant data that this basic test can reveal is imperative to monitoring the patient. Refer to Table 42-1 for a description of the data. See a general medical-surgical text for details of collecting urine samples correctly.

Nursing Diagnoses

- Pain, acute (indication)
- Incontinence, functional, stress, reflex, total, or urge urinary (indication)
- Infection (indication)
- Urinary retention (indication)

Planning

- Individualize the care plan to address the type of urinary tract disorder the individual has (e.g., retention, incontinence, or cystitis).
- Order medications prescribed and list on the medication administration record (MAR).
- Schedule diagnostic procedures ordered; transcribe orders relating to preparation for diagnostic procedures.
- Order laboratory studies (e.g., urinalysis, CBC with differential, and creatinine clearance).

Table 42-1 **Urinalysis**

PROPERTY	NORMAL DATA	ABNORMAL DATA
Color/appearance	Straw, clear yellow, or amber	Dark smoky color, reddish, or brown may indicate blood. White or cloudy may indicate urinary tract infection or chyluria. Dark yellow to amber may indicate dehydration. Green, deep yellow, or brown may indicate liver or biliary disease. Some drugs/food also alter the urine color: red or red brown: foods (e.g., beets, rhubarb); orange: phenazopyridine (Pyridium); dark yellow or brown: nitrofurantoin; blue: methylene blue; bright yellow: vitamin B complex; reddish-orange: rifampin.
Odor	Ammonia-like on standing	Foul smell may indicate infection. The dehydrated patient's urine is concentrated and the ammonia smell resulting from urea breakdown by bacteria is apparent. Sweet or fruity odor is associated with starvation or diabetic acidosis (ketoacidosis).
Protein	0 to trace	Foamy or frothy-appearing urine may indicate protein. Proteinuria is associated with kidney disease and toxemia of pregnancy. It is also found in leukemia, lupus erythematosus, cardiac disease.
Glucose	0 to trace	Presence is usually associated with diabetes mellitus or low renal threshold with glucose "spillage." Also seen at times of severe stress (e.g., major infection) or after high-carbohydrate intake.
Ketones	0	Associated with dehydration, starvation, ketoacidosis, and a diet high in protein and low in carbohydrates.
pH	4.5-8.0	A pH <4.5 indicates metabolic acidosis, respiratory acidosis, a diet high in meat protein and/or cranberries; medications can be prescribed to produce an alkaline or acidic urine pH. pH >8.0 is associated with bacteriuria (UTI due to *Klebsiella* or *Proteus*); diet high in fruits and/or vegetables.
Red blood cell count	0-3/HPF	Indicative of bleeding at some location in the urinary tract; infection, obstruction, calculi, renal failure, tumors, anticoagulants, excess aspirin, or menstrual contamination.
White blood cell count	0-5/HPF	An increase indicates an infection somewhere in the urinary tract. May also be associated with lupus nephritis and strenuous exercise.
Casts	0	May indicate dehydration, possible infection within renal tubules, or other types of renal disease.
Bacteria	0	May indicate urinary tract infection or a contaminated specimen collection.
Specific gravity	1.003-1.029	Used as indicator of hydration (in absence of renal pathology). Above 1.018 is an early sign of dehydration; below 1.010 is "dilute urine" and may indicate fluid accumulation. A fixed specific gravity (sp gr) at around 1.010 may indicate renal disease. Sp gr <1.005 may indicate diabetes insipidus, excess fluid intake or overhydration; sp gr >1.026 may indicate decreased fluid intake, vomiting, diarrhea, diabetes mellitus.

- Mark dietary orders on Kardex or enter data in the computer; indicate the amount of fluid to be taken every shift to maintain an adequate intake.
- Mark the Kardex or enter data into the computer for daily weights and accurate intake and output or enter data in the computer, and, as appropriate to diagnosis, indicate if bladder training, Kegel exercises, or others to be taught and encouraged.
- Indicate the level of activity or exercise permitted.
- Review treatment protocol and algorithms developed by the U.S. Department of Health and Human Services for the management of incontinence in adults.

Implementation

- Perform focused assessment of symptoms (e.g., retention, urinary frequency, and pain).
- Monitor the pain level and provide appropriate supportive and pharmacologic interventions.
- Administer prescribed medications; monitor response and side effects.
- Maintain adequate fluid intake and an accurate intake and output record. Instruct the patient to avoid foods known to be bladder irritants, such as spicy foods, citrus juices, alcohol, and caffeine.
- For inability to void, institute techniques to stimulate voiding (e.g., proper positioning to void, running water in sink, and pouring warm water over perineum).
- For incontinence, establish a regular toileting schedule, initiate bladder-training measures as appropriate and as ordered. Start measures to prevent perineal irritation. Apply external urinary diversion devices as ordered, such as an external condom (Texas catheter). Use incontinent pads as needed. Keep the urinal or bedpan readily available.
- Facilitate modifications of the environment that promote regular, easy access to toilet facilities, and pro-

mote the patient's safety with features such as better lighting, ambulatory assistance equipment, clothing alterations, timed voiding, and different toileting equipment.

- Implement measures to maintain the individual's dignity and privacy and to prevent embarrassment when incontinence is present.
- Maintain the activity and exercise level prescribed.

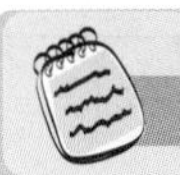

Patient Education and Health Promotion

For Incontinence

- Teach personal hygiene measures to keep the skin clean and dry and prevent perineal breakdown. Explore available appliances and incontinence products available for personal use.
- Teach Kegel exercises and bladder training, and stress importance of responding to the urge to void.
- Teach women the proper method of wiping after defecation or urination to prevent bacterial contamination.

For Urinary Tract Infections

- Teach women the following measures to avoid future urinary tract infections: avoid nylon underwear (use cotton) and tight, constrictive clothing in the perineal area; avoid frequent use of bubble bath; wash the perineal area immediately before and after sexual intercourse; and urinate immediately after intercourse.
- Explain the correct procedure for obtaining a clean-catch urine sample and the importance of having follow-up urine cultures collected as requested by the health care provider.
- Teach comfort measures such as the use of a sitz bath.
- Stress the importance of adequate fluid intake and its effect of diluting the urine, decreasing bladder irritability, and helping to remove organisms present in the bladder. Define "adequate intake of fluid" to the individual in terms of the number and size of glasses of liquid to be consumed during the day.
- Explain the signs of improvement or worsening of the urinary condition appropriate to the individual's diagnosis. Emphasize symptoms that should be reported to the health care provider.

For Urinary Retention. Teach self-examination to assess for bladder distention; Crede's maneuver (manual compression of the bladder through pressure on the lower abdomen) to aid in emptying the bladder; and, as appropriate, self-catheterization.

Medications

- For urinary retention, explain side effects to anticipate with the prescribed medications.
- For the urinary analgesic phenazopyridine hydrochloride, explain that the urine will be reddish orange. If discoloration of the skin or sclera occurs, contact the health care provider.
- For urinary tract infections, instruct patients to take the medicines exactly as prescribed for the entire course of medication. Discontinuing the antimicrobial agent when the symptoms improve may result in another infection after approximately 2 weeks that will be resistant to antimicrobial treatment. See individual drug monographs for specific instructions relating to acidification of the urine and instructions on taking medications with food or milk to avoid gastric irritation.
- See individual drug monographs regarding treatment of acute attacks and length of time before response can be anticipated. Stress the need for follow-up laboratory evaluation to evaluate response to therapy.

Fostering Health Maintenance

- Discuss medication information and how it will benefit the course of treatment to produce an optimal response. Stress maintenance of adequate urine volume as a part of the overall treatment of urinary tract disorders.
- Seek cooperation and understanding of the following points so that medication adherence is increased: name of medication, dosage, route and times of administration, side effects to expect, and side effects to report. See individual drug monographs for additional teaching.

Written Record. Enlist the patient's aid in developing and maintaining a written record of monitoring parameters for urinary antimicrobial agents (see Patient Self-Assessment Form on p. 684). Complete the Premedication Data column for use as a baseline to track response to therapy. Ensure that the patient understands how to use the form and instruct the patient to take the completed form to follow-up visits. During follow-up visits, focus on issues that will foster adherence with the therapeutic interventions prescribed.

DRUG THERAPY FOR URINARY TRACT INFECTIONS

URINARY ANTIMICROBIAL AGENTS

Actions

Urinary antimicrobial agents are substances that are secreted and concentrated in the urine in sufficient amounts to have an antiseptic effect on the urine and the urinary tract.

Uses

Selection of the product to be used is based on identification of the pathogens by the Gram stain or by urine culture in severe, recurrent, or chronic infections.

Cinoxacin, fosfomycin, norfloxacin, methenamine mandelate, nitrofurantoin, and nalidixic acid are used only for urinary tract infections. Examples of other antibiotics that are also used to treat urinary infections are ampicillin, sulfisoxazole, co-trimoxazole, ciproflox-

PATIENT SELF-ASSESSMENT FORM Urinary Antibiotics

MEDICATIONS	COLOR	TO BE TAKEN

Patient ____________________

Health Care Provider ____________________

Health Care Provider's phone ____________________

Next appt.* ____________________

What I Should Monitor			Premedication Data	Date	Date	Date	Date	Date	Date	Comments
Temperature										
Pain pattern and severity Severe (10) — Moderate (5) — Low (1) Description: On urination; without urination; flank area; suprapubic area										
Voiding and frequency	_____ times voiding/day									
	_____ times voiding/hour									
Fluid intake	_____ glasses/day									
	_____ cups/day									
Urine	Color (check one)	Straw								
		Dark								
		Red								
	Odor: Usual or unusual									
Other										

*Please bring this record with you to your next appointment.
Use the back of this sheet for additional information.

acin, lomefloxacin, ofloxacin, tetracycline, doxycycline, gentamicin, and carbenicillin. These agents are effective in a variety of tissue infections against many different microorganisms. Because of their use in multiple organ systems, they are discussed in detail (with nursing process) in Chapter 46.

Fluid intake should be encouraged so that there will be at least 2000 mL of urinary output daily. Duration of treatment depends on whether the infection is uncomplicated or complicated or acute, chronic, or recurrent; the pathogen being treated; the antimicrobial agent being used for treatment; and whether a follow-up culture can be collected to assess success of therapy.

DRUG CLASS: Fosfomycin Antibiotics

fosfomycin (fos foh my′ sin)

▶ MONUROL (mohn′ uhr ol)

Actions

Fosfomycin is the first of a new class of fosfomycin antibiotics. Fosfomycins act by inhibiting bacterial cell wall synthesis and by reducing adherence of bacteria to epithelial cells of the urinary tract.

Uses

Fosfomycin is the first antibiotic agent to be approved as a single-dose treatment for urinary tract infections. It is used to treat uncomplicated acute cystitis in women caused by susceptible strains of *E. coli* and *Enterococcus faecalis*. It is not indicated in the treatment of kidney infections such as pyelonephritis.

Therapeutic Outcomes

The primary therapeutic outcome associated with fosfomycin therapy is resolution of the urinary tract infection.

Nursing Process for Fosfomycin

Premedication Assessment

1. Record voiding characteristics (e.g., frequency, amount, color, odor, and associated symptoms such as burning and pain) to serve as a baseline for monitoring therapy.
2. Assess for and record any existing gastrointestinal complaints before initiating therapy.
3. Record baseline vital signs.

Planning

Availability. 3 g packets of fosfomycin granules.

Implementation

Dosage and Administration. *Adults:* PO: Pour the entire contents of a single-dose packet of fosfomycin into 90 to 120 mL (3 to 4 ounces) of water and stir to dissolve. Do not use hot water. Take immediately after dissolving in water. Fosfomycin may be taken with or without food.

Do not take additional packets of medicine without approval from the health care provider. More side effects develop with multiple doses, but there is little therapeutic gain.

Do not take in its dry form. Always mix fosfomycin with water before ingesting.

Evaluation

Side Effects to Expect

Nausea, Diarrhea, Abdominal Cramps, Flatulence. These side effects are usually mild and tend to resolve without need for therapy because only one dose of fosfomycin is administered.

Side Effects to Report

Perineal Burning, Dysuria. Burning with urination may be produced by the infection itself. Symptoms should improve in 2 to 3 days after taking fosfomycin; if not improved, the patient should contact the health care provider.

Drug Interactions

Metoclopramide. Metoclopramide has been reported to lower the serum concentrations and urinary excretion of fosfomycin by enhancing gastric motility. Other medicines that hasten gastrointestinal motility (e.g., cisapride) may produce a similar response.

DRUG CLASS: Quinolone Antibiotics

Actions

The antibacterial actions of the quinolones used more commonly for urinary tract infections (e.g., cinoxacin, nalidixic acid, and norfloxacin) act by inhibiting deoxyribonucleic acid (DNA) gyrase enzymes needed for DNA replication in bacteria.

Uses

Cinoxacin and nalidixic acid are effective in treating initial and recurrent urinary tract infections caused by *E. coli, P. mirabilis,* and other gram-negative microorganisms. They are not effective against *Pseudomonas* species, common pathogens in chronic urinary tract infections. Clinical studies indicate that cinoxacin may have milder side effects than nalidixic acid.

Norfloxacin has an advantage over other quinolones because it has a much broader spectrum of activity against gram-positive and gram-negative microorganisms. Because of expense, however, it should be reserved to treat resistant, recurrent urinary tract infections caused by *E. coli, P. mirabilis, Pseudomonas, Staphylococcus aureus, S. saprophyticus, Staphylococcus epidermidis,* and other gram-positive and gram-negative microorganisms no longer sensitive to the penicillins, cephalosporins, or sulfonamides. Because this antibiotic is administered orally, it also may be useful in treating patients on an outpatient basis who would have required hospitalization for parenteral therapy.

Therapeutic Outcomes

The primary therapeutic outcome associated with quinolone therapy is resolution of the urinary tract infection.

Nursing Process for Quinolones

Premedication Assessment

1. Record voiding characteristics (e.g., frequency, amount, color, odor, associated symptoms such as burning and pain) to serve as a baseline for monitoring therapy.
2. When using nalidixic acid, check for history of glucose-6-phosphate dehydrogenase deficiency; if present, withhold drug and contact health care provider.
3. When using cinoxacin or nalidixic acid, record any associated complaints of visual disturbances present before initiation of therapy (e.g., altered color perception, difficulty focusing, double vision).
4. Assess for and record any existing gastrointestinal complaints before initiating therapy.
5. Record baseline vital signs.

Planning

Availability. See Table 42-2.

Implementation

Dosage and Administration. See Table 42-2.

Evaluation

Side Effects to Expect

Nausea, Vomiting, Anorexia, Abdominal Cramps, Flatulence. These side effects are usually mild and tend to resolve with continued therapy. Encourage the

Drug Table 42-2 **QUINOLONE URINARY ANTIBIOTICS**

GENERIC NAME	BRAND NAME	AVAILABILITY	DOSAGE RANGE
cinoxacin		Capsules: 250, 500 mg	PO: 1 g daily in two to four divided doses for 7 to 14 days. Take with meals.
nalidixic acid	NegGram	Tablets: 500 mg	PO: 1 g four times daily for 7 to 14 days. Take with meals.
norfloxacin	Noroxin	Tablets: 400 mg	PO: 400 mg twice daily for 7 to 10 days. Take 1 hour before or 2 hours after meals with a large glass of fluid. Do not exceed 800 mg daily.

patient not to discontinue therapy without first consulting the health care provider.

Drowsiness, Headache, Dizziness. These side effects are usually mild and tend to resolve with continued therapy. Encourage the patient not to discontinue therapy without first consulting the health care provider.

Provide for patient safety during episodes of dizziness; report for further evaluation if recurrent.

Visual Disturbances. During the first few days of therapy with nalidixic acid, difficulty focusing, double vision, and changes in brightness and colors may occur shortly after each dose is given. If these symptoms persist or occur later in therapy, notify the health care provider for further evaluation.

Photosensitivity. Patients should avoid exposure to direct sunlight and wear sunshades and long-sleeved garments outdoors while taking this medication. A severe sunburn requires medical attention.

Side Effects to Report

Hematuria. Although rare, crystal formation has been reported when high doses of norfloxacin have been used or when the patient is dehydrated. The crystals may cause hematuria. Report bloody urine to the health care provider immediately. Encourage the patient to drink eight to twelve 8-oz glasses of water daily.

Perineal Burning, Urticaria, Pruritus, Hives. Burning with urination may be produced by the infection itself. However, a small percentage of patients receiving quinolones also develop these symptoms secondary to therapy.

Notify the health care provider if any of these symptoms develop. Symptomatic relief may be obtained by the use of cornstarch or baking soda in the bathwater. The use of antihistamines or topical steroids is rarely required.

Headache, Tinnitus, Dizziness, Tingling Sensations, Photophobia. Report these symptoms for further evaluation.

Drug Interactions

Probenecid. Probenecid may reduce urinary excretion of cinoxacin and norfloxacin, thereby causing inadequate antimicrobial therapy and the possibility of developing resistant strains of microorganisms.

Warfarin. The quinolones may enhance the anticoagulant effects of warfarin. Observe for the development of petechiae, ecchymoses, nosebleeds, bleeding gums, dark tarry stools, and bright red or "coffee ground" emesis. Monitor the prothrombin time, and reduce the dosage of warfarin if necessary.

Antacids, Sucralfate, Mineral Supplements Containing Iron, Magnesium, Calcium, or Aluminum. These ingredients will decrease absorption of the quinolones. Administer the quinolone 1 hour before or 2 hours after therapy with these agents.

Nitrofurantoin. Nitrofurantoin may antagonize the antibacterial effects of norfloxacin. Do not use concurrently.

Clinitest. Nalidixic acid may produce false-positive Clinitest results. Use Clinistix or Diastix to measure urine glucose.

DRUG CLASS: Other Urinary Antibacterial Agents

methenamine mandelate (meth en′ a meen man del′ ate)

MANDELAMINE (man del′ ah min)

Actions

Methenamine mandelate combines the action of methenamine and mandelic acid. Methenamine yields formaldehyde in the presence of an acidic urine. The formaldehyde released helps suppress the growth and multiplication of bacteria that may cause recurrent infection. Mandelic acid is present to help maintain the acidic urine. Ascorbic acid (vitamin C) also is often prescribed to help maintain the acidity of the urine.

Uses

Methenamine mandelate is used only in patients susceptible to chronic, recurrent urinary tract infections. It is not potent enough to be effective in patients suffering from a preexisting infection. The infection should be treated with antibiotics until the urine is sterile; methenamine should then be given to help prevent recurrence of the infection.

Therapeutic Outcomes

The primary therapeutic outcome associated with methenamine mandelate therapy is resolution of the urinary tract infection.

Nursing Process for Methenamine Mandelate

Premedication Assessment

1. Record voiding characteristics (e.g., frequency, amount, color, odor, and associated symptoms such as burning and pain) to serve as a baseline for monitoring therapy.
2. Check urine for acidification; give prescribed vitamin C; recheck urine for acidification.
3. Record baseline vital signs.

Planning

Availability. PO: 0.5 and 1 g enteric-coated tablets; 0.5 g per 5 mL suspension.

Implementation

Dosage and Administration. *Adult:* PO: 1 g four times daily after meals and at bedtime. Gastrointestinal symptoms may be minimized by administering with meals.

DO NOT crush the tablets! This will allow the formation of formaldehyde in the stomach, resulting in nausea and belching.

pH Testing: Perform urine testing for pH at regular intervals. Report values above 5.5.

Evaluation

Side Effects to Expect

Nausea, Vomiting, Belching. These side effects are usually mild and tend to resolve with continued therapy. Encourage the patient not to discontinue therapy without first consulting his or her health care provider.

Side Effects to Report

Hives, Pruritus, Rash. Report symptoms for further evaluation by the physician. Pruritus may be relieved by adding baking soda to the bathwater.

Bladder Irritation, Dysuria, Frequency. Notify the health care provider of these symptoms because they may indicate the presence of another urinary tract infection.

Drug Interactions

Acetazolamide, Sodium Bicarbonate. Acetazolamide and sodium bicarbonate produce alkaline urine, preventing the conversion of methenamine to formaldehyde, thereby inactivating the medication.

nitrofurantoin (ny tro fuhr' an toe in)
- FURADANTIN (fuhr ah dan' tin)
- MACRODANTIN (mak ro dan' tin)

Actions

Nitrofurantoin is an antibiotic that acts by interfering with several bacterial enzyme systems.

Uses

This antibiotic is not effective against microorganisms in the blood or in tissues outside the urinary tract. It is active against many gram-positive and gram-negative organisms, such as *Streptococcus faecalis, E. coli,* and *Proteus* species. It is not active against *P. aeruginosa* or *Serratia* species.

Therapeutic Outcomes

The primary therapeutic outcome associated with nitrofurantoin therapy is resolution of the urinary tract infection.

Nursing Process for Nitrofurantoin

Premedication Assessment

1. Record voiding characteristics (e.g., frequency, amount, color, odor, and associated symptoms such as burning and pain) to serve as a baseline for monitoring therapy.
2. Assess for and record any gastrointestinal complaints present before initiating drug therapy.
3. When using nitrofurantoin, check for history of glucose-6-phosphate dehydrogenase deficiency; if present, withhold drug and contact health care provider.
4. To serve as a baseline, assess for the presence of peripheral neuropathies before initiating therapy.
5. Record baseline vital signs.

Planning

Availability. PO: 25, 50, and 100 mg capsules; 25 mg per 5 mL suspension.

Implementation

NOTE: Nitrofurantoin must be in the bladder in sufficient concentrations to be therapeutically effective. Nitrofurantoin therapy is *not* recommended for use in patients with a creatinine clearance of less than 60 mL per minute.

Dosage and Administration. *Adult:* PO: 50 to 100 mg four times daily for 10 to 14 days. Administer with food or milk to reduce gastrointestinal side effects. To maintain adequate urine concentrations, space the doses at even intervals around the clock. *Pediatric:* Do not administer to infants younger than 1 month of age. PO: 5 to 7 mg/kg per 24 hours in four divided doses. Suspension: Store in a dark amber container away from bright light.

Evaluation

Side Effects to Expect

Nausea, Vomiting, Anorexia. Administer with food or milk to reduce gastric irritation.

Urine Discoloration. Tell the patient that urine may be tinted rust brown to yellow and that this discoloration should not be a cause for alarm.

Side Effects to Report

Dyspnea, Chills, Fever, Erythematous Rash, Pruritus. These symptoms are the early indications of an allergic reaction to nitrofurantoin.

Acute reactions usually occur within 8 hours in previously sensitized individuals and within 7 to 10 days in patients who develop sensitivity during the course of therapy.

Discontinue the drug and notify the health care provider.

Peripheral Neuropathies. Nitrofurantoin may cause peripheral neuropathies, particularly in patients with renal impairment, anemia, diabetes, electrolyte imbalance, or vitamin B deficiency. Nitrofurantoin should be discontinued at the first sign of numbness or tingling in the extremities.

Second Infection. Report immediately the development of dysuria, pungent-smelling urine, or fever. These symptoms may be the early indication of a second infection by an organism resistant to nitrofurantoin.

Drug Interactions

Clinitest. This drug may produce false-positive Clinitest results. Use Clinistix or Diastix to measure urine glucose.

Antacids. Discourage the patient from taking products containing magnesium trisilicate (e.g., Escot Capsules, Gaviscon, Gelusil) concurrently with nitrofurantoin because the antacid may inhibit absorption of the nitrofurantoin.

DRUG THERAPY FOR OVERACTIVE BLADDER SYNDROME

Overactive bladder (OAB) syndrome, also known as urge syndrome and urgency/frequency syndrome, is a common problem that is thought to affect more than 33 million Americans annually; it affects 30% to 40% of those older than the age of 75. OAB without urge incontinence is more common in men than women. It is defined by the International Continence Society (ICS) as "urgency, with or without urge incontinence, usually with frequency and nocturia. These symptoms are thought to be due to detrusor muscle [of the bladder] overactivity, but can also be due to other urinary dysfunction. The diagnosis of OAB can be made if there is no proven infection or other obvious pathology."

The three primary symptoms of OAB are frequency, urgency, and urinary incontinence. **Frequency** is the need to void eight or more times per day. **Urgency,** the most common symptom associated with OAB, is a sudden, compelling desire to pass urine that is very difficult to ignore. **Incontinence** is the inability to control urine from passing from the bladder. Incontinence can be subdivided into urge incontinence, stress incontinence, and overflow incontinence. **Urge incontinence** is the involuntary leakage of urine accompanied or immediately preceded by urgency. **Nocturia** is the need to void at night. Nocturia usually accompanies urgency with or without urge incontinence and is the complaint that the individual has to wake at night one or more times to void.

OAB and incontinence are frequently but erroneously used interchangeably. **Overactive bladder (OAB) syndrome** is the need to urinate with or without urge incontinence, and is usually accompanied by frequency during daytime and nighttime. About one third of OAB patients have urge incontinence, sometimes called "OAB wet," and two thirds have OAB without urge incontinence, or "OAB dry." Stress incontinence is generally not associated with urgency, frequency, or nocturia, and therefore does not fit the definition of OAB. However, it is not uncommon for patients with OAB also to have stress incontinence. Proper diagnosis of the underlying condition is important because treatments are different.

In males, an overlapping and often confusing problem is benign prostatic hyperplasia (BPH) (see Chapter 41). Patients with BPH are also susceptible to frequent urination, but unlike OAB, BPH can cause hesitancy and decreased flow during urination. Many men will have symptoms of both OAB and BPH and can be treated for both at the same time.

Overactive bladder syndrome cannot be cured, but a variety of nonpharmacologic and pharmacologic treatments can be used to reduce the symptoms associated with the disease. The goals of therapy are to decrease frequency by increasing voided volume, decrease urgency, and reduce incidents of urinary urge incontinence. A diary to record the pattern and type of urinary leakage and frequency and volume of fluid consumption ("ins and outs") can be very helpful in developing an awareness of contributors and improvement or deterioration of symptoms over time. Lifestyle changes such as spacing fluid consumption throughout the day instead of large intakes at one time, avoiding diuretic-like stimulants such as alcohol, caffeine, spicy foods, and avoiding fluid intake after 6:00 PM can help with symptoms. Note "hidden" sources of caffeine such as Excedrin, Midol, and Anacin. Kegel exercises are recommended to strengthen external sphincter function and increase resistance when there is sudden urinary urgency. Bladder training—the patient is initially taught to void every hour on the hour, then asked to increase the duration between voids by 15 minutes each week—can help increase volume and control urgency. A combination of bladder training and Kegel exercises helps the patient regain bladder control, increasing voided volumes and the time interval between voids. Absorbent undergarment products are helpful in allowing social mobility and maintaining dry skin. They also help promote self-confidence and dignity.

The first line of pharmacologic treatment of OAB is anticholinergic agents. Anticholinergic agents with more selective action on the bladder are darifenacin, oxybutynin, solifenacin, tolterodine, and trospium.

DRUG CLASS: Anticholinergic Agents for Overactive Bladder Syndrome

Actions

Anticholinergic agents, also known as urinary antispasmodic agents, block the cholinergic (muscarinic) receptors of the detrusor muscle of the bladder, causing relaxation. They decrease involuntary contractions of the detrusor muscle and improve bladder volume capacity.

Uses

The anticholinergic agents are used to reduce the urgency and frequency of bladder contractions and delay the initial desire to void in patients with overactive bladder. Cholinergic receptors are found throughout the body, particularly in the salivary glands, eyes, colon, and brain. Thus inhibition of these receptors can lead to adverse effects including dry mouth, blurred vision, constipation, confusion, and sedation. Each of these agents has some degree of selectivity for the cholinergic receptors in the bladder but are variable in whether they also block receptors in other parts of the body leading to more adverse effects. They should not be used in patients with narrow-angle glaucoma, myasthenia gravis, gastric retention, or bowel disease such as ulcerative colitis, or urinary retention caused by an obstructive uropathy such as prostatitis.

Therapeutic Outcomes

The primary therapeutic outcome expected from urinary anticholinergic agents is control of incontinence associated with overactive bladder.

Nursing Process for Urinary Anticholinergic Agents

Premedication Assessment

1. Record voiding characteristics (e.g., frequency, amount, color, odor, associated symptoms such as burning and pain) to serve as a baseline for monitoring therapy.
2. Obtain baseline vital signs.

Planning

Availability. See Table 42-3.

Drug Table 42-3 URINARY ANTICHOLINERGIC AGENTS

GENERIC NAME	BRAND NAME	AVAILABILITY	DOSAGE RANGE
darifenacin	Enablex	Tablets: 7.5 and 15 mg	Initial dose: 7.5 mg once daily. Based on individual response, the dose may be increased to 15 mg once daily, as early as 2 weeks after starting therapy. May be taken without regard to food.
oxybutynin	Ditropan	Tablets: 5 mg Syrup: 5 mg/5 mL	Initial dose: 5 mg (tablets or syrup) 2 or 3 times/day. Maximum dose: 20 mg daily.
	Ditropan XL	Extended release tablets: 5, 10, and 15 mg	Initial dose: 5 mg once daily. Dosage may be adjusted at weekly intervals in 5-mg increments. Maximum dose: 30 mg daily. May be administered with or without food and must be swallowed whole with the aid of liquids. Do not crush or chew. Pediatric (>5 years of age): PO: 5 mg twice daily, maximum dose 15 mg daily.
	Oxytrol	Transdermal patch: 36 mg (3.9 mg/day release)	Initial dose: Apply one patch every 3 to 4 days to dry, intact skin on the abdomen, hip, or buttock. Select a new application site with each new patch to avoid reapplication to the same site within 7 days.
solifenacin	Vesicare	Extended release tablets: 5 and 10 mg	Initial dose: 5 mg once daily. If well tolerated, the dose may be increased to 10 mg once daily. May be taken without regard to food.
tolterodine	Detrol	Tablets: 1 and 2 mg	Initial dose: 1-2 mg twice daily based on individual response and tolerance.
	Detrol LA	Extended release capsules: 2 and 4 mg	Initial dose: 2-4 mg once daily taken with liquids and swallowed whole.
trospium	Sanctura	Tablets: 20 mg	Initial dose: 20 mg twice daily at least 1 hour before meals on an empty stomach. For patients with a renal creatinine clearance <30 mL/min, the recommended dose is 20 mg once daily at bedtime.

Implementation

Dosage and Administration. See Table 42-3.

Evaluation

Side Effects to Expect

Dry Mouth, Urinary Hesitancy, Retention. These side effects are usually dose related and respond to a reduction in dosage.

Instruct the patient to relieve dry mouth by sucking on ice chips or hard candy, or by chewing gum.

Constipation, Bloating. Encourage balanced nutrition and inclusion of fresh fruits and vegetables for roughage and an adequate fluid intake to help alleviate this complication. If this approach is unsuccessful, suggest a stool softener or bulk-forming supplement. Avoid laxatives.

Blurred Vision. Caution patients not to drive or operate power equipment until they have adjusted to this side effect.

Side Effects to Report. If any of the aforementioned side effects intensify, it should be reported to the physician for evaluation.

Drug Interactions

Anticholinergic Agents. The concurrent use of the urinary anticholinergic agents with other anticholinergic agents may increase the frequency and severity of dry mouth, blurred vision, constipation, and other anticholinergic pharmacologic effects.

Fluoxetine, Erythromycin, Clarithromycin, Ketoconazole, Itraconazole, Miconazole, Vinblastine, Retonavir, Nefazodone. These agents inhibit the metabolism of tolterodine, darifenacin, and solifenacin. It is recommended that dosages not be raised above the initial starting dose in patients taking these medicines concurrently.

MISCELLANEOUS URINARY AGENTS

bethanechol chloride (beth an′ ek ol)

URECHOLINE (u reh ko′ leen)

Actions

Bethanechol is a parasympathetic nerve stimulant that causes contraction of the detrusor urinae muscle in the bladder, usually resulting in urination. It may also stimulate gastric motility, increase gastric tone, and restore impaired rhythmic peristalsis.

Uses

Bethanechol is used in nonobstructive urinary retention, particularly in postoperative and postpartum patients to restore bladder tone and urination.

Therapeutic Outcomes

The primary therapeutic outcome associated with bethanechol therapy is restoration of bladder tone and urination.

Nursing Process for Bethanechol

Premedication Assessment

1. Record voiding characteristics (e.g., frequency, amount, color, odor, and associated symptoms such as burning and pain) to serve as a baseline for monitoring therapy.
2. Record any gastrointestinal symptoms present to serve as a baseline for monitoring therapy.

Planning

Availability. PO: 5, 10, 25, and 50 mg tablets.

Implementation

Dosage and Administration. *Adult:* PO: 10 to 50 mg two to four times daily. The maximum daily dose is 120 mg. Subcutaneous: 2.5 to 5 mg. Atropine sulfate must be available to counteract serious adverse effects.

NOTE: If overdosage occurs, the pharmacologic actions of the drug can immediately be abolished by atropine.

Evaluation

Side Effects to Expect

Flushing of Skin, Headache. A pharmacologic property of the drug results in dilated blood vessels.

Side Effects to Report

Nausea, Vomiting, Sweating, Colicky Pain, Abdominal Cramps, Diarrhea, Belching, Involuntary Defecation. These effects are caused by a pharmacologic property of the drug. Consult the health care provider; a dosage adjustment may control these adverse effects.

Support the patient who develops diarrhea or involuntary defecation.

Drug Interactions

Quinidine, Procainamide. Do not use concurrently with bethanechol. The pharmacologic properties of these agents counteract those of bethanechol.

neostigmine (nee oh stig′ meen)

PROSTIGMIN (pro stig′ mihn)

Actions

Neostigmine is an anticholinesterase agent that binds to cholinesterase, preventing the destruction of acetylcholine. The acetylcholine accumulates at cholinergic synapses, and its effects become prolonged and exaggerated. This produces a general cholinergic response manifested by miosis; increased tone of intestinal, skeletal, and bladder muscles; bradycardia; stimulation of secretions of the salivary and sweat glands; and constriction of the bronchi and ureters.

Uses

From a urinary tract standpoint, neostigmine is used to prevent and treat postoperative distention and urinary retention.

Therapeutic Outcomes

The primary therapeutic outcome expected from neostigmine is prevention or treatment of postoperative or postdelivery urinary retention.

Nursing Process for Neostigmine

Premedication Assessment

1. Check for pregnancy, intestinal or urinary tract obstruction, and peritonitis; if present, withhold drug and contact health care provider.
2. Take baseline vital signs; if bradycardia is present, withhold drug and contact the health care provider.
3. Check for a recent coronary event, hyperthyroidism, epilepsy, asthma, or peptic ulcer; if present, this drug must be used with caution. Depending on symptoms, contact the health care provider for approval before administering the drug.
4. Record voiding characteristics (e.g., frequency, amount, color, odor, associated symptoms such as burning and pain) to serve as a baseline for monitoring therapy.

phenazopyridine hydrochloride (fen ay zoh peer' i deen)
PYRIDIUM (py rid' ee um)

Actions

Phenazopyridine is an agent that, as it is excreted through the urinary tract, produces a local anesthetic effect on the mucosa of the ureters and bladder. It acts within about 30 minutes after oral administration.

Uses

Phenazopyridine relieves burning, pain, urgency, and frequency associated with urinary tract infections. It also reduces bladder spasm, which relieves the resulting urinary retention. Phenazopyridine is also used for preoperative and postoperative surface analgesia in urologic surgical procedures and after diagnostic tests in which instrumentation is necessary. It is occasionally used to relieve the discomfort caused by the presence of an indwelling catheter.

Therapeutic Outcomes

The primary therapeutic outcome associated with phenazopyridine therapy is relief of burning, frequency, pain, and urgency associated with urinary tract infection.

Nursing Process for Phenazopyridine

Premedication Assessment

Record skin color before initiating therapy.

Planning

Availability. PO: 95, 97.2, 100, and 200 mg tablets.

Implementation

Dosage and Administration. *Adult:* PO: 200 mg three times daily. *Pediatric (6 to 12 years of age):* PO: 100 mg three times daily.

Evaluation

Side Effects to Expect

Reddish Orange Urine Discoloration. Be certain the patient understands that the color of the urine will become reddish orange when this drug is used and that the discoloration is not cause for alarm.

Side Effects to Report

Yellow Sclera or Skin. The patient should report any yellowish tinge developing in the sclera (white portion) of the eye.

Drug Interactions

Urine Colorimetric Procedures. This medication will interfere with colorimetric diagnostic tests performed on urine. Consult your hospital laboratory for alternative measures.

- Urinary tract infections are some of the most common types of infections and are found in all patient care settings.
- The nurse can provide significant care by understanding and reporting the early symptoms associated with acute and chronic infections.
- Nurses can also play a significant role in discretely assisting patients who have difficulty with urinary retention and incontinence.

Go to your Companion CD-ROM for Appendices, an Audio Glossary, animations, Drug Dosage Calculators, customizable Patient Self-Assessment forms, and Review Questions for the NCLEX® Examination.

evolve Be sure to visit the companion Evolve site at http://evolve.elsevier.com/Clayton for WebLinks and additional online resources.

MEDICATION SAFETY REVIEW

MATH REVIEW QUESTIONS

1. Order: Bethanechol chloride (Urecholine) 2.5 mg subcutaneously stat

   Available: Bethanechol chloride 5 mg/mL

   Give: _____ mL.

2. Order: Methenamine mandelate (Mandelamine) 750 mg PO

   Available: Methenamine mandelate 0.5 g per 5 mL suspension

   Give: _____ mL.

CRITICAL THINKING QUESTIONS

1. A 64-year-old female resident of Long-Meadow Nursing Home has developed her third urinary tract infection (UTI) in the past 4 months. What are the common organisms that cause UTIs? What assessments should be made? Discuss appropriate nursing actions during the treatment of the current UTI and measures to be instituted to prevent another episode.

2. Identify premedication assessments and actions associated with antimicrobial agents and bladder active drugs used to treat disorders of the urinary system.

CONTENT REVIEW QUESTIONS

1. A patient receiving methenamine mandelate (Mandelamine) has a urine pH of 5.2. The nurse knows that the _____ given has _____ the urine sufficiently for the medication to be active.
   1. probenecid (Benemid); acidified
   2. ascorbic acid; acidified
   3. ascorbic acid; alkalinized
   4. probenecid (Benemid); alkalinized

2. Fosfomycin (Monurol) is given:
   1. once.
   2. bid.
   3. tid.
   4. qid.

3. The use of _____ reduces the urinary excretion of cinoxacin and norfloxacin.
   1. formaldehyde in a medication
   2. probenecid (Benemid)
   3. nitrofurantoin (Furadantin, Macrodantin)
   4. bethanechol chloride (Urecholine)

4. _____ causes the urine to become reddish orange.
   1. Probenecid (Benemid)
   2. Nitrofurantoin (Furadantin, Macrodantin)
   3. Bethanechol chloride (Urecholine)
   4. Phenazopyridine hydrochloride (Pyridium)

5. Which of the following symptoms is not a component of OAB syndrome?
   1. Urge incontinence
   2. Stress incontinence
   3. Urgency
   4. Frequency
   5. Nocturia

6. Urge incontinence is defined as:
   1. leakage that occurs when the bladder is too full.
   2. the need to pass urine more than eight times a day.
   3. bladder leakage that occurs during exercise.
   4. sudden loss of bladder control.

7. First-line pharmacotherapy for OAB are the:
   1. beta-adrenergic blockers.
   2. anticholinergic (antimuscarinic) agents.
   3. muscle relaxants.
   4. calcium channel blockers.

CHAPTER

43 Drugs Used to Treat Glaucoma and Other Eye Disorders

evolve http://evolve.elsevier.com/Clayton

Chapter Content

Objectives

1. Describe the normal flow of aqueous humor in the eye.
2. Identify the changes in normal flow of aqueous humor caused by open-angle and closed-angle glaucoma.
3. Explain baseline data that should be gathered when an eye disorder exists.
4. Review the correct procedure for instilling eye drops or eye ointments.
5. Develop teaching plans for a person with an eye infection and a person receiving glaucoma medication.

Key Terms

cornea	near point
sclera	zonular fibers
iris	cycloplegia
sphincter muscle	lacrimal canaliculi
miosis	intraocular pressure
dilator muscle	closed-angle glaucoma
mydriasis	open-angle glaucoma
lens	

ANATOMY AND PHYSIOLOGY OF THE EYE

The eyeball has three coats, or layers: the protective external, or corneoscleral coat; the nutritive middle vascular layer, called the choroid; and the light-sensitive inner layer, or retina (Figure 43-1).

The **cornea,** or outermost sheath of the anterior eyeball, is transparent so that light can enter the eye. The cornea has no blood vessels; it receives its nutrition from the aqueous humor and its oxygen supply by diffusion from the air and surrounding vascular structures. There is a thin layer of epithelial cells on the external surface of the cornea that is quite resistant to infection. An abraded cornea, however, is highly susceptible to infection. The cornea has sensory fibers, and any damage to the corneal epithelium will cause pain. Seriously injured corneal tissue is replaced by scar tissue that is usually not transparent. The **sclera,** the eye's white portion, is continuous with the cornea and nontransparent.

The **iris** is a diaphragm that surrounds the pupil and gives the eye its color: blue, green, hazel, brown, or gray. The **sphincter muscle** within the iris encircles the pupil and is innervated by the parasympathetic nervous system. **Miosis** is contraction of the iris sphincter muscle, which causes the pupil to narrow. The

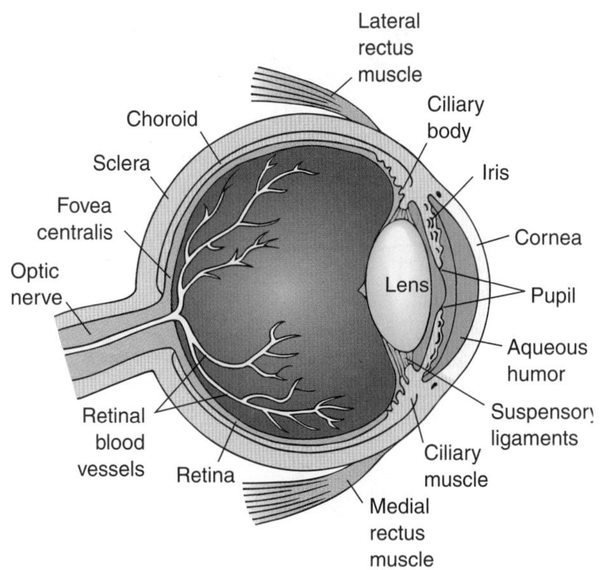

FIGURE **43-1** Cross section of the eye.

dilator muscle, which runs radially from the pupillary margin to the iris periphery, is sympathetically innervated. **Mydriasis** is contraction of the dilator muscle and relaxation of the sphincter muscle, which causes the pupil to dilate (Figure 43-2).

Constriction of the pupil normally occurs with light or when the eye is focusing on nearby objects. Dilation of the pupil normally occurs in dim light or when the eye is focusing on distant objects.

The **lens** is a transparent, gelatinous mass of fibers encased in an elastic capsule situated behind the iris. Its function is to ensure that the image on the retina is in sharp focus. It does this by changing shape (accommodation). This occurs readily in youth, but with age the lens becomes more rigid and the ability to focus close objects is lost. The **near point,** the closest point that can be seen clearly, recedes. With age, the lens may lose its transparency and become opaque, forming a cataract. Blindness can occur unless the cataract can be treated or surgically removed.

The lens has ligaments around its edge called **zonular fibers** that connect with the ciliary body. Tension on the zonular fibers helps change the shape of the lens. In the unaccommodated eye, the ciliary muscle is relaxed and the zonular fibers are taut. For near vision, the ciliary muscle fibers contract, relaxing the pull on the ligaments, and allowing the lens to become thick. Accommodation depends on two factors: the ability of the lens to assume a more biconvex shape when tension on the ligaments is relaxed and ciliary muscle contraction. Paralysis of the ciliary muscle is termed **cycloplegia.** The ciliary muscle is innervated by parasympathetic nerve fibers.

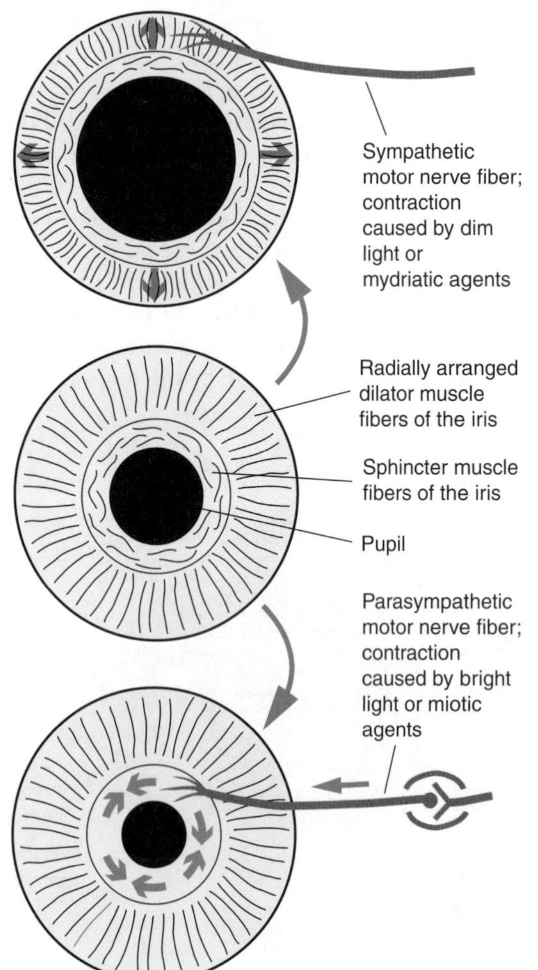

FIGURE **43-2** Effect of light or ophthalmic agents on the iris of the eye.

The ciliary body secretes aqueous humor, which bathes and feeds the lens, posterior surface of the cornea, and iris. After it is formed the fluid flows forward between the lens and the iris into the anterior chamber. It drains out of the eye through drainage channels located near the junction of the cornea and sclera into a meshwork that leads into Schlemm's canal and into the venous system of the eye.

Eyelids, eyelashes, tears, and blinking all protect the eye. There are about 200 eyelashes for each eye. The eyelashes cause a blink reflex whenever a foreign body touches them, closing the lids for a fraction of a second to prevent the foreign body from entering the eye. Blinking, which is bilateral, occurs every few seconds during waking hours. It keeps the corneal surface free from mucus and spreads the lacrimal fluid evenly over the cornea. Tears are secreted by lacrimal glands and contain lysozyme, a mucolytic lubrication for lid movements. They wash away foreign agents and form a thin film over the cornea, providing it with a good optical surface. Tear fluid is lost by drainage into two small ducts, the **lacrimal canaliculi,** at the inner corners of the eyelids and by evaporation.

GENERAL CONSIDERATIONS FOR TOPICAL OPHTHALMIC DRUG THERAPY

The most common route of administration for ophthalmic drugs is topical application. Advantages include convenience, simplicity, noninvasive nature, and the ability of the patient to self-administer. Topically administered medicines do not penetrate adequately for use with posterior eye diseases, so topical administration is not used for such diseases as with the optic nerve or retina.

Proper administration is essential to optimal therapeutic response. The administration technique used often determines drug safety and efficacy (see Chapter 8, p. 119).

- Based on the volume that the eye can retain, use of more than one drop per administration is questionable.
- If more than one drug is to be administered at about the same time, separate the administration of the different medicines by at least 5 minutes. This ensures that the first medicine is not washed away by the second, or that the second medication is not diluted by the first.

- Minimize systemic absorption of ophthalmic drops by compressing the lacrimal sac for 3 to 5 minutes after instillation. This reduces the passage of medicine via the nasolacrimal duct into areas of absorption such as the nasal and pharyngeal mucosa.
- Eyecup use is discouraged due to risk of contamination.
- Ophthalmic ointments may impede delivery of other ophthalmic drugs to the affected site by serving as a barrier to contact. Administer drops before ointments. Try not to administer drops for a few hours after the use of ointment.
- Ointments may blur vision during the waking hours. Use with caution in conditions in which visual clarity is critical (e.g., operating motor equipment, reading), or use at bedtime.
- Observe expiration dates closely. Do not use outdated medication.
- Solutions and ointments are frequently misused. Do not assume that patients know how to maximize safe and effective use of these agents. Combine appropriate patient education and counseling with prescribing and dispensing of ophthalmics.
- In an effort to enhance safety of ophthalmic medications, the ophthalmic medicine industry recommends the use of standard colors for drug labels and bottle caps (see chart below). Practitioners who dispense and administer ophthalmic solutions should become very familiar with these colors and medicines to help prevent inadvertently picking up and administering the wrong solution.

THERAPEUTIC CLASS	CAP AND LABEL COLOR
Antiinfectives	Brown or tan
Beta-adrenergic blocking agents	Yellow, blue, or both
Miotics	Green
Mydriatics and cycloplegics	Red
Nonsteroidal antiinflammatory agents	Gray

GLAUCOMA

Glaucoma is an eye disease characterized by abnormally elevated **intraocular pressure** (IOP), which may result from excessive production of the aqueous humor or from diminished ocular fluid outflow. Increased pressure, if persistent and sufficiently elevated, may lead to permanent blindness. There are three major types of glaucoma: primary, secondary, and congenital. Primary includes **closed-angle glaucoma** and **open-angle glaucoma.** These are diagnosed by the iridocorneal angle of the anterior chamber, where aqueous humor reabsorption takes place. Secondary glaucoma may result from previous eye disease or may occur after a cataract extraction and may require drug therapy for an indefinite period. Congenital glaucoma requires surgical treatment.

Open-angle glaucoma develops insidiously over the years as pathologic changes at the iridocorneal angle prevent the outflow of aqueous humor through the trabecular network to Schlemm's canal and into the veins of the eye. (See Figure 43-3 for the normal pathway of aqueous flow.) In cases of open-angle glaucoma, there is reduced outflow of aqueous humor through the trabecular network and Schlemm's canal because of resistance of the aqueous humor outflow; the iridocorneal angle is open (Figure 43-4).

Intraocular pressure builds up and, if not treated, will damage the optic disc. Initially, the patient has no symptoms, but over the years there is a gradual loss of peripheral vision. If untreated, total blindness may result.

Acute closed-angle glaucoma occurs when there is a sudden increase in IOP caused by a mechanical ob-

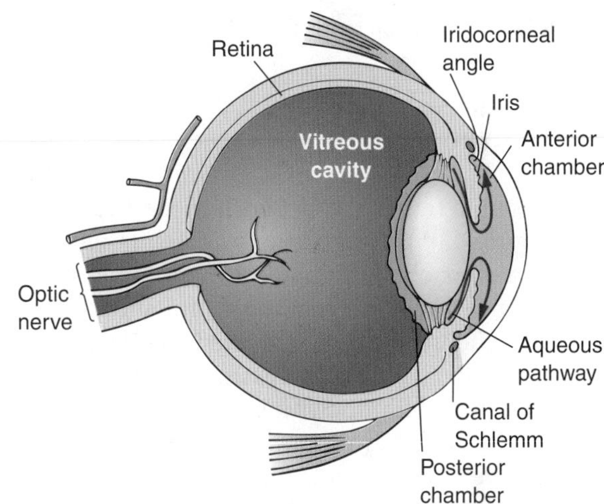

FIGURE 43-3 Anterior and posterior chambers of the eye. Arrows indicate the pathway of aqueous flow.

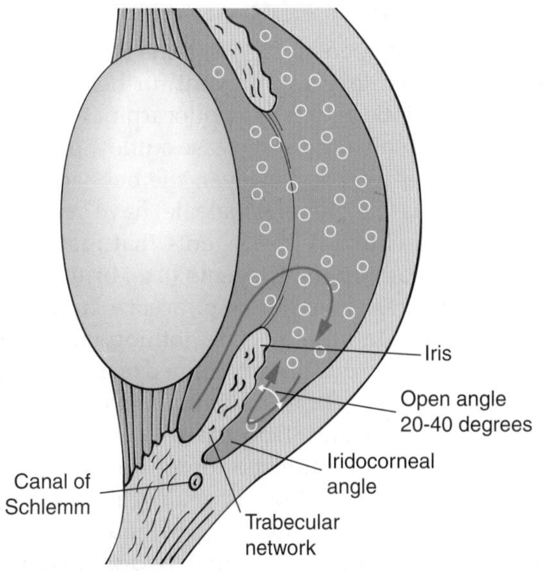

FIGURE 43-4 The flow of the aqueous humor is due to reduced outflow at Schlemm's canal in the trabecular network. There is no obstruction from closure of the iridocorneal angle.

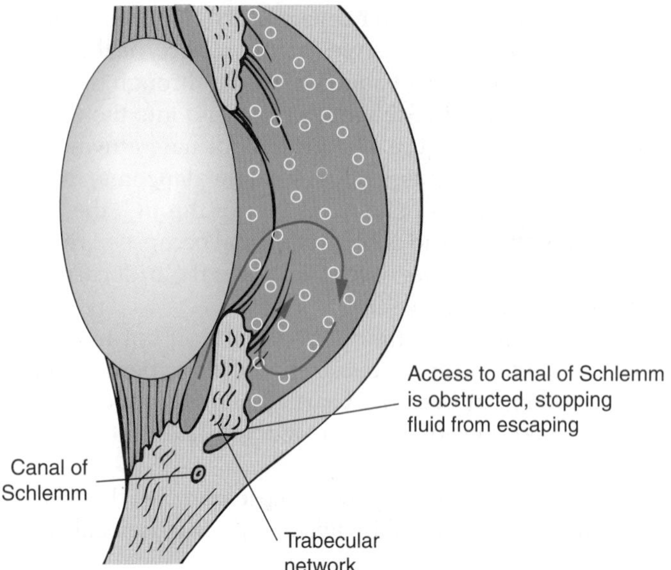

FIGURE **43-5** Obstruction to the flow of aqueous fluid, causing closed-angle glaucoma.

struction of the trabecular network in the iridocorneal angle (Figure 43-5). This occurs in patients who have narrow anterior chamber angles. Symptoms develop gradually and appear intermittently for short periods, especially when the pupil is dilated. (Dilation of the pupil pushes the iris against the trabecular meshwork, causing the obstruction.) Symptoms often reported are blurred vision, halos around white lights, frontal headache, and eye pain. Patients often associate the symptoms with stress or fatigue. An attack can also be precipitated by administration of a mydriatic agent such as atropine or scopolamine for eye examination.

DRUG THERAPY FOR GLAUCOMA

The treatment of open-angle glaucoma is maintenance of IOP at normal levels to prevent further blindness. Historically, miotic agents (e.g., pilocarpine) have been the most commonly used to increase outflow of aqueous humor. In recent years, however, the beta-adrenergic blocking agents (e.g., timolol maleate) have become the initial drug of choice. Other agents that may also be used are sympathomimetic agents (e.g., brimonidine), carbonic anhydrase inhibitors (e.g., acetazolamide), and cholinesterase inhibitors (e.g., echothiophate iodide). The selection of the drug is determined to a great extent by the requirements of the individual patient.

Acute angle-closure glaucoma requires immediate treatment with the administration of miotic agents to relieve the pressure of the iris against the trabecular network, and allow drainage of the aqueous humor. Mannitol, an osmotic diuretic, may be administered to draw aqueous humor from the eye, and acetazolamide may be administered to reduce formation of aqueous humor. Analgesics and antiemetics may be administered if pain and vomiting persist. Surgery is then required to correct the abnormality.

NURSING PROCESS *for Glaucoma and Other Eye Disorders*

The nurse has an important role in educating the public and promoting safety measures to protect the eye from potential sources of injury. Health professionals can participate in this role during their daily contacts with people in the community. The use of safety glasses in potentially hazardous situations, prevention of chemical burns from common household cleansing items or other agents at home or work, proper cleaning and wearing of contact lenses or glasses, and the selection of safe toys and play activities for children are examples of areas about which the nurse can teach the public. These safety measures can significantly reduce the number of injuries that occur annually.

Nurses also play an important role in detecting and implementing the treatment process. An example of this is in patients with diabetes mellitus. Encourage annual or more frequent eye examinations to detect and prevent complications associated with the disease.

The primary delivery of eye care is through self-administration of drugs. One of the greatest challenges in the care of chronic eye disorders such as glaucoma is convincing the patient of the need for long-term treatment and adherence to the therapeutic regimen.

Assessment

Eye Examination

- When an eye injury has occurred, document visual acuity by screening vision with the Snellen chart. Comparison screenings should be performed at each subsequent visit.
- Observe for eyelid edema. It may be an indication of a systemic disease process or tumor. Report if present.
- Assess pupils for equality of size, roundness, and response to light. Report irregular contour, unequal size, or decreased response to light.
- Observe for and report nystagmus.
- Observe for any redness or drainage in the eyes.
- Observe for complete closure of the eyelid. This is essential for protection of the cornea. Patients who have received corneal anesthesia, who have had fifth cranial nerve surgery, who have exophthalmos, or who are unconscious must have the cornea protected to prevent damage.
- Ask whether glasses or contact lenses are worn.
- Inspect the eye dressings and report immediately for evaluation if any drainage is observed. Never remove the dressing to inspect the eye.

History of Symptoms

- Ask the patient to describe the symptoms for which treatment is being sought. How do symptoms affect daily life? Do visual problems affect the ability to read?
- Is there a family history of cataracts, glaucoma, or macular degeneration?
- Are your activities limited in any way by your vision problem?
- Do you participate in any leisure activities that have the potential for eye injury?
- Has the person had any noticeable pain, burning, foreign body sensation, blurred or halo vision, or loss of vision?
- Ask whether there is any difficulty in adjusting vision when going from a dark to a brightly lighted area or vice versa.
- Are colors clear and crisp or do they lack clarity?
- Has there been an increase in tearing or discharge from the eye? If so, ask for details of appearance and amount of drainage.
- Has there been any recent nausea and vomiting?

Psychological. What type of response is the patient exhibiting to the disturbance in visual acuity? Is the patient withdrawing socially? Identify a support system available for at-home care and assistance.

Diagnostics. Ask the patient to describe what eye diagnostic procedures have been completed before admission (e.g., visual acuity measurement, tonometry, slit-lamp examination, visual fields). Normal intraocular pressure using an applanation tonometer is 10 to 21 mm Hg.

Medications. Ask for a list of all prescribed, over-the-counter (OTC) medications and herbal products being taken. Ask for details on medicines, dosage, schedule, and degree of compliance.

Nursing Diagnoses

- Injury, risk for (indication, side effects)
- Pain, acute (indication)
- Sensory perception, disturbed (visual) (indication, side effects)
- Self-care deficit (bathing/hygiene/dressing/grooming) (indication, side effects)
- Noncompliance (side effects)

Planning

- Schedule diagnostic procedures, surgery, and laboratory studies as ordered.
- List all ordered medications on the medication administration record (MAR). If beta blockers are being taken, list the pulse on the MAR as a preassessment to administration of the ophthalmic drops.
- Mark the Kardex or enter data in the computer with parameters relating to prevention of injury, activity and exercise level permitted, and diet orders.
- Plan a specific time to meet with patient and significant others to discuss at-home care and community resources available if assistance is indicated.

Implementation

- Perform assessments every shift consistent with the patient's status and diagnosis.
- Prepare the patient for eye examinations, diagnostics, or eye surgery.
- Administer cycloplegic and mydriatic medicines prescribed for dilation of the eye before an eye examination or ophthalmic surgery.
- Administer miotic medicine to produce constriction of the eye after eye examination or diagnostic procedures, as prescribed.
- Administer all ophthalmic medicines prescribed for identified disease process (e.g., glaucoma) after correct clinical procedure. Maintain aseptic technique to prevent the transfer of infection from one eye to the other.
- Protect the cornea from damage during anesthesia or in an unconscious patient through the use of ophthalmic ointment or artificial tears to prevent corneal drying.
- Assist with diagnostic procedures (e.g., visual fields, tonometry, visual acuity).
- Take baseline vital signs.
- Institute appropriate comfort measures.
- If eye surgery is performed (e.g., trabeculectomy), institute routine postoperative care measures. Position the patient as ordered, usually on the back or on the unoperated side. With the scleral buckling procedure, positioning orders may be extremely specific.
- Ensure that an eyepatch and shield are applied properly to protect the eye from further injury.
- Explain and enforce activity and exercise restrictions. To prevent an increase in IOP, instruct the patient to avoid heavy lifting, straining on defecation, coughing, or bending and placing the head in a dependent position.
- A blind or disoriented patient or a patient with both eyes patched may suffer from sensory deprivation.
- Always speak before touching the person with impaired vision.
- Check on the patient at frequent intervals; initiate conversations and regularly orient the patient to date, time, and place.
- Try to arrange for a semiprivate room with an alert roommate who can provide stimulation.
- If the patient is agitated, contact the physician; it may be necessary to obtain an order to remove one eyepatch or sedate the patient.
- Provide emotional support.

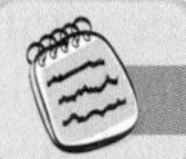

Patient Education and Health Promotion

After Eye Surgery

- Teach the patient and family proper hygiene and eye care techniques to ensure that medications, dressings, and/or surgical wounds are not contaminated during necessary eye care.

- Teach the patient and family about signs and symptoms of infections, and when and how to report them to allow early recognition and treatment of possible infection.
- Instruct the patient to comply with postoperative restrictions on head positioning, bending, coughing, and Valsalva maneuver to optimize visual outcomes and prevent increased intraocular pressure.
- Instruct the patient to instill eye medications using aseptic techniques and to comply with prescribed eye medication routine to prevent infection.
- Instruct the patient to monitor pain and take prescribed pain medication as directed; report pain not relieved by prescribed mediations.
- Instruct the patient about the importance of continued follow-up as recommended to maximize potential visual outcomes.

Disease or Disorder

- Reinforce the teaching of pertinent facts regarding the diagnosis and disease process.
- If the patient is being treated for glaucoma, stress the need for lifelong treatment and use of medications. Explain that adherence with the drug regimen can help prevent blindness.
- If an infectious process is present, teach personal hygiene measures to prevent introduction of an infection.
  1. Wash hands thoroughly each time the area is touched (before or after any eye treatments or instillation of medications).
  2. Use only sterile medications or dressings on the eye.
  3. Wipe the eye from the inner canthus outward; discard the tissue or cotton ball used; wash hands before proceeding to the second eye.
  4. When an infection is present, prevent cross-contamination; always use a separate source of medication and droppers for each eye.
  5. Never touch the eyeball or face with the tip of the dropper or opening of the ointment container. Demonstrate the proper way to set the lid down so that the inside is not contaminated.
  6. When inserting or removing contact lenses, wash hands first, and then follow the manufacturer's instructions regarding the cleansing and care of the lenses.
  7. Report any persistent redness or drainage from the eyes.

Visual Acuity. Provide for patient safety.

- Assess whether diminished visual acuity will reduce the ability of the patient to perform his or her usual activities of daily living. Teach adaptation methods appropriate to the situation.
- Restrict the operation of tools or power equipment, as appropriate, to the degree of alteration present.

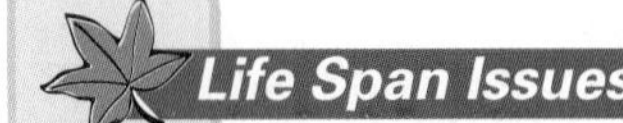

Diminished Visual Acuity

Diminished visual acuity has an effect on most aspects of an individual's life. Therefore, it is imperative that the person's ability to perform the usual activities of daily living be evaluated when visual impairment develops. Because many medicines used for other diseases reduce visual acuity, these side effects should be anticipated and their effect on the individual monitored. Every attempt must be made to assist the individual to adapt to the visual impairment while providing for personal safety.

Medications. Review the details of medication administration.

- Ensure that directions are printed in large, bold print that the individual is capable of reading.
- Have the patient store all medications in an area separate from other containers so that the person cannot inadvertently put things other than medicine in the eye.
- Have the person demonstrate the ability to self-administer the eye medications to ensure manual dexterity to perform the procedures.
- Keep an extra bottle of eye medications on hand, particularly those used to reduce IOP.

Fostering Health Maintenance

- Discuss medication information and how it will benefit the course of treatment (e.g., reduction of IOP, elimination of an infection).
- Seek cooperation and understanding of the following points so that medication compliance is increased: name of medication, dosage, route and times of administration, side effects to expect, and side effects to report. Verify ability to self-administer all medications. Additional health teaching is included in individual drug monographs.
- Encourage the patient to discuss any side effects the medications may produce to plan mutually with the health provider for ways to minimize these effects or make adaptation rather than reduce the frequency or eliminate the use of the medications.
- Enlist the patient's aid in developing and maintaining a written record (see p. 699) of monitoring parameters (e.g., blood pressure and pulse with adrenergic and beta-adrenergic blocking agents, degree of visual disturbance, progression of impairment) and response to prescribed therapies for discussion with the physician. Encourage the patient to take this record to all follow-up visits.

DRUG CLASS: Osmotic Agents

Actions

Osmotic agents are administered intravenously, orally, or topically to reduce IOP. These agents elevate the osmotic pressure of the plasma, causing fluid from the

PATIENT SELF-ASSESSMENT FORM Eye Medications

MEDICATIONS	COLOR	TO BE TAKEN

Patient ______

Health Care Provider ______

Health Care Provider's phone ______

Next appt.* ______

What I Should Monitor		Premedication Data	Date	Date	Date	Date	Date	Date	Comments
Blood pressure									
Pain in eye (right or left)									
No pain in eyes									
Vision (clarity)	Blurred all the time								
	Occasionally hazy								
	Clear								
Side vision	Must turn head to see								
	Can see without turning head								
Vision since starting eye medication No improvement (10) — Better (5) — Much better (1)									
Headache	None								
	If yes, location								
	What were you doing when it started?								
Eye color — Redness	Is redness improved by medication?								
Eye color — Burning	Is burning improved by medication?								
Itching, rash	None								
	Sometimes associated with medication								
	Always occurs with medication								
Other									

*Please bring this record with you to your next appointment.
Use the back of this sheet for additional information.

extravascular spaces to be drawn into the blood. The effect on the eye is reduction of volume of intraocular fluid, which produces a decrease in IOP.

Uses

The osmotic agents are used to reduce IOP in patients with acute narrow-angle glaucoma; before iridectomy; preoperatively and postoperatively in conditions such as congenital glaucoma, retinal detachment, cataract extraction, and keratoplasty; and in some secondary glaucomas.

Therapeutic Outcomes

The primary therapeutic outcome expected from osmotic agents is reduced intraocular pressure.

Nursing Process for Osmotic Agents

Premedication Assessment

1. Initiate an intravenous (IV) line for administration of the osmotic agent. Be certain the IV site is functional and not infiltrated before hanging the osmotic agent for infusion.
2. If a Foley catheter is used, ensure that it is functional; initiate strict intake and output monitoring.
3. Assess and record baseline weight, hydration status, lung sounds, and vital signs.
4. Record premedication IOP readings and visual acuity data.

Planning

Availability. See Table 43-1.

Implementation

Dosage and Administration. See Table 43-1.

- *Catheter:* Be certain the patient has an indwelling catheter if these drugs are used during an operative procedure; check with the physician before scrubbing for the procedure.
- *Intravenous:* Assess the IV site at regular intervals for any signs of infiltration. Tissue necrosis may occur from infiltration into the surrounding tissue. If it occurs, stop the IV, report, and then elevate the extremity and follow hospital protocol for extravasation. Note: Do not use veins in lower extremities for administration of these agents because this may cause phlebitis or thrombosis.

 **Drug Table 43-1 OSMOTIC AGENTS**

GENERIC NAME	BRAND NAME	AVAILABILITY	DOSAGE	COMMENTS
glycerin	Osmoglyn	50% solution	PO: 1-2 g/kg	An oral osmotic agent for reducing intraocular pressure Administer 60-90 min before surgery Use with caution in diabetic patients; monitor for hyperglycemia
isosorbide	Ismotic	100 g in 220 mL solution (45%)	PO: 1.5 g/kg (range: 1-3 g/kg) two to four times daily	An oral osmotic agent for reducing intraocular pressure Onset of action is 30 min, duration is 5-6 hr With repeated doses, monitor fluids and electrolytes The solution will taste better if poured over cracked ice and sipped
mannitol	Osmitrol	5%, 10%, 15%, 20%, 25% solutions for infusions	IV: 1.5-2 g/kg as a 20% solution over 30 min	Used intravenously when oral methods are unacceptable When used preoperatively, administer 60-90 min before surgery Use an in-line filter because mannitol has a tendency to crystallize
urea	Ureaphil	40 g in 150 mL	IV: 1-5 g/kg	Administer as a 30% solution at an infusion rate not to exceed 4 mL/min Used when mannitol and oral methods are not available Do not exceed 120 g daily Use extreme caution against extravasation; tissue necrosis may result Do not infuse in veins of lower extremities because of the possibility of thrombus formation

- *Mannitol crystals:* Check the mannitol solution for crystals; DO NOT administer if present. Follow directions in the literature accompanying the medication for a warm bath to dissolve the crystals, and then cool the solution before administration.

Evaluation

Side Effects to Report

Thirst, Nausea, Dehydration, Electrolyte Imbalance. The electrolytes most commonly altered are potassium (K^+), sodium (Na^+), and chloride (Cl^-).

Many symptoms associated with altered fluid and electrolyte balance are subtle and resemble general symptoms of drug toxicity or the disease process itself.

Gather data about changes in the patient's mental status (alertness, orientation, and confusion), muscle strength, muscle cramps, tremors, nausea, and general appearance (drowsy, anxious, and lethargic).

Always check the electrolyte reports for early indicators of electrolyte imbalance.

Keep accurate records of intake and output, daily weights, and vital signs.

Headache. This is an indication of cerebral dehydration. Keeping the patient in a supine position can minimize it.

Circulatory Overload. These medications act on the blood volume by pulling fluid from the tissue spaces into the general circulation (blood). Assess the patient at regularly scheduled intervals for signs and symptoms of fluid overload, pulmonary edema, or heart failure. Perform lung assessments; report the development of crackles and increasing dyspnea, frothy sputum, or cough.

Drug Interactions

Lithium. Mannitol increases the excretion of lithium. Patients being treated with lithium should be monitored for low lithium levels if treated with mannitol.

DRUG CLASS: Carbonic Anhydrase Inhibitors

Actions

These agents are inhibitors of the enzyme carbonic anhydrase. Inhibition of this enzyme results in a decrease in the production of aqueous humor, thus lowering IOP.

Uses

These agents are used in conjunction with other treatments to control IOP in cases of intraocular hypertension and closed-angle and open-angle glaucoma. Dorzolamide has the advantage of intraocular administration with less potential for systemic side effects.

Therapeutic Outcomes

The primary therapeutic outcome expected from carbonic anhydrase inhibitors is reduced IOP.

Nursing Process for Carbonic Anhydrase Inhibitors

Premedication Assessment

1. Establish whether the patient is pregnant; if pregnancy is suspected, withhold the medicine and contact the health care provider.
2. Check for allergy to sulfonamide antibiotics; withhold the medicine and contact the physician if allergy is present.
3. Ensure that contact lenses have been removed before the instillation of dorzolamide drops.
4. Ensure that baseline electrolyte laboratory studies have been drawn as ordered.
5. Assess and record baseline weight, hydration data, vital signs, and mental status.
6. Record premedication IOP readings and visual acuity data.
7. Assess for signs of gastric symptoms before initiating drug therapy. If present, schedule medications for administration with milk or food.

Planning

Availability. See Table 43-2.

Implementation

Dosage and Administration. See Table 43-2.

Sulfonamides. Do not administer to patients allergic to sulfonamide antibiotics without health care provider approval. Observe closely for the development of hypersensitivity.

Gastric Irritation. If gastric irritation occurs, administer with food or milk. If symptoms persist or increase in severity, report to the health care provider for evaluation.

Evaluation

Side Effects to Report

Electrolyte Imbalance, Dehydration. Although infrequent, treatment with carbonic anhydrase inhibitors may lead to excessive diuresis resulting in water dehydration and electrolyte imbalance. The electrolytes most commonly altered are K^+, Na^+, and Cl^-. Hypokalemia is most likely to occur.

Many symptoms associated with altered fluid and electrolyte balance are subtle and resemble general symptoms of drug toxicity or the disease process itself.

Gather data about changes in the patient's mental status (e.g., alertness, orientation, confusion), muscle strength, muscle cramps, tremors, nausea, and general appearance (e.g., drowsy, anxious, lethargic).

Always check the electrolyte reports for early indications of electrolyte imbalance.

Keep accurate records of intake and output, daily weight, and vital signs.

Drug Table 43-2 CARBONIC ANHYDRASE INHIBITORS

GENERIC NAME	BRAND NAME	AVAILABILITY	DOSAGE RANGE
acetazolamide	Diamox	Tablets: 125, 250 mg Capsules: 500 mg	PO: 250 mg to 1 g every 24 hr
brinzolamide	Azopt	Ophthalmic solution: 1% in 2.5, 5, 10, and 15 mL dropper bottles	Intraocular: 1 drop in affected eye(s) three times daily; if more than one ophthalmic agent is to be administered in the same eye, separate the administration by at least 10 min
dorzolamide	Trusopt	Ophthalmic solution: 2% in 5 and 10 mL droppers, bottles	Intraocular: 1 drop in affected eye(s) three times daily. If more than one ophthalmic agent is to be administered in the same eye, separate the administration by at least 10 min
methazolamide		Tablets: 25, 50 mg	PO: 50 to 100 mg, two or three times daily

Dermatologic, Hematologic, Neurologic Reactions. Carbonic anhydrase inhibitors are sulfonamide derivatives and thus have the potential to cause adverse effects similar to those associated with sulfonamide antimicrobial therapy. These adverse effects, although rare, include dermatologic, hematologic, and neurologic reactions. For further discussion see the section on sulfonamides in Chapter 46, p. 766).

Confusion. Perform a baseline assessment of the patient's degree of alertness and orientation to name, place, and time before initiating therapy. Make regularly scheduled subsequent mental status evaluations, and compare findings. Report changes in the patient's mental status.

Drowsiness. This side effect is usually mild and tends to resolve with continued therapy. Encourage the patient not to discontinue therapy without first consulting the health care provider.

People who work around machinery, drive, pour and give medicines, or perform any duties that require mental alertness should not take these medications while working.

Drug Interactions

Quinidine. These diuretics may inhibit quinidine excretion. If the patient is also receiving quinidine, monitor closely for signs of quinidine toxicity (e.g., tinnitus, vertigo, headache, confusion, bradycardia, visual disturbances).

Digoxin. Patients receiving these diuretics may excrete excess potassium, which leads to hypokalemia. If the patient is also receiving digoxin, monitor closely for signs of digoxin toxicity (e.g., anorexia, nausea, fatigue, blurred or colored vision, bradycardia, dysrhythmias).

Corticosteroids (Prednisone, Others). Corticosteroids may enhance the loss of potassium. Check potassium levels and monitor more closely for hypokalemia when these two agents are used concurrently.

DRUG CLASS: Cholinergic Agents

Actions

Cholinergic agents produce strong contractions of the iris (miosis) and ciliary body musculature (accommodation).

Uses

Cholinergic agents lower IOP in patients with glaucoma by widening the filtration angle, which permits outflow of aqueous humor. They also may be used to counter the effects of mydriatic and cycloplegic agents after surgery or ophthalmoscopic examination.

Cholinergic agents have several advantages: they are effective in many cases of chronic glaucoma, the side effects are less severe and less frequent than those of anticholinesterase agents, and they give better control of IOP with fewer fluctuations in pressure.

Therapeutic Outcomes

The primary therapeutic outcomes expected from cholinergic agents are as follows:

- Reduced IOP in patients with glaucoma
- Reversal of the mydriasis and cycloplegia secondary to ophthalmic agents used in surgery or ophthalmic examination

Nursing Process for Cholinergic Agents

Premedication Assessment

1. Obtain baseline vital signs.
2. Record premedication IOP readings and visual acuity data.

Planning

Availability. See Table 43-3.

Implementation

Dosage and Administration. See Table 43-3.

Drug Table 43-3 **CHOLINERGIC AGENTS**

GENERIC NAME	BRAND NAME	AVAILABILITY	DOSAGE	COMMENTS
acetylcholine chloride, intraocular	Miochol-E	1:100 solution	0.5-2 mL instilled into the eye during surgery	Used only during surgery to produce complete miosis within seconds; duration of action is only a few minutes, so pilocarpine may be added to maintain miosis
carbachol, intraocular	Miostat, Carbastat	0.01% solution	0.5 mL	Used only during surgery to produce complete miosis within 2-5 min
carbachol, topical	Isopto-Carbachol, Carboptic	0.75%, 1.5%, 2.25%, and 3% solution	1-2 drops into eye two to four times daily	Miotic action lasts 4-8 hr May be particularly useful in patients resistant to pilocarpine
pilocarpine	Isopto-Carpine, Pilocar, Akarpine, Pilopine HS	0.25%, 0.5%, 1%, 2%, 3%, 4%, 5%, 6%, 8%, 10% solutions; 4% gel	1-2 drops up to six times daily; 0.5%-4% solutions used most frequently	Safest, most commonly used miotic for glaucoma Also used to reverse mydriasis after eye examination Onset is 15 minutes to 1 hr; lasts for 2-3 hr
pilocarpine ocular therapeutic system	Ocusert Pilo-20	—	Inserted weekly, releases 20 mcg of pilocarpine per hr	A small reservoir containing pilocarpine that is placed in a corner of the eye *Advantages:* Convenience, once-weekly dosing Better continuous control of intraocular pressure Less medication used, lower incidence of toxicity *Disadvantages:* Cost Weekly insertion Conjunctival irritation Variable duration of action May fall out during sleep

Evaluation

Side Effects to Expect

Reduced Visual Acuity. A common side effect of cholinergic agents is difficulty in adjusting quickly to changes in light intensity. Reduced visual acuity may be most notable at night, particularly in areas of poor lighting, in older patients, and in patients developing lens opacities. Advise patients to use caution while driving at night or performing hazardous tasks in poor light.

Blurred vision occurs particularly during the first 1 to 2 hours after instilling the medication.

Be sure to keep eye medications separate from other solutions.

The ability to read for long periods is decreased because of impairment of near-vision accommodation.

Provide for patient safety when visual impairment exists. In hospitals, orient to the hospital unit, furniture placement, and call light; place the bed in a low position. At home, do not move furniture or the individual's household or personal belongings.

Conjunctival Irritation, Erythema, Headache. These side effects are usually mild and tend to resolve with continued therapy. Encourage the patient not to discontinue therapy without first consulting the health care provider.

Pain, Discomfort. Because of pupillary constriction, an increase in pain or discomfort may occur, particularly in bright light. Stress the need for adherence and assure the patient that this side effect will diminish with continued use.

Side Effects to Report

Systemic Side Effects. Rarely, a patient may develop signs of systemic toxicity manifested by diaphoresis, salivation, abdominal discomfort, diarrhea, bronchospasm, muscle tremors, hypotension, dysrhythmias, and bradycardia. These symptoms are indications of excessive administration.

Report to the health care provider for dosage adjustment. The adverse effects themselves usually do not need to be treated because they will resolve by withholding cholinergic therapy.

Prevent systemic effects by carefully blocking the inner canthus for 1 to 2 minutes after instilling the medication to prevent absorption via the nasolacrimal duct.

During drug therapy, assess the blood pressure every shift, and report significant changes from the baseline data.

If accidental overdose occurs during instillation, flush the affected eye with water or normal saline.

Drug Interactions. See the following section on cholinesterase inhibitors.

DRUG CLASS: Cholinesterase Inhibitors

echothiophate iodide (ek oh thi' oh fate)

▶ PHOSPHOLINE IODIDE (fos' foe lean)

Actions

Cholinesterase is an enzyme that destroys acetylcholine, the cholinergic neurotransmitter. The cholinesterase inhibitors prevent the metabolism of acetylcholine within the eye. This causes increased cholinergic activity, which results in decreased IOP and miosis.

Uses

Echothiophate is used in the treatment of open-angle glaucoma. Onset occurs within 10 to 45 minutes; duration may be several days. Tolerance may develop after prolonged use; a rest period will restore response. Because of the higher incidence of side effects, however, cholinesterase inhibitors are reserved for patients who do not respond well to cholinergic agents.

Therapeutic Outcomes

The primary therapeutic outcome expected from echothiophate is reduced IOP in patients with glaucoma.

Nursing Process for Cholinesterase Inhibitors

Premedication Assessment

1. Obtain baseline vital signs; withhold the medicine, and contact the health care provider if bradycardia or any type of respiratory disorder is present.
2. Record premedication IOP readings and visual acuity data.

Planning

Availability. Ophthalmic: 0.125% solution.

Implementation

Dosage and Administration. Glaucoma: 1 drop one or two times daily. NOTE: After reconstitution, use within 1 month. Properly dispose of any remaining medicine and reconstitute a fresh solution.

Evaluation

Side Effects to Expect

Reduced Visual Acuity. A common side effect of cholinesterase inhibitors (cholinergic agents) is difficulty in adjusting quickly to changes in light intensity. Reduced visual acuity may be most notable at night, particularly in areas of poor lighting, in older patients, and in patients developing lens opacities. Advise patients to use caution while driving at night or performing hazardous tasks in poor light.

Conjunctival Irritation, Erythema, Headache, Lacrimation. These side effects are usually mild and tend to resolve with continued therapy. Encourage the patient not to discontinue therapy without first consulting the health care provider.

Side Effects to Report

Systemic Side Effects. Rarely, a patient may develop signs of systemic toxicity manifested by diaphoresis, salivation, vomiting, abdominal cramps, urinary incontinence, diarrhea, dyspnea, bronchospasm, muscle tremors, hypotension, dysrhythmias, and bradycardia. These are indications of overdose or excessive administration. Report to the health care provider for treatment and dosage adjustment. If symptoms become severe, parenteral atropine should be administered.

If accidental overdose occurs during instillation, flush the affected eye with water or normal saline.

Drug Interactions

Carbamate and/or Organophosphate Insecticides and Pesticides. Gardeners, farmers, manufacturing employees, and others who are exposed to these pesticides and insecticides and who are receiving cholinesterase inhibitors should be warned of the added risk of systemic symptoms from absorption of these chemicals through the skin and respiratory tract. Respiratory masks and frequent washing and clothing changes are advisable.

Miotic Agents (e.g., Pilocarpine). The miotic and IOP lowering effects of the anticholinesterases is competitively inhibited by pilocarpine, carbachol, and acetylcholine.

Physostigmine. Physostigmine, a short-acting cholinesterase inhibitor, blocks the binding to receptors and therefore blocks the pharmacologic effect of subsequently administered long-acting cholinesterase inhibitors.

DRUG CLASS: Adrenergic Agents

Actions

Adrenergic agents have several uses in ophthalmology. Sympathomimetic agents cause pupil dilation, increased outflow of aqueous humor, vasoconstriction, relaxation of the ciliary muscle, and a decrease in the formation of aqueous humor.

Uses

Adrenergic agents are used to lower IOP in open-angle glaucoma, relieve congestion and hyperemia, and produce mydriasis for ocular examinations. Use with caution in patients with hypertension, diabetes mellitus, hyperthyroidism, heart disease, arteriosclerosis, or long-standing bronchial asthma.

Therapeutic Outcomes

The primary therapeutic outcomes expected from adrenergic agents are as follows:

- Mydriasis for ophthalmic examination
- Reduced IOP in open-angle glaucoma
- Reduced redness of the eyes from irritation

Nursing Process for Adrenergic Agents

Premedication Assessment

1. Obtain baseline vital signs, including blood pressure.
2. Record premedication IOP readings and visual acuity data.

Planning

Availability. See Table 43-4.

Implementation

Dosage and Administration. See Table 43-4.

Evaluation

Side Effects to Expect

Sensitivity to Bright Light. The mydriasis produced allows excessive amounts of light into the eyes, which causes the patient to squint. Sunglasses will help reduce the brightness. Caution the patient to temporarily avoid tasks that require visual acuity, such as driving or operating power machinery.

Conjunctival Irritation, Lacrimation. These side effects are usually mild and tend to resolve with continued therapy. Encourage the patient not to discontinue therapy without first consulting the health care provider.

Side Effects to Report

Systemic Side Effects. Systemic effects from ophthalmic instillation are uncommon and minimal. However, systemic absorption may occur via the lacrimal drainage system into the nasopharyngeal passages. Systemic effects are manifested by palpitations, tachycardia, dysrhythmias, hypertension, faintness, trembling, and diaphoresis. These are indications of overdose or excessive administration. Report to the health care provider for treatment and dosage adjustment.

Prevent systemic effects by carefully blocking the inner canthus for 1 to 2 minutes after instilling the medication to prevent absorption via the nasolacrimal duct.

Monitor the pulse rate and blood pressure, and instruct the patient to continue to do this at home; report significant changes from the baseline data.

Diaphoresis, Trembling. Touch the patient and bedding to assess for diaphoresis, particularly when these agents are used in surgery in which the patient is under sterile drapes, is anesthetized, and is unable to respond to verbal questioning.

Drug Interactions

Tricyclic Antidepressants. Tricyclic antidepressants (e.g., amitriptyline, imipramine, doxepin) may cause additive hypertensive effects. Monitor carefully for poor blood pressure control or a gradually increasing blood pressure.

Drug Table 43-4 ADRENERGIC AGENTS

GENERIC NAME	BRAND NAME	AVAILABILITY	DOSAGE	COMMENTS
apraclonidine	Iopidine	0.5%, 1% solution	1 drop 1 hr before surgery	Used to control intraocular pressure after laser surgery
brimonidine	Alphagan P	0.1%, 0.15%, 0.2% solution	1 drop every 8 hr in affected eye(s)	An alpha-2 adrenergic agent used to lower intraocular pressure in open-angle glaucoma or ocular hypertension
dipivefrin hydrochloride	Propine	0.1% solution	1 drop every 12 hr	This drug has no activity itself but is metabolized to epinephrine; used because it can penetrate the anterior chamber more readily than epinephrine and is less irritating
naphazoline hydrochloride	Vasoclear, Allerest, Naphcon, Albalon Liquifilm	0.012%, 0.02%, 0.03%, 0.1% solutions	1-2 drops every 3-4 hr	Used as a topical vasoconstriction
phenylephrine	Prefrin, Mydfrin	0.12%, 2.5%, 10% solution	1-2 drops two or three times daily	0.12% used as a decongestant for minor eye irritation; 2.5% and 10% solutions used for pupil dilation in uveitis, open angle glaucoma, and diagnostic procedures
tetrahydrozoline hydrochloride	Murine Plus, Optigene 3	0.05% solution	1-2 drops two or three times daily	Used as a topical vasoconstrictor

DRUG CLASS: Beta-Adrenergic Blocking Agents

Actions

The beta-adrenergic blocking agents are used in ophthalmology to reduce elevated IOP. The exact mechanism of action is not known, but these agents are thought to reduce the production of aqueous humor.

Uses

The beta-adrenergic blocking agents are used to reduce IOP in patients with chronic open-angle glaucoma or ocular hypertension. Unlike anticholinergic agents, there is no blurred or dim vision or night blindness because IOP is reduced with little or no effect on pupil size or visual acuity.

Therapeutic Outcomes

The primary therapeutic outcome expected from adrenergic blocking agents is reduced IOP.

Nursing Process for Beta-Adrenergic Blocking Agents

Premedication Assessment

1. Obtain baseline vital signs including blood pressure; withhold medicine and contact the physician if bradycardia, hypertension, or respiratory disorders are present.
2. Record the premedication IOP readings and visual acuity data.

Planning

Availability. See Table 43-5.

Implementation

Dosage and Administration. See Table 43-5.

Evaluation

Side Effects to Expect

Conjunctival Irritation, Lacrimation. These side effects are usually mild and tend to resolve with continued therapy. Encourage the patient not to discontinue therapy without first consulting the physician.

Side Effects to Report

Systemic Side Effects. Systemic effects are uncommon but may be manifested by bradycardia, dysrhythmias, hypotension, faintness, and bronchospasm. These adverse effects are more frequently observed in patients requiring higher doses of beta-adrenergic blocking agents and in patients with hypertension, diabetes mellitus, heart disease, arteriosclerosis, or long-standing bronchial asthma. Report to the health care provider for treatment and dosage adjustment.

Record the blood pressure and pulse rate at specific intervals.

Drug Interactions

Beta-Adrenergic Blocking Agents. Propranolol, atenolol, acebutolol, nadolol, pindolol, labetalol, and metoprolol may enhance the systemic therapeutic and toxic effects of ophthalmic beta-adrenergic blocking agents. Monitor for an increase in severity of side

Drug Table 43-5 BETA-ADRENERGIC BLOCKING AGENTS

GENERIC NAME	BRAND NAME	AVAILABILITY	INITIAL DOSAGE	COMMENTS
betaxolol hydrochloride	Betoptic	0.25%, 0.5% solutions in 2.5, 5, 10, and 15 mL dropper bottles	1 drop twice daily	A beta-1 blocking agent; onset in 30 min, duration is 12 hr; several weeks of therapy may be required to determine optimal dosage
carteolol	Ocupress	1% solution in 5, 10, 15 mL bottles	1 drop twice daily	A beta-1,2 blocking agent; duration is up to 12 hr
levobetaxolol	Betaxon	0.5% solution in 5, 10, 15 mL bottles	1 drop twice daily	A beta blocking agent; onset in 30 min, duration is 12 hr
levobunolol hydrochloride	Betagan	0.25% and 0.5% solution in 5, 10, and 15 mL dropper bottles	1 drop once or twice daily	A beta-1,2 blocking agent; onset within 60 min, duration is up to 24 hr
metipranolol	OptiPranolol	0.3% solution in 5 and 10 mL dropper bottles	1 drop twice daily in affected eye(s)	A beta-1,2 blocking agent; onset within 30 min, duration is 12-24 hr
timolol maleate	Timoptic	0.25%, 0.5% solutions in 5, 10, and 15 mL dropper bottles 0.25%, 0.5% solution, gel forming	1 drop of 0.25% solution twice daily 1 drop of solution once daily	A beta-1,2 blocking agent; onset within 30 min, duration is up to 24 hr Gel may be used once daily

effects such as fatigue, hypotension, bronchospasm, and bradycardia.

DRUG CLASS: Prostaglandin Agonists

Actions

Prostaglandin agonists reduce intraocular pressure by increasing the outflow of aqueous humor.

Uses

The prostaglandin agonists are used to reduce IOP in patients with chronic open-angle glaucoma or ocular hypertension who have not responded well to other IOP-lowering agents.

Therapeutic Outcomes

The primary therapeutic outcome expected from prostaglandin agonists is reduced IOP.

Nursing Process for Prostaglandin Agonists

Premedication Assessment

1. Obtain baseline vital signs.
2. Record the premedication IOP readings and visual acuity data.

Planning

Availability. See Table 43-6.

Implementation

Dosage and Administration. See Table 43-6. If more than one drug is to be instilled in the same eye, administer the drugs at least 5 minutes apart.

Do not administer prostaglandin agonists in eyes while wearing contact lenses. Lenses may be reinserted 15 minutes following administration.

Evaluation

Side Effects to Expect and Report

Conjunctival Irritation, Burning and Stinging, Lacrimation. These side effects are usually mild and tend to resolve with continued therapy. Encourage the patient not to discontinue therapy without first consulting the health care provider.

Eye Pigment Changes. The prostaglandin agonists may gradually cause changes to pigmented tissues, including change to eye color, increasing the amount of brown pigment in the iris. The change may take several months to years to develop and is thought to be permanent. Iris pigmentation changes may be more evident in patients with green-brown, blue/gray-brown or yellow-brown irises. The eyelids may also develop color changes. There may also be an increased growth of eyelashes.

Drug Interactions

Thimerosal. A precipitate occurs when eye drops containing thimerosal are mixed with latanoprost. Administer eye drops at least 5 minutes apart.

OTHER OPHTHALMIC AGENTS

DRUG CLASS: Anticholinergic Agents

Actions

Anticholinergic agents cause the smooth muscle of the ciliary body and iris to relax, producing mydriasis (extreme dilation of the pupil) and cycloplegia (paralysis of the ciliary muscle).

Uses

Ophthalmologists use these pharmacologic effects to examine the interior of the eye, measure the proper strength of lenses for eyeglasses (refraction), and rest the eye in inflammatory conditions of the uveal tract.

Therapeutic Outcomes

The primary therapeutic outcomes expected from anticholinergic ophthalmic use are as follows:

- Visualization of intraocular structures
- Reduced uveal tract inflammation

Nursing Process for Anticholinergic Agents

Premedication Assessment

1. Check for the existence of increased IOP. If present, withhold the medicine and contact the health care provider for approval before instillation of the anticholinergic agent.

Drug Table 43-6 PROSTAGLANDIN AGONISTS

GENERIC NAME	BRAND NAME	AVAILABILITY	DOSAGE RANGE	COMMENTS
bimatoprost	Lumigan	0.03% solution in 2.5 and 5 mL dropper bottles	1 drop in each affected eye in the evening	Do not exceed dosage because it may reduce IOP-lowering effect
latanoprost	Xalatan	0.005% solution in 2.5 mL dropper bottles	1 drop in each affected eye in the evening	Do not exceed dosage because it may reduce IOP-lowering effect
travoprost	Travatan	0.004% solution in 2.5 mL dropper bottles	1 drop in each affected eye in the evening	Do not exceed dosage because it may reduce IOP-lowering effect

2. Take vital signs; if the patient has hypertension, contact the health care provider for approval before instilling the anticholinergic agent.

Planning

Availability. See Table 43-7.

Implementation

NOTE: The pharmacologic effects of anticholinergic agents cause an increase in IOP. Use these agents with extreme caution in patients with narrow anterior chamber angle; in infants, children, and the elderly; and in patients with hypertension, hyperthyroidism, and diabetes. Discontinue therapy if signs of increased IOP or systemic effects develop.

Dosage and Administration. See Table 43-7.

Evaluation

Side Effects to Expect

Sensitivity to Bright Light. The mydriasis produced allows excessive light into the eyes, causing the patient to squint. Sunglasses will help reduce the brightness. Caution the patient to temporarily avoid tasks that require visual acuity, such as driving or operating power machinery.

Conjunctival Irritation, Lacrimation. These side effects are usually mild and tend to resolve with continued therapy. Encourage the patient not to discontinue therapy without first consulting the health care provider.

Side Effects to Report

Systemic Side Effects. Prolonged use may result in systemic effects manifested by flushing and dryness of the skin, dry mouth, blurred vision, tachycardia, dysrhythmias, urinary hesitancy and retention, vasodilation, and constipation. These are indications of overdose or excessive administration. Report to the health care provider for treatment and dosage adjustment. Children are particularly prone to develop systemic reactions.

Drug Interactions. No clinically significant drug interactions have been reported.

DRUG CLASS: Antifungal Agents

natamycin (na tah my′ sin)
NATACYN (na′ tah sin)

Actions

Natamycin acts by altering the cell wall of the fungus to prevent it from serving as a selective barrier, therefore causing loss of fluids and electrolytes.

Uses

Natamycin is an antifungal agent effective against a variety of yeasts, including *Candida, Aspergillus,* and *Fusarium.* It is effective in treating fungal blepharitis, conjunctivitis, and keratitis caused by susceptible organisms. If little or no improvement is noted after

Drug Table 43-7 ANTICHOLINERGIC AGENTS

GENERIC NAME	BRAND NAME	AVAILABILITY	DOSAGE	COMMENTS
atropine sulfate	Isopto-Atropine	1% ointment; 0.5%, 1%, 2% solution	Uveitis: 1-2 drops up to three times daily	Onset of mydriasis and cycloplegia is 30-40 min, duration is 7-12 days Do not use in infants
cyclopentolate hydrochloride	Cyclogyl, AK-Pentolate	0.5%, 1%, 2% solutions	Refraction: 1 drop followed by another drop in 5-10 min	For mydriasis and cycloplegia necessary for diagnostic procedures 1-2 drops of 1%-2% pilocarpine allows full recovery within 3-6 hr Central nervous system (CNS) disturbances of hallucinations, loss of orientation, restlessness, and incoherent speech have been reported in children
homatropine hydrobromide	Isopto-Homatropine	2%, 5% solutions	Uveitis: 1-2 drops every 3-4 hr	Onset of mydriasis and cycloplegia is 40-60 min; duration is 1-3 days
scopolamine hydrobromide	Isopto-Hyoscine	0.25% solution	Uveitis: 1-2 drops up to three times daily	Onset of mydriasis and cycloplegia is 20-30 min; duration is 3-7 days
tropicamide	Mydriacyl	0.5%, 1% solutions	Refraction: 1 or 2 drops, repeated in 5 min	Onset of mydriasis and cycloplegia is 20-40 min; duration is 6 hours CNS disturbances of hallucinations, loss of orientation, restlessness, and incoherent speech have been reported in children

7 to 10 days of treatment, resistance to the antifungal agent may have developed. Topical administration does not appear to result in systemic effects.

Therapeutic Outcomes

The primary therapeutic outcome expected from natamycin is eradication of fungal infection.

Nursing Process for Natamycin

Premedication Assessment

1. Collect ordered cultures or smears before initiating drug therapy.
2. Record baseline data relating to symptoms accompanying the fungal infection and the degree of visual impairment.

Planning

Availability. Ophthalmic: 5% suspension.

Implementation

Dosage and Administration. Fungal keratitis: one drop in the conjunctival sac at 1- or 2-hour intervals for the first 3 to 4 days. The dosage may then be reduced to one drop every 3 to 4 hours. Continue therapy for 14 to 21 days.

Evaluation

Side Effects to Expect

Sensitivity to Bright Light. The slight mydriasis produced allows an excessive amount of light into the eyes, causing the patient to squint. Sunglasses will help reduce the brightness. Caution the patient to temporarily avoid tasks that require visual acuity, such as driving or operating power machinery.

Blurred Vision, Lacrimation, Redness. Provide for patient safety during temporary visual impairment. Instruct the patient not to rub the eyes forcefully while tearing.

These side effects are usually mild and tend to resolve with continued therapy. Encourage the patient not to discontinue therapy without first consulting the physician.

Side Effects to Report

Eye Pain. If eye pain develops, discontinue use and consult an ophthalmologist immediately.

Therapeutic Effect. If, after several days of therapy, the symptoms do not improve or if they gradually worsen, consult the health care provider treating the patient.

Drug Interactions. No significant drug interactions have been reported.

DRUG CLASS: Antiviral Agents

Actions

The ophthalmic antiviral agents act by inhibiting viral replication.

Uses

Idoxuridine and trifluridine are chemically related compounds used to treat herpes simplex keratitis. Idoxuridine is particularly effective against initial infections but is not as effective against deep infections or chronic, recurrent infections. Trifluridine is used to treat recurrent infections in patients who are intolerant of or resistant to idoxuridine or vidarabine therapy; cross-sensitivity with these other agents has not been reported.

Vidarabine is used topically as an ophthalmic ointment to treat keratitis and keratoconjunctivitis caused by herpes simplex virus types 1 and 2. Vidarabine does not show cross-sensitivity to idoxuridine or trifluridine and may be effective in treating recurrent keratitis that is resistant to idoxuridine and trifluridine.

These antiviral agents are not effective against infections caused by bacteria, fungi, or *Chlamydia*.

Therapeutic Outcomes

The primary therapeutic outcome expected from antiviral agents is eradication of the viral infection.

Nursing Process for Antiviral Agents

Premedication Assessment

Record baseline data concerning the symptoms and the degree of visual impairment.

Planning

Availability. See Table 43-8.

Implementation

Dosage and Administration. See Table 43-8. NOTE: If significant improvement has not occurred in 7 to 14 days, other therapy should be considered. Do not exceed 21 days of continuous therapy because of potential ocular toxicity.

Storage: Trifluridine should be stored in the refrigerator.

Evaluation

Side Effects to Expect

Visual Haze, Lacrimation, Redness, Burning. Patients may notice a mild, transient stinging, burning, and redness of the conjunctiva and sclera on instillation. Provide for patient safety during temporary visual impairment. Instruct the patient not to rub the eyes forcefully while tearing.

These side effects are usually mild and tend to resolve with continued therapy. Encourage the patient not to discontinue therapy without first consulting the health care provider.

Sensitivity to Bright Light. The slight mydriasis produced allows excessive light into the eyes, causing the patient to squint. Sunglasses will help reduce the brightness. Caution the patient to temporarily avoid

Drug Table 43-8 ANTIVIRAL AGENTS

GENERIC NAME	BRAND NAME	AVAILABILITY	DOSAGE RANGE
fomivirsen	Vitravene	Injection: 6.6 mg/mL	Intravitreal injection to treat cytomegalovirus (CMV) retinitis in patients with AIDS who are intolerant of other treatments of CMV retinitis
ganciclovir	Vitrasert	Implant: 4.5 mg	A device surgically implanted to release drug over 5 to 8 mo to treat CMV retinitis in patients with AIDS
trifluridine	Viroptic	1% solution in 7.5 mL	Intraocular: Place 1 drop onto the cornea of the affected eye every 2 hr during waking hours. Do not exceed 9 drops daily. Continue for 7 more days to prevent recurrence, using 1 drop every 4 hr (5 drops daily)

Drug Table 43-9 OPHTHALMIC ANTIBIOTICS

ANTIBIOTIC	BRAND NAME	AVAILABILITY
bacitracin	Bacitracin Ophthalmic	Ointment
chloramphenicol	Chloromycetin Ophthalmic	Drops, ointment
ciprofloxacin	Ciloxan	Drops, ointment
erythromycin	Ilotycin Ophthalmic	Ointment
gentamicin	Garamycin Ophthalmic	Drops, ointment
levofloxacin	Quixin, Iquix	Drops
ofloxacin	Ocuflox	Drops
polymyxin B	Polymyxin B Sulfate	Drops
sulfacetamide	Cetamide, Ocusulf-10	Drops, ointment
tobramycin	Tobrex Ophthalmic	Drops, ointment
COMBINATIONS		
trimethoprim/Polymyxin B	Polytrim Ophthalmic	Drops
neomycin/Polymyxin B/Bacitracin	Neosporin Ophthalmic	Ointment
neomycin/Polymyxin B/Gramicidin	Ak-Spore Solution	Drops

tasks that require visual acuity, such as driving or operating power machinery.

Side Effects to Report

Allergic Reactions. Discontinue therapy and consult an ophthalmologist immediately.

Drug Interactions. No significant drug interactions have been reported.

DRUG CLASS: Antibacterial Agents

Uses

Antibacterial agents (Table 43-9) are used to treat superficial eye infections and for prophylaxis against gonorrhea infection in the eyes of newborn infants (ophthalmia neonatorum). Prolonged or frequent intermittent use of topical antibiotics should be avoided because of the possibility of hypersensitivity reactions and the development of resistant organisms, including fungi. If hypersensitivities or new infections appear during use, consult an ophthalmologist immediately. Refer to the Index for a discussion of these antibiotics.

DRUG CLASS: Corticosteroids

Uses

Corticosteroid therapy (Table 43-10) is used for allergic reactions of the eye and other acute, noninfectious inflammatory conditions of the conjunctiva, sclera, cornea, and anterior uveal tract. Corticosteroid therapy must not be used in bacterial, fungal, or viral infections

Drug Table 43-10 CORTICOSTEROIDS

GENERIC NAME	BRAND NAME	AVAILABILITY
dexamethasone	Decadron Maxidex	Ointment Suspension
fluorometholone	FML	Suspension
loteprednol	Lotemax	Suspension
medrysone	HMS	Suspension
prednisolone	Econopred Plus Inflamase Mild	Suspension Solution
rimexolone	Vexol	Suspension

of the eye because corticosteroids decrease defense mechanisms and reduce resistance to pathologic organisms. This therapy should be used for a limited time only, and the eye should be checked frequently for an increase in IOP. Prolonged ocular steroid therapy may cause glaucoma and cataracts. Refer to the Index for further discussion of the corticosteroids.

DRUG CLASS: Ophthalmic Antiinflammatory Agents

Flurbiprofen sodium, ketorolac tromethamine, suprofen, and diclofenac sodium are topical nonsteroidal antiinflammatory agents for ophthalmic use. These agents have been shown to have antiinflammatory, antipyretic, and analgesic activity by inhibiting the biosynthesis of prostaglandins that are responsible for an increase in intraocular inflammation and pressure. They also inhibit prostaglandin-mediated constriction of the iris (miosis) that is independent of cholinergic mechanisms. Flurbiprofen and suprofen are used primarily to inhibit miosis during cataract surgery. Diclofenac sodium is used to treat postoperative inflammation after cataract extraction. Flurbiprofen is available as a 0.03% solution (Ocufen) that should be used by instilling one drop in the appropriate eye every 30 minutes, beginning 2 hours before surgery (for a total of four drops). Suprofen (Profenal) is available as a 1% solution that is instilled (two drops) into the conjunctival sac at 3 hours, 2 hours, and 1 hour before surgery. Diclofenac sodium (Voltaren) is available as a 0.1% solution. One drop is applied to the affected eye four times daily beginning 24 hours after surgery and continued for 2 weeks. Ketorolac tromethamine is available as a 0.5% solution. One drop is applied to each eye four times daily to relieve ocular itching associated with seasonal allergic conjunctivitis.

DRUG CLASS: Antihistamines

Azelastine, emedastine, epinastine, ketotifen, and olopatadine are histamine H_2 antagonists that act by inhibiting release of histamine from mast cells. They are used for relief of signs and symptoms and prevention of itching associated with allergic conjunctivitis. For best results, they should be instilled in the eyes before exposure to allergens such as pollen (Table 43-11).

DRUG CLASS: Antiallergic Agents

Uses

Cromolyn sodium, lodoxamide, pemirolast, and nedocromil are stabilizing agents that inhibit the release of histamine and slow-reacting substance of anaphylaxis (SRS-A) from mast cells after exposure to specific antigens. They are used to treat allergic ocular disorders such as vernal keratoconjunctivitis, vernal keratitis, and allergic keratoconjunctivitis. Cromolyn sodium (Crolom) is available as a 4% solution; one or two drops are applied in each eye four to six times daily at regular intervals. Lodoxamide (Alomide) is available as a 0.1% solution; one or two drops in each affected eye four times daily. Pemirolast (Alamast) is available as a 0.1% solution; one or two drops in each affected eye four times daily. Nedocromil (Alocril) is available as a 2% solution; one or two drops in each eye twice daily at regular intervals.

Drug Table 43-11 OPHTHALMIC ANTIHISTAMINES

GENERIC NAME	BRAND NAME	AVAILABILITY	DOSAGE
azalastine	Optivar	Solution: 0.5 mg/mL in 6 mL dropper bottle	Instill 1 drop in each affected eye twice daily
emedastine	Emadine	Solution: 0.05% in 5 mL bottle	Instill 1 drop in each eye up to four times daily
epinastine	Elestat	Solution: 0.05% in 8 and 12-mL bottles	Instill 1 drop in each eye two times daily
ketotifen	Zaditor	Solution: 0.025% in 5 and 7.5 mL bottles	Instill 1 drop in each eye every 8-12 hours
olopatadine	Patanol	Solution: 0.1% in 5 mL bottle	Instill 1 or 2 drops in each affected eye two times daily at an interval of 6 to 8 hours
	Olopatadine	Solution: 0.2% in 2.5 mL bottle	Instill one drop in each affected eye once daily

DRUG CLASS: Sodium Fluorescein

Uses

Sodium fluorescein is used in fitting hard contact lenses and as a diagnostic aid in identifying foreign bodies in the eye and abraded or ulcerated areas of the cornea. It is also useful for evaluating retinal vasculature for abnormal circulation.

When sodium fluorescein is instilled in the eye, it stains the pathologic tissues green if observed under normal light and bright yellow if viewed under cobalt blue light. Sodium fluorescein sodium is available in 2% topical solution; 0.6- and 1-mg strips for topical application; and 10% and 25% solutions for injection into the aqueous humor. The strips have the advantage of being used once and then discarded. The solution carries the risk of bacterial contamination if used for several different patients. Product names include Fluorescite, AK-Fluor, Fluorets, and Ful-Glo.

DRUG CLASS: Artificial Tear Solutions

Uses

Artificial tear solutions mimic natural secretions of the eye. They provide lubrication for dry eyes and may be used as lubricants for artificial eyes. Most products contain variable concentrations of methylcellulose, polyvinyl alcohol, and polyethylene glycol. The dosage is one to three drops in each eye three or four times daily, as needed. Product names include Isopto Plain, Teargen, Tears Naturale, Murine, and Liquifilm Tears.

DRUG CLASS: Ophthalmic Irrigants

Uses

These products are sterile solutions used for soothing and cleansing the eye, for removing foreign bodies, in conjunction with hard contact lenses, or with fluorescein. Product names include Eye-Stream, Blinx, Dacriose, Collyrium, and Optigene.

DRUG CLASS: Vascular Endothelial Growth Factor Antagonist

Macular degeneration is a deterioration of the macula, a small area in the retina at the back of the eye that is required to see fine details clearly (such as reading or threading a needle), or to judge distances such as when driving an automobile. With macular degeneration, central vision is affected by blurriness, dark areas, and distortion. Peripheral vision is usually not affected.

Many older people develop macular degeneration as part of the body's natural aging process. The most common is age-related macular degeneration (AMD). Why it develops is unknown. Macular degeneration is the leading cause of severe vision loss in whites older than 65 years of age.

The two most common types of AMD are "dry" (atrophic) and "wet" (exudative).

- ***"Dry" macular degeneration (atrophic)*** is caused by the aging and thinning of the tissues of the macula. Vision loss is usually gradual. Most people have the "dry" form of AMD.
- ***"Wet" macular degeneration (exudative)*** accounts for about 10% of all AMD cases. It results when abnormal blood vessels form underneath the retina at the back of the eye. These new blood vessels leak fluid or blood and blur central vision. Vision loss may be rapid and severe.

Pegaptanib (Macugen) is a selective vascular endothelial growth factor (VEGF) antagonist. VEGF is secreted and binds to its receptors located primarily on the surface of endothelial cells of blood vessels. VEGF induces new blood vessel growth and increases vascular permeability and inflammation, all of which are thought to contribute to the progression of the wet form of AMD. Pegaptanib is an antagonist that binds to extracellular VEGF, preventing it from binding to VEGF receptors, thus preventing it from forming new blood vessels. It is injected into the vitreous humor of the affected eye once every 6 weeks. In the days following pegaptanib administration, patients are at risk for the development of endophthalmitis. Instruct the patient to seek immediate care with their ophthalmologist if the eye becomes red, sensitive to light, or painful, or a deterioration of vision is noted.

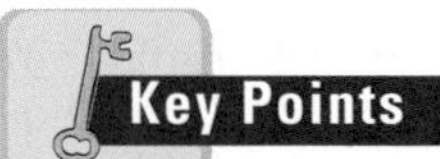

- The nurse has an important role in educating the public and promoting safety measures to protect the eyes from sources of injury.
- Examples of areas in which the nurse can teach the public are the use of safety glasses in hazardous situations, prevention of chemical burns from common household cleansing items or other agents at home or work, proper cleaning and wearing of contact lenses or glasses, and the selection of safe toys and play activities for children.
- These safety measures can significantly reduce the number of injuries that occur annually.

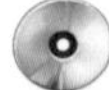

Go to your Companion CD-ROM for Appendices, an Audio Glossary, animations, Drug Dosage Calculators, customizable Patient Self-Assessment forms, and Review Questions for the NCLEX® Examination.

evolve Be sure to visit the companion Evolve site at http://evolve.elsevier.com/Clayton for WebLinks and additional online resources.

MEDICATION SAFETY REVIEW

MATH REVIEW QUESTIONS

1. Order: 1.5 g/kg mannitol 15% solution, IV over 30 minutes. The patient's weight is 156 pounds.

   The total dose of mannitol to administer would be:

   _____ g.

CRITICAL THINKING QUESTIONS

1. While working in the eye clinic, you observe that several of the patients being treated for glaucoma complain that the medications cause pain and headache and that reading ability is diminished. How would you respond to these statements?
2. Develop a teaching plan for a patient who is to self-administer Betoptic, one drop twice daily.
3. Examine premedication assessments and develop a list of contraindications to the administration of certain eye medications without first consulting the physician.

CONTENT REVIEW QUESTIONS

1. Osmotic agents act by:
   1. pulling fluid from the extravascular spaces into the blood.
   2. shifting fluid from the blood into the extravascular spaces.
   3. inhibiting enzymes from producing aqueous humor.
   4. causing pupil dilation and increased outflow of aqueous humor.
2. The therapeutic outcome when instilling an adrenergic agent in the eyes is to:
   1. produce miosis.
   2. produce mydriasis.
   3. act as an irritant.
   4. prevent production of aqueous humor.
3. Sodium fluorescein is used to:
   1. inhibit the release of histamine.
   2. treat an infection.
   3. stain the eye for examination.
   4. prevent production of aqueous humor.
4. Before administering a beta-adrenergic blocking agent for reduction of intraocular pressure, the nurse should check to see if the patient has a history of: *(Select all that apply.)*
   1. blood dyscrasias.
   2. diabetes mellitus or cardiac disease.
   3. hypertension or respiratory disorders.
   4. liver disease.
5. If more than one eye medication is to be administered, how long should you wait to administer the second medication?
   1. 1 minute
   2. 5 minutes
   3. 10 minutes
   4. You do not need to wait
6. How can systemic absorption be minimized after insertion of ophthalmic drops?
   1. Compress the lacrimal sac for 1 to 2 minutes after instillation.
   2. Compress the lacrimal sac for 1 to 2 minutes before instillation.
   3. This is not physiologically possible, so no action is needed.
   4. Have the patient close their eyes for 1 to 2 minutes after instillation.
7. Which of the following is an intervention to teach patients after eye surgery? *(Select all that apply.)*
   1. Notify the physician of pain not relieved by pain medication.
   2. Bending and coughing should not be a concern.
   3. Use aseptic technique when changing dressings or administering medications.
   4. The patient should notify the physician of any signs of infection.

CHAPTER

44 Drugs Affecting Neoplasms

evolve http://evolve.elsevier.com/Clayton

Chapter Content

Objectives

1. Cite the goals of chemotherapy.
2. Explain the normal cycle for cell replication and describe the effects of cell cycle–specific and cell cycle–nonspecific drugs within this process.
3. Cite the rationale for giving chemotherapeutic drugs on a precise time schedule.
4. State which types of chemotherapeutic agents are cell cycle–specific and those that are cell cycle–nonspecific.
5. Describe the role of targeted anticancer agents in treating cancer.
6. Describe the role of chemoprotective agents in treating cancer.
7. Describe the role of bone marrow stimulants in treating cancer.
8. Describe the nursing assessments and interventions needed for people experiencing adverse effects from chemotherapy.
9. Develop patient education objectives for a patient receiving chemotherapy.

Key Terms

cancer
metastases
cell cycle–specific
cell cycle–nonspecific
palliation
combination therapy
targeted anticancer agents
chemoprotective agents

CANCER AND THE USE OF ANTINEOPLASTIC AGENTS

Cancer is a disorder of cellular growth, life span, and death. It is a group of abnormal cells that generally proliferate (multiply) more rapidly than do normal cells, lose the ability to perform specialized functions, invade surrounding tissues, and develop growths in other tissues distant to the site of original growth (**metastases**). Many types of cancer cells also lose the ability to die properly as a part of their normal life cycle. Normal cells have a genetically programmed life cycle that includes a cell death known as apoptosis.

Cancer is a leading cause of death in the United States. Unfortunately, the number of people that die from malignant diseases increases each year. The American Cancer Society estimates new cancer cases in *Facts and Figures* annually as a means of projecting cancer incidence for the upcoming year (Figure 44-1). Early diagnosis and treatment is still one of the most important factors in providing a more optimistic prognosis for those patients stricken with the many forms of neoplastic disease.

Treatment of cancer often requires a combination of surgery, radiation, chemotherapy, and immunotherapy. Recent advancements in carcinogenesis, cellular and molecular biology, and tumor immunology have enhanced the role that antineoplastic agents may play in therapy. It is beyond the scope of this chapter to delve into the interrelationships of chemotherapy and neoplastic disease; however, a short discussion of the concepts of cancer chemotherapy will be presented. As a result of rapidly changing approaches to the treatment of specific malignancies and the changing nature of chemotherapeutic regimens, specific agents and dosages have not been discussed.

All cells, whether normal or malignant, pass through a similar series of phases during their lifetime, although duration of time spent in each phase differs with the type of cell (Figure 44-2). Mitosis is the phase of cellular proliferation in which the cell divides into two equal daughter cells. Cells either advance into a nonproliferative stage known as G_0, or advance to the first gap phase, G_1. G_0 is the largest variable in the cell cycle, and during this resting phase the cell is not actively replicating. Some stimulus results in the cell entering the G_1 phase. Phase G_1 is considered a presynthetic phase in which the cell prepares for DNA synthesis by manufacturing necessary enzymes. The S phase is the stage of active synthesis of two sets of DNA. Phase G_2 is a postsynthetic phase in which the cell prepares for mitosis by producing ribonucleic acid (RNA), specialized proteins, and the foundations for mitotic spindle apparatus needed for mitosis. The cell cycle begins again when the mitotic phase divides the cell into two daughter cells. The daughter cells may advance again to the G_1 phase or pass into G_0. The time required to complete one cycle is called the generation time.

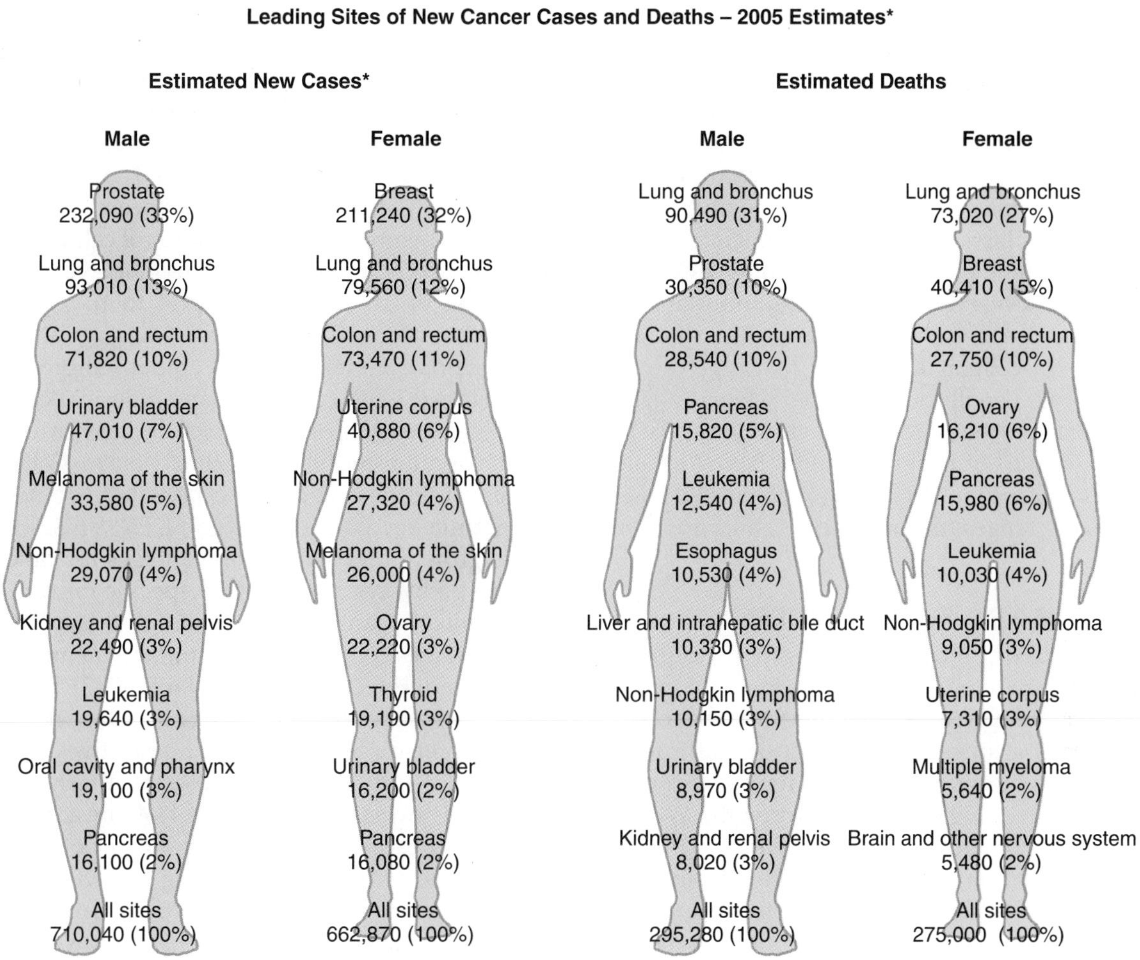

Leading Sites of New Cancer Cases and Deaths – 2005 Estimates*

Estimated New Cases*		Estimated Deaths	
Male	**Female**	**Male**	**Female**
Prostate 232,090 (33%)	Breast 211,240 (32%)	Lung and bronchus 90,490 (31%)	Lung and bronchus 73,020 (27%)
Lung and bronchus 93,010 (13%)	Lung and bronchus 79,560 (12%)	Prostate 30,350 (10%)	Breast 40,410 (15%)
Colon and rectum 71,820 (10%)	Colon and rectum 73,470 (11%)	Colon and rectum 28,540 (10%)	Colon and rectum 27,750 (10%)
Urinary bladder 47,010 (7%)	Uterine corpus 40,880 (6%)	Pancreas 15,820 (5%)	Ovary 16,210 (6%)
Melanoma of the skin 33,580 (5%)	Non-Hodgkin lymphoma 27,320 (4%)	Leukemia 12,540 (4%)	Pancreas 15,980 (6%)
Non-Hodgkin lymphoma 29,070 (4%)	Melanoma of the skin 26,000 (4%)	Esophagus 10,530 (4%)	Leukemia 10,030 (4%)
Kidney and renal pelvis 22,490 (3%)	Ovary 22,220 (3%)	Liver and intrahepatic bile duct 10,330 (3%)	Non-Hodgkin lymphoma 9,050 (3%)
Leukemia 19,640 (3%)	Thyroid 19,190 (3%)	Non-Hodgkin lymphoma 10,150 (3%)	Uterine corpus 7,310 (3%)
Oral cavity and pharynx 19,100 (3%)	Urinary bladder 16,200 (2%)	Urinary bladder 8,970 (3%)	Multiple myeloma 5,640 (2%)
Pancreas 16,100 (2%)	Pancreas 16,080 (2%)	Kidney and renal pelvis 8,020 (3%)	Brain and other nervous system 5,480 (2%)
All sites 710,040 (100%)	All sites 662,870 (100%)	All sites 295,280 (100%)	All sites 275,000 (100%)

*Excludes basal and squamous cell skin cancers and in situ carcinoma except urinary bladder.
Note: Percentages may not total 100% due to rounding.

FIGURE **44-1** Leading sites of new cancer cases and deaths—2005 estimates. (From American Cancer Society: Cancer facts and figures—2005, www.cancer.org; accessed January 28, 2006).

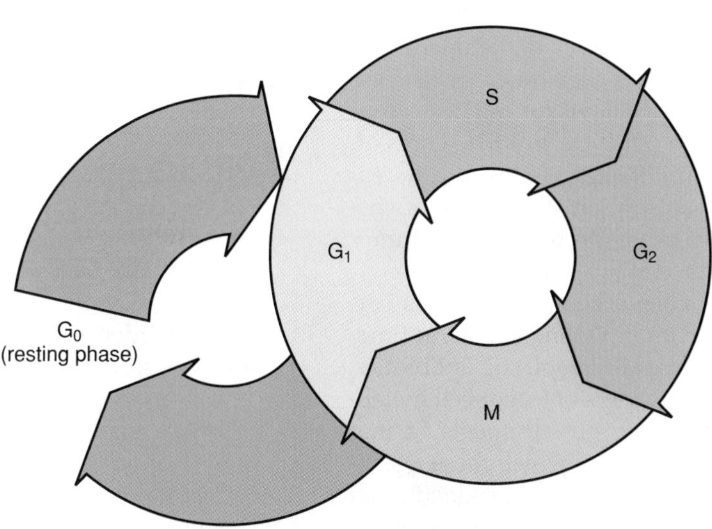

FIGURE **44-2** The cell cycle. G_0, resting phase; G_1, gap 1 phase; G_2, gap 2 phase; *M*, mitosis; *S*, synthesis.

Many antineoplastic agents are **cell cycle–specific** (i.e., the drug is selectively toxic when the cell is in a specific phase of growth, and therefore is schedule dependent). Malignancies most amenable to cell cycle–specific chemotherapy are those that proliferate rapidly. **Cell cycle–nonspecific** drugs are active throughout the cell cycle and may be more effective against slowly proliferating neoplastic tissue. These medicines are not schedule dependent, but are dose dependent. One implication of cell cycle specificity is the importance of correlating the dosage schedule of anticancer therapy with the known cellular kinetics of that type of neoplasm. Drugs are usually administered when the cell is most susceptible to the cytotoxic effects of the agent for a greater "kill rate" of neoplastic cells. Table 44-1 lists the more common commercially available drugs, their general dosage ranges, major toxicities, and major indications.

DRUG THERAPY FOR CANCER

The overall goal of cancer chemotherapy is to give a dose large enough to be lethal (cytotoxic) to the cancer cells, but small enough to be tolerable for normal cells. It is hoped that a long-term survival or cure can be achieved by this means. A second goal may be control of the disease (arresting of the tumor growth). When a cancer is beyond control, the goal of treatment may be **palliation** (alleviation) of symptoms. Finally, in some types of cancer in which no tumor is detectable yet the patient is known to be at risk of developing a particular cancer or having reoccurrence of a cancer, prophylactic chemotherapy may be administered.

Chemotherapy is most effective when the tumor is small and the cell replication is rapid. Cancer cells are the most sensitive to chemotherapy when the cells are dividing rapidly. This is when phase-specific drugs are most effective. As a tumor enlarges, more of the cells are in the resting G_0 phase. These cells respond better to phase-nonspecific chemotherapeutic agents. **Combination therapy,** using cell cycle–specific and cell cycle–nonspecific agents, is superior in therapeutic effect than the use of single-agent chemotherapy. The use of combination drug therapy allows for cell death during different phases of the cell cycle, but the agents often have toxic effects on different organs at different time intervals after administration. The choice of chemotherapeutic agents depends on the types of tumor cells, their rate of growth, and the size of the tumor.

The major groups of chemotherapeutic agents currently used are classified as alkylating agents, antimetabolites, natural products, antineoplastic antibiotics, and hormones. As new pathways of tumor cell metabolism are identified, however, not all agents fit into these classes. The mechanisms by which these agents cause cell death have not been fully determined in all cases. Guidelines for the safe handling of chemotherapeutic agents by health care providers include measures to prevent inhalation of aerosols, prevention of drug absorption through the skin, safe disposal, and prevention of contamination of body fluids.

Three other groups of medicines, targeted anticancer agents, chemoprotective agents and bone marrow stimulants have become available to help fight cancers from different directions. Targeted anticancer agents (Table 44-2) have evolved from research that indicates that cell membrane receptors control cell proliferation, cell migration, angiogenesis (new blood vessel growth), and cell death that are integral to the growth and spread of cancer. **Targeted anticancer agents** are those that act on receptors such as epidermal growth factor receptors (EGFRs) (e.g., human epidermal growth factor receptor-2 [HER-2]), platelet-derived growth factor, and vascular endothelial growth factor (VEGF). Targeted anticancer agents are noncytotoxic drugs that target the key pathways (e.g., EGFR, VEGF) that provide growth and survival advantages for cancer cells. These pathways are relatively specific for cancer cells; theoretically, targeted agents are not associated with the toxicities common with cytotoxic chemotherapy.

Chemoprotective agents (Table 44-3) help reduce the toxicity of chemotherapeutic agents to normal cells. Both targeted agents and chemoprotective agents allow the use of full therapeutic doses to attack the cancer. Bone marrow stimulants (Table 44-4) are another recent stride in treating cancers. Several types of cancer (e.g., leukemias, lymphomas) are being treated either by chemotherapeutic agents that kill bone marrow cells while killing the cancer cells, or by bone marrow transplantation of healthy cells. The bone marrow stimulants trigger the recovery of bone marrow cells several days earlier than would be the natural course of recovery. The major benefit to this earlier recovery is that patients' immune systems are able to respond to and stop infections from being so pathological, and patients are able to be released from isolation rooms several days earlier. Cancers and other diseases (chronic renal failure, anemia of chronic disease) also cause anemia, which can be very debilitating to the patient. Darbepoetin and epoetin stimulate the bone marrow to produce red blood cells to treat anemia.

NURSING PROCESS *for Chemotherapy*

Assessment

History of Risk Factors

- Ask age, gender, and race. Take family history of the incidence of cancer.
- Ask about job-related exposure to known chemical carcinogens (e.g., benzene, vinyl chloride, asbestos, soot, tars, oils).
- Ask about exposure to tobacco smoke. Obtain a history of the number of cigarettes or cigars smoked daily. How long has the person smoked? Has the person ever tried to stop smoking? How does the person feel about modifying the smoking

Text continued on p. 724

Drug Table 44-1 CANCER CHEMOTHERAPEUTIC AGENTS

DRUG	USUAL DOSAGE	TOXICITY: ACUTE	TOXICITY: DELAYED	MAJOR INDICATIONS
ALKYLATING AGENTS				
busulfan (Myleran)	2-8 mg/day for 2-3 wk PO; stop for recovery; then maintenance	None	Bone marrow depression	Chronic myelogenous leukemia
carboplatin (Paraplatin)	360 mg/m² every 4 wk	Nausea, vomiting	Bone marrow suppression, anemia, nephrotoxicity	Ovarian carcinoma
carmustine (BCNU)	As single agent: 100-200 mg/m² IV; over 1-2 hr infusion every 6-8 wk In combination: 30-60 mg/m² IV Use gloves because solution may cause skin discoloration	Nausea and vomiting; pain along vein of infusion	Granulocyte and platelet suppression Hepatic, pulmonary, and renal toxicity	Brain, Hodgkin's disease, lymphosarcoma, myeloma, malignant melanoma
chlorambucil (Leukeran)	Start 0.1-0.2 mg/kg/day PO; adjust for maintenance	None	Bone marrow depression (anemia, leukopenia, thrombocytopenia) can be severe with excessive dosage	Chronic lymphocytic leukemia, Hodgkin's disease, non-Hodgkin's lymphoma, trophoblastic neoplasms
cisplatin (Platinol-AQ)	20-100 mg/m² IV; frequency highly variable	Nausea, vomiting	Nephrotoxicity, ototoxicity, blurred vision, changes in color perception	Testicular and ovarian cancers; bladder cancer
cyclophosphamide (Cytoxan)	40-50 mg/kg IV divided in 2-8 daily doses or 2-4 mg/kg/day PO for 10 days; adjust for maintenance	Nausea and vomiting	Bone marrow depression, alopecia, cystitis	Hodgkin's disease and other lymphomas, multiple myeloma, lymphocytic leukemia, many solid cancers
ifosfamide (Ifex)	1.2 g/m²/day for 5 days IV	Nausea, vomiting, diarrhea	Hematuria, alopecia, confusion, coma	Testicular, lung, breast, ovarian, pancreatic, gastric cancer
lomustine (CCNU, CeeNU)	130 mg/m² PO once every 6 wk	Severe nausea and vomiting; anorexia	Thrombocytopenia, leukopenia, alopecia, confusion, lethargy, ataxia	Brain, Hodgkin's disease
mechlorethamine (nitrogen mustard; Mustargen)	0.4 mg/kg IV in single or divided doses	Nausea and vomiting	Moderate depression of peripheral blood count	Hodgkin's disease and other lymphomas, bronchogenic carcinoma
melphalan (Alkeran)	0.2 mg/kg/day for 5 days PO; 2-4 mg/day as maintenance or 0.1-0.15 mg/kg/day for 2-3 wk	Nausea, vomiting, diarrhea	Bone marrow depression	Multiple myeloma, ovarian carcinoma, testicular seminoma
streptozocin (Zanosar)	As single agent: 1.0-1.5 mg/m²/wk for 6 consecutive wk with 4 wk of observation In combination: 400-500 mg/m² for 4-5 consecutive days with 6 wk of observation	Hypoglycemia, severe nausea, and vomiting	Moderate but transient renal and hepatic toxicity, hypoglycemia, mild anemia, leukopenia	Pancreatic islet cell carcinoma

Continued

Drug Table 44-1 CANCER CHEMOTHERAPEUTIC AGENTS—cont'd

DRUG	USUAL DOSAGE	TOXICITY: ACUTE	TOXICITY: DELAYED	MAJOR INDICATIONS
ALKYLATING AGENTS—cont'd				
temozolomide (Temodar)	Variable for regimen being used	Headache, nausea, vomiting, constipation	Bone marrow depression, seizures	Glioblastoma, astrocytoma
thiotepa (Thioplex)	0.2 mg/kg IV for 5 days	Dizziness, headache, anorexia	Bone marrow depression	Hodgkin's disease, ovary and breast carcinomas, bladder cancer
ANTIMETABOLITES				
capecitabine (Xeloda)	2500 mg/m^2 daily for 2 wk followed by 1 wk of rest	Nausea and vomiting, diarrhea, constipation, fatigue	Bone marrow depression, dermatitis, hand-and-foot syndrome lymphopenia	Breast cancer, colorectal cancer
cladribine (Leustatin)	0.09 mg/kg/day IV infused over 24 hr for 7 consecutive days	Headache, dizziness, rash, nausea	Bone marrow depression, purpura	Hairy cell leukemia, lymphomas
clofarabine (Clolar)	52 mg/m^2 IV over 2 hr daily for 5 days	Flushing, hypotension, hypertension, headache, nausea, vomiting	Bone marrow depression, dermatitis	Acute lymphocytic leukemia
cytarabine hydrochloride (Cytosar)	Highly variable for condition being treated	Nausea and vomiting, anorexia, oral ulceration	Bone marrow depression, megaloblastosis	Acute leukemias
fludarabine (Fludara)	25 mg/m^2 daily for 5 days; start each 5-day cycle every 28 days	Nausea, vomiting, diarrhea, anorexia, myalgia	Edema, rash, weakness, cough, dyspnea, hemolytic anemia	Chronic lymphocytic leukemia, other leukemias
fluorouracil (5-FU, FU)	12.5 mg/kg/day IV for 3-5 days or 15 mg/kg/wk for 6 wk	Nausea	Oral and GI ulceration, stomatitis and diarrhea, bone marrow depression	Breast, large bowel, ovarian, pancreatic, stomach carcinoma
gemcitabine (Gemzar)	1000 mg/m^2 IV once weekly for 7 wk	Nausea, vomiting	Bone marrow suppression, rashes, edema	Pancreatic, breast, lung cancer
mercaptopurine (6-MP, Purinethol)	2.5 mg/kg/day PO	Occasional nausea and vomiting, usually well tolerated	Bone marrow depression, occasional hepatic damage	Acute lymphocytic and granulocytic leukemia
methotrexate (MTX)	Highly variable for condition being treated	Occasional diarrhea, hepatic necrosis	Oral and GI ulceration, bone marrow depression (anemia, leukopenia, thrombocytopenia), cirrhosis	Acute lymphocytic leukemia, choriocarcinoma, carcinoma of cervix and head and neck area, mycosis fungoides, solid cancers
pemetrexed (Alimta)	500 mg/m^2 IV over 10 min	Nausea, vomiting, diarrhea	Bone marrow depression, renal dysfunction	Malignant pleural mesothelioma, non–small cell lung cancer

GI, Gastrointestinal.

Drug Table 44-1 **CANCER CHEMOTHERAPEUTIC AGENTS—cont'd**

DRUG	USUAL DOSAGE	TOXICITY ACUTE	TOXICITY DELAYED	MAJOR INDICATIONS
ANTIMETABOLITES—cont'd				
pentostatin (Nipent)	4 mg/m² IV over 20-30 min every other wk	Nausea, vomiting, muscle pain, headache, bloating, constipation, diarrhea	Bone marrow, depression, renal dysfunction	Hairy cell leukemia, lymphomas
thioguanine (TG, Tabloid)	2 mg/kg/day PO	Occasional nausea and vomiting, usually well tolerated	Bone marrow depression	Acute nonlymphocytic leukemia
NATURAL PRODUCTS				
etoposide (VePesid, Toposar)	50-100 mg/m² daily for 5 days IV; cycles of therapy are given every 3-4 wk	Nausea (15%), vomiting, stomatitis, diarrhea	Leukopenia, nadir in 10-14 days, recovery in 3 wk; thrombocytopenia; alopecia	Testicular tumors, small cell carcinoma of the lung, Hodgkin's disease and non-Hodgkin's lymphoma, acute nonlymphocytic leukemia, ovarian carcinoma, Kaposi's sarcoma
docetaxel (Taxotere)	60 to 100 mg/m² every 3 wk IV	Nausea, vomiting, diarrhea	Bone marrow suppression, rashes, hypersensitivity	Breast cancer, prostate cancer
paclitaxel (Taxol)	135 to 175 mg/m² every 3 wk IV	Nausea, vomiting, hypotension, diarrhea	Bone marrow suppression, mucositis, peripheral neuropathy	Ovarian carcinoma, breast carcinoma, AIDS-related Kaposi's sarcoma, lung cancer
vinblastine sulfate (Velban)	0.1-0.2 mg/kg/wk IV or every 2 wk	Nausea and vomiting, local irritant	Alopecia, stomatitis, bone marrow depression, loss of reflexes	Hodgkin's disease and other lymphomas, solid cancers
vincristine sulfate (Oncovin)	1.4 mg/m²/wk IV	Local irritant	Areflexia, peripheral neuritis, paralytic ileus, mild bone marrow depression	Acute lymphocytic leukemia, Hodgkin's disease and other lymphomas, solid cancers
vinorelbine (Navelbine)	30 mg/m²/wk IV	Nausea, vomiting, constipation, diarrhea	Bone marrow suppression, hepatotoxicity, bronchospasm	Non–small cell lung cancer, breast cancer, cervical carcinoma, Kaposi's sarcoma
ANTIBIOTICS				
bleomycin (Blenoxane)	0.25-0.5 units/kg once or twice a wk, IV, IM, subcutaneous	Nausea and vomiting, fever, very toxic	Edema of hands, pulmonary fibrosis, stomatitis, alopecia	Hodgkin's disease, non-Hodgkin's lymphoma, squamous cell carcinoma of head and neck, testicular carcinoma
dactinomycin (Actinomycin D; Cosmegen)	Highly variable for condition being treated	Nausea and vomiting, local irritant	Stomatitis, oral ulcers, diarrhea, alopecia, mental depression, bone marrow depression	Testicular carcinoma, Wilms' tumor, rhabdomyosarcoma, Ewing's and osteogenic sarcoma, and other solid tumors

Continued

Drug Table 44-1 CANCER CHEMOTHERAPEUTIC AGENTS—cont'd

DRUG	USUAL DOSAGE	TOXICITY: ACUTE	TOXICITY: DELAYED	MAJOR INDICATIONS
ANTIBIOTICS—cont'd				
daunorubicin (Cerubidine)	30-45 mg/m²/day for 2 or 3 days of combination therapy; never give IM or subcutaneous	Nausea, vomiting, diarrhea, fever, chills	Bone marrow suppression, reversible alopecia	Acute nonlymphocytic leukemia in adults; acute lymphocytic leukemia in children and adults
doxorubicin (Adriamycin)	60-90 mg/m² IV, single dose or over 3 days; repeat every 3 wk up to total dose 500 mg/m²	Nausea, red urine (not hematuria)	Bone marrow depression, cardiotoxicity, alopecia, stomatitis	Soft tissue, osteogenic and miscellaneous sarcomas, Hodgkin's disease, non-Hodgkin's lymphoma, bronchogenic and breast carcinoma, thyroid cancer, leukemias
epirubicin (Ellence)	Variable	Nausea, vomiting, red urine (not hematuria), rash, diarrhea	Bone marrow depression, cardiotoxicity, alopecia, stomatitis	Breast cancer
idarubicin (Idamycin)	12 mg/m²/day for 3 days by slow (10-15 min) IV; do not give IM or subcutaneous	Nausea, vomiting, diarrhea	Bone marrow suppression, cardiotoxicity, mucositis, hemorrhage	Acute myelocytic leukemia
mitomycin C (Mutamycin)	0.05 mg/kg/day IV for 5 days	Nausea and vomiting, flu-like syndrome	Bone marrow depression, skin toxicity; pulmonary, renal, CNS effects	Squamous cell carcinoma of cervix; adenocarcinoma of the stomach, pancreas, bladder cancer
mitoxantrone (Novantrone)	12 mg/m²/day for 3 days by IV infusion	Nausea, vomiting, diarrhea	Heart failure; GI bleeding; cough, dyspnea	Acute nonlymphocytic leukemia, prostate cancer
valrubicin (Valstar)	800 mg weekly via urethral catheter into bladder	Bladder spasm, hematuria, abdominal pain	Rash	Carcinoma-in-situ of the urinary bladder
OTHER SYNTHETIC AGENTS				
aldesleukin (Proleukin)		Confusion, dyspnea, nausea, diarrhea	Bone marrow depression, liver dysfunction	Melanoma, renal cell carcinoma, T-cell lymphoma
altretamine (Hexalen)	260 mg/m²/day for 14 or 21 days in a 28-day cycle; give daily doses as four divided oral doses	Nausea, vomiting	Anemia, leukopenia, thrombocytopenia, peripheral neuropathy	Ovarian cancer
dacarbazine (DTIC-Dome; DIC)	2-4.5 mg/kg/day IV for 10 days; repeated every 28 days	Nausea and vomiting, flu-like syndrome	Bone marrow depression (rare)	Metastatic malignant melanoma, Hodgkin's disease
hydroxyurea (Hydrea)	80 mg/kg PO single dose every 3 days or 20-30 mg/kg/day PO	Mild nausea and vomiting	Bone marrow depression	Chronic granulocytic leukemia, ovarian cancer, melanoma
interferon alfa-2a (Roferon-a)	3 million units daily IM or subcutaneously	Flu-like syndrome	Bone marrow depression	Hairy cell leukemia, Kaposi's sarcoma

CNS, central nervous system.

Drug Table 44-1 **CANCER CHEMOTHERAPEUTIC AGENTS—cont'd**

DRUG	USUAL DOSAGE	TOXICITY: ACUTE	TOXICITY: DELAYED	MAJOR INDICATIONS
OTHER SYNTHETIC AGENTS—cont'd				
interferon alfa-2b (Intron a)	2 million mcg/m^2 IM or subcutaneous three times/wk	Flu-like syndrome	Bone marrow depression	Hairy cell leukemia, Kaposi's sarcoma, malignant melanoma
levamisole (Ergamisol)	50 mg PO every 8 hr for 3 days every 2 wk	Nausea, diarrhea	Dermatitis, alopecia, leukopenia	Colon cancer
leuprolide acetate (Lupron)	1 mg subcutaneously daily	Hot flashes; initial exacerbation of symptoms	Dysrhythmias, edema	Prostatic carcinoma, breast carcinoma
mitotane (Lysodren)	2-6 mg/day in 3-4 divided doses	Nausea and vomiting	Dermatitis, diarrhea, mental depression	Adrenal cortical carcinoma
procarbazine hydrochloride (Matulane)	Start 1-2 mg/kg/day PO; increase over 1 wk to 3 mg/kg; maintain for 3 wk, then reduce to 1-2 mg/kg/day until toxicity	Nausea and vomiting	Bone marrow depression, CNS depression	Hodgkin's disease, non-Hodgkin's lymphoma, lung cancer, melanoma
HORMONES				
abarelix (Plenaxis)	100 mg IM in buttock	Sleep disturbance, headache	Gynecomastia, hot flashes	Prostate cancer
anastrozole (Arimidex)	1 mg daily PO	Nausea, vomiting, headache	Hot flashes, diarrhea, constipation, pelvic pain, edema	Breast cancer in postmenopausal women with disease progression following tamoxifen therapy
bicalutamide (Casodex)	50 mg daily PO (use with luteinizing hormone–releasing hormone [LHRH])	Nausea, constipation, peripheral edema, diarrhea	Hepatitis, gynecomastia, dyspnea	Prostate cancer
estramustine (Emcyt)	14 mg/kg/day in three to four divided doses Take with water, no calcium-rich products	Nausea, diarrhea	Thrombosis, hyperglycemia, hepatic dysfunction, breast tenderness	Prostate cancer
Ethinyl estradiol	3 mg/day PO	None	Fluid retention, hypercalcemia, feminization, uterine bleeding	Breast and prostate carcinomas
exemestane (Aromasin)	25 mg daily PO	Nausea, fatigue, insomnia	Depression, anxiety, hot flashes, dyspnea	Breast cancer in postmenopausal women with disease progression following tamoxifen therapy
fluoxymesterone	10-40 mg/day PO in divided doses	None	Fluid retention, masculinization, cholestatic jaundice	Breast carcinoma
flutamide (Eulexin) ✱ (Euflex)	2 capsules PO three times daily at 8-hr intervals	Nausea, vomiting	Hot flashes, loss of libido, impotence, gynecomastia, hepatotoxicity	Metastatic prostatic carcinoma

✱ Available in Canada.

Continued

Drug Table 44-1 CANCER CHEMOTHERAPEUTIC AGENTS—cont'd

		TOXICITY		
DRUG	**USUAL DOSAGE**	**ACUTE**	**DELAYED**	**MAJOR INDICATIONS**
HORMONES—cont'd				
fulvestrant (Faslodex)	250 mg IM in buttock once monthly	Nausea, headache, constipation	Dyspnea, rash	Breast cancer
goserelin (Zoladex)	3.6 mg subcutaneously every 28 days in upper abdominal wall; local anesthesia may be used	Anorexia, dizziness, pain	Hot flashes, sexual dysfunction	Prostate and breast cancer
histrelin (Vantas)	50 mg subcutaneously implanted in inner aspect of upper arm	Insertion site reaction	Hot flashes, gynecomastia, fatigue	Prostate cancer
letrozole (Femara)	2.5 mg daily PO	Nausea, vomiting, headache	Muscle aches, hot flashes, constipation, diarrhea, fatigue	Breast cancer in postmenopausal women with disease progression following antiestrogen therapy
medroxyprogesterone acetate	400-1000 mg IM/wk	None	None	Endometrial carcinoma, renal cell, breast cancer
nilutamide (Nilandron)	300 mg PO once daily for 30 days, then 150 mg daily	Insomnia, headache, nausea, constipation	Hot flashes, impaired adaptation to dark	Prostate cancer
tamoxifen (Nolvadex)	20-40 mg daily in two divided doses	Nausea, vomiting, hot flashes	Increased bone and tumor pain, thrombocytopenia, leukopenia, edema, hypercalcemia	Breast cancer (estrogen sensitive)
testolactone (Teslac)	250 mg four times daily PO	None	Fluid retention, masculinization	Breast carcinoma
testosterone enanthate	200-400 mg every 2-4 wk IM	None	Fluid retention, masculinization	Breast carcinoma
toremifene (Fareston)	60 mg daily PO	Nausea, vomiting	Hot flashes, sweating, vaginal discharge	Metastatic breast cancer in postmenopausal women with estrogen positive tumors
triptorelin (Trelstar)	Depot: 3.75 mg IM every 28 days LA: 11.25 mg IM every 84 days	Vomiting, fatigue	Hot flashes, impotence, insomnia	Prostate cancer
DNA TOPOISOMERASE INHIBITORS				
irinotecan (Camptosar)	Variable depending on regimen	Nausea, vomiting, anorexia, diarrhea, constipation, shortness of breath	Diarrhea, bone marrow suppression, alopecia	Carcinoma of the colon and rectum
topotecan (Hycamtin)	1.5 mg/m^2 IV over 30 min	Nausea, vomiting, diarrhea, shortness of breath	Alopecia, bone marrow depression, stomatitis	Ovarian cancer, small cell lung cancer

 Drug Table 44-2 **TARGETED ANTICANCER AGENTS**

GENERIC NAME	BRAND NAME	MAJOR INDICATIONS
MONOCLONAL ANTIBODIES		
alemtuzumab	Campath	Alemtuzumab is a monoclonal antibody (alemtuzumab-1H) that binds to CD52, an antigen that is present on the surface of essentially all B and T lymphocytes, most monocytes, macrophages, natural killer cells, and some granulocytes. It is thought that the binding of the antibody to the cell-surface antigen kills leukemic cells. Alemtuzumab is used to treat B-cell chronic lymphocytic leukemia in patients who have been treated with alkylating agents and have failed fludarabine therapy.
bevacizumab	Avastatin	Bevacizumab is an antibody that is a vascular endothelial growth factor (VEGF) antagonist. VEGF is secreted and binds to its receptors located primarily on the surface of endothelial cells of blood vessels, inducing new blood vessel growth. Bevacizumab binds to VEGF, preventing attachment of VEGF to its receptors on endothelial cells. Administration of bevacizumab causes a reduction of new blood vessel growth, inhibiting metastatic disease progression. Bevacizumab is used in combination with chemotherapy for treating patients with metastatic carcinoma of the colon or rectum. It is also used to treat metastatic renal cell carcinoma and non–small cell lung cancer. Do not administer or mix bevacizumab infusions with dextrose solutions.
cetuximab	Erbitux	Cetuximab is a monoclonal antibody that binds specifically to the human epidermal growth factor receptor (EGFR) on normal and tumor cells, inhibiting attachment of epidermal growth factor (EGF). This results in inhibition of cell growth and eventual cell death. The addition of cetuximab to irinotecan or irinotecan plus 5-fluorouracil in animal studies resulted in an increase in antitumor effects compared with chemotherapy alone. Cetuximab is used to treat certain types of colon and rectal cancer and head and neck cancer.
gemtuzumab ozogamicin	Mylotarg	Gemtuzumab ozogamicin is an engineered anti-CD33 monoclonal antibody that is linked to calicheamicin, a potent antitumor antibiotic. The anti-CD33 antibody portion of gemtuzumab binds specifically to the CD33 antigen of acute myelogenous leukemia (AML) cells and is transported into the cells. In the cell, the calicheamicin is released and binds to DNA, causing DNA strand cleavage and cell death. The major benefit of gemtuzumab is that it selectively targets cancer cells containing CD33 antigen and spares other cells from toxicity.
ibritumomab tiuxetan	Zevalin	Ibritumomab tiuxetan is a radioimmunotherapeutic agent. It is the bonding of a monoclonal antibody ibritumomab to tiuxetan, a chelator that provides a binding site for radioactive indium-111 or yttrium-90. The antibody ibritumomab induces apoptosis (programmed cell death) by attaching to the CD20 antigen found on the surface of normal and malignant B lymphocytes. The chelate tiuxetan is used to carry radioactive Y-90 which emits beta rays, inducing cellular damage by the formation of free radicals in the target and neighboring cells. Ibritumomab tiuxetan is used to treat relapsed or refractory B-cell non-Hodgkin's lymphoma that is refractory to rituximab therapy. Patients must receive a predose of rituximab before receiving the ibritumomab tiuxetan radioactive product. Because this is a radioactive medicinal agent, it must be prepared in a nuclear pharmacy before administration, and personnel must be aware of radioactive precautions when handling the product.
rituximab	Rituxan	Rituximab is a genetically engineered monoclonal antibody that binds specifically to the CD20 antigen found on the surface of normal and malignant B lymphocytes and on B-cell non-Hodgkin's lymphomas. Binding of the antibody to the antigen causes normal body defense mechanisms to kill the cell. Rituximab is used to treat patients with relapsed or refractory low-grade or follicular, CD20-positive, B-cell non-Hodgkin's lymphoma.
trastuzumab	Herceptin	Trastuzumab is an engineered monoclonal antibody that binds to the human epidermal growth factor receptor-2 protein (HER-2), inhibiting growth of tumor cells. The HER-2 protein is present in 25% to 30% of primary breast cancers. Trastuzumab is used to treat metastatic breast cancer with HER-2–positive tumors either as a single agent in patients who have received one or more chemotherapy regimens, or in combination with paclitaxel in patients who have not received chemotherapy for their metastatic disease.

Continued

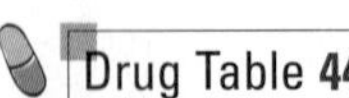

Drug Table 44-2 TARGETED ANTICANCER AGENTS—cont'd

GENERIC NAME	BRAND NAME	MAJOR INDICATIONS
TYROSINE KINASE INHIBITORS		
imatinib	Gleevec	Imatinib is a tyrosine kinase inhibitor that inhibits a specific protein (Bcr-Abl tyrosine kinase) secreted by the Philadelphia chromosome abnormality associated with chronic myelogenous leukemia (CML). Because Bcr-Abl is secreted only in cancer cells and not in normal cells, imatinib selectively inhibits abnormal cell growth in cancer cells, generally sparing normal cells. It inhibits cell multiplication and induces apoptosis in leukemic cells. It is also used to treat gastrointestinal stromal tumors (GIST).
gefitinib	Iressa	Gefitinib inhibits tyrosine kinases associated with epidermal growth factor receptors (EGFR). It is thought that by inhibiting the epidermal growth factors, the malignant cells cannot multiply and will die. Gefitinib is used to treat non–small cell lung cancer.
erlotinib	Tarceva	See gefitinib.
sunitinib	Sutent	Sunitinib inhibits tyrosine kinases associated with platelet-derived growth factor receptors, vascular endothelial growth receptors, stem cell factor receptors, colony-stimulating factor receptors, and neurotrophic factor receptors. Sunitinib is used to treat GIST and advanced renal cell carcinoma.
PROTEASOME INHIBITORS		
bortezomib	Velcade	Proteasomes are enzymes that play an important role in the production and metabolism of proteins. Specific types of cancer cells depend on proteasomes for rapid growth that are not part of normal cell growth. Bortezomib selectively inhibits NF-kappa-B, a proteasome important in the growth and proliferation of multiple myeloma cells.

Drug Table 44-3 CHEMOPROTECTIVE AGENTS

GENERIC NAME	BRAND NAME	MAJOR INDICATIONS
amifostine	Ethyol	Amifostine is a prodrug that is metabolized by enzymes in tissues to a free thiol metabolite that can reduce the toxic effects of cisplatin. Normal tissue has a higher affinity for the free thiol. The higher concentration of free thiol in normal tissues is available to bind to and detoxify the reactive metabolites of cisplatin, reducing damage to normal tissues. Amifostine is used to reduce the cumulative renal toxicity associated with the repeated administration of cisplatin in patients with advanced ovarian cancer.
dexrazoxane	Zinecard	Dexrazoxane is an intracellular chelating agent used in conjunction with doxorubicin. It is used to reduce the incidence and severity of cardiomyopathy associated with doxorubicin in women with metastatic breast cancer who have received a cumulative doxorubicin dose of 300 mg/m^2 and who would benefit from continuing doxorubicin therapy.
mesna	Mesnex	Mesna is a prodrug that is metabolized by enzymes in kidney tissue to a free thiol metabolite that can reduce the toxic effects of ifosfamide and cyclophosphamide. The free thiol binds and deactivates the toxic metabolites of ifosfamide and cyclophosphamide. Mesna is used as a prophylactic agent to reduce the incidence of ifosfamide- and cyclophosphamide-induced hemorrhagic cystitis.

habit? Is there chronic exposure to secondhand smoke at home or at work?

- Obtain a drug history to acquire information on pharmacologic agents that have the potential to become carcinogens (e.g., diethylstilbestrol, cyclophosphamide, melphalan, azathioprine).
- Ask about a history of viral diseases suspected of being associated with carcinogenesis (e.g., Epstein-Barr virus, hepatitis B virus, human immunodeficiency virus [HIV]).
- Is there a history of exposure to or treatment with radiation?

Dietary Habits

- Take a dietary history. Ask specific questions to obtain data relating to foods eaten that are high in fat, animal protein (especially red meats; salt-cured, smoked, or charcoaled foods; and nitrate and nitrite additives). Are whole grains included in the diet? How many servings of fruits and vegetables are eaten daily? What types of vegetables are eaten daily? Estimate the number of calories consumed per day.
- Ask the patient about normal eating patterns, food likes and dislikes, and elimination pattern.

Drug Table 44-4 BONE MARROW STIMULANTS

GENERIC NAME	BRAND NAME	MAJOR INDICATIONS
darbepoetin	Aranasep	Darbepoetin stimulates erythropoiesis (production of red blood cells [RBCs]). It is used to treat anemia in patients receiving chemotherapy. Increased hemoglobin levels are not generally observed until 2-6 weeks after initiating treatment with darbepoetin. Darbepoetin is administered by weekly subcutaneous injection.
epoetin alpha	Procrit, Epogen	Stimulates production of RBCs. It is used to treat anemia in patients receiving chemotherapy. Epoetin is administered by subcutaneous or IV injection three times per week.
filgrastim	Neupogen	Also known as a human granulocyte colony-stimulating factor (G-CSF). It stimulates production of neutrophilic white blood cells. It is used to reduce the neutropenia interval in bone marrow transplantation, to stimulate white cell production in patients receiving myelosuppressive chemotherapy, and to treat neutropenia in acute myelogenous leukemia.
oprelvekin	Neumega	Stimulates platelet production at the stem cell level. Oprelvekin is used to prevent severe chemotherapy-induced thrombocytopenia in nonmyeloid malignancies, and to decrease the need for platelet transfusions.
pegfilgrastim	Neulasta	Pegfilgrastim and filgrastim have the same mechanism of action. Pegfilgrastim has reduced renal clearance and prolonged duration of action compared with filgrastim.
sargramostim	Leukine	Also known as granulocyte macrophage colony–stimulating factor (GM-CSF); it stimulates production of granulocytes and macrophages, increases the cytotoxicity of monocytes toward certain neoplastic cell lines, and activates polymorphonuclear neutrophils to inhibit the growth of tumor cells. Sargramostim is used to accelerate bone marrow transplant recovery, correct neutropenia in patients with aplastic anemia, and stimulate bone marrow recovery in patients receiving myelosuppressive chemotherapy.

- Ask whether certain foods cause bloating, indigestion, or diarrhea, and how much seasoning and spices are put on food.
- What is the usual fluid intake daily? How much coffee, tea, soft drinks, and fruit juices are consumed? Determine the frequency and volume of alcoholic beverages consumed.
- Is the person experiencing anorexia, nausea, and vomiting? If so, what measures are being used to control these symptoms?
- Obtain a baseline height and weight. Has there been a weight gain or loss in the past year?
- Obtain details of any symptoms that are affecting the individual's ability to eat (e.g., anorexia, vomiting, diarrhea, smells that deter eating, pain).

Preexisting Health Problems. Ask about any preexisting health problems for which the patient is or has been receiving treatment.

Diagnosis

- Ask the patient to explain his or her understanding of the current diagnosis and plan of treatment.
- Review the admission notes or old charts to determine the details relating to the diagnostic test data, type of cancer, the staging of the disease, laboratory values, and treatments to date.

Adaptation to the Diagnosis

- Determine whether this is the initial or a subsequent cycle of chemotherapy. Gather data regarding the patient's and significant others' understanding of the disease and the planned course of treatment.
- Ask how the patient normally copes with stressful situations. Does the patient have a confidante who is supportive and understanding?
- Observe both the verbal and nonverbal messages conveyed during the interview. Take note of the patient's general appearance, tone of voice, inflections, and gestures. Try to pick up on subtle clues and confirm their meanings with the patient.
- Inquire regarding psychological issues that the patient is perceiving—loss of control; self-esteem; loss of body parts; lifestyle; guilt; and so on.
- Review the health care provider's progress notes for information being imparted to the patient and family throughout the course of treatment.

Psychomotor Functions

- Type of lifestyle. Ask the patient to describe exercise level in terms of amount tolerated, the degree of fatigue present, and the ability to perform activities of daily living.
- Is the patient having difficulty performing normal roles (e.g., homemaker, provider, mother, father)?

Safety. Assess for weakness, confusion, orthostatic hypotension, or similar symptoms that could signal impending potential for injury problems.

Symptoms of Pharmacologic Side Effects. Ask specific questions to determine whether the individual has been or is experiencing symptoms associated with the type of drugs being administered, such as myelosuppression, anemia, bleeding, stomatitis (mucositis), altered bowel patterns (e.g., diarrhea, constipation), alopecia, neurotoxicity, anorexia, nausea, or vomiting.

Physical Assessment

- Perform a baseline physical, psychosocial, and spiritual assessment of the individual to serve as the database for ongoing assessments throughout the course of care.
- Throughout the course of therapy perform daily assessments of the physical, psychosocial, and spiritual needs of the individual and family. Perform a focused assessment on the body systems affected by the disease process and those likely to be affected by metastasis (e.g., lungs, brain, bone, liver).

Sexual Assessment. Discuss birth control and reproductive counseling issues at the time of initiation of therapy. Male patients may wish to use a sperm bank. Female patients may wish to harvest eggs. A contraceptive method should be discussed.

Pain. Ask whether the person is having any pain and what interventions are being used to manage the pain. Obtain a rating of pain level and the degree of relief being gained from current medications and supportive practices (e.g., relaxation or guided imagery).

Nursing Diagnoses

- Infection, risk for (side effect)
- Nutrition, imbalanced: less than body requirements (side effect)
- Activity intolerance (side effect)
- Injury, risk for (side effect)
- Deficient knowledge (chemotherapy treatment, side effects)
- Body image, disturbed (side effect)

Planning

History of Risk Factors. Review assessment data to determine needed interventions for the individual and support personnel.

Dietary Habits. After obtaining the dietary history, develop a plan to meet the individual's nutritional needs based on the number of calories being eaten, current weight, and calculated needs to meet the demands of the disease process. Consult with dietitian, as appropriate to circumstances.

Smoking. Discuss smoking habits with the patient, and plan a mutually agreeable way to handle this habit, both while hospitalized and when at home. Does the patient wish to modify the habit?

Preexisting Health Problems. Plan interventions to continue treatment of any preexisting health problems (e.g., angina, heart failure, asthma).

Diagnosis and Adaptation to Diagnosis. Analyze data to determine effectiveness of current coping strategies used to adapt to the diagnosis. Attempt to identify adaptive coping strategies that could replace unsuitable or unsuccessful strategies.

Psychomotor Functions

- Schedule nursing care needs so the individual will have adequate rest periods between needed care delivery.
- Plan a referral to social services for needed guidance for the patient or support personnel to assist in the management of problems relating to inability to work, home care, and so forth.

Safety. Determine the amount of assistance needed with self-care, ambulation, and so on, and mark the Kardex or document in the computer clearly so that all caregivers will provide adequately for the individual's safety needs.

Symptoms of Pharmacologic Side Effects. Research the specific drugs prescribed to identify the usual side effects to expect, and plan to institute measures to minimize or prevent their occurrence.

Physical Assessment. Schedule physical, psychosocial, and spiritual assessments on a regular basis. Usually these are done once per shift while hospitalized and more frequently when specific problems exist. Read the drug monograph and perform a focused assessment on body systems likely to be affected by a particular chemotherapeutic agent prescribed (e.g., drugs known to be cardiotoxic should have a thorough cardiovascular assessment to detect early symptoms).

Always plan to assess body weight and height, as dosages of many chemotherapy agents are based on body surface area (BSA).

Laboratory Studies. Order prescribed laboratory studies as requested (e.g., electrolytes, leukocyte counts, arterial blood gases, serum transferrin, albumin).

Medication Administration

- Plan drug administration exactly at the time intervals prescribed to promote maximum cytotoxicity of the chemotherapy agents and maximum effectiveness of drug therapy. See individual drug monographs.
- Review drug orders for any premedication or hydration prescribed and schedule initiation at appropriate intervals in advance of the chemotherapy.
- Schedule oral hygiene measures using prescribed local anesthetic and antimicrobial solutions. Perform before and after meals and at bedtime if symptoms are mild. With moderate lesions, increase the frequency to every 2 hours. In patients with severe symptoms, the mouth is rinsed hourly while the patient is awake.
- Chemotherapy administration should be performed by qualified registered nurses or physicians with specific skills in the correct handling and administration techniques for chemotherapeutic agents. For more information on advanced education required for administering chemotherapeutic agents, consult *The Oncology Nursing Society* guidelines.

Implementation

- Implement planned interventions consistent with assessment data and identified individual needs of the patient (e.g., nutritional support, blood component therapy, growth factor therapy, fatigue, alopecia, anemia, constipation, diarrhea, nausea and vomiting, neutropenia, pain, and thrombocytopenia).

- Examine laboratory data on a continuum. Monitor for the development of cancer emergencies (e.g., hypercalcemia, superior vena cava syndrome, disseminated intravascular coagulation).
- Monitor vital signs, including temperature, pulse, respirations, and blood pressure, at least every shift or more frequently depending on recommended monitoring parameters of specific drugs prescribed.
- *Hydration:* Monitor the patient's state of hydration. Check skin turgor, mucous membranes, and softness of the eyeballs. Electrolyte reports require vigilant observation; report abnormal findings to the health care provider. Fluid replacement via intravenous (IV) administration or total parenteral nutrition may be appropriate in some circumstances. Some chemotherapeutic agents require prehydration before the chemotherapeutic agent is administered to prevent damage to the kidneys or bladder. Prehydration is also planned for highly emetogenic chemotherapy (see Chapter 34, p. 546) to prevent dehydration from vomiting. Regardless of the agents administered, always monitor 24-hour urine output and read the urinalysis to detect abnormalities.
- *Infection:* Report even the slightest sign of infection for evaluation (e.g., elevating temperature, chills, malaise, hypotension, pallor).
- *Nausea, vomiting:* There are three patterns of emesis associated with antineoplastic therapy: acute, delayed, and anticipatory. (See Chapter 34 for the treatment of nausea and vomiting associated with chemotherapy.) The goal of treatment is to prevent nausea and vomiting. Many chemotherapy regimens require prechemotherapy administration of an antiemetic followed by PRN orders for breakthrough nausea and vomiting.
  1. Chart the degree of effectiveness achieved when antiemetics are given. Report poor control to the health care provider. Changing the antiemetic medication ordered or the route of administration may improve control. Patients experiencing nausea and vomiting must be weighed daily and monitored for electrolyte values and accurate intake and output.
- *Positioning:* Hospitalized patients may be sedated. Position the patient on one side to prevent aspiration. Position changes should be scheduled to prevent alterations in skin integrity.
- *Diarrhea:* Record the color, frequency, and consistency of stool. Include an estimate of the volume of watery stools in the output record. Check for occult blood. Provide for adequate hydration and administer any drugs ordered to relieve the symptoms.
  1. Encourage adequate fluid intake and dietary alterations, such as eliminating spicy foods and those high in fat content. It may be necessary to switch to a clear liquid diet followed by a diet low in roughage. Diarrhea may require high-protein foods with high caloric value and vitamin and mineral supplements. Patients with diarrhea should be weighed daily and monitored for fluid intake and output and electrolyte values.
  2. Check the anal area for irritation, provide for hygiene measures, and protect from excoriation with products such as A&D ointment or zinc oxide ointment.
- *Constipation:* Compare this symptom with the patient's usual pattern of elimination. Many people do not normally defecate daily.
- Perform daily assessment of bowel sounds when the patient is hospitalized. When a patient is constipated, the health care provider usually orders stool softeners or laxatives, fluids, and a diet that enhances normal defecation. Observe carefully for signs of an impaction (the urge to defecate with little to no stool or seepage of watery stool).
- *Stomatitis (mucositis):* Use meticulous oral hygiene measures (see Chapter 32, p. 522).
- *Bleeding:* Observe and report signs and symptoms of bleeding, for example, epistaxis, hematuria, bruises, petechiae, dark tarry stools, "coffee ground" emesis, or blurred vision. Instruct female patients to report menstrual flow that is excessive, bright colored, or lasts for a prolonged period. Check laboratory reports for changes in hematologic status, electrolytes, and so on; report abnormal or changing values to the health care provider.
- *Pain:* Administer pain medications prescribed at scheduled intervals to maintain a constant blood level of the analgesic and thereby promote maximum pain control. Maintain a record of pain medications administered and the patient's rating of the degree of pain relief achieved (see Chapter 20, p. 327).
  1. Report insufficient pain relief. Obtain orders for the treatment of the pain, or institute PRN analgesics prescribed for breakthrough pain episodes.
- *Neurotoxicity:* Monitor for disorientation, confusion, fine motor activity alterations, gait alterations, and paresthesias.
- *Anxiety:* Monitor the degree of anxiety being exhibited, and intervene appropriately to alleviate. Give prescribed medications; discuss issues about which the patient or significant others are concerned. Keep the patient involved in making appropriate decisions regarding self-care to give some degree of control over the situation; discuss when prescribed treatments are to be performed.

1. Implement relaxation techniques (use of biofeedback, visual imagery) as prescribed. Deal with stress-related issues that arise within the support or family group.

- Administration of intravenous medications (see Chapter 12 for IV administration principles, administration of drugs via venous access devices and care and handling of venous catheters). It is essential to wear latex or nitrite gloves and disposable, nonpermeable fabric when handling any body fluids.

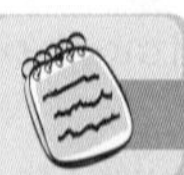

Patient Education and Health Promotion

Nutrition

- Teach the patient specific ways to implement dietary needs (e.g., ways to support increased protein and caloric intake such as adding powdered milk to puddings, creamed soups). Suggest using nutritional supplements such as Ensure or Carnation Instant Breakfast. When using nutritional supplements, try different brands and add freshly squeezed orange or lemon juice to help alter the aftertaste frequently cited by postchemotherapy patients using nutritional supplements.
- If the patient is receiving enteral tube feedings, peripheral parenteral nutrition, or total parenteral nutrition, arrange for necessary at-home support for administration and monitoring of therapy. Suggest obtaining educational materials from the American Cancer Society on dietary interventions during the treatment of cancer.

Preexisting Health Problems. Continue prescribed medications and regimens for preexisting health problems.

Diagnosis and Adaptation to Diagnosis

- Encourage the patient and support group to discuss concerns about the disease, prognosis, and treatment.
- Present the patient with appropriate choices that allow involvement in the decisions concerning selection of care. Encourage the patient to maintain the best health possible. Include the patient in selection of diet, planning activities, scheduling rest periods, and personal care. Stress what the patient *can* do, not what the patient cannot do.
- Limit the amount of information to the facts that are significant at this point in the care plan and to the degree of symptoms present. Emphasize the prevention of complications through maintenance of nutrition and hydration and commitment to hygiene practices.

Sexual Needs. Patients should discuss methods of birth control to be used during chemotherapy and/or sperm storage and fertilization counseling.

Vascular Access Devices. Instruction should be provided on the self-care and frequency of required follow-up care for central lines or ports.

Skin Care. Have the patient bathe in lukewarm water and use mild soap. Gently pat the skin dry. Discuss the use of skin moisturizer with the physician. Instruct the patient to report rashes or areas that appear sunburned or blistered. Stress the need to avoid sunlight for patients receiving drugs that may produce a photosensitivity reaction.

Psychomotor. Discuss activities the patient is able to perform independently and those requiring assistance. Provide for patient safety on a continuum. Include the support group in the development of a plan to provide for self-care at home. Arrange appropriate referrals to support the self-care needs of the person in the home environment.

Nausea and Vomiting

- Teach the person when and how to take prescribed antiemetics.
- Make suggestions for comfort measures to minimize nausea (e.g., rinsing mouth frequently, cool cloth to wash face, relaxation and distraction techniques).
- Teach the patient to take weight daily and give parameters of weight loss that must be reported to the health care provider.

Diarrhea or Constipation

- Teach the patient the proper use of PRN medications prescribed to treat either constipation or diarrhea.
- Explain measures to prevent constipation, such as drinking sufficient fluids daily, eating high-fiber foods, and avoiding foods that cause constipation. Instruct the individual to report failure to have stools in a usual pattern of elimination, or seeping, loose watery stools while feeling the need to defecate (may be an indication of an impaction).
- When diarrhea is present, instruct the patient to avoid foods that irritate or stimulate peristalsis, for example, coffee, tea, and hot or cold beverages. Encourage the increased intake of potassium-containing foods. Teach personal hygiene measures to provide for skin care and to prevent skin breakdown.

Neutropenia

- Explain the measures the individual should initiate to minimize the chance of infection when neutropenia is present (e.g., handwashing; avoidance of exposure to individuals known to have an infection; no fresh flowers, vegetables, or receptacles with freestanding water such as denture cups or humidifiers; and avoidance of pets and patients receiving immunizations).
- Teach signs and symptoms of infection and when to report symptoms present. Be certain the person understands how to take a temperature and that even minor elevations should be reported.
- Teach self-care of central lines, when present, consistent with the patient or significant others'

ability to perform the procedure while maintaining strict aseptic technique. Arrange for referral to community or home care agency as indicated.

- See Table 44-4 for bone marrow stimulants used to treat neutropenia.

Pain

- Discuss beliefs about pain with the patient and significant others as a baseline for health teaching needed.
- Instruct the patient to record the intensity of the pain being experienced and degree of pain relief being obtained from prescribed medications (see Chapter 20, p. 322 for a pain scale).
- Emphasize the need to report pain that is not being controlled or new symptoms of pain being felt.
- Stress the importance of taking pain medications at prescribed intervals to obtain maximum relief.
- Determine whether the patient has access to medications for pain. (Does the patient have sufficient money to purchase or obtain prescribed medication?)
- Stress the need to start stool softeners and to take them regularly to prevent constipation when morphine or codeine therapy is used.
- Oral medications are often used to provide pain relief. Several analgesics are also available as rectal suppositories. (Pain control must be achieved. When oral and rectal forms of pain management no longer suffice, patients may require hospitalization for stabilization on parenteral forms of narcotic analgesics. Infusion pumps are frequently used, and spinal morphine may be delivered effectively via epidural or intrathecal catheters. Patients must understand that they can be kept comfortable!)

Anemia. Teach the patient the possible causes and related self-care needed when anemia is present (e.g., management of fatigue by spacing of activities and prevention of orthostatic hypotension by rising slowly, sitting and resting, and then standing). Instruct the patient not to drive or operate power equipment for safety reasons. See Table 44-4 for bone marrow stimulants used to treat anemia.

Thrombocytopenia

- Teach self-monitoring for other blood-related symptoms (e.g., bleeding, bruising, hematuria, epistaxis, "coffee ground" emesis, or excessive or prolonged menstrual flow).
- Suggest safety measures when at home (e.g., avoiding use of sharp knives, shaving with an electric razor, wearing a thimble when sewing).
- Stress that the patient should not take any aspirin or aspirin-containing products.
- See Table 44-4 for bone marrow stimulants used to treat thrombocytopenia.

Home Care. While receiving chemotherapy, wash soiled linens separate from other household linens; place in washable pillow cases and wash fabric twice. Since most chemotherapeutic agents are excreted in the urine and feces, it is best to flush the toilet two or three times after each voiding or defecation. If emesis occurs, dump waste in toilet and flush two or three times.

Anxiety. Assist the patient to practice stress reduction techniques, and make the patient aware of cancer support resources available (e.g., Make Today Count).

Fostering Health Maintenance

- Throughout the course of treatment, discuss medication information and how the medication will benefit the patient.
- Drug therapy will be individualized for the patient and type of cancer being treated. The need to follow the established regimen precisely must be emphasized to obtain maximum cytotoxic effects while minimizing side effects. Side effects to the drug therapy should be expected and the patient and significant others must be educated in the management of the side effects to expect and those that should be reported. Additional teaching must be individualized to the patient for equipment used to administer drug therapy or nutritional support.
- Seek cooperation and understanding of the following points so that medication compliance is increased: name of medication, dosage, route and times of administration, side effects to expect, and side effects to report.
- Patients should be encouraged to maintain basic good health practices throughout treatment (e.g., adequate rest, exercise consistent with abilities, stress management or stress reduction techniques, and maintenance of usual spiritual beliefs).

Written Record. Enlist the patient's aid in developing and maintaining a written record of monitoring parameters (e.g., nausea, vomiting, pain relief, constipation, diarrhea) (see Patient Self-Assessment Form on p. 730). Complete the Premedication Data column for use as a baseline to track response to drug therapy. Ensure that the patient understands how to use the form and instruct the patient to take the completed form to follow-up visits. During follow-up visits, focus on issues that will foster adherence with the therapeutic interventions prescribed.

DRUG CLASS: Alkylating Agents

Actions

The alkylating agents are highly reactive chemical compounds that bond with DNA molecules, causing cross-linking of DNA strands. The interstrand binding prevents the separation of the double-coiled DNA molecule that is necessary for cellular division. Alkylating agents are cell cycle–nonspecific, which means they are capable of combining with cellular components at any phase of the cell cycle. Generally, the development of resistance to one alkylating agent imparts cross-resistance to other alkylators.

PATIENT SELF-ASSESSMENT FORM Antineoplastic Agents

MEDICATIONS	COLOR	TO BE TAKEN

Patient ______

Health Care Provider ______

Health Care Provider's phone ______

Next appt.* ______

What I Should Monitor		Premedication Data	Date	Date	Date	Date	Date	Date	Comments
Temperature	AM / PM								
Pain level Severe — Moderate — None 10 — 5 — 1	8 AM								
	Noon								
	6 PM								
	Night								
Fatigue level Exhausted with minimal activities — Tired with performance of activities of daily living — Normal 10 — 5 — 1									
Fear and anxiety Anxious — Calm 10 — 5 — 1									
Nausea: Degree of relief Good — Moderate — Poor 10 — 5 — 1	Time of day								
Appetite Good — Normal — Poor 10 — 5 — 1									
Oral hygiene Normal — Moderate Pain — Severe pain 10 — 5 — 1									
Bleeding (Yes/No)	Nosebleeds								
	Bruising								
Bowel movements	Color: brown, tarry								
	Diarrhea: Number of stools								
	Normal								
Other									

*Please bring this record with you to your next appointment.
Use the back of this sheet for additional information.

Uses

See Table 44-1.

Therapeutic Outcomes

The primary therapeutic outcome from alkylating agent therapy is eradication of malignant cells.

Nursing Process for Alkylating Agents

Premedication Assessment

1. Check laboratory reports for baseline data reflecting hepatic and renal function.
2. Assess the patient's state of hydration and review health care provider's orders for oral and intravenous hydration instructions before drug therapy (e.g., cisplatin). Initiate intake and output monitoring if not already in effect.
3. Administer prechemotherapy drugs prescribed at time intervals specified (e.g., mesna).
4. Review laboratory data for baseline hematologic studies that reflect the degree of myelosuppression present before initiating chemotherapy.
5. Discuss birth control methods, sperm storage, and egg harvesting before beginning therapy.

DRUG CLASS: Antimetabolites

Actions

The antimetabolites (subclassified as folic acid, purine, and pyrimidine antagonists) inhibit key enzymes in the biosynthetic pathways of DNA and ribonucleic acid (RNA) synthesis. Many of the antagonists are cell cycle–specific, killing cells during the S phase of cell maturation.

Uses

See Table 44-1.

Therapeutic Outcomes

The primary therapeutic outcome from antimetabolite therapy is eradication of malignant cells.

Nursing Process for Antimetabolites

Premedication Assessment

1. Check laboratory reports for baseline data reflecting hepatic and renal function.
2. Assess gastrointestinal symptoms before initiating therapy to serve as baseline data, for example, status of mouth (ulcerations and mucositis), bowel pattern (diarrhea), anorexia, nausea, and vomiting.
3. Review baseline laboratory data for degree of myelosuppression present.
4. Discuss birth control methods and sperm storage before initiating therapy.

DRUG CLASS: Natural Products

Actions

Vinca Alkaloids

Vincristine and vinblastine are natural derivatives of the periwinkle plant. They are cell cycle–specific agents that block the formation of the mitotic spindle during mitosis, thus inhibiting cell division. Even though there is close structural similarity, cross-resistance does not usually develop between the two agents.

Antibiotics

Through various mechanisms, the antibiotics bind with cellular DNA, preventing its replication as well as RNA synthesis, which is required for subsequent protein synthesis.

Uses

See Table 44-1.

Therapeutic Outcomes

The primary therapeutic outcome from natural product therapy is eradication of malignant cells.

Nursing Process for Natural Products

Premedication Assessment

1. Check laboratory reports for baseline data reflecting hepatic function.
2. Assess for peripheral neuropathy, mentation, orientation, gait, and motor weakness before initiation of therapy with the natural products.
3. Review baseline laboratory data for degree of myelosuppression present.
4. Discuss birth control methods, sperm storage, and egg harvesting before initiating therapy.

DRUG CLASS: Antineoplastic Antibiotics

Actions

The antineoplastic antibiotics bind to DNA, inhibiting DNA or RNA synthesis. This eventually inhibits protein synthesis, preventing cell replication. Dactinomycin, daunorubicin, doxorubicin, and possibly mitomycin are cell cycle–nonspecific agents. It is not known whether bleomycin and plicamycin are cycle-specific or cycle-nonspecific agents.

Uses

See Table 44-1.

Therapeutic Outcomes

The primary therapeutic outcome from antineoplastic antibiotic therapy is eradication of malignant cells.

Nursing Process for Antineoplastic Antibiotics

Premedication Assessment

1. Check laboratory reports for baseline data reflecting hepatic and renal function.
2. Assess the patient's history for cardiac disease before use of antineoplastic antibiotics. Report presence to the health care provider before initiation of therapy.
3. Assess gastrointestinal symptoms before initiation of therapy to serve as baseline data for example, status of mouth (ulcerations and mucositis), bowel pattern (diarrhea), anorexia, nausea, and vomiting.
4. Assess respiratory function and review the chart for any tests that may indicate compromised respiratory function before treatment with bleomycin.
5. Review baseline laboratory data for degree of myelosuppression present.
6. Review medical records for indications of allergies.
7. Discuss birth control methods, sperm storage, and egg harvesting before initiating therapy.

DRUG CLASS: Hormones

Actions

Corticosteroids (usually prednisone) may be beneficial in treating lymphomas and acute leukemia because of their lympholytic effects and their ability to suppress mitosis in lymphocytes. Steroids are also used to help reduce edema secondary to radiation therapy and as palliative therapy in temporarily suppressing fever, diaphoresis, and pain and in restoring, to some degree, appetite, weight, strength, and a sense of well-being in critically ill patients. With symptomatic relief, it is hoped that the patient's general physical condition may be improved sufficiently to permit further definitive therapy.

Uses

Estrogens and androgens are used in malignancies of sexual organs based on the assumption that these malignancies have hormonal requirements similar to those of nonmalignant sexual organs. Estrogens (usually diethylstilbestrol) may be used in prostatic carcinoma. There are regressions in the primary tumor and in soft tissue metastases, with significant symptomatic relief from the point of view of the patient. Androgens may be used in the treatment of metastatic breast cancer in any age-group, and estrogens may be used in postmenopausal women with metastatic breast cancer (see Table 44-1).

Therapeutic Outcomes

The primary therapeutic outcome from hormone therapy is reduction in rate of growth and proliferation of malignant cells.

Nursing Process for Hormones

Premedication Assessment

1. Obtain baseline weight vital signs, especially blood pressure.
2. Discuss birth control methods and sperm storage before initiation of therapy.
3. Check baseline electrolytes (e.g., calcium with diethylstilbestrol, tamoxifen, testosterone).

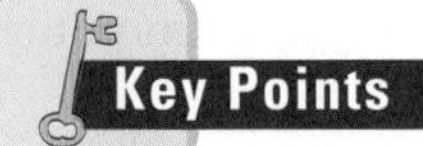

- Nurses play a crucial role in the treatment of patients with cancer. No other disease seems to evoke fear and anxiety equal to the effect that the diagnosis of cancer has on the patient and family. Nurses are often the contact between the health care provider, patient and family in helping with adaptation to the diagnosis and entry into the health care system for treatment.
- Nurses are often first to identify complications of therapy, such as recognizing and reporting early symptoms of infection in an immunocompromised patient. Early recognition and prompt action often reduce the severity of the complications.
- It is important for nurses caring for cancer patients to research all drugs prescribed for the patient and to perform focused assessments on body systems known to be affected by the specific agents administered.
- Health teaching for the patient and significant others is essential to achieving the best response to the therapeutic regimen prescribed. Everyone involved in the patient's care need to understand the purpose of the medications prescribed and when to contact the physician for any problems encountered. The patient and significant others must feel like integral parts of the team, whose members desire the best possible quality of life for those affected by the disease.
- Nurses are active providers of public information on wellness. They also coordinate screening programs for the early detection of cancer.

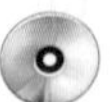

Go to your Companion CD-ROM for Appendices, an Audio Glossary, animations, Drug Dosage Calculators, customizable Patient Self-Assessment forms, and Review Questions for the NCLEX® Examination.

evolve Be sure to visit the companion Evolve site at http://evolve.elsevier.com/Clayton for WebLinks and additional online resources.

MEDICATION SAFETY REVIEW

MATH REVIEW QUESTIONS

1. Order: Cefazolin 1 g IV q8h

   Available: Cefazolin 1 g diluted in 50 mL D5W

   To administer this medication over a 30-minute period on a pump that is calibrated in milliliters per hour, what rate would the pump be set?

2. Order: PCA morphine sulfate 1 mg per dose with 6-minute lockout. Maximum 30 mg q4h.

   Discuss how to initiate the PCA setup on this patient, how to set up the initial settings on the PCA pump, and when and how to record the amount of morphine sulfate used each shift.

CRITICAL THINKING QUESTIONS

Situation: A 65-year-old patient has small cell cancer of the lung with brain and liver metastases. He has had several grand mal seizures in the past month. His orders read:

- Daily weight
- Assist with ambulation as tolerated
- Routine vitals
- Seizure precautions
- Intake and output
- Heparin lock the IV
- Physical therapy consult to assist with plan for self-care at home
- IV site dressing change every 72 hours

Medications:

Folic acid 1 mg PO daily

Multivitamin 1 PO daily

Ensure, 1 can tid

KCl 20 mEq PO bid

NS flush 2.5 mL, heparin lock after medications

ranitidine 300 mg PO at bedtime

ondansetron 32 mg IV 30 minutes before chemotherapy

dexamethasone 10 mg IV before chemotherapy, then 6 mg q6h for a total of four doses

phenytoin 300 mg PO daily

lorazepam 1 mg PO q12h

1. Develop a Kardex for this patient and a medication administration record (MAR) that includes the scheduling of each medication.
2. For each medication prescribed, state the action, side effects to expect, and side effects to report.
3. For IV medications prescribed, state the action, rate of administration, dilution for administration, monitoring required, and what type of IV setup would be required to initiate the IV delivery of the medications.

Situation: A 68-year-old patient has metastatic cervical cancer. She has the following medication orders:

- D5W/0.45% NS at 100 mL/hr
- ondansetron 32 mg IV in 50 mL D5W to run for 15 minutes
- dexamethasone 5 mg IV prior to chemotherapy, then 4 mg q6h for a total of four doses.
- Aprepitant 125 mg PO 1 hour before chemotherapy on day 1, followed by 80 mg once daily in the morning on days 2 and 3 of the treatment regimen
- cisplatin 100 mg in 2 L D5W/0.45% NS to run for 8 hours
- Add mannitol 37.5 g to cisplatin

4. Chemotherapy is usually given through a central venous access device for maximum dilution because it is an irritating medication. As a chemotherapy-certified nurse, what would be your responsibilities during the execution of these orders? (You may need to refer to Chapter 12 for this information.) What is the action of each medication, side effects to expect, and side effects to report?
5. How would you set a pump to deliver the ondansetron in 15 minutes? (The pump is calibrated in mL/hr.) At what rate would the same type of pump be set to administer the cisplatin?
6. Study the targeted anticancer agents, chemoprotective agents, and bone marrow stimulants to identify the major indications for use.

Continued

CONTENT REVIEW QUESTIONS

1. When the drug monograph says that a particular chemotherapeutic agent may cause thrombocytopenia, it is important that the nurse teach the patient to:
   1. avoid having fresh flowers, vegetables, or fruit.
   2. rise slowly from a sitting or lying position to avoid hypotension.
   3. report "coffee ground" emesis, hematuria, or epistaxis.
   4. obtain adequate daily exercise.
2. The purpose of administering epoetin alfa (Procrit) to a patient receiving chemotherapy is to:
   1. stimulate WBC production.
   2. stimulate RBC production.
   3. prevent thrombocytopenia.
   4. protect the kidneys from toxic chemotherapy.
3. The drug mesna (Mesnex) is given to:
   1. stimulate WBC production.
   2. stimulate RBC production.
   3. prevent thrombocytopenia.
   4. protect the bladder from toxic chemotherapy.
4. The purpose of androgens in the treatment of cancer is to:
   1. alter the female hormone environment to prevent cancer cell growth.
   2. facilitate the development of testosterone to prevent cancer cell growth.
   3. inhibit RNA synthesis.
   4. provide a cell cycle–specific chemotherapeutic agent.
5. What is the overall goal of cancer chemotherapy?
   1. To give a dose large enough to kill the cancer cells but tolerable enough for normal cells
   2. To kill all fast-growing cells without harmful side effects
   3. To alleviate symptoms of cancer
   4. To destroy cellular proliferation
6. Corticosteroids may be beneficial in treating what type of cancer?
   1. Ovarian and uterine cancer
   2. Breast cancer
   3. Lymphomas and acute leukemia
   4. Lung cancer
7. Which of the following interventions would be helpful to the patient who is experiencing diarrhea related to chemotherapy?
   1. Increase high-fiber foods
   2. Increase amounts of hot and cold beverages
   3. Increase intake of potassium-containing foods
   4. Avoid foods that cause constipation

CHAPTER 45

Drugs Used to Treat the Muscular System

evolve http://evolve.elsevier.com/Clayton

Chapter Content

Objectives

1. Prepare a list of assessment data needed to evaluate a patient with a skeletal muscle disorder.
2. State the nursing assessments needed to monitor therapeutic response and the development of side effects to expect and report from skeletal muscle relaxant therapy.
3. Develop a health teaching plan for patients with skeletal muscle relaxant therapy.
4. Describe the effect of centrally acting skeletal muscle relaxants on the central nervous system and the safety precautions required during use.
5. Describe essential components of patient assessment used for patients receiving neuromuscular blocking agents.
6. State where information on the use of these agents is found in the patient's chart.
7. List the equipment that should be available in the immediate patient care area when neuromuscular blocking agents are to be administered.
8. Describe the physiologic effects of neuromuscular blocking agents.
9. Cite four uses of neuromuscular blocking agents.
10. Identify the effect of neuromuscular blocking agents on consciousness, memory, and the pain threshold.
11. Describe disease conditions that may affect the patient's ability to tolerate the use of neuromuscular blocking agents.
12. List steps required to treat respiratory depression.

Key Terms

cerebral palsy
multiple sclerosis
hypercapnia
muscle spasticity
hyperreflexia
clonus
stroke syndrome
neuromuscular blocking agents

MUSCLE RELAXANTS AND NEUROMUSCULAR BLOCKING AGENTS

NURSING PROCESS *for Skeletal Muscle Relaxants and Neuromuscular Blocking Agents*

Assessment

Assessment for Skeletal Muscle Disorders. Musculoskeletal disorders may produce varying degrees of pain and immobility, impairing the individual's ability to perform the activities of daily living. The nursing assessments performed are individualized to the muscles affected and the underlying disease.

Current History

- What is the reason for seeking treatment now? Request a brief history of any symptoms present.
- What is the degree of impairment present (e.g., strength, gait, conservation effect, compensatory action)? What is the effect on usual daily activities (e.g., dressing, preparing meals, eating, performing basic hygiene, maintaining home)?
- Assess the pain level and extent, frequency of analgesic use, precipitating factors, and any measures the patient has identified that alleviate pain.
- Assess the extent of muscle spasticity and the muscle groups affected. Are there impairments that affect the patient's self-care, activities of daily living, or ability to fulfill work responsibilities?

History

- Ask the patient to describe diagnoses that cause musculoskeletal impairment (e.g., scoliosis, poliomyelitis, rickets, osteoarthritis, cerebral palsy, multiple sclerosis, muscular dystrophy, spinal cord injury, stroke).
- Have there been any injuries to or surgeries on the musculoskeletal system (e.g., dislocations, sprains, fractures, joint replacements)? If so, obtain details.

Medication History

- Ask the patient to list all prescribed and over-the-counter (OTC) medications taken within the past 6 months. Are any herbal medicines being taken? Ask specifically about antiinflammatory or corticosteroid use.

- What has been the response to the medications taken (e.g., antiinflammatory, analgesics, skeletal muscle relaxants)?
- What are the medications most recently taken and when were they taken?
- What nonpharmacologic treatments are being used (e.g., heating pad, massage therapy, acupuncture, cupping)?

Activity and Exercise

- What is the extent of usual daily exercise?
- Determine which activities of daily living can be performed independently and which require assistance.
- Ask about any assistive devices used (e.g., cane, walker).

Sleep and Rest. Does the pain of repositioning at night awaken the patient? Seek further information regarding the positions that initiate pain, the type of padding or additional pillows or devices being used for positioning.

Elimination. Ask specifically about the ability to toilet independently. Does mobility interfere with this function? Is constipation, diarrhea, or incontinence a problem? If so, how is it managed?

Nutrition

- Take a diet history. Are the four food groups included? Are supplemental vitamins and minerals (e.g., calcium) taken daily?
- Weigh the individual and ask whether there has been a weight gain or loss over the past 6 months. If so, obtain details.

Physical Examination

- Inspect the affected part for swelling, edema, bruises, redness, localized tenderness, deformities, or malalignments. (Be gentle during the inspection.)
- During examination, note differences in circumference, symmetry, or length of limbs.
- Record any abnormalities present (e.g., scoliosis, contractures, atrophy).
- Record range of motion present in joints, gait, and degree of mobility.

Laboratory and Diagnostic Studies

- Review diagnostic studies performed (e.g., x-rays, magnetic resonance imaging [MRI], computed tomography [CT], arthroscopic reports, bone scan, bone mass measurements, endoscopy).
- Examine laboratory reports associated with the disease process present (e.g., calcium, phosphorus, lupus testing, rheumatoid factor, uric acid level, C-reactive protein, human leukocyte antigen, aldolase, aspartate, creatine kinase).

Assessment for Neuromuscular Blocking Agents

- Assessment of the patient's vital signs, mental status, and particularly, respiratory function is mandatory for people having received neuromuscular blocking agents. The side effects associated with these drugs may occur 48 hours or more after administration. Close observation of respiratory function, ability to swallow secretions, and the presence of a cough reflex is necessary. Suction, oxygen, mechanical ventilators, and resuscitation equipment should be available in the immediate area.
- Monitor blood pressure, pulse, and respirations. Review the baseline readings of the patient's vital signs before administration of anesthetic and neuromuscular blocking agents. Generally, changes from the baseline should be reported.
- Monitor the patient closely for clinical signs of hypoxia and **hypercapnia** (tachycardia, hypotension, and cyanosis). Arterial blood gases (ABGs; see Table 31-1) may be drawn to accurately confirm the clinical observations.

Detection of Respiratory Depression

- Early signs of diminished ventilation are difficult to detect, particularly in the immediate postoperative period. Often the signs of restlessness, anxiety, lethargy, decreased mental alertness, and headache are early, subtle clues to distress.
- Use of the abdominal, intercostal, or neck muscles is an indication of respiratory distress. Flaring of the nostrils may be present in severe cases.
- As respiratory distress progresses, respirations become shallow and rapid. Assess for asymmetric chest movements.
- The development of cyanosis is a late sign of respiratory complications. Respiratory distress should be detected early through close observation before cyanosis develops.
- Assess muscle strength by asking the patient to lift his or her head off the pillow and hold a few seconds.

Pain Assessment. Assess the degree of pain present because neuromuscular blocking agents paralyze the muscles but do NOT relieve pain.

Nursing Diagnoses

- Pain, acute or chronic (indication)
- Activity intolerance (indication, side effect)
- Body image, disturbed (indication)
- Self-care deficit (bathing, hygiene, others) (indication)
- Injury, risk for (indication, side effect)
- Physical mobility, impaired (indication)

Planning

Planning must be done cooperatively with the patient and significant others. Adaptations in care needs must be based on the individual's ability to perform the activities of daily living and self-care.

Medications. When on an inpatient service, the prescribed medications and schedule are listed on the medication administration record (MAR). For patients being instructed in self-care at home, obtain prescriptions and perform health teaching.

Activity and Exercise

- Discuss the specifics of the prescribed regimen (e.g., degree of exercise allowed, bed rest, immobilization).
- Review treatments prescribed, such as hot and cold applications.

Psychosocial

- Plan with the patient for at-home management of the musculoskeletal problems and needed supportive services or referrals.
- When self-care is no longer possible, involve appropriate resource personnel in patient placement in a care facility.

Implementation

Nursing Interventions with Musculoskeletal Disorders

- Assist with physical examination, drawing of blood samples, obtaining vital signs, and weighing for preparation for diagnostic procedures.
- Adapt procedures to meet the self-care abilities of the individual patient.
- Administer prescribed medications (e.g., antiinflammatory drugs, analgesics, muscle relaxants).
- Provide specific instructions on the application of hot or cold packs. Generally, ice packs alleviate swelling immediately after muscle injury. Later in the course of treatment, heat application provides comfort.
- Elevating the extremity immediately after injury decreases swelling and to some degree alleviates pain.
- Maintain the activity level prescribed (e.g., bed rest, immobilization of muscle group or limb). During the initial phase of treatment, immobilizing the affected part will decrease muscle spasms and therefore decrease pain. Maintenance of proper alignment of the affected part will also relieve pain and swelling. Various approaches may be used for immobilization, including elastic bandages, splinting, casts, bed rest, or modified activity levels.
- Range-of-motion exercises may be prescribed to maintain joint function and to prevent muscle atrophy and contractures. The activity plan prescribed must be individualized to the diagnosis and should be carefully followed for maximum effectiveness.
- Increased anxiety produces stress on the body's muscles. Implement measures to produce relaxation and provide for the psychological needs of the individual.

Nursing Interventions with Neuromuscular Blockers

- Neuromuscular blockers are used during anesthesia and surgery to relax muscle groups and during the use of mechanical ventilation to improve airflow and oxygenation of the patient. See a general medical-surgical nursing text for a detailed discussion of nursing care while the patient is receiving mechanical ventilation. The patient must be intubated and receiving mechanical ventilation before administration of neuromuscular blocking agents.
- Monitor airway patency, respiratory rate, and tidal volume in accordance with hospital policy.
- The histamine release caused by these drugs may produce increased salivation. In patients who are paralyzed or who have incomplete return of control over swallowing, coughing, and deep breathing, these secretions may obstruct the airway.
- Assess for dyspnea and loud or gurgling sounds with respirations. Suction secretions according to hospital policies and procedures. If qualified, palpate for coarse chest wall vibrations and listen for rales or rhonchi.
- Deep-breathing exercises can allow the opportunity to assess the patient's cough reflex. Assist the patient by splinting any abdominal or thoracic incisions. Have the patient take three or four deep breaths and then cough. During this process, assess the patient's ability to breathe deeply. Cupping your hand and holding it a few inches from the patient's mouth while the patient breathes allows you to feel the air being exhaled.
- Patients can usually cough better in a semi-Fowler's or high Fowler's position; therefore depending on the situation and stability of the patient's vital signs, elevating the head of the bed may assist coughing and breathing. For unconscious or semiconscious individuals, position on the side, using good body alignment. Keep the bed's side rails up.
- People still paralyzed by the effects of these agents may experience pain and be unable to speak to request medication. Ensure that analgesics are scheduled on a regular basis and administered on time.
- Deal calmly with the patient experiencing respiratory dysfunction. The inability to breathe may cause the patient to panic. Give reassurance while initiating measures to assist the patient.
- Question antibiotic orders that prescribe aminoglycosides or tetracycline when neuromuscular blockers have been used. These drugs may potentiate the neuromuscular blocking activity.

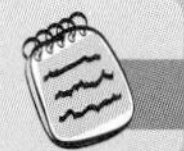

Patient Education and Health Promotion

Pain Relief

- The degree of musculoskeletal pain relief with and without activity must be discussed. Make modifications appropriate to the diagnosis and degree of impairment.
- Teach procedures designed to relieve pain (e.g., application of cold or heat, elevation of body part, proper body alignment).

Activities and Exercise. The patient must resume activities of daily living within the boundaries set by the health care provider. (Activities such as regular

PATIENT SELF-ASSESSMENT FORM Muscle Relaxants

MEDICATIONS	COLOR	TO BE TAKEN

Patient ____________________

Health Care Provider ____________________

Health Care Provider's phone ____________________

Next appt.* ____________________

What I Should Monitor			Premedication Data	Date	Date	Date	Date	Date	Date	Comments
Muscle areas affected	List areas 1. 2. 3. 4.		AM	AM	AM	AM	AM	AM	AM	
Chart areas affected two times per day	Example: 1. Arm, lower 2. Lower back 3. 4.	AM 1, 2 PM 1, 2	PM	PM	PM	PM	PM	PM	PM	
Exercise and range of motion pain No improvement 10 — Moderate improvement 5 — Much improvement 1										
Pattern of pain	Location									
	Time of day pain occurs									
	Relieved by									
	Made worse by									
Impairment(s) and improvement	Example: Could not comb hair—can now; could not turn head—can now									
Physical therapy prescribed	Example: Application of cold packs at 8 AM, 4 PM, and bedtime	Therapy								
		Time of day								
		Feeling, response								
Other										

*Please bring this record with you to your next appointment.
Use the back of this sheet for additional information.

moderate exercise, meal preparation, resumption of usual sexual activities, and social interaction must all be encouraged once specific orders are obtained.)

Psychosocial. For chronic disorders, encourage the patient to express feelings regarding chronic illness. The adjustment to this situation involves working through great personal fears, frustrations, hostilities, and resentments associated with the loss of personal control within one's life.

Medications. Many of the medications used in the treatment of musculoskeletal disorders produce sedation. Teach the patient about maintaining safety precautions such as avoiding power equipment or driving while taking these medications.

Fostering Health Maintenance

- Throughout the course of treatment discuss medication information and the individual's expectations of therapy. Ensure that the individual understands the activity level prescribed, pain relief methods and safety precautions to ensure personal safety during mobility.
- Seek cooperation and understanding of the following points so that medication compliance is increased: name of medication, dosage, route and

times of administration, side effects to expect, and side effects to report.

Written Record. Enlist the patient's aid in developing and maintaining a written record of monitoring parameters (e.g., level, location and duration of pain; areas or muscles affected; degree of impairment with improvement in mobility; exercise tolerance) (see Patient Self-Assessment Form on p. 738). Complete the Premedication Data column for use as a baseline to track response to drug therapy. Episodes of nausea, vomiting, or diarrhea should also be reported for the physician's evaluation if it is a new symptom. Ensure that the patient understands how to use the form and instruct the patient to take the completed form to follow-up visits. During follow-up visits, focus on issues that will foster adherence with the therapeutic interventions prescribed. ■

DRUG THERAPY FOR MUSCLE DISORDERS

DRUG CLASS: Centrally Acting Skeletal Muscle Relaxants

Actions

The centrally acting skeletal muscle relaxants belong to a class of compounds used to relieve acute muscle spasm. The exact mechanism of action of the centrally acting skeletal muscle relaxants is not known, except that they act by central nervous system (CNS) depression. They do not have any direct effect on muscles, nerve conduction, or neuromuscular junctions. All of these muscle relaxants produce some degree of sedation, and most health care providers believe that the benefits of these agents come from their sedative effects rather than from actual muscle relaxation.

Uses

The centrally acting skeletal muscle relaxants are used in combination with physical therapy, rest, and analgesics to relieve muscle spasm associated with acute, painful musculoskeletal conditions. They should not be used in **muscle spasticity** associated with cerebral or spinal cord disease because they may reduce the strength of remaining active muscle fibers and produce further impairment and debilitation.

Therapeutic Outcomes

The primary therapeutic outcome expected from centrally acting skeletal muscle relaxant therapy is relief from muscle spasm.

Nursing Process for Centrally Acting Skeletal Muscle Relaxants

Premedication Assessment

1. Obtain baseline vital signs and mental status of patient.
2. Have ordered laboratory studies drawn (e.g., liver function studies, complete blood count [CBC]).

Planning

Availability. See Table 45-1.

Implementation

Dosage and Administration. See Table 45-1.

Drug Table 45-1 CENTRALLY ACTING MUSCLE RELAXANTS

GENERIC NAME	BRAND NAME	ADULT DOSAGE (PO)	COMMENTS
carisoprodol	Soma	350 mg four times daily	Onset of action: 30 min; duration: 4 to 6 hr
chlorphenesin carbamate	Maolate	400-800 mg three or four times daily	Recommended only for short-term treatment (8 wk) of muscle spasm induced by trauma or inflammation; may cause blood dyscrasias
chlorzoxazone	Paraflex	250-750 mg three or four times daily	Commonly causes gastrointestinal discomfort; may be hepatotoxic
cyclobenzaprine	Flexeril	10 mg three times daily; do not exceed 60 mg	Recommended only for short-term treatment (2-3 wk) of painful musculoskeletal conditions; very sedating
metaxalone	Skelaxin	800 mg three or four times daily	Use with caution in patients with liver disease; causes false-positive Clinitest reaction
methocarbamol	Robaxin	1-1.5 g four times daily	Parenteral forms also available
orphenadrine citrate	Norflex	100 mg two times daily	Also has analgesic properties; do not use in patients with glaucoma or prostatic hyperplasia
tizanidine	Zanaflex	4-8 mg every 6 to 8 hours; do not exceed 36 mg daily	Peak effects at 1 to 2 hr and dissipates between 3 to 6 hr. Used for management of increased muscle tone associated with spasticity

Evaluation

Side Effects to Expect

Sedation, Weakness, Lethargy, Gastrointestinal Complaints. These side effects are usually mild and tend to resolve with continued therapy. Encourage the patient not to discontinue therapy without first consulting the health care provider.

Provide for patient safety for the duration of these symptoms. Patients must avoid operating power equipment or driving.

Dizziness. Provide for patient safety during episodes of dizziness; report for further evaluation.

Side Effects to Report

Hepatotoxicity. The symptoms of hepatotoxicity are anorexia, nausea, vomiting, jaundice, hepatomegaly, splenomegaly, and abnormal liver function tests (e.g., elevated bilirubin, aspartate aminotransferase [AST], alanine aminotransferase [ALT], gamma-glutamyltransferase [GGT], alkaline phosphatase, prothrombin time).

Blood Dyscrasias. Routine laboratory studies (e.g., red blood cell [RBC], white blood cell [WBC], differential counts) are scheduled for patients taking these agents for 30 days or longer. Stress the importance of returning for this laboratory work.

Monitor for the development of sore throat, fever, purpura, jaundice, or excessive progressive weakness.

Drug Interactions

CNS Depressants. Alcohol, narcotics, barbiturates, anticonvulsants, sedative-hypnotics, tranquilizers, phenothiazines, and antidepressants. People who work around machinery, drive a car, pour and give medicines, or perform other duties that require mental alertness should not take these medications while working.

baclofen (bak′ lo fen)

▶ LIORESAL (ly or′ e sahl)

Actions

Baclofen is a skeletal muscle relaxant that acts somewhat differently from the centrally acting musculoskeletal agents. Its complete mechanism of action is unknown, although reflex activity at the spinal cord is partially inhibited.

Uses

Baclofen is used in the management of muscle spasticity resulting from multiple sclerosis, spinal cord injuries, and other spinal cord diseases. It is not recommended for use in spasticity associated with Parkinson's disease, cerebral palsy, stroke, or rheumatic disorders. Use with caution in patients who must use spasticity to maintain an upright posture and balance in moving.

Therapeutic Outcomes

The primary therapeutic outcome expected from baclofen therapy is relief from muscle spasm.

Nursing Process for Baclofen

Premedication Assessment

1. Check history for any spastic disorders (e.g., Parkinson's disease, cerebral palsy, stroke, rheumatic disorders). If present, withhold medication and check with physician.
2. Perform a baseline mental status examination.

Planning

Availability. PO: 10 and 20 mg tablets; 10 and 20 mg orally disintegrating tablets; intrathecal: 0.05 mg/mL, 0.5 mg/mL, 2 mg/mL ampules.

Implementation

Dosage and Administration. *Adult:* PO: Initially 5 mg three times daily. Increase the dosage by 5 mg every 3 to 7 days based on response. Optimum effects are usually noted at dosages of 40 to 80 mg daily but may take several weeks to achieve. Orally disintegrating tablets are available for more rapid onset of action and for patients who have difficulty swallowing.

NOTE: Do not abruptly discontinue therapy. Severe exacerbation of spasticity and hallucinations may result.

Evaluation

Side Effects to Expect

Nausea, Fatigue, Headache, Drowsiness. These side effects are usually mild and tend to resolve with continued therapy. Encourage the patient not to discontinue therapy without first consulting the health care provider.

Dizziness. Provide for patient safety during episodes of dizziness; report for further evaluation.

Drug Interactions

CNS Depressants. CNS depressants, including sleep aids, analgesics, tranquilizers, and alcohol, potentiate the sedative effects of baclofen. Persons who are working around machinery, driving a car, pouring and giving medicines, or performing other duties in which they must remain mentally alert should not take these medications while working.

DRUG CLASS: Direct-Acting Skeletal Muscle Relaxant

dantrolene (dan′ tro leen)

▶ DANTRIUM (dan′ tree um)

Actions

Dantrolene is a muscle relaxant that acts directly on skeletal muscle. It produces generalized mild weakness of skeletal muscles and decreases the force of reflex muscle contractions, **hyperreflexia, clonus,** muscle stiffness, involuntary muscle movements, and spasticity.

Uses

Dantrolene is used to control the spasticity of chronic disorders such as cerebral palsy, multiple sclerosis, spinal cord injury, and stroke syndrome. It is also used to treat neuroleptic malignant syndrome associated with the use of antipsychotic agents (see p. 292).

Therapeutic Outcomes

The primary therapeutic outcome expected from dantrolene therapy is relief from muscle spasm.

Nursing Process for Dantrolene

Premedication Assessment

1. When used for neuroleptic malignant syndrome, perform a baseline assessment of vital signs, especially temperature.
2. Establish a baseline of degree of muscle symptoms present.

Planning

Availability. PO: 25, 50, and 100 mg capsules; IV: 0.32 mg/mL in 70 mL vials.

Implementation

Dosage and Administration. *Adult:* PO: Initially 25 mg daily. Increase to 25 mg two, three, or four times daily at 4- to 7-day intervals, then gradually increase the dosage up to 100 mg two, three, or four times daily. A small number of patients may require 200 mg four times daily.

Evaluation

Side Effects to Expect

Weakness, Diarrhea, Drowsiness. These side effects are usually mild and tend to resolve with continued therapy. They can often be minimized by starting therapy with low doses. Encourage the patient not to discontinue therapy without first consulting the health care provider.

Dizziness, Lightheadedness. Provide for patient safety during episodes of dizziness; report for further evaluation.

Response to Therapy. Tell the patient that effectiveness of the drug may not be apparent for 1 week or longer. Encourage the patient not to discontinue therapy without first consulting the health care provider.

Side Effects to Report

Photosensitivity. The patient should be cautioned to avoid exposure to sunlight and ultraviolet light. Suggest wearing long-sleeved clothing, hat, and sunglasses while exposed to sunlight. The patient must not use tanning lamps. The patient should not discontinue therapy without notifying the health care provider.

Hepatotoxicity. The symptoms of hepatotoxicity are anorexia, nausea, vomiting, jaundice, hepatomegaly, splenomegaly, and abnormal liver function tests (e.g., elevated bilirubin, AST, ALT, GGT, alkaline phosphatase, prothrombin time).

Drug Interactions

CNS Depressants. CNS depressants, including sleeping aids, analgesics, tranquilizers, and alcohol, will potentiate the sedative effects of dantrolene. People who work around machinery, drive a car, pour and give medicines, or perform other duties that require mental alertness should not take these medications while working.

DRUG CLASS: Neuromuscular Blocking Agents

Actions

Neuromuscular blocking agents act by interrupting transmission of impulses from motor nerves to muscles at the skeletal neuromuscular junction. Neuromuscular blocking agents have no effect on consciousness, memory, or the pain threshold. Reassurance by nursing personnel is essential to paralyzed patients (e.g., those on ventilators), and analgesics and sedatives must be administered on schedule. These patients may suffer extreme pain and may be unable to ask for analgesics.

Uses

Neuromuscular blocking agents are important skeletal muscle relaxants. These agents are used to produce adequate muscle relaxation during anesthesia to reduce the use (and side effects) of general anesthetics, ease endotracheal intubation and prevent laryngospasm, decrease muscular activity in electroshock therapy, and aid in the muscle spasms associated with tetanus.

Therapeutic Outcomes

The primary therapeutic outcome expected from neuromuscular blocking therapy is smooth and skeletal muscle relaxation.

Nursing Process for Neuromuscular Blocking Agents

Premedication Assessment

1. These drugs are administered by an anesthetist or anesthesiologist during surgical anesthesia or when a patient is placed or being maintained on a ventilator. Check hospital policy for who may administer these drugs and specific monitoring parameters.
2. Check history for hepatic, pulmonary, renal disease or neurologic disorders such as myasthenia gravis, spinal cord injury, or multiple sclerosis. If present, tag the chart appropriately before administration of anesthesia.
3. Have oxygen, suction, and artificial respiration equipment available in the immediate area whenever these drugs are to be used. Also have antidotes (e.g., neostigmine methylsulfate [Prostigmin], pyridostigmine

bromide [Mestinon, Regonol], edrophonium chloride [Tensilon]) available.

Planning

Availability. See Table 45-2.

Implementation

Administration. These agents are usually given intravenously (IV) but may also be given intramuscularly (IM). Because they are potent drugs, they should be used only by people thoroughly familiar with their effects, such as an anesthetist or anesthesiologist, and under conditions in which the patient can receive constant, close attention for signs of respiratory failure. Adequate equipment for artificial respiration, antidotes, and other measures for prompt treatment of toxicity must be readily available.

Patients with hepatic, pulmonary, or renal disease or neurologic disorders such as myasthenia gravis, spinal cord injury, or multiple sclerosis must be fully evaluated to assess their ability to tolerate neuromuscular blocking agents. Much smaller doses are often necessary when these diseases are present. Neonates and elderly patients also require adjustments in dosage because of the insensitivity of their neuromuscular junction.

Treatment of Overdose. Treatment of overdose includes artificial respiration with oxygen and antidotes such as neostigmine methylsulfate (Prostigmin), pyridostigmine bromide (Mestinon, Regonol), and edrophonium chloride (Tensilon). Atropine sulfate is usually administered with neostigmine or pyridostigmine to block bradycardia, hypotension, and salivation induced by these agents. There is no antidote for the early blockade induced by succinylcholine. Fortunately, it is of short duration and does not require reversal.

Evaluation

Side Effects to Expect

Salivation. Neuromuscular blocking agents cause histamine release, which may cause bronchospasm, bronchial and salivary secretions, flushing, edema, and urticaria. Ensure that the airway is patent and that secretions are suctioned regularly to prevent obstruction. Report evidence of bronchospasm, edema, and urticaria immediately.

Mild Discomfort. Mild to moderate discomfort, particularly in the neck, upper back, and lower intercostal and abdominal muscles, will be noted when the patient first ambulates after use.

Side Effects to Report

Signs of Respiratory Distress. Monitor vital signs for a prolonged period after administration of neuromuscular blocking agents.

Diminished Cough Reflex, Inability to Swallow. Assess deep breathing and coughing at regular intervals. Have suction and oxygen equipment available, and be familiar with emergency code practices at your hospital.

Drug Interactions

Drugs That Enhance Therapeutic and Toxic Effects. General anesthetics (e.g., ether, fluroxene, methoxyflurane, enflurane, halothane, cyclopropane), aminoglycoside antibiotics (e.g., kanamycin, gentamicin, neomycin, streptomycin, netilmicin, tobramycin, amikacin), clindamycin, tetracycline, quinidine, quinine, procainamide, lidocaine, beta-adrenergic blocking agents (e.g., propranolol, timolol, pindolol, nadolol), aprotinin, tacrine, metoclopramide, lithium, and agents that deplete potassium (e.g., thiazide diuretics, furosemide, torsemide, bumetanide, ethacrynic acid, chlorthalidone, amphotericin B, corticosteroids), inhibit neuromuscular transmission, thus prolonging neuromuscular blockade.

Label charts of patients scheduled for surgery who are taking any of these agents. These combinations may potentiate respiratory depression. Check the anesthetist's records of surgical patients; monitor postoperative patients for respiratory depression for a prolonged period. This may occur 48 hours or more after drug administration.

Drugs That Reduce Therapeutic Effects. Neostigmine methylsulfate, pyridostigmine bromide, and

Drug Table 45-2 NEUROMUSCULAR BLOCKING AGENTS

GENERIC NAME	BRAND NAME	AVAILABILITY
atracurium besylate	Tracrium	10 mg/mL in 5 and 10 mL ampules
cisatracurium besylate	Nimbex	2 mg/mL in 5 and 10 mL vials; 10 mg/mL in 20 mL vials
mivacurium chloride	Mivacron	2 mg/mL in 5 and 10 mL vials
pancuronium bromide	Pancuronium	1 mg/mL in 10 mL vials; 2 mg/mL in 2 and 5 mL ampules
rocuronium bromide	Zemuron	10 mg/mL in 5 mL and 10 mL vials
succinylcholine	Anectine, Quelicin	20 mg/mL in 10 mL vials, 50 mg/mL in 10 mL ampules, 500 mg and 1 g powder in vials
tubocurarine chloride	Tubocurarine Chloride	3 mg/mL in 10 and 20 mg vials
vecuronium bromide	Norcuron	10 mg in 10 mL vials, 20 mg in 20 mL vials

edrophonium chloride. These agents are used as antidotes in case of overdosage of the neuromuscular blocking agents.

Carbamazepine hastens recovery time from neuromuscular blocking agents. Higher or more frequent doses of the neuromuscular blocking agent may be necessary.

Respiratory Depressants. Analgesics, sedatives, and tranquilizers, in combination with muscle relaxants, may potentiate respiratory depression. Check the anesthetist's records of surgical patients. Monitor postoperative patients for respiratory depression for a prolonged period. This may occur 48 hours or more after drug administration.

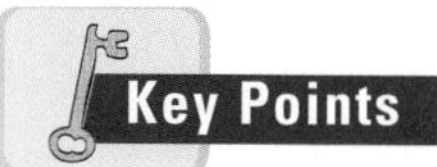

- Nurses can play an important role in providing counseling and guidance to patients and family in understanding muscle spasticity and pain and how to maintain an appropriate balance between daily activities and timing of analgesics to optimize quality of life.
- Nurses also play a crucial role in providing comfort and monitoring to patients who have received neuromuscular blocking agents. It is mandatory that nurses know how to recognize and respond quickly when respiratory emergencies arise.

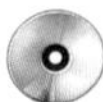

Go to your Companion CD-ROM for Appendices, an Audio Glossary, animations, Drug Dosage Calculators, customizable Patient Self-Assessment forms, and Review Questions for the NCLEX® Examination.

evolve Be sure to visit the companion Evolve site at http://evolve.elsevier.com/Clayton for WebLinks and additional online resources.

MEDICATION SAFETY REVIEW

MATH REVIEW QUESTIONS

1. Order: Methocarbamol (Robaxin) 1.5 g qid

   Convert 1.5 g to ______ mg.

2. Order: Pancuronium 2 mg

   Available: Pancuronium 1 mg/mL in 10-mL vial

   How many mL would you give? _____ mL

CRITICAL THINKING QUESTIONS

1. A patient presents with a "pulled muscle" in his back. The doctor prescribed cyclobenzaprine 10 mg three times daily for 1 week. Before the patient leaves the health care provider's office, what health teaching should you provide for the medication and temporary lifestyle changes?

Situation: After an extensive major surgical procedure, the patient is transferred to the postanesthesia recovery unit with an endotracheal tube in place. During the surgical procedure the anesthesia record notes the administration of tubocurarine chloride.

2. What criteria should be used to determine when to remove the endotracheal tube?
3. What monitoring of the patient should be done to check for residual effects of the neuromuscular blocking agent?
4. Examine the drug monographs to identify premedication assessments used with musculoskeletal agents.
5. Review drug monographs to identify the specific use of direct-acting and centrally acting skeletal muscle relaxants.
6. Research the cost of three of the centrally acting muscle relaxants at a local drug store or online.

CONTENT REVIEW QUESTIONS

1. Centrally acting skeletal muscle relaxant drugs should NOT be given to patients having:
   1. muscle spasms.
   2. cerebral or spinal cord disease.
   3. a sprained ankle.
   4. pulled back muscles.
2. Neuromuscular blocking agents require the availability of _____ to treat an overdose.
   1. dantrolene (Dantrium)
   2. baclofen (Lioresal)
   3. neostigmine methylsulfate (Prostigmin)
   4. carisoprodol (SOMA)

Continued

CONTENT REVIEW QUESTIONS—cont'd

3. Which of the following is an early sign of respiratory depression? *(Select all that apply.)*
   1. Restlessness
   2. Confusion
   3. Anxiety
   4. Cyanosis
4. Which antibiotics can potentiate neuromuscular blocking activity?
   1. Tetracyclines and aminoglycosides
   2. Cephalosporins and primaxin
   3. Macrolides
   4. Penicillins
5. Lioresal is used for the management of spasticity for which disease process?
   1. Multiple sclerosis
   2. Parkinson's disease
   3. Cerebral palsy
   4. Stroke
6. Dantrolene is used to treat spasticity of which of the following chronic diseases? *(Select all that apply.)*
   1. Cerebral palsy
   2. Multiple sclerosis
   3. Stroke syndrome
   4. Parkinson's disease
7. Neuromuscular blocking agents paralyze the muscles, but do NOT relieve pain.
   1. True
   2. False

CHAPTER

46 Antimicrobial Agents

evolve http://evolve.elsevier.com/Clayton

Chapter Content

Objectives

1. Identify significant data in a patient history that could alert the medical team that a patient is more likely to experience an allergic reaction.
2. Identify baseline data the nurse should collect on a continual basis for comparison and evaluation of antimicrobial drug effectiveness.
3. Describe basic principles of patient care that can be implemented to enhance an individual's therapeutic response during an infection.
4. Identify criteria used to select an effective antimicrobial agent.
5. Differentiate between gram-negative and gram-positive microorganisms and between anaerobic and aerobic properties of microorganisms.
6. Explain the major action and effects of drugs used to treat infectious diseases.
7. Describe the nursing assessments and interventions for the common side effects associated with antimicrobial agents: allergic reaction; direct tissue damage (e.g., nephrotoxicity, ototoxicity, hepatotoxicity); secondary infection; and other considerations such as photosensitivity, peripheral neuropathy, and neuromuscular blockage.
8. Review parenteral administration techniques and the procedure for vaginal insertion of drugs.
9. Develop a plan for implementing patient education for patients receiving aminoglycosides, carbapenems, cephalosporins, glycyclines, ketolides, penicillins, quinolones, streptogramins, sulfonamides, tetracyclines, antifungal agents, and antiviral agents.

Key Terms

pathogenic
antibiotics
nephrotoxicity
ototoxicity
gram-positive microorganisms
gram-negative microorganisms
hypoprothrombinemia
thrombophlebitis
penicillinase-resistant penicillins

ANTIMICROBIAL AGENTS

Antimicrobial agents are chemicals that eliminate living microorganisms that are **pathogenic** to the patient. Antimicrobial agents may be of chemical origin, such as the sulfonamides, or they may be derived from other living organisms. Those derived from other living microorganisms are called **antibiotics;** for example, penicillin was first derived from the mold *Penicillium notatum*. Most antibiotics used today are harvested from large colonies of microorganisms, which are then purified and chemically modified into semisynthetic antimicrobial agents. The chemical modification makes the antibiotic more effective against certain specific pathogenic organisms. Antimicrobial agents are often first classified according to the type of pathogen to be destroyed, such as bacteria (antibacterial agents), fungus (antifungal agents), or virus (antiviral agents). The antimicrobial agents are then subdivided by chemical families into drug classes such as the penicillins, tetracyclines, and aminoglycosides.

The selection of the antimicrobial agent must be based on the sensitivity of the pathogen and the possible toxicity to the patient. If at all possible, infecting organisms should first be isolated and identified. Culture and sensitivity tests should be completed. The antimicrobial therapy is then started based on the sensitivity results and the clinical judgment of the health care provider.

NURSING PROCESS *for Antimicrobial Therapy*

Nurses must consider the entire patient when administering and monitoring antimicrobial therapy. It is essential that the nurse be knowledgeable about the drugs, including physiologic parameters for monitoring expected therapeutic activity and adverse effects. It is important to teach the individual with an infection the basic principles of self-care, which will enhance the recovery process, and measures to prevent the spread of infection. With communicable diseases, exposed individuals must be contacted for follow-up testing and appropriate treatment.

Assessment

History of Current Infection

What symptoms are described by the patient? Which of the symptoms described potentially relate to an infectious process? Extend questioning to help the patient focus, e.g., when did the symptoms begin? Have they worsened? Is there fever, night sweats, malaise, chronic fatigue, weight loss, arthralgia, cough (type of secretions), diarrhea, painful urination, nausea, vomiting, lesions or skin rash, discharge, or drainage? Is there any swelling, pain, or heat in a particular area or discharge from a site? Has the patient been treated previously for a similar infection? Ask questions specific to the body systems affected by the infection (e.g., pain and burning with urination for a urinary tract infection [UTI]).

When treating patients with sexually transmitted diseases, ask about the number of sexual partners, sexual orientation, and use of precautions during intercourse. (See Chapter 41 for further details.)

Past History. Ask the patient about previously treated conditions. What treatments were used, and what was the response to therapy? Focus on areas that may impinge on antimicrobial therapy, such as reduced renal or hepatic function, immunocompromised conditions, blood dyscrasias, partial deafness, and gastrointestinal complaints.

Allergies. Is the patient allergic to certain medicines, dust, weeds, foods, or other environmental substances?

Medication History

- Ask the patient to list all current prescribed and over-the-counter (OTC) medications or those taken in the past 6 months. Ask specifically about any medicines, such as corticosteroids, chemotherapy, or transplant suppressants, that may affect the immune status of the individual.
- Does the person take any type of allergy injections or medications?
- Is the person immunized against childhood diseases (see Appendix E)?
- Has the person been treated for an infection recently? If yes, what medications were taken and were there any allergic responses? If so, ask for details of the symptoms of the allergic reaction.
- Has the patient taken this medication before? If so, what symptoms (such as nausea, vomiting, diarrhea, rash, itching, or hives) developed when taking it that led the patient to state that there is an allergy? Ask the patient to describe the appearance of a rash, where it started, and the course of recovery. How soon after starting the medication did the symptoms develop?
- Ask if the patient has ever developed a secondary infection (black hairy tongue; white patches [plaques] in mouth; or a vaginal infection) when taking an antibiotic. For example, women taking antibiotics may develop a vaginal infection because of suppression of normal flora.

Physical Examination

- Perform a head-to-toe body or functional assessment, focusing on the areas pertinent to the admitting diagnosis.
- Assess for risk factors that may contribute to development of infection, such as extensive surgical procedures, obesity, underlying contributory conditions (e.g., chronic obstructive pulmonary disease, diabetes), immunotherapy drugs, malnutrition, and age extremes (infant or older adults).

Psychosocial. For an individual with a serious communicable disease, assess the response and adaptive processes used to cope with the disease and its treatments.

Laboratory and Diagnostic Studies

- Review laboratory reports on the chart (e.g., complete blood count [CBC], urinalysis, creatinine clearance, blood urea nitrogen [BUN], aspartate aminotransferase [AST], alanine aminotransferase [ALT], gamma-glutamyl transferase [GGT], culture reports, electrolytes, screening tests for sexually transmitted diseases).
- Tuberculin skin testing and chest x-rays screen for exposure to tuberculosis. Sputum cultures are collected to confirm the presence of *Mycobacterium tuberculosis*.

Assessments during Antimicrobial Therapy

Read each drug monograph for specific side effects to expect and side effects to report, and individualize the assessments for the drugs prescribed. Nausea, vomiting, diarrhea, allergies, anaphylaxis, nephrotoxicity, hepatotoxicity, ototoxicity, hematologic dyscrasias, secondary infection, and photosensitivity are found with recurring frequency in the antimicrobial drug monographs.

- *Nausea, vomiting, and diarrhea:* These conditions are the "big three" side effects associated with antimicrobial drug therapy. When they occur, gather data such as the following:
  1. Did the patient have a history of nausea, vomiting, or diarrhea before starting the drug therapy?
  2. How soon after starting the medication did the symptoms start?

3. Since starting the medication, has the diet or water source changed in any way?
4. Was the patient taking other drugs, either prescription or OTC medications, before initiating antibiotic therapy?
5. How much fluid is the patient consuming when taking medications? Inadequate fluid intake sometimes causes gastritis manifested by nausea.
6. For diarrhea, what was the pattern of elimination before drug therapy? Report diarrhea, and the character and frequency of stools as well as any abdominal pain promptly. Nausea, vomiting, and diarrhea are often dose related and result from changes in normal bacterial flora in the bowel, irritation, and secondary infection. Symptoms resolve within a few days, and discontinuation of therapy is rarely required.

- *Secondary infection:* Assess for symptoms of secondary infection such as oral infection. Observe for a black hairy tongue, white patches (plaques) in the oral cavity, cold sores, canker sores, and glossitis. There may be lesions and itching in the vaginal and anal areas. Secondary infection of the intestine can produce severe life-threatening diarrhea.
- *Allergies and anaphylaxis:* The severity of allergic reaction ranges from a mild rash to fatal anaphylaxis. Allergic reactions may develop within 30 minutes of administration (e.g., anaphylaxis, laryngeal edema, shock, dyspnea, skin reactions) or may occur several days after discontinuing therapy (e.g., skin rashes, fever). All patients must be questioned for previous allergic reactions, and allergy-prone patients must be observed closely. It is important that a patient not be labeled "allergic" to a particular medication without adequate documentation. The medication to which a patient claims an allergy may be a lifesaving drug for that patient.
- *Nephrotoxicity:* Assess **nephrotoxicity** through an increasing BUN and creatinine, decreasing urine output, decreasing urine specific gravity, casts or protein in the urine, frank blood or smoky-colored urine, or red blood cells (RBCs) in excess of 0 to 3 RBC/HPF (see Table 42-1) on the urinalysis report.
- *Hepatotoxicity:* Assess for preexisting hepatic disease such as cirrhosis or hepatitis. Review laboratory studies (e.g., bilirubin, AST, ALT, GGT, alkaline phosphatase, prothrombin time) and report abnormal findings to the health care provider.
- *Ototoxicity:* Damage to the eighth cranial nerve, **ototoxicity**, can occur from drug therapy, particularly from aminoglycosides. This may initially be manifested by dizziness, tinnitus, and progressive hearing loss. Assess the patient for difficulty in walking unaided, and assess the level of hearing daily. Intentionally speak to patients softly; note if they are aware that you said anything. Take particular notice of the patient who repeatedly asks, "What did you say?" or who starts talking more loudly or progressively increases the volume on the television or radio.
- *Blood dyscrasias*
  1. Ask specifically about any history of blood disorders diagnosed and treatments prescribed.
  2. Ask specifically about any types of anemia (e.g., aplastic, hemolytic, megaloblastic) or deficiencies of folic acid, vitamin B_{12}, or glucose-6-phosphate dehydrogenase (G6PD).
  3. Ask whether the individual has received chemotherapy, radiation therapy, or transplant therapy, all of which may induce an immunocompromised state and changes in the blood.
  4. Has the patient received blood cell stimulator drugs such as Epogen or Neupogen?
  5. Does the patient have any bleeding disorders, such as hemophilia or thrombocytopenia?
  6. Observe for bleeding gums, prolonged bleeding at an injection site, petechiae, and epistaxis (nosebleeds).
  7. Review admission laboratory studies and report abnormalities (e.g., CBC with differential, BUN, creatinine).
- *Photosensitivity:* Assess for the development of dermatologic symptoms such as exaggerated sunburn, itching, rash, urticaria, pruritus, and scaling.

Nursing Diagnoses

- Infection, risk for (indication; side effect)
- Body temperature, imbalanced (indication)
- Fluid volume, deficient (indication, side effect)
- Injury, risk for (side effect)
- Fatigue (indication)

Planning

Medication Assessment

- Order medications prescribed and schedule these on the medication administration record (MAR).
- When scheduling the times of administration of antibiotic therapy, the other drugs prescribed and their potential interactions (e.g., antacids) should be taken into consideration. Antibiotics are usually given at even intervals over 24 hours to maintain cyclic blood levels of the medication. Orders such as four times daily (qid) should be clarified to determine whether the health care provider meant 8-12-4-8 o'clock or 12-6-12-6 o'clock administration times.
- Have any cultures been ordered before initiation of antimicrobial therapy? Mark the Kardex or enter data in computer when blood draws for serum level peak or trough are ordered.

- Request necessary infusion equipment for administration of prescribed antimicrobials (e.g., syringe pump or infusion pump).
- If a definite drug allergy is identified, the patient's chart, unit Kardex, and an identification bracelet should be carefully marked to alert all personnel to the specific drugs the patient should not receive.

Laboratory Tests. Order any stat or subsequent laboratory studies (e.g., culture and sensitivity, urinalysis, CBC, baseline electrolytes, renal or hepatic function tests).

Nursing Care. Individualize the nursing care plan for the type and severity of the infectious process. Monitor symptoms present, vital signs, and response to therapy including side effects to expect and to report as listed in individual drug monographs. Perform premedication assessments before administering prescribed antibiotic. Provide supportive nursing measures appropriate to the type of infection. Plan to provide health teaching to the patient and significant others regarding the patient's basic care, preventing spread of the infection, and medication regimen.

Implementation

- Routine monitoring of all individuals receiving antimicrobial therapy should include status of hydration, temperature, pulse, respirations, and blood pressure. Monitor at least every 4 hours and more frequently as the patient's clinical status warrants.
- Use Centers for Disease Control and Prevention (CDC) recommended precautions for infection transmission: universal precautions. Consult the CDC's website as well as clinical policies and procedures to prevent transmission of infection. Always remember the importance of adequate handwashing!
- Always monitor for phlebitis when antimicrobials are administered intravenously.
- Administer antimicrobials as prescribed on the time schedule established.
- In some instances a second drug, (e.g., probenecid) may be administered concurrently to inhibit the excretion of the antibiotic (e.g., penicillin, cephalosporin). When this is done, monitor extremely closely for adverse effects.
- Some oral antimicrobials can be administered without regard to meals; others should be given 1 hour before or 2 hours after meals.
- Always give oral antibiotics with sufficient water, and maintain adequate hydration throughout therapy. Drugs such as sulfonamides require forcing fluids unless contraindicated by coexisting medical conditions.
- Check the drug monograph for drug-drug or drug-food interactions and establish administration times accordingly. For example, tetracyclines need to be administered 1 hour before or 2 hours after ingesting antacids, milk and other dairy products, or products containing calcium, aluminum, magnesium, or iron (such as vitamins).
- Monitor for adaptive or maladaptive responses to the diagnosis and intervene appropriately by providing support and information and by making appropriate referrals.

Nausea, Vomiting, and Diarrhea. When drug therapy causes nausea and vomiting, the health care provider may elect to give the antibiotic with food to decrease irritation even though absorption may be slightly decreased, or may choose to switch to a parenteral dosage form. When reporting any incidence of nausea and vomiting, all significant data should be collected and reported. Administer prescribed antiemetics or antidiarrheal agents (see also Chapters 34 and 35).

Secondary Infection. Secondary infection may occur in patients receiving broad-spectrum antibiotic therapy, particularly those who are immunosuppressed. Monitor for the development of symptoms of secondary infection, and notify the health care provider if this occurs. Initiate prescribed treatment consistent with the etiology of the symptoms. Obtain cultures as ordered, and administer additional antibiotics effective against the new organism. Instruct the patient to minimize exposure to people known to have an infection, and to practice good personal hygiene measures.

Allergies and Anaphylaxis. Closely monitor all patients, particularly those with histories of allergies, asthma, or rhinitis and those who are taking multiple drug preparations, for an allergic response during antimicrobial therapy. All patients should be watched carefully for possible allergic reactions for at least 20 to 30 minutes after administration of a medication. However, some drug reactions may not occur for several days.

Hold the prescribed antimicrobial medication if the person reports a possible allergy; share all information obtained with the health care provider, who will decide whether to administer the drug. Older adults, because of the physiologic changes of aging, require close observation for therapeutic response and for drug toxicity. Learn the location of the hospital emergency cart and the procedure for summoning it. In the event of suspected anaphylaxis, summon the health care provider and the emergency cart immediately.

Although a serious reaction may occur with the first administration of a drug, repeated exposures to a previously sensitized substance can be fatal. Respond immediately to any signs of reaction, including swelling, redness, or pain at the site of injection; hives; nasal congestion and discharge; wheezing progressing to dyspnea; pulmonary edema; stridor; and sternal retractions.

When symptoms of an allergic response occur, follow hospital protocol, which will usually include the following steps:

- Activate the patient emergency care system.
- Establish and maintain a patent airway; administer oxygen, and elevate the head of the bed.

- Monitor the patient's vital signs continually and lung sounds frequently. Report hypotension, increasing pulse, respirations that become labored and shallow, and abnormal breath sounds.
- Have emergency equipment and drugs available for administration.
- An intravenous infusion should be initiated if not already available.

Nephrotoxicity. Report abnormal laboratory results relating to kidney function (BUN, serum creatinine). Maintain an accurate intake and output record; report declining output, or output below 30 mL per hour.

Many antimicrobial agents are potentially nephrotoxic (e.g., aminoglycosides, tetracyclines, cephalosporins). Concomitant therapy with diuretics enhances the likelihood of toxicity, particularly in the elderly or debilitated patient. When renal function is impaired, most drug dosages must be decreased or alternate drug therapy used.

Hepatotoxicity. Several drugs to be studied in this unit are potentially hepatotoxic (e.g., isoniazid, sulfonamides). The liver is active in the metabolism of many drugs, and drug-induced hepatitis may occur. The actual liver damage may occur shortly after exposure to the pharmacologic agent or may not appear for several weeks after initial exposure. The symptoms of hepatotoxicity are anorexia, nausea, vomiting, jaundice, hepatomegaly, splenomegaly, and abnormal liver function tests (e.g., elevated bilirubin, AST, ALT, GGT, alkaline phosphatase, prothrombin time). Patients with preexisting hepatic disease such as cirrhosis or hepatitis will require lower dosages of drugs metabolized by the liver.

Ototoxicity. Report preexisting hearing impairment or symptoms of developing hearing deficits to the health care provider and initiate orders prescribed. Provide for patient safety if tinnitus or dizziness accompanies the symptoms of hearing impairment.

Blood Dyscrasias. Individualize care to the type of blood dyscrasia present. When hypoprothrombinemia is present the usual treatment is administration of vitamin K. Serious and possibly fatal bone marrow suppression may occur after therapy is initiated with some antibiotics (e.g., chloramphenicol). Monitor for signs and symptoms including sore throat, fatigue, elevated temperature, small petechial hemorrhages, and bruises on the skin. If present, report immediately.

Photosensitivity. This adverse effect is seldom evident during hospitalization. It is more commonly seen in ambulatory practice.

When the drug monograph mentions this as a potential side effect to report, the nurse should provide health teaching to prevent its occurrence. Instruct the patient to avoid exposure to sunlight and ultraviolet light (e.g., sunlamps, suntanning beds); to wear long-sleeved clothing, a hat, and sunglasses; and to apply a sunscreen when going out into the sunlight.

Medication History

- Ask the patient to list all prescribed or OTC medications being taken. Ask specifically about the recent use of corticosteroids, chemotherapy, or transplant suppressants.
- Does the patient have any allergies? If so, obtain details of medications and actual symptoms that occur during an allergic reaction. What treatment was used for any past allergic responses? What antibiotics have been taken? Were there any problems during antibiotic therapy?

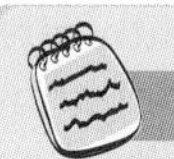

Patient Education and Health Promotion

The following basic principles of patient care should not be overlooked when treating a patient with infections:

- Adequate rest with as little stress as possible. Rest decreases metabolic needs and enhances the physiologic repair process.
- Nutritional management, including attention to hydration, proteins, fats, carbohydrates, minerals, and vitamins, to support the body's needs during an inflammatory response. Adequate nutrients to meet the energy needs, especially during times of fever, are essential so that the body will not break down its protein stores to meet energy requirements. The dietary teaching must be individualized to the patient's diagnosis and point of recovery. Unless contraindicated by coexisting disease, encourage adequate fluid intake of 2000 to 3000 mL per 24 hours and simultaneously monitor the patient for signs and symptoms of fluid volume deficit or fluid volume overload.
- Extensive teaching, individualized to the circumstances and mode of transmission of the disease, should be given to individuals with communicable infection. This should include contacting exposed individuals in accordance with institutional policies for disease screening, treatment, and follow-up counseling.
- Explain personal hygiene measures, such as handwashing techniques, management of excretions such as sputum, and wound care.
- Instruct the patient to refrain from sexual intercourse during therapy for sexually transmitted disease infections.

Medications

- Drug therapy specific for the type of microorganism causing the infection should be explained in detail so the patient will realize the need for adherence with the prescribed regimen.
- Examine each drug monograph to identify suggestions to the patient for how to handle the common side effects associated with antimicrobial therapy. The patient also must be taught the signs and symptoms that must be reported to the health

care provider. Stress to the patient the importance of not discontinuing the prescribed medication until the side effects have been discussed with the health care provider.

- Develop a medication schedule with the patient for at-home medications prescribed. Make sure that the patient understands why it is important to take antimicrobials for the entire course of drug therapy and not to discontinue them when feeling improved. Also, patients must know self-monitoring parameters for the prescribed drug therapy.
- Nursing mothers should remind their health care provider that they are breastfeeding so that antibiotics may be selected that will have no effect on the infant.
- After an allergic reaction the patient and family should be alerted to inform anyone treating the patient in the future of the allergy to a specific drug.
- Follow recommendations for annual influenza vaccine and pneumococcal vaccine for high-risk individuals (e.g., older adults, health care workers, people with chronic or debilitating diseases). Always check with the health care provider if in doubt about advisability of administering vaccine.

Fostering Health Maintenance

- Throughout the course of treatment, discuss medication information. Continue to emphasize those factors the patient can control to alter the progression of the disease: maintenance of general health and nutritional needs, adequate rest and appropriate exercise, and taking the prescribed medication until the entire course of therapy has been completed.
- Discuss expectations of therapy so that the patient understands whether a satisfactory response to drug therapy is being achieved, such as the relief of symptoms for which treatment was sought (e.g., relief of burning with urination and frequency of urination, relief of cough, and end of drainage and healing of a wound).

Written Record

Enlist the patient's aid in developing and maintaining a written record of monitoring parameters (e.g., list presenting symptoms: cough with a large amount of phlegm, wound drainage, temperature, exercise tolerance) (see Patient Self-Assessment Form on p. 751). Complete the Premedication Data column for use as a baseline to track response to drug therapy. Ensure that the patient understands how to use the form and instruct the patient to take the completed form to follow-up visits. During follow-up visits, focus on issues that will foster adherence with the therapeutic interventions prescribed. ■

DRUG THERAPY FOR INFECTIOUS DISEASE

DRUG CLASS: Aminoglycosides

Actions

Aminoglycoside antibiotics kill bacteria primarily by inhibiting protein synthesis. Other mechanisms of action are not yet fully defined.

Uses

The aminoglycosides are used primarily against gram-negative microorganisms that cause urinary tract infections, meningitis, wound infections, and life-threatening septicemias. They are the mainstays in the treatment of nosocomial gram-negative infections (e.g., *Acinetobacter, Citrobacter, Enterobacter, Escherichia coli, Klebsiella, Providencia, Pseudomonas, Salmonella,* and *Shigella*). Kanamycin and neomycin may also be used before surgery to reduce the normal flora content of the intestinal tract.

Therapeutic Outcomes

The primary therapeutic outcome expected from aminoglycoside therapy is elimination of bacterial infection.

Nursing Process for Aminoglycosides

Premedication Assessment

1. Obtain baseline assessments of presenting symptoms.
2. Record temperature, pulse, respirations, blood pressure, and hydration status.
3. Assess for any allergies and symptoms of hearing loss or renal disease. If present, withhold drug and report findings to health care provider.
4. If the patient has had anesthesia within the past 48 to 72 hours, check to see if skeletal muscle relaxants were administered. If used, withhold the drug and notify the health care provider.
5. Check for scheduled time of laboratory aminoglycoside serum level testing. After levels are determined, assess whether results are normal or toxic. Contact the health care provider as appropriate.
6. Obtain baseline laboratory studies ordered (e.g., CBC with differential, BUN, creatinine).

Planning

Availability. See Table 46-1.

Implementation

Dosage and Administration. See Table 46-1.

Compatibilities. DO NOT mix other drugs in the same syringe or infuse together with other drugs. See Drug Interactions for incompatibilities.

Laboratory. Check with the hospital laboratory regarding timing of aminoglycoside blood level tests.

PATIENT SELF-ASSESSMENT FORM Antibiotics

MEDICATIONS	COLOR	TO BE TAKEN

Patient ______

Health Care Provider ______

Health Care Provider's phone ______

Next appt.* ______

What I Should Monitor			Premedication Data	Date	Date	Date	Date	Date	Date	Comments
Temperature	On arising	12 noon								
	5 PM	9 PM								
Aspirin	Time; # tabs, e.g.	8AM2								
Acetaminophen	Time; # tabs, e.g.	12N2								
Site of infection	Redness									
Scale	Pain									
(+ Small ++++ Severe)	Drainage									
Cough and sputum	Color									
Productive	Thickness									
	No cough									
Mouth and throat	Sore throat									
	No problem									
Dizziness	Walk unaided									
	Must use support									
	Walk with help									
Hearing	Had to ↑ volume of radio or TV									
	No difficulty									
Skin	Rash with itching									
	Rash: Fine red									
	No itching									
	No rash									
Vaginal itching (Yes/No)										
Rectal itching (Yes/No)										
Other										

*Please bring this record with you to your next appointment.
Use the back of this sheet for additional information.

Drug Table 46-1 **AMINOGLYCOSIDES**

GENERIC NAME	BRAND NAME	AVAILABILITY	ADULT DOSAGE RANGE
amikacin	Amikin	50 and 250 mg/mL in 2 and 4 mL vials	IM, IV: 15 mg/kg/24 hr
gentamicin	Garamycin	10, 40 mg/mL in 2 and 20 mL vials 60 mg/1.5 mL in cartridge-needle units	IM, IV: Up to 240 mg/24 hr
kanamycin	Kantrex	75, 500 mg, 1 g vials	IM, IV: Up to 15 mg/kg/24 hr, not to exceed 1.5 g/24 hr
neomycin	Neo-fradin	500 mg tablets 125 mg/5 mL in 480 mL bottle	PO: 4-12 g daily in four divided doses
streptomycin	Streptomycin	400 mg/mL in 2.5-mL vials; 1 g vials	IM: 1-4 g/24 hr
tobramycin	Tobramycin	10 mg/mL in 2 mL vials 40 mg/mL in 1.5 mL syringes and 2 and 30 mL vials 1.2 g in 1.2 g vials 300 mg/5 mL nebulizer solution	IM, IV: Up to 5 mg/kg/24 hr

After levels have been determined, assess whether results are normal or toxic.

Rate of Infusion. Consult with a pharmacist or see the individual package literature.

Evaluation

Side Effects to Report

Ototoxicity. Damage to the eighth cranial nerve can occur as a result of aminoglycoside therapy. This may initially be manifested by dizziness, tinnitus, and progressive hearing loss. Continue to observe patients for ototoxicity after therapy has been discontinued. These adverse effects may appear several days later.

Assess each patient for difficulty in walking unaided and assess the level of hearing daily. Intentionally speak softly: Note if the patient is aware that you said anything. Take particular notice of the patient who repeatedly asks, "What did you say?" or who starts talking more loudly or progressively increases the volume on the television or radio.

Nephrotoxicity. Monitor urinalysis and kidney function tests for abnormal results. Report an increasing BUN and creatinine, decreasing urine output or decreasing specific gravity (despite amount of fluid intake), casts or protein in the urine, frank blood or smoky-colored urine, or RBCs in excess of 0 to 3 RBC/HPF (see Table 42-1) on the urinalysis report.

Drug Interactions

Nephrotoxic Potential. Cephalosporins, enflurane, methoxyflurane, vancomycin, and diuretics, when combined with aminoglycosides, may increase the nephrotoxic potential. Monitor the urinalysis and kidney function tests for abnormal results.

Ototoxic Potential. Aminoglycosides, when combined with ethacrynic acid, torsemide, bumetanide, and furosemide, may increase ototoxicity. Therefore nursing assessments for tinnitus, dizziness, and decreased hearing should be done regularly every shift.

Neuromuscular Blockade. Aminoglycoside antibiotics in combination with skeletal muscle relaxants may produce respiratory depression.

Check the anesthesia record in postoperative patients to determine if skeletal muscle relaxants such as succinylcholine or pancuronium bromide were administered during surgery.

The nurse should monitor and assess the respiratory rate, depth of respirations, and chest movement and report apnea immediately. Because these effects may be seen for up to 48 hours after administration of skeletal muscle relaxants, continue monitoring respirations, pulse, and blood pressure beyond the usual postsurgical vital signs routine.

Heparin. Gentamicin and heparin are physically incompatible. DO NOT mix together before infusion.

Ampicillin, Piperacillin, Ticarcillin. These penicillins rapidly inactivate aminoglycoside antibiotics. DO NOT mix together or administer together at the same IV site.

DRUG CLASS: Carbapenems

Actions

The carbapenems are extremely potent broad-spectrum antibiotics resistant to beta-lactamase enzymes secreted by bacteria. They act by inhibiting bacterial cell wall synthesis.

Uses

Imipenem/cilastatin (Primaxin) is a combination product containing a carbapenem antibiotic called imipenem and cilastatin, an inhibitor of the renal

Drug Table 46-2 **CARBAPENEMS**

GENERIC NAME	BRAND NAME	AVAILABILITY	DOSAGE RANGE
ertapenem	Invanz	Injection: 1 g vials	IM, IV: 1 g daily. Infuse IV solution over 30 min for up to 14 days. Limit IM injection to 7 days.
imipenem/ cilastatin	Primaxin	Injection: IM: 500 and 750 mg vials; IV: 250 and 500 mg vials	IV: 125, 250, or 500 mg by IV infusion over 20 to 30 min. Infuse 750 mg or 1 g dose over 40 to 60 min. If nausea develops, slow the infusion rate. Do not exceed 50 mg/kg/day or 4 g/day. IM: 500 to 750 mg every 12 hr, depending on the severity of infection. Do not exceed 1500 mg/day.
meropenem	Merrem IV	Injection: 500 mg and 1 g vials	IV: 1 g IV every 8 hr. Infuse over 15-30 min or as a bolus over 3-5 min.

dipeptidase enzyme dehydropeptidase I. Cilastatin has no antimicrobial activity; it prevents the inactivation of imipenem by the renal enzyme. It is used in the treatment of lower respiratory tract and intraabdominal infections; infections of the urinary tract, bones, joints, and skin; gynecologic infections; endocarditis; and bacterial septicemia caused by gram-negative or gram-positive organisms. A primary therapeutic role of imipenem/cilastatin is in the treatment of severe infections caused by multiresistant organisms and in mixed anaerobic-aerobic infections, primarily those involving intraabdominal and pelvic sepsis in which *Bacteroides fragilis* is a common pathogen. It should be used in combination with antipseudomonal agents because of resistance of *Pseudomonas cepacia* and *P. aeruginosa* to imipenem.

Meropenem is a carbapenem antibiotic that has a chemical structure that protects it against dehydropeptidase I, so that cilastatin is not necessary. It has a broad spectrum of activity similar to imipenem, but is more active against Enterobacteriaceae and less active against gram-positive bacteria. It is used alone IV for the treatment of intraabdominal infections caused by *Escherichia coli, Klebsiella pneumoniae, P. aeruginosa, B. fragilis,* and *Peptostreptococcus.* It is also used alone IV in the treatment of bacterial meningitis caused by *Streptococcus pneumoniae, Haemophilus influenzae,* and *Neisseria meningitidis.*

Ertapenem is a carbapenem antibiotic that has a chemical structure that protects it against dehydropeptidase I, so that cilastatin is not necessary. It has a broad spectrum of activity and is approved to treat infections caused by aerobic and anaerobic gram-positive and gram-negative bacteria causing complicated intraabdominal infections, skin and skin structure infections, community-acquired pneumonia, urinary tract infections (including pyelonephritis), and acute pelvic infections. It is effective against susceptible strains of *Staphylococcus aureus, S. agalactiae, S. pneumoniae, Streptococcus pyogenes, E. coli, K. pneumoniae, Moraxella catarrhalis, H. influenzae, Bacteroides* species, *Clostridium,* and *Peptostreptococcus.*

Therapeutic Outcomes

The primary therapeutic outcome expected from carbapenem therapy is elimination of bacterial infection.

Nursing Process for Carbapenems

Premedication Assessment

1. Obtain baseline assessments of presenting symptoms.
2. Record temperature, pulse, respirations, blood pressure, and hydration status.
3. Assess for and record any gastric symptoms before initiating therapy.
4. Assess for any allergies. Ask specifically about penicillin and cephalosporin allergies.
5. Obtain baseline laboratory studies ordered (e.g., CBC with differential).
6. Perform a baseline assessment of the patient's degree of alertness and orientation to name, place, and time before beginning therapy.
7. Ask whether there is a history of seizure activity before initiating therapy.

Planning

Availability. See Table 46-2.

Implementation

Hypersensitivity. Although these antibiotics are carbapenems rather than penicillins or cephalosporins, they also contain a beta-lactam nucleus. Cross-hypersensitivity may develop between these classes. Complete a history of hypersensitivity before starting therapy. If an allergic reaction to a carbapenem occurs, discontinue the infusion. Serious reactions may require epinephrine and other emergency measures.

Dosage and Administration. See Table 46-2.

Evaluation

Side Effects to Report

Severe Diarrhea. Severe diarrhea may develop from using carbapenems. Blood and mucus in the stool may also be present. This may be an indication of drug-induced pseudomembranous colitis and should be reported immediately. Withhold the next dose of antibiotic until the health care provider gives approval for administration.

Dizziness. Provide for patient safety during episodes of dizziness; report for further evaluation.

Confusion, Seizures. Seizure activity, including myoclonic activity, focal tremors, confusional states, and other seizures, has been reported with the carbapenems. These episodes occurred most commonly in patients with histories of previous seizure activity.

Perform a baseline assessment of the patient's degree of alertness and orientation to name, place, and time before initiating therapy. Make regularly scheduled subsequent mental status evaluations, and compare findings. Report alterations.

Implement seizure precautions. Make sure the patient continues with anticonvulsant therapy. If seizures develop, provide for patient safety and then record the exact time of seizure onset and duration of each phase, a description of the specific body parts involved, and any progression in the affected parts. Describe automatic responses during the clonic phase: altered, jerky respirations or frothy salivation; dilated pupils and any eye movements; cyanosis; diaphoresis; or incontinence.

Phlebitis. Carefully assess patients for thrombophlebitis. Inspect the IV area frequently when providing care; inspect visually during dressing changes and whenever the IV is changed to a new site. Report redness, warmth, tenderness to touch, and edema in the affected part; if in the lower extremities, dorsiflexion of the foot may cause pain in the calf area (Homans' sign). Compare the affected limb with the unaffected limb.

Drug Interactions

Probenecid. Probenecid inhibits the urinary excretion of carbapenems. Do not administer probenecid concurrently.

Ganciclovir. Concurrent administration of ganciclovir and imipenem/cilastatin has resulted in an increased incidence of seizures. Avoid concurrent use if at all possible.

Admixture Compatibility. The carbapenems require special care regarding mixing and administration.

- Imipenem/cilastatin should not be mixed with or physically added to other antibiotics, but it may be administered concomitantly with other antibiotics such as aminoglycosides.
- Meropenem should not be mixed with or physically added to solutions containing other medicines.
- Ertapenem for IV use should be reconstituted with water for injection, bacteriostatic water for injection, or 0.9% sodium chloride (normal saline) for injection. Do not reconstitute or dilute with dextrose solutions.
- Ertapenem for IM use should be reconstituted with 1% lidocaine injection (without epinephrine). Administer the injection within 1 hour of reconstitution.

DRUG CLASS: Cephalosporins

Actions

The cephalosporins are chemically related to the penicillins and have a similar mechanism of activity. The cephalosporins act by inhibiting cell wall synthesis in bacteria. The cephalosporins may be divided into groups, or "generations," based primarily on antimicrobial activity. The first-generation cephalosporins have effective activity against gram-positive microorganisms *(S. aureus, S. epidermidis; S. pyogenes, S. pneumoniae)* and relatively mild activity against gram-negative microorganisms *(E. coli, K. pneumoniae, Proteus mirabilis).* Second-generation cephalosporins have somewhat increased activity against gram-negative bacteria but are much less active than the third-generation agents, which are generally less active than first-generation agents against gram-positive cocci, although they are much more active against penicillinase-producing bacteria. Some of the third-generation cephalosporins also are active against *P. aeruginosa*, a potent gram-negative microorganism. Fourth-generation cephalosporins are broad spectrum, with both gram-negative and gram-positive coverage.

Uses

Cephalosporins may be used with caution as alternatives when patients are allergic to the penicillins, unless they are also allergic to the cephalosporins. The cephalosporins are used for certain urinary and respiratory tract infections, abdominal infections, bacteremia, meningitis, and osteomyelitis.

Therapeutic Outcomes

The primary therapeutic outcome expected from cephalosporin therapy is elimination of bacterial infection.

Nursing Process for Cephalosporins

Premedication Assessment

1. Obtain baseline assessments of presenting symptoms.
2. Record temperature, pulse, respirations, blood pressure, and hydration status.
3. Assess for any allergies, symptoms of renal disease, or bleeding disorders. If present, withhold drug and report findings to the health care provider.
4. Obtain baseline laboratory studies ordered (e.g., CBC with differential).

Planning

Availability. See Table 46-3.

Drug Table 46-3 CEPHALOSPORINS

GENERIC NAME	BRAND NAME	GENERATION	AVAILABILITY	ADULT DOSAGE RANGE
cefaclor	Ceclor	2	250, 500 mg capsules 375, 500 mg extended release tablets 125, 187, 250, 375 chewable tablets 125, 187, 250, 375 mg/5 mL suspension	PO: 250-500 every 8 hr; do not exceed 4 g/day
cefadroxil	Duricef	1	500 mg capsules 1000 mg tablets 125, 250, 500 mg/5 mL suspension	PO: 1-2 g daily in 1-2 doses daily
cefdinir	Omnicef	3	300 mg capsules 125 mg/5 mL oral suspension 250 mg/mL oral suspension	PO: 300-600 mg every 12 hr
cefepime	Maxipime	4	500 mg in 1, 2 g vials	IM, IV: 0.5-2 g every 12 hr
cefixime	Suprax	3	100 mg/5 mL suspension	PO: 200 mg every 12 hr or 400 mg once daily
cefmetazole	Zefazone	2	1, 2 g vials	IV: 2 g every 6-12 hr
cefoperazone	Cefobid	3	1, 2, 10 g vials	IV: 1-3 g every 6-8 hr
cefotaxime	Claforan	3	500 mg; 1, 2, 10 g vials	IV: 1-2 g every 4-8 hr; do not exceed 12 g/day
cefotetan	Cefotan	3	1, 2, 10 g vials	IM, IV: 1-2 g every 12 hr; do not exceed 6 g/day
cefoxitin	Mefoxin	2	1, 2, 10 g vials	IM, IV: 1-2 g every 6-8 hr; do not exceed 12 g/day
cefpodoxime	Vantin	3	100, 200 mg tablets 50, 100 mg/5 mL suspension	PO: 200 mg every 12 hr for 7-14 days
cefprozil	Cefzil	2	250, 500 mg tablets 125, 250 mg/5 mL suspension	PO: 250-500 mg every 12 hr for 10 days
ceftazidime	Fortaz, Tazidime	3	500 mg; 1, 2, 6, 10 g vials	IM, IV: 1-2 g every 12 hr
ceftibuten	Cedax	3	400 mg capsules 90 mg/5 mL suspension	PO: 400 mg once daily 2 hr before or 1 hr after meals for 10 days
ceftizoxime	Cefizox	3	500 mg; 1, 2, 10 g vials	IV: 1-2 g every 8-12 hr
ceftriaxone	Rocephin	3	250, 500 mg; 1, 2, 10 g vials	IM, IV: 1-2 g once daily; do not exceed 4 g daily
cefuroxime	Zinacef, Ceftin	2	125, 250, 500 mg tablets; 750 mg; 1.5, 7.5 g vials 125, 250 mg/5 mL suspension	PO: 250-500 mg every 12 hr IV: 750 mg to 1.5 g every 8 hr
cephalexin	Keflex, ✱Novolexin	1	250, 500 mg capsules, tablets 125, 250 mg/5 mL suspension	PO: 250-1000 mg every 6 hr
cephradine	Velosef	1	250, 500 mg capsules 125, 250 mg/5 mL suspension	PO: 250-500 mg every 6 hr; do not exceed 8 g/day
loracarbef	Lorabid	2	200, 400 mg capsules 100 mg/5 mL suspension 200 mg/5 mL suspension	PO: 200-400 mg every 12 hr 1 hr before or 2 hr after a meal for 7-14 days

✱ Available in Canada.

Implementation

Dosage and Administration. See Table 46-3.

Evaluation

Side Effects to Report

Diarrhea. Cephalosporins cause diarrhea by altering the bacterial flora of the gastrointestinal (GI) tract. The diarrhea is usually not severe enough to warrant discontinuing medication. Encourage the patient not to discontinue therapy without consulting the health care provider. When diarrhea persists, monitor the patient for signs of dehydration.

Secondary Infections. Oral thrush, genital and anal pruritus, vaginitis, and vaginal discharge may occur with cephalosporin therapy. Report promptly because these infections are resistant to the original antibiotic used.

Teach the importance of meticulous oral and perineal personal hygiene.

Abnormal Liver and Renal Function Tests. Transient elevations of liver function tests (e.g., AST, ALT, alkaline phosphatase) and renal function tests (e.g., BUN, serum creatinine) have been reported. Renal toxicity, as evidenced by proteinuria, hematuria, casts, decreased creatinine clearance, and decreased urine output, also has developed.

Monitor returning laboratory data and report abnormal findings to the health care provider.

Hypoprothrombinemia. Hypoprothrombinemia, with and without bleeding, has been reported. These rare occurrences are most frequent in older adult, debilitated, or otherwise compromised patients with borderline vitamin K deficiency. Treatment with broad-spectrum antibiotics eliminates enough gastrointestinal flora to cause a further reduction in vitamin K synthesis.

Assess your patient for ecchymosis after minimal trauma, prolonged bleeding at an infusion site or from a surgical wound, or the development of petechiae, bleeding gums, or nosebleeds. Notify the health care provider of any of the signs of hypoprothrombinemia. The usual treatment is administration of vitamin K.

Thrombophlebitis. Phlebitis and thrombophlebitis are recurrent problems associated with intravenous (IV) administration of cephalosporins. Use small IV needles, large veins, and alternate infusion sites, if possible, to minimize irritation.

Carefully assess patients receiving IV cephalosporins for the development of thrombophlebitis.

Inspect the area frequently when providing care; inspect during dressing changes and at times when the IV is changed to a new site. Always investigate pain at the IV site. Report redness, warmth, tenderness to touch, or edema in the affected part. If in the lower extremities, dorsiflexion of the foot may cause pain in the calf area (Homans' sign). Compare findings in the affected limb with those in the unaffected limb.

Electrolyte Imbalance. If a patient develops hyperkalemia or hypernatremia, consider the electrolyte content of the antibiotics. Most of the cephalosporins have a high electrolyte content.

Drug Interactions

Nephrotoxic Potential. Patients receiving cephalosporins, aminoglycosides, polymyxin B, vancomycin, and loop diuretics concurrently should be assessed for signs of nephrotoxicity. Monitor urinalysis and kidney function tests for abnormal results. Report an increasing BUN and creatinine, decreasing urine output or decreasing specific gravity (despite amount of fluid intake), casts or protein in the urine, frank blood or smoky-colored urine, or red blood cells (RBCs) in excess of 0 to 3 RBC/HPF (see Table 42-1) on the urinalysis report.

Antacids. Antacids inhibit the absorption of cefaclor, cefdinir, and cefpodoxime. If antacids must be taken, the antibiotic should be taken 2 hours before or after the antacid.

H_2 Antagonists. H_2 antagonists (i.e., cimetidine, famotidine, nizatidine, ranitidine) inhibit the absorption of cefpodoxime and cefuroxime, decreasing the antibiotic effect. Because of the long duration of action of the H_2 antagonists, it is recommended that they not be administered when these cephalosporins are prescribed.

Iron Supplements. Iron supplements and food fortified with iron inhibit the absorption of cefdinir. If iron supplements must be taken, the antibiotic should be taken 2 hours before or after the iron supplement.

Probenecid. Patients receiving probenecid in combination with cephalosporins are more susceptible to toxicity because of the inhibition of excretion of the cephalosporins by probenecid. Monitor closely for adverse effects.

Alcohol. Instruct the patient to avoid alcohol consumption during cefmetazole, cefoperazone, cefotetan, and possibly ceftizoxime therapy. Patients ingesting alcohol during and for 24 to 72 hours after administration of these cephalosporins will become flushed, tremulous, dyspneic, tachycardic, and hypotensive. Also tell the patient not to use OTC preparations containing alcohol, such as mouthwash (e.g., Cepacol, Listerine) or cough preparations.

Oral Contraceptives. Cephalosporins may interfere with the contraceptive activity of oral contraceptives. Oral contraceptives should not be discontinued, but counseling regarding use of additional methods of contraception (e.g., condoms and foam) should be planned.

DRUG CLASS: Glycyclines

Tigecycline (tie geh cyc' lean)

TYGACIL (tig' ah sil)

Actions

Tigecycline is the first of a new family of antimicrobial agents known as the glycyclines. Tigecycline is chemically related to the tetracyclines, but is not susceptible to the mechanisms that cause resistance to the tetracyclines. It acts by binding to the 30S ribosome, preventing protein synthesis. It is a bacteriostatic antibiotic effective against a broad spectrum of gram- positive, gram-negative, and anaerobic microorganisms. It is not effective against viruses.

Uses

Tigecycline is used to treat complicated skin and skin structure infections (cSSSI) caused by *E. coli, Enterococcus faecalis, S. aureus* (methicillin-susceptible and methicillin-resistant isolates), *S. agalactiae,* and *Bacteroides fragilis.* It may also be used to treat complicated intraabdominal infections (cIAI) caused by *Citrobacter freundii, Enterobacter cloacae, E. coli, Klebsiella oxytoca, K. pneumoniae, E. faecalis, S. aureus* (methicillin-susceptible isolates only), *B. fragilis, B. vulgaris, C. perfringens,* and *Peptostreptococcus micros.* In an effort to slow the development of strains of bacteria resistant to tigecycline, it should be used only when the pathogen is resistant to other available antibiotics.

Tigecycline is not approved for use in people younger than the age of 18. As with tetracyclines, tigecycline administered during the ages of tooth development (the last half of pregnancy through 8 years of age) may cause enamel hypoplasia and permanent yellow, gray, or brown staining of the teeth.

Therapeutic Outcomes

The primary therapeutic outcome expected from tigecycline therapy is elimination of bacterial infection.

Nursing Process for Tigecycline Therapy

Premedication Assessment

1. Obtain baseline assessments of presenting symptoms.
2. Record temperature, pulse, respirations, blood pressure, and hydration status.
3. Assess for and record any gastric symptoms before initiating therapy.
4. Assess for any allergies.
5. Obtain baseline laboratory studies ordered (e.g., CBC with differential).

Planning

Availability. IV: 50 mg in 5-mL vials.

Implementation

Dosage and Administration. IV: Initial: 100 mg followed by 50 mg every 12 hours. Administer by IV infusion over 30 to 60 minutes. Therapy is continued for 5 to 14 days, depending on the severity and site of the infection and the patient's clinical progress.

Evaluation

Side Effects to Report

Gastric Irritation. The most common side effects of tigecycline therapy are nausea and vomiting (30% and 20%, respectively). These side effects are usually mild and moderate in the first 1 to 2 days of therapy, but tend to resolve with continued therapy.

Severe Diarrhea. Rarely, severe diarrhea may develop from the use of tigecycline. Report diarrhea of five or more stools per day to the health care provider. This may be an indication of drug-induced pseudomembranous colitis.

Blood or mucus in the stool should also be reported to the health care provider. *Warn patients not to treat diarrhea themselves when taking this drug.* The use of diphenoxylate, loperamide, or paregoric may prolong or worsen the condition. Large doses of attapulgite (Kaopectate) may be effective in diminishing the diarrhea.

Photosensitivity. Photosensitivity resulting in an exaggerated sunburn after short exposure has been reported. The patient should be cautioned to avoid exposure to sunlight and ultraviolet light. Suggest wearing long-sleeved clothing, a hat, and sunglasses when outdoors. Discourage the use of tanning lamps. Consult the health care provider about the advisability of discontinuing therapy.

Drug Interactions

Warfarin. This medication may enhance the anticoagulant effects of warfarin. Observe for petechiae, ecchymoses, nosebleeds, bleeding gums, dark tarry stools, and bright red or "coffee ground" emesis. Monitor the prothrombin time (INR) and reduce the dosage of warfarin if necessary.

Oral Contraceptives. Tigecycline may interfere with the contraceptive activity of oral contraceptives. Oral contraceptives should not be discontinued, but counseling regarding use of additional methods of contraception (e.g., condoms and foam) should be planned.

DRUG CLASS: Ketolides

telithromycin (tel ith roh my' sin)
▶ KETEK (kee' tec)

Actions

Telithromycin is the first of a new family of antimicrobial agents known as the ketolides. They are chemically related to the macrolide antibiotics and have a similar mechanism of bactericidal action by preventing bacterial ribosomes from translating its mRNA, preventing the synthesis of new proteins.

Uses

Telithromycin is used to treat acute bacterial sinusitis, bronchitis, and lung (pneumonia) infections caused by susceptible strains of gram-positive bacteria such as: *S. pneumoniae, H. influenzae, M. catarrhalis, S. aureus, Chlamydophila pneumoniae,* or *Mycoplasmia pneumoniae.* It can be used as an alternative to macrolide, oral cephalosporin, or fluoroquinolone antibiotic therapy. In an effort to slow the development of strains of bacteria resistant to telithromycin, it should be used only when the pathogen is resistant to other available antibiotics.

Therapeutic Outcomes

The primary therapeutic outcome expected from telithromycin therapy is elimination of bacterial infection.

Nursing Process for Telithromycin Therapy

Premedication Assessment

1. Obtain baseline assessments of presenting symptoms.
2. Record temperature, pulse, respirations, blood pressure, and hydration status.
3. Assess for and record any gastric symptoms before initiating therapy.
4. Assess for and record any visual acuity issues before initiating therapy.
5. Assess for any allergies.
6. Obtain baseline laboratory studies ordered (e.g., CBC with differential).

Planning

Availability. PO: 400 mg tablets

Implementation

Dosage and Administration. PO: 800 mg once daily for 5, 7, or 10 days, depending on the type of infection. In general, bacterial bronchitis and sinusitis are treated for 5 days, and pneumonia is treated for 7 to 10 days.

Evaluation

Side Effects to Expect

Gastric Irritation. The most common side effects of oral telithromycin therapy are diarrhea, nausea, and vomiting. These side effects are usually mild and tend to resolve with continued therapy. Encourage the patient not to discontinue therapy without first consulting the health care provider.

Dizziness. Although uncommon, ciprofloxacin may cause these disturbances. They tend to be self-limiting, and therapy should not be discontinued until the patient consults a health care provider.

Caution the patient against driving or performing hazardous tasks until adjusted to the effects of the medication.

Side Effects to Report

Visual Disturbances. Visual disturbances (e.g., blurred vision, difficulty focusing, double vision) may occur after the first or second dose and last for several hours. If visual difficulties occur, patients should be advised to avoid driving a motor vehicle, operating heavy machinery, or engaging in otherwise hazardous activities. If the visual disturbances interfere with daily activities, the patient should contact the health care provider.

Drug Interactions

Toxicity Caused by Telithromycin. Telithromycin is a strong inhibitor of the CYP 3A4 system. It may inhibit the metabolism of several drugs, causing accumulation and potential toxicity. These drugs are benzodiazepines (e.g., midazolam, triazolam), cisapride, buspirone, carbamazepine, digoxin, HMG-CoA reductase inhibitors (e.g., atorvastatin, lovastatin, simvastatin), and metoprolol. Read individual monographs for monitoring parameters of toxicity from these agents.

Pimozide. Coadministration of telithromycin with pimozide is contraindicated.

Rifampin, Rifabutin, Carbamazepine, Phenobarbital. The coadministration of telithromycin with any of these medicines may cause a reduction in antimicrobial effect while increasing the frequency of GI adverse effects.

Oral Contraceptives. Telithromycin may interfere with the contraceptive activity of oral contraceptives. Oral contraceptives should not be discontinued, but counseling regarding use of additional methods of contraception (e.g., condoms and foam) should be planned.

DRUG CLASS: Macrolides

Actions

The macrolide antibiotics act by inhibiting protein synthesis in susceptible bacteria. They are bacteriostatic and bacteriocidal, depending on the organism and the concentration of medicine present. Erythromycin is effective against gram-positive microorganisms and gram-negative cocci. Azithromycin is less active against gram-positive organisms than erythromycin but has greater activity against gram-negative organisms that are resistant to erythromycin. Clarithromycin has a spectrum of activity similar to that of erythromycin, but has considerably greater potency. Dirithromycin is a prodrug, the active metabolite of which is erythromycylamine. Erythromycylamine has a spectrum of activity somewhat similar to that of erythromycin. Dirithromycin also has a tentative advantage over the other macrolide antibiotics in that it does not affect liver metabolism of other drugs; thus it has fewer interactions.

Uses

The macrolides are used for respiratory, GI tract, skin, and soft tissue infections; and for sexually transmitted diseases, especially when penicillins, cephalosporins, and tetracyclines cannot be used.

Therapeutic Outcomes

The primary therapeutic outcome expected from macrolide therapy is elimination of bacterial infection.

Nursing Process for Macrolide Therapy

Premedication Assessment

1. Obtain baseline assessments of presenting symptoms.
2. Record temperature, pulse, respirations, blood pressure, and hydration status.
3. Assess for and record any gastric symptoms before initiating therapy.
4. Assess for any allergies.
5. Obtain baseline laboratory studies ordered (e.g., CBC with differential).

Planning

Availability. See Table 46-4.

Implementation

Dosage and Administration. See Table 46-4. PO: Azithromycin and erythromycin should be administered at least 1 hour before or 2 hours after meals. Clarithromycin may be taken without regard to meals. IM: Because of pain on injection and the possibility of sterile abscess formation, IM administration of erythromycin is generally not recommended for multiple-dose therapy. IV: Dilute the dosage of erythromycin in 100 to 250 mL of saline solution or 5% dextrose and administer over 20 to 60 minutes. Thrombophlebitis after IV infusion is a relatively common side effect.

Evaluation

Side Effects to Expect

Gastric Irritation. The most common side effects of oral macrolide therapy are diarrhea, nausea and vomiting, and abnormal taste. These side effects are usually mild and tend to resolve with continued therapy. Encourage the patient not to discontinue therapy without first consulting the health care provider.

Side Effects to Report

Thrombophlebitis. Carefully assess patients receiving IV erythromycin for thrombophlebitis. Inspect the IV area frequently when providing care; inspect during dressing changes and when the IV is changed to a new site. Always investigate pain at the IV site. Report redness and edema in the affected part. If in lower extremities, dorsiflexion of the foot may cause pain in the calf area (Homans' sign). Compare the affected limb with the unaffected limb.

Drug Interactions

Toxicity Caused by Macrolides. Macrolide antibiotics may inhibit the metabolism of several drugs, causing accumulation and potential toxicity. These drugs are alfentanil, astemizole, benzodiazepines (e.g., alprazolam, diazepam, midazolam, triazolam), bromocriptine, cisapride, buspirone, carbamazepine, cyclosporine, digoxin, disopyramide, felodipine, HMG-CoA reductase inhibitors (e.g., atorvastatin, lovastatin, simvastatin), omeprazole, sparfloxacin, tacrolimus, theophyllines, vinblastine, and warfarin. Read indi-

Drug Table 46-4 MACROLIDES

GENERIC NAME	BRAND NAME	AVAILABILITY	ADULT DOSAGE RANGE
azithromycin	Zithromax	PO: 250, 500, 600 mg tablets; 100, 167, 200, 1000 mg/5 mL suspension 500 mg in 10 mL vial for injection	PO: 500 mg as a single dose on day 1, followed by 250 mg once daily on days 2-5 for a total dose of 1.5 g IV: As for PO dose Dilute powder to a concentration of 1-2 mg/mL; infuse 1 mg/mL concentration over 3 hr or the 2 mg/mL concentration over 1 hr. Do *NOT* administer as an IV bolus or IM
clarithromycin	Biaxin	PO: 250, 500 mg tablets; 125, 250 mg/5 mL suspension;	PO: 250-500 mg every 12 hr for 7-14 days
	Biaxin XL	PO: 500 and 1000 mg extended release tablets	
dirithromycin	Dynabac	PO: 250 mg extended release tablets	PO: 500 mg as a single dose daily; take with food or within 1 hr of having eaten; take for 7-14 days
erythromycin	Eryc, Ilosone, E-Mycin, many others	PO: 333, 500 mg enteric-coated tablets; 250, 500 mg chewable tablets; 250, 500 mg film-coated tablets; 333, 500 mg enteric-coated pellets in capsules; 125, 200, 250, 400 mg/5 mL suspension, 100 mg/mL and 100 mg/2.5 mL drops IV: 500, 1000 mg vials for reconstitution	PO: 250 mg four times daily for 10-14 days IM: 100 mg every 4-6 hr IV: 15-20 mg/kg/24 hr; up to 4 g/24 hr

vidual monographs for monitoring parameters of toxicity from these agents.

Pimozide. Coadministration of a macrolide antibiotic with pimozide is contraindicated. Death has resulted from this combination of drug therapy.

Rifampin, Rifabutin. The coadministration of a macrolide antibiotic with rifampin or rifabutin may cause a reduction in antimicrobial effect while increasing the frequency of GI adverse effects.

Oral Contraceptives. Macrolides may interfere with the contraceptive activity of oral contraceptives. Oral contraceptives should not be discontinued, but counseling regarding use of additional methods of contraception (e.g., condoms and foam) should be planned.

DRUG CLASS: Penicillins

Actions

Penicillins were the first true antibiotics to be grown and used against pathogenic bacteria in human beings. They currently remain one of the most widely used classes of antibiotics.

The penicillins act by interfering with the synthesis of bacterial cell walls. The resulting cell wall is weakened because of defective structure, and the bacteria are subsequently destroyed by osmotic lysis. The penicillins are most effective against bacteria that multiply rapidly. They do not hinder growth of human cells because human cells have protective membranes but no cell wall.

Many bacteria that are initially sensitive to penicillins develop a protective mechanism and become resistant to penicillin therapy. These bacteria produce the enzyme penicillinase (beta-lactamase), which can destroy the antibacterial activity of most penicillins. Penicillinase inactivates the penicillin antibiotics by splitting open the beta-lactam ring of the penicillin molecule. Researchers have developed two mechanisms to prevent this inactivation. The first is to modify the penicillin molecule to "protect" the ring structure while retaining antimicrobial activity. This mechanism culminated in the development of the **penicillinase-resistant penicillins** (e.g., nafcillin, oxacillin, dicloxacillin). The second method is to add another chemical with similar structure that will more readily bond to the penicillinase enzymes than the penicillin, leaving the free penicillin to inhibit cell wall synthesis. Potassium clavulanate is now added to amoxicillin (Augmentin) and ticarcillin (Timentin) to bond to penicillinases that would normally destroy these antibiotics. Sulbactam has been added to ampicillin (Unasyn) and tazobactam to piperacillin (Zosyn) for similar reasons.

Uses

Penicillins are used to treat middle ear infections (otitis media), pneumonia, meningitis, urinary tract infections, syphilis, and gonorrhea, and as a prophylactic antibiotic before surgery or dental procedures for patients with histories of rheumatic fever.

Therapeutic Outcomes

The primary therapeutic outcome expected from penicillin therapy is elimination of bacterial infection.

Nursing Process for Penicillins

Premedication Assessment

1. Obtain baseline assessments of presenting symptoms.
2. Record temperature, pulse, respirations, blood pressure, and hydration status.
3. Assess for and record any allergies, symptoms of diarrhea, and abnormal liver or renal function tests. If present, withhold drug and report findings to the health care provider.
4. Obtain baseline laboratory studies ordered (e.g., CBC with differential).

Planning

Availability. See Table 46-5.

Implementation

Dosage and Administration. See Table 46-5.

Compatibilities. DO NOT mix with other drugs in the same syringe or infuse with other drugs. See under Drug Interactions for incompatibilities.

Rate of Infusion. Consult with a pharmacist or see package literature.

Evaluation

Side Effects to Report

Diarrhea. Penicillins cause diarrhea by altering the bacterial flora of the GI tract. The diarrhea is usually not severe enough to warrant discontinuation. Encourage the patient not to discontinue therapy without first consulting the health care provider. If diarrhea persists, monitor the patient for signs of dehydration.

Abnormal Liver and Renal Function Tests. Monitor returning laboratory data and report abnormal findings to the health care provider.

Thrombophlebitis. Carefully assess patients receiving IV penicillins for the development of thrombophlebitis.

Inspect the IV area frequently when providing care; inspect during dressing changes and at times the IV is changed to a new site. Always investigate pain at the IV site. Report redness, warmth, tenderness to touch, and edema in the affected part. If in the lower extremities, dorsiflexion of the foot may cause pain in the calf area (Homans' sign). Compare the affected limb with the unaffected limb.

Electrolyte Imbalance. The electrolyte content of the antibiotics may cause hyperkalemia or hypernatremia. Some of the penicillins (e.g., penicillin G IV, piperacillin, ticarcillin) have a high electrolyte content.

Drug Table 46-5 **PENICILLINS**

GENERIC NAME	BRAND NAME	AVAILABILITY	ADULT DOSAGE RANGE
amoxicillin	Amoxil, Trimox	500, 875 mg tablets 125, 200, 250, 400 mg chewable tablets 250, 500 mg capsules 50, 125, 200, 250, 400 mg/5 mL suspension 200, 400 mg tablets for suspension	PO: 250-500 mg/8 hr
ampicillin	Principen, ✱ Apo-Ampi, Ampicin	0.25, 0.5, 1, 2 g vials 250, 500 mg capsules 125, 250 mg/5 mL suspension	IM, IV: 0.5 to 1 g/4-6 hr PO: 250-500 mg/6 hr
carbenicillin	Geocillin	382 mg tablets	PO: 382-764 mg four times daily
dicloxacillin	Dicloxacillin	250, 500 mg capsules 62.5 mg/5 mL suspension	PO: 250-500 mg/6 hr
nafcillin	Nafcillin	1, 2 g powder for injection 1, 2 g premixed containers	IV: 500-1000 mg q4h
oxacillin	Oxacillin	0.5, 1, 2, 10 g vials 250 mg/5 mL suspension	IM, IV: 0.5-1 g/4-6 hr PO: 250-500 mg/4-6 hr
penicillin G, potassium or sodium	Pfizerpen, ✱ Novopen G	Vials of 1, 2, 3, 5, 20 million units	IM, IV: 600,000 to 30 million units daily
penicillin V potassium	Penicillin VK, Veetids	250, 500 mg tablets 125, 250 mg/5 mL suspension	PO: 250-500 mg/6 hr
piperacillin	Piperacillin	2, 3, 4, 40 g vials	IM, IV: 3-4 g/4-6 hr, not to exceed 24 g/24 hr
ticarcillin	Ticar	3 g vials	IM: Do not exceed 2 g/injection site IV: Up to 18 g/24 hr
COMBINATION PRODUCTS			
amoxicillin and potassium clavulanate (co-amoxiclav)	Augmentin, ✱ Clavulin	125, 200, 250, 400 mg chewable tablets 250, 500, 875 mg tablets 1000 mg extended release tablets 125, 200, 250, 400, 600 mg/5 mL suspension	PO: 250-600 mg/8 hr
ticarcillin and potassium clavulanate	Timentin	3 g ticarcillin/100 mg clavulanate/vial	IV: Up to 18 g/24 hr Infuse over 30 minutes
ampicillin and sulbactam sodium	Unasyn	1.5, 3, 15 g bottles and vials	IM, IV: 1.5-3 g/6 hr
piperacillin and tazobactam	Zosyn	2, 3, 4, 36 g vials	IV: 3 g/6 hr

✱ Available in Canada.

Drug Interactions

Probenecid. Patients receiving probenecid in combination with penicillins are more susceptible to toxicity because probenecid inhibits excretion of the penicillins. Monitor closely for adverse effects.

This combination may be used to advantage in the treatment of gonorrhea and other infections in which high levels are indicated.

Ampicillin and Allopurinol. When used concurrently, these two agents are associated with a high incidence of rash. Do not label the patient as allergic to penicillins until further skin testing has verified that there is a true hypersensitivity to penicillins.

Antacids. Excessive use of antacids may diminish the absorption of oral penicillins.

Oral Contraceptives. Penicillins may interfere with the contraceptive activity of oral contraceptives. Oral contraceptives should not be discontinued, but counseling regarding use of additional methods of contraception (e.g., condoms and foam) should be planned.

DRUG CLASS: Quinolones

Actions

Quinolone antibiotics are rapidly emerging as an important class of therapeutic agents. This class is not new; the original members—nalidixic acid and cinoxacin—have been available for the treatment of urinary tract infections (see Chapter 42, p. 685) for well over two decades. A new subclass known as the fluoroquinolones is showing great promise against a wide range of gram-positive and gram-negative bacteria, including some anaerobes. The fluoroquinolones act by inhibiting the activity of deoxyribonucleic acid (DNA) gyrase, an enzyme that is essential for the replication of bacterial DNA.

Uses

- Ciprofloxacin is the first well-tolerated, broad-spectrum oral antibiotic in the quinolone series. It demonstrates rapid bactericidal activity against the pathogens that cause nosocomial and community-acquired urinary tract infections; most of the strains that cause enteritis; gonococci, meningococci, *Legionella, Pasteurella, H. influenzae*, and methicillin-resistant staphylococci; and some gram-negative bacteria, including *P. aeruginosa*. The activity of ciprofloxacin against gram-positive and gram-negative cocci is equal to or better than that of the penicillins, cephalosporins, and aminoglycosides, but most anaerobic organisms are resistant.
- Gemifloxacin is similar in spectrum of activity and use to levofloxacin and moxifloxacin. It also has an advantage of once-daily oral dosing.
- Levofloxacin has broad-spectrum activity against gram-negative, gram-positive, and anaerobic bacteria. It is used to treat maxillary sinusitis, acute bacterial exacerbations of chronic bronchitis, community-acquired pneumonia, skin and soft tissue infections, urinary tract infections, and acute pyelonephritis. It has an advantage of once-daily oral dosing.
- Lomefloxacin is used to treat adults with mild to moderate lower respiratory infections *(H. influenzae* and *M. catarrhalis)* and urinary tract infections *(E. coli, K. pneumoniae, P. mirabilis*, and *Enterobacter cloacae)*. Lomefloxacin should not be used empirically to treat acute exacerbations of chronic bronchitis when it is probable that *S. pneumoniae* is the pathogen. This organism is resistant to lomefloxacin. Lomefloxacin is not active against anaerobes. Photosensitivity reactions have been reported in patients exposed to sunlight or sunlamps. Advise patients to seek medical attention at the first signs of a sensation of skin burning, redness, swelling, blisters, rash, itching or dermatitis.
- Moxifloxacin is active against gram-positive microorganisms such as *S. pneumoniae* and *S. aureus*, gram-negative organisms such as *H. influenzae*, and atypical causes of pneumonia such as *C. pneumoniae* and *M. pneumoniae*. It is approved for use in patients with acute bacterial sinusitis, acute bacterial exacerbation of chronic bronchitis, and community-acquired pneumonia caused by susceptible organisms.
- Ofloxacin has broad-spectrum activity against gram-negative, gram-positive, and anaerobic bacteria. It differs from ciprofloxacin in that it has less activity against *P. aeruginosa* but greater activity against sexually transmitted diseases such as *N. gonorrhoeae, C. trachomatis*, and genital ureaplasma. Ofloxacin is also less susceptible to drug interactions than other fluoroquinolones. Ofloxacin is used to treat urinary tract infections, prostatitis, skin infections (e.g., cellulitis and impetigo), lower respiratory pneumonia, and sexually transmitted diseases other than syphilis.
- Sparfloxacin is used to treat adults with community-acquired pneumonia and acute bacterial exacerbations of bronchitis caused by *H. influenzae, C. pneumoniae, K. pneumoniae, S. pneumoniae, S. aureus*, and *M. catarrhalis*.
- Cinoxacin, nalidixic acid, and norfloxacin are used to treat urinary tract infections (see Chapter 42, p. 686).

Therapeutic Outcomes

The primary therapeutic outcome expected from quinolone therapy is elimination of bacterial infection.

Nursing Process for Quinolones

Premedication Assessment

1. Obtain baseline assessments of presenting symptoms.
2. Record temperature, pulse, respirations, blood pressure, and hydration status.
3. Assess for and record any gastric symptoms before initiation of therapy.
4. Assess for any allergies.
5. Obtain baseline laboratory studies ordered (e.g., CBC with differential).
6. Ensure that the patient is not pregnant.
7. Warn patients of possible phototoxicity to lomefloxacin (see under Side Effects to Report).

Planning

Availability. See Table 46-6.

Implementation

Dosage and Administration. See Table 46-6.

Children. Pediatric therapy is not recommended because of the potential for permanent cartilage damage.

Pregnancy. Quinolone therapy is not recommended during pregnancy unless the benefit of therapy outweighs the risk. No studies have been completed in human patients, but animal studies have demonstrated various teratogenic effects.

Drug Table **46-6** **QUINOLONES**

GENERIC NAME	BRAND NAME	AVAILABILITY	DOSAGE RANGE
cinoxacin	Cinobac	Capsules: 250, 500 mg	PO: 1 g daily in two to four divided doses for 7 to 14 days. Take with meals.
ciprofloxacin	Cipro	Tablets: 100, 250, 500, 750 mg Tablets: Extended release: 500, 1000 mg Suspension: 250, 500 mg/5 mL Injection: 200, 400 mg vials	PO: 0.5-1.5 g daily in two divided doses 2 hr after meals. IV: 400-800 mg daily in two divided doses every 12 hr.
gemifloxacin	Factive	Tablets: 320 mg	PO: 320 mg once daily. It may be taken without regard to meals.
levofloxacin	Levaquin	Tablets: 250, 500, 750 mg Suspension: 25 mg/mL Injection: 250, 500, 750 mg vial	PO: 500 mg once daily. IV: 250-500 mg infused slowly over at least 60 min.
lomefloxacin	Maxaquin	Tablets: 400 mg	PO: 400 mg once daily. It may be taken without regard to meals.
moxifloxacin	Avelox	Tablets: 400 mg Injection: 400 mg	IV, PO: 400 mg once daily. It may be taken without regard to meals.
nalidixic acid	NegGram	Tablets: 500 mg	PO: 1 g four times daily for 7-14 days. Take with meals.
norfloxacin	Noroxin	Tablets: 400 mg	PO: 400 mg twice daily for 7-10 days. Take 1 hr before or 2 hr after meals with a large glass of fluid. Do not exceed 800 mg daily.
ofloxacin	Floxin	Tablets: 200, 300, 400 mg	PO: 600-800 mg daily in two divided doses every 12 hr, 1 hr before or 2 hr after meals, with a large glass of fluid.
sparfloxacin	Zagam	Tablets: 200 mg	PO: 200-400 mg once daily. It may be taken with or without meals.

Evaluation

Side Effects to Expect

Nausea, Vomiting, Diarrhea, Discomfort. These side effects are usually mild and tend to resolve with continued therapy. Encourage the patient not to discontinue therapy without first consulting the health care provider. If the patient should become debilitated, contact the health care provider.

Dizziness, Lightheadedness. Although uncommon, ciprofloxacin may cause these disturbances. They tend to be self-limiting, and therapy should not be discontinued until the patient consults a health care provider.

Caution the patient against driving or performing hazardous tasks until adjusted to the effects of the medication.

Side Effects to Report

Phototoxicity. Phototoxic reactions have been reported in patients treated with lomefloxacin. Exposure to direct and indirect sunlight and the use of sunlamps should be avoided. These reactions have occurred with and without the use of sunblocks and sunscreens and with single doses of lomefloxacin. The patient should not take additional doses and should contact the health care provider if a sensation of skin burning, redness, swelling, blisters, rash, itching, or dermatitis develops. Suggest wearing long-sleeved clothing, a hat, and sunglasses when exposed to sunlight.

Rash. Report a rash or pruritus immediately and withhold additional doses pending approval by the health care provider.

Abnormal Laboratory Tests. Monitor returning laboratory data and report abnormal findings to the health care provider.

Neurologic Effects. Report the development of tinnitus, headache, dizziness, mental depression, drowsiness, or confusion.

Drug Interactions

Iron, Antacids, Sucralfate. Iron salts, zinc salts, sucralfate, and antacids containing magnesium hydroxide or aluminum hydroxide decrease the absorption of quinolones. Administer at least 4 hours before or 4 hours after ingestion of antacids, sucralfate, or iron-containing products.

Probenecid. Patients receiving probenecid in combination with norfloxacin or lomefloxacin are more susceptible to toxicity because probenecid inhibits excretion of the quinolones. Monitor closely for toxic effects.

The combination may be used advantageously in treating serious or resistant infections in which high serum levels of a quinolone are required.

Nonsteroidal Antiinflammatory Drugs (NSAIDs). The concurrent administration of NSAIDs with fluoroquinolones (e.g., levofloxacin, ofloxacin) may increase the risk of CNS stimulation with seizures. Use with extreme caution. Consider the use of other analgesics or antiinflammatory agents.

Didanosine. Do not administer quinolone antibiotics within 4 hours of administration of didanosine tablets or pediatric powder for oral solution. The antacid present in these formulations inhibits the absorption of the quinolones.

Theophylline. The fluoroquinolones (e.g., ciprofloxacin, norfloxacin, ofloxacin), when given with theophylline, may produce theophylline toxicity. Observe for vomiting, dizziness, restlessness, and cardiac dysrhythmias. Monitor theophylline serum levels. The dosage of theophylline may need to be reduced.

Toxicity Induced by Sparfloxacin. Sparfloxacin may induce life-threatening dysrhythmias when used with the following agents: antidysrhythmics (e.g., amiodarone, bretylium, disopyramide, procainamide, quinidine, sotalol), antihistamines (e.g., astemizole, terfenadine) and bepridil, erythromycin, phenothiazines, and tricyclic antidepressants. Use of sparfloxacin with any of these agents is contraindicated.

Toxicity Induced by Moxifloxacin. Moxifloxacin may induce life-threatening dysrhythmias when used with the following antidysrhythmic agents: amiodarone, bretylium, disopyramide, procainamide, quinidine, and sotalol. Use of moxifloxacin with any of these agents is contraindicated.

DRUG CLASS: Streptogramins

quinupristin/dalfopristin (qwin u pris′ tin) (dal foh pris′ tin)
SYNERCID (sin′ erh sid)

Actions

Quinupristin/dalfopristin is the first of a new class of antimicrobial agents known as streptogramins. These two agents are developed from pristamycin. When used in combination, they are synergistic and act by inhibiting protein synthesis in bacterial cells.

Uses

Quinupristin/dalfopristin are agents that can be used in the treatment of serious or life-threatening infections associated with vancomycin-resistant *Enterococcus faecium* bacteria and complicated skin and skin structure infections caused by methicillin-susceptible *S. aureus* or *S. pyogenes*. As a representative of a new class of antibiotics, quinupristin/dalfopristin use should be reserved for those cases in which other antibiotics such as vancomycin are ineffective so that resistant strains of bacteria do not rapidly develop.

Therapeutic Outcomes

The primary therapeutic outcome expected from quinupristin/dalfopristin therapy is elimination of bacterial infection.

Nursing Process for Streptogramins

Premedication Assessment

1. Obtain baseline assessments of presenting symptoms.
2. Record temperature, pulse, respirations, blood pressure, and hydration status.
3. Assess for and record any gastric symptoms before initiating therapy.
4. Assess for any allergies.
5. Obtain baseline laboratory studies ordered (e.g., CBC with differential, platelets, blood glucose, electrolytes, creatine kinase, liver function tests).

Planning

Availability. IV: 500 mg (150 mg quinupristin and 350 mg dalfopristin) in 10-mL vial. All dosage recommendations are based on total quinupristin and dalfopristin milligrams.

Implementation

Dosage and Administration. *Adult:* IV: 7.5 mg/kg every 8 hours for the treatment of vancomycin-resistant *E. faecium* bacteremia or every 12 hours for treatment of complicated skin infections. Infuse the dose over 60 minutes. Reconstitute only with 5% dextrose or sterile water for injection and then dilute with 5% dextrose to a final concentration of 100 mg/mL. A precipitate will form if reconstituted with other standard diluents. If infused in IV tubing being used for other medicines, flush with 5% dextrose. Do not flush with heparin or sodium chloride.

Evaluation

Side Effects to Report

Pain, Infusion Site Inflammation. The most frequent adverse venous events include pain at the administration site, edema, infusion site reaction, and thrombophlebitis.

Nausea, Vomiting, Anorexia, Abdominal Cramps, Diarrhea. These side effects are usually mild and tend to resolve with continued therapy.

Arthralgia, Myalgia. Arthralgias and myalgias may occur during therapy. Decreasing the frequency of administration to every 12 hours may minimize recurrence.

Hepatotoxicity. The symptoms of hepatotoxicity are anorexia, nausea, vomiting, jaundice, hepatomegaly, splenomegaly, and abnormal liver function tests (e.g., elevated bilirubin, AST, ALT, GGT, alkaline phosphatase, prothrombin time).

Drug Interactions

Toxicity Induced by Quinupristin/Dalfopristin. Quinupristin/dalfopristin may decrease the metabolism of HMG-CoA reductase inhibitors (e.g., atorvastatin, cerivastatin, lovastatin, pravastatin, fluvastatin, simvastatin), cyclosporine, delavirdine, nevirapine, indinavir, ritonavir, vincristine, paclitaxel, docetaxel, tamoxifen, diazepam, midazolam, cisapride, methylprednisolone, carbamazepine, nifedipine, verapamil, diltiazem, quinidine, lidocaine, and disopyramide. Serum concentrations of these agents should be monitored closely if used concurrently with quinupristin/dalfopristin.

DRUG CLASS: Sulfonamides

Actions

The sulfonamides are not true antibiotics because they are not synthesized by microorganisms. However, they are highly effective antibacterial agents. Sulfonamides act by inhibiting bacterial biosynthesis of folic acid, which eventually results in bacterial cell death. Human cells do not synthesize folic acid and therefore are not affected.

Uses

Sulfonamides are used primarily to treat urinary tract infections and otitis media. They may also be used to prevent streptococcal infection or rheumatic fever in people who are allergic to penicillin.

Because of an increasing incidence of organisms resistant to sulfonamide therapy and the unreliability of in vitro sulfonamide sensitivity tests, patients should be monitored closely for continued therapeutic response to treatment. This is particularly important in patients being treated for chronic and recurrent urinary tract infections.

The sulfonamide most commonly used today is actually a combination of trimethoprim and sulfamethoxazole (e.g., co-trimoxazole, TMP-SMX). This combination blocks two steps in the pathway of folic acid production; therefore, fewer resistant strains of microorganisms have developed. Co-trimoxazole is often used for treatment of urinary tract infections, otitis media in children, traveler's diarrhea, acute exacerbations of chronic bronchitis in adults, and prophylaxis and treatment of *Pneumocystis jiroveci (carinii)* pneumonia (PJP, formerly PCP) in immunocompromised patients.

Therapeutic Outcomes

The primary therapeutic outcome expected from sulfonamide therapy is elimination of bacterial infection.

Nursing Process for Sulfonamides

Premedication Assessment

1. Obtain baseline assessments of presenting symptoms.
2. Record temperature, pulse, respirations, blood pressure, and hydration status.
3. Assess for and record any gastric symptoms before beginning therapy.
4. Assess for any allergies.
5. Obtain baseline laboratory studies ordered (e.g., CBC with differential).

Planning

Availability. See Table 46-7.

Drug Table 46-7 SULFONAMIDES

GENERIC NAME	BRAND NAME	AVAILABILITY	ADULT DOSAGE RANGE
sulfadiazine	Sulfadiazine	500 mg tablets	PO: Initial dose: 2-4 g, then 4-8 g/24 hr in divided doses
sulfasalazine	Azulfidine	500 mg tablets 500 mg delayed-release tablets	PO: Initial therapy: 3-4 g daily in divided doses; maintenance dosage is 2 g daily
sulfisoxazole	Sulfisoxazole, Gantrisin	500 mg tablets 500 mg/5 mL suspension	PO: Initial dose: 2-4 g; maintenance dose is 4-8 g/24 hr divided into three to six doses
co-trimoxazole	Bactrim, Septra, Bactrim DS, Septra DS	Tablets, suspension, infusion	PO: two to four tablets daily, depending on strength, disease being treated IV: 15-20 mg/kg/24 hr (based on trimethoprim) in three or four divided doses for up to 14 days
erythromycin-sulfisoxazole	Pediazole, Eryzole	Suspension	PO: 2.5-10 mL every 6 hr, depending on weight of patient

Implementation

Dosage and Administration. See Table 46-7. NOTE: Patients should be encouraged to drink water several times daily while receiving sulfonamide therapy. In rare situations, crystals form in the urinary tract if the patient becomes too dehydrated.

Evaluation

Side Effects to Report

Nausea, Vomiting, Anorexia, Diarrhea. These side effects are usually mild and tend to resolve with continued therapy. Encourage the patient not to discontinue therapy without first consulting the health care provider.

If the patient becomes debilitated, contact the health care provider.

Dermatologic Reactions. Report a rash or pruritus immediately and withhold additional doses pending approval by the health care provider.

Photosensitivity. The patient should be cautioned to avoid exposure to sunlight and ultraviolet light. Suggest wearing long-sleeved clothing, a hat, and sunglasses when outdoors. Discourage the use of tanning lamps.

Hematologic Reactions. Routine laboratory studies (e.g., CBC with differential) are scheduled for patients taking sulfonamides for 14 days or longer. Stress the importance of returning for this laboratory work.

Monitor for the development of a sore throat, fever, purpura, jaundice, or excessive and progressive weakness.

Neurologic Effects. Report the development of tinnitus, headache, dizziness, mental depression, drowsiness, or confusion.

Drug Interactions

Oral Hypoglycemic Agents. Sulfonamides may displace sulfonylurea oral hypoglycemic agents (e.g., tolbutamide, acetohexamide, tolazamide, chlorpropamide) from protein-binding sites, resulting in hypoglycemia.

Monitor for hypoglycemia, headache, weakness, decreased coordination, general apprehension, diaphoresis, hunger, and blurred or double vision.

The dosage of the hypoglycemic agent may need to be reduced. Notify the health care provider if any of the above-mentioned symptoms appear.

Clinitest. A false-positive reaction for glucose in the urine may occur with Clinitest tablets, but will not occur with Diastix.

Warfarin. Sulfonamides may enhance the anticoagulant effects of warfarin. Observe for petechiae, ecchymoses, nosebleeds, bleeding gums, dark tarry stools, and bright red or "coffee ground" emesis. Monitor the prothrombin time (INR) and reduce the dosage of warfarin if necessary.

Methotrexate. Sulfonamides may produce methotrexate toxicity when given simultaneously. Monitor patients on concurrent therapy for oral stomatitis and for signs of nephrotoxicity (e.g., oliguria, hematuria, proteinuria, casts).

Phenytoin. Sulfisoxazole may displace phenytoin from protein-binding sites, resulting in phenytoin toxicity.

Monitor patients on concurrent therapy for signs of phenytoin toxicity (e.g., nystagmus, sedation, lethargy); serum levels may be ordered. A reduced dosage of phenytoin may be required.

DRUG CLASS: Tetracyclines

Actions

Tetracyclines are a class of antibiotics that are effective against gram-negative and gram-positive bacteria. They act by inhibiting protein synthesis by bacterial cells.

Uses

The tetracyclines are often used in patients allergic to the penicillins for the treatment of certain venereal diseases, urinary tract infections, upper respiratory tract infections, pneumonia, and meningitis. They are particularly effective against skin (acne), rickettsial, and mycoplasmic infections.

Tetracyclines administered during the ages of tooth development (the last half of pregnancy through 8 years of age) may cause enamel hypoplasia and permanent yellow, gray, or brown staining of the teeth. Tetracyclines are secreted in breast milk, so nursing mothers on tetracycline therapy are advised to feed their infants formula or cow's milk, as appropriate.

Therapeutic Outcomes

The primary therapeutic outcome expected from tetracycline therapy is elimination of bacterial infection.

Nursing Process for Tetracyclines

Premedication Assessment

1. Obtain baseline assessments of presenting symptoms.
2. Record temperature, pulse, respirations, blood pressure, and hydration status.
3. Assess for and record any gastric symptoms present before beginning therapy.
4. Assess for any allergies.
5. Obtain baseline laboratory studies ordered (e.g., CBC with differential).

Planning

Availability. See Table 46-8.

Implementation

Dosage and Administration. See Table 46-8. PO: Emphasize the importance of taking medication 1 hour before or 2 hours after ingesting antacids, milk, or other dairy products, or products containing calcium, aluminum, magnesium, or iron (e.g., vitamins). *Exception:* Food and milk do not interfere with the absorption of doxycycline.

Drug Table 46-8 **TETRACYCLINES**

GENERIC NAME	BRAND NAME	AVAILABILITY	ADULT DOSAGE RANGE
demeclocycline	Declomycin	150, 300 mg tablets	PO: 150 mg four times daily or 300 mg twice daily
doxycycline	Vibramycin	100, 200 mg vials 50, 100 mg tablets 50, 100 mg capsules 25, 50 mg/5 mL syrup	IV: 100-200 mg once or twice daily PO: 200 mg on day 1, then 100 mg divided in two doses
minocycline	Minocin	100 mg vial 50, 75, 100 mg capsules 50, 75, 100 mg tablets 50 mg/5 mL suspension	PO, IV: 200 mg, followed by 100 mg/12 hr
oxytetracycline	Terramycin	50, 125 mg/mL with 2% lidocaine for injection	IM: 250 mg every 24 hr or 300 mg every 8-12 hr.
tetracycline	Sumycin	250, 500 mg capsules and tablets 125 mg/5 mL suspension	PO: 250-500 mg four times daily

Evaluation

Side Effects to Report

Nausea, Vomiting, Anorexia, Abdominal Cramps, Diarrhea. These side effects are usually mild and tend to resolve with continued therapy. Encourage the patient not to discontinue therapy without first consulting the health care provider.

Photosensitivity. Photosensitivity resulting in an exaggerated sunburn after short exposure has been reported. The patient should be cautioned to avoid exposure to sunlight and ultraviolet light. Suggest wearing long-sleeved clothing, a hat, and sunglasses when outdoors. Discourage the use of tanning lamps. Consult the health care provider about the advisability of discontinuing therapy.

Drug Interactions

Warfarin. This medication may enhance the anticoagulant effects of warfarin. Observe for petechiae, ecchymoses, nosebleeds, bleeding gums, dark tarry stools, and bright red or "coffee ground" emesis. Monitor the prothrombin time (INR) and reduce the dosage of warfarin if necessary.

Methoxyflurane. If patients are receiving tetracycline and are scheduled for surgery, label the front of the chart "taking tetracycline." Fatal nephrotoxicity has been reported when methoxyflurane is administered to a person taking tetracycline.

Impaired Absorption. Iron; calcium-containing foods (milk and dairy products); calcium, aluminum, or magnesium preparations (antacids); H_2 antagonists (cimetidine, famotidine, nizatidine, ranitidine), and alkaline products (sodium bicarbonate) decrease absorption of tetracycline. Administer all tetracycline products 1 hour before or 2 hours after ingestion of these foods or products. *Exception:* Food and milk do not interfere with the absorption of doxycycline.

Phenytoin, Carbamazepine. These agents reduce the half-life of doxycycline. Monitor patients for lack of clinical improvement from the infection.

Tooth Development. Do not administer tetracyclines to pregnant patients or to children younger than 8 years of age. The infant's or child's tooth enamel may be permanently stained yellow, gray, or brown.

Lactation. Nursing mothers must switch their babies to formula while taking tetracyclines because tetracyclines are present in the breast milk.

Oral Contraceptives. Tetracyclines may interfere with the contraceptive activity of oral contraceptives. Oral contraceptives should not be discontinued, but counseling regarding use of additional methods of contraception (e.g., condoms and foam) should be planned.

Didanosine. Do not administer tetracycline antibiotics within 2 hours of taking didanosine tablets or pediatric powder for oral solution. The antacid present in these formulations inhibits the absorption of the quinolones.

DRUG CLASS: Antitubercular Agents

ethambutol (e tham' bu tol)
MYAMBUTOL (my am' bu tol)

Actions

Ethambutol inhibits tuberculosis bacterial growth by altering cellular ribonucleic acid (RNA) synthesis and phosphate metabolism.

Uses

Ethambutol is an antitubercular agent. It must be used in combination with other antitubercular agents to prevent the development of resistant organisms.

Therapeutic Outcomes

The primary therapeutic outcome expected from ethambutol therapy is elimination of tuberculosis.

Nursing Process for Ethambutol

Premedication Assessment

1. Obtain baseline assessments of presenting symptoms.
2. Record temperature, pulse, respirations, blood pressure, and hydration status.
3. Assess for and record any gastric symptoms before initiating therapy.
4. Assess for any allergies.
5. Perform baseline mental status assessment (e.g., orientation and alertness), assess for GI symptoms, and test color vision (e.g., red-green discrimination) before initiating therapy.
6. Review laboratory data of tuberculin testing on the patient's chart.

Planning

Availability. PO: 100 and 400 mg tablets.

Implementation

Dosage and Administration. *Adults:* PO: Initial treatment: 15 mg/kg administered as a single dose every 24 hours. Retreatment: 25 mg/kg as a single daily dose. After 60 days reduce the dosage to 15 mg/kg and administer as a single dose every 24 hours. Administer once daily with food or milk to minimize gastric irritation.

Counseling. The patient should be warned that omission or interrupted intake may result in drug resistance, reversal of clinical improvement, and increased susceptibility of family members and others to tuberculosis.

Evaluation

Side Effects to Expect

Nausea, Vomiting, Anorexia, Abdominal Cramps. These side effects are usually mild and tend to resolve with continued therapy. Encourage the patient not to discontinue therapy without first consulting the health care provider. Administer daily dose with food to minimize nausea and vomiting.

Side Effects to Report

Confusion, Hallucinations. Perform a baseline assessment of the patient's degree of alertness and orientation to name, place, and time before initiating therapy. Make regularly scheduled subsequent mental status evaluations, and compare findings. Report development of alterations. Provide for patient safety during episodes of altered behavior or periods of dizziness.

Blurred Vision, Red-Green Vision Changes. Before initiating therapy, check for any visual alterations using a color vision chart. Schedule subsequent evaluations on a regular basis. Report the development of visual disturbances for the health care provider's evaluation. These adverse effects disappear within a few weeks after therapy is discontinued.

Drug Interactions

Antacids. Aluminum salts may delay and reduce absorption of ethambutol. Separate administration by at least 2 hours.

isoniazid (i so ny' ah zid)

INH, NYDRAZID (ny' dra zid)

Actions

Isoniazid has been a mainstay for many years in the prevention and treatment of tuberculosis. Despite this, its mechanism of action is still not fully known. It appears to disrupt the *M. tuberculosis* cell wall and inhibit replication.

Uses

Isoniazid is used for the prophylaxis and treatment of tuberculosis. It should be used in combination with other antitubercular agents for therapy of active disease.

Therapeutic Outcomes

The primary therapeutic outcomes expected from isoniazid therapy are as follows:

- Prevention of tuberculosis in people with a positive skin test.
- Elimination of tuberculosis in people with active disease

Nursing Process for Isoniazid

Premedication Assessment

1. Obtain baseline assessments of presenting symptoms.
2. Record temperature, pulse, respirations, blood pressure, and hydration status.
3. Assess for and record any gastric symptoms, abnormal liver function tests, or paresthesias present before initiation of therapy.
4. Assess for any allergies.
5. Check medication orders for concurrent administration of other antitubercular drugs and for an order for pyridoxine.

Planning

Availability. PO: 100 and 300 mg tablets; 50 mg/mL syrup; IM: 100 mg/mL in 10 mL vials.

Implementation

Dosage and Administration. *Adult:* PO: Treatment of active tuberculosis is 5 mg/kg to a maximum of 300 mg daily. Isoniazid should be used in conjunction with other effective antitubercular agents. Prophylactic therapy: 300 mg daily in single or divided doses. Administer on an empty stomach for maximum effectiveness. It is usually given as a single daily dose but may be given in divided doses. Pyridoxine, 25 to 50 mg daily, is often given concurrently with isoniazid to diminish peripheral neuropathies, dizziness, and ataxia. IM: As for PO administration.

Pediatric: PO: 10 to 30 mg/kg per 24 hours in single or divided doses. Infants and children tolerate larger doses than adults. Maximum dose is 500 mg daily.

Evaluation

Side Effects to Expect and Report

Tingling, Numbness, Nausea, Vomiting. Tingling and numbness of the hands and feet and nausea and vomiting are relatively common side effects of isoniazid and are dosage related. Concurrent use of pyridoxine, 25 to 50 mg daily, will usually prevent these symptoms.

When paresthesias are present, the patient must be cautioned to inspect the extremities for any skin breakdown because of the diminished sensation.

Caution patients not to immerse feet or hands in water without first testing the temperature.

Monitor patients with paresthesias for adequate nutrition.

Dizziness, Ataxia. Provide for patient safety and assistance in ambulation until either a dosage adjustment or addition of pyridoxine provides symptomatic relief.

Hepatotoxicity. The incidence of hepatotoxicity increases with age and with the consumption of alcohol. This reaction usually occurs within the first 3 months of therapy and is thought to be an allergic reaction.

The symptoms of hepatotoxicity are anorexia, nausea, vomiting, jaundice, hepatomegaly, splenomegaly, and abnormal liver function tests (e.g., elevated bilirubin, AST, ALT, GGT, alkaline phosphatase, prothrombin time).

Drug Interactions

Disulfiram. Patients may experience changes in physical coordination and mental affect and behavior. Provide for patient safety and monitor the patient's mental status before and during therapy. If possible, avoid concomitant therapy.

Carbamazepine. Isoniazid may inhibit the metabolism of carbamazepine. Monitor patients receiving concurrent therapy for signs of carbamazepine toxicity (e.g., ataxia, headache, vomiting, blurred vision, drowsiness, confusion).

Theophylline. Isoniazid may inhibit the metabolism of theophylline. Monitor patients receiving concurrent therapy for signs of theophylline toxicity (e.g., anxiety, tachycardia, nausea, headache, vomiting).

Phenytoin. Isoniazid may inhibit the metabolism of phenytoin. Monitor patients receiving concurrent therapy for signs of phenytoin toxicity (e.g., nystagmus, sedation, lethargy). Serum levels may be ordered and the dosage of phenytoin reduced.

Clinitest. This drug may produce false-positive Clinitest results. Use Diastix to measure urine glucose.

rifampin (rif am' pin)
RIFADIN (rif' ah din)

Actions

Rifampin prevents RNA synthesis in mycobacterium by inhibiting DNA-dependent RNA polymerase. This action blocks key metabolic pathways needed for mycobacterium cells to grow and replicate.

Uses

Rifampin is used in combination with other agents in the treatment of tuberculosis. Rifampin is also used to eliminate meningococci from the nasopharynx of asymptomatic *N. meningitidis* carriers and to eliminate *H. influenzae* type b (Hib) from the nasopharynx of asymptomatic carriers.

Therapeutic Outcomes

The primary therapeutic outcomes expected from rifampin therapy are as follows:

- Elimination of tuberculosis
- Eradication of meningococci or Hib from asymptomatic carriers of these diseases

Nursing Process for Rifampin

Premedication Assessment

1. Obtain baseline assessments of presenting symptoms.
2. Record temperature, pulse, respirations, blood pressure, and hydration status.
3. Assess for and record any gastric symptoms present before beginning therapy.
4. Assess for any allergies.
5. Obtain baseline laboratory studies ordered (e.g., CBC with differential, tuberculin tests, chest radiograph).

Planning

Availability. PO: 150 and 300 mg capsules; IV: 600 mg vials.

Implementation

Dosage and Administration. *Adult:* PO: 600 mg once daily either 1 hour before or 2 hours after a meal; IV: as for PO.

Pediatric: PO: 10 to 20 mg/kg per 24 hours, with a maximum daily dose of 600 mg; IV: as for PO.

NOTE: Patients should be warned that omission or interrupted intake may result in drug resistance, reversal of clinical improvement, and increased susceptibility of family members to tuberculosis.

Evaluation

Side Effects to Expect

Reddish Orange Secretions. Urine, feces, saliva, sputum, sweat, and tears may be tinged reddish orange. The effect is harmless and will disappear after discontinuing therapy. Rifampin may permanently discolor soft contact lenses.

Side Effects to Report

Nausea, Vomiting, Anorexia, Abdominal Cramps. These side effects are usually mild and tend to resolve with continued therapy. Encourage the patient not to discontinue therapy without first consulting the health care provider. If these symptoms are accompanied by fever, chills, or muscle and bone pain, or if unusual bruising or a yellowish discoloration of the skin or eyes appears, contact the patient's health care provider.

Drug Interactions

Warfarin. This medication may diminish the anticoagulant effects of warfarin. Monitor the prothrombin time (INR) and increase the dosage of warfarin if necessary.

Isoniazid. Concurrent therapy may rarely result in hepatotoxicity. Patients on combined therapy should have liver function tests monitored periodically.

Benzodiazepines (Diazepam, Midazolam, Triazolam) Quinidine, Amiodarone, Verapamil, Nifedipine, Mexiletine, Enalapril, Tocainide, Theophylline, Beta Blocking Agents (Bisoprolol, Metoprolol, Propranolol), Disopyramide, Barbiturates, Fluoroquinolones, Ondansetron, Haloperidol, Losartan, Protease Inhibitors, Oral Antidiabetic Agents, Many Other Drugs. Rifampin stimulates the metabolism of these agents. Long-term combined therapy may require an increase in dosages for therapeutic effect.

Ketoconazole. Administration of rifampin and ketoconazole decreases serum levels of both drugs. Avoid concurrent use if possible.

Oral Contraceptives. Rifampin interferes with the contraceptive activity of oral contraceptives. Counseling regarding alternative methods of birth control should be planned.

DRUG CLASS: Miscellaneous Antibiotics

aztreonam (aze tree′ on am)

AZACTAM (aze ak′ tam)

Actions

Aztreonam is the first in a new class of synthetic, bactericidal antibiotics called the monobactams, which act by inhibiting cell wall synthesis.

Uses

The monobactams have a high degree of activity against beta-lactamase–producing aerobic gram-negative bacteria, including *P. aeruginosa*. Aztreonam has essentially no activity against anaerobes or gram-positive microorganisms. It is used to treat urinary tract, lower respiratory tract, skin, intraabdominal, gynecologic, and bacteremic infections and meningitides, caused by *P. aeruginosa, Salmonella, Shigella, N. gonorrhoeae,* and ampicillin-resistant *H. influenzae*. It is recommended that aztreonam be combined with a broad-spectrum antibiotic in the initial treatment of an infection of unknown cause to treat susceptible anaerobes or gram-positive organisms.

Therapeutic Outcomes

The primary therapeutic outcome expected from aztreonam therapy is elimination of bacterial infection.

Nursing Process for Miscellaneous Antibiotics

Premedication Assessment

1. Obtain baseline assessments of presenting symptoms.
2. Record temperature, pulse, respirations, blood pressure, and hydration status.
3. Assess for and record any gastric symptoms before initiating therapy.
4. Assess for any allergies.
5. Obtain baseline laboratory studies ordered (e.g., CBC with differential).

Planning

Availability. Injection: 500 mg, 1 and 2 g powders in 15 mL, 30 mL, and 100 mL bottles for reconstitution.

Implementation

Dosage and Administration. *Adult:* IM or IV: Urinary tract infections: 0.5 to 1 g every 8 to 12 hours. Moderately severe systemic infections: 1 to 2 g every 8 to 12 hours. Life-threatening infections: 2 g every 6 to 8 hours. IM: Reconstitute a 15-mL vial with at least 3 mL of diluent per gram of aztreonam. After adding diluent to container, shake immediately and vigorously. Inject deeply into the large muscle mass of the gluteus maximus. Discard unused portion of vial. IV bolus: Reconstitute a 15-mL vial with 6 to 10 mL of diluent. Immediately shake vigorously. Inject directly into a vein or into the tubing of a suitable IV set over 3 to 5 minutes. Discard any unused portion of the vial. IV infusion: Reconstitute the 100-mL bottle with at least 50 mL of diluent. Shake immediately and vigorously. Infuse over the next 30 to 60 minutes.

Evaluation

Side Effects to Expect

Nausea, Vomiting, Diarrhea. These side effects are usually mild and tend to resolve with continued therapy.

Side Effects to Report

Phlebitis. Avoid IV infusion in the lower extremities or in areas with varicosities. Use proper technique in starting the IV solution.

Carefully assess at regularly scheduled intervals for signs of developing phlebitis. Inspect for redness, warmth, tenderness to touch, edema, or pain.

Always assess complaints of pain at the infusion site. If signs of inflammation accompany complaints, discontinue and restart elsewhere.

Secondary Infections. Oral thrush, genital and anal pruritus, vaginitis, and vaginal discharge may occur. Report promptly because these infections are resistant to the original antibiotic used. Teach the importance of meticulous oral and perineal hygiene measures.

Drug Interactions

Cefoxitin, Imipenem. These antibiotics induce beta-lactamase production in some gram-negative organisms, resulting in possible antagonism with a beta-lactam antibiotic such as aztreonam. It is recommended that beta-lactamase–stimulating antibiotics not be used concurrently with aztreonam.

chloramphenicol (klo ram fen' i kol)

▶ CHLOROMYCETIN (klo ro my see' tin)

Actions

Chloramphenicol is an antibiotic that acts by inhibiting bacterial protein synthesis of a variety of gram-positive and gram-negative organisms.

Uses

Chloramphenicol is particularly effective in treating rickettsial infections, meningitis, and typhoid fever. It must not be used in the treatment of trivial infections or when it is not indicated, such as in colds, influenza, throat infections, or as a prophylactic agent to prevent bacterial infection.

Therapeutic Outcomes

The primary therapeutic outcome expected from chloramphenicol therapy is elimination of bacterial infection.

Nursing Process for Chloramphenicol

Premedication Assessment

1. Obtain baseline assessments of presenting symptoms.
2. Record temperature, pulse, respirations, blood pressure, and hydration status.
3. Assess for and record any gastric symptoms before initiating therapy.
4. Assess for any allergies.
5. Obtain baseline laboratory studies ordered (e.g., CBC with differential).

Planning

Availability. IV: 100 mg/mL in 1-g vials.

Implementation

Dosage and Administration. *Adult:* IM: not recommended due to poor absorption and clinical response; IV: 50 to 100 mg/kg every 6 hours. Reconstitute by adding 10 mL of sterile water for injection or 5% dextrose to 1 g of chloramphenicol to make a solution containing 100 mg/mL. Administer the calculated dose intravenously over 1 minute.

Pediatric: IM: Not recommended. IV: Neonates: 25 mg/kg per 24 hours in four equally divided doses. Infants over 2 weeks of age: 50 mg/kg per 24 hours in four equally divided doses. Administer over 1 minute. Use only chloramphenicol sodium succinate IV in children.

Evaluation

Side Effects to Report

Hematologic. Serious and possibly fatal bone marrow suppression may occur after therapy is initiated with chloramphenicol. Early signs include sore throat, fatigue, elevated temperature, and small petechial hemorrhages and bruises on the skin. If patients describe any of these symptoms, report them to the health care provider immediately. Routine laboratory studies (RBC, white blood cells [WBC], and differential counts) are scheduled for patients taking chloramphenicol for 14 days or longer. Stress the importance of returning for this laboratory work.

Monitor for the development of sore throat, fever, purpura, jaundice, or excessive or progressive weakness.

Secondary Infections. Oral thrush, genital and anal pruritus, vaginitis, and vaginal discharge may occur. Report promptly because these infections are resistant to the original antibiotic used.

Teach the importance of meticulous oral and perineal hygiene.

Drug Interactions

Warfarin. This medication may enhance the anticoagulant effects of warfarin. Observe for the development of petechiae, ecchymoses, nosebleeds, bleeding gums, dark tarry stools, and bright red or "coffee ground" emesis. Monitor prothrombin time (INR) and reduce the dosage of warfarin if necessary.

Oral Hypoglycemic Agents. Monitor for hypoglycemia: headache, weakness, decreased coordination, general apprehension, diaphoresis, hunger, and blurred or double vision.

The dosage of the hypoglycemic agent may need to be reduced. Notify the health care provider if any of these symptoms appear.

Clinitest. Chloramphenicol may cause a false-positive urinary glucose reaction when Clinitest is used. Diastix may be used instead to test for the presence of urine glucose.

Phenytoin. Chloramphenicol inhibits the metabolism of phenytoin. Monitor patients with concurrent therapy for signs of phenytoin toxicity: nystagmus, sedation, and lethargy. Serum levels may be ordered and the dosage of phenytoin reduced.

clindamycin (klin dah my′ sin)
CLEOCIN (klee o′ sin)
DALACIN C (dahl′ ah sin C) ✱

Actions

Clindamycin is an antibiotic that acts by inhibiting protein synthesis.

Uses

Clindamycin is useful against infections caused by gram-negative aerobic organisms and a variety of gram-positive and gram-negative anaerobes.

Therapeutic Outcomes

The primary therapeutic outcome expected from clindamycin therapy is elimination of bacterial infection.

Nursing Process for Clindamycin

Premedication Assessment

1. Obtain baseline assessments of presenting symptoms.
2. Record temperature, pulse, respirations, blood pressure, and hydration status.
3. Record pattern of bowel elimination before initiating drug therapy.
4. Assess for any allergies.
5. Obtain baseline laboratory studies ordered (e.g., CBC with differential).

Planning

Availability. PO: 75, 150 and 300 mg capsules, 75 mg/5 mL suspension; IV: 150 mg/mL in 2, 4, and 6 mL ampules.

Implementation

Dosage and Administration. *Adult:* PO: 150 to 450 mg every 6 hours. DO NOT refrigerate the suspension. It is stable at room temperature for 14 days. IM: 600 to 2700 mg per 24 hours. DO NOT exceed 600 mg per injection. Pain, induration, and sterile abscesses have been reported. Deep IM injection is recommended to help minimize this reaction. IV: 600 to 2700 mg per 24 hours. Dilute to less than 6 mg/mL, and administer at a rate less than 30 mg per minute. Administration by IV push is not recommended.

Pediatric: PO: suspension: 8 to 25 mg/kg per 24 hours in four divided doses. Capsules: 8 to 20 mg/kg per 24 hours in four divided doses. Capsules should be taken with a full glass of water to prevent esophageal irritation. IM: 15 to 40 mg/kg per 24 hours in four divided doses; IV: as for IM use. Dilute to less than 6 mg/mL and administer at a rate less than 30 mg per minute.

Evaluation

Side Effects to Report

Diarrhea. These side effects are usually mild and tend to resolve with continued therapy. Encourage the patient not to discontinue therapy without first consulting the health care provider.

Severe Diarrhea. Severe diarrhea may develop from the use of clindamycin. Report diarrhea of five or more stools per day to the health care provider. This may be an indication of drug-induced pseudomembranous colitis.

Blood or mucus in the stool should also be reported to the health care provider. *Warn patients not to treat diarrhea themselves when taking this drug.* The use of diphenoxylate, loperamide, or paregoric may prolong or worsen the condition.

Drug Interactions

Neuromuscular Blockade. Label charts of patients scheduled for surgery who are taking clindamycin. When combined with surgical muscle relaxants or aminoglycosides, neuromuscular blockade may result.

These combinations may potentiate respiratory depression. Check the anesthesia record of surgical patients. Monitor postoperative patients (for respiratory depression) for a prolonged period. This can occur 48 hours or more after the drug administration.

Theophylline Toxicity. Clindamycin, when given with theophylline, may result in theophylline toxicity. Observe for vomiting, dizziness, restlessness, and cardiac dysrhythmias. The dosage of theophylline may need to be reduced.

Erythromycin. Therapeutic antagonism has been reported between clindamycin and erythromycin. Do not administer concurrently.

daptomycin (dap toe my′ sin)
CUBICIN (cube′ ih sin)

Actions

Daptomycin is the first of a new class of antibiotics known as the cyclic lipopeptide antibiotics. It has a unique mechanism of action among the antibiotics. It binds to bacterial membranes and causes a rapid depolarization of membrane potential leading to inhibition of protein, RNA, and DNA synthesis, leading to cell death. Due to its unique mechanism of action, is effective against microorganisms that have developed resistance to other commonly used antibiotics.

Uses

Daptomycin has been approved for the treatment of complicated skin and skin structure infections (cSSSI) caused by *S. aureus*, *S. pyogenes*, *S. agalactiae*, and *E. faecalis*. It is particularly valuable in cases of gram-positive organisms becoming resistant to the beta-lactam (penicillins and cephalosporins) antibiotics and vancomycin. In an effort to slow the development of strains of bacteria resistant to daptomycin, it should be used only when the pathogen is resistant to other available antibiotics.

Therapeutic Outcomes

The primary therapeutic outcome expected from daptomycin therapy is elimination of bacterial infection.

Nursing Process for Daptomycin Therapy

Premedication Assessment

1. Obtain baseline assessments of presenting symptoms.
2. Record temperature, pulse, respirations, blood pressure, and hydration status.
3. Assess for any allergies.
4. Assess the bowel elimination patterns and record before initiating therapy.
5. Ensure that a baseline creatine phosphokinase (CPK, CK) has been drawn and sent to the laboratory before daptomycin is started. Also inquire and record whether the patient has any particular muscle weakness or pains, particularly in the extremities.
6. Obtain other baseline laboratory studies ordered (e.g., CBC with differential).

Planning

Availability. IV: 250 and 500 mg vials.

Implementation

Dosage and Administration. NOTE: Daptomycin is not compatible with dextrose-containing diluents, and additives or other medications should not be added to daptomycin or infused simultaneously through the same IV line. If the same IV line is used for sequential infusion of several different drugs, the line should be flushed with a compatible infusion solution before and after infusions with daptomycin.

IV: 4 mg/kg infused over 30 minutes every 24 hours for 7 to 14 days. Patients who have reduced renal function with a creatinine clearance of less than 30 mL per minute should have the same dose administered every 48 hours.

Evaluation

Side Effects to Expect

Gastric Irritation. The most common side effects of daptomycin therapy are diarrhea, constipation, nausea, and vomiting. These side effects are usually mild and tend to resolve with continued therapy.

Side Effects to Report

Severe Diarrhea. Severe diarrhea may develop from using daptomycin. Blood and mucus in the stool also may be present. This may be an indication of drug-induced pseudomembranous colitis and should be reported immediately. Withhold the next dose of antibiotic until the health care provider gives approval for administration.

Skeletal Muscle Weakness and Pain. Patients should be monitored for the development of muscle pain or weakness, particularly in the distal extremities. It is recommended that CPK concentrations be monitored weekly in patients treated with daptomycin, and more frequently in those who develop unexplained elevations of CPK during therapy.

Drug Interactions

HMG-CoA Reductase Inhibitors. The statins (e.g., atorvastatin, lovastatin, simvastatin, others) may infrequently cause skeletal muscle myopathy and potentially rhabdomyolysis. It is therefore suggested that statin therapy be discontinued in patients who are being treated with daptomycin. Statin therapy may be reinitiated after daptomycin therapy is complete.

metronidazole (met row nyd′ a zol)

FLAGYL (fla′ jil)

Actions

Metronidazole is a nitroimidazole. It is a somewhat unusual medication in that it has bactericidal, trichomonacidal, and protozoacidal activity. Its mechanism of action is unknown.

Uses

Metronidazole is used to treat trichomoniasis, giardiasis, amebic dysentery, amebic liver abscess, and anaerobic bacterial infections.

Therapeutic Outcomes

The primary therapeutic outcome expected from metronidazole therapy is elimination of infection.

Nursing Process for Metronidazole

Premedication Assessment

1. Obtain baseline assessments of the presenting symptoms.
2. Record temperature, pulse, respirations, blood pressure, and hydration status.

3. Assess for and record any gastric symptoms, peripheral neuropathy, or seizure disorders before initiating therapy.
4. Assess for any allergies.
5. Perform a baseline assessment of the patient's degree of alertness and orientation to name, place, and time before initiating therapy.
6. Obtain baseline laboratory studies ordered (e.g., CBC with differential).

Planning

Availability. PO: 250 and 500 mg tablets; 375 mg capsules; 750 mg extended release tablets; injection: 500 mg powder per vial.

Implementation

Dosage and Administration. PO:

- *Trichomoniasis:* Men and women: 250 mg three times daily for 7 days. Sexual partners must be treated concurrently to prevent reinfection. Single doses of 2 g or two doses of 1 g each administered the same day appear to provide adequate treatment for trichomoniasis in both sexes.
- *Amebic dysentery:* 750 mg three times daily for 5 to 10 days.
- *Amebic liver abscess:* 500 to 750 mg three times daily for 5 to 10 days.
- *Giardiasis:* 250 mg two or three times daily for 5 to 10 days.
- *Anaerobic bacterial infections:* Start with parenteral therapy initially. The usual oral dosage is 7.5 mg/kg every 6 hours. Do not exceed 4 g per 24 hours. The usual duration is 7 to 10 days. Infections of the bone and joint, lower respiratory tract, and endocardium may require longer treatment.

IV: *Anaerobic bacterial infections:* Loading dose: 15 mg/kg infused over 1 hour. Maintenance dosage: 7.5 mg/kg infused over 1 hour every 6 hours. Do not exceed 4 g per 24 hours. Convert to oral dosages when clinical condition is stable. Dosage reduction is necessary in patients with hepatic impairment but not renal impairment.

Pediatric: PO: trichomoniasis: 35 to 50 mg/kg per 24 hours in three divided doses for 7 days. Amebiasis: 35 to 50 mg/kg per 24 hours in three divided doses for 10 days. Giardiasis: 35 to 50 mg/kg per 24 hours in three divided doses for 7 days.

Evaluation

Side Effects to Expect

Nausea, Vomiting, Diarrhea. These side effects are usually mild and tend to resolve with continued therapy.

Side Effects to Report

Dizziness. Provide for patient safety during episodes of dizziness; report for further evaluation.

Confusion, Seizures. Patients receiving high doses, those with histories of seizure activity, and those with significant hepatic impairment are at greater risk of confusion and seizures. Perform a baseline assessment of the patient's degree of alertness and orientation to name, place, and time before initiating therapy. Make regularly scheduled subsequent mental status evaluations and compare findings. Report development of alterations.

Implement seizure precautions. Make sure the patient continues with anticonvulsant therapy. If seizures develop, provide for patient safety and then record the exact time of seizure onset and duration of each phase, a description of the specific body parts involved, and any progression in the affected parts. Describe the automatic responses seen during the clonic phase: altered, jerky respirations; frothy salivation; dilated pupils and eye movements; cyanosis; diaphoresis; or incontinence.

Phlebitis. Carefully assess patients for thrombophlebitis. Inspect the IV area frequently when providing care; visually inspect during dressing changes and whenever the IV is changed to a new site. Report redness, warmth, tenderness to touch, and edema in the affected part. If in lower extremities, dorsiflexion of the foot may cause pain in the calf area (Homans' sign). Compare the affected limb with the unaffected limb.

Drug Interactions

Alcohol. Use of alcohol and alcohol-containing preparations, such as OTC cough medications and mouthwashes (e.g., Listerine, Cepacol), should be avoided during therapy and up to 48 hours after discontinuation of metronidazole therapy. Metronidazole inhibits enzymes required to metabolize alcohol, resulting in mild symptoms of abdominal cramping, flushing, headache, nausea, vomiting, and sweating.

Warfarin. This medication may enhance the anticoagulant effects of warfarin. Observe for the development of petechiae, ecchymoses, nosebleeds, bleeding gums, dark tarry stools, and bright red or "coffee ground" emesis. Monitor the prothrombin time (INR) and reduce the dosage of warfarin if necessary.

Disulfiram. Combined use of disulfiram and metronidazole may result in mental confusion and psychoses. Concurrent therapy is not recommended.

Lithium. Patients receiving higher dosages of lithium are more susceptible to lithium toxicity and potential renal damage. Metronidazole should be initiated only if absolutely necessary. Frequently monitor serum lithium and creatinine concentrations when metronidazole and lithium are administered concurrently.

Phenytoin, Fosphenytoin. Metronidazole inhibits phenytoin metabolism. Monitor patients with concurrent therapy for signs of phenytoin toxicity: nystagmus, sedation, and lethargy. Serum levels may be ordered and the dosage of phenytoin reduced.

spectinomycin (spek ti no my' sin)
TROBICIN (tro' bi sin)

Actions

Spectinomycin is a bacteriostatic agent thought to inhibit protein synthesis.

Uses

Spectinomycin is used specifically to treat gonorrhea in both men and women. It has the particular advantage that most bacterial strains of gonorrhea respond to one administration of the recommended dosage. It is not effective in the treatment of syphilis. Serology testing for syphilis should be done before beginning therapy and should be repeated 3 months after spectinomycin therapy. This drug will mask the symptoms of syphilis.

Therapeutic Outcomes

The primary therapeutic outcome expected from spectinomycin therapy is elimination of gonorrhea.

Nursing Process for Spectinomycin

Premedication Assessment

1. Obtain baseline assessments of presenting symptoms.
2. Record temperature, pulse, respirations, blood pressure, and hydration status.
3. Assess for any allergies.

Planning

Availability. IM: 400 mg/mL in 2-g vials.

Implementation

Dosage and Administration. *Adult:* IM: A 20-gauge needle is recommended. Injections should be made deep into the upper outer quadrant of the gluteal muscle. The usual dose for both men and women is 2 g. In geographic areas in which penicillin-resistant gonorrhea is common, a dose of 4 g is recommended (2 g in each gluteal muscle).

Evaluation

Side Effects to Expect

Pain at Injection Site. Pain at the injection site is common. Give deeply in a large muscle mass. Devise a plan for rotation of injection sites if more than one injection is administered.

Drug Interactions. No significant drug interactions have been reported.

tinidazole (tin id′ a zol)

TINDAMAX (tin dah′ max)

Actions

Tinidazole is a nitroimidazole similar to metronidazole. Its mechanism of action is unknown.

Uses

Tinidazole is used to treat parasites such as trichomoniasis caused by *T. vaginalis* in both female and male patients, giardiasis caused by *Giardia lamblia*, and intestinal amebiasis and amebic liver abscess caused by *Entamoeba histolytica*.

Therapeutic Outcomes

The primary therapeutic outcome expected from tinidazole therapy is elimination of parasitic infection.

Nursing Process for Tinidazole

Premedication Assessment

1. Obtain baseline assessments of the presenting symptoms.
2. Record temperature, pulse, respirations, blood pressure, and hydration status.
3. Assess for and record any gastric symptoms, peripheral neuropathy, or seizure disorders before initiating therapy.
4. Assess for any allergies.
5. Perform a baseline assessment of the patient's degree of alertness and orientation to name, place, and time before initiating therapy.
6. Obtain baseline laboratory studies ordered (e.g., CBC with differential).

Planning

Availability. PO: 250 and 500 mg tablets

Implementation

Dosage and Administration. PO: NOTE: Tinidazole should be administered with food to reduce the incidence of gastrointestinal effects.

- *Trichomoniasis:* Men and women: 2 g one time. Sexual partners must be treated concurrently to prevent reinfection.
- *Amebic dysentery and amebic liver abscess:* 2 g once daily for 3 days.
- *Giardiasis:* 2 g one time.

Evaluation

Side Effects to Expect

Nausea, Vomiting, Diarrhea. These side effects are usually mild and tend to resolve with continued therapy.

Side Effects to Report

Dizziness. Provide for patient safety during episodes of dizziness; report for further evaluation.

Confusion, Seizures. Patients receiving high doses, those with histories of seizure activity, and those with significant hepatic impairment are at greater risk of confusion and seizures. Perform a baseline assessment of the patient's degree of alertness and orientation to name, place, and time before initiating therapy. Make regularly scheduled subsequent mental status evaluations and compare findings. Report development of alterations.

Implement seizure precautions. Make sure the patient continues with anticonvulsant therapy. If seizures develop, provide for patient safety and then record the exact time of seizure onset and duration of each phase, a description of the specific body parts involved, and any progression in the affected parts. Describe the automatic responses seen during the clonic phase: altered, jerky respirations; frothy salivation; dilated pupils and eye movements; cyanosis; diaphoresis; or incontinence.

Drug Interactions

Alcohol. Use of alcohol and alcohol-containing preparations, such as OTC cough medications and mouthwashes (e.g., Listerine, Cepacol), should be avoided during therapy and for 72 hours after discontinuation of tinidazole therapy. Tinidazole inhibits enzymes required to metabolize alcohol, resulting in mild symptoms of abdominal cramping, flushing, headache, nausea, vomiting, and sweating.

Warfarin. This medication may enhance the anticoagulant effects of warfarin during and up to 8 days after taking tinidazole. Observe for the development of petechiae, ecchymoses, nosebleeds, bleeding gums, dark tarry stools, and bright red or "coffee ground" emesis. Monitor the prothrombin time (INR) and reduce the dosage of warfarin if necessary.

Lithium. Patients receiving higher dosages of lithium are more susceptible to lithium toxicity and potential renal damage. Tinidazole should be initiated only if absolutely necessary. Frequently monitor serum lithium and creatinine concentrations when tinidazole and lithium are administered concurrently.

Phenytoin, Fosphenytoin. Tinidazole inhibits phenytoin metabolism. Monitor patients with concurrent therapy for signs of phenytoin toxicity: nystagmus, sedation, and lethargy. Serum levels may be ordered and the dosage of phenytoin reduced.

vancomycin (van ko my′ sin)
▶ VANCOCIN (van ko′ sin)

Actions

Vancomycin is an antibiotic that prevents the synthesis of bacterial cell walls. This site of action is different from the sites sensitive to penicillin and other antibiotics interfering with cell wall synthesis.

Uses

Vancomycin is effective against only gram-positive bacteria such as streptococci, staphylococci, *Clostridium difficile, Listeria monocytogenes*, and *Corynebacterium* that may cause endocarditis, osteomyelitis, meningitis, pneumonia, or septicemia. It may be used orally against staphylococcal enterocolitis and antibiotic-associated pseudomembranous colitis produced by *C. difficile*. Because of potential adverse effects, vancomycin therapy is reserved for patients with potentially life-threatening infections who cannot be treated with less toxic agents such as penicillins or cephalosporins.

The most prominent and severe adverse effects associated with vancomycin are nephrotoxicity and ototoxicity. These occur with greater frequency and severity in patients with renal impairment or when large doses are administered. Hearing loss may be preceded by tinnitus and high-tone hearing loss and is often permanent. Elderly patients appear to be particularly susceptible to the ototoxic effects.

Therapeutic Outcomes

The primary therapeutic outcome expected from vancomycin therapy is elimination of bacterial infection.

Nursing Process for Vancomycin

Premedication Assessment

1. Obtain baseline assessments of presenting symptoms.
2. Record temperature, pulse, respirations, blood pressure, and hydration status.
3. Assess for normal renal function and hearing before initiating therapy.
4. Assess for any allergies.
5. Obtain baseline laboratory studies ordered (e.g., CBC with differential).

Planning

Availability. PO: 125 and 250 mg capsules; 1 g powder per vial for oral solution; IV: 0.5, 1, 5 and 10 g powder per vial.

Implementation

Red Man Syndrome. Rapid intravenous administration may result in a severe hypotensive episode. Patients develop a *redneck syndrome*, or *red man syndrome*, characteristic of vancomycin. It is manifested by a sudden and profound hypotension with or without a maculopapular rash over the face, neck, upper chest, and extremities. The rash generally resolves within a few hours after terminating the infusion. In rare cases the administration of fluids, antihistamines, or corticosteroids may be necessary. Administer the solution diluted to less than 5 mg/mL over at least 60 minutes. Monitor blood pressure during infusion.

PO Reconstitution. Add 30 mL of distilled water to the contents of the 500 mg IV container.

Dosage and Administration. *Adult:* PO: 500 mg every 6 hours or 1 g every 12 hours. Pseudomembranous colitis produced by *C. difficile:* 250 mg to 1 g per day in three or four divided doses for 7 to 10 days; IM: not recommended because of poor absorption and clinical response; IV: 500 mg every 6 hours or 1 g every 12 hours. Dosage must be adjusted for patients with impaired renal function. Check serum concentrations.

Pediatric: PO: neonates: 10 mg/kg/day in divided doses; children: 40 mg/kg/day in four divided doses, not to exceed 2 g per day; IM: not recommended because of poor absorption and clinical response; IV: neonates: initial dose of 15 mg/kg followed by 10 mg/kg every 12 hours until 1 month of age, then every 8 hours thereafter; children: 40 mg/kg/day in divided doses.

Evaluation

Side Effects to Report

Ototoxicity. This may initially be manifested by dizziness, tinnitus, and progressive hearing loss. Assess patients for difficulty in walking unaided and assess the level of hearing daily. Intentionally speak to patients softly; note if they are aware that you said anything. Take particular notice of the patient who repeatedly asks, "What did you say?" or who starts talking more loudly or progressively increases the volume on the television or radio.

Nephrotoxicity. Monitor urinalysis and kidney function tests for abnormal results. Report an increasing BUN and creatinine, decreasing urine output or decreasing urine specific gravity (despite amount of fluid intake), casts or protein in the urine, frank blood or smoky-colored urine, or RBCs in excess of 0 to 3 RBC/HPF (see Table 42-1) on the urinalysis report.

Serum Levels. Serum levels of vancomycin should be routinely ordered to minimize these adverse effects. Notify the health care provider of any abnormal serum levels reported so that dosage adjustments may be made. Consult laboratory reports for normal range.

Secondary Infections. Oral thrush, genital and anal pruritus, vaginitis, and vaginal discharge may occur. Report promptly because these infections are resistant to the original antibiotic used. Teach the importance of meticulous oral and perineal personal hygiene.

Drug Interactions

Nephrotoxicity, Ototoxicity. Concurrent and sequential use of other ototoxic or nephrotoxic agents such as neomycin, streptomycin, kanamycin, gentamicin, paromomycin, polymyxin B, colistin, tobramycin, amikacin, cisplatin, furosemide, torsemide, and bumetanide requires careful monitoring.

Neuromuscular Blockade. Vancomycin, in combination with skeletal muscle relaxants, may produce respiratory depression.

Check the anesthesia record in postoperative patients to determine if skeletal muscle relaxants such as succinylcholine or pancuronium bromide were administered during surgery. The nurse should monitor and assess the respiratory rate, depth of respirations, and chest movement and report apnea immediately. Because these effects may be seen for up to 48 hours after administration of skeletal muscle relaxants, continue monitoring respirations, pulse, and blood pressure beyond the usual postsurgical vital signs routine.

DRUG CLASS: Topical Antifungal Agents

Actions

The exact mechanisms by which antifungal agents act are unknown. However, it is known that cell membranes are altered, resulting in increased permeability, leakage of amino acids and electrolytes, and impaired uptake of essential nutrients needed for cell growth.

Uses

The common topical fungal infections caused by several different dermatophytes are tinea pedis (athlete's foot), tinea cruris (jock itch), tinea corporis (ringworm), and tinea versicolor. *Candida albicans* is the most common cause of oral candidiasis (thrush), cutaneous candidiasis (e.g., diaper rash), and vaginal candidiasis (i.e., moniliasis, or "yeast infection").

Therapeutic Outcomes

The primary therapeutic outcome expected from topical antifungal therapy is elimination of fungal infection.

Nursing Process for Topical Antifungal Therapy

Premedication Assessment

1. Obtain baseline assessments of presenting symptoms.
2. Assess for any allergies.

Planning

Availability. See Table 46-9.

Implementation

Dosage and Administration. See Table 46-9.

- *Topical:* Wash hands thoroughly before and immediately after application. Cleanse skin with soap and water and dry thoroughly.

For athlete's foot, the powder is most effective in intertriginous areas and in cases in which a dry environment may enhance the therapeutic response. Instruct patients to wear cotton socks (avoid nylon) if possible, and change them two or three times daily. Treatments may be required for 6 weeks or more with long-standing infections and in areas of thickened skin.

For jock itch or ringworm, wear well-fitting, nonconstrictive, ventilated clothing.

For all fungal infections, instruct patients to avoid tight-fitting clothing and occlusive dressings unless otherwise instructed by the health care provider.

- *Eye contact:* Instruct patients to avoid contact with the eye and wash eyes immediately if contact should occur.
- *Intravaginal:* Give the patient the following instructions:
  1. Wash the applicator in warm soapy water after each use so that it does not become a vehicle for reinfection.
  2. A pad may be used to protect clothing.
  3. Use the number of doses prescribed even if symptoms disappear or menstruation begins.
  4. Refrain from sexual intercourse during therapy (or the male should wear a condom to avoid reinfection).
  5. Contraception other than a diaphragm or condom should be used when the patient is being

Drug Table 46-9 TOPICAL ANTIFUNGAL AGENTS

GENERIC NAME	BRAND NAME	AVAILABILITY	ADULT DOSAGE RANGE
butenafine	Lotrimin Ultra, Mentax	Cream 1%	For ringworm, jock itch, athlete's foot: Apply topically to affected area once or twice daily for 1-4 wk.
butoconazole	Gynazole-1 Mycelex-3	Vaginal cream: 2%	For vaginal candidiasis: Gynazole-1: one applicatorful intravaginally at bedtime once. Mycelex-3: one applicatorful intravaginally at bedtime for 3 days; may be extended to 6 days, if needed
ciclopirox	Loprox	Cream: 0.77% Lotion: 0.77% Shampoo 1% Solution for nails: 8%	For ringworm, jock itch, athlete's foot, cutaneous candidiasis, and tinea versicolor: Massage cream or lotion into affected skin twice daily for at least 4 weeks Shampoo: Twice weekly for 4 weeks
clotrimazole	Gyne-Lotrimin	Vaginal tablets: 200 mg	For vaginal candidiasis: Cream: one applicatorful at bedtime for 3-7 nights
	Mycelex-7	Vaginal cream: 1%	Tablets: Insert one 200 mg tablet intravaginally at bed time for 3-7 nights
	Desenex Lotrimin AF Mycelex	Cream: 1% Solution: 1% Oral lozenges: 10 mg (troches)	For ringworm, jock itch, athlete's foot: Apply topically to affected skin morning and evening; gently rub in For oral candidiasis: Allow one lozenge to dissolve slowly in mouth five times daily for 14 consecutive days.
econazole	Spectazole	Cream: 1%	For ringworm, jock itch, athlete's foot, tinea versicolor: Apply over affected area once daily For cutaneous candidiasis: Apply twice daily, morning and evening
ketoconazole	Nizoral	Cream: 2%	For ringworm, jock itch, athlete's foot, cutaneous candidiasis, and tinea versicolor: Massage in cream to affected and surrounding tissue once daily; may require 2-4 weeks of treatment For seborrheic dermatitis: Massage in cream to affected area twice daily for 4 wk
		Shampoo: 2%	For dandruff: Moisten hair and scalp with water; apply shampoo and lather gently for 1 min; rinse and reapply, leaving lather on scalp for 3 min; rinse thoroughly and dry hair; apply shampoo twice weekly for 4 wk with at least 3 days between shampooing
miconazole	Monistat 3	Vaginal suppositories: 200 mg	For vaginal candidiasis: Monistat 3: insert one suppository intravaginally at bedtime for 3 days
	Monistat 7	Vaginal suppositories: 100 mg Vaginal cream: 2%	Monistat 7: insert one applicatorful or one suppository at bedtime for 3-7 days.
	Micatin	Cream: 2% Powder: 2% Spray: 2%	For ringworm, jock itch, athlete's foot, cutaneous candidiasis, and tinea versicolor: Cover affected areas twice daily, morning and evening; treatment may require 2-4 weeks
naftifine	Naftin	Cream: 1% Gel: 1%	For ringworm, jock itch, athlete's foot: Cream: massage into affected area once daily Gel: massage into affected area twice daily

Drug Table 46-9 **TOPICAL ANTIFUNGAL AGENTS—cont'd**

GENERIC NAME	BRAND NAME	AVAILABILITY	ADULT DOSAGE RANGE
nystatin	Mycostatin	Vaginal tablets: 100,000 U	For vaginal candidiasis: one tablet intravaginally daily for 2 weeks
	Mycostatin, Nilstat	Oral suspension: 100,000 U/mL	For oral candidiasis: 4-6 mL four times daily; retain in mouth as long as possible before swallowing
	Mycostatin pastilles	Oral lozenges: 200,000 U (troches)	One or two tablets four or five times daily; do not chew or swallow
	Mycostatin, Nilstat	Cream, ointment, powder	For cutaneous candidiasis: Apply to affected area two or three times daily
oxiconazole nitrate	Oxistat	Cream: 1% Lotion: 1%	For ringworm, jock itch, athlete's foot: Massage into affected areas once daily at bedtime
sertaconazole	Ertaczo	Cream 2%	For athlete's foot: Apply twice daily for 4 weeks
sulconazole	Exelderm	Cream: 1% Solution: 1%	For ringworm, jock itch, athlete's foot: Massage into affected area twice daily
terbinafine	Lamisil AT	Cream: 1% Spray: 1%	Massage into affected area twice daily; treatment may require 2-4 weeks
terconazole	Terazol 7 Terazol 3	Vaginal cream: 0.4% Vaginal cream: 0.8%	For vaginal candidiasis: Insert one applicatorful intravaginally daily at bedtime for 3 (Terazol 3) or 7 (Terazol 7) consecutive days
		Vaginal suppository: 80 mg	Insert one suppository intravaginally once daily at bedtime for 3 consecutive days
tioconazole	Vagistat-1 Monistat-1	Vaginal ointment: 6.5%	For vaginal candidiasis: Insert one applicatorful intravaginally at bedtime once
tolnaftate	Tinactin	Cream: 1% Solution: 1% Gel: 1% Spray: 1% Powder: 1%	For ringworm, jock itch, athlete's foot, cutaneous candidiasis, and tinea versicolor: Cover affected areas twice daily, morning and evening; treatment may require 2-4 weeks

treated with the vaginal ointment (e.g., Vagistat). Prolonged contact with petrolatum-based products may cause the diaphragm and condom to deteriorate.

Evaluation

Side Effects to Expect and Report

Irritation. Some patients experience vulvar or vaginal burning, vulvar itching, discharge, soreness, or swelling from the intravaginal products. These side effects are usually mild and tend to resolve with continued therapy. Encourage the patient not to discontinue therapy without first consulting the health care provider.

Redness, Swelling, Blistering, Oozing. These signs may be an indication of hypersensitivity. Inform the health care provider.

Drug Interactions. No clinically significant drug interactions have been reported.

DRUG CLASS: Systemic Antifungal Agents

amphotericin B (am fo tair' ih sin), **amphotericin B sodium desoxycholate ("conventional")**

▶ FUNGIZONE IV

amphotericin B cholesteryl sulfate complex

▶ AMPHOTEC

amphotericin B lipid complex

▶ ABELCET

amphotericin B liposomal

▶ AMBISOME

Actions

Amphotericin B is a fungistatic agent that disrupts the cell membrane of fungal cells, resulting in a loss of cellular contents.

Uses

Amphotericin B is used primarily in treating systemic life-threatening fungal infections. It should not be used to treat noninvasive fungal infections such as oral thrush, vaginal candidiasis, and esophageal candidiasis in immunocompetent patients with normal neutrophil counts. There are four dosage forms of amphotericin B, each with different brand names and somewhat different approval for use. Each has different requirements for reconstitution, dilution, filtration, and administration rate. Work closely with the pharmacy department to ensure that the correct dosage form is being reconstituted and diluted properly, and that proper administration technique including the use of appropriate inline filters and rate of infusion is being used.

Therapeutic Outcomes

The primary therapeutic outcome expected from amphotericin B therapy is elimination of fungal infection.

Nursing Process for Amphotericin B

Premedication Assessment

1. Obtain baseline assessments of presenting symptoms.
2. Record temperature, pulse, respirations, blood pressure, and hydration status.
3. Assess for normal renal function and normal electrolytes before initiating therapy.
4. Assess for any allergies.
5. Gather baseline data about the patient's mental status (e.g., alertness, orientation, confusion); muscle strength; presence of muscle cramps, tremors, and nausea; and general appearance (e.g., drowsy, anxious, lethargic).

Planning

Availability. IV:

- Amphotericin B sodium desoxycholate ("conventional" amphotericin B) (Fungizone) IV: 50 mg per vial
- Amphotericin B cholesteryl sulfate complex (Amphotec): 50 and 100 mg per vial
- Amphotericin B lipid complex (Abelcet): 5 mg/mL in 100 mg concentrate
- Amphotericin B liposomal (AmBisome): 50 mg per vial

Implementation

Dosage and Administration

- Dosage varies depending on the dosage form and the organism for which the medicine is being used. Consult the physician, laboratory results, and pharmacist to provide checks on the appropriate dose and administration of the antifungal agent.

Evaluation

Side Effects to Expect and Report

Nephrotoxicity. Nephrotoxicity may be manifested by increases in excretion of uric acid, potassium, and magnesium; oliguria; granular casts in the urine; proteinuria; and increased BUN and serum creatinine levels.

Monitor urinalysis and kidney function tests for abnormal results. Report an increasing BUN and creatinine, decreasing urine output or decreasing urine specific gravity (despite amount of fluid intake), casts or protein in the urine, frank blood or smoky-colored urine, or RBCs in excess of 0 to 3 RBC/HPF (see Table 42-1) on the urinalysis report. Report input and output, as well as a progressive decrease in daily urine volume or changes in visual characteristics.

Electrolyte Imbalance. The electrolytes most commonly altered are potassium (K^+) and magnesium (Mg^{++}). Hypokalemia is most likely to occur.

Many symptoms associated with altered fluid and electrolyte balance are subtle and resemble general symptoms of drug toxicity or the disease process itself.

Gather data about changes in the patient's mental status (e.g., alertness, orientation, confusion), muscle strength, muscle cramps, tremors, nausea, and general appearance (e.g., drowsy, anxious, lethargic).

Always check the electrolyte reports for early indications of electrolyte imbalance.

Keep accurate records of input and output, daily weights, and vital signs.

Malaise, Fever, Chills, Headache, Nausea, Vomiting. These adverse effects tend to be dose related and may be minimized by slow infusion, reduction of dosage, and alternate-day administration. Check PRN and standing orders for drugs (e.g., antihistamines, aspirin, antiemetics) that may alleviate these symptoms.

Thrombophlebitis. Carefully assess patients receiving IV amphotericin B for the development of thrombophlebitis.

Inspect the IV area often when providing care; inspect during dressing changes and whenever the IV is changed to a new site. Always investigate pain at the IV site. Report redness, warmth, tenderness to touch, and edema in the affected part. If in lower extremities, dorsiflexion of the foot may cause pain in the calf (Homans' sign). Compare the affected limb with the unaffected one.

Drug Interactions

Corticosteroids (e.g., Prednisone). Corticosteroids may enhance the loss of potassium. Check potassium levels and monitor more closely for hypokalemia when these agents are used concurrently.

Nephrotoxic Potential. Combining amphotericin B with other nephrotoxic agents such as aminoglycosides, diuretics, or cisplatin should be done with extreme caution. Monitor closely for signs of nephrotoxicity.

Digoxin. Because amphotericin B may induce hypokalemia, use cautiously in patients receiving digoxin.

Hypokalemia may induce digoxin toxicity. Monitor patients for dysrhythmias, nausea, and bradycardia.

Diuretics. Thiazide and loop diuretics may induce hypokalemia. Monitor patients receiving amphotericin B and diuretic therapy very closely for hypokalemia.

fluconazole (flu kon′ a zol)
▶ DIFLUCAN (dye′ flu can)

Actions

Fluconazole is an antifungal agent chemically related to ketoconazole and itraconazole. It acts by inhibiting certain metabolic pathways in fungi, thus interfering with cell wall synthesis.

Uses

Fluconazole is used for oral and IV treatment of cryptococcal meningitis and oropharyngeal, esophageal, vulvovaginal, or systemic candidiasis. Fluconazole therapy is usually reserved for patients in whom other antifungal therapy was not tolerated or was ineffective. Fluconazole is also used prophylactically to prevent candidiasis in bone marrow transplant patients who are receiving radiation or chemotherapy treatment and in patients with human immunodeficiency virus (HIV) infection. Fluconazole is also approved as a single-dose treatment of vaginal candidiasis in immunocompetent patients.

Therapeutic Outcomes

The primary therapeutic outcomes expected from fluconazole therapy are as follows:

- Prevention of systemic fungal infections.
- Elimination of fungal infection.

Nursing Process for Fluconazole

Premedication Assessment

1. Obtain baseline assessments of presenting symptoms.
2. Record temperature, pulse, respirations, blood pressure, and hydration status.
3. Assess for and record any gastric symptoms and abnormal liver and renal function before initiating therapy.
4. Assess for any allergies.
5. Obtain baseline laboratory studies ordered (e.g., CBC with differential).

Planning

Availability. PO: 50, 100, 150, and 200 mg tablets; 50 and 200 mg per 5 mL suspension; IV: 200 and 400 mg vials.

Implementation

Dosage and Administration. PO: 100 to 400 mg daily, dosage must be individualized to type of infection being treated; IV: as for PO.

Evaluation

Side Effects to Expect

Nausea, Vomiting, Diarrhea. These side effects are usually mild and tend to resolve with continued therapy. Encourage the patient not to discontinue therapy without first consulting the health care provider.

Side Effects to Report

Rash. Report symptoms for further evaluation by the health care provider. Do not administer any further doses until so ordered by the health care provider.

Hepatotoxicity. The symptoms of hepatotoxicity are anorexia, nausea, vomiting, jaundice, hepatomegaly, splenomegaly, and abnormal liver function tests (e.g., elevated bilirubin, AST, ALT, GGT, alkaline phosphatase, prothrombin time).

Drug Interactions

Cimetidine. Cimetidine inhibits the absorption of fluconazole. Concurrent use is not recommended.

Diuretics. Diuretics inhibit the excretion of fluconazole. Monitor patients for an increase in frequency of side effects. The dosage of fluconazole may need to be decreased if concurrent therapy with diuretics is required.

Toxicity Induced by Fluconazole. Fluconazole can increase serum concentrations of alfentanil, benzodiazepines, buspirone, cyclosporine, losartan, phenytoin, vincristine, zidovudine, zolpidem, tricyclic antidepressants, and oral sulfonylurea hypoglycemic agents (tolbutamide, glipizide, and glyburide). Fluconazole can also potentiate the anticoagulant effects of warfarin. Read individual monographs for monitoring parameters of toxicity from these agents.

flucytosine (flu sy′ toe seen)
▶ ANCOBON (on′ ko bon)

Actions

Flucytosine is an antifungal agent. Its mechanism of action is thought to be inhibition of RNA and protein synthesis.

Uses

Flucytosine is effective against susceptible candidal septicemia, endocarditis, urinary tract infections, cryptococcal meningitis, and pulmonary infections.

Therapeutic Outcomes

The primary therapeutic outcome expected from flucytosine therapy is elimination of fungal infection.

Nursing Process for Flucytosine

Premedication Assessment

1. Obtain baseline assessments of presenting symptoms.
2. Record temperature, pulse, respirations, blood pressure, and hydration status.

3. Assess for and record any gastric symptoms or abnormal liver or renal function before initiating therapy.
4. Assess for any allergies.
5. Record baseline mental status assessment data.

Planning

Availability. PO: 250 and 500 mg capsules.

Implementation

Dosage and Administration. *Adult:* PO: 50 to 150 mg/kg/day divided into doses every 6 hours. Doses up to 250 mg/kg/day may be required in cryptococcal meningitis. Nausea may be reduced if the capsules are given a few at a time over 20 to 30 minutes.

Evaluation

Side Effects to Expect

Nausea, Vomiting, Diarrhea. These side effects are usually mild and tend to resolve with continued therapy. Encourage the patient not to discontinue therapy without first consulting the health care provider.

Side effects may be reduced by administering a few capsules at a time over 30 minutes.

Side Effects to Report

Hematologic, Rash. Monitor for sore throat, fever, purpura, jaundice, or excessive and progressive weakness.

Nephrotoxicity. Monitor urinalysis and kidney function tests for abnormal results. Report an increasing BUN and creatinine, decreasing urine output or decreasing urine specific gravity (despite amount of fluid intake), casts or protein in the urine, frank blood or smoky-colored urine, or RBCs in excess of 0 to 3 RBC/HPF (see Table 42-1) on the urinalysis report.

Hepatotoxicity. The symptoms of hepatotoxicity are anorexia, nausea, vomiting, jaundice, hepatomegaly, splenomegaly, and abnormal liver function tests (e.g., elevated bilirubin, AST, ALT, GGT, alkaline phosphatase, prothrombin time).

Drug Interactions

Amphotericin B. Flucytosine and amphotericin B display enhanced activity when used concurrently.

griseofulvin (griz ee o ful′ vin)
- FULVICIN (ful′ vi sin)
- GRIFULVIN (gri ful′ vin)

Actions

Griseofulvin is a fungistatic agent that acts by stopping cell division and new cell growth.

Uses

Griseofulvin is used to treat ringworm of the scalp, body, nails, and feet. After griseofulvin is absorbed, it is incorporated into the keratin of the nails, skin, and hair in therapeutic amounts. The infecting fungus is not killed, but its growth into new cells is prevented. Once the cells are shed or removed, they are replaced by new cells that are free from the infection. Because of slow nail growth, treatment is often required for several months.

Therapeutic Outcomes

The primary therapeutic outcome expected from griseofulvin therapy is elimination of fungal infection.

Nursing Process for Griseofulvin

Premedication Assessment

1. Obtain baseline assessments of presenting symptoms.
2. Record temperature, pulse, respirations, blood pressure, and hydration status.
3. Assess for and record any gastric symptoms or abnormal hematologic, liver, or renal function tests before initiating therapy.
4. Assess for any allergies.
5. Obtain baseline laboratory studies ordered (e.g., CBC with differential, liver and renal function tests).
6. Record results of baseline mental status examination.

Planning

Availability. PO: 125, 250, and 500 mg tablets; 125 mg per 5 mL oral suspension.

Implementation

Dosage and Administration. *Adult:* PO: depending on the specific organism and the location of the infection, 500 mg to 4 g in single or divided doses daily. Absorption from the gastrointestinal tract may be increased by administering griseofulvin with a high-fat meal.

Evaluation

Side Effects to Expect

Nausea, Vomiting, Anorexia, Abdominal Cramps. These side effects are usually mild and tend to resolve with continued therapy. Encourage the patient not to discontinue therapy without first consulting the health care provider.

Side Effects to Report

Urticaria, Rash, Pruritus. Hypersensitivity reactions, manifested by itching, urticaria, and rash, are relatively common. Report symptoms for further evaluation by the health care provider.

Pruritus may be relieved by adding baking soda to the bathwater.

Confusion. Perform a baseline assessment of the patient's degree of alertness and orientation to name, place, and time before initiating therapy. Make regularly scheduled subsequent mental status evaluations, and compare findings. Report development of alterations.

Dizziness. Provide for patient safety during episodes of dizziness; report for further evaluation.

Secondary Infections. With griseofulvin, oral thrush, genital and anal pruritus, vaginitis, and vaginal discharge may occur. Report promptly because these infections are resistant to the original antimicrobial agent.

Teach the importance of meticulous oral and perineal personal hygiene.

Photosensitivity. The patient should be cautioned to avoid exposure to sunlight and ultraviolet light. Suggest wearing long-sleeved clothing, hat, and sunglasses when outdoors. Discourage the use of tanning lamps. Notify the health care provider for the advisability of continuing therapy.

Hematologic. Routine laboratory studies (e.g., RBC, WBC, differential counts) are scheduled for patients taking griseofulvin 30 days or longer. Stress the importance of returning for this laboratory work. Monitor for sore throat, fever, purpura, jaundice, or excessive and progressive weakness.

Nephrotoxicity. Monitor urinalysis and kidney function tests for abnormal results. Report an increasing BUN and creatinine, decreasing urine output or decreasing urine specific gravity (despite amount of fluid intake), casts or protein in the urine, frank blood or smoky-colored urine, or RBCs in excess of 0 to 3 RBC/HPF (see Table 42-1) on the urinalysis report.

Hepatotoxicity. The symptoms of hepatotoxicity are anorexia, nausea, vomiting, jaundice, hepatomegaly, splenomegaly, and abnormal liver function tests (e.g., elevated bilirubin, AST, ALT, GGT, alkaline phosphatase, prothrombin time).

Drug Interactions

Warfarin. Griseofulvin may diminish the anticoagulant effects of warfarin. Monitor the prothrombin time (INR) and increase the dosage of warfarin if necessary.

Barbiturates. The absorption of griseofulvin is impaired when combined with barbiturates. If concurrent therapy cannot be avoided, administer the griseofulvin in divided doses three times daily.

Oral Contraceptives. Griseofulvin may cause amenorrhea, increased breakthrough bleeding, and possibly decreased contraceptive efficacy when used concomitantly with oral contraceptives. Other methods of contraception such as condoms and foam should be considered during griseofulvin therapy.

itraconazole (it rah kon′ a zol)
SPORANOX (spor′ ahn ox)

Actions

Itraconazole is an antifungal agent chemically related to fluconazole and ketoconazole. It acts by interfering with cell wall synthesis, causing leakage of cellular contents.

Uses

Itraconazole is used orally to treat candidiasis, chronic mucocutaneous candidiasis, oral thrush, onychomycosis, candiduria, coccidioidomycosis, histoplasmosis, chromomycosis, blastomycosis, and paracoccidioidomycosis. It is also effective against *Aspergillus.*

NOTE: Do not administer itraconazole to patients with a history of heart failure. Itraconazole is a negative inotropic agent and may seriously aggravate heart failure.

NOTE: Itraconazole has many drug interactions because it is a potent inhibitor of metabolizing enzymes in the liver (see Drug Interactions, later). Coadministration of itraconazole with cisapride, pimozide, dofetilide, or quinidine is *contraindicated*. Fatal reactions may result.

Therapeutic Outcomes

The primary therapeutic outcome expected from itraconazole therapy is elimination of fungal infection.

Nursing Process for Itraconazole

Premedication Assessment

1. Obtain baseline assessments of presenting symptoms.
2. Record temperature, pulse, respirations, blood pressure, and hydration status.
3. Assess for and record any gastric symptoms, abnormal liver function tests, or heart failure before beginning therapy.
4. Assess for any allergies.
5. Obtain baseline laboratory studies ordered (e.g., liver function tests).

Planning

Availability. PO: 100 mg capsules, 10 mg/mL oral solution in 150 mL containers; IV: 250 mg ampule.

Implementation

NOTE: Do not use capsules and oral solution interchangeably. Capsules are used to treat systemic fungal infections. The oral solution should only be used to treat oral or esophageal candidiasis in adult HIV-positive or other immunocompromised patients.

Dosage and Administration. *Adults:* PO: 100 to 400 mg daily. Doses of more than 200 mg should be given in two divided doses. Instruct the patient to take with a full meal to ensure maximum absorption.

Evaluation

Side Effects to Expect

Nausea, Vomiting. These side effects are usually mild and tend to resolve with continued therapy. Encourage the patient not to discontinue therapy without first consulting the health care provider. Administer after a full meal for maximum absorption.

Side Effects to Report

Hepatotoxicity. Liver function tests are recommended before initiating therapy, with follow-up tests biweekly to monthly.

The symptoms of hepatotoxicity are anorexia, nausea, vomiting, jaundice, hepatomegaly, splenomegaly, and abnormal liver function tests (e.g., elevated bilirubin, AST, ALT, GGT, alkaline phosphatase, prothrombin time).

Heart Failure. Monitor the six cardinal signs of heart disease and individualize care to deal with the degree of impairment: dyspnea, chest pain, fatigue, edema, syncope, and palpitations (see also Chapter 28).

Pruritus, Rash. Report symptoms to the health care provider for further evaluation. Pruritus may be relieved by adding baking soda to the bathwater.

Drug Interactions

H_2 Antagonists, Antacids, Indinavir, Ritonavir. H_2 antagonists (e.g., cimetidine, famotidine, ranitidine, nizatidine), antacids, indinavir, and ritonavir inhibit the absorption of itraconazole. Concurrent use is not recommended.

Carbamazepine, Phenytoin, Rifampin. Concurrent administration of itraconazole and these agents has resulted in a significant decrease in itraconazole activity and clinical failure. The mechanism is unknown, but it is suspected that these agents stimulate the metabolism of itraconazole. If these agents are to be used concurrently, itraconazole levels must be monitored to ensure therapeutic effect.

Toxicity Induced by Itraconazole. Itraconazole can increase serum concentrations of alfentanil, benzodiazepines (e.g., triazolam, midazolam, alprazolam), buspirone, calcium channel blockers (e.g., felodipine, nisoldipine, nifedipine, verapamil), carbamazepine, cisapride, cyclosporine, digoxin, dofetilide, haloperidol, HMG-CoA reductase inhibitors (e.g., atorvastatin, lovastatin), isoniazid, pimozide, quinidine, tacrolimus, tolterodine, vincristine, zolpidem, and oral sulfonylurea hypoglycemic agents (e.g., tolbutamide, glipizide, glyburide). Itraconazole can also potentiate the anticoagulant effects of warfarin. Read individual monographs for monitoring parameters of toxicity from these agents.

ketoconazole (key toe kon′ a zol)
▶ NIZORAL (nis′ o ral)

Actions

Ketoconazole is an antifungal agent chemically related to fluconazole and itraconazole. It acts by interfering with cell wall synthesis, causing leakage of cellular contents.

Uses

Ketoconazole is used orally to treat candidiasis, chronic mucocutaneous candidiasis, oral thrush, candiduria, coccidioidomycosis, histoplasmosis, chromomycosis, and paracoccidioidomycosis. It is also used topically to treat seborrheic dermatitis, ringworm, athlete's foot, and cutaneous tinea versicolor (see Table 46-9).

Therapeutic Outcomes

The primary therapeutic outcome expected from ketoconazole therapy is elimination of fungal infection.

Nursing Process for Ketoconazole

Premedication Assessment

1. Obtain baseline assessments of presenting symptoms.
2. Record temperature, pulse, respirations, blood pressure, and hydration status.
3. Assess for and record any gastric symptoms or abnormal liver function tests before initiating therapy.
4. Assess for any allergies.
5. Obtain baseline laboratory studies ordered (e.g., liver function tests).

Planning

Availability. PO: 200 mg tablets

Implementation

NOTE: Administer at least 2 hours before giving drugs that reduce stomach acidity.

Dosage and Administration

Adult: PO: 200 to 400 mg once daily. Absorption is improved when administered with food.

Pediatric: PO: 44 pounds or less, 50 mg once daily; 44 to 88 pounds, 100 mg once daily; more than 88 pounds, 200 mg once daily.

Evaluation

Side Effects to Expect

Nausea, Vomiting. These side effects are usually mild and tend to resolve with continued therapy. Encourage the patient not to discontinue therapy without first consulting the health care provider.

Administer with food or milk to reduce irritation.

Side Effects to Report

Hepatotoxicity. Liver function tests are recommended before initiating therapy with follow-up tests biweekly to monthly.

The symptoms of hepatotoxicity are anorexia, nausea, vomiting, jaundice, hepatomegaly, splenomegaly, and abnormal liver function tests (e.g., elevated bilirubin, AST, ALT, GGT, alkaline phosphatase, prothrombin time).

Pruritus, Rash. Report symptoms to the health care provider for further evaluation. Pruritus may be relieved by adding baking soda to the bathwater.

Drug Interactions

Drugs That Reduce Therapeutic Effects. Isoniazid, rifampin, sucralfate, and proton pump inhibitors (e.g., omeprazole, esomeprazole, lansoprazole) alter the absorption of ketoconazole, reducing therapeutic effect. Avoid concurrent use, if possible.

Anticholinergic agents (e.g., dicyclomine, Donnatal, propantheline), antacids, didanosine, and H_2 antagonists (e.g., cimetidine, ranitidine, nizatidine, famotidine) diminish stomach acidity and decrease absorption of ketoconazole. Administer ketoconazole at least 2 hours before these medications.

Administration of rifampin and ketoconazole decreases serum levels of both drugs. Avoid concurrent use if possible.

Alcohol. Instruct patients to avoid alcohol consumption during ketoconazole therapy. Patients ingesting alcohol during and for 24 to 72 hours after administration of ketoconazole will become flushed, tremulous, dyspneic, tachycardic, and hypotensive. Tell patients to avoid use of OTC preparations containing alcohol, such as mouthwash (e.g., Cepacol, Listerine) or cough preparations, because of their alcohol content.

Toxicity Induced by Ketoconazole. Ketoconazole can increase serum concentrations of benzodiazepines (i.e., triazolam, midazolam, alprazolam), buspirone, calcium channel blockers (i.e., nisoldipine), carbamazepine, cisapride, cyclosporine, donepezil, quinidine, tacrolimus, tricyclic antidepressants, vincristine, zolpidem, and oral sulfonylurea hypoglycemic agents (tolbutamide, glipizide, glyburide). Ketoconazole can also potentiate the anticoagulant effects of warfarin. Read individual monographs for monitoring parameters of toxicity from these agents.

terbinafine (ter bin′ ah feen)
LAMISIL (lahm′ ih sil)

Actions

Terbinafine is an allylamine derivative that acts by inhibiting squalene epoxidase, a key enzyme required in sterol biosynthesis in fungi. This action causes accumulation of squalene and a deficiency of ergosterol, resulting in fungal cell death.

Uses

Terbinafine is used in the treatment of onychomycosis of the toenail or fingernail due to dermatophytes. Maximum clinical effect is observed months after the fungus has been eradicated when a new nail has grown.

Therapeutic Outcomes

The primary therapeutic outcome expected from terbinafine therapy is elimination of fungal infection in toenails and fingernails.

Nursing Process for Terbinafine Therapy

Premedication Assessment

1. Obtain baseline assessments of presenting symptoms.
2. Record temperature, pulse, respirations, blood pressure, and hydration status.
3. Assess for and record any gastric symptoms before initiating therapy.
4. Assess for any allergies.
5. Obtain baseline laboratory studies ordered (e.g., CBC with differential, liver function tests, and electrolyte levels).

Planning

Availability. PO: 250 mg tablets.

Implementation

Dosage and Administration. *Adult:* PO: 250 mg daily for 6 weeks to treat fungal infections of the fingernail and 12 weeks for treatment of infections of the toenail.

Evaluation

Side Effects to Report

Pruritus, Rash, Fever, Chills. Report symptoms to the health care provider for further evaluation. Pruritus may be relieved by adding baking soda to the bathwater.

Nephrotoxicity. Assess for an increasing BUN and creatinine, decreasing urine output, decreasing urine specific gravity, casts or protein in the urine, frank blood or smoky-colored urine, or RBCs in excess of 0 to 3 RBC/HPF (see Table 42-1) on the urinalysis report.

Hepatotoxicity. Review laboratory studies (e.g., bilirubin, AST, ALT, GGT, alkaline phosphatase, prothrombin time) and report abnormal findings to the health care provider.

Neutropenia, Lymphopenia. Neutropenia (neutrophil count less than 1000 cells/mm^3) and lymphopenia have been observed in patients receiving terbinafine. Monitor the CBC with differential in patients receiving treatment for greater than 6 weeks.

Drug Interactions

Cyclosporine. Terbinafine can increase serum concentrations of cyclosporine. Monitor patients for nephrotoxicity, hepatotoxicity, leukopenia, and thrombocytopenia.

Caffeine. Terbinafine can increase serum concentrations of caffeine. Monitor patients for excitability, agitation, irritability, and tachycardia.

Dextromethorphan. Terbinafine can increase serum concentrations of dextromethorphan. Monitor patients for dizziness, drowsiness, GI disturbances, altered sensory perception; ataxia; slurred speech; dysphoria.

Rifampin. Rifampin reduces serum levels of terbinafine. Use of another antifungal agent whose metabolism is not induced by rifampin may be necessary.

Cimetidine. Cimetidine may inhibit the metabolism of terbinafine, increasing the potential for toxicity from terbinafine. Switching to another H_2 antagonist such as famotidine that is not likely to inhibit metabolism may resolve the interaction. Continue to monitor for terbinafine toxicity.

DRUG CLASS: Antiviral Agents

abacavir (ah bak′ ah veer)
ZIAGEN (ziy′ ah jen)

Actions

Abacavir (ABC) is the first guanosine nucleoside analog reverse transcriptase inhibitor (NRTI) and a member of the NRTI class. Abacavir is a prodrug that is converted in cells to carbovir. Carbovir inhibits the activity of HIV-1 reverse transcriptase, preventing viral DNA growth.

Uses

Abacavir (ABC) is used in combination with zidovudine and lamivudine for the treatment of HIV-1 infection. Abacavir should always be used in conjunction with other antiretroviral agents. A benefit of abacavir is that it is not metabolized by the cytochrome P-450 enzyme system like the protease inhibitors and the nonnucleoside reverse transcriptase inhibitors. This is particularly useful in patients who must also take medicines whose metabolism is induced by this enzyme system (e.g., rifampin, phenytoin, carbamazepine).

Therapeutic Outcomes

The primary therapeutic outcomes expected from abacavir therapy are as follows:

- Slowed clinical progression of HIV-1 infection
- Reduced frequency of opportunistic secondary infections

Nursing Process for Abacavir

Premedication Assessment

1. Obtain baseline assessments of presenting symptoms.
2. Record temperature, pulse, respirations, blood pressure, and hydration status.
3. Assess for and record any gastric symptoms before initiating therapy.
4. Assess for any allergies.
5. Obtain baseline laboratory studies ordered (e.g., blood glucose, triglycerides, creatine kinase, liver function tests)

Planning

Availability. PO: 300 mg tablets; 20 mg per mL oral solution in 240 mL bottles.

Implementation

Dosage and Administration. *Adult:* PO: 300 mg twice daily with other antiretroviral agents. Ensure that the patient understands the Medication Guide and Hypersensitivity Warning card that is dispensed with each prescription.

Transmission of HIV. Abacavir therapy has not been shown to reduce the risk of transmission of HIV to others through sexual contact or blood contamination.

Evaluation

Side Effects to Report

Hypersensitivity. A hypersensitivity reaction has been reported in approximately 5% of patients receiving abacavir therapy. It does not seem to be dose related and usually appears several days to 6 weeks (median of 11 days) after starting therapy. The reaction involves several organ systems, resulting in multiple symptoms including fever, nausea, vomiting, diarrhea, malaise, and rash. A rash is not seen in all cases of hypersensitivity, but when present is usually urticarial or maculopapular. Development of these symptoms should be reported to the health care provider immediately. Patients should not be rechallenged with abacavir because more severe symptoms will recur within hours and may include life-threatening hypotension and death.

Lactic Acidosis and Hepatotoxicity. Lactic acidosis and severe hepatomegaly with steatosis have been reported with the use of nucleoside analogs, including abacavir. Women appear to be more susceptible to this adverse effect than men. Obesity and prolonged nucleoside exposure may be risk factors. The symptoms of hepatotoxicity are anorexia, nausea, vomiting, jaundice, hepatomegaly, splenomegaly, and abnormal liver function tests (e.g., elevated bilirubin, AST, ALT, GGT, alkaline phosphatase, prothrombin time). Symptoms should be reported to the health care provider immediately.

It is crucial that patients understand the importance of returning periodically for blood tests while receiving therapy.

Drug Interactions

Alcohol. Metabolism of abacavir is inhibited by ethanol. Coadministration of ethanol and abacavir results in increased occurrence of adverse effects associated with abacavir therapy.

acyclovir (a sy′klo veer)
▶ ZOVIRAX (zoh′ ve rahx)

Actions

Acyclovir is an antiviral agent that acts by inhibiting viral cell replication.

Uses

Acyclovir is used topically to treat initial infections of herpes genitalis and non–life-threatening cases of mucocutaneous herpes simplex virus infections in patients with suppressed immune systems. The oral form is used to treat initial episodes and for management of recurrent episodes of genital herpes in certain patients. The intravenous form is used to treat initial and recurrent mucosal and cutaneous herpes simplex types 1 and 2 infections in immunosuppressed adults and children and to treat severe initial clinical episodes of herpes genitalis in patients who are not immunosuppressed.

Therapeutic Outcomes

The primary therapeutic outcome expected from acyclovir therapy is elimination of symptoms of viral infection.

Nursing Process for Acyclovir

Premedication Assessment

1. Obtain baseline assessments of presenting symptoms.
2. Record temperature, pulse, respirations, blood pressure, and hydration status.
3. Assess for and record any abnormal renal function before beginning therapy.
4. Assess for any allergies.
5. Obtain baseline laboratory studies ordered (e.g., renal function tests).
6. Perform baseline mental status examination (e.g., orientation).

Planning

Availability. Topical: 5% ointment and cream. PO: 200 mg capsules; 400 and 800 mg tablets; 200 mg per 5 mL suspension. IV: 500, 1000 mg per vial.

Implementation

Dosage and Administration. *Adult:* Topical: apply to each lesion every 3 hours, six times daily for 7 days. A finger cot or rubber gloves should be used to avoid the spread of virus to other tissues and people. Use meticulous handwashing technique before and after applying the ointment. DO NOT apply to the eyes. It is not an ophthalmic ointment. IV: Note: Bolus or rapid IV infusions may result in renal tubular damage. Acyclovir is reconstituted with 10 mL of preservative-free sterile water for injection to provide a solution concentration of 50 mg/mL. The solution is stable for 12 hours. This solution should be further diluted by a glucose and electrolyte IV fluid to a concentration of 1 to 7 mg/mL before administration (stable for 24 hours). Infuse over at least 1 hour to well-hydrated patients to prevent renal damage. Observe for phlebitis at the infusion site.

Dose for patients with normal renal function: 5 mg/kg every 8 hours for 5 to 7 days.

PO: Initial treatment of genital herpes: 200 mg every 4 hours while the patient is awake, for a total of 1000 mg daily for 10 days. Chronic suppressive therapy for recurrent disease: 400 mg two times daily for up to 12 months. Some patients require 200 mg five times daily. Intermittent therapy: 200 mg every 4 hours while the patient is awake for a total of 1000 mg for 5 days. Therapy should be initiated at the earliest sign or symptom (prodrome) of recurrence.

Pediatric: Topical: As for adult patients. IV: Patients older than 12 years of age: 250 mg/m^2 every 8 hours for 7 days at a constant infusion rate over 1 hour.

Evaluation

Side Effects to Report

Pruritus, Rash, Burning. Report symptoms to the health care provider for further evaluation. Pruritus may be relieved by adding baking soda to the bathwater.

Intravenous Therapy. Avoid IV infusion in the lower extremities and areas with varicosities. Use proper technique in starting the IV solution.

Carefully assess at regularly scheduled intervals for signs of developing phlebitis. Inspect for redness, warmth, tenderness to touch, edema, or pain.

Rash, Hives. Assess, describe, and chart the location and extent of these presenting symptoms. Report for further evaluation.

Diaphoresis. Diaphoresis can be serious if the patient is not well hydrated. Assess hydration state, monitor electrolytes, and provide nursing interventions (e.g., clean, dry linens; adequate fluid intake).

Nephrotoxicity. Monitor urinalysis and kidney function tests for abnormal results. Report an increasing BUN and creatinine, decreasing urine output or decreasing urine specific gravity (despite amount of fluid intake), casts or protein in the urine, frank blood or smoky-colored urine, or RBCs in excess of 0 to 3 RBC/HPF (see Table 42-1) on the urinalysis report.

Hypotension. Record the blood pressure in both supine and sitting positions before and during administration of this drug. Caution the patient to rise slowly from a supine or sitting position.

Confusion. Perform a baseline assessment of the patient's degree of alertness and orientation to name, place, and time *before* initiating therapy. Make regularly scheduled subsequent mental status evaluations, and compare findings. Report development of alterations.

Drug Interactions

Probenecid. Probenecid may reduce urinary excretion of acyclovir. Monitor closely for signs of toxicity from acyclovir.

Zidovudine. Patients may complain of severe drowsiness and lethargy when acyclovir and zidovudine are used concurrently. Observe for patient safety.

amantadine hydrochloride (ah man' tah deen)
▸ SYMMETREL (sim' eh trel)

Uses

Amantadine is an antiviral agent that has specific activity against the influenza A virus. Its current primary use, however, is as an antiparkinsonian agent. It does not treat the underlying disease but reduces its clinical manifestations. It is described in greater detail in Chapter 15 (see p. 236).

amprenavir (am pren' ah veer)
▸ AGENERASE (a jen' er ace)

Actions

Amprenavir (APV) prevents maturation of viral particles by inhibiting HIV-1 protease. Immature viral particles are not infectious. Amprenavir is classified as a protease inhibitor.

Uses

Amprenavir is used in combination with other antiretroviral agents in treating HIV-1 infection. Amprenavir should always be used in conjunction with other antiretroviral agents.

Therapeutic Outcomes

The primary therapeutic outcomes expected from amprenavir therapy are as follows:

- Slowed clinical progression of HIV-1 infection
- Reduced incidence of opportunistic secondary infections

Nursing Process for Amprenavir

Premedication Assessment

1. Obtain baseline assessments of presenting symptoms.
2. Record temperature, pulse, respirations, blood pressure, and hydration status.
3. Assess for and record any gastric symptoms before initiating therapy.
4. Assess for any allergies.
5. Obtain baseline laboratory studies ordered (e.g., blood glucose, triglycerides, cholesterol, liver function tests).

Planning

Availability. PO: 50 mg capsules; 15 mg/mL oral solution in 240 mL bottles.

Implementation

Dosage and Administration. Adult: PO: 1200 mg (eight capsules) twice daily in combination with other antiretroviral agents. Amprenavir oral solution is approximately 14% less bioavailable than capsules. Amprenavir may be taken with food or milk, but high fat content should be avoided because it reduces the drug's absorption. Amprenavir is a sulfonamide. Cross-reactivity in patients with sulfonamide hypersensitivity is unknown. Patients allergic to sulfonamides should be treated with caution. Advise patients not to take supplemental vitamin E because the vitamin E content of amprenavir capsules (109 international units) and oral solution (46 international units) exceeds the Dietary Reference Intake recommendations (adults = 30 international units). The effects of long-term, high-dose vitamin E administration in humans is not well described and has not been specifically studied in HIV-infected patients.

Transmission of HIV. Amprenavir therapy has not been shown to reduce the risk of transmission of HIV to others through sexual contact or blood contamination.

Evaluation

Side Effects to Expect

Fat Distribution. Redistribution or accumulation of body fat including central obesity, dorsocervical fat enlargement (buffalo hump), peripheral wasting, breast enlargement, and "cushingoid appearance" has been reported in patients receiving protease inhibitors. The causes and long-term consequences are unknown.

Side Effects to Report

Nausea, Vomiting, Diarrhea. Many patients develop mild to moderate GI disturbances. These symptoms generally resolve with continued therapy.

Rash. Approximately one fourth of patients treated with amprenavir develop mild to moderate maculopapular skin eruptions, some with pruritus. Rashes had onsets ranging from 7 to 73 days (median, 10 days) after starting amprenavir therapy. Report to the health care provider as soon as possible. In most patients, the rash resolves within 1 month with continued therapy. Amprenavir can be restarted in patients who have therapy interrupted because of rash. Antihistamines or corticosteroids are recommended when amprenavir is restarted. Amprenavir should be discontinued in patients who develop severe rash accompanied by blistering, desquamation, mucosal involvement, or fever.

Hyperglycemia. As with other protease inhibitors, amprenavir may induce hyperglycemia, aggravate preexisting diabetes mellitus, and induce new-onset diabetes. Diabetic ketoacidosis has been reported. Insulin or oral hypoglycemic therapy may be necessary to treat hyperglycemia. Ensure that the patient understands how to monitor blood glucose using a glucometer, and knows when to seek medical attention when hyperglycemia persists.

Hepatotoxicity. The symptoms of hepatotoxicity are anorexia, nausea, vomiting, jaundice, hepatomegaly, splenomegaly, and abnormal liver function tests (e.g., elevated bilirubin, AST, ALT, GGT, alkaline phosphatase, prothrombin time).

It is crucial that patients understand the importance of returning periodically for blood tests while receiving therapy.

Drug Interactions

Toxicity Induced by Amprenavir. Amprenavir is contraindicated and should not be administered concurrently with astemizole, bepridil, cisapride, dihydroergotamine, ergotamine, midazolam, and triazolam. Serious, life-threatening complications may result.

Amprenavir may inhibit metabolism of the following agents: antidysrhythmics (amiodarone, quinidine, lidocaine), calcium channel blockers (diltiazem, nicardipine, nifedipine, nimodipine), benzodiazepines (alprazolam, clorazepate, diazepam, clonazepam) antiseizure medicines (carbamazepine), tricyclic antidepressants, pimozide, loratadine, dapsone, and clozapine. Serum concentrations of these agents should be monitored closely if used concurrently with amprenavir.

Drugs That Increase Therapeutic and Toxic Effects. The following drugs may increase serum levels of amprenavir, resulting in a greater incidence of toxicity: itraconazole, ketoconazole, cimetidine, indinavir, retonavir, delavirdine, zidovudine, clarithromycin, and erythromycin.

Drugs That Decrease Therapeutic Effects. Nelfinavir, efavirenz, nevirapine, phenobarbital, phenytoin, carbamazepine, and rifampin may decrease amprenavir concentrations by enhancing metabolism.

HMG-CoA Reductase Inhibitors. Concurrent administration of protease inhibitors and HMG-CoA reductase inhibitors is not recommended. Amprenavir may increase serum concentrations of HMG-CoA reductase inhibitors (e.g., atorvastatin, lovastatin, pravastatin, simvastatin), which may increase the risk of myopathy, including rhabdomyolysis. Read individual monographs for monitoring parameters of toxicity from these agents.

Antacids. Antacids may inhibit the absorption of amprenavir. Separate times of administration by at least 1 hour.

Oral Contraceptives. Amprenavir has variable effects on estrogens and progestins that may decrease the contraceptive efficacy of these hormones. Other methods of contraception such as condoms and foam should be considered during amprenavir therapy.

Sildenafil. Amprenavir may inhibit the metabolism of sildenafil. This may result in an increased risk of sildenafil-associated adverse effects, including hypotension, visual changes, and priapism. These symptoms should be reported promptly to the patient's health care provider. The dose of sildenafil should not exceed a maximum single dose of 25 mg in a 48-hour period. There is no drug interaction between amprenavir and tadalafil or vardenafil.

Warfarin. Amprenavir may increase serum concentrations of warfarin. The vitamin E in amprenavir capsules and solution may also exacerbate the blood coagulation defect of vitamin K deficiency caused by warfarin therapy. The patient's INR must be monitored closely.

atazanavir (at ah zan′ ah veer)
REYATAZ (ray′ ah taz)

Actions

Atazanavir (ATV) is an HIV protease inhibitor. It prevents maturation of viral particles by inhibiting HIV-1 protease. Immature viral particles are not infectious.

Uses

Atazanavir is used in combination with other antiretroviral agents in treating HIV-1 infection. It should always be used in conjunction with other antiretroviral agents. It has an advantage of once-daily dosage and does not cause hyperlipidemia as other protease inhibitors do.

Therapeutic Outcomes

The primary therapeutic outcomes expected from amprenavir therapy are as follows:

- Slowed clinical progression of HIV-1 infection
- Reduced incidence of opportunistic secondary infections

Nursing Process for Atazanavir

Premedication Assessment

1. Obtain baseline assessments of presenting symptoms.
2. Record temperature, pulse, respirations, blood pressure, and hydration status.
3. Assess for and record any gastric symptoms before initiation of therapy.
4. Assess for any allergies.
5. Obtain baseline laboratory studies ordered (e.g., viral load, CD4 cell count, blood glucose, triglycerides, cholesterol, liver function tests).

Planning

Availability. PO: 100, 150, and 200 mg capsules

Implementation

Dosage and Administration. *Adult:* PO: 400 mg once daily with food.

Transmission of HIV. Amprenavir therapy has not been shown to reduce the risk of transmission of HIV to others through sexual contact or blood contamination.

Evaluation

Side Effects to Expect

Fat Distribution. Redistribution or accumulation of body fat including central obesity, dorsocervical fat enlargement (buffalo hump), peripheral wasting, breast enlargement, and "cushingoid appearance" has been reported in patients receiving protease inhibitors. The causes and long-term consequences are unknown.

Hyperbilirubinemia. About one third of patients taking atazanavir develop jaundice and scleral icterus. Atazanavir blocks the metabolic pathway of bilirubin, causing its accumulation. It is not a sign of hepatic toxicity, although some patients object to the cosmetic effect. Encourage the patient not to discontinue therapy, but to speak with the health care provider to change to another protease inhibitor. The jaundice is reversible on discontinuation of atazanavir.

Side Effects to Report

Nausea, Vomiting, Diarrhea. Many patients develop mild to moderate GI disturbances. These symptoms generally resolve with continued therapy.

Rash. Approximately 20% of patients treated with atazanavir develop mild to moderate maculopapular skin eruptions, some with pruritus. Rashes have a median onset of 8 weeks after starting atazanavir therapy. Report to the health care provider as soon as possible. In most patients, the rash resolves within 1 to 2 weeks of continued therapy. Atazanavir should be discontinued in patients who develop severe rash accompanied by blistering, desquamation, mucosal involvement, or fever.

Hyperglycemia. As with other protease inhibitors, atazanavir may induce hyperglycemia, aggravate preexisting diabetes mellitus, and induce new-onset diabetes. Diabetic ketoacidosis has been reported. Insulin or oral hypoglycemic therapy may be necessary to treat hyperglycemia. Ensure that the patient understands how to monitor blood glucose using a glucometer, and knows when to seek medical attention when hyperglycemia persists.

Hepatotoxicity. The symptoms of hepatotoxicity are anorexia, nausea, vomiting, jaundice, hepatomegaly, splenomegaly, and abnormal liver function tests (e.g., elevated bilirubin, AST, ALT, GGT, alkaline phosphatase, prothrombin time).

It is crucial that patients understand the importance of returning periodically for blood tests while receiving therapy.

Drug Interactions

Toxicity Induced by Atazanavir. Atazanavir is contraindicated and should not be administered concurrently with bepridil, cisapride, dihydroergotamine, ergotamine, midazolam, and triazolam. Serious life-threatening complications may result.

Atazanavir may inhibit metabolism of the following agents: antidysrhythmics (amiodarone, quinidine, lidocaine), calcium channel blockers (diltiazem, verapamil, felodipine, nicardipine, nifedipine, nimodipine), antiseizure medicines (carbamazepine), tricyclic antidepressants, pimozide, irinotecan, rifabutin, and clozapine. Serum concentrations of these agents should be monitored closely if used concurrently with atazanavir.

Drugs That Increase Therapeutic and Toxic Effects. The following drugs may increase serum levels of atazanavir, resulting in a greater incidence of toxicity: itraconazole, ketoconazole, voriconazole, cimetidine, indinavir, ritonavir, clarithromycin, and erythromycin.

Drugs That Decrease Therapeutic Effects. Nelfinavir, efavirenz, buffered didanosine, tenofovir, nevirapine, phenobarbital, phenytoin, carbamazepine, St. John's wort, and rifampin may decrease atazanavir concentrations by enhancing metabolism.

Prolongation of the PR Interval. Atazanavir has been reported to prolong the PR interval of the electrocardiogram, rarely developing first-degree atrioventricular block. Use atazanavir cautiously in patients with heart disease, or in patients who are taking other medicines that prolong the PR interval, such as beta blockers, digoxin, diltiazem, and verapamil.

HMG-CoA Reductase Inhibitors. Concurrent administration of protease inhibitors and HMG-CoA reductase inhibitors is not recommended. Atazanavir may increase serum concentrations of HMG-CoA reductase inhibitors (e.g., atorvastatin, lovastatin, simvastatin), which may increase the risk of myopathy, including rhabdomyolysis. Read individual monographs for monitoring parameters of toxicity from these agents.

Antacids. Antacids may inhibit the absorption of atazanavir. Separate times of administration by at least 1 hour.

Proton Pump Inhibitors. Proton pump inhibitors (e.g., esomeprazole, lansoprazole, omeprazole, pantoprazole, rabeprazole) elevate the pH of the stomach, reducing absorption of atazanavir and its antiviral therapeutic effects. Do not administer proton pump inhibitors to patients receiving atazanavir.

Oral Contraceptives. Atazanavir has variable effects on estrogens and progestins that may decrease the contraceptive efficacy of these hormones. Other methods of contraception such as condoms and foam should be considered during atazanavir therapy.

Phosphodiesterase-5 Inhibitors. Atazanavir may inhibit the metabolism of sildenafil, tadalafil, and vardenafil. This may result in an increased risk of sildenafil-associated adverse effects, including hypotension, visual changes, and priapism. These symptoms should be reported promptly to the patient's health care provider. The dose of sildenafil should not exceed a maximum single dose of 25 mg in a 48-hour period, tadalafil 10 mg every 72 hours, or vardenafil up to 2.5 mg every 72 hours.

Warfarin. Atazanavir may increase serum concentrations of warfarin. The patient's prothrombin time (INR) must be monitored closely.

didanosine (die dahn' oh seen)
▶ VIDEX (vye' dex)

Actions

Didanosine (ddI) is an antiviral agent that acts by inhibiting viral cell replication. It is classified as a nucleoside reverse transcriptase inhibitor (NRTI).

Uses

Didanosine is used to treat pediatric and adult patients with advanced HIV-1 infection who have received prolonged courses of zidovudine and have deteriorated clinically or who cannot tolerate zidovudine therapy. Zidovudine is still considered drug of choice in HIV-1 disease because it has been shown to prolong survival and decrease the incidence of secondary infections in patients with acquired immunodeficiency syndrome (AIDS).

Therapeutic Outcomes

The primary therapeutic outcomes expected from didanosine therapy are as follows:

- Slowed clinical progression of HIV-1 infection
- Reduced incidence of opportunistic secondary infections

Nursing Process for Didanosine

Premedication Assessment

1. Obtain baseline assessments of presenting symptoms.
2. Record temperature, pulse, respirations, blood pressure, and hydration status.
3. Assess for and record any peripheral neuropathies or gastrointestinal symptoms before initiating therapy.
4. Assess for any allergies.
5. Obtain baseline laboratory studies ordered (e.g., CBC with differential, serum amylase).

Planning

Availability. PO: 25, 50, 100, and 200 mg chewable/dispersible buffered tablets; 125, 200, 250, and 400 mg delayed release capsules; 100 and 250 mg buffered powder for oral solution; and 2 and 4 g powder for pediatric oral solution.

Implementation

Dosage and Administration. *Adult:* Chewable/dispersible tablets: PO: for patients more than 60 kg, 200-mg tablets every 12 hours. For patients less than 60 kg, 125-mg tablets every 12 hours. Tablets should be thoroughly chewed or crushed and well dispersed in at least 1 ounce of water.

Capsules, delayed release (Videx EC): PO: for patients more than 60 kg, 400-mg capsules once daily. For patients less than 60 kg, 250-mg capsules once daily.

Powder, buffered: PO: for patients more than 60 kg, 250 mg of buffered powder every 12 hours. For patients less than 60 kg, 167 mg of buffered powder every 12 hours. The buffered powder should be mixed with at least 4 ounces of water and thoroughly dispersed. Instruct the patient to drink the entire solution immediately. Do not mix with fruit juice or other acid-containing liquid.

NOTE: For all dosage forms, food significantly reduces absorption. Administer on an empty stomach 1 hour before or 2 hours after meals.

Transmission of HIV. Didanosine therapy has not been shown to reduce the risk of transmission of HIV to others through sexual contact or blood contamination.

Evaluation

Side Effects to Expect

Diarrhea. There appears to be a higher incidence of diarrhea associated with the buffered powder. If diarrhea develops, try switching to the oral tablet form.

Side Effects to Report

Abdominal Pain, Nausea, Vomiting. Patients receiving didanosine are susceptible to developing pancreatitis. If these symptoms develop, withhold further administration of didanosine and report to the health care provider.

Numbness, Tingling. Patients receiving didanosine are susceptible to developing peripheral neuropathies characterized by numbness, tingling, or pain in the feet or hands. Report to the health care provider for further evaluation.

Drug Interactions

Drugs That Increase Therapeutic and Toxic Effects. The following drugs may increase serum levels of didanosine, resulting in a greater incidence of toxicity: allopurinol and ganciclovir.

Quinolone and Tetracycline Antibiotics, Dapsone. Do not administer quinolone or tetracycline antibiotics within 2 hours of administering didanosine tablets or pediatric powder for oral solution. The antacid present in these formulations inhibits the absorption of the quinolones, tetracyclines, and dapsone.

efavirenz (ef ahv′ er enz)
Sustiva (sus tee′ vha)

Actions

Efavirenz (EFV) is a nonnucleoside reverse transcriptase inhibitor (NNRTI) antiviral agent that acts by inhibiting replication of HIV-1. It does not inhibit HIV-2 reverse transcriptase.

Uses

Efavirenz (EFV) is used in combination with a protease inhibitor or NRTI for the treatment of HIV-1 infection. Efavirenz must not be used as a single agent to treat HIV-1 or added as a sole agent to a failing regimen, because resistant virus emerges rapidly when NNRTIs are administered as monotherapy. A particular benefit of efavirenz is its once-daily dosage.

Therapeutic Outcomes

The primary therapeutic outcomes expected from efavirenz therapy are as follows:

- Slowed clinical progression of HIV-1 infection
- Reduced frequency of opportunistic secondary infections

Nursing Process for Efavirenz

Premedication Assessment

1. Obtain baseline assessments of presenting symptoms.
2. Record temperature, pulse, respirations, blood pressure, and hydration status.
3. Assess for and record any gastric symptoms before initiating therapy.
4. Assess for any allergies.
5. Obtain baseline laboratory studies ordered (e.g., cholesterol, liver function tests).

Planning

Availability. PO: 50, 100, and 200 mg capsules; 600 mg capsules.

Implementation

Dosage and Administration. *Adult:* PO: 600 mg once daily with other antiretroviral agents. It is recommended that efavirenz be taken on an empty stomach, preferably at bedtime. Food increases absorption and increases the incidence of toxic effects.

Transmission of HIV. Efavirenz therapy has not been shown to reduce the risk of transmission of HIV to others through sexual contact or blood contamination.

Teratogenic Effects. There is positive evidence of fetal defects associated with efavirenz therapy when taken in the first trimester of pregnancy. Women who are or may become pregnant should not take efavirenz.

Evaluation

Side Effects to Report

CNS Symptoms. Approximately half of patients taking efavirenz develop symptoms of drowsiness, dizziness, impaired concentration, vivid dreams, depression, or delusions. These symptoms are likely to improve 2 to 4 weeks following therapy initiation. Taking the once-daily dosage at bedtime may minimize these adverse effects.

Rash. Approximately one fourth of patients treated with efavirenz develop mild to moderate maculopapular skin eruptions within the first 2 weeks of treatment. Report to the health care provider as soon as possible. In most patients, the rash resolves within 1 month with continued therapy. Efavirenz can be restarted in patients interrupting therapy because of rash. Antihistamines or corticosteroids are recommended when efavirenz is restarted. Efavirenz should be discontinued in patients who develop severe rash accompanied by blistering, desquamation, mucosal involvement, or fever.

Hepatotoxicity. The symptoms of hepatotoxicity are anorexia, nausea, vomiting, jaundice, hepatomegaly, splenomegaly, and abnormal liver function tests (e.g., elevated bilirubin, AST, ALT, GGT, alkaline phosphatase, prothrombin time).

It is crucial that patients understand the importance of returning periodically for blood tests while receiving therapy.

Drug Interactions

Toxicity Induced by Efavirenz. Efavirenz may inhibit metabolism and can increase serum concentrations of warfarin, retonavir, phenytoin, cisapride, midazolam, triazolam, and ergot derivatives, creating the potential for serious or life-threatening adverse effects (e.g., cardiac dysrhythmias, prolonged sedation, respiratory depression). Read individual monographs for monitoring parameters of toxicity from these agents.

Drugs That Decrease Therapeutic Effects. The following drugs may enhance the metabolism of efavirenz: carbamazepine, phenobarbital, phenytoin, rifampin, rifabutin, retonavir, St. John's wort.

Indinavir, Amprenavir, Atazanavir. Efavirenz stimulates the metabolism of indinavir, atazanavir, and amprenavir. Dosages of these agents must be increased to maintain therapeutic effect.

Alcohol. Ingestion of ethanol may aggravate CNS adverse effects associated with efavirenz therapy.

Oral Contraceptives. Efavirenz has variable effects on the metabolism of ethinyl estradiol that may decrease the contraceptive efficacy of this estrogen. Other methods of contraception such as condoms and foam should be considered during efavirenz therapy.

emtricitabine (em tree sit′ a bean)
EMTRIVA (em tree′ vah)

Actions

Emtricitabine (FTC) is a nucleoside reverse transcriptase inhibitor that acts by inhibiting replication of viruses such as HIV-1.

Uses

Emtricitabine is used in combination with other antiviral agents in treating HIV-1 infection.

Therapeutic Outcomes

The primary therapeutic outcomes expected from emtricitabine therapy are as follows:

- Slowed clinical progression of HIV-1 infection
- Reduced incidence of opportunistic secondary infections

Nursing Process for Emtricitabine

Premedication Assessment

1. Obtain baseline assessments of presenting symptoms.
2. Record temperature, pulse, respirations, blood pressure, and hydration status.
3. Assess for and record any gastric symptoms before initiating therapy.
4. Assess for any allergies.
5. Obtain baseline laboratory studies ordered (e.g., CBC with differential, CD4 cell count).

Planning

Availability. PO: 200 mg capsules.

Implementation

Dosage and Administration. *Adult:* 200 mg once daily without regard to food. Dosage must be reduced for patients with impaired renal function. For patients with a creatinine clearance of:

- 30 to 49 mL per minute, administer the dose every 48 hours

- 15 to 19 mL per minute, administer the dose every 72 hours
- Less than 15 mL per minute, administer the dose every 96 hours

Transmission of HIV. Emtricitabine therapy has not been shown to reduce the risk of transmission of HIV to others through sexual contact or blood contamination.

Evaluation

Side Effects to Report

Lactic Acidosis, Hepatotoxicity. Lactic acidosis and severe hepatomegaly with steatosis have been reported with the use of nucleoside analogs, including emtricitabine. Women appear to be more susceptible to this adverse effect than men. Obesity and prolonged nucleoside exposure may be risk factors. The symptoms of hepatotoxicity are anorexia, nausea, vomiting, jaundice, hepatomegaly, splenomegaly, and abnormal liver function tests (e.g., elevated bilirubin, AST, ALT, GGT, alkaline phosphatase, prothrombin time). Symptoms should be reported to the health care provider immediately.

Skin Hyperpigmentation. Although uncommon, skin discoloration manifested by hyperpigmentation on the palms and/or soles has been reported. It is mild and asymptomatic, and the mechanism by which it is caused is unknown.

Other Common Side Effects. Diarrhea (23%), nausea (18%), rhinitis (18%), rash (17%), asthenia (16%), cough (14%), and headache (13%). Report to the health care provider for further evaluation.

Drug Interactions. No clinically significant drug interactions have been reported.

enfuvirtide (en fu′ vear tide)

FUZEON (few′ ze on)

Actions

Enfuvirtide (T-20) is the first of a new class of antiviral agents that interfere with the entry of viruses into host cells. This new class is titled entry inhibitors or fusion inhibitors. The fusion of HIV with host CD4 cells is an important step in viral replication. Enfuvirtide interferes with the entry of HIV into cells by inhibiting fusion of viral and cellular membranes.

Uses

Enfuvirtide is used in combination with other antiviral agents for the treatment of HIV-1 infection in patients with evidence of HIV-1 replication even while receiving ongoing antiviral therapy that depends on other mechanisms of action. Clinical indications of continued HIV-1 replication are increasing plasma HIV RNA concentrations and reduced CD4 cell counts. When enfuvirtide is added to current therapy, there are greater reductions of plasma HIV RNA and greater increases in CD4 cell count. Enfuvirtide should not be used alone because combination regimens are more effective and resistance will develop sooner.

Therapeutic Outcomes

The primary therapeutic outcomes expected from enfuvirtide therapy are as follows:

- Slowed clinical progression of HIV-1 infection
- Reduced incidence of opportunistic secondary infections

Nursing Process for Enfuvirtide

Premedication Assessment

1. Obtain baseline assessments of presenting symptoms.
2. Record temperature, pulse, respirations, blood pressure, and hydration status.
3. Assess for any allergies.
4. Obtain baseline laboratory studies ordered (e.g., CBC with differential, CD4 cell count).

Planning

Availability. Subcutaneous: 90 mg/mL single-use vials.

Implementation

Dosage and Administration. *Adult:* Subcutaneous: 90 mg (1 mL) in the arm, thigh or abdomen two times daily. Rotate injection sites.

NOTE: Vials may be stored at room temperature until reconstituted. Both daily doses may be prepared at the same time. For reconstitution, slowly inject 1.1 mL of sterile water of injection (supplied) so that it drips down the side of the vial into the powder. Gently tap the vial with a fingertip for 10 seconds to start dissolution of the powder. Gently roll the vial between the hands, but do not shake, because the resultant foaming will increase the time needed for the powder to dissolve. When the powder starts to dissolve, set the vial aside until the powder completely dissolves, which may take 45 minutes. If the drug is to be administered later, store in the refrigerator and then warm to room temperature before injection. Use within 24 hours of reconstitution.

Transmission of HIV. Enfuvirtide therapy has not been shown to reduce the risk of transmission of HIV to others through sexual contact or blood contamination.

Evaluation

Side Effects to Report

Injection Site Reactions. Most patients develop mild to moderate reactions at the site of injection. Patients report pain, induration, erythema, and nodules or cyst formation. Most reactions resolve within 1 week. Rotation of sites and massaging the area after injection may help reduce the incidence of reactions. Pain and discomfort at the injection site may be managed with NSAIDs or acetaminophen.

Pneumonia. Patients receiving enfuvirtide may be more susceptible to developing bacterial pneumonia. Patients with a low initial CD4 lymphocyte count, a high initial viral load, IV drug use, cigarette use, and a history of lung disease are at a higher risk of pneumonia. Report signs of pneumonia (e.g., cough, shortness of breath, chest pain upon inspiration, and fever) to a health care provider as soon as possible.

Nausea, Vomiting, Diarrhea. These side effects are usually mild and tend to resolve with continued therapy. Encourage the patient not to discontinue therapy without first consulting the health care provider.

Other Common Side Effects. Fatigue (16%), insomnia (11%), peripheral neuropathy (9%), cough (7%), decreased appetite (6%). Report to the health care provider for further evaluation.

Drug Interactions

No clinically significant drug interactions have been reported.

famciclovir (pham sik′ lo veer)
FAMVIR (pham′ veer)

Actions

Famciclovir is a prodrug of penciclovir, an antiviral agent that acts by inhibiting viral cell replication.

Uses

Famciclovir is used orally to treat recurrent infections of genital herpes and in the management of acute herpes zoster (shingles). In patients with genital herpes, famciclovir reduces the time of viral shedding, the duration of symptoms, and the time of healing if started within 6 hours of the onset of symptoms and continued for 5 days. In patients with shingles, if therapy is begun within 72 hours and continued for 7 days, famciclovir reduces the times to full crusting, loss of vesicles, loss of ulcers, and loss of crusts more effectively than placebo treatment. Early treatment with famciclovir can also reduce the duration of postherpetic neuralgia.

Therapeutic Outcomes

The primary therapeutic outcome expected from famciclovir therapy is elimination of symptoms of viral infection.

Nursing Process for Famciclovir

Premedication Assessment

1. Obtain baseline assessments of presenting symptoms.
2. Record temperature, pulse, respirations, blood pressure, and hydration status.
3. Assess for and record any abnormal renal function before initiating therapy.
4. Assess for any allergies.
5. Perform baseline mental status exam (e.g., orientation).

Planning

Availability. PO: 125, 250, and 500 mg tablets.

Implementation

Dosage and Administration. *Adult:* PO: Treatment of genital herpes: 125 mg two times daily for 5 days. Therapy should be started within 6 hours of the first sign or symptom of herpes breakout. Treatment of herpes zoster (shingles): 500 mg every 8 hours for 7 days. To be effective, therapy must be started within 72 hours of the onset of symptoms.

Evaluation

Side Effects to Expect

Nausea, Vomiting, Headache. These side effects are usually mild and tend to resolve with continued therapy. Encourage the patient not to discontinue therapy without first consulting the health care provider. Administer with food or milk to reduce irritation.

Side Effects to Report

Confusion. Perform a baseline assessment of the patient's degree of alertness and orientation to name, place, and time before initiating therapy. Make regularly scheduled subsequent mental status evaluations, and compare findings. Report development of alterations.

Drug Interactions

Probenecid. Probenecid may reduce urinary excretion of penciclovir. Monitor closely for signs of toxicity from penciclovir.

lamivudine (lahm ih′ vu deen)
EPIVIR (ep′ i vihr)
EPIVIR-HBV

Actions

Lamivudine (3TC) is a nucleoside reverse transcriptase inhibitor that acts by inhibiting replication of viruses such as HIV-1 and hepatitis B virus (HBV).

Uses

Lamivudine (3TC) is used in combination with zidovudine in treating HIV-1 infection. Laboratory studies indicate that the two medicines work synergistically to prolong life expectancy in HIV-positive patients and reduce the incidence of secondary infections associated with AIDS. (It is available in a combination with lamizudine in a product called Combivir.)

Lamivudine is also approved for use in the treatment of chronic hepatitis B associated with evidence of hepatitis B viral replication and active liver inflammation.

Therapeutic Outcomes

The primary therapeutic outcomes expected from lamivudine therapy are as follows:

- Slowed clinical progression of HIV-1 infection
- Slowed clinical progression of HBV infection
- Reduced incidence of opportunistic secondary infections

Nursing Process for Lamivudine

Premedication Assessment

1. Obtain baseline assessments of presenting symptoms.
2. Record temperature, pulse, respirations, blood pressure, and hydration status.
3. Assess for and record any gastric symptoms before initiation of therapy.
4. Assess for any allergies.
5. Obtain baseline laboratory studies ordered (e.g., CBC with differential, amylase, liver function tests).

Planning

Availability. PO: 100, 150, and 300 mg tablets; 5 and 10 mg/mL oral solution in 240 mL bottles.

Implementation

Dosage and Administration. *Adult:* HIV infection: PO: 150 mg twice daily with zidovudine. HBV infection: PO: 100 mg once daily.

Transmission of HIV. Lamivudine therapy has not been shown to reduce the risk of transmission of HIV to others through sexual contact or blood contamination.

Evaluation

Side Effects to Report

Anemia, Granulocytopenia. Monitor hematologic indices every 2 weeks to detect serious anemia or granulocytopenia. In patients developing bone marrow suppression, reduction in hemoglobin may occur as early as 2 to 4 weeks; granulocytopenia usually occurs after 6 to 8 weeks.

It is crucial that patients understand the importance of returning periodically for blood counts while receiving therapy.

Lactic Acidosis, Hepatotoxicity. Lactic acidosis and severe hepatomegaly with steatosis have been reported with the use of nucleoside analogs, including lamivudine. Women appear to be more susceptible to this adverse effect than men. Obesity and prolonged nucleoside exposure may be risk factors. The symptoms of hepatotoxicity are anorexia, nausea, vomiting, jaundice, hepatomegaly, splenomegaly, and abnormal liver function tests (e.g., elevated bilirubin, AST, ALT, GGT, alkaline phosphatase, prothrombin time). Symptoms should be reported to the health care provider immediately.

Abdominal Pain, Nausea, Vomiting. Patients receiving lamivudine are susceptible to developing pancreatitis. If these symptoms develop, withhold further administration of lamivudine and report to the health care provider.

Numbness, Tingling. Patients receiving lamivudine are susceptible to developing peripheral neuropathies characterized by numbness, tingling, or pain in the feet or hands. Report to the health care provider for further evaluation.

Drug Interactions

Co-trimoxazole. Concurrent administration of lamivudine and co-trimoxazole results in a significant increase in lamivudine levels and potential for toxicity. Dosage levels of lamivudine may need to be reduced.

Zalcitabine. Concurrent administration of lamivudine and zalcitabine results in inactivation of both drugs. Use of lamivudine in combination with zalcitabine is not recommended.

Zidovudine. Concurrent administration of lamivudine and zidovudine results in a significant increase in zidovudine levels and potential for toxicity. Dosage levels of zidovudine may need to be reduced.

oseltamivir (oh sel tahm′ ah veer)
TAMIFLU (tahm′ ih fluh)

Actions

Oseltamivir is an antiviral agent that acts by inhibiting neuraminidase, an enzyme on the viral cell coat necessary for reproduction and spread of viral cell particles.

Uses

Oseltamivir is the first neuraminidase inhibitor approved for oral use in treating uncomplicated acute illness due to influenza. Studies show that the duration of symptoms of influenza infection (e.g., nasal congestion, sore throat, cough, myalgia, fatigue, headache, chills, sweats) will be reduced by about 1 day (4 days versus 5 days) if the patient has been symptomatic for no more than 2 days when treatment is started. The severity of symptoms and potential for complications from secondary infection are also significantly reduced. It is not known whether oseltamivir is effective in preventing influenza infection, and it should not be used as a substitute for annual influenza vaccination. Oseltamivir has not been shown to reduce the risk of transmission of influenza to others.

Therapeutic Outcomes

The primary therapeutic outcome expected from oseltamivir therapy is reduced symptomatology caused by influenzavirus infection. It may also reduce the incidence of opportunistic secondary infections such as pneumonia.

Nursing Process for Oseltamivir

Premedication Assessment

1. Obtain baseline assessments of presenting symptoms.
2. Record temperature, pulse, respirations, blood pressure, and hydration status.
3. Assess for and record any gastric symptoms before initiating therapy.
4. Assess for any allergies.

Planning

Availability. PO: 75 mg capsules; 12 mg/mL oral suspension.

Implementation

Dosage and Administration. *Adult:* PO: 75 mg twice daily for 5 days. Treatment should begin within 2 days after the onset of symptoms of influenza. Patients may also take decongestants, analgesics, and antipyretic agents to reduce symptomatology.

Evaluation

Side Effects to Report

Nausea, Vomiting. Patients receiving oseltamivir may develop nausea and vomiting within the first 2 days of treatment. Administering with food or milk will minimize incidence of nausea and vomiting. If these symptoms continue, report to the health care provider for evaluation of other potential complications.

Cough, Sore Throat, Fever, Continuing Symptoms. If the patient starts coughing up yellow or green sputum; if a sore throat worsens and becomes severe; if fever returns after going away; or if symptoms last for more than 1 or 2 weeks, report to the health care provider for evaluation of other potential complications.

Drug Interactions. No clinically significant drug interactions have been reported.

ribavirin (ribe ah vi' rihn)
- VIRAZOLE (vi' rah zohl) (aerosol)
- REBETOL (rehb et' ohl) (oral capsules and suspension)

Actions

The mechanism of action of ribavirin is unknown.

Uses

Ribavirin has been shown to have inhibitory activity against members of the DNA-type viral families of Adenoviridae, Herpesviridae, and Poxviridae. The RNA viruses for which ribavirin exerts inhibitory activity are the influenza, parainfluenza, and respiratory syncytial virus (RSV).

Ribavirin has been given FDA approval to be used by aerosol administration to treat severe lower respiratory tract infections caused by RSV in infants and young children. Ribavirin aerosol should not be used in adults.

Ribavirin has also been given FDA approval to be used in oral capsular form in combination with interferon alfa-2b, recombinant (Intron A) injection for the treatment of chronic hepatitis C in patients with compensated liver disease previously untreated with alpha interferon or in those who have relapsed following alpha interferon therapy. Due to the potential for hemolytic anemia, patients with a history of heart disease should not be treated with ribavirin.

Therapeutic Outcomes

The primary therapeutic outcome expected from ribavirin therapy is elimination of viral infection: RSV in infants and children, and chronic hepatitis C in adults.

Nursing Process for Ribavirin

Premedication Assessment

1. Obtain baseline assessments of presenting symptoms.
2. Record temperature, pulse, respirations, blood pressure, and hydration status.
3. Assess for and record any gastric symptoms before initiating therapy.
4. Assess for any allergies.
5. Obtain baseline laboratory studies ordered (e.g., pulmonary function tests, hemoglobin, hematocrit, CBC with differential, platelets, liver function tests [GGT, AST, ALT]).
6. Determine if the patient is pregnant; if pregnancy is suspected, check with the health care provider before administering the drug.

Planning

Availability. PO: 200 mg capsules and 40 mg/mL oral solution. Inhalation: aerosol powder: 6 g vials of powder for reconstitution.

Implementation

Dosage and Administration. Capsules: Less than 75 kg: 400 mg in the morning; 600 mg in the evening daily. Greater than 75 kg: 600 mg in the morning; 600 mg in the evening daily.

Aerosol powder: ribavirin must be administered through a specific, small-particle aerosol generator (SPAG-2).

1. Using aseptic technique, reconstitute 6 g of drug by adding at least 75 mL of sterile water for injection to the 100-mL vial. Shake well.
2. When dissolved, transfer the contents to a clean, sterilized 500-mL widemouth Erlenmeyer flask (SPAG-2 reservoir) and further dilute with sterile water for injection to a final volume of 300 mL. The final concentration is 20 mg/mL.

3. Administer ribavirin at an initial concentration of 20 mg/mL through the reservoir of the small-particle aerosol generator. Treatment is carried out for 12 to 18 hours per day for at least 3 and no more than 7 days. The aerosol is delivered from the generator to the patient via an oxygen hood or face mask. It should not be administered concurrently with any other aerosolized medication.
4. The liquid in the reservoir should not have any other substances (e.g., antibiotics) added to it. Discard and replace ribavirin solution in the SPAG-2 at least every 24 hours.

Pregnancy. Ribavirin is contraindicated in women who are or may become pregnant during exposure to the drug. It is also contraindicated in the male partners of women who are pregnant or who may become pregnant. Ribavirin has been reported to cause birth defects in several animal species. It is not completely eliminated from human blood for at least 4 weeks after administration. It is recommended that at least two reliable forms of effective contraception be used during treatment and during the 6-month posttreatment follow-up to prevent pregnancy.

Patients on Respirators. Ribavirin is not recommended for patients requiring assisted ventilation because precipitation of the drug in the respiratory equipment may interfere with safe and effective use of the ventilator by these patients. If it is deemed necessary to treat a patient with ribavirin who is also receiving ventilatory support, prefilters must be placed in the equipment to prevent precipitation in the endotracheal tube or on the valves and tubing.

Evaluation

Side Effects to Expect

Rash, Conjunctivitis. These adverse effects tend to occur because of local irritation from poorly placed inhalation equipment. Work with the patient for optimal fit. Methylcellulose eye drops may be applied to reduce conjunctival irritation.

Side Effects to Report

Diminishing Pulmonary Function. Perform baseline pulmonary function tests to assess whether the patient shows deterioration after therapy is initiated. If initiation of treatment appears to produce sudden deterioration of respiratory function, treatment should be discontinued immediately and reinstituted only with extreme caution and continuous monitoring. Immediately report complaints of chest soreness, shortness of breath, or other adverse effects.

Anemia. The primary toxicity of capsule ribavirin is hemolytic anemia, which develops in about 10% of patients treated with ribavirin/Intron A after 1 to 2 weeks of therapy. It is recommended that a baseline hemoglobin or hematocrit be obtained and at weeks 2 and 4 of therapy. Fatal and nonfatal myocardial infarctions have been reported in patients who develop anemia secondary to ribavirin therapy.

Drug Interactions

Antacids. Antacids containing aluminum, magnesium, and simethicone may inhibit absorption of ribavirin when taken orally. Take the capsule at least 1 hour before or 2 hours after taking antacids.

stavudine (stav′ u deen)
Zerit (zair′ it)
Zerit XR

Actions

Stavudine (d4T) is a thymidine nucleoside analog reverse transcriptase inhibitor (NRTI). It is a prodrug that converts to stavudine triphosphate, the active antiviral agent against HIV-1.

Uses

Stavudine is used in combination with other antiviral agents for the treatment of HIV-1 infection.

Therapeutic Outcomes

The primary therapeutic outcomes expected from stavudine therapy are as follows:

- Slowed clinical progression of HIV-1 infection
- Reduced frequency of opportunistic secondary infections

Nursing Process for Stavudine

Premedication Assessment

1. Obtain baseline assessments of presenting symptoms.
2. Record temperature, pulse, respirations, blood pressure, and hydration status.
3. Assess for and record peripheral neuropathic symptoms (numbness, tingling, pain in the feet and hands) before initiating therapy.
4. Assess for and record any gastric or abdominal symptoms before beginning therapy.
5. Assess for any allergies.
6. Obtain baseline laboratory studies ordered (e.g., CD4 cell count, amylase, triglycerides, serum creatinine, liver function tests)

Planning

Availability. PO: 15, 20, 30, 40 mg capsules; 37.5, 50, 75, and 100 mg extended-release capsules; 1 mg/mL powder for oral solution.

Implementation

Dosage and Administration. *Adult:* PO: Immediate release capsules:

- Less than 60 kg: 30 mg every 12 hours
- More than 60 kg: 40 mg every 12 hours

Extended release capsules:

- Less than 60 kg: 75 mg once daily
- More than 60 kg: 100 mg once daily

NOTE:
- Dosage adjustment is required for patients with a creatinine clearance less than 50 mg/mL.
- If peripheral neuropathy, manifested by numbness, tingling, and pain in the hands and feet develops, stop stavudine therapy. Symptoms may resolve if therapy is quickly discontinued.

Transmission of HIV. Abacavir therapy has not been shown to reduce the risk of transmission of HIV to others through sexual contact or blood contamination.

Evaluation

Side Effects to Expect

Fat Distribution. Redistribution or accumulation of body fat including central obesity, dorsocervical fat enlargement (buffalo hump), peripheral wasting, facial wasting, breast enlargement, and "cushingoid appearance" has been reported in patients receiving nucleoside reverse transcriptase inhibitors. The causes and long-term consequences are unknown.

Side Effects to Report

Lactic Acidosis and Hepatotoxicity. Lactic acidosis and severe hepatomegaly with steatosis have been reported with the use of nucleoside analogs, including abacavir. Women appear to be more susceptible to this adverse effect than men. Obesity and prolonged nucleoside exposure may be risk factors. The symptoms of hepatotoxicity are anorexia, nausea, vomiting, jaundice, hepatomegaly, splenomegaly, and abnormal liver function tests (e.g., elevated bilirubin, AST, ALT, GGT, alkaline phosphatase, prothrombin time). Symptoms should be reported to the health care provider immediately.

It is crucial that patients understand the importance of returning periodically for blood tests while receiving therapy.

Abdominal Pain, Nausea, Vomiting. Patients receiving stavudine are susceptible to developing pancreatitis. If these symptoms develop, withhold further administration of didanosine and report to the health care provider.

Numbness, Tingling. Patients receiving stavudine are susceptible to developing peripheral neuropathies characterized by numbness, tingling, or pain in the feet or hands. Report immediately to the health care provider for further evaluation. Quick discontinuation of therapy may prevent ongoing peripheral neuropathy.

Drug Interactions

Drugs That Decrease Therapeutic Effects. The following agents may reduce the therapeutic effects of stavudine and should not be used concurrently: doxorubicin, ribavirin, methadone, and zidovudine.

Didanosine, Hydroxyurea. Administering didanosine or hydroxyurea concurrently with stavudine may result in a higher incidence of lactic acidosis, hepatotoxicity, pancreatitis, or peripheral neuropathy. Use with extreme caution.

valacyclovir (vahl ah syk' lo veer)
VALTREX (vahl' trex)

Actions

Valacyclovir is a prodrug of acyclovir, an antiviral agent that acts by inhibiting viral cell replication.

Uses

Valacyclovir is used orally to treat acute herpes zoster (shingles) in immunocompetent patients.

Therapeutic Outcomes

The primary therapeutic outcome expected from valacyclovir therapy is elimination of symptoms of viral infection.

Nursing Process for Valacyclovir

Premedication Assessment

1. Obtain baseline assessments of presenting symptoms.
2. Record temperature, pulse, respirations, blood pressure, and hydration status.
3. Assess for and record any abnormal renal function before initiating therapy.
4. Assess for any allergies.
5. Perform baseline mental status exam (e.g., orientation).

Planning

Availability. PO: 500 mg and 1 g caplets.

Implementation

Dosage and Administration. *Adult:* PO: treatment of herpes zoster (shingles): 1 g three times daily for 7 days. To be effective, therapy must be started within 48 hours of the onset of the herpes rash.

Evaluation

See acyclovir.

zanamivir (zahn am' ah veer)
RELENZA (rehl en' zah)

Actions

Zanamivir is an antiviral agent that acts by inhibiting neuraminidase, an enzyme on the viral cell coat necessary for replication and spread of viral cell particles.

Uses

Zanamivir is the first neuraminidase inhibitor marketed for use in the treatment of uncomplicated acute illness due to influenza. Studies show that the duration of symptoms (nasal congestion, sore throat, cough, myalgia, fatigue, headache, chills, and sweats) of influenza infection will be reduced by about 1 day (4 days versus 5 days) if the patient has been symptomatic for no more than 2 days when treatment is started. The severity of symptoms and potential for complications from secondary infection are also significantly reduced. It is not known whether zanamivir is effective in preventing influenza infection, and it should not be used as a substitute for annual influenza vaccination. Zanamivir has not been shown to reduce the risk of transmission of influenza to others.

Therapeutic Outcomes

The primary therapeutic outcome expected from zanamivir therapy is reduced symptomatology caused by influenzavirus infection. It may also reduce the incidence of opportunistic secondary infections such as pneumonia.

Nursing Process for Zanamivir

Premedication Assessment

1. Obtain baseline assessments of presenting symptoms.
2. Record temperature, pulse, respirations, blood pressure, and hydration status.
3. Assess for any allergies.
4. Obtain baseline laboratory studies ordered (e.g., pulmonary function tests).

Planning

Availability. Inhaler: 5 mg blisters of powder for inhalation.

Implementation

Dosage and Administration. *Adult:* Inhalation: two inhalations (one 5-mg blister per inhalation for a total of 10 mg) two times daily (approximately 12 hours apart) for 5 days. Treatment should begin within 2 days after the onset of symptoms of influenza. On the first day of treatment, two doses should be taken, provided there are at least 2 hours between doses. On subsequent days, doses should be approximately 12 hours apart at approximately the same time each day.

Patients who are scheduled to use an inhaled bronchodilator should use the bronchodilator before taking zanamivir. Patients may also take decongestants, analgesics, and antipyretic agents to reduce symptomatology.

Evaluation

Side Effects to Report

Asthma, Bronchospasm, Diminishing Pulmonary Function. Perform baseline pulmonary function tests to assess whether the patient shows deterioration after therapy is started. If starting inhalation treatment appears to produce sudden bronchospasm or deterioration of respiratory function, treatment should be discontinued immediately and the health care provider contacted. Immediately report complaints of chest soreness, shortness of breath, or other adverse effects.

Cough, Sore Throat, Fever, Continuing Symptoms. If the patient starts coughing up yellow or green sputum; if a sore throat worsens and becomes severe; if fever returns after going away; or if symptoms last for more than 1 or 2 weeks, report to the health care provider for evaluation of other potential complications.

Drug Interactions. No clinically significant drug interactions have been reported.

zidovudine (zid ohv′ u deen)
RETROVIR (ret′ roh veer)

Actions

Zidovudine (AZT; ZDV) is the first of a series of antiviral agents that have been shown to be effective for certain patients with HIV-1 infection. It acts by inhibiting replication of the virus. It is classified as a nucleoside reverse transcriptase inhibitor. In controlled clinical trials, zidovudine was shown to prolong the lives of patients with AIDS and AIDS-related complex (ARC), reduce the risk and severity of opportunistic infections, and improve immune status.

Uses

Zidovudine is indicated for patients who have confirmed absolute CD4 lymphocyte counts of less than 500/mm^3 in the peripheral blood before therapy. Unfortunately, zidovudine is not a cure for HIV-1 infection, and patients may continue to acquire illnesses associated with AIDS. (It is available in a combination with lamivudine in a product called Combivir.)

Therapeutic Outcomes

The primary therapeutic outcomes expected from zidovudine therapy are as follows:

- Slowed clinical progression of HIV-1 infection
- Reduced incidence of opportunistic secondary infections

Nursing Process for Zidovudine

Premedication Assessment

1. Obtain baseline assessments of presenting symptoms.
2. Record temperature, pulse, respirations, blood pressure, and hydration status.
3. Assess for any allergies.
4. Obtain baseline laboratory studies ordered (e.g., CBC with differential, platelets, hemoglobin, hematocrit, amylase, and liver function tests).

Planning

Availability. PO: 100 mg capsules; 300 mg tablets; 50 mg per 5 mL syrup. IV: 10 mg/mL in 20-mL vial.

Implementation

Dosage and Administration. *Adult:* PO: asymptomatic HIV infection: 100 mg every 4 hours while the patient is awake (500 mg/day). Patients must understand the importance of taking the medication every 4 hours around the clock, even though this may interrupt normal sleep. Patients must also understand that the drug is taken orally and must not be shared with other people and that they must not exceed the recommended dose. Fatal adverse effects may result. Symptomatic HIV infection: 200 mg every 4 hours in a 24-hour period. After 1 month reduce to 100 mg every 4 hours. IV: 1 to 2 mg/kg infused over 1 hour; administer every 4 hours six times daily.

Transmission of HIV. Zidovudine therapy has not been shown to reduce the risk of transmission of HIV to others through sexual contact or blood contamination.

Evaluation

Side Effects to Report

Anemia, Granulocytopenia. Monitor hematologic indices every 2 weeks to detect serious anemia or granulocytopenia. In patients developing bone marrow suppression, reduction in hemoglobin may occur as early as 2 to 4 weeks; granulocytopenia usually occurs after 6 to 8 weeks.

It is crucial that patients understand the importance of returning periodically for blood counts while receiving therapy.

Numbness, Tingling. Patients receiving zidovudine are susceptible to developing peripheral neuropathies characterized by numbness, tingling, or pain in the feet or hands. Report to the health care provider for further evaluation.

Drug Interactions

Drugs That Increase Therapeutic and Toxic Effects. These agents may inhibit the metabolism and excretion of zidovudine, enhancing the potential for toxicity: ganciclovir, methadone, atovaquone, valproic acid, phenytoin, trimethoprim, and fluconazole. Patients must be warned not to use these agents while receiving zidovudine therapy.

Drugs That Decrease Therapeutic Effects. The following agents may induce metabolism and/or excretion of zidovudine, thus reducing therapeutic effects: nelfinavir, ritonavir, stavudine, ribavirin, acetaminophen, doxorubicin, and rifamycin.

Nephrotoxic, Cytotoxic, Hepatotoxic Agents. Use of drugs such as dapsone, pentamidine, amphotericin B, flucytosine, vincristine, vinblastine, adriamycin, or interferon may increase the risk of toxicity.

Hematologic Toxicity. The following agents may induce hematologic toxicity when administered concurrently with zidovudine: ganciclovir, interferon alfa, and interferon beta-1b.

Acyclovir. Acyclovir and zidovudine used concurrently may cause severe drowsiness and lethargy. Ensure patient safety.

DRUG THERAPY FOR URINARY TRACT INFECTIONS

The urinary antiinfective agents, including cinoxacin, methenamine mandelate, nalidixic acid, nitrofurantoin, and norfloxacin, are mainstays in urinary antimicrobial therapy. They are discussed in greater detail in Chapter 42.

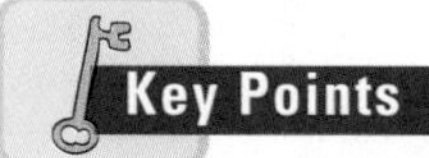

- Antimicrobial agents are chemicals that eliminate living microorganisms that are pathogenic to the patient.
- If at all possible, the infecting organisms should first be isolated and identified. The antimicrobial therapy is then started based on the sensitivity results and the clinical judgment of the health care provider.
- Nurses must consider the entire patient when administering and monitoring antimicrobial therapy.
- It is essential that the nurse be knowledgeable about the drugs, including physiologic parameters for monitoring expected therapeutic activity and for potential adverse effects.
- Beginning nursing students need to focus on the commonality of the premedication assessments and side effects that may occur with the various drugs prescribed for infectious disease. Because of the numerous drug interactions listed within the monographs, it is essential to consult a drug reference before administering a prescribed antimicrobial.
- It is important to teach the individual with an infection basic principles of self-care that will enhance the recovery process and measures to prevent the spread of the infection. In the case of communicable diseases, exposed individuals must be contacted for follow-up testing and appropriate treatment.

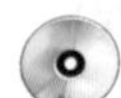

Go to your Companion CD-ROM for Appendices, an Audio Glossary, animations, Drug Dosage Calculators, customizable Patient Self-Assessment forms, and Review Questions for the NCLEX® Examination.

evolve Be sure to visit the companion Evolve site at http://evolve.elsevier.com/Clayton for WebLinks and additional online resources.

MEDICATION SAFETY REVIEW

MATH REVIEW QUESTIONS

1. Order: An antibiotic 50 mg/kg per 24 hours intravenously (IV) in four equally divided doses for an infant 12 weeks old weighing 13 pounds.

   The infant's weight in kg is: ______.

   The amount of antibiotic to be administered in a 24-hour period is _____ mg.

   Each of the four divided doses is _____ mg.

   Available: Antibiotic 100 mg/mL.

   Give _____ mg for each single dose.

2. Order: Amoxicillin 150 mg q8h PO. After establishing that this dose is safe for the weight of the infant, you proceed to prepare it:

   Available: amoxicillin oral suspension 125 mg/5 mL.

   Give ______ mL.

3. Order: An antibiotic oral suspension 320 mg to be administered two times daily

   Available: 400 mg/5 mL

   Give _____ mL.

4. Order: An IV antibiotic for administration over 30 minutes. The volume to be given is 50 mL. The administration set delivers 15 gtt/mL.

   Set the drip rate at _____ gtt/min.

5. Order: Vancomycin 1 g in 150 mL D5W over 1.5 hours.

   Using an infusion pump to deliver this IVPB, set the pump at _____ mL/hr.

CRITICAL THINKING QUESTIONS

1. A 6-month-old infant in the hospital is to have an antibiotic injection before discharge. After calculating the drug dosage, what type of syringe and what size needle would you use to administer the prescribed medication? What site of administration would be best in an infant of this age? Give the rationale. Explain the correct technique for administration, including landmark identification.

2. When providing care to a patient diagnosed 3 months ago with tuberculosis, you suspect nonadherence with the prescribed regimen. How would you proceed to verify this, and what interventions would you attempt?

3. Examine the antimicrobial drug monographs to identify commonality in the premedication assessments for the different classifications of drugs used to treat infectious diseases.

4. Identify assessments needed during the administration of antimicrobial therapy.

5. Drugs within a class of antibiotics often have similar adverse effects. It helps to remember the adverse effects associated with a class of antibiotics rather than having to remember the adverse effects of individual agents. Complete the following table by identifying which adverse effects tend to occur with which classes of antibiotics. The first row has been completed for you.

DRUG CLASS	OTOTOXICITY	HEPATOTOXICITY	NEPHROTOXICITY	NEUROMUSCULAR BLOCKADE	PHOTOSENSITIVITY	SEIZURES	PHLEBITIS	OTHER
Aminoglycosides	Y		Y	Y				Serum levels often required
Carbapenems								
Cephalosporins								
Glycyclines								
Ketolides								
Macrolides								
Penicillins								
Quinolones								
Streptogramins								
Sulfonamides								
Tetracyclines								
Vancomycin								

Continued

CONTENT REVIEW QUESTIONS

1. Probenecid, when given with antibiotics that are excreted in the urine, causes:
   1. photosensitivity.
   2. increased serum levels by blocking urinary excretion of the prescribed antiinfective agent.
   3. increased incidence of nephrotoxicity.
   4. increased incidence of ototoxicity.

2. Ototoxicity is seen with:
   1. systemic antifungals.
   2. quinolones
   3. carbapenems.
   4. aminoglycosides.

3. Cephalosporins, carbapenems, and _____ have the potential for cross-sensitivity.
   1. penicillins
   2. tetracyclines
   3. chloramphenicol
   4. quinolones

4. Photosensitivity may be seen with the administration of quinolones, sulfonamides, and ______.
   1. tetracyclines
   2. aminoglycosides
   3. choramphenicol
   4. cephalosporins

5. Many drugs are known to interact with antimicrobial agents by decreasing the absorption of the prescribed medication. When antacids are prescribed, it is safest to schedule antimicrobial drugs how many hours before or after the antacid?
   1. 1 to 2
   2. 2 to 3
   3. 3 to 4
   4. 4 to 5

6. When looking at drugs within each classification in the various antimicrobial tables throughout the chapter, note that the quinolones all end in "-oxacin" except for:
   1. cephalexin.
   2. neomycin.
   3. nalidixic acid.
   4. piperacillin.

7. Which of the following drugs is an active antiviral agent against HIV-1?
   1. Zerit
   2. Valtrex
   3. Zovirax
   4. Lamisil

8. Which of the following drugs is used to treat parasites such as trichomoniasis caused by *T. vaginalis* in both male and female patients?
   1. Trobicin
   2. Flagyl
   3. Vancocin
   4. Tinidazole

CHAPTER

47 Nutrition

evolve http://evolve.elsevier.com/Clayton

Chapter Content

Objectives

1. Differentiate between information found in the dietary reference intake tables and the Recommended Dietary Allowances table.
2. Identify the function of macronutrients in the body.
3. Compare and contrast the Estimated Energy Requirement for a healthy male and female of similar height, weight, and level of activity.
4. Research good dietary sources of fiber.
5. Identify the exercise guidelines currently recommended for people with different daily patterns of physical activity (sedentary, low active, active, and very active).
6. Differentiate between fat-soluble and water-soluble vitamins.
7. List five functions of minerals in the body.
8. Describe nutritional assessments essential before administration of tube feedings and parenteral nutrition.
9. Describe physical changes associated with a malnourished state.
10. Cite common laboratory and diagnostic tests used to monitor a patient's nutritional status.
11. Discuss nursing assessments and interventions required during the administration of enteral nutrition.
12. Discuss home care needs of a patient being discharged on any form of enteral or parenteral nutrition.

Key Terms

macronutrients
Dietary Reference Intakes (DRIs)
Estimated Average Requirement (EAR)
Recommended Dietary Allowances (RDAs)
Adequate Intake (AI)
Tolerable Upper Intake Level (UL)
kilocalories
Estimated Energy Requirement (EER)
carbohydrates
monosaccharides
disaccharides
polysaccharides
fiber
fats
lipids
essential fatty acids
proteins
gluconeogenesis
vitamins
minerals
water
physical exercise
marasmus
kwashiorkor
mixed kwashiorkor-marasmus
enteral nutrition
tube feedings
parenteral nutrition
peripheral parenteral nutrition (PPN)
total parenteral nutrition (TPN)

"For the two out of three adult Americans who do not smoke and do not drink excessively, one personal choice seems to influence long-term health prospects more than any other: what we eat."

Surgeon General's Report on Nutrition and Health, 1988

PRINCIPLES OF NUTRITION

It is no coincidence that eating is one of life's greatest pleasures. The body needs a regular source of energy to sustain its various functions, including respiration, nerve transmission, circulation, physical work, and maintenance of core temperature. There are many environmental, cultural, and behavioral reasons for what and how we eat, but the most basic is to sustain life. Because the body cannot make most of the needed nutrients, these chemicals must be supplied from external sources. For the most part they are supplied from the food we eat. Other chemicals are supplied by the air we breathe, such as oxygen; by the water we drink; and by sunlight, which helps the body manufacture vitamin D. The energy derived from external sources is converted by the body to chemical energy, which sustains the body's functions. The heat produced during these chemical reactions maintains body temperature. Energy sources required for balanced metabolism are the **macronutrients:** fats, carbohydrates, fiber, and proteins, which are measured in calories (see Macronutrients, p. 807). Other essential nutrients include vitamins, minerals, and water. Imbalances between energy intake (food) and energy expenditure result in gain or loss of body composition, primarily in the form of fat, which determines changes in weight.

Nutritional requirements vary based on level of activity, age of the individual (e.g., infant, preschool child, adolescent, adult, and older adult), and the individual's gender. Among females are differences in nutritional requirements for a pregnant teenager, an adult woman, and a lactating mother. The presence of disease, wound healing, and the degree of catabolism also can influence one's nutritional needs. Therefore the reader should consult a reliable nutritional textbook for up-to-date, detailed information.

No one food source can meet all of our basic nutritional requirements. Foods from a variety of groups are required to provide an optimal nutrient balance and to minimize naturally occurring toxic substances from a single food source. Two federal agencies, the U.S. Food and Drug Administration (FDA) of the Department of Health and Human Services (HHS) and the U.S. Department of Agriculture (USDA), collaborate to publish *Dietary Guidelines for Americans* every 5 years. These are based on research of nutrients within foods, and recommend how to make the best food choices to promote good health. There is controversy, however, about the use of the latest scientific evidence and of selection of committee members who make the final recommendations. There is intense lobbying by the agricultural industry and other special interest groups for committee appointments.

As an educational tool, foods are grouped into the Food Guide Pyramid first published in 1991. The USDA recently retired the old Food Guide Pyramid and replaced it with MyPyramid, a new symbol, and interactive website (www.mypyramid.gov) (Figure 47-1). The

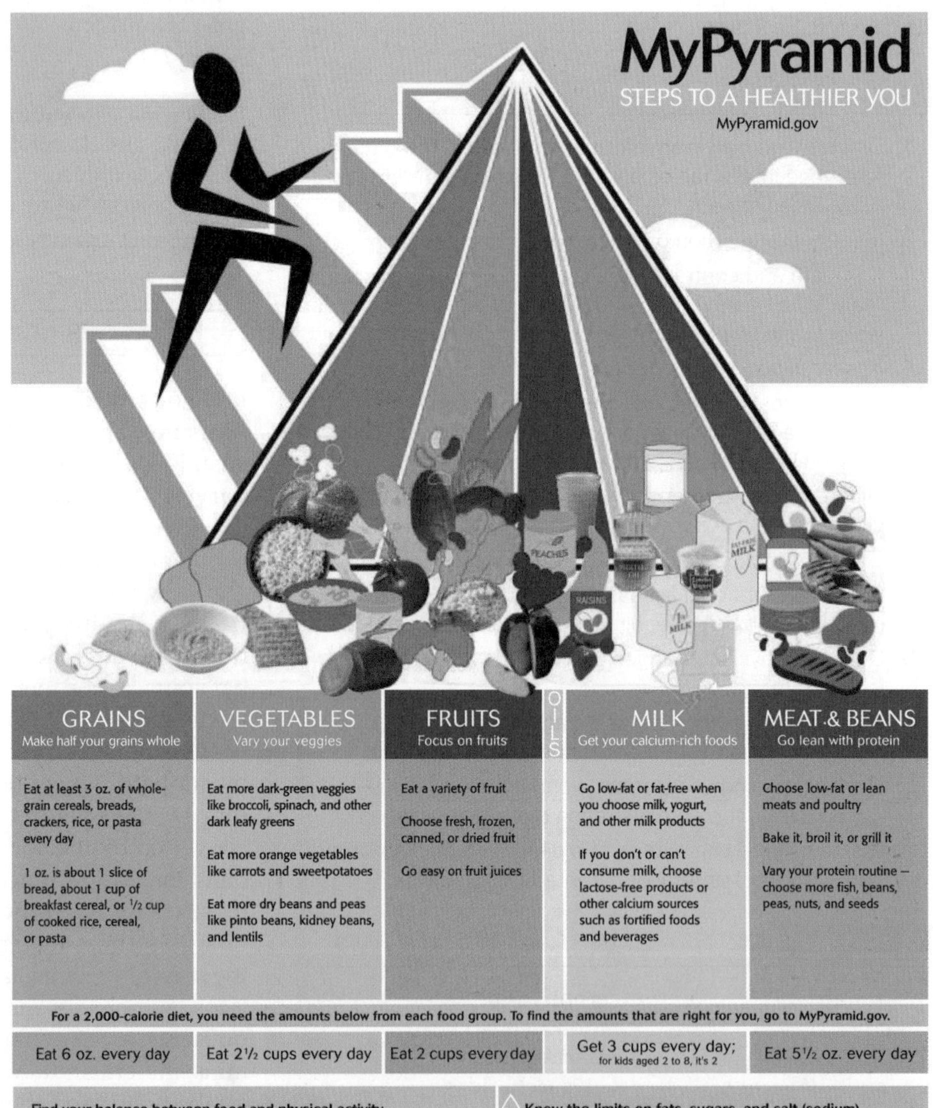

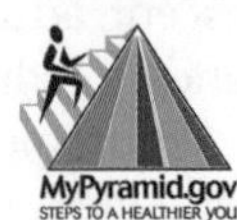

FIGURE 47-1 Sample MyPyramid guideline of a 2000-calorie diet. Individual personalized dietary guidelines can be accessed at MyPyramid.gov. (From U.S. Department of Agriculture, Center for Nutrition Policy and Promotion, April 2005.)

new pyramid is basically the old pyramid turned on its side. The pyramid recommends eating a variety of foods per day to receive the necessary nutrients while consuming an appropriate amount of calories to maintain health and weight. Triangles of color making up the face of the pyramid represent daily servings for food groups: orange for grains, green for vegetables, red for fruits, yellow for oils, blue for milk, and purple for meat and beans. The stairs and human image running up the side of the pyramid serve as a reminder of the importance of physical activity. The new guidelines also emphasize the importance of controlling weight. For consumers who want to track nutritional value of foods eaten each day and physical activity performed, the website provides a detailed comparison to the 2005 Dietary Guidelines, nutrient intake, and energy balance. A history function tracks progress over time, up to 1 year.

With the frequency of obesity, metabolic syndrome, and type 2 diabetes mellitus in the American population reaching epidemic proportions over the past decade, and with recent research findings raising questions of concern, MyPyramid has undergone substantial scrutiny.

- There is a concern that the guidelines overemphasize the intake of carbohydrates such as bread, pasta, cereal, potatoes, and rice, and that the American public is consuming too many refined carbohydrates (i.e., those grains that have been milled [leaving "white flour"] to eliminate the outer bran shell that contains vitamins, minerals, and fiber). The new guidelines encourage the use of whole grains and suggest that people limit sugar intake.
- Another concern in the average American diet is the consumption of *trans* fatty acids (also called hydrogenated fats) and saturated fats that have no known nutritional benefit but increase cholesterol and the frequency of heart disease. The primary sources of *trans* fats are commercially fried foods, stick margarine, processed and ready-to-eat foods, and snack foods. The new guidelines now emphasize that intake of *trans* fats should be as low as possible. (As of January 2006, food labels are required to list *trans* fat content to help consumers become aware of and reduce their intake of *trans* fats.)
- In the previous pyramid, all fats were considered harmful and total fat intake was fairly restricted. Research indicates that monounsaturated and polyunsaturated fats have some health benefits, so the latest guidelines recommend getting between 20% and 35% of daily calories from fats, and recognize the potential health benefits of monounsaturated and polyunsaturated fats. Saturated fats should continue to be limited. Primary sources of saturated fats are red meats, butter, and high-fat dairy products (e.g., whole milk) (Table 47-1 and Figure 47-2).
- The new guidelines recommend drinking three glasses of low-fat milk or eating three servings of other dairy products per day to prevent osteoporosis. Research has not demonstrated that eating dairy products will reduce the incidence of osteoporosis, and consumption of dairy products adds 300 calories daily to the diet. Calcium supplements have been shown to reduce the incidence of osteoporosis and do not add calories to the diet.

Nutrition experts at Harvard University School of Public Health have proposed a new Healthy Eating Pyramid (Figure 47-3) that reflects recent research on an optimal diet. Some highlights of this pyramid are as follows:

- Daily activity and weight control serve as the foundation for the pyramid.
- Whole grain foods, fruits, and vegetables (sources of fiber, vitamins, and minerals) are emphasized.
- Vegetable oils and nuts (sources of unsaturated fats) and legumes have greater emphasis as a source of protein, fiber, vitamins, and minerals. Good sources of healthy unsaturated fats include olive, canola, soy, corn, sunflower, and peanut oils.
- Red meat should be consumed sparingly because of saturated fat content. Switching to fish or chicken several times a week can improve cholesterol levels.
- Food sources high in refined carbohydrates (e.g., white rice, white bread, potatoes, pasta, sweets) should be consumed only sparingly. They can cause rapid increases in blood sugar that can lead to weight gain, diabetes, and heart disease. Whole-grain carbohydrates cause slower, steadier

Table 47-1 ***Dietary Fat Sources***

MONOUNSATURATED FATS	POLYUNSATURATED FATS	SATURATED FATS	*TRANS* FATS
Olives	Corn oil	Whole milk	Stick margarines
Olive oil	Soybean oil	Cheese	Vegetable shortening
Canola oil	Safflower oil	Ice cream	Deep-fried chips
Peanut oil	Cottonseed oil	Red meat	French fries
Cashews	Fish	Chocolate	Many fast foods
Peanuts		Coconuts	Most commercial baked goods
Avocados		Coconut oil	

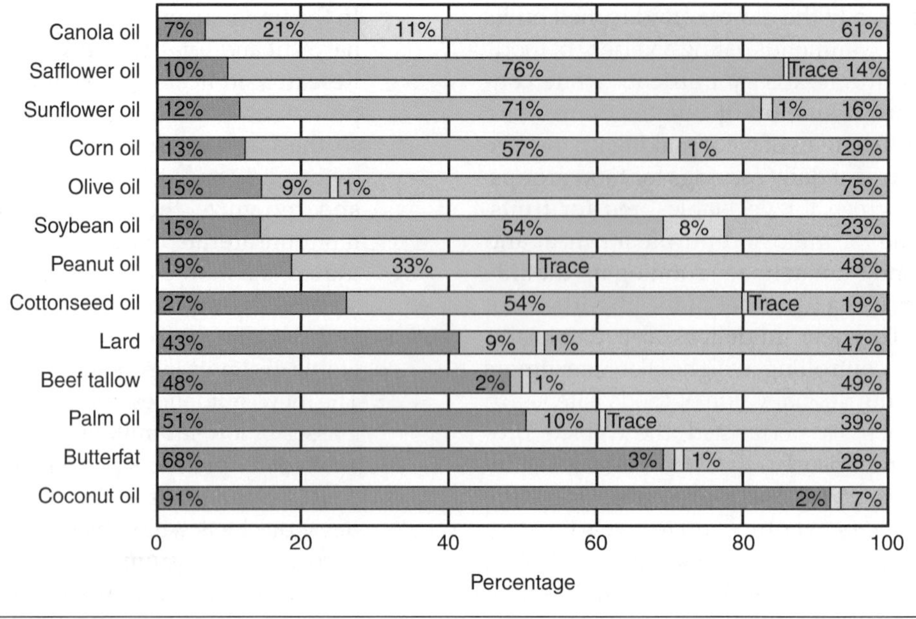

FIGURE **47-2** All plant oils used in food preparation contain saturated, monounsaturated, and polyunsaturated fatty acids. It is recommended that we minimize the use of those oils higher in saturated fatty acids. (From Brown KM, Thomas DQ, Kotecki JE: *Physical activity and health: an interactive approach,* Sudbury, Mass, 2002, Jones and Bartlett. Reprinted with permission.)

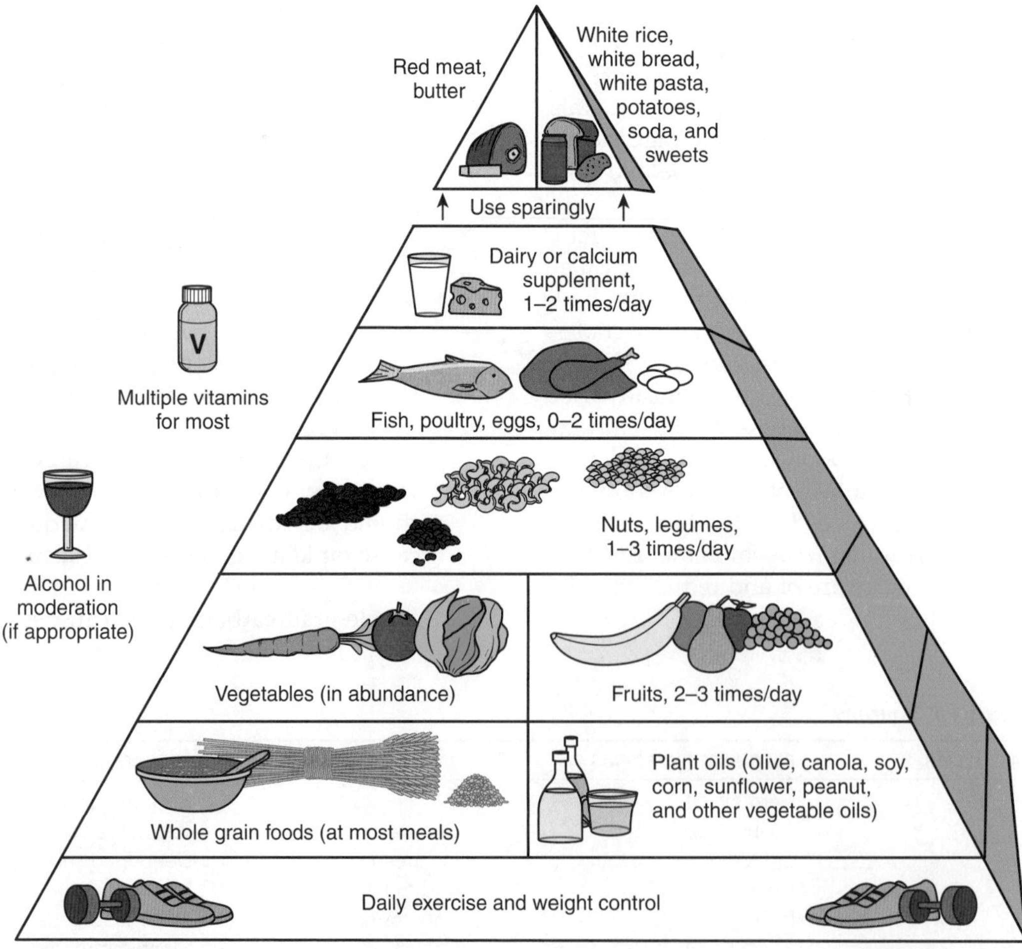

FIGURE **47-3** An alternative Food Guide Pyramid based on the latest research on optimal nutrition. (Redrawn from Willett WC: Eat, drink, and be healthy. Copyright © 2001, 2005 by the President and Fellows of Harvard College. Reprinted by permission of Free Press/Simon & Schuster, Inc.)

increases in blood sugar that don't overwhelm the body's ability to metabolize sugars.

- Dairy products are de-emphasized and placed in their own category (it is felt that dairy products being consumed as a calcium source could be replaced with a calcium supplement to avoid unneeded calories and saturated fats).
- A daily multiple vitamin is recommended for most people.
- Moderate daily alcohol may be a healthy option unless contraindicated for specific people. A good balance for men is one or two drinks daily. Women should limit alcohol to no more than one drink per day.

Another excellent source of healthy nutritional information is Oldways (www.oldwayspt.org), a nutritional foods think tank. Oldways develops education programs to help consumers make informed choices about eating, drinking, and lifestyle. Their principles are grounded in a combination of science, strong social conscience, and culinary excellence. Oldways promotes Asian, Latin, Mediterranean, and vegetarian evidence-based food pyramids for healthy eating.

DIETARY REFERENCE INTAKES

The National Academy of Sciences is collecting data and publishing a series of tables known as **Dietary Reference Intakes (DRIs)** that provide quantitative estimates of nutrient intakes for planning and assessing diets for healthy people. The DRIs are actually a set of four reference values: Estimated Average Requirement (EAR), Recommended Dietary Allowances (RDAs), Adequate Intake (AI), and Tolerable Upper Intake Level (UL) that have replaced the 1989 RDAs. Dietary intakes for the macronutrients are shown in Table 47-2 and some of the vitamins, minerals, and trace elements are shown in Table 47-3.

The **Estimated Average Requirement (EAR)** is a nutrient intake value that is estimated to meet the requirement of half of the healthy individuals in a group. The most well-known component of the DRIs is the **Recommended Dietary Allowances (RDAs)** table. It lists the average daily dietary intake level that is sufficient to meet the nutrient requirements of nearly all (97%-98%) of healthy individuals in a group. (Groups are based on gender, age, and, if applicable, pregnancy or lactation.) Recommended daily allowances are goals in meeting nutritional needs. RDAs do not meet the nutritional needs of ill patients and do not account for nutritional value that may be lost in cooking.

The RDA is based on the EAR plus twice the standard deviation:

$$RDA = EAR + 2SD$$

The RDA for a nutrient is a value to be used as a goal for dietary intake by healthy individuals. There is no established benefit for healthy individuals if they consume nutrient intakes greater than the RDA or AI.

Adequate Intake (AI) is a value based on observed or experimentally determined approximations of nutrient intake by a group of healthy people. The AI is used when the RDA cannot be determined.

Another category in the DRI tables is the **Tolerable Upper Intake Level (UL).** This level is defined as the highest level of daily nutrient intake that is likely to pose no risk of adverse health effects to almost all individuals in the general population. As intake increases above the UL, the risk of adverse effects increases. The UL is not intended to be a recommended level of intake. For many nutrients there are insufficient data on which to develop a UL. This does not mean that there is no potential for adverse effects resulting from high intake. Over time these data will help establish the value of megadoses of vitamins and nutrients and whether there are therapeutic and toxic effects to ingestion of large doses of these chemicals.

Macronutrients

The metabolism of the macronutrients, carbohydrates, fiber, fats, and proteins provides energy for the body to maintain life (respiration, circulation, physical work, nerve transmission, core body temperature) and to repair damage induced by illness or injury. Energy is measured in **kilocalories** (kcal). The heat generated during these processes is reflected as body temperature. Energy balance in an individual depends on dietary energy intake and energy expenditure. An excess of energy (food) intake over that which is burned results in weight gain. Body weight is lost through burning more kilocalories than are consumed. A pound of body weight is approximately 3500 kilocalories.

The **Estimated Energy Requirement (EER)** is defined as the average dietary energy intake that is predicted to maintain energy balance in a healthy adult of a defined age, gender, weight, height, and level of physical activity consistent with good health (see Table 47-4).

The National Academy of Sciences published the *Dietary Reference Intakes for Energy, Carbohydrate, Fiber, Fat, Fatty Acids, Cholesterol, Protein and Amino Acids* in 2005. This report on macronutrients was sponsored for both the United States and Canada through several governmental agencies including Health Canada, the Department of Health and Human Services, FDA, National Institutes of Health, Centers for Disease Control and Prevention, the Department of Agriculture, and private sources. These guidelines are based on research of nutrients within foods and how the body uses energy from foods. The report recommends that to meet the body's energy and nutritional needs while minimizing risk for chronic disease, adults should get 45% to 65% of their calories from carbohydrates, 20% to 35% from fat, and 10% to 35% from protein.

Carbohydrates, often referred to as "sugars" because many of them taste sweet, are the major source of energy for body activities and metabolism. They

Text continued on p. 813

Table 47-2 ***Dietary Reference Intakes: Macronutrients***

NUTRIENT	FUNCTION	GROUP	RDA/AI* g/d	AMDR†	SELECTED FOOD SOURCES	ADVERSE EFFECTS OF EXCESSIVE CONSUMPTION
Carbohydrate: total digestible	RDA based on its role as the primary energy source for the brain; AMDR based on its role as a source of kilocalories to maintain body weight	*Infants*			Starch and sugar are the major types of carbohydrates. Grains and vegetables (e.g., corn, pasta, rice, potatoes, breads) are sources of starch. Natural sugars are found in fruits and juices. Sources of added sugars are soft drinks, candy, fruit drinks, and desserts.	Although no defined intake level at which potential adverse effects of total digestible carbohydrate was identified, the upper end of the adequate macronutrient distribution range (AMDR) was based on decreasing risk of chronic disease and providing adequate intake of other nutrients. It is suggested that the maximal intake of added sugars be limited to providing no more than 25% of energy.
		0–6 mo	60*	ND‡		
		7–12 mo	95*	ND		
		Children				
		1–3 yr	**130**	45–65		
		4–8 yr	**130**	45–65		
		Men	**130**	45–65		
		Women	**130**	45–65		
		Pregnancy	**175**	45–65		
		Lactation	**210**	45–65		
Total fiber	Improves laxation, reduces risk of coronary heart disease, assists in maintaining normal blood glucose levels	*Infants*			Includes dietary fiber naturally present in grains (e.g., oats, wheat, or unmilled rice) and functional fiber synthesized or isolated from plants or animals and shown to be of benefit to health.	Dietary fiber can have variable compositions and therefore it is difficult to link a specific source of fiber with a particular adverse effect, especially when phytate is also present in the natural fiber source. It is concluded that as part of an overall healthy diet, a high intake of dietary fiber will not produce deleterious effects in healthy individuals. Although occasional adverse gastrointestinal symptoms are observed when consuming some isolated or synthetic fibers, serious chronic adverse effects have not been observed. Because of the bulky nature of fibers, excess consumption is likely to be self-limiting. Therefore, an upper limit was not set for individual functional fibers.
		0–6 mo	ND			
		7–12 mo	ND			
		Children				
		1–3 yr	19*			
		4–8 yr	25*			
		Men				
		9–13 yr	31*			
		14–50 yr	38*			
		50–70 yr	30*			
		>70 yr	30*			
		Women				
		9–18 yr	26*			
		19–50 yr	25*			
		>50 yr	21*			
		Pregnancy				
		≤18–50 yr	28*			
		Lactation				
		≤18–50 yr	29*			

From *Dietary Reference Intakes for Energy, Carbohydrate, Fiber, Fat, Fatty Acids, Cholesterol, Protein, and Amino Acids (2002)*. This report may be accessed via www.nap.edu

NOTE: The table is adapted from the DRI reports, see www.nap.edu. It represents recommended dietary allowances (RDAs) in **bold type,** adequate intakes (AIs) in ordinary type followed by an asterisk (*). RDAs and AIs may both be used as goals for individual intake. RDAs are set to meet the needs of almost all (97% to 98%) individuals in a group. For healthy breastfed infants, the AI is the mean intake. The AI for other life stage and gender groups is believed to cover the needs of all individuals in the group, but lack of data prevent being able to specify with confidence the percentage of individuals covered by this intake.

†Acceptable Macronutrient Distribution Range (AMDR) is the range of intake for a particular energy source that is associated with reduced risk of chronic disease while providing intakes of essential nutrients. If an individual consumes in excess of the AMDR, there is a potential of increasing the risk of chronic diseases and/or insufficient intake of essential nutrients.

‡ND = Not determinable because of lack of data of adverse effects in this age group and concern with regard to lack of ability to handle excess amounts. Source of intake should be from food only to prevent high levels of intake.

Table 47-2 Dietary Reference Intakes: Macronutrients—cont'd

NUTRIENT	FUNCTION	GROUP	RDA/AI* g/d	AMDR†	SELECTED FOOD SOURCES	ADVERSE EFFECTS OF EXCESSIVE CONSUMPTION
Total fat	Energy source and when found in foods, is a source of *n*-6 and *n*-3 polyunsaturated fatty acids; its presence in the diet increases absorption of fat soluble vitamins and precursors such as vitamin A and pro-vitamin A carotenoids	*Infants*			Butter, margarine, vegetable oils, whole milk, visible fat on meat and poultry products, invisible fat in fish, shellfish, some plant products such as seeds and nuts, and bakery products.	Although no defined intake level at which potential adverse effects of total fat was identified, the upper end of AMDR is based on decreasing risk of chronic disease and providing adequate intake of other nutrients. The lower end of the AMDR is based on concerns related to the increase in plasma triacylglycerol concentrations and decreased HDL cholesterol concentrations seen with very low-fat (and thus high-carbohydrate) diets.
		0–6 mo	31*			
		7–12 mo	30*			
		Children				
		1–3 yr		30–40		
		4–8 yr		25–35		
		Men		25–35		
		Women		25–35		
		Pregnancy				
		≤18–50 yr		20–35		
		Lactation				
		≤18–50 yr		20–35		
n-6 Polyunsaturated fatty acids (linoleic acid)	Essential component of structural membrane lipids, involved with cell signaling, and precursor of eicosanoids; required for normal skin function	*Infants*			Nuts, seeds, and vegetable oils such as soybean, safflower, and corn oil.	Although no defined intake level at which potential adverse effects of *n*-6 polyunsaturated fatty acids was identified, the upper end of the AMDR is based on the lack of evidence that demonstrates long-term safety and human in vitro studies which show increased free-radical formation and lipid peroxidation with higher amounts of *n*-6 fatty acids. Lipid peroxidation is thought to be a component of the development of atherosclerotic plaques.
		0–6 mo	4.4*	ND‡		
		7–12 mo	4.6*	ND		
		Children				
		1–3 yr	7*	5–10		
		4–8 yr	10*	5–10		
		Men				
		9–13 yr	12*	5–10		
		14–18 yr	16*	5–10		
		19–30 yr	17*	5–10		
		31–50 yr	17*	5–10		
		50–70 yr	14*	5–10		
		>70 yr	14*	5–10		
		Women				
		9–13 yr	10*	5–10		
		14–18 yr	11*	5–10		
		19–30 yr	17*	5–10		
		31–50 yr	17*	5–10		
		50–70 yr	14*	5–10		
		>70 yr	14*	5–10		
		Pregnancy				
		≤18–50 yr	13*	5–10		
		Lactation				
		≤18–50 yr	13*	5–10		

Continued

Table 47-2 Dietary Reference Intakes: Macronutrients—cont'd

NUTRIENT	FUNCTION	GROUP	RDA/AI* g/d	AMDR†	SELECTED FOOD SOURCES	ADVERSE EFFECTS OF EXCESSIVE CONSUMPTION
n-3 Polyunsaturated fatty acids (alpha-linolenic acid)	Involved with neurologic development and growth; precursor of eicosanoids	*Infants*			Vegetable oils such as soybean, canola, and flax seed oil, fish oils, fatty fish, with smaller amounts in meats and eggs.	Although no defined intake level at which potential adverse effects of *n*-3 polyunsaturated fatty acids was identified, the upper end of AMDR is based on maintaining the appropriate balance with *n*-6 fatty acids and on the lack of evidence that demonstrates long-term safety, along with human in vitro studies which show increased free-radical formation and lipid peroxidation with higher amounts of polyunsaturated fatty acids. Lipid peroxidation is thought to be a component in the development of atherosclerotic plaques.
		0–6 mo	0.5*	ND‡		
		7–12 mo	0.5*	ND		
		Children				
		1–3 yr	0.7*	0.6–1.2		
		4–8 yr	0.9*	0.6–1.2		
		Men				
		9–13 yr	1.2*	0.6–1.2		
		14–>70 yr	1.6*	0.6–1.2		
		Women				
		9–>70 yr	1.1*	0.6–1.2		
		Pregnancy				
		≤18–50 yr	1.4*	0.6–1.2		
		Lactation				
		≤18–50 yr	1.3*	0.6–1.2		
Saturated and *trans* fatty acids, and cholesterol	No required role for these nutrients other than as energy sources was identified; the body can synthesize its needs for saturated fatty acids and cholesterol from other sources	*Infants* *Children* *Men* *Women* *Pregnancy* *Lactation*	ND		Saturated fatty acids are present in animal fats (meat fats and butter fat), and coconut and palm kernel oils. Sources of cholesterol include liver, eggs, and foods that contain eggs such as cheesecake and custard pies. Sources of *trans* fatty acids include stick margarines and foods containing hydrogenated or partially-hydrogenated vegetable shortenings.	There is an incremental increase in plasma total and low-density lipoprotein cholesterol concentrations with increased intake of saturated or *trans* fatty acids or with cholesterol at even very low levels in the diet. Therefore, the intakes of each should be minimized while consuming a nutritionally adequate diet.

Table 47-2 ***Dietary Reference Intakes: Macronutrients—cont'd***

NUTRIENT	FUNCTION	GROUP	RDA/AI* g/d	AMDR†	SELECTED FOOD SOURCES	ADVERSE EFFECTS OF EXCESSIVE CONSUMPTION
Protein and amino acids	Serves as the major structural component of all cells in the body, and functions as enzymes, in membranes, as transport carriers, and as some hormones. During digestion and absorption dietary proteins are broken down to amino acids, which become the building blocks of these structural and functional compounds. Nine of the amino acids must be provided in the diet; these are termed indispensable amino acids. The body can make the other amino acids needed to synthesize specific structures from other amino acids	*Infants*			Proteins from animal sources, such as meat, poultry, fish, eggs, milk, cheese, and yogurt, provide all nine indispensable amino acids in adequate amounts, and for this reason are considered "complete proteins." Proteins from plants, legumes, grains, nuts, seeds, and vegetables tend to be deficient in one or more of the indispensable amino acids and are called "incomplete proteins." Vegan diets adequate in total protein content can be "complete" by combining sources of incomplete proteins which lack different indispensable amino acids.	Although no defined intake level at which potential adverse effects of protein was identified, the upper end of AMDR is based on complementing the AMDR for carbohydrate and fat for the various age groups. The lower end of the AMDR is set at approximately the RDA.
		0–6 mo	9.1*	ND‡		
		7–12 mo	**11.0**	ND		
		Children				
		1–3 yr	**13**	5–20		
		4–8 yr	**19**	10–30		
		Men				
		9–13 yr	**34**	10–30		
		14–18 yr	**52**	10–30		
		19–>70 yr	**56**	10–35		
		Women				
		9–13 yr	**34**	10–30		
		14–>70 yr	**46**	10–30		
		Pregnancy				
		≤18–50 yr	**71**	10–35		
		Lactation				
		≤18–50 yr	**71**	10–35		

NUTRIENT	FUNCTION	IOM/FNB 2002 SCORING PATTERN*	mg/g PROTEIN	ADVERSE EFFECTS OF EXCESSIVE CONSUMPTION
INDISPENSABLE AMINO ACIDS				
Histidine	The building blocks of all proteins in the body and some hormones. These nine amino acids must be provided in the diet and thus are termed indispensable amino acids. The body can make the other amino acids needed to synthesize specific structures from other amino acids and carbohydrate precursors.	Histidine	18	Since there is no evidence that amino acids found in usual or even high intakes of protein from food present any risk, attention was focused on intakes of the L-form of these and other amino acid found in dietary protein and amino acid supplements. Even from well-studied amino acids, adequate dose-response data from human or animal studies on which to base an upper limit were not available. Although no defined intake level at which potential adverse effects of protein was identified for any amino acid, this does not mean that there is no potential for adverse effects resulting from high intakes of amino acids from dietary supplements. Since data on the adverse effects of high levels of amino acid intakes from dietary supplements are limited, caution may be warranted.
Isoleucine		Isoleucine	25	
Lysine		Lysine	55	
Leucine		Leucine	51	
Methionine and cysteine		Methionine and cysteine	25	
Phenylalanine and tyrosine		Phenylalanine and tyrosine	47	
Threonine		Threonine	27	
Tryptophan		Tryptophan	7	
Valine		Valine	32	

Table 47-3 ***Dietary Reference Intakes (DRIs)***

FOOD AND NUTRITION BOARD, INSTITUTE OF MEDICINE-NATIONAL ACADEMY OF SCIENCES
DIETARY REFERENCE INTAKES: RECOMMENDED LEVELS FOR INDIVIDUAL INTAKE[a]

LIFE-STAGE GROUP	CALCIUM (mg/d)	PHOSPHORUS (mg/d)	MAGNESIUM (mg/d)	VITAMIN D[bc] (mcg/d)	FLUORIDE (mg/d)	THIAMINE (mg/d)	RIBOFLAVIN (mg/d)	NIACIN[d] (mg/d)	VITAMIN B_6 (mg/d)	FOLATE[e] (mcg/d)	VITAMIN B_{12} (mcg/d)	PANTOTHENIC ACID (mg/d)	BIOTIN (mcg/d)	CHOLINE[f] (mg/d)
INFANTS														
0-6 mo	210*	100*	30*	5*	0.01*	0.2*	0.3*	2*	0.1*	65*	0.4*	1.7*	5*	125*
7-12 mo	270*	275*	75*	5*	0.5*	0.3*	0.4*	4*	0.3*	80*	0.5*	1.8*	6*	150*
CHILDREN														
1-3 yr	500*	460	80	5*	0.7*	0.5	0.5	6	0.5	150	0.9	2*	8*	200*
4-8 yr	800*	500	130	5*	1*	0.6	0.6	8	0.6	200	1.2	3*	12*	250*
MALES														
9-13 yr	1300*	1250	240	5*	2*	0.9	0.9	12	1.0	300	1.8	4*	20*	375*
14-18 yr	1300*	1250	410	5*	3*	1.2	1.3	16	1.3	400	2.4	5*	25*	550*
19-30 yr	1000*	700	400	5*	4*	1.2	1.3	16	1.3	400	2.4	5*	30*	550*
31-50 yr	1000*	700	420	5*	4*	1.2	1.3	16	1.3	400	2.4	5*	30*	550*
51-70 yr	1200*	700	420	10*	4*	1.2	1.3	16	1.7	400	2.4[g]	5*	30*	550*
>70 yr	1200*	700	420	15*	4*	1.2	1.3	16	1.7	400	2.4[g]	5*	30*	550*
FEMALES														
9-13 yr	1300*	1250	240	5*	2*	0.9	0.9	12	1.0	300	1.8	4*	20*	375*
14-18 yr	1300*	1250	360	5*	3*	1.0	1.0	14	1.2	400[h]	2.4	5*	25*	400*
19-30 yr	1000*	700	310	5*	3*	1.1	1.1	14	1.3	400[h]	2.4	5*	30*	425*
31-50 yr	1000*	700	320	5*	3*	1.1	1.1	14	1.3	400[h]	2.4	5*	30*	425*
51-70 yr	1200*	700	320	10*	3*	1.1	1.1	14	1.5	400	2.4[g]	5*	30*	425*
>70 yr	1200*	700	320	15*	3*	1.1	1.1	14	1.5	400	2.4[g]	5*	30*	425*
PREGNANCY														
<18 yr	1300*	1250	400	5*	3*	1.4	1.4	18	1.9	600[i]	2.6	6*	30*	450*
19-30 yr	1000*	700	350	5*	3*	1.4	1.4	18	1.9	600[i]	2.6	6*	30*	450*
31-50 yr	1000*	700	360	5*	3*	1.4	1.4	18	1.9	600[i]	2.6	6*	30*	450*
LACTATION														
<18 yr	1300*	1250	360	5*	3*	1.5	1.6	17	2.0	500	2.8	7*	35*	550*
19-30 yr	1000*	700	310	5*	3*	1.5	1.6	17	2.0	500	2.8	7*	35*	550*
31-50 yr	1000*	700	320	5*	3*	1.5	1.6	17	2.0	500	2.8	7*	35*	550*

From the Food and Nutrition Board-National Academy of Sciences, 1998.

[a]Recommended Dietary Allowances (RDAs) are presented in bold type and Adequate Intakes (AIs) in ordinary type followed by an asterisk (*). RDAs and AIs may both be used as goals for individual intake. RDAs are set to meet the needs of almost all (97% to 98%) individuals in a group. For healthy breast-fed infants, the AI is the mean intake. The AI for other life-stage and gender groups is believed to cover needs of all individuals in the group, but lack of data or uncertainty in the data prevent being able to specify with confidence the percentage of persons covered by this intake. Source: The Natural Academy of Sciences, Copyright 1998.

[b]As cholecalciferol. 1 mcg cholecalciferol = 40 IU vitamin D.

[c]In the absence of adequate esposure to sunlight.

[d]As niacin equivalents (NE). 1 mg niacin = 60 mg tryptophan; 0 to 6 mo = preformed niacin (not NE).

[e]As dietary folate equivalent (DFE). 1 DFE = 1 mcg food folate = 0.6 mcg folic acid (from fortified food or supplement) consumed with food = 0.5 mcg synthetic (supplemental) folic acid taken on an empty stomach.

[f]Although AIs have been set for choline, there are few data to assess whether a dietary supply of choline is needed at all stages of the life cycle, and it may be that the choline requirement can be met by endogenous synthesis at some of these stages.

[g]Because 10% to 30% of older people may malabsorb food-bound vitamin B_{12}, it is advisable for those older than 50 years to meet their RDA mainly by consuming foods fortified with vitamin B_{12} or a supplement containing vitamin B_{12}.

[h]In view of evidence linking folate intake with neural tube defects in the fetus, it is recommended that all women capable of becoming pregnant consume 400 mcg synthetic folic acid from fortified foods and/or supplements in addition to intake of food folate from a varied diet.

[i]It is assumed that women will continue consuming 400 mcg folic acid until their pregnancy is confirmed and they enter prenatal care, which ordinarily occurs after the end of the periconceptional period—the critical time for formation of the neural tube.

Table 47-4 *Calculation of Estimated Energy Requirements (EER)*

MEN AGES 19 YEARS AND OLDER:
EER = 662 − (9.53 × age [y]) + PA × (15.91 × weight [kg] + 539.6 × height [m])

WOMEN AGES 19 YEARS AND OLDER:
EER = 354 − (6.91 × age [y]) + PA × (9.36 × weight [kg] + 726 × height [m])

LIFESTYLE	MEN	WOMEN
Sedentary	1.00	1.00
Low active	1.11	1.12
Active	1.25	1.27
Very active	1.48	1.45

PA, Physical activity coefficient.
Source: Dietary Reference Intakes for Energy, Carbohydrate, Fiber, Fat, Fatty Acids, Cholesterol, Protein, and Amino Acids/Panel on Macronutrients, Panel on the Definition of Dietary Fiber, Subcommittee on Upper Reference Levels of Nutrients, Subcommittee on Interpretation and Uses of Dietary Reference Intakes, and the Standing Committee on the Scientific Evaluation of Dietary Reference Intakes, Food and Nutrition Board, Institute of Medicine of the National Academies. Washington DC, National Academies Press, 2005, p. 185. Accessed from http://fermat.nap.edu/books/0309085373/html/185.html.

occur in nature as simple and complex molecules and are water soluble. The simple carbohydrates are also known as monosaccharides and disaccharides. **Monosaccharides** such as glucose (also known as dextrose), fructose, and galactose are the only sugars that can be absorbed directly from the gastrointestinal (GI) tract into the blood. They are the most rapidly available sources of energy and are the only sugars capable of being used directly to produce energy for the body. **Disaccharides** such as sucrose (common table sugar), maltose, and lactose are the most common sugars in foods, but must be metabolized to monosaccharides before being absorbed into the bloodstream. For example, a molecule of lactose is metabolized by the enzyme lactase into a molecule each of glucose and galactose, which are then absorbed through the gut wall into the blood. Complex carbohydrates such as starch, dextrin, and fiber, are also known as **polysaccharides.** Complex carbohydrates must also be metabolized into simple sugars in the intestine before being absorbed. The carbohydrates provide about 4 kcal of energy per gram. Daily caloric needs from carbohydrates range from 3 to 5.5 g/kg/day, depending on energy requirements for daily living, stress, and wound healing. Fruits, grains, and vegetables are excellent sources of carbohydrates. Candies and carbonated beverages are very commonly used sources of calories, but contain no other nutrients. End products of carbohydrate metabolism are carbon dioxide, excreted primarily through the lungs, and water.

A by-product of some complex carbohydrate metabolism is **fiber.** Until recently, fiber was thought to be only a by-product of carbohydrate metabolism that needed to be eliminated from the body. It is now recognized as a macronutrient, a separate factor necessary for complete nutrition and wellness. *Dietary fiber* is derived from plant sources and consists of undigestible carbohydrates and lignin and digestible macronutrients (carbohydrates, proteins) such as cereal brans, sweet potatoes, and legumes that contribute to overall nutrition. Another category of fiber is *functional fiber,* which consists of undigestible carbohydrates that have a beneficial physiologic effect on humans. An excellent example of a functional fiber is psyllium, an undigestible fiber that adds bulk to fecal content, which helps timely passage of fecal contents in the GI tract, preventing constipation. Functional fiber content may delay gastric emptying, giving a sense of fullness, which may contribute to weight control. Delayed gastric emptying may also reduce postprandial blood glucose concentrations, potentially preventing excessive insulin secretion and insulin sensitivity. Fibers can reduce the absorption of dietary fat and cholesterol as well as enterohepatic recirculation of cholesterol and bile acids, which may also reduce blood cholesterol concentrations. *Total fiber* is the sum of dietary fiber and functional fiber.

Fats, also known as **lipids,** serve as the body's major form of stored energy and are key components of membranes, prostaglandins, and many hormones. They are not water soluble. Examples of lipids are cholesterol, fatty acids, triglycerides, and phospholipids. Excess dietary carbohydrates and proteins are converted to fat for storage. When used as an energy source, fats generate 9 kcal of energy per gram. Fat intake usually constitutes 25% to 40% of total caloric intake, although the DRIs recommend limits of 20% to 35% from fat. Healthy adults require 1 to 1.5 g/kg/day. Even when patients severely restrict intake for dieting purposes, 4% to 10% of total calories must be supplied in the form of fats to prevent essential fatty acid deficiency.

Essential fatty acids (EFAs) are not produced by the body and must be obtained from dietary sources. The most prominent EFAs are omega-3 and omega-6 fatty acids. They are polyunsaturated fatty acids also known as alpha-linolenic and linoleic acid, respectively. Both fatty acids are required for eicosanoid and prostaglandin production and cell membrane structure.

Dietary fats can be subdivided into four categories: monounsaturated, polyunsaturated, saturated, and *trans* fats (see Table 47-1 for sources of dietary fats). Monounsaturated fats decrease low-density lipoproteins (LDLs) and increase high-density lipoproteins (HDLs) and are considered to be cardioprotective. Polyunsaturated fats also lower LDL and raise HDL. Saturated fats raise both LDL and HDL and are thought to increase atherosclerotic plaque formation in the arteries. Only recently has it been recognized that *trans* fats may induce more heart disease than saturated fats because, in addition to raising LDL cholesterol, *trans* fats *decrease* HDL cholesterol and increase triglycerides as well as another undesirable blood fat, lipoprotein (a). Saturated fats and *trans* fats have no known beneficial nutritional effect and should be eliminated as much as possible from the diet. Note in Figure 47-2 how all plant oils used in food preparation contain saturated, monounsaturated, and polyunsaturated fatty acids. It is recommended that we minimize the use of those oils higher in saturated fatty acids. (See also Chapter 22, p. 352 for further discussion of lipoproteins and cholesterol.) End products of fat metabolism are water and carbon dioxide and insoluble substances excreted in sweat, bile, and feces.

Proteins are complex molecules composed of amino acid chains. Amino acids can be subclassified as essential and nonessential. The essential amino acids must be provided from external sources to sustain life; nonessential amino acids can be synthesized to meet metabolic requirements. Before absorption, proteins must be metabolized in the gut to the individual amino acids. Once absorbed, the amino acids are used to build new proteins, such as muscle and other vital tissues, or are used as an energy source if other energy sources are depleted. Amino acids generate 4 kcal of energy per gram, similar to carbohydrates. Sources of highest protein value are dairy products (e.g., milk, eggs, cheese), fish, and meat. Grains and beans have less protein value. End products of amino acid metabolism are nitrogenous products such as urea, uric acid and ammonium, carbon dioxide, and water. Protein requirements for healthy people are 0.5 to 1 g/kg/day. Depending on the amount of stress the patient is undergoing and the amount of tissue building and wound healing required, protein requirements may range from 1.5 to 2.5 g/kg/day. Calories from proteins generally constitute 12% to 20% of total calorie intake, but the Academy of Sciences recommends 10% to 35% for healthy nutrition.

It is crucial that calorie intake be balanced among carbohydrates, proteins, and fats. If there is an inadequate amount of carbohydrates to provide energy to break down the proteins and carbohydrates, the body will actually metabolize body proteins and fats through a process called **gluconeogenesis** to provide glucose energy to use the incoming proteins and fats. Even though patients are receiving adequate total calories, they may actually develop a protein-wasting condition.

Vitamins

Vitamins, whose name originally derived from the term "vital amines," are a specific set of chemical molecules that regulate human metabolism necessary to maintain health. To be classified as a vitamin, a chemical must be ingested because the human body does not make sufficient quantities to maintain health, and the lack of a vitamin in the diet produces a specific vitamin deficiency disease (e.g., beriberi is a thiamine deficiency; scurvy is an ascorbic acid deficiency). To date, 13 compounds have been identified as vitamins, 9 of which are classified as water soluble, and four as fat soluble (Table 47-5). Vitamins were originally named according to letters of the alphabet, but as a result of the diversity of actions of different vitamins, they are commonly referred to by their generic names (e.g., phytonadione is vitamin K, thiamine is vitamin B_1).

Minerals

Minerals (Table 47-6) are inorganic chemicals found in nature. Minerals are essential to life, serving as components of enzymes, hormones, and bone and tooth structure. They help regulate acid-base and water balance, osmotic pressure and cell membrane permeability, nerve conduction, muscle contractility, metabolism of nutrients in foods, oxygen transport, and blood clotting, to name a few.

Water

Water is another nutrient essential for life. As noted in Table 3-1 (p. 27), water accounts for 60% to 83% of total body weight and plays a crucial role in transport of nutrients, temperature regulation, and metabolic reactions. Normal water losses occur through urination, perspiration, defecation, and vaporization through the lungs. Normal daily intake is highly variable, depending on climate, activity level, and presence of a fever,

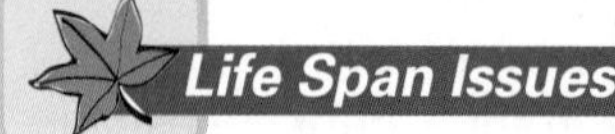

Life Span Issues

Food for Thought

Because a pound of stored fat represents about 3500 excess kilocalories:

- An average excess of only 10 kcal per day in energy intake over energy expenditure can result in about a 1-pound weight gain in 1 year (10 kcal/day × 365 days = 3650 kcal).
- Cutting back on only 100 kcal per day (e.g., 1 soft drink) results in approximately a 10-pound weight loss in 1 year (100 kcal/day × 365 days = 36,500 kcal), or an extra 100 kcal per day will result in a 10-pound gain!

For weight gain: add 500 calories per day to gain approximately 1 pound per week.

For weight loss: subtract 500 calories per day for a loss of approximately 1 pound per week.

Table 47-5 ***Vitamins***

FAT-SOLUBLE VITAMINS	ACTIONS	SOURCES
Vitamin A (Retinol)	Essential to proper vision, growth, cellular differentiation, healthy skin and mucous membranes, reproduction, and immune system integrity. Needed to maintain healthy skin and mucous membranes *Deficiency:* night blindness, conjunctival xerosis	Liver, fish-liver oils, eggs, whole milk, sweet potatoes, cantaloupe, carrots, spinach, broccoli, raw apricots
Vitamin D (ergocalciferol (D_2); cholecalciferol (D_3)	Regulates calcium and phosphorous metabolism *Deficiency:* rickets	Liver, cod-liver oil, egg yolks, butter and oily fish. Produced in skin by exposure to sunlight
Vitamin E (alpha-tocopherol)	Acts as an antioxidant and protects essential cellular components from oxidation	Wheat germ oil, sunflower oil, cottonseed oil, safflower oil, corn oil, soybean oil, almonds, peanuts, green leafy vegetables
Vitamin K (phytonadione)	Used for synthesis of prothrombin and factors VII, IX, and X needed for blood coagulation	Needs bile salts to be adequately absorbed in the intestines. Malabsorptive disease processes can lead to decreased vitamin K absorption. Vitamin K is synthesized by intestinal flora; severe diarrhea or the use of antibiotics that kill the intestinal flora may result in a deficiency. A deficiency exists in newborn infants
WATER-SOLUBLE VITAMINS		
Vitamin C (ascorbic acid)	Antioxidant Aids in formation and maintenance intracellular cement substances *Deficiency:* scurvy	Found in citrus fruits and juices, fruits, and vegetables such as broccoli, cabbage
Niacin (nicotinic acid, vitamin B_3)	Used to decrease cholesterol levels. Regulates energy metabolism, helps maintain the health of the skin, tongue, and digestive system *Deficiency:* pellegra	Organ meats, poultry, fish, meats, yeast, bran cereal, peanuts, brewer's yeast
Riboflavin (vitamin B_2)	Affects fetal growth and development. Is a co-enzyme for production of mitochondrial energy	Green leafy vegetables, fruit, eggs and dairy products, enriched cereal products, organ meats, peanuts and peanut butter
Thiamine (vitamin B_1)	Co-enzyme for carbohydrate metabolism; used for nerve conduction and energy production *Deficiency:* beriberi	Pork products, whole grains, wheat germ, meats, peas, cereal, dry beans, peanuts
Pyridoxine (vitamin B_6)	Metabolism of amino acids and proteins. May be important in red blood cell regeneration and normal nervous system functioning. *Deficiency:* anemia, spotty hair loss, paresthesias	Milk, meats, whole grain cereals, fish, vegetables
Cyanocobalamin (vitamin B_{12})	Needed as co-enzyme for red blood cell synthesis. *Deficiency:* megaloblastic anemia	Seafood, egg yolks, organ meats, milk, most cheeses
Folic acid (folacin)	Essential for cell growth and reproduction, synthesis of DNA in red blood cells *Deficiency:* impaired development of central nervous system; anencephaly and spina bifida	Liver, beans, green vegetables, yeast, nuts, fruit
Biotin	Essential for gluconeogenesis, fatty acid synthesis, and metabolism of branched-chain amino acids	Soy flour, cereals, egg yolk, liver; also synthesized in lower GI tract by bacteria and fungi
Pantothenic acid (vitamin B_5)	Essential for fat, carbohydrate, and protein metabolism	Organ meats, beef, and egg yolk

Table 47-6 *Essential Minerals*

MINERAL	ACTIONS	SOURCES
Calcium	Nerve transmission, bone and tooth formation, blood clotting; most abundant mineral in body	Milk, cheese, vegetables
Chlorine	Acid-base balance, gastric acid	Table salt
Chromium	Glucose and energy metabolism	Vegetables, oils, meats, fats, brewer's yeast, cheddar cheese, wheat germ
Cobalt	Component of cyanocobalamin (B_{12})	Meats, milk
Copper	Component of enzymes needed for iron metabolism	Meats, drinking water
Fluorine	Bone and tooth structure	Drinking water, seafood, tea
Iodine	Component of thyroid hormones	Seafood, vegetables, dairy products, iodized salt
Iron	Component of hemoglobin for oxygen transport; enzymes for energy metabolism	Meats, legumes, grains, leafy vegetables, eggs, clams, prunes, raisins
Magnesium	Component of bones, enzymes; protein synthesis, nerve transmission	Grains, green leafy vegetables, nuts, legumes, oysters, crab, cornmeal
Manganese	Component of enzymes; fat synthesis, bone and connective tissue synthesis	Whole grains, cereals, green vegetables, tea, ginger, cloves
Molybdenum	Component of enzymes; metabolize iron and uric acid	Cereals, legumes, meat, sunflower seeds, wheat germ
Phosphorus	Acid-base balance, bone and tooth structure, energy production	Milk, cheese, grains, meats, green leafy vegetables, fish
Potassium	Acid-base balance, nerve conduction, body water balance, muscle contractions	Citrus fruits, meat, milk, bananas, liver
Selenium	Antioxidant	Seafood, meat, grains, liver, kidney
Sodium	Water balance, membrane transport, muscle contraction, acid-base balance	Table salt, soy sauce, cured meats
Sulfur	Component of many tissue types such as tendons and cartilage, metabolic pathways, blood clotting	Sulfur-containing amino acids (e.g., methionine, cystine), garlic, onion, seafood, asparagas
Ultratrace minerals		
Nickel	Cofactor in enzyme reactions	Chocolate, nuts, fruits
Silicon	Bone calcification, collagen	Chicken skin, whole grains
Tin	Exact functions unknown	General diet
Vanadium	Cofactor in enzyme reactions	Olives, shellfish, mushrooms
Zinc	Component of enzymes required for digestion, wound healing, vision, sexual development	Oysters, liver, milk, fish, meats, carrots, oatmeal, peas

but ranges from 1.5 to 3 L daily for the average adult. Intake should slightly exceed losses so that the person maintains adequate urine output to help flush waste products through the kidneys, and to minimize constipation.

PHYSICAL ACTIVITY

Balanced nutrition plays a key role in health and wellness, but another equally important component is physical activity and exercise. Throughout history, it has long been known that the intake of food was necessary to meet the physical energy needs to sustain life. The balance of dietary energy intake and energy expenditure was accomplished almost subconsciously by most individuals because of the need for manual labor in everyday life. Since the beginning of the industrial revolution in the mid-800s, the invention of many labor-saving devices (manufacturing assembly lines, telegraph, telephone, e-mail, cell phone, automobile, remote control) and new forms of entertainment (radio, television) has reduced our energy expenditure through physical activity. Today, despite common knowledge that regular exercise is healthful, more than 60% of Americans are not regularly physically active, and 25% are not active at all. In the past 50 years our society has welcomed an immense variety of new types of foods made from basic food sources (animals, plants). Ease and convenience of food preparation (e.g., fast-food restaurants, drive-throughs; use of a microwave versus a convection oven), and increases in portion sizes ("Supersize it, please!") to increase commercial market share have placed too many easily consumed calories on the table of the American public. Consequently, reduced physical activity and increased caloric intake have resulted in a national epidemic of obesity, causing metabolic syndrome (see Chapter 21), and premature death.

The latest report from the Academy of Sciences (2002) stresses the importance of balancing diet with physical activity and makes recommendations about daily maximum caloric intake of food to be consumed based on height, weight, and gender for four different levels of physical activity (sedentary, low active, active, and very active). The report illustrates how difficult it is to lose weight based just on reduction of calories alone, and how important it is to maintain a level of physical activity to prevent reduction in lean body mass (muscle or protein wasting). The report now recommends 60 minutes of moderate intensity physical activity (e.g., walking at a rate of 4 to 5 miles per hour) or high-intensity activity (e.g., jogging at a rate of 4 to 5 miles in 20 to 30 minutes) four to seven times weekly, in addition to the activities of daily living, to maintain body weight (in adults) in the recommended body mass index range (18 to 25 kg/m^2).

MALNUTRITION

Nutrition plays a vital role in helping a patient recover from illness. Adequate intake of nutrients is critical to restoring normal homeostasis and rebuilding damaged tissue. If nutritional needs are not adequately addressed, malnutrition results. Malnutrition is a major source of morbidity and mortality in patients who suffer from disease, because they are much more susceptible to infections and organ failure. Malnutrition generally results from inadequate intake of protein and calories, or from a deficiency of one or more vitamins and minerals.

Malnutrition resulting from inadequate ingestion of proteins and calories may be subdivided into three types: marasmus, kwashiorkor, and mixed kwashiorkor-marasmus. **Marasmus,** the most common form of malnutrition in hospitalized patients, results from a lack of both total energy calories and protein. Marasmus occurs most commonly in patients who suffer from chronic disease and who do not ingest or utilize adequate amounts of proteins and calories. These patients, in essence, are starving, and have a cachectic appearance. Laboratory tests indicate normal serum albumin and transferrin concentrations, but delayed cutaneous hypersensitivity. In severe cases, muscle function is diminished. **Kwashiorkor** is a protein deficiency that develops when the patient receives adequate fats and carbohydrates in the diet, but little or no protein. These patients are often difficult to recognize because they appear well nourished. They are often edematous and laboratory tests may show hypoalbuminemia. **Mixed kwashiorkor-marasmus** results from inadequate protein building combined with a wasting of fat stores and skeletal muscle. This most often results in a patient with marasmus who is suddenly stressed with a new insult such as infection. The additional stress causes a greater energy need, leading to a greater loss of fat stores, muscle mass, and serum proteins. These patients often have lower immunocompetence, are hypoalbuminemic, and heal wounds very slowly.

A patient's nutritional status must be assessed to diagnose a nutritional deficiency. Nutrition assessment requires completion of a medical history, dietary history, physical examination, anthropometric measurements (height, weight, skinfold thickness, limb size, and wrist circumference), and laboratory data. Laboratory tests used to assess lean body mass include albumin, prealbumin, retinol-binding protein, and transferrin. Tests commonly used to assess immune function are total lymphocyte count and delayed cutaneous hypersensitivity reactions. Skin tests such as mumps, purified protein derivative (PPD), and *Candida albicans* are used to test for anergy because it is associated with malnutrition.

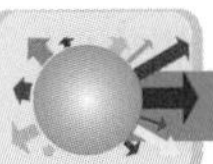

Clinical Landmine

Total parenteral nutrition (TPN) orders are formulated daily based on the patient's status, weight, and fluid and electrolyte balance. It is essential to check all aspects of the health care provider's order against the actual container of TPN solution with a second qualified nurse and initiate the flow rate specified using an infusion pump. Follow clinical practice guidelines for changing of TPN container and tubing, generally every 24 hours.

Therapy for Malnutrition

During illness, patients may require partial or full supplementation of their nutritional needs to prevent metabolic imbalances and starvation. One of two forms of supplementation is often used, depending on the patient's requirements. **Enteral nutrition** is administered orally, either by drinking or instillation into the stomach by way of a feeding tube **(tube feedings)** (i.e., nasogastric, nasoduodenal, nasojejunal tube) or feeding gastrostomy port. (See Administration of Enteral Feedings, p. 138.) Administration of nutrients directly into veins is known as **parenteral nutrition.** Parenteral nutrition may be subdivided into **peripheral parenteral nutrition (PPN)** and **total parenteral nutrition (TPN).** (See pp. 179 to 181 for a discussion of central venous access and implantable vascular access devices that may be used to administer parenteral nutrition.)

NURSING PROCESS *for Nutritional Support*

The purpose of enteral or parenteral nutrition is to supply the patient with an adequate intake of nutrients to meet the body's metabolic needs. Enteral and parenteral forms of nutritional support are undertaken for individuals who are unable to eat, have altered absorptive processes, or are unable to meet the body's required nutritional demands resulting from coexisting disease.

Assessment

History of Nutritional Deficit. Review the patient's history to identify the rationale for use of nutritional support (e.g., protein-calorie malnutrition [kwashiorkor and marasmus]), burn, surgery, cancer, acquired immunodeficiency syndrome (AIDS), hyperemesis gravidarum, infection, radiation therapy, chemotherapy, malabsorptive disorders, anorexia).

Nutritional History

- Are socioeconomic factors influencing the individual's dietary practices?
- Are cultural or religious practices affecting the individual's food intake pattern? What are the patient's food preferences and food customs?
- Ask the patient to describe the pattern of the developing nutritional problem (e.g., amount of weight loss and period of time over which it has occurred; any concurrent symptoms).
- Ask the patient to do a 24-hour recall of foods eaten and fluids ingested, including an estimate of serving sizes.
- As time permits and condition of the patient warrants, have the individual keep a record of all foods eaten and fluids ingested over a specific time, usually 3 days. It may be useful to have the patient record the times of meals and any activities that coincide with the food intake. This will help establish a pattern of the daily eating cycle.
- Are there any physical conditions that alter the patient's ability to ingest food? Examine the oral cavity for dentition or chewing problems, observe swallowing, and check history regarding any incidence of aspiration.

Physical Changes Related to a Malnourished State

- Obtain height, weight, arm muscle circumference, and triceps skinfold thickness.
- Check the skin integrity, skeletal muscle mass, and subcutaneous fat distribution. When performing an examination, take into consideration normal alterations in fat distribution throughout the life cycle.
- *Skin integrity, muscle mass, and fat distribution:* Starvation may be manifested by depletion of skeletal muscle mass; however, this may also be due to muscle atrophy from disease or lack of use. Another indication of starvation is fat depletion in the waist, arms, and legs. Dry, dull hair that can be easily pulled from the scalp is associated with protein deficiency. With advanced protein deficiency, known as kwashiorkor, the skin may become dry and flaky. Observe for edema in the abdomen and subcutaneous tissues, another sign of possible protein deficiency.
- *Cardiovascular alterations:* Caloric deficiencies over a long period may cause hypotension, generalized weakness, and low energy levels. A thiamine deficiency can increase heart rate and heart size and may be recognized by a widened pulse pressure.
- *Respiratory alterations:* Obese patients may have an increase in fat sufficient to restrict expansion and contraction of the chest, thereby compromising pulmonary function. Patients need to have lung sounds assessed to detect crackling sounds, an indication of overhydration and excessive fluid intake.
- *Neurologic alterations:* Vitamin B deficiencies may be related to abnormal findings with accompanying symptoms such as decreased position sense and diminished vibratory sense, decreased tendon reflexes, weakness, paresthesias, or decreased tactile sensations require a more thorough neurologic evaluation. Thiamine deficiency may result in neurologic deficit.
- *Abdominal alterations:* Proceed to perform an examination of the abdomen by inspection, auscultation, percussion, light palpation, and deep palpation as dictated by the nurse's level of knowledge and assessment skills.
- Obtain a history of gastrointestinal symptoms such as diarrhea, vomiting, constipation, and abdominal pain and its relationship to food consumption; ask specifically for details on how any of these conditions have been self-treated or treated by a health care provider.
- *Thyroid function:* The thyroid gland and its hormones influence all body cells. Be aware of the signs and symptoms of hypothyroidism (e.g., weight gain, dry brittle hair, facial edema, enlarged breasts, slowed pulse, coarse dry skin, deepening of the voice, lethargy, slowed speech and impaired memory, muscle weakness, altered reflexes). Conversely, be aware of the signs and symptoms of hyperthyroidism (e.g., goiter, hyperactive reflexes, weight loss, increased pulse rate, dysrhythmias, elevated blood pressure, emotional lability, heat intolerance).

Laboratory and Diagnostic Tests. A variety of laboratory tests may be used to assess nutritional status: blood prealbumin, albumin, urea nitrogen, creatinine, electrolytes, hemoglobin, hematocrit, lipids, liver function studies, glucose, total lymphocyte count, ferritin, transferrin, and urine specific gravity and ketones.

Nursing Diagnoses

- Nutrition, imbalanced: less than body requirements (indications)
- Nutrition, imbalanced: more than body requirements (indications)
- Injury, risk for (side effects)
- Fluid volume, deficient, excess (indication, side effects)

Planning

- The dietary history is reviewed by the health team and specific recommendations are made to alleviate the dietary problems or to treat the disease process.
- Transcribe the health care provider's orders for parenteral fluids, supplements, and tube feedings or total parenteral nutrition.
- Order prescribed nutritional therapy and equipment for administration.

- Label the Kardex or enter in the computer dietary and nutritional orders and with fluid restrictions or other pertinent parameters.
- Label the Kardex or enter in the computer aspiration precautions.
- Place the patient on intake and output (I&O) and daily weights.
- Order laboratory studies and schedule glucose checks as prescribed by the health care provider.
- Schedule central line care as appropriate.
- Schedule oral hygiene and comfort measures.
- Initiate and continue I&O flow record.
- Review clinical practice policies relating to enteral and parenteral nutrition (e.g., checking feeding tube placement, ordering nutritional supplements, procedures for setting up and changing pumps/tubing/equipment).

Implementation

- Implement orders for diet, nutritional supplements, vitamins, minerals, tube feedings, intravenous therapy or total parenteral nutrition.
- Perform assessments for nutritional and fluid deficits and excess.
- Implement proper administration and monitoring for complications associated with enteral, parenteral, or total parenteral administration.
- Perform verification of tube placement including pH testing in accordance with clinical site policies.
- Implement institutional policies for flushing and administration of medications via feeding tubes.
- Document all aspects of patient care relating to nutritional therapy and the patient's response to therapy.

Monitoring Tube Feedings

- Check tube placement and gastric pH according to clinical guidelines or health care provider orders.
- In general, tube placement and residual volumes are checked before administration of each bolus tube feeding, or every 4 or 8 hours for continuous feedings. When residual volumes exceed 100 mL, or another limit specified by the health care provider's order, further tube feeding is held and residual volume is rechecked in 1 hour. Most clinical settings then resume the prescribed ordered volume if the repeat residual volume is less than 100 mL. Because higher residual volumes may indicate obstruction, the health care provider should be notified if the residual amount has not diminished to less than 100 mL.
- Follow the health care provider's orders for the amount, type, strength of solution, and rate of administration, as well as the method of administration prescribed (e.g., continuous, intermittent, bolus, cyclic). Enteral feedings are often initiated at half strength to determine how well the patient's GI tract tolerates the solution. If diarrhea or cramping starts, discontinue administration and notify the health care provider for further orders.
- Initiate enteral feeding at a lower rate of about 50 mL per hour. Every 12 to 24 hours increase the rate by about 25 mL per hour until the appropriate hourly volume is attained.
- Record intake and output; vital signs; check for gastric residuals and the individual patient response to the formula (e.g., abdominal distention, nausea, vomiting, diarrhea).
- Perform daily serum blood and urine tests for glucose ketones as dictated by the health care provider's orders or clinical site policies.
- Perform daily weights and monitor for signs of dehydration or overhydration and laboratory or diagnostic test results (notify health care provider of abnormal results).
- Change tube feeding apparatus in accordance with clinical facility policy, usually every 24 hours.
- Handle enteral feedings carefully to prevent bacterial contamination. Store in a clean, cool place and wash lids before opening the ready-to-use preparations. Check manufacturer's recommendations for the length of time a formula is considered safe at room temperature (usually 12 hours). Many clinical sites suggest placing only enough formula for 4 or 8 hours in the delivery apparatus; check individual clinical site guidelines.

Monitoring Peripheral Parenteral Nutrition (PPN)

- Observe IV site for signs of infiltration, phlebitis, or local reaction.
- Monitor actual IV infusion rate and all aspects of the IV order (type/strength of solution, rate of administration). Check date on IV container and tubing for need to be changed, usually every 72 hours.
- Monitor the patient for signs and symptoms of fluid overload (e.g., bounding pulse rate, hoarseness, dyspnea, cough, venous distention).
- Monitor for pyrogenic reaction (e.g., fever, chills, general malaise, vomiting) usually within 30 minutes of initiating therapy.
- Monitor for anaphylactic reaction to proteins (e.g., wheezing, itching, hypotension, tightness in chest).

Monitoring Total Parenteral Nutrition (TPN)

- Monitor daily weights and laboratory or diagnostic test results (notify health care provider of abnormal results).
- Check all aspects of the health care provider's order against the actual container of TPN solution with a second qualified nurse and initiate the flow rate specified using an infusion pump. Follow clinical practice guidelines for changing of TPN container and tubing, generally every 24 hours.
- Provide site care for central venous access in accordance with clinical site policy. Assess site for redness, swelling or drainage, elevated temperature, or fatigue (signs of infection).

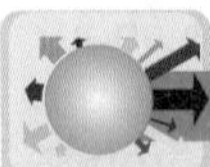

Clinical Landmine

Do not speed up TPN solution infusion to "catch up" if the amount delivered is "behind schedule." This practice may cause significant hyperglycemia and metabolic imbalance.

- Perform glucose and ketone tests as specified by health care provider's orders and administer regular insulin according to orders. Check patient for signs of hypoglycemia (e.g., nausea, weakness, thirst, rapid respirations, headache).
- Assess parenteral setup to be sure all connections are secure to prevent an air embolism or contamination.
- Assess for signs of "refeeding syndrome" during the first 24 to 48 hours after initiation of TPN (e.g., changes in electrolytes, respiratory depression, confusion, weakness, irritability, generalized lethargy).
- Observe for fluid and electrolyte imbalances and hyperglycemia resulting from high glucose content of solution. Do not speed up TPN solution to "catch up" if amount delivered is "behind schedule." This practice may overload the individual's system with glucose.
- Individuals are "tapered" from TPN by gradually slowing the infusion rate of the TPN while simultaneously increasing oral intake over a few days. This procedure ensures that the patient's gastrointestinal system can tolerate adequate oral feedings without diarrhea developing.

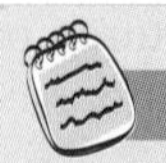

Patient Education and Health Promotion

- Patients being discharged with enteral nutrition for home use require considerable education for themselves and family or significant others.
- Give specific written instructions on the administration procedures, type, rate and frequency, storage, and handling of tube feedings ordered. Include in the description when to call the health care provider (e.g., diarrhea, nausea, vomiting, signs of infection).
- Teach the patient or primary caregiver the procedure used in the hospital to administer the enteral or parenteral solutions.
- Ask the appropriate individuals to demonstrate competency in performing the procedures before discharge. As appropriate, request a referral to a community agency, such as visiting nurses, for assistance in the home with the feedings.
- Give specific instructions on changing tubing and apparatus used and the importance of adhering to the techniques taught in the hospital to prevent infection.
- Have the patient role-play the resolution of common problems associated with the prescribed nutritional therapy (e.g., tube obstruction, cramping diarrhea, nausea).
- Teach the person with a central IV line the proper care of the line and dressing changes, as permitted by the employing institution.
- Teach the individual to perform daily weights at the same time of day in similar clothing on the same scale.
- Teach appropriate oral hygiene measures and include ways to alleviate thirst and mouth dryness (e.g., rinsing the mouth frequently, use of hard candy or sugarless gum).
- Give written instructions of what to do if the patient aspirates or the tube comes out.
- Explain techniques that can be used to self-administer tube feedings ordered for intermittent administration.
- Explain the importance of having the prescribed laboratory tests done as scheduled to evaluate the response to the nutritional therapy.
- Teach the patient to maintain a record of temperature, pulse, respirations, blood pressure, and defined monitoring parameters.

Fostering Health Maintenance

- Provide the patient and significant others with important information for specific medicines prescribed. For instance when iron preparations are prescribed the patient should understand it is best taken between meals; however, as a result of stomach irritation, it may be best to take it with food or immediately after meals. Liquid iron should be taken with a straw placed well back on the tongue and the mouth should be rinsed immediately after administration to prevent staining of the teeth. When vitamins and minerals are prescribed it is necessary to continue their use for the period specified by the health care provider and to adhere to the prescribed dosage.
- Ensure that the patient understands the care, handling, and storage of all enteral, supplemental, or parenteral solutions and the need to prevent infection through use of the proper administration techniques.
- Discuss ways that the individual who is to be maintained on enteral or TPN for a long time can be involved, as appropriate, with other household members during mealtimes.
- Seek cooperation and understanding of the following points so that medication compliance is increased: name of medication, dosage, route of administration, side effects to expect, and side effects to report. For all supplemental, enteral, or TPN solutions, the individual must understand all components of the health care provider's orders.

Written Record. Enlist the patient's aid in developing and maintaining a written record of monitoring parameters (see Patient Self-Assessment Form below). Complete the Premedication Data column for use as a baseline to track response to drug therapy. Ensure that the patient understands how to use the form and instruct the patient to take the completed form to follow-up visits. During follow-up visits, focus on issues that will foster adherence with the therapeutic interventions prescribed.

Enteral Nutrition

Actions

Enteral nutrition is the provision of nutrients through the GI tract. Formulas may be administered orally or by nasogastric, nasoduodenal, or nasojejunal tube; feeding gastrostomy; or needle-catheter jejunostomy.

Uses

There is an adage often used in medicine: "When the gut works, and can be safely used, use it." Supplementation with enteral food formulas is indicated when oral consumption is either inadequate or contraindicated. Examples of when tube feedings might be necessary are head and neck surgery, esophageal obstruction, stroke resulting in inability to chew or swallow food, and dementia. Advantages to enteral nutrition, when compared with parenteral nutrition, are that it avoids risks associated with IV therapy, provides GI stimulation, and is physiologic; protocols for administration are much less stringent because there is less risk of infection, and enteral feeding is less expensive. Enteral feedings are contraindicated when there is intractable vomiting, a paralyzed ileum, and in the presence of certain types of fistulas. See Table 47-7 for examples of oral supplements,

PATIENT SELF-ASSESSMENT FORM Nutritional Therapy

MEDICATIONS	COLOR	TO BE TAKEN

Patient ____________

Health Care Provider ____________

Health Care Provider's phone ____________

Next appt.* ____________

What I Should Monitor	Premedication Data	Date	Date	Date	Date	Date	Date	Comments
Weight								
Blood pressure								
Pulse								
Temperature								
Blood glucose								
Insulin (regular)								
Nausea, vomiting								
Diarrhea								
Constipation								
Date tubing/apparatus changed								
Energy level								
Control of secretions								
Strength of formula								
ml received/day								
Other								

*Please bring this record with you to your next appointment.
Use the back of this sheet for additional information.

Table 47-7 ***Enteral Formulas****

FORMULA TYPE	BRAND NAMES	CALORIES (kcal/mL)	PROTEIN CONTENT (g/L)	OSMOLALITY (Mosm/kg water)	COMMENTS
Oral supplements	Ensure Liquid	1.06	37.0	590	These products are dietary supplements and are available in a variety of flavors for oral use. Requires full digestive capability by gut. At recommended dosages, these formulas provide 100% of the RDA for vitamins and minerals.
	Ensure Plus HN	1.50	59.2	650	
	Ensure Plus	1.50	52.0	680	
	ProSure	1.27	70.8	635	
	Boost	1.01	37.0	610-670	
Standard isotonic formulas	Isocal	1.06	34.0	270	These products are standard formulas used for tube feeding. The formulas are lactose-free to prevent bloating and flatulence and are low residue and low viscosity. At recommended dosages, these formulas provide 100% of the RDA for vitamins and minerals.
	Isocal HN	1.06	44.0	270	
	Osmolite 1 cal	1.06	37.0	300	
	Osmolite 1.2	1.2	55.5	360	
	Nutren 1.0	1.00	40.0	315	
	Isosource	1.20	43.0	490	
Pediatric formulas	Isomil	1.0	24.0	200	Soy-based infant formula; for allergy to cow's milk or lactose-intolerant or galactosemic infants
	Similac	1.0	20.0	300	Milk-based infant formula
	Alimentum	0.67	19.0	NA	For severe food allergies, protein maldigestion, and fat malabsorption
	Pregestimil	0.67	18.7	280	Predigested; for patients with severe malabsorption
	Phenex-1	0.48	15.0	NA	Phenylalanine free; for phenylketonuria
Specialized formulas	Glucerna Liquid	1.00	41.8	355	High-fat, low-carbohydrate formula for glucose-intolerant patients
	NovaSource Pulmonary	1.50	75.0	650	High-fat, low-carbohydrate formula for pulmonary patients
	Peptamen	1.00	40.0	270	Predigested; for protein maldigestion
	NovaSource Renal	1.5	7.5	650	Essential amino acids for renal failure
	Nutri-Hep	1.5	40.0	790	High in branched-chain and low in aromatic amino acids; for patients with hepatic encephalopathy

*Formulas listed are representative examples and are not intended to be a complete list.

standard feeding tube formulas, pediatric formulas, and formulas for special cases such as hepatic, renal or pulmonary failure, or malabsorption syndrome.

Therapeutic Outcomes

The primary therapeutic outcomes expected from enteral nutrition are:

- Stabilization of weight within identified parameters
- Sufficient intake of nutrients to maintain age-appropriate growth and development
- Improvement of laboratory assessments of nutrition

Nursing Process for Enteral Nutrition

Assessment

1. Assess for underlying diseases such as heart disease or renal or liver impairment that may limit the rate of administration and type of enteral formula to be used.
2. Assess for food allergies and lactose intolerance.
3. Review and record daily weights, changes in gastric motility, and stool characteristics.
4. Before administration of oral supplements, assess for swallowing difficulty and whether aspiration precautions should be ordered.
5. Monitor for signs and symptoms of aspiration (e.g., respiratory rate and depth, lung sounds) and elevation in body temperature.
6. Check tube placement and residual volume present according to policy. (See Chapter 9, pp. 138 to 140.)
7. Check all aspects of the health care provider's order for a tube feeding: type, amount, rate of administration, method of administration (bolus or continuous); and for specific orders regarding additional water intake.
8. Check to ensure that laboratory tests have been completed before starting enteral therapy (e.g., se-

rum prealbumin, albumin, urea nitrogen, creatinine, electrolytes, hemoglobin, hematocrit, lipids, liver function studies, glucose, total lymphocyte count, ferritin, transferrin, urine specific gravity and ketones).

9. Be prepared to monitor for potential signs and symptoms of enteral nutrition complications throughout the shift (e.g., tube obstruction, skin and mucous membrane breakdown, nausea, diarrhea, constipation, pulmonary complications, hyperglycemia, hypercapnia, fluid volume excess or deficits).

Planning

Availability. See Table 47-7.

Implementation

Dosage and Administration. NOTE: Tube feedings, especially those that have an osmolality of 300 mOsm/L water or greater, need to be started with a quarter- or half-strength formula to prevent diarrhea from a hypertonic solution.

Tube feedings are administered by one of the following three methods:

1. *Bolus feeding:* Administer 200 mL or more of formula over 3 to 5 minutes. Formula is advanced using a syringe. Used primarily for patients with feeding gastrostomy.
2. *Intermittent feeding:* Administer 200 mL or more of formula over 20 to 30 minutes using a reservoir bottle or bag. Formula is advanced by gravity.
3. *Continuous drip:* Formula is slowly administered continuously over 12 to 24 hours using an infusion pump. This method is recommended when feeding is infused into the jejunum.

Administration of Medicines to the Tube-Fed Patient. NOTE: Do not add prescribed medications directly to the formula being administered.

- Do not crush and administer any enteric-coated, chewable, or sublingual tablets via the feeding tube. Obtain a liquid form of the medication. Do not crush slow-release tablets and give via the tube. If the size of the tube is sufficient, the slow-release capsules may be opened, added to water, and given via the tube with adequate water to clear the tubing completely following administration.
- Administer each drug separately; do not combine. Give a small amount of water between different medications.
- Medicines should be administered on an empty stomach.
  1. Stop formula, flush tubing with 15 to 30 mL water.
  2. Wait 30 to 60 minutes, then administer prescribed medication on an empty stomach.
  3. Flush tube with 15 to 30 mL of water, then clamp.
  4. Do not reinitiate tube feeding for 15 to 30 minutes or as stated in clinical guidelines.

Evaluation

Side Effects to Expect

Hyperglycemia. Hyperglycemia may develop easily, especially when feeding is started for a malnourished person. Check health care provider's orders for frequency of blood glucose monitoring and whether insulin has been ordered for elevated glucose levels.

Side Effects to Report

Pulmonary Complications. Assess for symptoms of aspiration.

Diarrhea or Constipation. Changes in bowel pattern and consistency often develop when enteral nutrition is initiated. If diarrhea starts, discontinue feedings immediately and await further health care provider's orders.

Nausea, Vomiting, Increased Residual Volumes. These signs are an indication of bowel obstruction. Discontinue feedings and await further health care provider's orders.

Rash, Chills, Fever, Respiratory Difficulty. These signs are an indication of allergy to formula. Provide emergency care, as needed. Immediately discontinue feedings and await further health care provider's orders.

Drug Interactions. Food can affect medicines by altering absorption, metabolism, and excretion; conversely, medicines can affect nutrition by similar pathways. Interactions between drugs and nutrients are particularly significant in elderly patients who often have several chronic diseases requiring long-term multiple drug therapy, and who may often have poor nutrition. The following list is a synopsis of the more common potential food-drug interactions.

Alcohol versus Disulfiram, Metronidazole, Tinidazole. Alcohol interacts with these three medicines, causing nausea, vomiting, abdominal cramps, headache, sweating, and flushing of the face. Use of alcohol and alcohol-containing preparations, such as OTC cough medications and mouthwashes (e.g., Listerine, Cepacol) should be avoided during therapy and for 72 hours after discontinuation of metronidazole or tinidazole therapy. The interaction with disulfiram may last several weeks.

Tetracycline, Doxycycline, Ciprofloxacin, Levofloxacin. Avoid taking these antibiotics within 2 hours before or after antacids, iron, zinc, and dairy products (e.g., milk, ice cream, cheese, yogurt). If taken close together, the absorption of the antibiotic is inhibited.

Itraconazole (Capsules), Ganciclovir, Ritonavir. These medicines should be taken with food to increase absorption and therapeutic effect.

Itraconazole (Suspension), Didanosine, Indinavir. Take these medicines at least 1 hour before or 2 hours after meals. They need to be taken on an empty stomach to increase absorption and therapeutic effect.

Alendronate, Residronate, Ibandronate, Tiludronate. Take alendronate at least 30 minutes (for residronate, ibandronate, tiludronate, 2 hours) before the first food, beverage, or medication of the day. The patient should take with a full glass of plain water and not lie down for at least 30 minutes with alendronate or residronate, or 60 minutes with ibandronate.

Monoamine Oxidase Inhibitors (MAOIs) (Tranylcypromine, Phenelzine, Isocarboxazid). A major potential complication with MAOI therapy is hypertensive crisis, particularly with tranylcypromine. Because MAOIs block amine metabolism in tissues outside the brain, patients who consume foods or medications containing indirect sympathomimetic amines are at considerable risk for a hypertensive crisis. Foods containing significant quantities of tyramine include well-ripened cheeses (e.g., Camembert, Edam, Roquefort, Parmesan, mozzarella, cheddar); yeast extract; red wines; pickled herring; sauerkraut; overripe bananas, figs, and avocados; chicken livers; and beer. Other foods containing vasopressors include fava beans, chocolate, coffee, tea, and colas. Common prodromal symptoms of hypertensive crisis include severe occipital headache, stiff neck, sweating, nausea, vomiting, and sharply elevated blood pressure. This drug-food interaction may occur for up to 2 weeks after discontinuation of the MAOI.

Warfarin. Patients receiving warfarin should avoid extreme changes in diet and daily consumption of large amounts of dark green vegetables. Herbal medicines (e.g., ginseng, ginkgo biloba, garlic) inhibit platelet aggregation. Monitor patients for signs of bleeding.

Grapefruit Juice. Fresh and frozen grapefruit juice inhibits the metabolism of several drugs. The severity of the interaction varies among people, among drugs, and the quantity of grapefruit juice consumed. The more potentially serious interactions are listed below:

- Calcium channel blockers (dihydropyridine class: felodipine, nifedipine, nimodipine, amlodipine, isradipine, nicardipine): Monitor for signs of toxicity such as flushing, headache, tachycardia, and hypotension.
- Verapamil: Monitor for signs of toxicity such as bradycardia, atrioventricular block, constipation, and hypotension.
- Cyclosporine: Monitor for signs of toxicity such as nephrotoxicity, hepatotoxicity, and increased immunosuppression.
- Triazolam: Monitor for increased sedation.
- Caffeine: Monitor for signs of toxicity such as nervousness and overstimulation.

Herbal Interactions

- Patients receiving warfarin should avoid herbal medicines (e.g., ginseng, ginkgo biloba, garlic) that inhibit platelet aggregation.

PARENTERAL NUTRITION

Actions

Parenteral nutrition is the administration of nutrients by intravenous infusion. Parenteral nutrient solutions provide a balanced combination of carbohydrates, amino acids, and essential fats, along with appropriate minerals, vitamins, and electrolytes.

Uses

Parenteral nutrition is used for patients who are unable to take nutrition enterally for more than 7 days. Parenteral nutrition is generally used for intractable vomiting and diarrhea, malabsorption syndromes, bowel surgery, coma, bowel rest, and for conditions requiring additional nutrition such as massive wound healing secondary to trauma or major infection.

The type of parenteral nutrition prescribed depends on the patient's status, metabolic needs, disease process, and the length of time that the individual will not be able to meet metabolic demands through normal oral intake.

PPN is used for patients requiring support for a limited time, usually lasting less than 3 to 4 weeks. It is appropriate for the patient who is anticipated to be having normal GI functioning reestablished within a short time. PPN administration generally requires relatively high fluid volume of approximately 2000 mL per day and therefore may not be tolerated well or indicated for some coexisting disease processes such as heart failure. PPN solutions consist of 2% to 5% crystalline amino acid preparations with 5% or 10% dextrose and added electrolytes and vitamins.

TPN consists of glucose (15% to 25%), amino acids (3.5% to 15%), fat emulsion (10% to 20%), and electrolytes, vitamins, and minerals. The Harris-Benedict equation may be used to estimate caloric and nutritional requirements. Special hepatic, renal, and stress formulations are also available.

Therapeutic Outcomes

The primary therapeutic outcomes expected from parenteral nutrition are:

- Stabilization of weight within identified parameters
- Sufficient intake of nutrients to maintain age-appropriate growth and development
- Improvement of laboratory assessments of nutrition

Nursing Process for Parenteral Nutrition

Assessment

1. Assess for underlying disorders such as heart disease or renal or liver impairment that may limit the rate of administration and type of parenteral formula to be used.
2. Review and record daily weight; note hydration of mucous membranes.

3. Check to ensure that laboratory tests have been completed before starting parenteral therapy (e.g., serum prealbumin, albumin, urea nitrogen, creatinine, electrolytes, hemoglobin, hematocrit, lipids, liver function studies, glucose, total lymphocyte count, ferritin, transferrin, and urine specific gravity and ketones).
4. Compare the entire health care provider's order with the actual contents of the TPN container before initiating or adding it to the running access site.
5. Check the patient's identification and the expiration date and time on the TPN to be hung.
6. Discard any TPN solution that remains at the end of 24 hours. Have the next container of TPN ready. In the event it is not ready, hang a solution of 10% dextrose. Do NOT simply shut off the infusion, because of the danger of rebound hypoglycemia.
7. Take vital signs at least every 4 hours while TPN is being administered.
8. Be prepared to monitor for potential signs and symptoms of parenteral nutrition complications throughout the shift (e.g., pulmonary complications, hyperglycemia, hypercapnia, and fluid volume excess or deficits).

Planning

Availability. Check at least 1 to 2 hours in advance of needing the next container of TPN to be certain it will be ready.

Always use an infusion pump for administration of TPN. Do not "speed up" TPN if it gets behind schedule. Speeding it up could result in hyperglycemia, seizures, coma, or death.

Schedule blood glucose monitoring as prescribed by the health care provider, generally every 4 hours during initiation, or every 6 hours thereafter.

Schedule daily electrolyte studies as prescribed.

Implementation

Dosage and Administration. NOTE: Do not use total parenteral nutrition IV lines or central venous catheters for delivery of any other medications or solutions.

Side Effects to Expect

Hyperglycemia. Hyperglycemia may develop easily, especially when TPN is initiated for a malnourished person. Symptoms include headache, nausea and vomiting, abdominal pain, dizziness, rapid pulse, rapid shallow respirations, and a fruity odor to the breath from acetone. Check the health care provider's orders for frequency of blood glucose monitoring and whether insulin has been ordered for elevated glucose levels.

Side Effects to Report

Hypoglycemia. Nervousness, tremors, headache, apprehension, sweating, cold clammy skin, and hunger. This may progress to blurred vision, lack of coordination, incoherence, coma, and death.

Fluid Imbalance. Overhydration may be recognized by weight gain, neck vein distention, change in mental status, edema, dyspnea, rales and rhonchi, tachycardia, and bounding pulses.

Dehydration may be noted by loss of skin turgor, sticky oral mucous membranes, a shrunken or deeply furrowed tongue, crusted lips, weight loss, deteriorating vital signs, soft or sunken eyeballs, weak pedal pulses, delayed capillary refill, excessive thirst, and mental confusion.

Rash, Chills, Fever, Respiratory Difficulty. These signs are an indication of allergy to formula. Provide emergency care, as needed. Immediately discontinue feedings and await further health care provider's orders.

Electrolyte Imbalances. Check for indications of electrolyte imbalance (e.g., mental status [alertness, orientation, confusion], muscle strength, muscle cramps, tremors, nausea, decline in general appearance). Check laboratory values and report abnormal values to health care provider.

Vitamin Deficiencies. Fat-soluble (vitamins A, D, E, K):

- *A:* Diarrhea; dry, scaly, rough, cracked skin; alterations in adaptation to light and dark
- *D:* Involuntary spasms and twitching, decreased calcium and phosphorus demineralization of bones
- *E:* Hemolysis of red blood cells; in older children, neurologic syndrome of vitamin E deficiency
- *K:* Symptoms of bleeding and/or delayed clotting

Water-soluble (cyanocobalamin, folic acid, niacin, pyridoxine, riboflavin, thiamine, and vitamin C):

- *Cyanocobalamin:* Anorexia, ataxia, diarrhea, constipation, irritability, paresthesia, delirium, hallucinations
- *Folic acid:* Diarrhea, glossitis, macrocytic anemia, low serum levels
- *Niacin:* Glossitis, diarrhea, rashes, weakness, anorexia, indigestion; as deficiency progresses central nervous system involvement is manifested by confusion, disorientation, neuritis
- *Pyridoxine:* Anemia, dyspnea, cheilosis, glossitis, convulsions
- *Riboflavin:* Cheilosis, glossitis, seborrheic dermatitis, photophobia, poor wound healing
- *Thiamine:* Anorexia, constipation, indigestion, confusion, edema, muscle weakness, cardiomegaly, heart failure
- *Vitamin C:* Anemia, petechiae, depression, delayed wound healing

Hepatotoxicity. Fatty liver may develop. Check liver function tests (elevated bilirubin, aspartate aminotransferase [AST], alanine aminotransferase [ALT], gamma-glutamyltransferase [GGT], alkaline phosphatase, prothrombin time) and report abnormal laboratory values to health care provider.

Drug Interactions. No other drugs should be administered concurrently with TPN. Consult a pharmacist for parenteral nutrition solutions and compatibility with specific medicines.

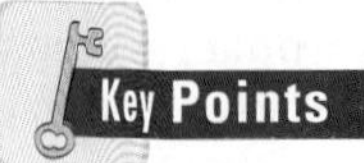

- Energy sources required for balanced metabolism are the macronutrients: fats, carbohydrates, and proteins. Other essential nutrients include vitamins, minerals, fiber, and water. Nutritional requirements vary based not only on the age of the individual but also on the gender and level of activity.
- No one food source can meet all of our basic nutritional requirements. Healthful diets provide a balance of carbohydrates, fiber, fat, protein, and essential nutrients to reduce risks of chronic diseases and support a full and productive lifestyle. Healthful nutrition must also be accompanied with regular mild to moderate physical activity to help maintain muscle tone and agility.
- Nutrition plays a vital role in helping a patient recover from illness. Adequate intake of nutrients is critical to restoring normal homeostasis and rebuilding damaged tissue. If nutritional needs are not adequately addressed, malnutrition results. Malnutrition is a major source of morbidity and mortality in patients who are suffering from disease because they are much more susceptible to infections and organ failure.
- During illness, patients may require partial or full supplementation of their nutritional needs. One of two forms of supplementation is often used. Enteral nutrition is administered orally, either by the patient drinking the liquid or by administration into the GI tract by way of a feeding tube. Administration of nutrients directly into veins is known as parenteral nutrition.
- Nurses need to understand the importance of cultural beliefs whenever special diets are prescribed. Because the nurse may not have knowledge of the cultural aspects of dietary adaptations, it is essential to involve a nutritionist in the dietary planning process.

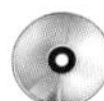

Go to your Companion CD-ROM for Appendices, an Audio Glossary, animations, Drug Dosage Calculators, customizable Patient Self-Assessment forms, and Review Questions for the NCLEX® Examination.

evolve Be sure to visit the companion Evolve site at http://evolve.elsevier.com/Clayton for WebLinks and additional online resources.

MEDICATION SAFETY REVIEW

MATH REVIEW QUESTIONS

1. The patient has an order to receive Osmolite, full strength, at 80 mL per hour around the clock. The feeding is shut off for 1 hour three times per day when medications are administered that interact with the nutritional product. What adjustment in the rate of administration would need to be made to administer the full amount of prescribed formula during the hours it is running?
2. A patient is receiving intermittent bolus feedings of Ensure, 250 mL every 4 hours, followed by a water bolus of 150 mL per bolus feeding. What is the individual's total fluid intake over a 24-hour period?

CRITICAL THINKING QUESTIONS

1. A patient's TPN solution has gotten behind in the rate of administration. As the nurse you realize the client needs the nutrients. What interventions could be initiated and what actions would be contraindicated? (Give rationale for your interventions.)
2. In the long-term care home, the patient on a continuous tube feeding could have the tube feeding scheduled to run at night, thus leaving greater mobility during the daytime. If the client has to have an intake of 80 mL per hour over a 24-hour span, how would the hourly intake be adjusted to administer the enteral product between 8:00 PM and 8:00 AM?
3. Explain teaching for an adult being discharged on bolus enteral feedings. How would you teach the person to administer the enteral product and what monitoring for complications should be done before discharge home?
4. It is time to hang the next bag of TPN and it has not arrived from the pharmacy. What would be appropriate actions for the nurse to take?
5. While caring for an older adult client receiving continuous tube feedings using a kangaroo feeding pump, you suspect the patient has aspirated some of the formula. What symptoms would you assess for and what immediate nursing actions should you take?
6. Research clinical practice guidelines for performing enteral and parenteral nutrition procedures.

CONTENT REVIEW QUESTIONS

1. Select good food sources of dietary fiber.
   1. Lettuce salad with dressing
   2. Potatoes, pasta, and white bread
   3. Cereal brans, sweet potatoes, vegetables, and fruits
   4. Beef, chicken, fish, and tofu

2. Sources of the type of dietary fats that are cardioprotective include: *(Select all that apply.)*
   1. Corn oil
   2. Soybean oil
   3. Safflower oil
   4. Coconut oil
   5. Olive oil
   6. Peanut oil
   7. Canola oil
   8. Stick margarine

3. The Harvard Health Eating Pyramid base is composed of:
   1. breads, cereal, rice, and pasta.
   2. dairy products.
   3. whole grains, fruits, and vegetables.
   4. activity and weight control.

4. Medications known to interact with grapefruit juice include: *(Select all that apply.)*
   1. Calcium channel blockers
   2. Barbiturates
   3. Cyclosporine
   4. Sulfonamides
   5. Angiotensin-converting enzyme (ACE) inhibitors
   6. Triazolam
   7. Prokinetic agents

5. The National Academy of Sciences recommendations for daily nutritional distribution of carbohydrates (CHO), fats, and proteins to minimize chronic disease include:
   1. CHO 40% to 63%, fats 25% to 50%, proteins 12% to 20%.
   2. CHO 35% to 45%, fats 10% to 15%, proteins 30% to 50%.
   3. CHO 50% to 60%, fats 30%, proteins 10% to 20%.
   4. CHO 45% to 65%, fats 20% to 35%, proteins 10% to 35%.

6. When introducing a feeding to a client with an indwelling gastrostomy tube for enteral nutrition, the nurse should first:
   1. irrigate the tube with normal saline solution.
   2. check to see that the tube is properly placed.
   3. place the client in a supine position.
   4. introduce some water before giving the liquid nourishment.

7. A client has a gastrostomy tube in place and is receiving tube feedings. While the nurse is administering the feeding, the client begins to experience abdominal cramping and nausea. The nurse should:
   1. cool the formula.
   2. remove the tube.
   3. use a more concentrated formula.
   4. decrease the administration rate.

8. A nasogastric tube is inserted for the client to receive intermittent tube feedings. An initial chest radiograph is done to confirm placement of the tube in the stomach. After the radiograph confirmation, the most reliable method of checking for tube placement is for the nurse to:
   1. place the end of the tube in water and observing for bubbling.
   2. auscultate while introducing air into the tube.
   3. measure the pH of the secretions aspirated.
   4. ask the client to speak.

CHAPTER

48 Herbal and Dietary Supplement Therapy

evolve http://evolve.elsevier.com/Clayton

Chapter Content

Objectives

1. Summarize the primary actions, uses, and interactions of the herbal and dietary supplement products cited.
2. Describe the possible impact of the use of herbal and dietary supplement products on cultural/ethnic beliefs.

Key Terms

dietary supplements
herbal medicines
botanicals
phytomedicine
phytotherapy

HERBAL MEDICINES, DIETARY SUPPLEMENTS, AND RATIONAL THERAPY

Over the past two decades we have witnessed a tremendous resurgence in the popularity of self-care and alternative therapies, including acupuncture, aromatherapy, homeopathy, vitamin and other supplement therapy, and herbal medicine. We have been attracted to "all natural" products because we have placed a greater emphasis on health, wellness and disease prevention, and the general perception that all natural is synonymous with "better" and not harmful. Some of the more than 250 herbal medicines and hundreds of combinations of other supplements may be beneficial, but unfortunately, the whole field of complementary medicine is fraught with false claims, lack of standardization, and adulteration and misbranding of products.

In the early 1990s, the U.S. Food and Drug Administration (FDA) threatened to ban herbal medicines and other types of supplements that were being touted as good for health from the U.S. market until appropriate scientific studies were completed to prove that these products were safe and effective. Such an uproar was created by this threat that Congress passed the Dietary Supplement Health and Education Act (DSHEA) of 1994. Under this act almost all herbal medicines, vitamins, minerals, amino acids, and other supplemental chemicals used for health were reclassified legally as **dietary supplements,** a food category. The legislation also allows manufacturers to include information on the label and through advertisements about the ways that these products affect the human body. These labels and advertisements also must contain a statement that the product has not yet been evaluated by the FDA for treating, curing, or preventing any disease. The law does not prevent other people (e.g., nutritionists, health food store clerks, herbalists, strength coaches, or other unlicensed individuals) from making claims (founded or unfounded) about the therapeutic effects of supplement ingredients. The result of the new law is that dietary supplements are not required to be safe and effective, and unfounded claims of therapeutic benefit abound. Hundreds of herbal medicines and other dietary supplements are marketed in the United States as single- and multiple-ingredient products for an extremely wide variety of uses, all implying that they will improve one's health. The vast majority of the popular claims made for herbal medicines and dietary supplements are unproven. There are also no standardized manufacturing practices that control the manufacture of most of these products as there are with medicines approved by the FDA. Since 1999 ConsumerLab.com has been

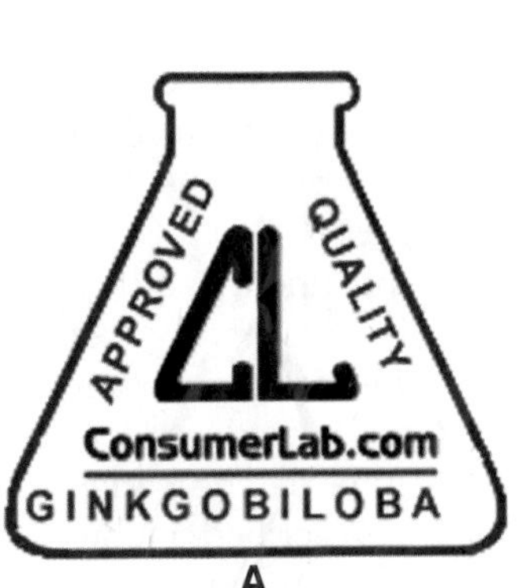

A

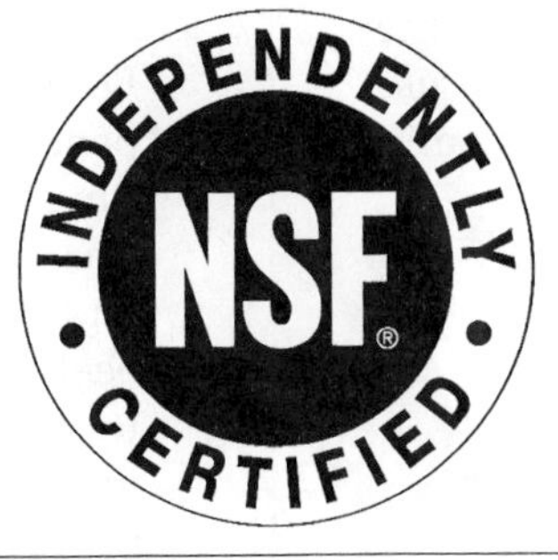

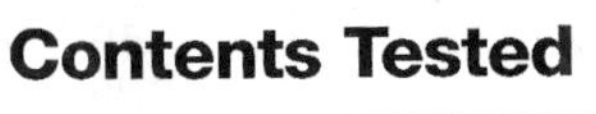

B

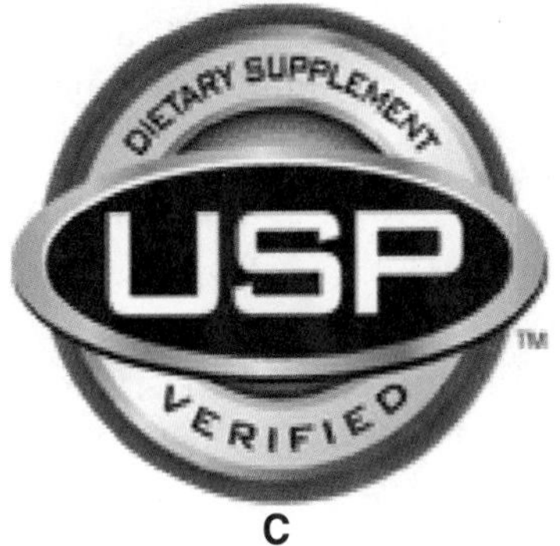

C

FIGURE **48-1** The certification marks signify that the dietary supplements to which their mark is affixed contain ingredients as listed on the label and that they were manufactured using good manufacturing practices, but they do not certify whether the products are safe and effective for the labeled use. (**A,** Used with permission from ConsumerLab.com; **B,** used with permission from NSF International; **C,** used with permission from the USP.)

testing dietary supplements, and the U.S. Pharmacopeia (USP) launched DSVP in 2001 and began testing products that year. In 2003 the **National Sanitation Foundation** (NSF) International began testing dietary supplements. Products that pass testing are eligible to bear the mark of approval from the testing agency (Figure 48-1). It is important to remember that the products are tested for labeled potency, good manufacturing practices, and contamination, but they are not tested for safety and efficacy or for manufacturer's claims on the label. Dietary supplement therapy, under the current legal standards, creates an ethical dilemma for nurses and other health care professionals. Licensed health care professionals have a moral and ethical responsibility to recommend only medicines that are proven to be safe and effective. They should be aware of a medicine's legal use versus its popular use, its potential for toxicity, and its potential for interactions with other medicines. Box 48-1 lists the factors to consider when recommending dietary supplements.

Box 48-1 ***Factors to Consider When Recommending Herbal Medicines and Other Dietary Supplements***

1. Diet supplements are not miraculous cure-alls. Most of those intended for therapeutic use are technically unapproved drugs. They may have been used for centuries, but substantial data on safety and efficacy of long-term use are often lacking.
2. Prospective consumers may be seriously misinformed about the value of certain diet supplements as a result of false advertising and unsubstantiated claims made by advocacy literature.
3. Diet supplements are generally mild medications and should not be endorsed for the treatment of human immunodeficiency virus infection, cancer, self-diagnosed heart disease, or other serious conditions.
4. Quality control of diet supplement products is often deficient in this country. Purchase them only from the most reliable producers. Purchase standardized products when possible.
5. Do not recommend diet supplement use by pregnant women, lactating mothers, infants, or young children without approval from the patient's health care provider.
6. Advise patients to cease taking a diet supplement immediately if adverse effects (e.g., allergy, stomach upsets, skin rashes, headache) occur.
7. Products containing many different ingredients such as herbs should be carefully examined to determine whether the ingredients are present in therapeutic amounts. Some contain only a few milligrams of each ingredient in quantities insufficient for any beneficial effect.
8. Be cautious in recommending any product that does not indicate, or permit calculation of, the quantity of individual ingredients contained in it.
9. The labels of dietary supplement products should also show the scientific name of the ingredients, the name and address of the actual manufacturer, a batch or lot number, the date of manufacture, and the expiration date.
10. Do not confuse herbal medicine, which employs therapeutic doses of botanical drugs, with homeopathy, which uses products containing few or no active ingredients.

Adapted from Tyler VE: What pharmacists should know about herbal remedies, *J Am Pharm Assoc (Wash)* NS36(1):29, 1996.

NURSING PROCESS *for Herbal and Diet Supplement Therapy*

Assessment

- Discuss specific dietary supplement products and the patient's reasons for using these products.
- Obtain a listing of the specific symptoms the patient is treating with the supplement products and details of whether the symptoms have improved (or worsened) since beginning therapy. Ask whether the use of supplement products has been shared with the patient's health care provider.
- Did anyone in particular recommend herbal products? If yes, what was the basis of the recommendations? Ask whether the patient's health care provider and other health team members know of the supplement products being self-administered.

- Obtain a detailed listing of all prescribed, over-the-counter (OTC), and supplemental products in use. Have any prescribed medications been discontinued in lieu of initiating supplements?
- What cultural or ethnic beliefs does the individual espouse?

Nursing Diagnoses

- Knowledge, deficient related to dietary supplement products (indications, side effects)
- Noncompliance, drug therapy (indication)

Planning

History of Symptoms. Examine data to determine the individual's understanding of the symptoms or the disease process for which the individual began taking supplements.

Medication History

- Check the history and physical (H&P) assessment by the health care provider to determine whether any supplement products are listed.
- Research supplement products being taken and identify drug interactions, actions, and side effects that may occur.
- Check the hospital policy regarding the administration and recording of the products. Because they are not medications, but rather are classified legally as dietary supplements, a food category, how are the orders for their use handled? Are they self-administered? If so, how often and in what quantity?

Cultural and Ethnic Beliefs. If cultural issues are involved in the use of the supplement products, research the belief system and ways the nurse can appropriately be involved in supporting the individual.

Implementation

- Perform detailed nursing assessments of the symptoms for which the products are being taken, including any side effects.
- Record data in the nursing notes regarding the use, response, or lack of response to the products.
- Label the front of the chart with a listing of supplement products being used in the event the physician does not have knowledge of their use.
- Discuss cultural and ethnic beliefs with the individual patient, and consult other members of the health care team regarding appropriate approaches for patient care and education.

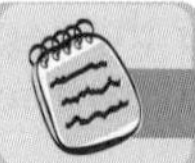

Patient Education and Health Promotion

Expectations of Therapy. Discuss the expectations of therapy with the patient and why self-treatment needs to be discussed with other members of the health care team. Emphasize to the patient that supplement products can and do interact with other medications.

Fostering Health Maintenance

- Discuss medication information and how it will benefit the course of treatment to produce an optimal response. Have the health care provider or pharmacist discuss implications of medications and products being used.
- Seek cooperation and understanding of the following points so that medication compliance is increased: name of medication, dosage, route and times of administration, side effects to expect, and side effects to report. The patient must understand not only prescribed medication data, but that of the supplement products as well. The individual must believe in the prescribed regimen in order for compliance to be enhanced.

Written Record. Enlist the patient's aid in developing and maintaining a written record of monitoring parameters (e.g., blood pressure, pulse, daily weight, degree of pain relief) (see Patient Self-Assessment Form in Appendix I). Complete the Premedication Data column for use as a baseline to track response to drug therapy. Ensure that the patient understands how to use the form and instruct the patient to take the completed form to follow-up visits. During follow-up visits, focus on issues that will foster adherence with the therapeutic interventions prescribed. The health care team members must understand that simply telling the patient not to take supplements may result in the patient's hiding the use of these products, creating myriad additional problems.

HERBAL THERAPY

Herbal medicine is as old as the human race. For thousands of years civilizations have depended on substances found in nature to treat illnesses. **Herbal medicines** are defined as natural substances of botanical or plant origin. Other names for herbal medicines are **botanicals, phytomedicine,** and **phytotherapy.**

Common name: aloe (al' oh)

- OTHER NAMES: aloe vera, salvia, burn plant
- BOTANICAL SOURCE: *Aloe barbadensis*
- PARTS USED: aloe gel: clear, jelly-like secretion obtained from the thin-walled, sticky cells of the inner portion of the leaf; aloe latex: cells just below the outer skin of the aloe plant

Actions

Two products derived from aloe plant leaves are aloe gel and aloe latex. Aloe gel (commonly known as aloe vera), is a gelatinous extract from the sticky cells lining the inner portion of the leaf. Aloe gel is composed of polysaccharides and lignin, salicylic acid, saponin, sterols, triterpenoids, and a variety of enzymes. Aloe gel may possibly inhibit bradykinin and histamine, reducing pain and itching. Aloe latex (resin), also known as aloins, contains pharmacologically active anthraquinone derivatives that, when taken orally, act as a laxative by irritating the intestinal lining, increasing peristalsis and fluid and electrolyte secretions.

Uses

Aloe has been used as a medicinal agent for more than 5000 years for a vast array of internal and external illnesses, including arthritis, colitis, the common cold, ulcers, hemorrhoids, seizures, and glaucoma. Aloe gel is the form most commonly used in the cosmetic and health food industries. Most recently, aloe gel has been marketed for topical use to treat pain, inflammation and itching, and as a healing agent for sunburn, skin ulcers, psoriasis, and frostbite. The FDA has reviewed studies of aloe gel and has not found adequate scientific evidence to support these claims. Therefore aloe gel is not classified as a drug, but is allowed to remain on the market as a cosmetic for topical use. It is frequently used as a coingredient in skin-care products, but the product labeling should not make therapeutic claims of the aloe gel because none have been substantiated through scientific studies.

Aloe latex contains anthraquinone derivatives that, when taken orally, act as a laxative. There is a concern, however, about carcinogenicity, so aloe latex has been removed from the pharmaceutical market because it is not proven to be safe and effective.

Aloe, as cited in the Bible, is a fragrant wood used as incense and is unrelated to aloe vera.

Availability

- *Aloe gel:* moisturizing lotion, shampoo, hair conditioner, gels, toothpaste, aloe juice for topical application. Capsules and tinctures are also available for oral use. There are no proven therapeutic effects from these products.
- *Aloe latex:* aloe juice drinks for catharsis; whole leaf aloe vera: juice

Side Effects

When applied to the skin, no adverse effects have been reported. When taken orally, aloe products may cause diarrhea due to anthraquinone content.

Drug Interactions

Diabetic Therapy. Monitor blood glucose levels closely due to claims that when taken orally aloe may have hypoglycemic effects.

Common name: black cohosh (koh' hawsh)

- OTHER NAMES: squawroot, black snakeroot, bugbane, bugwort
- BOTANICAL SOURCE: *Cimicifuga racemosa*
- PARTS USED: fresh and dried root

Actions

The active ingredients in black cohosh are complex triterpenes and flavonoids. It is thought that these agents have estrogen-like effects by suppressing release of luteinizing hormone and by binding to estrogen receptors in peripheral tissue.

Herbal Interactions

Black Cohosh

Hormone Replacement Therapy

- Women already receiving hormone replacement therapy (usually estrogen and progestin) to treat symptoms associated with menopause and to prevent osteoporosis should be cautious about receiving additional estrogenic effects from concurrent use of black cohosh.

Antihypertensive Therapy

- Black cohosh may cause added antihypertensive effects when taken with other antihypertensive agents. If black cohosh is being taken, monitor the blood pressure response to the cumulative effects. Take blood pressures in the supine and erect positions.

Uses

Black cohosh is used to reduce symptoms of premenstrual syndrome (PMS), dysmenorrhea, and menopause. Therapy is not recommended for longer than 6 months. Black cohosh should not be used in the first two trimesters of pregnancy because of its uterine-relaxing effects.

Availability

Elixirs, tablets, capsules.

Side Effect

Upset stomach is a rare side effect.

Comments

Do not confuse black cohosh with blue cohosh. Although blue cohosh is used as an antispasmodic and uterine stimulant to promote menstruation or labor, it is quite different and potentially more toxic than black cohosh. Beware of commercial products that contain both black and blue cohosh when only black cohosh is sought.

Common name: chamomile (kam' oh mile)

- OTHER NAMES: German or Hungarian chamomile: pin heads, chamomilla, genuine chamomile; Roman or English chamomile: ground apple, whig plant, common chamomile
- BOTANICAL SOURCE: *Matricaria recutita* (German or Hungarian chamomile); *Chamaemelum nobile* (Roman or English chamomile)
- PARTS USED: predominantly flower heads, but other aboveground parts also contain the volatile oils

Actions

Two herbs are known as chamomile: German and Roman chamomile. The therapeutic effects of chamomile derive from a complex mixture of different compounds. The antiinflammatory and antispasmodic effects come from a volatile oil containing matricin, bisabolol, and bisabololoxides A and B, and flavonoids such as apigenin and luteolin. Coumarins, herniarin, and umbelliferone exhibit antispasmodic properties. Chamazulene has also been shown to possess antiinflammatory and antibacterial properties.

Uses

Both chamomiles are used in herbalism and medicine; however, German chamomile is the species most commonly used in the United States and Europe, whereas Roman chamomile is favored in Great Britain. Chamomile is used as a digestive aid for bloating, an antispasmodic and antiinflammatory in the gastrointestinal (GI) tract, an antispasmodic for menstrual cramps, an antiinflammatory for skin irritation, and a mouthwash for minor mouth irritation or gum infections. Plant extracts are used in cosmetic and hygiene products in the form of ointments, lotions, and vapor baths for topical application. For internal use, chamomile is taken in the form of a strong tea.

Availability

German chamomile is available as ointment and gel in strengths of 3% to 10%. As a bath additive, 50 g is added to 1 L of water. For internal use as a tea: Pour 150 mg of boiling water over 3 g of chamomile (1 teaspoon = 1 g of chamomile), cover for 5 to 10 minutes, then strain.

Side Effects

Rare hypersensitivity reactions may occur in patients who are allergic to ragweed, asters, chrysanthemums, or daisies.

Drug Interactions

No clinically significant drug interactions have been reported with chamomile.

Common name: echinacea (ek ihn ace′ eah)

- OTHER NAMES: purple coneflower, coneflower, black sampson
- BOTANICAL SOURCE: *Echinacea angustifolia, E. purpurea,* and other related species
- PARTS USED: roots, rhizomes, aboveground parts

Actions

Echinacea is a nonspecific stimulator of the innate (nonspecific) immune system. It stimulates phagocytosis and effector cell activity. There is an increased release of tumor necrosis factors and interferons from macrophages and T lymphocytes, which increases the body's resistance to bacterial and viral infection. It may have antiinflammatory effects by inhibiting hyaluronidase, a potent inflammatory. Echinacea has no direct bactericidal or bacteriostatic effects.

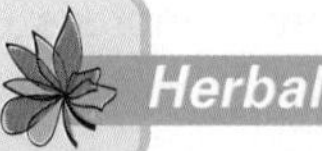

Herbal Interactions

Echinacea

- Echinacea may interfere with immunosuppressive therapy. Concurrent use with immunosuppressants (e.g., azathioprine, cyclosporine) is not recommended.

Uses

As a nonspecific immunostimulant, echinacea may prevent or treat viral respiratory tract infections such as the common cold or flu. Symptoms of the common cold may be reduced if echinacea is taken during the early, acute phase. It has also been used to treat urinary tract infections and may be applied externally to difficult-to-heal superficial wounds. Because of its immunomodulating effects, it is recommended that it not be used for more than 8 weeks at a time.

Availability

Echinacea is available as dried roots, teas, tinctures, and dry powder extracts.

Side Effects

Rare hypersensitivity reactions may occur in patients who are allergic to ragweed, asters, chrysanthemums, or daisies.

Comments

Because echinacea appears to be an immunomodulator, it is not recommended in patients with autoimmune diseases such as multiple sclerosis or lupus erythematosus, or in diseases affecting the immune system such as acquired immunodeficiency syndrome (AIDS).

Common name: ephedra (ee fed′ rah)

- OTHER NAMES: ma-huang, desert herb, ephedrine
- BOTANICAL SOURCE: *Ephedra sinica*
- PARTS USED: stems, rhizomes with roots

Action

The active ingredient in ephedra is the alkaloid ephedrine.

Uses

Ephedra was perhaps the first Chinese herbal medicine to be used in Western medicine. It is used as a bronchodilator for asthma, as a nasal decongestant, and as a central nervous system (CNS) stimulant. It is contraindicated in patients with heart conditions, hypertension, diabetes, and thyroid disease.

Side Effects

Ephedra elevates systolic and diastolic blood pressure and heart rate, causing palpitations. It also causes nervousness, headache, insomnia, and dizziness.

Herbal Interactions

Ephedra

Drugs That Enhance Toxic Effects

- Beta adrenergic–blocking agents (e.g., propranolol, timolol, atenolol, nadolol) and monoamine oxidase inhibitors (e.g., isocarboxazid, tranylcypromine, phenelzine).
- Excessive use may result in significant hypertension.
- Patients already receiving antihypertensive therapy should not use decongestants, such as ephedrine, because they raise blood pressure.

Methyldopa, Reserpine

- Frequent use of decongestants inhibits the antihypertensive activity of these agents. Concurrent therapy is not recommended.

Comments

- In recent years, popular culture has touted ephedra as a weight-loss product, an energy booster, an aphrodisiac, and a mental stimulant. There is no substantial evidence that supports these claims. It is commonly found in OTC weight-loss products. Deaths have been reported from its overuse and in those patients who may have underlying cardiovascular disease.
- Because ephedrine can serve as a precursor to the synthesis of illegal methamphetamine (speed), several states have passed laws regulating the sale of products containing ephedrine.
- Ephedrine is a medicine approved as safe and effective by the FDA and is readily available commercially. There are several other medicines that are safer, with fewer side effects (e.g., pseudoephedrine). There is really no need to use herbal ephedra for rational medical therapy.

Common name: feverfew (fee′ ver few)

- OTHER NAMES: featherfoil, flirtwort, bachelor's buttons
- BOTANICAL SOURCE: *Tanacetum parthenium*
- PARTS USED: leaves

Actions

There is significant controversy as to which ingredients in feverfew are therapeutic. Several sesquiterpene lactones are smooth-muscle relaxants in the walls of the cerebral blood vessels and may be the source of antimigraine activity. Feverfew has also been shown to inhibit the release of arachidonic acid, which serves as a substrate for production of prostaglandins and leukotrienes. Feverfew also inhibits release of serotonin and histamine from platelets and white cells, which helps prevent or control migraine headaches. Parthenolide, long thought to be the primary active ingredient, has been shown by one well-controlled study to be of minimal therapeutic effect. Perhaps additional compounds work synergistically with parthenolide to prevent migraine headaches.

Uses

Feverfew is used to reduce the frequency and severity of migraine headaches. Its antiinflammatory effects have also been used to treat rheumatoid arthritis.

Availability

Leaf powder for making tea; tablets.

Side Effects

Fresh feverfew leaves appear to be most effective in reducing the frequency and the pain associated with migraine headaches. Ulcerations of the oral mucosa and swelling of the lips and tongue have been reported by 7% to 12% of patients. Feverfew therapy should be discontinued if these lesions develop. Rare hypersensitivity reactions may occur in patients who are allergic to ragweed, asters, chrysanthemums, or daisies.

Herbal Interactions

Feverfew

Nonsteroidal Antiinflammatory Drugs (NSAIDs)

- Even though feverfew has antiinflammatory properties, it has been reported that concurrent use with NSAIDs may reduce the effectiveness of feverfew.

Anticoagulants

- Because feverfew reduces platelet aggregation, it should be used with extreme caution in patients who are also receiving platelet inhibitors (e.g., aspirin, ticlopidine, dipyridamole, clopidogrel), anticoagulants (e.g., warfarin), and herbal medicines (e.g., ginkgo, garlic, ginger, ginseng). Monitor patients for signs of bleeding.

Comments

The sesquiterpene lactone content is higher in the flowering tops than in leaves, stalks, and roots. The sesquiterpene lactone content diminishes with time and with exposure to light. Because the active ingredients are not known, there are no standards established for purity. Many products sold in the United States have been found to have low, variable quantities of sesquiterpene lactones.

Common name: garlic (gahr′ lik)

- OTHER NAMES: none
- BOTANICAL SOURCE: *Allium sativum*
- PARTS USED: bulb

Actions

Garlic contains a large variety of chemicals, making it difficult to determine which ingredients are responsible for its biologic effects. Alliin is a major component of garlic that, when crushed, is acted on by the enzyme allinase, to produce allicin. Allicin is thought to have the greatest pharmacologic activity, but it is also responsible for garlic's characteristic odor. A metabolite of allicin, ajoene (ah′ ho ween) is also thought to have biologic activity.

Uses

Garlic has been one of the most widely used herbal medicines for centuries. At various times, claims have been made for it curing almost all diseases as well as being an excellent aphrodisiac. It also has been widely used in folklore to ward off vampires, demons, and witches. Its most frequent use supported by scientific literature is in reducing cholesterol and triglycerides. Garlic has been shown to lower serum cholesterol by 9% to 12% and triglycerides by as much as 17%. Garlic also demonstrates antiplatelet activity similar to aspirin, and may also modestly lower high blood pressure.

Availability

Cloves, oil, enteric-coated tablets, capsules, elixirs.

Side Effects

The most common adverse effect of garlic is its characteristic taste and odor. Enteric-coated oral preparations minimize this problem. There are rare reports of patients developing nausea and vomiting, and burning of the mouth and stomach after ingesting various commercial preparations.

Comments

Fresh garlic is the most potent from a biologic standpoint, releasing the active ingredients in the mouth when chewed. The enzyme allinase, necessary for conversion of alliin to the active principles of allicin and ajoene, is inactivated in stomach acid. The active ingredients of garlic are easily destroyed by freeze-drying or heat-drying, and commercial products are of variable potency. Dried garlic preparations are most effective if they are enteric coated, allowing them to pass into the intestine before dissolution. These products tend to have less of the characteristic odor associated with garlic because the allicin is released in the intestine. One fresh clove daily or a daily dose of 8 mg of alliin from a product standardized for alliin content is the current dosage recommendation to treat hypercholesterolemia. Diet and exercise will aid the garlic in reducing high blood pressure and cholesterol.

Common name: ginger (gihn′ jer)

- OTHER NAMES: African ginger, Jamaica ginger, race ginger
- BOTANICAL SOURCE: *Zingiber officinale*
- PARTS USED: roots and rhizomes

Actions

The active ingredients in ginger roots and rhizomes are known as gingerols. They increase the rate of gastrointestinal motility, act as serotonin antagonists, and inhibit cyclooxygenase pathways.

Uses

Ginger has been used for centuries to alleviate nausea and vomiting from a variety of causes. It is thought to act as an antiemetic by increasing gastroduodenal motility and by blocking serotonin receptors that when stimulated may trigger nausea and vomiting. Ginger is possibly safe when used in pregnancy, and a few controlled studies indicate that it may reduce the frequency of morning sickness. The use of ginger in pregnancy is controversial, however, because it has never been thoroughly studied for safety in this patient population.

Ginger has also been shown to be modestly effective in reducing inflammation and pain in patients with rheumatoid arthritis, osteoarthritis, and muscle discomfort because it is a cyclooxygenase-2 (COX-2) inhibitor.

The rhizome is used as the source for the dried powder used in food preparation.

Availability

Powdered gingerroot; ginger tea made from gingerroot; tinctures. The dosages are quite variable, but it is recommended that doses not exceed 4 g daily.

Side Effects

Generally, ginger is quite well tolerated. There have been reports of heartburn, diarrhea, and irritation to the mouth and throat.

Herbal Interactions

Garlic

Anticoagulants

- Because garlic reduces platelet aggregation, it should be used with extreme caution in patients who are also receiving platelet inhibitors (e.g., aspirin, ticlopidine, dipyridamole, clopidogrel), anticoagulants (e.g., warfarin), and herbal medicines (e.g., ginkgo, ginger, feverfew, ginseng). Monitor patients for signs of bleeding

Herbal Interactions

Ginger

Anticoagulants

- Because ginger reduces platelet aggregation, it should be used with extreme caution in patients who are also receiving platelet inhibitors (e.g., aspirin, ticlopidine, dipyridamole, clopidogrel), anticoagulants (e.g., warfarin), and herbal medicines (e.g., garlic, ginkgo, ginseng, feverfew). Monitor for signs of bleeding.

Comments

Ginger is generally recognized as safe (GRS) when used in food preparation. The dosages used for nausea, vomiting, and analgesia are substantially higher and have not been proven to be safe or effective.

Common name: ginkgo (gihnk' ho)

- OTHER NAMES: maidenhair tree
- BOTANICAL SOURCE: *Ginkgo biloba*
- PARTS USED: green-picked leaves

Actions

The active ingredients in ginkgo leaves are flavonoids and terpenes. Because higher concentrations of these chemicals are necessary for biologic activity, the green-picked leaves are processed to form a concentrated ginkgo biloba extract (GBE). GBE is standardized to a potency of 24% flavonoids (primarily flavonoid glycosides and quercetin) and 6% terpenes (primarily composed of ginkgolides A, B, C, and J, and bilobalide). GBE is a smooth muscle relaxant and vasodilator that improves blood flow in arteries and capillaries. It may also be a free-radical scavenger, preventing endothelial cell damage. Ginkgolides inhibit platelet-activating factor, inhibiting platelet aggregation.

Uses

Ginkgo biloba extract is used primarily for increasing cerebral blood flow, particularly in geriatric patients. Conditions treated are short-term memory loss, headache, dizziness, tinnitus, and emotional instability with anxiety. Patients with Alzheimer's disease may show modest improvement in cognitive performance and social functioning. Other uses include improved walking distance in patients with intermittent claudication, improvement in erectile dysfunction secondary to antidepressant therapy, improved peripheral blood flow in patients with diabetes mellitus, and improved hearing in patients whose hearing is impaired secondary to poor circulation to the ears. Therapy must be continued for up to 6 months to assess optimal response.

Availability

40 mg GBE in liquid, tablets, and capsules. Dosages range from 120 to 240 mg of GBE twice daily.

Herbal Interactions

Ginkgo

Anticoagulants

- Because ginkgo reduces platelet aggregation, it should be used with extreme caution in patients who are also receiving platelet inhibitors (e.g., aspirin, ticlopidine, dipyridamole, clopidogrel), anticoagulants (e.g., warfarin), and herbal medicines (e.g., ginger, garlic, feverfew, ginseng). Monitor patients for signs of bleeding.

Side Effects

Large doses of GBE may cause mild restlessness, diarrhea, nausea, vomiting, and dizziness. Adverse effects may be minimized by slowly titrating the dose upward as tolerated.

Common name: ginseng (gihn' sehng)

- OTHER NAMES: aralia cinquefoil, five fingers, tartar root, red berry
- BOTANICAL SOURCE: *Panax ginseng* (Chinese or Korean ginseng)
- PARTS USED: root

Actions

Ginseng contains a large variety of chemicals, making it difficult to determine which components are responsible for its biologic effects. The ingredients believed to be responsible are triterpenoid saponins that are classified into panaxosides, ginsenosides, and chikusetsusaponins. Unfortunately, the literature is extremely difficult to interpret because of differences in composition between Asian and American ginseng species, different scientific terminologies for active ingredients, and the lack of well-controlled scientific studies.

Uses

Ginseng is not used to cure a disease but is an "adaptogen" in maintaining health. Current claims for ginseng are that it increases the body's resistance to stress, overcomes disease by building up defenses, and strengthens general vitality. It has also been used for centuries as an aphrodisiac. There is no scientific basis for its claims as an aphrodisiac and little scientific evidence as an adaptogen.

Availability

Teas, powders, capsules, tablets, liquids. There are no standardized methods of purity. Commercial ginseng extract products range from 100 to 600 mg standardized to a percent of ginsenosides.

Side Effects

Many adverse effects have been reported with the use of ginseng, but most are single case reports, and may be the pharmacologic effect of adulterants added to ginseng. Adverse effects most commonly attributed to ginseng are insomnia, diarrhea, and skin eruptions.

Comments

- Even though thousands of articles have been written lauding its praises, very few scientific studies have been completed on ginseng. Most of the literature is based on superstition and anecdotal reports. Many of the reports have been written by governments and companies making claims for financial gain. It is an herbal medicine that is commonly adulterated so it is difficult to know whether the results

Herbal Interactions

Ginseng

Anticoagulants

- Ginseng may affect platelet aggregation and blood coagulation. Ginseng should be used with extreme caution in patients who are also receiving platelet inhibitors (e.g., aspirin, ticlopidine, dipyridamole, clopidogrel), anticoagulants (e.g., warfarin), and herbal medicines (e.g., garlic, feverfew, ginger, ginkgo). Monitor for signs of bleeding.

Insulin

- Ginseng has been shown to raise insulin levels in laboratory animals. It may have the potential to induce hypoglycemia. Blood glucose levels of patients with type 1 or type 2 diabetes mellitus should be monitored closely if the patient insists on taking ginseng.

of studies are because of the ginseng content or the added ingredients.

- Siberian ginseng (*Eleutherococcus senticosus;* also known as eleuthero) is different than American or Asian ginseng and should not be substituted. It has been marketed as a cheaper form of ginseng, but is known to have many adulterants, and there are no scientific studies to support its claims as an immune system stimulant and enhancer of endurance.

Common name: goldenseal

- OTHER NAMES: yellow root, Indian dye, Indian paint, jaundice root
- BOTANICAL SOURCE: *Hydrastis canadensis*
- PARTS USED: rhizomes with root fibers

Actions

The active ingredients in goldenseal are contained in a group of plant alkaloids, the most active of which are hydrastine and berberine. Berberine gives the herb its characteristic golden color.

Uses

Goldenseal is popular in herbal medicine as an antiseptic and astringent, reducing inflammation of mucous membranes. It is used topically as a tea for treatment of canker sores, sore mouth, and cracked and bleeding lips. Goldenseal may have weak antibacterial properties and may stimulate the immune system to help fight viral upper respiratory infections such as a cold or flu. Goldenseal is sometimes marketed in combination with echinacea to ward off bouts of the common cold. No controlled studies have been completed to validate this combined therapy. In high doses, goldenseal may have uterine stimulant effects and should not be taken during pregnancy. In recent years there has been a common myth that goldenseal, when taken as tea, or put into urine, will mask assays for street drugs (see Comments).

Availability

Powder for tea, tincture, fluid extract, freeze-dried root.

Side Effects

The alkaloids in goldenseal are not absorbed to any extent when swallowed, producing no systemic effects. High doses may cause nausea, vomiting, diarrhea, and CNS stimulation.

Comments

One of the more recent popular uses for goldenseal is the masking of the presence of illicit drugs in urine samples. Contrary to popular belief, goldenseal does not prevent detection of drugs by urine tests, nor does it "flush" illicit drugs from the body. When goldenseal is present, the urine takes on a distinctive dark amber or brown color.

Drug Interactions

There are no drug interactions of clinical significance.

Common name: green tea

- OTHER NAMES: Chinese tea, teagreen
- BOTANICAL SOURCE: *Camellia sinensis*, evergreen shrub
- PARTS USED: leaf, leaf bud, and stem

Actions

When steamed, green tea leaves and stems yield high concentrations of polyphenols such as gallic acid and catechins and caffeine, which are thought to be the active ingredients of green tea. Mechanisms of action are unknown. Green tea also contains B vitamins and ascorbic acid.

Uses

Green tea has been used as a very common beverage in Asian cultures for centuries. The caffeine produces CNS stimulation and is thought to improve cognitive performance. It raises blood pressure, heart rate, and contractility, and acts as a diuretic. Green tea has been shown to lower cholesterol, triglycerides, and low-density lipoprotein (LDL) and raise high-density lipoprotein (HDL). There is some evidence that green tea might reduce the risk of bladder, esophageal, and pancreatic cancers, and reduce or prevent the onset of parkinsonism. Green tea is also used to treat diarrhea.

Availability

Green tea is readily available in premade tea bags and in bulk form for brewing. Moderate consumption of 1 to 4 cups daily appears to provide therapeutic benefits. Consumption of 5 or more cups daily has significantly more side effects that are associated with excessive caffeine.

Herbal Interactions

Green Tea

Increased Therapeutic and Toxic Effects

- The following drugs, when used concurrently with green tea, may significantly increase the stimulant effects and the adverse effects of the caffeine in green tea by inhibiting its metabolism: ephedrine, cimetidine, disulfiram, grapefruit juice, monoamine oxidase (MAO) inhibitors (tranylcypromine, phenelzine, isocarboxazid), mexiletine, oral contraceptives, quinolones (e.g., ciprofloxacin, enoxacin, norfloxacin, sparfloxacin), theophylline, and verapamil.

Beta-Adrenergic Agents (e.g., Albuterol, Metoproterenol, Terbutaline)

- Concurrent consumption of green tea (caffeine) with beta agonists can increase the heart rate and the potential for dysrhythmias. Use with caution. Discontinue green tea consumption if palpitations develop.

Ephedra

- Concurrent consumption of ephedra and the caffeine in green tea results in significantly more stimulant effects with greater possibility of adverse effects.

Warfarin

- Concurrent consumption of large quantities of green tea with warfarin may antagonize the anticoagulant effects of warfarin. Monitor the patient's International Normalized Ratio (INR) for therapeutic effect of warfarin.

Side Effects

Many of the adverse effects of green tea are an extension of the pharmacologic effects of caffeine: anxiety, nervousness, headache, diuresis, insomnia, tremor, irritability, palpitations, and dysrhythmias. The chronic use of high quantities can produce tolerance, habituation, and psychologic dependence. The abrupt discontinuation may cause withdrawal headaches, irritation, and nervousness.

Common name: saw palmetto

- OTHER NAMES: palmetto scrub, sabal, American dwarf palm tree, cabbage palm
- BOTANICAL SOURCE: *Serenoa repens*
- PARTS USED: seeds

Actions

The chemical constituents that are responsible for the pharmacologic activity of saw palmetto have not been fully identified. Ingredients within saw palmetto act as an androgen hormone inhibitor by inhibiting the enzyme 5-alpha reductase. The conversion of testosterone to dihydrotestosterone (DHT) is catalyzed by 5-alpha reductase. Reduction in DHT levels reduces the hyperplastic cell growth associated with prostatic hyperplasia.

Uses

Saw palmetto is used to treat the symptoms associated with benign prostatic hyperplasia (BPH), to reduce the risks associated with urinary retention, and to minimize the need for surgery associated with BPH. (See Chapter 41 for further discussion of the treatment of BPH.)

Availability

Saw palmetto extract is standardized to contain 85% to 95% fatty acids and sterols. Saw palmetto is sold in the United States only as a dietary supplement and is not available as an OTC or prescription product. The usual dose is 160 mg of saw palmetto extract twice daily.

Side Effects

Upset stomach is a rare side effect. High doses have been reported to cause diarrhea.

Comments

- Although saw palmetto is marketed to promote hair regrowth in men, there is no clinical evidence to support the claim of the herb preventing hair loss or promoting regrowth.
- Saw palmetto tea made from the berries is ineffective because the active ingredients are not water soluble.

Drug Interactions

Finasteride. The mechanism of action of both finasteride and saw palmetto is inhibition of the enzyme 5-alpha reductase. The two drugs should not be used concurrently.

Common name: St. John's wort

- OTHER NAMES: klamath weed, hardhay, amber
- BOTANICAL SOURCE: *Hypericum perforatum*
- PARTS USED: fresh buds and flowers

Actions

The active ingredients of St. John's wort are unknown. Studies indicate that it is a reuptake inhibitor, prolonging the effect of serotonin, dopamine, and norepinephrine.

Uses

St. John's wort is used orally to treat mild depression and to heal wounds.

Availability

St. John's wort is available as powder, tablets, capsules, and liquid. It is also found in semisolid preparations for topical use. It is commonly standardized to hypericin content, but it has been shown that hypericin content is not related to antidepressant effect, so this standard is of little value. Therapeutic effects are variable between various products and different batches of the same product. Because the therapeutic ingredients are unknown, there is no effective standardization for St. John's wort products. The average

Herbal Interactions

St. John's Wort

Serotonin Stimulants

- Selective serotonin reuptake inhibitors (e.g., paroxetine, sertraline, fluoxetine), tricyclic antidepressants (e.g., amitriptyline, imipramine, doxepin), monoamine oxidase inhibitors (e.g., isocarboxazid, phenelzine, tranylcypromine), and dopamine agonists (e.g., bromocriptine) may induce a serotonin syndrome when taken concurrently with St. John's wort. Patients should contact their health care provider immediately if they start noticing symptoms of this syndrome (see Side Effects).

daily dose for internal use is 2 to 4 g of herb or 0.2 to 1 mg of total hypericin.

Side Effects

St. John's wort may cause photosensitivity. Patients should discontinue the herbal medicine and report excessive sunburn, pruritus, and edema immediately.

There is concern about St. John's wort contributing to the development of serotonin syndrome. The seriousness of this adverse effect warrants that patients be informed of this complication of therapy. Serotonin syndrome may result from taking two or more drugs that affect serotonin levels. Symptoms associated with the syndrome are confusion, agitation, shivering, fever, diaphoresis, nausea, diarrhea, muscle spasms, and tremor. These symptoms have a sudden onset, somewhat like a panic attack, and may progress to a coma. The syndrome is life threatening. When switching between serotonergic agents and St. John's wort, a 5- to 7-day washout period is recommended (see Drug Interactions).

Comments

- Folklore tells us that St. John's wort received its name because its golden flower is particularly abundant on June 24, the day celebrated as the birthday of John the Baptist.
- St. John's wort products are light and heat sensitive. Exposure to light and excessive heat for 2 weeks will alter the content of the chemical constituents.
- Depression is a serious, potentially fatal illness. It is important that patients discuss their symptoms and the use of St. John's wort before starting self-treatment.

Common name: valerian

- OTHER NAMES: amantilla, setwall, heliotrope, vandal root
- BOTANICAL SOURCE: *Valeriana officinalis*
- PARTS USED: dried roots and rhizomes

Actions

The chemical constituents that are responsible for the therapeutic effects of valerian have not been fully identified.

Uses

Valerian has been used for more than 1000 years as a mild tranquilizer. Valerian is used for restlessness and may promote sleep.

Availability

Valerian may be administered in the form of a tea, tincture, extract, tablets, or capsules. Some preparations are standardized for valepotriate content, but it is not known whether these compounds are the active ingredients.

Side Effects

Side effects with valerian are rare. Chronic users may experience excitability, uneasiness, and headache.

Comments

Because of similarity in names, valerian and Valium have sometimes been confused. Valerian is a mild tranquilizer, whereas Valium is the brand name of a much more potent tranquilizer more appropriately known by the generic name of diazepam. Diazepam is a member of the benzodiazepines (see the Index).

Drug Interactions

No clinically significant drug interactions have been reported, but concurrent use of other medicines with sedative properties such as antihistamines, benzodiazepines, alcohol, and barbiturates should be avoided.

OTHER DIETARY SUPPLEMENTS

Common name: coenzyme Q_{10}

- OTHER NAMES: CoQ_{10}, ubiquinone
- SOURCES: commercial sources: fermentation of cane sugar and beets using special strains of yeast; natural sources: beef, soy oil, sardines, peanuts

Description and Actions

Coenzyme Q_{10} is a provitamin found in every living cell and is essential for energy production in the mitochondria. Organs with high energy requirements contain highest levels of CoQ_{10}: heart muscle, liver, kidney, and pancreas. Human cells synthesize CoQ_{10} from the amino acid tyrosine in a series of chemical reactions that also require folic acid, niacin, riboflavin, and pyridoxine. A deficiency of any of these vitamins may result in a deficiency in CoQ_{10}. Deficiency of CoQ_{10} also results from diminished dietary intake, impairment of biosynthesis, and increased usage of CoQ_{10} by the body.

Uses

CoQ_{10} has been used to treat a variety of disorders. Its primary use is as an adjunctive therapy for chronic heart failure. It has also been tested with varying degrees of success in other cardiovascular diseases (e.g., ischemic heart disease [angina], hypertension, dysrhythmias, toxin-induced cardiomyopathy, surgery for heart valve replacement), cancer (breast, lung, prostate, pancreatic, colon), muscular dystrophy, periodontal disease, and acquired immunodeficiency syndrome (AIDS). Additional studies are required to determine degree of therapeutic benefit in these diseases.

Availability

Powder-filled capsules, tablets, liquid-filled gel capsules, chewable wafers, intraoral spray.

Dosage

Prevention of deficiency: 30 to 60 mg daily; treatment of deficiency: 100 to 200 mg daily. Administer with meals that contain some fat to enhance absorption. Doses more than 100 mg daily should be divided into two or three dosages.

The safety of CoQ_{10} in pregnancy and lactation has not been established and its use is not recommended.

Side Effects

No serious adverse effects have been reported. Less than 1% of patients describe symptoms of nausea, upset stomach, diarrhea, and appetite suppression. Doses of 100 mg or greater taken at bedtime may cause mild insomnia. Patients taking 300 mg daily for extended periods demonstrate mild elevations of liver e[nzymes] but no cases of hepatotoxicity have been reported.

Herbal Interactions

Coenzyme Q_{10}

HMG-CoA, Gemfibrozil

- These antilipemic agents appear to reduce total body levels of CoQ_{10} by inhibiting its synthesis by the body. The clinical significance of this interaction is not known at this time.

Beta-Adrenergic Blocking Agents

- Beta-adrenergic blocking agents appear to reduce total body levels of CoQ_{10} by inhibiting its synthesis. The clinical significance of this interaction is not known at this time.

Insulin, Oral Hypoglycemic Agents

- CoQ_{10} supplementation has been reported to reduce insulin requirements in diabetes mellitus. Oral hypoglycemic agents (tolazamide, glyburide, acetohexamide) have also been reported to reduce total body levels of CoQ_{10}; therefore patients with diabetes who are taking CoQ_{10} require close monitoring of blood glucose with adjustment in dosages of antidiabetic medicines as needed.

Warfarin

- The chemical structure of CoQ_{10} and vitamin K are quite similar. There are reports that administration of CoQ_{10} to patients receiving warfarin causes a decrease in the INR. Monitor the INR closely for therapeutic effect.

Common name: creatine

- OTHER NAMES: creatine monohydrate
- SOURCES: natural sources: meat and fish (muscle)

Description and Actions

Creatine is a naturally occurring, energy-producing substance in the human body that is synthesized from amino acids. It plays a key role in providing energy to muscles for short duration, high-intensity exercise. About 95% of the body's creatine is in skeletal muscle, of which 60% is in the form of creatine phosphate. Muscle adenosine triphosphate (ATP) provides immediate energy for muscle contraction, after which it is replenished by creatine phosphate. The rapidity with which creatine phosphate is replenished depends on the amount of free creatine available.

Uses

Creatine is used as an ergonomic aid (i.e., a performance-enhancing substance). Creatine supplementation is thought to enhance muscle performance for short bouts of repeated, intense exercise such as sprinting, jumping, and power lifting. Increasing creatine phosphate stores enhances rapid replenishment of ATP, and increased supplies of free creatine shorten muscle recovery time by rebuilding depleted creatine phosphate stores faster. Many small studies have attempted to document the benefits of creatine supplementation, but with mixed results. At best, some studies indicate a 1% to 3% improvement in performance for brief periods.

Small clinical studies also indicate that patients with heart failure and muscular dystrophy might benefit from creatine supplementation by preserving energy stores in the myocardium and skeletal muscle, respectively. Additional studies are needed to assess long-term benefits of creatine therapy in these and other conditions.

Availability

Powder, candy, gum, and liquid. It is often combined with other supplements for "energy."

Dosage

1. A loading dose of 5 to 6 g four times daily for 5 to 7 days, followed by doses of 2 g per day to maintain elevated creatine concentrations in the muscle

OR

2. 3 g per day for 28 days.

   NOTE:

- It is recommended that at least eight 8-ounce glasses of water be consumed daily while taking creatine supplements.

- Creatine supplementation should be avoided by people who have impaired renal function or who are taking potentially nephrotoxic medicines.
- The safety of creatine in pregnancy and lactation has not been established and use is not recommended.

Side Effects

No serious adverse effects have been reported, but long-term studies have not been completed that might document adverse effects. Creatine causes weight gain of 3 to 6 pounds because of water retention. Other side effects of creatine may include muscle cramping, dehydration, and GI bloating and diarrhea.

Drug Interactions

No drug interactions have been reported.

Common name: gamma-hydroxybutyrate (GHB)

OTHER NAMES: Georgia home boy (GHB), liquid ecstasy, salty water, many others

Description and Actions

GHB occurs naturally in the brain, kidneys, heart, and skeletal muscle. It is a metabolite of gamma aminobutyric acid (GABA), an inhibitory neurotransmitter. A wide variety of physiologic responses occur when GHB receptors are stimulated, including dopamine release, growth hormone release, and induction of sleep.

Uses

In the late 1980s, GHB was marketed and sold in the health food industry as a "growth hormone stimulator" to help bodybuilders promote muscle mass and maintain weight, and as an OTC sedative. The drug was banned by the FDA in 1990 after several reports of adverse reactions in individuals using nutritional and weight-loss supplements containing GHB. Despite the FDA ban, GHB continues to be marketed as a dietary supplement. Home manufacturing kits can be purchased and recipes are readily available on Internet websites.

GHB is usually abused for its intoxicating, sedative, and euphoric properties. GHB is an increasingly popular drug of abuse, particularly at rave parties where it is used as a euphoriant and as a "date rape" drug that is added to alcoholic drinks. Like alcohol, GHB's intoxicating effects begin 10 to 20 minutes after ingestion. The effects typically last up to 4 hours, depending on the dose. In progressively higher doses, the sedative effects may progress from sleep to coma to death. As with other commonly abused substances, repeated exposure leads to reinforcement, tolerance, and dependence. Dependence may be manifested by withdrawal symptoms such as the need to continue to take the drug, anxiety, insomnia, and abnormal thinking.

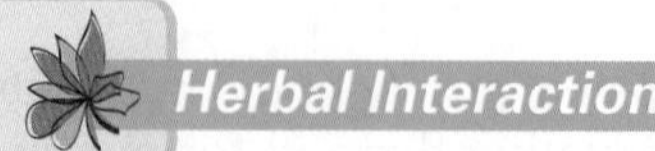

Herbal Interactions

Gamma-hydroxybutyrate

Drugs That Increase Toxic Effects

- Alcohol, antihistamines, analgesics, anesthetics, tranquilizers, antidepressants, valproic acid, phenytoin, and sleep aids will increase the sedative-hypnotic effects of GHB.

GHB is available as a prescription product (sodium oxybate, Xyrem) for treating a small population of patients with narcolepsy who experience episodes of cataplexy, a condition characterized by weak or paralyzed muscles. Because of safety concerns associated with the use of the drug, sodium oxybate is a Schedule III controlled substance and the distribution of Xyrem is tightly restricted. The medicine is to be used only at bedtime because it induces sleep very quickly.

Side Effects

Adverse effects related to GHB ingestion are highly variable among individuals, possibly relating to contaminating chemicals from home manufacturing kits. A wide range of effects have been reported, including impairment of judgment, aggression, and hallucinations, but those that are potentially life threatening are vomiting (with aspiration into the lungs), respiratory depression, bradycardia, and hypotension.

Common name: lycopene

SOURCES: natural: tomatoes, watermelon, pink grapefruit

Description and Actions

Lycopene is a carotenoid, a family of more than 50 nutrients from yellow, red, and orange plant pigments that act as antioxidants to protect the body against free radicals (unstable molecules that are released when the body uses oxygen).

Uses

There is some evidence to suggest that diets high in lycopene may reduce the risk of prostate cancer (and possibly lung, colon, and breast cancer). Small studies also indicate that the antioxidant properties have a lowering effect on LDL cholesterol and can protect against heart attack and stroke. Lycopene may also help prevent ophthalmic conditions such as macular degeneration and cataracts.

Availability

Research indicates that lycopene in tomatoes can be absorbed more efficiently by the body if processed into tomato juice, sauce, paste, and ketchup. Most products are sold as carotenoid complex containing natural tomato powder and tomato extract.

Dosage

Optimal dosages of lycopene have not been established. Analysis of major studies indicate that 5 to 10 servings per week of tomato-based sauces and other products (juices, extracts) may have a protective effect against developing prostate cancer. Tablets: a common dosage is 1 to 15 mg tablet two or three times daily with meals.

Side Effects

No serious adverse effects have been reported.

Drug Interactions

No drug interactions have been reported.

Common name: melatonin

OTHER NAMES: sleep hormone, MEL, MLT

Description and Actions

Melatonin is a human hormone synthesized from serotonin and secreted by the pineal gland. Its secretion is increased by dark and suppressed by light through the retina.

Uses

Melatonin is best known as a sleep aid and treatment for jet lag. It may also be helpful in patients withdrawing from benzodiazepine therapy. Melatonin has also been recommended as an antiaging medicine, but good clinical studies do not support this claim.

Availability

Tablets: 200 mcg, 1, 1.3, 2, 3 mg; liquid: 1 mg/mL.

Dosage

- *Insomnia:* 1 to 3 mg about 30 minutes before going to bed. Drowsiness develops within 30 to 40 minutes, and lasts about 4 hours.
- *Jet lag prevention:* 1 to 3 mg at bedtime on the day before travel, and 1 to 3 mg for the first 2 to 3 days after arrival. Stay awake during the daytime hours after arrival to help adjust to changes in time zones.

NOTE: The safety of melatonin in children and during pregnancy and lactation has not been established and use is not recommended.

Side Effects

Drowsiness, Sedation, Lethargy. Because melatonin causes drowsiness, people who work around machinery, drive a car, pour and give medicines, or perform other duties in which they must remain mentally alert should not take melatonin while working.

Paradoxical Response. Occasionally melatonin causes a paradoxical reaction such as agitation and insomnia. Provide supportive care and safety during these responses. Assess the level of excitement and deal calmly with the individual. During periods of excitement, protect the patient from harm and provide for physical channeling of energy (e.g., walking). See a change in the medication order.

Herbal Interactions

Melatonin

CNS Depressants

- Melatonin may add to CNS depression caused by alcohol, benzodiazepines, sleep aids, and other sedative-hypnotics. Do not administer melatonin to patients already receiving any of these medications without health care provider approval.

Common name: policosanol

OTHER NAMES: polycosanol, N-octacosanol, octacosyl alcohol, octacosanol, wheat germ oil

Description and Actions

Policosanol is a plant sterol that contains a mixture of waxy-type alcohols derived from plant sources including sugarcane and wheat germ oil. The alcohols that comprise policosanol are primarily octacosanol, tetracosanol, hexacosanol, heptacosanol, nonacosanol, triacosanol, dotriacontanol, and tetratriacontanol. Policosanol appears to lower cholesterol levels by inhibiting hepatic cholesterol synthesis, and by increasing the degradation of LDL cholesterol. Policosanol also reduces platelet aggregation but does not seem to significantly affect coagulation time.

Uses

Plant sterols are included in the National Cholesterol Education Program guidelines as part of the Therapeutic Lifestyle Changes (TLC) program. Orally, policosanol is used to treat dyslipidemia, lowering LDL cholesterol 17% to 27% and increasing HDL 7% to 10%. It has no effect on triglycerides. Clinical studies indicate that policosanol has similar efficacy in treating dyslipidemias as lower doses of the statins. As a platelet inhibitor, policosanol is used to treat intermittent claudication in patients with peripheral artery disease and myocardial ischemia in patients with coronary heart disease.

Availability

10 and 20 mg tablets

Dosage

5 to 10 mg two times daily in a product containing at least 60% octacosanol. Two months of therapy may be required to see significant changes in cholesterol levels. Doses of 40 mg daily do not appear to have added benefit.

Side Effects

No serious adverse effects have been reported. Only mild side effects such as nervousness, headache, diarrhea, and insomnia were reported. In long-term studies of 2 to 4 years, adverse effects occurred in less than 1% of patients. Weight loss, excessive urination, and insomnia were reported.

Drug Interactions

Aspirin, Warfarin, Heparin, Clopidogrel, Ticlopidine, Pentoxyphyline. The blood-thinning properties of policosanol may enhance the anticoagulant effects of these agents. Use with extreme caution and monitor closely for bruising and bleeding.

Garlic, Ginkgo, High-Dose Vitamin E. The blood-thinning properties of policosanol may enhance the blood-thinning effects of these agents. Use with extreme caution and monitor closely for bruising and bleeding.

Common name: S-adenosylmethionine (SAM-e)

OTHER NAMES: Sammy, SAM, ademetionine

Description and Actions

SAM-e is a naturally occurring substance found in all cells of the human body, particularly in the brain and liver. It is produced from adenosine triphosphate, an energy-producing compound, and methionine, an amino acid. SAM-e is involved in a wide range of essential biochemical reactions including synthesis, activation, and metabolism of hormones, neurotransmitters, proteins, and phospholipids, and in the deactivation of toxic substances.

Uses

As a supplement, SAM-e has been proposed for treating depression, osteoarthritis, and fibromyalgia. It is thought that SAM-e may have a dopaminergic effect in treating depression, but study results have been highly variable and inconclusive. In small studies for the treatment of osteoarthritis, SAM-e has been compared with NSAIDs (i.e., ibuprofen, naproxen, indomethacin) and placebo, and showed mild symptomatic improvement after 2 weeks. Other small studies suggest possible benefit in relieving symptoms associated with liver disease (e.g., chronic fatigue) and fibromyalgia (e.g., pain, depression, morning stiffness). SAM-e is relatively expensive, so other more conventional treatments of osteoarthritis and depression for several weeks are warranted before considering courses of SAM-e treatment.

Availability

A variety of tablet and capsule dosage forms are available, but it is recommended that the enteric forms that dissolve in the intestines (not the stomach) are more effective. There are two forms of SAM-e: the preferred form is S-adenosylmethionine 1,4 butanedisulfonate (sulfate form) over the toluensulfonate (tosylate) form. There are cases of misleading labeling; for example, 400 mg SAM-e tosylate-disulfate actually contains only 200 mg or less of the preferred sulfate form.

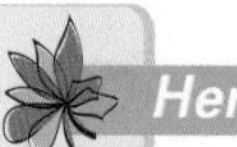

Herbal Interactions

S-Adenosylmethionine

Antidepressants (Tricyclic Antidepressants, SSRIs, MAO Inhibitors)

- SAM-e may interfere with the actions of these antidepressants or magnify their side effects. Combined use of antidepressants and SAM-e should be recommended only by a health care provider.

Levodopa

- It is reported that SAM-e may reduce some of the side effects of levodopa used to treat parkinsonism, but it is also felt that SAM-e may reduce the beneficial effects of levodopa in the treatment of parkinsonism over time.

Dosage

400 mg three or four times daily is recommended. Patients should start with lower dosages and work up to avoid mild stomach distress.

NOTE:

- Do not administer to patients diagnosed with manic depression. SAM-e has been reported to trigger manic episodes in patients with bipolar disease.
- The safety of SAM-e in pregnancy and lactation and in children has not been established and use is not recommended.

Side Effects

No serious adverse effects have been reported. Mild stomach distress has been reported when starting doses at 400 mg three or four times daily.

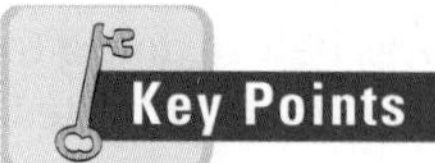

Key Points

- Herbal therapies are as old as the human race. Herbal medicines are defined as those natural substances derived from botanical or plant origin.
- Over the past two decades we have witnessed a tremendous resurgence in the popularity of self-care and alternative therapies, including acupuncture, aromatherapy, homeopathy, vitamin therapy, and herbal therapy. Some of the more than 250 herbal medicines may be beneficial, but unfortunately, the whole field of herbal therapy is fraught with false claims, lack of standardization, and adulteration and misbranding of products.
- Dietary supplement therapy under the current legal standards creates an ethical dilemma for nurses and other health care professionals. Licensed health care professionals have a moral and ethical responsibility to recommend only medicines that are proven to be safe and effective. Regarding dietary supplements, including herbal medicines, the health care professional should be aware of their legal uses versus their popular uses; their potential for toxicity; and their potential for interaction with other medicines.

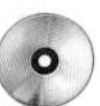

Go to your Companion CD-ROM for Appendices, an Audio Glossary, animations, Drug Dosage Calculators, customizable Patient Self-Assessment forms, and Review Questions for the NCLEX® Examination.

evolve Be sure to visit the companion Evolve site at http://evolve.elsevier.com/Clayton for WebLinks and additional online resources.

MEDICATION SAFETY REVEIW

CRITICAL THINKING QUESTIONS

1. Discuss the pros and cons of allowing a patient to use herbal products for self-treatment of such things as premenstrual syndrome (black cohosh), especially if the woman is using an estrogen/progestin replacement therapy hormone as well. What if the individual also has hypertension?
2. What recommendations should a nurse make to an immunocompromised patient who asks you about taking echinacea as an antiinflammatory "for my arthritis."
3. Research the law in your state. What does it say about the use of ephedrine?
4. What health teaching would need to be done for a patient taking NSAIDs and feverfew concurrently?
5. Discuss herbal products listed in this chapter that interact with anticoagulants.

CONTENT REVIEW QUESTIONS

1. Saw palmetto is used to treat:
   1. gastrointestinal symptoms.
   2. cholesterol.
   3. benign prostatic hyperplasia.
   4. rheumatoid arthritis.
2. Coenzyme Q_{10} is used primarily as adjunctive therapy for:
   1. chronic heart failure.
   2. insomnia.
   3. depression.
   4. antiviral treatment of human immunodeficiency virus (HIV).
3. Melatonin has become best known for use for/as:
   1. euphoriant.
   2. prostate cancer.
   3. colds.
   4. sleep alterations.
4. SAM-e should not be used in patients diagnosed with:
   1. fibromyalgia.
   2. manic depression.
   3. osteoarthritis.
   4. eating disorders.
5. Policosanol is used to treat which of the following?
   1. Hypertension
   2. Dyslipidemia
   3. Ulcers
   4. Viral infections
6. Goldenseal will mask the presence of drugs in urine tests.
   1. True
   2. False
7. Which of the following is used to treat mild depression?
   1. St. John's wort
   2. Goldenseal
   3. Green tea
   4. Saw palmetto

CHAPTER

49 Substance Abuse

evolve http://evolve.elsevier.com/Clayton

Chapter Content

Objectives

1. Differentiate among the key terms associated with substance abuse.
2. Explore biologic, psychological, and sociocultural models that influence the assessment and treatment of substance abuse.
3. Describe the different types of screening tools used to assess alcohol and substance abuse.
4. Cite the responsibilities of professionals who suspect substance abuse by a colleague.
5. Explain the primary long-term goals in the treatment of substance abuse.
6. Study the withdrawal symptoms and approaches to treatment and relapse prevention for major substances that are commonly abused.

Key Terms

substance abuse
impairment
dependence
addiction
illicit substance
intoxication

DEFINITIONS OF SUBSTANCE ABUSE

The Diagnostic and Statistical Manual of Mental Disorders (DSM-IV-TR) defines substance-related disorders as those that arise from (1) taking a drug of abuse, (2) the side effects of a medication, and (3) toxin exposure. The DSM-IV-TR groups substances of abuse into 11 categories (Box 49-1). Many other medications taken for therapeutic purposes can induce Substance-Related Disorders as a side effect, especially when large doses of the medications are taken (Box 49-2). Symptoms usually disappear when the dosage is lowered or the medication is stopped. Volatile substances are classified as "inhalants" if they are used for the purpose of becoming intoxicated, but are defined as "toxins" if exposure is accidental or part of intentional poisoning.

Box 49-1 ***Substances of Abuse***

- Alcohol (ethanol)
- Amphetamine or similarly acting sympathomimetics
- Caffeine
- Cannabis (marijuana)
- Cocaine
- Hallucinogens
- Inhalants
- Nicotine
- Opioids
- Phencyclidine (PCP) or similarly acting arylcyclohexylamines
- Sedatives, hypnotics, and anxiolytics

From the American Psychiatric Association: *Diagnostic and statistical manual of mental disorders,* ed 4, Washington, DC, 2000, American Psychiatric Association.

Box 49-2 ***Substances Whose Side Effects May Induce Substance Abuse***

- Anesthetics
- Analgesics
- Anticholinergic agents
- Anticonvulsants
- Antihistamines
- Antihypertensive and cardiovascular medications
- Antimicrobial medications
- Antiparkinsonian medications
- Chemotherapeutic agents
- Corticosteroids
- Gastrointestinal medications
- Muscle relaxants
- Nonsteroidal antiinflammatory agents
- Antidepressants

From the American Psychiatric Association: *Diagnostic and statistical manual of mental disorders,* ed 4, Washington, DC, 2000, American Psychiatric Association; and US Department of Health and Human Services, Substance Abuse and Mental Health Services Administration: *2001 National Household Survey on Drug Abuse (NHSDA),* available at www.samhsa.gov/oas/nhsda/2k1nhsda.

Impairments in cognition or mood are the most common symptoms associated with toxic substances, although anxiety, hallucinations, delusions, or seizures also can occur. The symptoms usually disappear when exposure stops, but resolution of symptoms may take up to several months of treatment.*

*American Psychiatric Association: Diagnostic and statistical manual of mental disorders, ed 4, Washington, D.C., 2000, American Psychiatric Association.

SUBSTANCES OF ABUSE

Substance abuse is defined as the periodic purposeful use of a substance that leads to clinically significant impairment. The **impairment** results in failure to fulfill major obligations at work, school, or home (e.g., absenteeism, poor work performance, neglect of responsibilities); places the person in physically hazardous situations (e.g., operating a vehicle or machinery when impaired); and creates legal problems (e.g., arrests for intoxication, disorderly conduct) or social problems that are aggravated by the substance (e.g., physical fights, spousal arguments). If substance abuse behavior is not stopped, substance abuse may lead to another more serious medical condition known as substance **dependence** (commonly known as **addiction**) that includes symptoms of overwhelming compulsive use, tolerance, and withdrawal on discontinuation. A phrase that characterizes chemical dependency is "using a substance to live and living to use." The amount of drug exposure and the frequency of use necessary to develop dependence are unknown and highly individual, based on the pharmacology of the drug, emotional condition, heredity, and environmental factors. A term frequently associated with substance abuse is **illicit substance**—any chemical or mixture of chemicals that alters biologic function and is not required to maintain health. "Illicit substances" applies primarily to illegal substances. Any chemical that can produce a pleasurable state of mind has potential for abuse. Commonly abused substances, their pharmacologic effects, street names, and potential long-term consequences are described in Table 49-1.

Substance abuse is a societal issue that plagues many cultures and all races throughout the world, including the United States. In the United States, as many as one in four individuals meets the criteria for a substance use disorder at some time in their lives. According to the National Survey on Drug Use and Health (NSDUH) (formerly the National Household Survey on Drug Abuse), an estimated 22.5 million Americans (9.4% of the U.S. population) ages 12 or older in 2004 were classified with dependence on or abuse of either alcohol or illicit drugs. Of these, 3.4 million were classified with dependence on or abuse of both alcohol and illicit drugs, 3.9 million were dependent on or abused illicit drugs but not alcohol, and 15.2 million were dependent on or abused alcohol but not illicit drugs. The number of people with substance dependence or abuse increased from 14.5 million (6.5% of the U.S. population) in 2000.*

THEORIES ON WHY SUBSTANCES ARE ABUSED

Even though substance abuse has been a condition of the human mind since prehistoric times and very extensively studied, there is no one theory that accounts for why individuals abuse chemicals. The major theories of substance abuse are classified as biologic, psychological, and sociocultural models.* Belief in any particular theory influences assessment and treatment.

The *biologic model* hypothesizes that substance abuse is caused by a person's genetic profile, making a predisposition to substance abuse a hereditary condition. Specific genes have been found that appear to be associated with alcoholism and possibly other types of substance abuse. It is thought that these genetic aberrations block feelings of well-being, resulting in anxiety, anger, low self-esteem, and other negative feelings, leaving a feeling of craving for a substance that will suppress the bad feelings. Genes may also play a role in alteration of metabolic enzyme systems within the body that enhance or detract from pleasurable responses to chemical substances.

Many *psychological theories* have been studied that attempt to explain why people abuse chemicals. Psychoanalytic theories see alcoholics as fixated at the oral stage of development, thus seeking need satisfaction through oral behaviors such as drinking. Behavior or learning theories view addictive behaviors as overlearned, maladaptive habits that can be examined and changed in the same way as other habits. Cognitive theories suggest that addiction is based on a distorted way of thinking about substance use. Family system theory emphasizes the pattern of relationships among family members through the generations as an explanation of substance abuse.

Substance abuse has been linked to several psychological traits (e.g., depression, anxiety, antisocial personality, dependent personality), but there is no particular evidence that these traits cause the substance abuse. It is quite possible that long-term substance abuse causes these traits. There also does not appear to be a specific type of addictive personality because there is a wide variety of personality types among those who become alcoholics. Unfortunately, after long-term substance abuse, personality patterns emerge from the effects of alcohol and/or drugs on previously normal psychological functions, combined with ineffective responses to these effects.

Sociocultural factors play a role in a person's choice of whether to use drugs, which drugs to use, how much to use, and treatment for substance abuse. Attitudes, values, norms, and sanctions differ according to nationality, religion, gender, family background, and social environment. Combinations of factors may make a person more susceptible to drug abuse and interfere with recovery. Assessment of these factors is necessary to understand the whole person.

*U.S. Department of Health and Human Services, Substance Abuse and Mental Health Services Administration, 2004, National Survey on Drug Use and Health (NSDUH), available at http://oas.samhsa.gov/nsduh.htm#NSDUHinfo.

*Jefferson LV: Chemically mediated responses and substance-related disorders. In Stuart GW, Laraia MT, eds: *Principles and practice of psychiatric nursing*, ed 7, St. Louis, 2001, Mosby.

Drug Table 49-1 SUBSTANCES OF ABUSE

PSYCHOACTIVE DRUGS IDENTIFICATION CHART

DRUGS	MEDICAL USES	MEDICAL NAMES	SLANG NAMES	FORMS	USUAL ADMINISTRATION	EFFECTS SOUGHT
STIMULANTS						
Nicotine	None	Nicotine	Butt, chew, smoke, cig	Pipe, tobacco, cigarettes, snuff	Sniff, chew, smoke	Relaxation
Caffeine	Hyperkinesis, stimulant	Caffeine	None	Chocolates, tea, soft drinks, coffee	Swallow	Alertness
Amphetamines	Hyperkinesis, narcolepsy, weight control, mental disorders	Dexedrine, benzedrine	Speed, bennies, dexies, pep pills	Capsules, liquid, tablets, powder	Inject, swallow	Alertness, activeness
Cocaine	Local anesthetic	Cocaine	Coke, rock, crack, blow, tool, white, blast, snow, flake	Powder, rock	Inject, smoke, inhale	Excitation, euphoria
DEPRESSANTS						
Alcohol	None	Ethyl alcohol	Booze	Liquid	Swallow	Sense alteration, anxiety reduction
Sedatives	Anesthetic, sedative hypnotic, anticonvulsant	Secobarbital, phenobarbital, seconal	Barbs, reds, downers, sopors	Capsules, tablets, powder	Inject, swallow	Anxiety reduction, euphoria, sleep
Tranquilizers	Antianxiety, sedative hypnotic	Valium, Miltown, Librium	Downers	Capsules, tablets	Swallow	Anxiety reduction, euphoria, sleep
NARCOTICS						
Opium	Analgesic, antidiarrheal	Paregoric	None	Powder	Smoke, swallow	Euphoria, prevent withdrawal, sleep
Morphine	Analgesic, antitussive	Morphine, pectoral syrup	None	Powder, tablet, liquid	Inject, smoke, swallow	Euphoria, prevent withdrawal, sleep
Heroin	Research	Diacetylmorphine	China white, smack, junk, H, horse	Powder	Inject, swallow	Euphoria, prevent withdrawal, sleep
Codeine	Analgesic, Antitussive	Codeine, Empirin compound with codeine, Robitussin AC	None	Capsules, tablets, liquid	Inject, swallow	Euphoria, prevent withdrawal, sleep
CANNABIS						
THC	Research, cancer chemotherapy antinauseant	Tetrahydrocannabinol	THC	Tablets, liquid	Swallow	Relaxation, euphoria, increased perception

From the Center for Substance Abuse Prevention, *Curriculum Modules on Alcohol and Other Drug Problems for Schools of Social Work.*
For more information, contact the Florida Alcohol and Drug Abuse Association Resource Center, 1030 E. Lafayette St., Suite 100, Tallahassee, FL, 32301.

POSSIBLE EFFECTS	OVERDOSE	LONG-TERM EFFECTS
Respiratory difficulties, fatigue, high blood pressure	None	Dependency, lung cancer, heart attacks, respiratory ailments
Increased alertness, pulse rate, and blood pressure; excitation, insomnia, loss of appetite	Irritability	Dependency may aggravate organic actions
Increased alertness, pulse rate, and blood pressure; excitation, insomnia, loss of appetite	Agitation, increase in body temperature, hallucinations, convulsions, possible death	Severe withdrawal, possible convulsions, toxic psychosis
Increased alertness, pulse rate, and blood pressure; excitation, insomnia, loss of appetite	Agitation, increase in body temperature, hallucinations, convulsions, possible death	Dependency, depression, paranoia, convulsions
Loss of coordination, sluggishness, slurred speech, disorientation, depression	Total loss of coordination, nausea, unconsciousness, possible death	Dependency, toxic psychosis, neurologic damage
Loss of coordination, sluggishness, slurred speech, disorientation, depression	Cold clammy skin, dilated pupils, shallow respiration, weak and rapid pulse, coma, possible death	Dependency, severe withdrawal, possible convulsions, toxic psychosis
Loss of coordination, sluggishness, slurred speech, disorientation, depression	Cold clammy skin, dilated pupils, shallow respiration, weak and rapid pulse, coma, possible death	Dependency, severe withdrawal, possible convulsions, toxic psychosis
Euphoria, drowsiness, respiratory depression, constricted pupils, sleep, nausea	Clammy skin, slow and shallow breathing, convulsions, coma, possible death	Dependency, constipations, loss of appetite, severe withdrawal
Euphoria, drowsiness, respiratory depression, constricted pupils, sleep, nausea	Clammy skin, slow and shallow breathing, convulsions, coma, possible death	Dependency, constipations, loss of appetite, severe withdrawal
Euphoria, drowsiness, respiratory depression, constricted pupils, sleep, nausea	Clammy skin, slow and shallow breathing, convulsions, coma, possible death	Dependency, constipations, loss of appetite, severe withdrawal
Euphoria, drowsiness, respiratory depression, constricted pupils, sleep, nausea	Clammy skin, slow and shallow breathing, convulsions, coma, possible death	Dependency, constipation, loss of appetite, severe withdrawal
Relaxed inhibitions, euphoria, increased appetite, distorted perceptions, disoriented behavior	Fatigue, paranoia, possible psychosis	Amotivational syndrome, respiratory difficulties, lung cancer, interference with physical and emotional development

Continued

Drug Table 49-1 SUBSTANCES OF ABUSE—cont'd

PSYCHOACTIVE DRUGS IDENTIFICATION CHART						
DRUGS	**MEDICAL USES**	**MEDICAL NAMES**	**SLANG NAMES**	**FORMS**	**USUAL ADMINISTRATION**	**EFFECTS SOUGHT**
CANNABIS—cont'd						
Hashish	None	Tetrahydro-cannabinol	Hash	Solid resin	Smoke	Relaxation, euphoria, increased perception
Marijuana	Research	Tetrahydro-cannabinol	Pot, grass, sin, semilla, dobie, ganja, dope, gold, herb, weed, reefer	Plant particles	Smoke, swallow	Relaxation, euphoria, increased perception
HALLUCINOGENS						
PCP	None	Phencyclidine	Angel dust, zoot, peace pill, hog	Tablets, powder	Smoke, swallow	Distortion of sense, insight, exhilaration
LSD	Research	Lysergic acid diethylamide	Acid, sugar	Capsules, tablets, liquid	Swallow	Distortion of sense, insight, exhilaration
Organics	None	Mescaline, psilocybin	Mesc, mushrooms	Crude preparations, tablets, powder	Swallow	Distortion of sense, insight, exhilaration
INHALANTS						
Aerosols and solvents	None	None	Glue, benzene, toluene, freon	Solvents, aerosols	Inhale	Intoxication

SIGNS OF IMPAIRMENT

When signs of impairment start showing, it is usually not one sign alone but a cluster that raise questions of an impairment problem. The disease is usually first manifested in family life (e.g., domestic violence, separation, financial problems, problem behavior in children), then in social life (e.g., overt public intoxication; isolation from friends, peers, church). Physical and mental changes may be manifested by excessive tiredness, multiple illnesses, frequent injuries or accidents, and emotional crises. Deterioration in physical status is an important sign, but occurs late in the disease. Flagrant evidence of impairment at the worksite is relatively rare and usually occurs after the disease is quite advanced. In many cases, the workplace is the source of the drug of choice, so the impaired person will strive to protect the source with appropriate behavior.

SCREENING FOR ALCOHOL AND SUBSTANCE ABUSE

Because of the large number of health problems associated with alcohol and substance abuse, *Healthy People 2010*, the U.S. Preventive Services Task Force, the American Medical Association, and the American Nurses Association support and encourage screening patients for alcohol and other substance abuse. Screening instruments for substance abuse can be divided into the following four categories: (1) comprehensive drug abuse screening and assessment; (2) brief drug abuse screening; (3) alcohol abuse screening; and (4) drug and alcohol abuse screening for use with adolescents (Table 49-2). All of the screening instruments listed have been validated for accuracy for specific purposes (e.g., differentiating between early detection of excessive drinking vs. alcoholism, the potential for substance abuse vs. substance addiction). Another example of assessment for specific purposes is the Drug Abuse Screening Test (DAST), which can be used to differentiate among alcohol problems only, drug problems only, and both drug and alcohol problems. Some instruments are designed to be administered through an interview by a trained health professional, whereas others are designed for self-assessment by the patient using pencil and paper or computer entry. It is crucial that the proper assessment instrument be selected for use with a specific patient to attain meaningful results for an appropriate diagnosis. A disadvantage of some of the comprehensive screening instruments is the length of time

POSSIBLE EFFECTS	OVERDOSE	LONG-TERM EFFECTS
Relaxed inhibitions, euphoria, increased appetite, distorted perceptions, disoriented behavior	Fatigue, paranoia, possible psychosis	Amotivational syndrome, respiratory difficulties, lung cancer, interference with physical and emotional development
Relaxed inhibitions, euphoria, increased appetite, distorted perceptions, disoriented behavior	Fatigue, paranoia, possible psychosis	Amotivational syndrome, respiratory difficulties, lung cancer, interference with physical and emotional development
Illusions and hallucinations, distorted perception of time and distance	Longer and more intense "trips" or episodes, psychosis, convulsions, possible death	May intensify existing psychosis, flashbacks, panic reactions
Illusions and hallucinations, distorted perception of time and distance	Longer and more intense "trips" or episodes, psychosis, convulsions, possible death	May intensify existing psychosis, flashbacks, panic reactions
Illusions and hallucinations, distorted perception of time and distance	Longer and more intense "trips" or episodes, psychosis, convulsions, possible death	May intensify existing psychosis, flashbacks, panic reactions
Exhilaration, confusion, poor concentration	Heart failure, unconsciousness, asphyxiation, possible death	Impaired perception, coordination, and judgment; neurologic damage

required to administer the assessment and the availability of a qualified data interpreter. Many of the comprehensive instruments have been modified to be used as quick-screening instruments. A four-question assessment for alcohol abuse commonly used in the primary care setting because of its ease of administration is the CAGE questionnaire (Box 49-3). CAGE stands for Cut down, *A*nnoyed, *G*uilty, and *E*ye-opener, an acronym that provides the interviewer with a quick reminder of questions to be asked. A disadvantage of many of the instruments is that they were developed using adult male patients and have not been validated in special populations (e.g., women, the elderly, and adolescents).

HEALTH PROFESSIONALS AND SUBSTANCE ABUSE

Although the prevalence of substance abuse among physicians, nurses, pharmacists, and other health professionals is not precisely known, it is probably similar to that of the general population. There is thought to be more prescription drug and less street drug use because of easier access to prescription drugs. It is a misperception that education somehow protects health professionals from addiction because "they know better." Stress brought on by intense patient care practice, managing more patients with the same resources, zero tolerance for making a mistake in association with the expectation of 100% perfection, and financial debt are thought to be major contributors leading to substance abuse among health professionals.

Health professionals are responsible for maintaining a code of ethics and standards of care, and the inappropriate use of substances puts both of these principles in jeopardy. Signs that raise suspicion of substance abuse include behavioral changes (e.g., wearing long-sleeved garments all the time, diminished alertness, lack of attention to hygiene, mood swings) and performance deterioration (e.g., requests for frequent schedule changes, errors in clinical judgment, excessive absenteeism, frank odor of alcohol on the breath—often with an attempt to camouflage it with breath fresheners, frequent or long breaks, or deterioration in professional practice and patient care).

If a health professional suspects that a colleague is impaired, a confidential report should be made to an appropriate supervisor familiar with institutional policy. An investigation should be initiated; observation

Table 49-2 Screening Instruments for Substance Abuse

TITLE	ACRONYM
COMPREHENSIVE DRUG ABUSE SCREENING AND ASSESSMENT INSTRUMENTS	
Addiction Severity Index	ASI
Alcohol Use Disorders Identification Test	AUDIT
Alcohol, Smoking and Substance Involvement Screening Test	ASSIST
Composite International Diagnostic Interview Substance Abuse Module	CIDI-SAM
Drug Abuse Screening Test	DAST
Drug Use Screening Inventory	DUSI
Individual Assessment Profile	IAP
Millon Clinical Multiaxial Inventory	MCMI
Minnesota Multiphasic Personality Inventory	MMPI
MacAndrew Scale	MAC
Minnesota Multiphasic Personality Inventory-2	MMPI-2
BRIEF DRUG ABUSE SCREENING INSTRUMENTS	
CAGE-Adapted to Include Drugs	CAGE-AID
Millon Clinical Multiaxial Inventory	MCMI
Drug Dependence Scale	MCMI-III
Minnesota Multiphasic Personality Inventory-2	
Addiction Potential Scale	API
Addiction Acknowledgement Scale	AAS
Screening Instrument of Substance Abuse Potential	SISAP
Short Michigan Alcohol Screening Test-Adapted to Include Drugs	SMAST-AID
ALCOHOL ABUSE SCREENING INSTRUMENTS	
CAGE	CAGE
Michigan Alcohol Screening Test	MAST
Short Michigan Alcohol Screening Test	SMAST
Millon Clinical Multiaxial Inventory	MCMI
Alcohol Dependence Scale	MCMI-III
DRUG AND ALCOHOL SCREENING INSTRUMENTS FOR ADOLESCENTS	
Adolescent Alcohol Involvement Scale	AAIS
Adolescent Drug Involvement Scale	ADIS
Adolescent Drug Abuse Diagnosis	ADAD
Adolescent Drinking Inventory	ADI
Comprehensive Adolescent Severity Inventory	CASI
Drug and Alcohol Quick Screen	DAP
Home, Education/Employment, Activities, Drugs, Sexuality, Suicide/Depression	HEADSS
Home, Education, Abuse, Drugs, Safety, Friends, Image, Recreation, Sexuality and Threats	HEADS FIRST
Problem Oriented Screening Instrument for Teenagers	POSIT

Adapted from McPherson TL, Hersch PK: Brief substance use screening instruments for primary care settings: a review, *J Subst Abuse Treat* 18:193, 2000.

Box 49-3 CAGE Questionnaire

Have you ever felt you ought to **C**ut down on your drinking?
Have people **A**nnoyed you by criticizing your drinking?
Have you ever felt bad or **G**uilty about your drinking?
Have you ever had a drink first thing in the morning to steady your nerves or get rid of a hangover (**E**ye-Opener)?

From Ewing JA: Detecting alcoholism: the CAGE questionnaire, *JAMA* 252:1905, 1984.
A medical diagnosis of alcoholism should not be based solely on this questionnaire. The purpose of the questionnaire is to raise an index of suspicion that alcoholism might exist. Even one affirmative answer calls for further evaluation.

and documentation are crucial to building a record of repeat instances over time to support the suspicion of impairment. Because faulty memory is easily attacked by the impaired individual, examples of inappropriate actions need to be well documented over time. An accurate record can also be quite useful in helping the impaired individual recognize the problem and submit voluntarily to treatment.

When considering whether to report a colleague for suspected drug abuse, remember the following:

- Clinical practice is a privilege, not a right.
- Good-faith reporting should not be considered unfair or disloyal to a colleague; you may be protecting patients and the profession from harm.
- It is very unlikely that an individual making a confidential report to a supervisor will be sued if a reasonable effort is made to establish that the concerns are legitimate and it is clear that patient safety is the primary concern.
- An unreported colleague is more likely than a reported one to die as a result of the impairment (from suicide, accidental overdose, other accident, disease, or violence).
- Colleagues who are reported to licensing authorities (especially those who self-report) have a very good chance of retaining their license and salvaging their careers.
- If a health professional has knowledge of suspected impairment of another health professional but fails to report it, the health professional may potentially be named in a civil lawsuit or be named as a contributor in a malpractice suit against the impaired health provider.
- In some states, if impairment of a colleague is suspected, filing a report with the licensing authority is mandatory. Failure to do so may result in a reprimand or probation from the licensing authority.

Legal Considerations of Substance Abuse and Dependence

All states have laws pertaining to the reporting of impairment of health care workers. Some require that suspected impairment be reported to the health professional's licensure or disciplinary board. Other states allow referral to a professional society's impairment committee, which then contracts with the impaired individual to participate in a recovery program. As long as the health professional continues to participate, the committee can refrain from notifying the licensure board.

The health professional who makes a conscious effort to be treated for an addictive disorder has a variety of legal protections that can be helpful to reestablishing a career. The Americans with Disabilities Act (ADA) that went into effect in 1992 defines a disabled person as one "with a physical or mental impairment seriously limiting one or more major life activities." People dependent on drugs, but who are no longer using drugs illegally and are receiving treatment for chemical dependence or who have been rehabilitated successfully, are protected by the ADA from discrimination on the basis of past drug addiction. However, a substance abuser whose current use of chemicals impairs job performance or conduct may be disciplined, discharged, or denied employment to the extent that this person is not a "qualified individual with a disability." An individual who is currently engaging in the illegal use of drugs is not an "individual with a disability" under the ADA. State and federal handicap laws also mandate that every employer, including health care institutions, ensure each recovering chemically impaired individual who applies for employment or reinstatement be afforded the same protection received by anyone with a handicap.

Once a chemically dependent person has been through treatment, an ongoing monitoring program is routinely established to help ensure that the person is free of the abused substance. Urinalysis for drugs is the most common form of drug testing. The Drug-Free Workplace Act of 1988 encourages (but does not require) drug screening in an effort to provide drug-free workplaces. The Drug-Free Schools and Communities Act Amendments of 1989 extends this act to all educational institutions.

The Supreme Court has ruled that drug screening does not violate one's constitutional right to privacy or represent unreasonable search. Drug screening may be required for employment and can be requested for cause (e.g., suspicious behavior; arrest; after an accident), or a random test can be requested as a part of a return-to-work agreement for people in recovery. A positive drug test means that the reported drug is present in the specimen. It does not establish that the person is dependent on the drug, and it does not by itself prove the drug was the cause of an impaired performance.

Educating Health Professionals about Substance Abuse

The curricula of health profession educational programs should ensure that all students have multiple opportunities during their development of professional attitudes and behaviors to consider and formulate values about self-medication and substance abuse that are consistent with professional and legal standards. Employers should make available drug abuse resources, such as information about employee assistance programs and policies, professional recovery assistance (e.g., recovery networks), and educational opportunities. Prevention of drug misuse, whether it is illegal or inappropriate use or drug abuse, is an important priority in the practice of every health profession.

PRINCIPLES OF TREATMENT FOR SUBSTANCE ABUSE

It is important to recognize that substance abuse and addiction are diseases as described in DSM-IV-TR and are treatable disorders. This focus is essential to successful treatment. The American Psychiatric Association lists long-term goals in treating substance abuse as follows:

- Reduction or abstinence in the use and effects of substances
- Reduction in the frequency and severity of relapse
- Improvement in psychological and social functioning

By the time a person seeks treatment for substance abuse or is ordered into a treatment program by the courts, the illness has become very complex, affecting nearly every aspect of the person's life. Treatment requires lifelong effort with a combination of psychosocial support and sometimes pharmacologic treatment. Key factors associated with long-term recovery are negative consequences of substance use (e.g., deteriorating health; divorce; loss of job, family and friends) and social and community support, particularly with participation with self-help organizations whose goals include total abstinence of substances being abused (e.g., Alcoholics Anonymous, Narcotics Anonymous, Women for Sobriety, Rational Recovery). The types of social support given by the 12-step programs (e.g., Alcoholics Anonymous, Narcotics Anonymous), such as 24-hour availability when cravings arise, networking, role modeling and advice on abstinence based on direct, personal experiences appear to be primary characteristics for success in maintaining recovery (Figure 49-1).

Diagnostic criteria for assessment of substance abuse and related disorders are defined in the DSM-IV-TR. A combination of interviews, screening tools (see Table 49-2), information from colleagues, and laboratory tests will determine whether there is a single diagnosis of abuse of one or more substances or if there are multiple diagnoses. Other psychiatric (e.g., depression, psychosis, delirium, dementia) and medical conditions (e.g., anemia, cirrhosis, hepatic encephalopathy, nutrition deficiencies, cardiomyopathy) may be induced by substance abuse. Based on the findings, priorities must be assigned. Immediate medical needs must be addressed first (e.g., thiamine deficiency, withdrawal and detoxification, safety). Detoxification programs are an important first step in substance abuse treatment. Detoxification initiates abstinence, reduces the severity of withdrawal symptoms, and retains the

The Twelve Steps of Alcoholics Anonymous
1. We admitted we were powerless over alcohol—that our lives had become unmanageable. 2. Came to believe that a Power greater than ourselves could restore us to sanity. 3. Made a decision to turn our will and our lives over to the care of God as we understood Him. 4. Made a searching and fearless moral inventory of ourselves. 5. Admitted to God, to ourselves and to another human being the exact nature of our wrongs. 6. Were entirely ready to have God remove all these defects of character. 7. Humbly asked Him to remove our shortcomings. 8. Made a list of all persons we had harmed, and became willing to make amends to them all. 9. Made direct amends to such people wherever possible, except when to do so would injure them or others. 10. Continued to take personal inventory and when we were wrong promptly admitted it. 11. Sought through prayer and meditation to improve our conscious contact with God as we understood Him, praying only for knowledge of His will for us and the power to carry that out. 12. Having had a spiritual awakening as the result of these steps, we tried to carry this message to alcoholics and to practice these principles in all our affairs.
Alcoholics Anonymous World Services, Inc.

FIGURE **49-1** The Twelve Steps of Alcoholics Anonymous. (The Twelve Steps are reprinted with permission of Alcoholics Anonymous World Services, Inc. [AAWS]. Permission to reprint the Twelve Steps does not mean that AAWS has reviewed or approved the contents of this publication, or that AAWS necessarily agrees with the views expressed herein. AA is a program of recovery from alcoholism *only*; use of the Twelve Steps in connection with programs and activities patterned after AA but that address other problems or in any other non-AA context, does not imply otherwise.)

person in treatment to forestall relapse. During detoxification, behavioral interventions (e.g., contingency management, motivational enhancement, and cognitive therapies) can also be started.

Alcohol

In the United States, the Behavior Risk Factor Surveillance System sponsored by the CDC* reports that binge drinking, defined as 5 or more drinks on one or more occasions in the past month, is reported to have occurred in approximately 15% of the survey population from 1990 to 2002. Recent studies indicate that the frequency of binge drinking appears to be rising on college campuses. Chronic drinking, defined as 2 or more drinks per day, or more than 60 drinks per month, is rising. The median in 1990 was 3.2% of the survey population, but has grown to 5.9% in 2002. A common characteristic of alcohol abusers is denial of a problem. Individuals who abuse alcohol may continue to consume alcohol despite the knowledge that continued consumption poses a significant social and health hazard to themselves.

Research over the past two decades indicates that with *acute* ingestion of alcohol, the central nervous system (CNS) depressant effects of alcohol come from release of the major inhibitory neurotransmitter gamma-aminobutyric acid (GABA) and suppression of the major excitatory neurotransmitter, glutamate, a by-product of the *N*-methyl-D-aspartate (NMDA) receptors. With long-term *chronic* ingestion, the reverse occurs; tolerance to alcohol leads to reduced GABAergic activity and higher levels of NMDA activity. There are also inconsistent effects on the serotonin, dopamine, and opioid receptors of the CNS that may also account for some of the acute and chronic effects of alcohol ingestion. Stimulation of opioid and dopamine receptors appears to be related to the alcohol "high," or the rewarding aspects of drinking alcohol.

- *Intoxication:* Alcohol abuse, or more appropriately ethanol abuse, is commonly called alcohol intoxication. **Intoxication** is defined as the ingestion of ethanol to the point of clinically significant maladaptive behavioral or psychological changes (e.g., inappropriate sexual or aggressive behavior, mood lability, impaired judgment, impaired social or occupational functioning). These changes are accompanied by evidence of slurred speech, incoordination, unsteady gait, nystagmus, impairment in attention or memory, or stupor or coma.*
- *Withdrawal:* When alcohol is ingested in quantities leading to intoxication, symptoms of overindulgence (e.g., "hangover" queasy stomach, headache) are common over the next several hours because of direct toxic effects on body cells. If a person frequently drinks to intoxication over long periods (i.e., months to years), a physical dependence (i.e., addiction) develops and a decrease in the blood alcohol level over 4 to 12 hours may cause symptoms of alcohol withdrawal. Development of withdrawal symptoms and craving often induces the person to continue to abuse alcohol. See Figure 49-2 for symptoms and a time

*Centers for Disease Control and Prevention: *Behavioral risk factor surveillance system survey data*, Atlanta, Ga, 2005, U.S. Department of Health and Human Services. Available at www.cdc.gov/brfss.

*American Psychiatric Association: *Diagnostic and statistical manual of mental disorders*, ed 4, Washington, D.C., 2000, American Psychiatric Association.

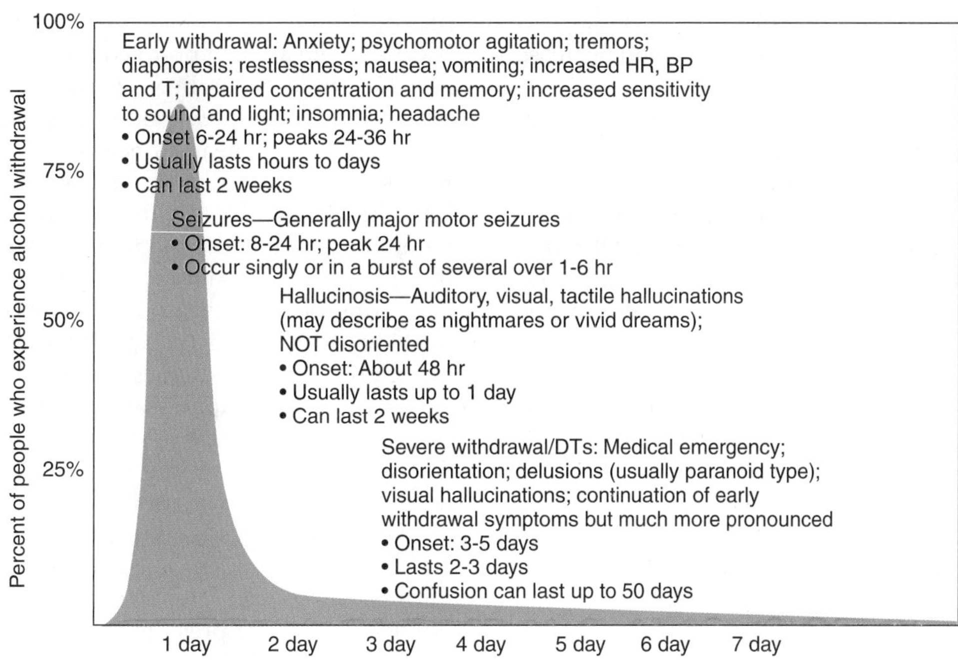

FIGURE **49-2** Alcohol withdrawal syndrome. (From Stuart GW, Laraia MT: *Principles and practice of psychiatric nursing,* ed 7, St. Louis, 2001, Mosby.)

sequence of alcohol withdrawal. The person may no longer get much effect from the alcohol other than its ability to prevent withdrawal.

Alcohol withdrawal symptoms can begin within a few hours of discontinuation of drinking and may continue for 3 to 10 days. Withdrawal can progress to more severe symptoms, including visual and auditory hallucinations, and seizures (usually tonic-clonic type). Less than 1% of patients develop delirium tremens (the DTs), the worst of withdrawal symptoms. This syndrome is manifested by hyperactivity, delirium, and severe hyperthermia. The mortality rate of patients who progress to delirium tremens is 20%, most commonly as a result of stroke or cardiovascular collapse. Because it is difficult to predict who may have severe withdrawal, anyone experiencing alcohol withdrawal should be observed closely and treated if necessary.

- *Treatment:* Patients who appear to be developing withdrawal symptoms should be quickly assessed for hydration and electrolyte and nutritional status. Excessive loss of fluids and electrolytes may occur through vomiting, sweating, and hyperthermia. Dehydration also may be due to inadequate fluid intake and diuresis during prolonged and heavy alcohol consumption. Thiamine and multiple vitamins should routinely be administered to patients in alcohol withdrawal. Intravenous fluid therapy for rehydration may be necessary, but thiamine must be administered before glucose infusion to prevent Wernicke's encephalopathy.

If a person addicted to alcohol seeks treatment for withdrawal symptoms, benzodiazepines (e.g., diazepam, chlordiazepoxide, clorazepate, oxazepam, lorazepam) are commonly used for detoxification because they enhance GABA activity that has been suppressed by chronic alcohol ingestion.

There are two approaches for benzodiazepine dosing in treating withdrawal symptoms. The fixed-dose schedule uses a set dose of benzodiazepine administered at specific intervals. Usually about the second day, smaller tapering doses of benzodiazepines are administered on a fixed schedule. The symptom-triggered schedule depends on the use of a rating scale such as the Clinical Institute Withdrawal Assessment–Alcohol, Revised (CIWA-AR). The CIWA-AR protocol calls for administration of a benzodiazepine when the patient shows certain symptoms (symptom-triggered regimen) rather than a fixed schedule regimen. It is hypothesized that the symptom-triggered medication regimen significantly reduces the amount of medication given and may shorten the length of treatment necessary.

The longer-acting benzodiazepines (e.g., chlordiazepoxide, diazepam, clorazepate) offer advantages of less fluctuation in blood levels and appear to be associated with fewer rebound effects and withdrawal seizures on discontinuation. Due to the longer half-lives and active metabolites, they taper themselves off just by discontinuing the dosage. The short-acting benzodiazepines (e.g., oxazepam, lorazepam) have the advantage of having no active metabolites that may produce additional adverse effects in the elderly or people with concurrent liver disease. They do, however, have to be administered more often, and tapering may be required. Carbamazepine is also effective in decreasing seizure frequency and some of the psychiatric symptoms associated with withdrawal (e.g., anxiety, agitation). Beta blockers (e.g., atenolol, propranolol) and an alpha agonist such as clonidine may reduce craving and decrease severity of withdrawal symptoms.

- *Relapse prevention:* Lifelong effort with a combination of psychosocial support and sometimes pharmacologic treatment is necessary to prevent relapse. Key factors associated with long-term recovery are social and community support through participation with self-help organizations and negative consequences of substance use (e.g., job loss, divorce, loss of child custody). Current treatments are effective for about 50% of patients and significantly reduce the cost of health care, morbidity, and mortality associated with alcoholism.

Three medicines have been approved for use in helping promote abstinence. Disulfiram (Antabuse) (see p. 865) helps reduce the desire for alcohol by inducing nausea and vomiting (disulfiram reaction) if alcohol is ingested while disulfiram is being taken. Reactions can be quite severe, so it is essential that the patient understand the consequences of drinking alcohol while taking the medicine. It also means the patient must avoid alcohol taken in the form of medicines (e.g., cough and cold elixirs, nighttime sedatives, mouthwashes), soups and sauces containing cooking sherry, and aftershave lotions or perfumes that contain alcohol that can be absorbed through the skin. Success with disulfiram very much depends on adherence to the medication regimen, and many alcoholics become lax in taking their medication as prescribed.

Naltrexone (ReVia) (see p. 334) is an opioid antagonist prescribed to block the pharmacologic effects of the "high" associated with opioids and alcohol. Studies report less alcohol craving and fewer drinking days, especially when naltrexone is combined with psychosocial treatment. Success is somewhat limited with naltrexone because, although it blocks the "high" from drinking, it provides no relief or promise of reward against the emotions that trigger the desire to drink in the first place.

Acamprosate (Campral) (p. 863) is the newest agent available to help maintain abstinence from alcohol. It enhances abstinence and reduces drinking rates in alcohol-dependent patients who are abstinent at the beginning of treatment. It is neither a sedative nor anxiolytic, and it is not addictive. It does not reduce the rewarding effects of alcohol like naltrexone does, nor does it cause nausea and vomiting when alcohol is consumed, like disulfiram. Studies indicate similar rates of success with naltrexone and acamprosate and a slightly higher success rate when used together.

Opioids

Commonly abused opiates (i.e., derived from opium) are heroin, morphine, hydromorphone (Dilaudid), codeine, oxycodone, and hydrocodone, as well as the synthetic opiate-like (opioid) substances such as meperidine, fentanyl, pentazocine, buprenorphine, and butorphanol. Heroin is a "street" drug derived from opium because there are no approved medicinal uses for heroin. Heroin use has been growing in recent years because it is now available in a more pure form. Improved purity means a heroin user can get "high" from smoking or sniffing heroin, avoiding intravenous injection. There is also a misperception that inhaling heroin does not lead to addiction. As many as 40% of those who initially sniff heroin become an intravenous user of heroin. The other opioids are made by legitimate manufacturers in specific concentrations for prescription use as anesthetics, analgesics, antidiarrheal agents, and cough suppressants, but have been diverted from medicinal use into the illicit drug market for pleasure and profit. Obtaining prescriptions from one or more health care providers simultaneously for faked or exaggerated medical conditions (e.g., "severe" pain, back injury) is another mechanism for acquisition for illicit use by abusers. Health care providers who abuse opioids may write prescriptions for self-use, or steal medicines intended for other patients or from pharmacy or floor stock.

- *Intoxication:* Indications of opioid intoxication are the presence of inappropriate behaviors after administration such as an initial euphoria ("high") followed by apathy, dysphoria, agitation, impaired judgment, and/or impaired social and occupational functioning. Additional signs are pupillary constriction (miosis) and one or more of the following: drowsiness ("on the nod"), slurred speech, and impairment of attention and memory. Intoxicated people also may show an indifference to placing themselves in potentially hazardous situations. The extent to which an intoxicated person shows these signs and symptoms depends on the dosage taken, the route of administration, frequency of use, and acquired tolerance. Intoxication will usually last for several hours, but depends on the half-life of the drug taken and the frequency of readministration of the opioid. Overdosage, especially with street drugs in which the concentration of drug is not known, can lead to severe intoxication manifested by coma, respiratory depression, pupillary dilation (mydriasis), and death.
- *Withdrawal:* All opioids produce similar signs and symptoms of withdrawal. Onset of withdrawal symptoms in opioid-dependent people is somewhat predictable based on the half-life of the drug being abused; the symptoms begin two or three half-lives after the last dose was taken. Onset of withdrawal symptoms from heroin or morphine is usually within 6 to 12 hours after the last dose, whereas it may take 2 to 4 days following discontinuation of longer-acting drugs such as methadone. Onset of withdrawal for people who abuse a variety of drugs and alcohol is extremely variable. Physical signs

and symptoms associated with withdrawal are anxiety and restlessness, increased blood pressure and pulse, pupillary dilation, rhinorrhea, sweating, nausea, vomiting, and diarrhea. In severe cases, piloerection and fever may be present. Subjectively, the person may complain of an "achy feeling" often located in the back and legs, an increased sensitivity to pain, and drug-seeking behavior (craving). Acute withdrawal symptoms from short-acting opiates (e.g., heroin) usually peak in 1 to 3 days, and dissipate over the next 5 to 7 days. Chronic withdrawal symptoms (e.g., insomnia, anxiety, drug craving, apathy toward the pleasures in life [anhedonia]) may require weeks to months to dissipate.

- *Treatment:* Withdrawal from opioids is very uncomfortable, but usually not life-threatening unless there are coexisting medical conditions. Treatment is focused on relieving the acute symptoms. Clonidine (see p. 383) is useful in decreasing tremors, sweating, and agitation; cyclobenzaprine (see Table 45-1 on p. 739) reduces skeletal muscle spasms, and dicyclomine (see p. 216) reduces gastrointestinal cramping and diarrhea. A protocol such as the Clinical Institute Narcotic Assessment (CINA) rating scale is helpful in assessing and monitoring a patient undergoing opioid withdrawal.
- Another approach to treatment of opioid dependence is the substitution of another opioid, usually long-acting methadone, to reduce the severity of withdrawal symptoms. Once the person is detoxified from the abused opiate substance, the methadone can be gradually tapered to allow the person to be drug-free. The long half-life of the methadone requires that the taper be prolonged over several weeks.

Another treatment alternative is an opioid maintenance program. As mentioned, the patient is started on methadone to minimize withdrawal symptoms. Instead of being tapered off the methadone, however, the person is maintained on a daily dose to prevent the development of withdrawal symptoms. The benefits to this approach are that the person can be maintained on a stable dosage without tolerance and substantial craving developing and can function more normally in the work and home environment, although still addicted to an opiate. Opioid maintenance programs have been shown to reduce opioid use, criminal activity, and the transmission of human immunodeficiency virus (HIV) and hepatitis among opioid-dependent people.

- *Relapse prevention:* As with alcoholism, lifelong effort with a combination of psychosocial support and sometimes pharmacologic treatment is necessary to prevent relapse. Key factors associated with long-term recovery are social and community support through participation with self-help organizations (e.g., Narcotics Anonymous) and negative consequences of substance use. Current treatments are effective for maintaining abstinence for some patients and significantly reduce the cost of health care, morbidity, and mortality associated with opioid addiction.

Naltrexone (ReVia) (see Chapter 20) is an opioid antagonist prescribed to block the pharmacologic effects of the "high" associated with opioids and alcohol. Studies report less drug craving and a reduced use of illicit drugs, especially when naltrexone is combined with psychosocial treatment. Success is somewhat limited with naltrexone because, although it blocks the "high" from opioid use, it provides no relief or promise of reward against the emotions that trigger the desire to "get high" in the first place.

Another approach to reducing the abuse of opioids is the methadone long-term maintenance program described as a treatment option. A disadvantage of this program is that the drug is available only through specially registered clinics, and patients often have to travel long distances to the clinics as often as six times per week. The Drug Addiction Treatment Act of 2000 (DATA) opened up the possibility of physician office–based management of addicted patients who meet certain criteria by legalizing the prescribing of Schedule III, IV, and V medications for the treatment of opioid dependence. A drug that has been well studied in office practice is buprenorphine (see Chapter 20), a partial opioid agonist. Because it has opioid agonist as well as antagonist properties, it has a "ceiling effect" on analgesia and respiratory depression, giving it a much greater safety profile. Two new dosage forms of buprenorphine have been approved for maintenance opioid programs: buprenorphine-only (Subutex) and buprenorphine-naloxone (Suboxone). The naloxone in the Suboxone product is to prevent abuse of the buprenorphine as a narcotic antagonist (similar in concept to Talwin NX, see Chapter 20). Specifically trained physicians administer the buprenorphine-only sublingual tablets directly to the patient in their offices, usually for 2 days. After dosage adjustment, the patient is switched to Suboxone for maintenance therapy.

Cocaine

Cocaine is obtained from the leaves of trees indigenous to Bolivia, Colombia, Peru, Indonesia, and other parts of the world. For centuries, workers who traveled in mountainous South American countries have chewed coca leaves to improve stamina and suppress hunger. It has been used in Western medicine as a topically applied local anesthetic particularly in ophthalmic, nasal, oral, and laryngeal procedures for more than 100 years. Pharmacologically, cocaine blocks the transmission of nerve impulses when applied to tissues in these areas. When injected intravenously, inhaled as smoke, or sniffed onto the mucous membranes of the nose (snorted using a straw), it blocks the reuptake of catecholamines in the brain, causing sudden CNS stimulation with euphoria (the "rush").

Popular as a recreational drug for its euphoric efforts, cocaine use soared in the United States through the 1970s and 1980s. When treated with hydrochloric acid, cocaine becomes cocaine hydrochloride, which can be dried to a powder for sniffing or dissolved in water for intravenous injection for an immediate "rush." Another method of extraction of cocaine led to the creation of the more potent "free-base" and "crack" cocaine. Freebase is formed when cocaine hydrochloride is mixed with ammonia to form a base, which then is dissolved in ether. The ether evaporates, leaving a powder residue. The powder is then smoked for the "rush," but ether vapors remaining are extremely flammable and can ignite, causing a small explosion with severe burns to the face and airways if inhaled. Crack cocaine is formed when the cocaine hydrochloride is mixed with baking soda and then heated. The resulting mass that forms is left to harden into slabs of cocaine. Chunks of the slab are sold as "rocks" of cocaine. This form of cocaine is the cheapest and most potent. When smoked, it makes a crackling sound, hence its name. Other drugs (e.g., nicotine, alcohol, heroin) are frequently used at the same time to enhance and prolong the euphoria. Cocaine smoking and intravenous use tend to be particularly associated with a rapid progression from use to abuse to dependence, often occurring over weeks to months. Intranasal use is associated with a more gradual progression, usually occurring over months to years. With continued use, tolerance and dependence develop, leading to increases in dosage and a reduction in the pleasurable effects of the euphoria.

- *Intoxication:* Acute cocaine intoxication usually begins with a euphoric feeling with a variety of other behaviors including enhanced vigor, hyperactivity, restlessness, hypervigilance, talkativeness, anxiety, tension, alertness, grandiosity, anger and impaired judgment. Signs and symptoms that develop are tachycardia or bradycardia, pupillary dilation, hyper- or hypotension, sweating or chills, and nausea and vomiting. With chronic use, fatigue, sadness, social withdrawal, respiratory depression, chest pain, cardiac dysrhythmias, and confusion may be more manifest. Severe intoxication can lead to hyperpyrexia, seizures (primarily tonic-clonic), respiratory depression, coma, and death.
- *Withdrawal:* Because cocaine has a short half-life, withdrawal symptoms (a "crash") may begin within a few hours of a reduction in dosage, frequency of administration, or a discontinuation of cocaine. Acute withdrawal symptoms are more likely to be seen after periods of repetitive high-dose use ("runs" or "binges"). People often complain of fatigue, vivid and unpleasant dreams, extreme depression, insomnia or hypersomnia, and increased appetite. There is often an intense craving and drug-seeking behavior. These symptoms cause significant distress and social withdrawal with the inability to continue work. Several days of rest and recuperation are required for symptoms to resolve. Depression with suicidal ideation is generally the most serious problem associated with cocaine withdrawal.
- *Treatment:* There are no medicines approved to treat cocaine dependence. Many classes of drugs (e.g., dopamine agonists, antidepressants, anticonvulsants, calcium channel blockers, serotonin reuptake inhibitors) have been tested in controlled studies with minimal effect. Studies are ongoing with GABA, the inhibitory neurotransmitter. Two additional areas of investigation are vaccines and maintenance drugs. Animal studies have shown that vaccines trigger the formation of antibodies that might increase the metabolism of cocaine. Long-acting maintenance medicines similar to methadone or buprenorphine for opioid addiction are also under investigation. Unfortunately, the rate of relapse for patients who develop a cocaine dependency is very high.

NURSING PROCESS *for Substance Abuse*

Assessment

Despite early detection of an overdose of a substance, the adverse effects of the ingested substance on multiple body systems may result in death. Assess the ABCs—airway, breathing, and circulation—immediately on admission. A thorough physical and neurologic examination must be taken to detect life-threatening symptoms. Care must be prioritized, based on the individual patient's care needs.

Refer to Table 49-1 for a listing of substances abused and symptoms associated with each substance. Table 49-2 can serve as a reference for Screening Instruments for Substance Abuse and Box 49-3 for the CAGE questionnaire used as an index of individuals suspected of alcoholism. Screening instruments will have to be administered in a manner appropriate to circumstances and the overall condition of the patient.

History of the Event, Accident, or Behavior. For the person who appears to be intoxicated, ask simple, direct questions with regard to whether the person has been drinking or using drugs. "Do you drink alcohol?" If yes, ask, "When was your last drink (time)?" "How much have you had to drink?" "Approximately how much alcohol have you consumed over the past week or month?" This would be an appropriate time to administer the CAGE questionnaire (see Box 49-3) if other more urgent care is not needed. If the answer to the question regarding drug and alcohol use is "no," ask whether the individual has a history of drinking alcohol, treatment for alcohol abuse, or has lost a driver's license, been fined, or ordered to a treatment program as a result of either alcohol or drug abuse. Ask specific questions regarding the use of any "street drugs" or prescription drugs. Be direct and name examples such as cocaine, marijuana, amphetamines, crack cocaine, barbiturates, tranquilizers, narcotics, phencyclidine (PCP), and lysergic acid diethylamide (LSD).

People with symptoms of bizarre or inappropriate behavior and who are combative, violent, and possibly hallucinating should be screened for not only substance abuse but for possible psychiatric disorders that may be either the primary cause of the presenting symptoms or a result of substance abuse, or a combination of both. (See also Chapters 16, 17, and 18 for further information.) Know how to summon security personnel or have them present to provide for patient and personnel safety.

If the patient has been injured, follow emergency department policies regarding forms and legal documents that need to be completed (e.g. screening toxicology, rape kit procedures) to meet the medicolegal requirements.

Vital Signs. Persistent abnormal vital signs during routine testing should raise suspicion of substance abuse. Vital signs should be taken as often as necessary to monitor the patient's status.

- *Blood pressure:* Blood pressure may be elevated from the use of stimulants and other coexisting conditions. Blood pressure readings should be performed at least twice daily and more often if indicated by the patient's symptoms or the health care provider's orders. Use the proper-sized blood pressure cuff and position the patient's arm at heart level.
- Record the blood pressure in both arms. A systolic pressure variance of 5 to 10 mm Hg is normal; readings reflecting a variance of more than 10 mm Hg should be reported for further evaluation. ALWAYS REPORT A NARROWING PULSE PRESSURE (difference between systolic and diastolic readings).
- *Pulse:* Assess bilaterally the rhythm, quality, equality, and strength of the pulses (i.e., carotid, brachial, radial, femoral, popliteal, posterior tibial, dorsalis pedis). If any pulse is diminished or absent, record the level at which initial changes are noted. The usual words to describe the pulse are "absent," "diminished," or "average," "full and brisk," or "full bounding, frequently visible." *Report irregular rate, rhythm, and palpitations.* Check for delayed capillary refill.
- *Respirations:* Table 49-1 notes that respirations are affected by narcotics and depressants; however, because the patient may have coexisting medical conditions, respiratory rate cannot be relied on as a definitive observation for substance abuse. Lungs also may have substantial damage from smoking or prolonged inhalations of drugs, aerosols, and solvents, making the patient susceptible to respiratory abnormalities. Observe and chart the rate and depth of respirations. Check breath sounds at least every shift, making specific notations regarding the presence of abnormal breath sounds (e.g. crackles, wheezes). Observe the degree of dyspnea that occurs and whether it happens with or without exertion.
- *Temperature:* Record temperature at least every shift.

Basic Mental Status. Be particularly alert for fluctuating levels of consciousness; lack of awareness or attention; paranoid thoughts; visual, auditory, or tactile hallucinations; and confusion about the immediate surroundings.

Identify the person's level of consciousness and clarity of thought—both are indicators of cerebral perfusion. Terms frequently used to chart levels of consciousness include the following: alert (mentally functioning), confused (poor mental coordination), obtunded (sleepy, can respond appropriately when aroused or stimulated), stuporous (difficult to arouse, responds only to vigorous stimulation), light coma (grimaces and withdraws to painful stimulation), or deep coma (no observable response to painful stimulation). Assess regularly for improvement or deterioration. Always report declining mental status to the health care provider.

Appearance. Describe the individual's gait, coordination, and physical appearance.

Neurologic Assessment. Administer the Glasgow Coma Scale if appropriate.

GLASGOW COMA SCORE*

Eye-Opening (E)	Verbal Response (V)	Motor Response (M)
4 = Spontaneous	5 = Normal conversation	6 = Normal
3 = To voice	4 = Disoriented conversation	5 = Localizes to pain
2 = To pain	3 = Words, but not coherent	4 = Withdraws to pain
1 = None	2 = No words, only sounds	3 = Decorticate posture
	1 = None	2 = Decerebrate posture
		1 = None

*Total = E + V + M.

Heart Assessment. Heart palpitations and irregularity may occur during withdrawal. Cocaine is associated with causing cardiotoxicity that can be fatal to a first-time user or to an individual who already has cardiovascular disease. (See Chapters 24, 25, and 28 for further details relating to heart assessments.)

Auscultation and Percussion. Nurses with advanced skills can perform auscultation and percussion to note changes in heart size and heart and lung sounds. (See a medical-surgical nursing text for details of performing these advanced skills.) As appropriate to nursing skill level, note changes in cardiac rate and rhythm, heart sounds, and murmurs.

Eyes. Check pupil size, equality, light reaction, and accommodation (i.e., normal: equal, round, react to light, and react to accommodation). Note ptosis, nystagmus, or other abnormal eye movements. Abnormal pupil changes include either enlarged, dilated pupils (mydriasis); very small, pinpoint pupils (miosis); or nonreactive pupils (do not respond to light).

Dry eyes may be a problem in a person with alcoholism. Blurred vision is common with alcoholism, and the condition may resolve after approximately 3 to 4 months of sobriety, but if the condition persists or increases, an eye examination should be scheduled.

Ears, Oral Cavity, Nose, and Throat. The range of symptoms associated with substance abuse is extensive in these tissues. Ringing, buzzing, and roaring in the ears are most common among benzodiazepine users.

The oral cavity, which is often ignored by people who abuse drugs, may have bleeding gums, canker sores, cold sores, dental caries, and infections. During withdrawal the mouth may be very dry. The long-term use of alcohol, especially when combined with smoking, increases the risk of oral cancer so a thorough examination of the mouth and throat should be completed.

Snorting of cocaine and heroin can seriously damage the tissues in the nose, showing evidence of inflammation, ulceration, and perforation of the nasal septum. Nosebleeds are common.

Skin Assessment. Check skin color (jaundice may indicate hepatitis, which is common in drug abusers who share needles) and for rashes, abscesses, and for evidence of "tracking" along veins on forearm, wrist, dorsum of hand, antecubital area, ankle, scrotal area, between the toes, and under the tongue. Is the skin dry, moist, or clammy? Sweating may be observed during withdrawal.

Musculoskeletal Assessment. Alcohol depletes calcium from the bones, making them more susceptible to fractures. Osteoporosis also may be prevalent in alcoholics. Muscle pains (myalgia) and weakness in the muscles may be associated with withdrawal.

Medication History. Ask specific questions relating to the use of prescription, over-the-counter, and "street" or illicit drugs. Does the individual also use any herbal products?

Coexisting Diseases and Disorders. Is the individual currently under treatment for other diseases? Is there a history of any cardiac, respiratory, renal, endocrine, or neurologic disorders? Is there a history of head trauma or seizures?

Sexually Transmitted Diseases. The individual will need examination and testing for the entire scope of sexually transmitted diseases. Sexual activity is common during drug and alcohol intoxication. Prostitution is commonly used to support a substance abuse habit.

Pregnancy. Ask the female patient if she is pregnant. Use of drugs and alcohol while pregnant has a strong likelihood of harming not only the mother but also the baby before and after birth. Alcohol and drug use during pregnancy may cause preterm birth, low birthweight, birth defects, fatal bleeding disorders, and behavioral problems later in life. Intravenous (IV) drug abusers who share needles may expose the fetus to hepatitis B, HIV, or acquired immunodeficiency syndrome (AIDS). Sexually transmitted diseases also place both the mother and the fetus at risk. Infants of drug addicts must be monitored closely for symptoms of withdrawal after delivery.

Laboratory Tests. Urine and/or blood toxicology screening, complete blood cell count, electrolyte studies, renal and liver function tests, thyroid levels, serologic tests for hepatitis (HBV), venereal disease, HIV; chest x-ray, tuberculosis (TB) skin test, and an electrocardiogram are a routine panel for most individuals suspected of substance abuse.

The sensitivity of the blood and urine testing for drugs depends on the amount, frequency of use, and when the drug was last used. The presence of any drug depends on the drug's half-life and metabolites. Hallucinogens may be detected in urine for up to 28 days after last use in regular users, whereas opiates and narcotics may be detectable for only 12 to 36 hours after the last use.

Nursing Diagnoses

- Ineffective coping (indication)
- Family processes, alcoholism, dysfunctional (indication)
- Injury, risk for (indication)
- Sensory perception, disturbed (indication)
- Thought processes, disturbed (indication)

Planning

Emergency Treatment. The nurse should be aware of the policy for calling codes, location of the emergency cart, and procedures used to check the emergency cart supplies, as well as understand the procedure for defibrillation and cardioversion. The nurse should also be familiar with the medicolegal components of providing care to injured or impaired patients.

Safety. Provide for patient safety during and following detoxification until the individual is able to assume self-responsibility.

Medications. Order medications prescribed and schedule these on the medication administration record (MAR). (See Principles of Treatment for Substance Abuse earlier in this chapter.)

Basic Mental Status. Schedule basic neurologic checks at least once per shift.

Physical and Psychological Status. Perform physical and psychological assessments at least once per shift or as indicated by the patient's condition and/or health care provider's orders.

Goal Setting for the Patient. Establish goals and outcomes for the immediate needs of an individual who has had an injury or has inflicted injury to others.

Plan for the patient's immediate care needs and arrange for follow-up in an inpatient or outpatient detoxification and rehabilitation program designed to assist the individual to reach the goal of long-term abstinence. Involve the patient in goal setting as the ability to assume responsibility for one's own actions evolves.

In a rehabilitation program the individual will be given factual information regarding the harmful use of drugs and/or alcohol. The individual will often not acknowledge that he or she has a problem (denial); when the problem is recognized, the person does not have insight into how to overcome the problem. Throughout the program the patient will need to explore positive and negative aspects of his or her behavior to develop new behaviors that do not include the use of drugs and alcohol. The person will evolve through the following five stages of change: precontemplation, contemplation, preparation, action, and maintenance* as he or she advances through the rehabilitation program (Figure 49-3).

Family/Support Involvement. Integrate family/support personnel into the long-term planning for treatment and support. Encourage them to become involved in the rehabilitation program. Family members and friends need guidance in appropriate ways to be involved in the recovery of an individual who exhibits symptoms of a dysfunctional family relationship. Enrollment in community groups (e.g., Al-Anon, Nar-Anon) designed to provide support for family and friends will assist the support personnel to understand the addiction problem and provide them with guidance in coping with potential problems.

Laboratory Tests. Order stat and subsequent laboratory studies.

*Prochaska J, DiClemente C: Towards a comprehensive model of change. In Miller W, Heather N, eds: *Treating addictive behaviors: a process of change,* New York, 1986, Plenum.

Implementation

- In an emergency department setting, the immediate care needs of the individual must be met to stabilize the individual and provide for patient safety. Deliver physical care while providing for psychological support of the individual and significant others. Orient the patient to date, time, place, person, and situation. Once stabilized, the patient may be admitted to an intensive care, acute care, psychiatric, or rehabilitation facility designed to provide treatment of the presenting problems.
- The nurse needs to be familiar with the protocol and health care provider orders used during detoxification. Refer to the earlier section, Principles of Treatment for Substance Abuse, and to other textbooks with more extensive coverage of substance abuse for details regarding detoxification for specific agents being abused.
- During withdrawal, patient care needs include providing a quiet, safe care environment with staff who are experienced in detoxification methods.
- Provide for patient and staff safety. Have emergency equipment available at all times and be particularly vigilant for seizure activity.
- Perform physical assessments of the patient in accordance with the clinical policies (e.g., every 2, 4, or 8 hours, or as indicated by the patient's status).

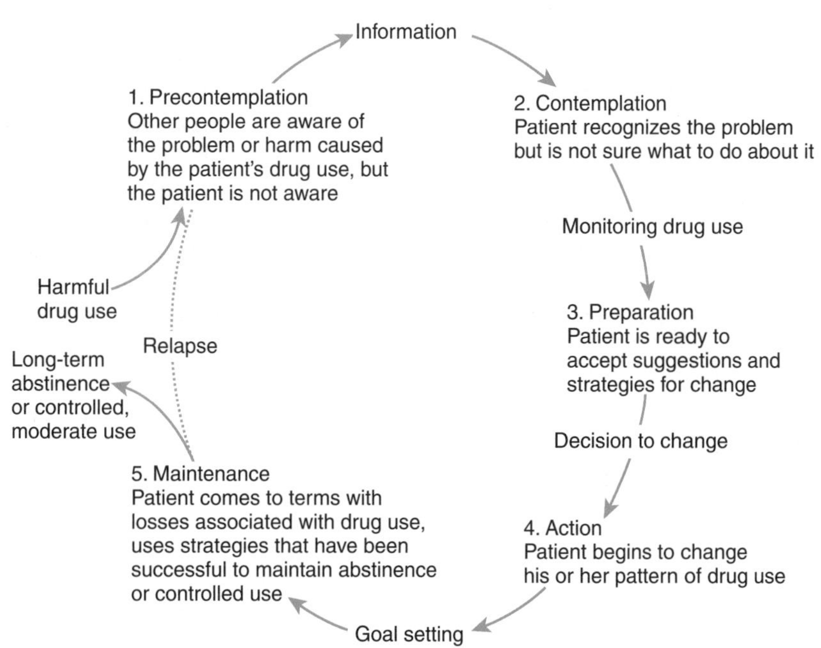

FIGURE **49-3** A model for change in substance use disorders. (Modified from Prochaska J, DiClemente C: Towards a comprehensive model of change. In Miller W, Heather N, eds: *Treating addictive behaviors: a process of change,* New York, 1986, Plenum.)

- Have medications listed in the protocol or health care provider's orders readily available for administration (e.g., benzodiazepines, clonidine, beta blockers for treatment of withdrawal; carbamazepine for seizures; cyclobenzaprine for muscle spasms; naltrexone to reduce craving).
- Implement measures to reduce anxiety, including administering prescribed medications that can best alleviate the patient's symptoms and provide maximum level of comfort. Support the patient in a calm manner even if the patient responds in a hostile or confrontational way. React appropriately to the patient's expressions of resistance (e.g., arguing, denying, ignoring).
- As the patient progresses, encourage the patient to make choices and take responsibility for the decisions made. See discussion earlier in chapter of intoxication, withdrawal, treatment, and relapse prevention.

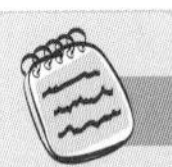

Patient Education and Health Promotion

Design an individualized approach to assist the patient to modify factors that are within the patient's control.

Ongoing Health Care. The patient must place himself or herself under the care of a health care provider who is trained to treat substance abuse and who can guide the patient through the challenges of withdrawal and recovery. The rehabilitation center or abuse counselor may have a list of health care providers, or can contact the American Society of Addiction Medicine at 4601 North Park Avenue, Upper Arcade #101, Chevy Chase, MD 20815; phone: (301) 656-3920; fax: (301) 656-3815 for a list of health care providers experienced in treating people with addictions.

The patient should inform all health care providers (e.g., physician, dentist, psychiatrist, podiatrist) of the history of addictive behavior so that a comprehensive plan can be derived for medication when it is necessary.

If planning to get pregnant, it is wise for the patient to consult with a health care provider about planning for a pregnancy that can be safe for the recovering addict and the baby.

Nutrition Status. Encourage a well-balanced diet. Consultation with a dietitian may be necessary. The B vitamins, especially thiamine, are vital to the repair of the nervous system, calcium may be needed for weakened bones, and excessive vitamin A and D may be harmful. If the patient is anemic, an iron preparation may also be prescribed. Consult the health care provider or a pharmacist about an appropriate vitamin supplement.

Have the patient drink eight to ten 8-ounce glasses of water daily, unless coexisting medical problems prohibit it.

Sugars may affect the mood of some individuals. If mood swings are a problem it may be wise to limit the patient's sugar intake.

Stress Management. Identify stress-producing situations in the patient's life and seek means to significantly reduce these factors. In some cases, referral for training in stress management, relaxation techniques, mediation, or biofeedback may be necessary. If stress is produced in the work setting, it may be appropriate to involve the nurse at the patient's place of employment.

Financial Status. What is the financial status of the individual? Has the individual borrowed money from everyone? Are legal charges pending for theft or for writing bad checks? As part of the rehabilitation process involve a social worker or counselor to assist the individual to create a plan for assuming responsibility for social and financial debts.

Job or Employment. The person may need assistance to establish a plan for how to integrate back into the work environment. Many fears are associated with the work environment (e.g., fear of being fired; fear of being tempted to use again because of stress at work; fear of not being able to perform the job duties satisfactorily).

The individual may need to contact the employer to see if returning to the job held before admission is acceptable. Many times the person may have displayed poor work habits while using alcohol or drugs and may have been terminated. The employer may also have an assistance program that can provide support to the employee in recovery.

Drug testing may be a requirement of court order, rehabilitation program, or returning to employment. The individual needs to understand the policies in place.

If it is necessary to find a new job, the individual may need guidance in how to go about finding job leads, how to apply for a new position, and how to interview.

Career Changes. Depending on the circumstances, the individual may need to make a career change to a less demanding work environment or to one that is better suited to his or her abilities.

Licenses and Insurance. If a driver's license has been revoked, the state licensing agency should be contacted for guidance in steps to be taken for reinstatement. Once the license is reinstated, the person must also hold insurance to license and drive a car. Contact the auto insurance company for a list of companies that may sell automobile insurance to "at risk" individuals. Understand that even with a valid driver's license, the cost of insurance is usually "rated," based on the previous driving violations.

If the patient holds a license to practice a profession, and if employment requires licensure, contact the state agency that issued the license to determine eligibility for continued licensure and potential employment in the field. Licensing boards usually require participation in a recovery program with urine testing as well as periodic reports to the licensing agency to maintain a license and practice a profession.

Fostering Health Maintenance. Seek the patient's cooperation and understanding of the following points so that medication adherence is increased: name of medication, dosage, route and times of administration, side effects to expect, and side effects to report. The person who has an alcohol or drug abuse problem needs to reveal his or her history to all health care providers so the prescriber can take this into account when selecting agents for use. At the supermarket, pharmacy, or nutrition center, the patient should always read labels thoroughly to avoid food and medicinal products that contain alcohol.

Written Record. Enlist the patient's aid in developing and maintaining a written record of monitoring parameters for coexisting medical problems (e.g., pulse rate, blood pressure, degree of dyspnea and what precipitates it, chest pain, edema) (see Patient Self-Assessment Form in Appendix I). Complete the Premedication Data column for use as a baseline to track response to drug therapy. Ensure that the patient understands how to use the form and instruct the patient to take the completed form to follow-up visits. During follow-up visits, focus on issues that will foster adherence with the therapeutic interventions prescribed.

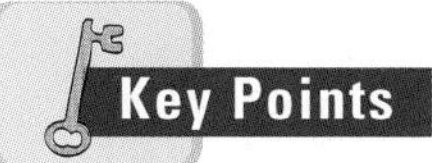

Key Points

- Substance abuse is defined as the periodic purposeful use of a substance that leads to clinically significant impairment.
- Major theories relating to why substances are abused include biologic, psychological, and sociocultural models that influence whether substances are abused.
- Table 49-2 summarizes several assessment instruments.
- Frequency of substance abuse among health care providers is probably similar to that of the general population.
- Health professionals suspecting a colleague of substance abuse need to observe, document, and report relevant data to the supervisor and to the licensing agency or disciplinary board in states where mandatory reporting is required. Many states have licensee assistance programs and procedures for reporting or seeking counseling from this resource.
- The DSM-IV-TR recognizes substance abuse and addiction as treatable diseases. Treatment needs to be individualized to the person's needs.
- Professionals providing health care to people with a substance abuse problem need to be vigilant for coexisting medical or psychiatric problems.
- People with a substance abuse problem must be encouraged to assume responsibility for their own actions and to focus not only on the need for a change in the abuse behavior but also on strategies for self-management of their lives and approaches that will make it possible to cope more effectively with life situations.
- Group support for the individual and for family/significant others need to be established. Many rehabilitation programs involve family as part of the treatment regimen. Others suggest community resources such as Alcoholics Anonymous or Narcotics Anonymous for the person in recovery and Al-Anon for family members.

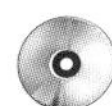

Go to your Companion CD-ROM for Appendices, an Audio Glossary, animations, Drug Dosage Calculators, customizable Patient Self-Assessment forms, and Review Questions for the NCLEX® Examination.

evolve Be sure to visit the companion Evolve site at http://evolve.elsevier.com/Clayton for WebLinks and additional online resources.

MEDICATION SAFETY REVIEW

MATH REVIEW QUESTIONS

1. Order: Chlordiazepoxide (Librium) 100 mg IM
   Available: Chlordiazepoxide (Librium) 100 mg/mL
   Give: ____ mL.
2. Order: Lorazepam (Ativan) 2 mg IM every hour until patient is moderately sedated.
   Available: Lorazepam (Ativan) 4 mg/mL
   Give: _____ mL.
3. Order: Lorazepam (Ativan) 2 mg PO stat
   Available: Lorazepam (Ativan) 1-mg tablet
   Give: _____ tablet.

Continued

CRITICAL THINKING QUESTIONS

1. Investigate the community resources available in your area for alcoholics, drug users, and families or significant others. Then attend a meeting to observe:
   - **a.** how participants are guided to accept responsibility for their actions.
   - **b.** how participants deal with the problem of relapse.
   - **c.** what problems with sobriety participants discuss.
   - **d.** the incidence of alcohol and drug use in teens, adults, and older adults.
2. Research the protocol used for treatment of alcohol withdrawal in the nursing units where assigned.
3. What medicolegal requirements are incorporated into emergency department procedures for people admitted with suspected substance abuse?

CONTENT REVIEW QUESTIONS

1. The __________ theory of substance abuse focuses on the patterns of relationships between family members through the generations.

2. The theory that attributes alcohol abuse to a person being fixed in the oral stage of development is an example of a(n) __________ theory.

3. Symptoms of alcohol withdrawal include: *(Select all that apply.)*
   1. nausea.
   2. vomiting.
   3. psychomotor agitation.
   4. diaphoresis.

4. Which of the following should be assessed in an individual with signs and symptoms of alcohol withdrawal syndrome (AWS)?
   1. Nutritional status
   2. Hydration
   3. Electrolytes

5. The nurse concludes that the client has learned an important fact about cocaine use when he says:
   1. "Cocaine is not addictive."
   2. "Cocaine withdrawal is relatively easy."
   3. "Since cocaine is a depressant, one should not drive."
   4. "I know a young person can have a heart attack from using cocaine."

6. The nurse teaching a client taking disulfiram (Antabuse) should focus on:
   1. emotional support.
   2. abstaining from alcohol ingestion.
   3. daily exercise.
   4. hygiene.

7. Signs and symptoms that would raise suspicion of substance abuse by a health professional include which of the following? *(Select all that apply.)*
   1. Wearing long-sleeved garments all the time
   2. Diminished alertness
   3. Requests for frequent schedule changes
   4. Rarely being absent from work

CHAPTER

50 Miscellaneous Agents

evolve http://evolve.elsevier.com/Clayton

Chapter Content

MISCELLANEOUS AGENTS

acamprosate (a kamp′ roh sait)
CAMPRAL (kam′ prahl)

Actions

Acamprosate is classified as a weak *N*-methyl-D-aspartate (NDMA) receptor antagonist. It is a synthetic compound structurally related to gamma-aminobutyric acid (GABA). A variety of mechanisms have been proposed, but none are well proven.

Uses

Acamprosate is used in alcohol rehabilitation programs for chronic alcoholic patients who want to maintain sobriety. It should be used only in conjunction with other rehabilitative therapy. It enhances abstinence and reduces drinking rates in alcohol-dependent patients who are abstinent at the beginning of treatment. It is neither a sedative nor an anxiolytic, and it is not addictive. It does not reduce the rewarding effects of alcohol like naltrexone does, nor does it cause nausea and vomiting when alcohol is consumed, like disulfiram. Studies indicate similar rates of success with naltrexone and acamprosate, and a slightly higher success rate when used together. Acamprosate may also be used in cases when naltrexone is contraindicated, such as in patients with liver disease or in those receiving concurrent opioid therapy or methadone maintenance therapy. Acamprosate does not treat withdrawal symptoms.

Therapeutic Outcomes

The primary therapeutic outcome expected from acamprosate is improved adherence with an alcohol treatment program by abstinence from alcohol.

NURSING PROCESS *for Acamprosate*

Premedication Assessment

1. Perform baseline neurologic assessment (e.g., orientation to date, time, and place; mental alertness; bilateral handgrip; motor functioning).
2. Take vital signs (i.e., temperature, blood pressure, pulse, respirations).
3. Check laboratory values for urine screen for alcohol use, blood urea nitrogen (BUN) and serum creatinine for renal function.
4. Monitor for gastrointestinal symptoms before and during therapy.

Planning

Availability. PO: 333-mg delayed release tablets.

Implementation

Dosage and Administration

Behavior Modification. Acamprosate therapy in combination with behavioral therapy has been shown to be more effective than acamprosate or behavioral therapy alone in prolonging alcohol cessation in patients who were formerly physically dependent on alcohol.

NOTE: Acamprosate is contraindicated in patients with severe renal failure as indicated by a creatinine clearance of less than 30 mL per minute.

Adult: PO: Two 333-mg tablets (666 mg) three times daily. Tablets may be taken without regard to meals. Acamprosate should be started as soon as possible after the period of alcohol withdrawal, when the patient has become abstinent.

Patients with moderate renal function as indicated by a creatinine clearance of 30 to 50 mL per minute should take one 333-mg tablet three times daily.

Evaluation

Side Effects to Expect

Diarrhea. Diarrhea may occur in 10% to 20% of patients taking acamprosate, but rarely is it a cause for discontinuing therapy. Symptoms are usually mild and tend to resolve with continued therapy. Encourage the patient not to discontinue therapy without first consulting the health care provider and treatment program.

Side Effects to Report

Suicidal Actions. In clinical studies with acamprosate, suicidal ideation, suicide attempts, and completed suicides were infrequent, but were more common in acamprosate-treated patients than in patients treated with placebo (2.4% versus 0.8%). The interrelationship of alcohol dependence, depression, and suicide is well recognized and complex. Monitor alcohol-dependent patients, including those patients being treated with acamprosate, for symptoms of negative thoughts, feelings, behaviors, depression, or suicidal thinking. Alert families and caregivers of patients being treated with acamprosate of the need to monitor patients for the emergence of these symptoms, and to report such symptoms to the patient's health care provider.

Drug Interactions. No clinically significant drug interactions have been reported.

allopurinol (al oh pur' in ol)
ZYLOPRIM (zy' lo prim)
ALOPRIM (ahl' oh prim)

Actions

Allopurinol blocks the terminal steps in uric acid formation by inhibiting the enzyme xanthine oxidase.

Uses

This agent can be used to treat primary gout or gout secondary to antineoplastic therapy. It is not effective in treating acute attacks of gouty arthritis. Allopurinol has an advantage over uricosuric agents in that gouty nephropathy and the formation of urate stones are less likely because the drug inhibits the production of uric acid. It may also be used in patients with renal failure. Uricosuric agents should not be used in this case.

Therapeutic Outcomes

The primary therapeutic outcome associated with allopurinol therapy is reduced serum uric acid levels with a lower frequency of acute gouty attacks.

Nursing Process for Allopurinol

Premedication Assessment

1. Inquire about the time of onset of gouty attack; do not start the medication during an acute attack.
2. Assess for and record any gastrointestinal complaints before initiating drug therapy.
3. Obtain baseline blood studies, blood counts, renal and liver function studies as requested.

Planning

Availability. PO: 100 and 300 mg tablets; IV: 500 mg in 30 mL vial.

Implementation

Dosage and Administration. *Adult:* IV: 200 to 400 mg/m^2 per day, up to a maximum of 600 mg per day. Infuse at a concentration no greater than 6 mg/mL. When possible, allopurinol therapy should be started 24 to 48 hours before chemotherapy known to cause tumor lysis. PO: initially 100 mg daily. Increase the daily dosage by 100 mg per week until the serum urate level falls to 6 mg/100 mL or a maximum dosage of 800 mg daily is achieved. The average maintenance dose is 300 mg daily. Dosage must be reduced in patients with a creatinine clearance of 20 mL/min or lower.

Gastric Irritation. If gastric irritation occurs, administer with food or milk. If symptoms persist or increase in severity, report for health care provider evaluation.

Fluid Intake. Maintain fluid intake at eight to twelve 8-ounce glasses daily.

Evaluation

Side Effects to Expect

Acute Gout Attacks. Patients should be told that the frequency of gout attacks may increase for the first few months of therapy. The patient should continue therapy without changing the dosage during the attacks.

Nausea, Vomiting, Diarrhea, Dizziness, Headache. These side effects are usually mild and tend to resolve with continued therapy. Encourage the patient not to discontinue therapy without first consulting the health care provider.

Side Effects to Report

Hepatotoxicity. The symptoms of hepatotoxicity are anorexia, nausea, vomiting, jaundice, hepatomegaly, splenomegaly, and abnormal liver function tests (elevated bilirubin, aspartate aminotransferase [AST], alanine aminotransferase [ALT], gamma-glutamyl transferase [GGT], alkaline phosphatase, prothrombin time).

Blood Dyscrasias. Routine laboratory studies (red blood cells [RBC], white blood cells [WBC], differential counts) should be scheduled. Stress the importance of returning for this laboratory work. Monitor for sore throat, fever, purpura, jaundice, or excessive and progressive weakness.

Fever, Pruritus, Rash. Report symptoms for further evaluation by the health care provider. Pruritus may be relieved by adding baking soda to the bathwater.

Drug Interactions

Theophylline Derivatives. Allopurinol, when given with theophylline derivatives, may cause theophylline toxicity. Observe for vomiting, dizziness, restlessness, and cardiac arrhythmias. The dosage of theophylline may need to be reduced.

Chlorpropamide. Allopurinol may reduce the metabolism of chlorpropamide. Monitor for hypoglycemia (headache, weakness, decreased coordination, general apprehension, diaphoresis, hunger, and blurred or double vision). The dosage of the hypoglycemic agent may need to be reduced. Notify the health care provider if any of these symptoms appear.

Azathioprine, Mercaptopurine. When initiating therapy with azathioprine or mercaptopurine, start at one fourth to one third of the normal dosage and adjust subsequent dosages according to the patient's response.

Ampicillin, Amoxicillin. There is a high incidence of rash when patients are taking both allopurinol and ampicillin or amoxicillin. Do not consider the patient allergic to either drug until sensitivity tests identify a hypersensitivity reaction.

Cyclophosphamide. There is a greater incidence of bone marrow depression in patients receiving these agents concurrently. Monitor for sore throat, fever, purpura, jaundice, or excessive and progressive weakness.

colchicine (kol' chi sin)

Actions

The exact mechanism of action is not known, but colchicine does interrupt the cycle of urate crystal deposition in the tissues that results in an acute attack of gout. It does not affect the amount of uric acid in the blood or urine; therefore it is not a uricosuric agent.

Uses

Colchicine is an alkaloid that has been used for hundreds of years to prevent or relieve acute attacks of gout. Joint pain and swelling begin to subside within 12 hours and are usually gone within 48 to 72 hours after initiating therapy.

Therapeutic Outcomes

The primary therapeutic outcome expected from colchicine therapy is elimination of joint pain secondary to acute gout attack.

Nursing Process for Colchicine

Premedication Assessment

1. Assess for and record any gastrointestinal complaints present before initiation of drug therapy.
2. Obtain baseline complete blood count (CBC) and differential, uric acid level, and so on as requested by health care provider for future comparison and to monitor for development of blood dyscrasias and track progress in control of uric acid level.

Planning

Availability. PO: 0.5 and 0.6 mg tablets; IV: 1 mg per 2-mL ampules.

Implementation

Dosage and Administration. NOTE: Use with extreme caution in older adults or debilitated patients and in those patients with impaired renal, cardiac, or gastrointestinal function. *Adult:* PO: Acute gout: Initially 0.5 to 1.3 mg, followed by 0.6 mg every 1 to 2 hours until pain subsides or nausea, vomiting, and diarrhea develop. A total dose of 4 to 10 mg may be required. After the acute attack, 0.5 to 0.6 mg should be administered every 6 hours for a few days to prevent relapse. Do not repeat high-dose therapy for at least 3 days. Prophylaxis for recurrent gout: 0.5 to 0.6 mg every 1 to 3 days depending on the frequency of gouty attacks. IV: Acute gout: Initially 2 mg diluted in 20 mL of saline solution and administer slowly over 5 minutes. Follow with 0.5 mg every 6 to 12 hours to a maximum of 4 mg in 24 hours. If pain recurs, daily doses of 1 to 2 mg may be administered for several days. Do not repeat high-dose therapy for at least 3 days. Avoid extravasation! Observe IV site for any change in color, size, or skin integrity. Pain, swelling, or erythema signifies infiltration.

DO NOT ADMINISTER SUBCUTANEOUSLY OR IM!

Extravasation. Clamp, report, and follow hospital protocol for extravasation. Elevate the infiltrated area. Prepare to assist with administration of drugs to counteract the necrotizing effects.

Fluid Intake. Monitor intake and output during therapy. Maintain fluid intake at 8 to 12, 8-ounce glasses daily.

Evaluation

Side Effects to Expect

Nausea, Vomiting, Diarrhea. These are common adverse effects of colchicine therapy. Discontinue therapy when gastrointestinal symptoms develop. Always report bright red blood in vomitus, "coffee ground" vomitus, or dark tarry stools.

Side Effects to Report

Blood Dyscrasias. Serious, potentially fatal blood dyscrasias, including anemia, agranulocytosis, and thrombocytopenia, have been associated with colchicine therapy. Although the development of blood dyscrasias is rare, periodic differential blood counts are recommended if the patient requires prolonged treatment. Routine laboratory studies (e.g., RBC, WBC, differential counts) should be scheduled. Stress to the patient the importance of returning for this laboratory work. Monitor for the development of sore throat, fever, purpura, jaundice, or excessive and progressive weakness. Report immediately.

Drug Interactions. No clinically significant drug interactions have been reported.

disulfiram (di sul' fur am)
ANTABUSE (an' ah byuse)

Actions

Disulfiram is an agent that, when ingested before any form of alcohol is consumed, produces a very unpleasant reaction to the alcohol. Disulfiram blocks the metabolism of acetaldehyde, a metabolite of alcohol. Elevated levels of acetaldehyde produce the disulfiram-alcohol reaction, which is manifested by nausea, severe vomiting, sweating, throbbing headache, dizziness, blurred vision, and confusion. The intensity of the reaction somewhat depends on the sensitivity of the individual and the amount of alcohol consumed. The duration of the reaction depends on the presence of alcohol in the blood. Mild reactions may last from 30 to 60 minutes, whereas more severe reactions may last for several hours. Prolonged administration of disulfiram does not produce tolerance; indeed, the longer a patient remains on therapy, the more exquisitely sensitive the person becomes to alcohol.

Uses

Disulfiram is used in alcohol rehabilitation programs for chronic alcoholic patients who want to maintain sobriety. It should be used only in conjunction with other rehabilitative therapy. Patients must be fully informed of the consequences of drinking alcohol while receiving disulfiram therapy. As little as 10 to 15 mL of alcohol may produce a reaction. Patients must not drink or apply alcohol in any form, including over-the-counter products such as sleep aids, cough and cold products, aftershave lotions, mouthwashes, and rubbing alcohol. Dietary sources, such as sauces and vinegars containing alcohol, are prohibited. A disulfiram-alcohol reaction may occur with the ingestion of any alcohol for 1 to 2 weeks after discontinuing disulfiram therapy. Disulfiram must never be administered to a patient who is intoxicated. Because of the consequence of a disulfiram-alcohol reaction on other disease states, use disulfiram therapy very cautiously in patients with diabetes mellitus, hypothyroidism, epilepsy, cerebral damage, chronic or acute nephritis, hepatic cirrhosis, or hepatic failure.

Therapeutic Outcomes

The primary therapeutic outcome expected from disulfiram is improved adherence with an alcohol treatment program by abstinence from alcohol.

Nursing Process for Disulfiram

Premedication Assessment

1. Perform baseline neurologic assessment (e.g., orientation to date, time, and place; mental alertness; bilateral handgrip; motor functioning).
2. Take vital signs (i.e., temperature, blood pressure, pulse, respirations).
3. Check laboratory values for hepatotoxicity; screen urine for alcohol use.
4. Monitor for gastrointestinal symptoms before and during therapy.
5. The manufacturer recommends that baseline determinations of liver function should be performed in all patients before initiation of therapy and repeated in 10 to 14 days. A baseline CBC count and serum chemistries also are recommended and should also be repeated every 6 months along with the liver function tests.

Planning

Availability. PO: 250 mg tablets.

Implementation

Dosage and Administration

Behavior Modification. Disulfiram therapy in combination with behavioral therapy has been shown to be more effective than disulfiram or behavioral therapy alone in prolonging alcohol cessation in patients who were formerly physically dependent on alcohol.

- Disulfiram must never be administered to patients when they are in a state of intoxication or when they are unaware they are receiving therapy. Family members should also be told about the treatment to help provide motivation and support and to help avoid accidental disulfiram-alcohol reactions.
- Do not administer disulfiram until the patient has abstained from alcohol for at least 12 hours.
- It is recommended that all patients receiving disulfiram carry a patient identification card stating the use of disulfiram and describing the symptoms most likely to occur as a result of the disulfiram-alcohol reaction. This card also should indicate the health care provider or institution to be contacted in an emergency.

Adult: PO: Initially a maximum of 500 mg once daily for 1 to 2 weeks. The maintenance dosage is usually 250 mg daily (range 125-500 mg). Do not exceed 500 mg daily. Administer at bedtime to avoid the complications of sedative effects.

Evaluation

Side Effects to Expect

Drowsiness, Fatigue, Headache, Impotence, Metallic Taste. These side effects are usually mild and tend to resolve with continued therapy. Encourage the patient not to discontinue therapy without first consulting the health care provider and treatment program.

Side Effects to Report

Hepatotoxicity. The symptoms of hepatotoxicity are jaundice, nausea, vomiting, anorexia, hepatomegaly, splenomegaly, and abnormal liver function tests (e.g., elevated bilirubin, aspartate aminotransferase [AST], alanine aminotransferase [ALT], alkaline phosphatase, and prothrombin time [PT]). Because many of these patients do not develop clinical symptoms but do develop abnormal liver function test results, strongly encourage patients to report for blood tests as scheduled. Report abnormal values to the appropriate health care provider.

Hives, Pruritus, Rash. Report symptoms for further evaluation by the health care provider. Pruritus may be relieved by taking antihistamines and adding baking soda to the bathwater.

Drug Interactions

Warfarin. Disulfiram may enhance the anticoagulant effects of warfarin. Observe for the development of petechiae, ecchymoses, nosebleeds, bleeding gums, dark tarry stools, and bright red or "coffee ground" emesis. Monitor the prothrombin time (INR) and reduce the dosage of warfarin if necessary.

Phenytoin. Disulfiram inhibits the metabolism of phenytoin. Monitor patients with concurrent use for signs of phenytoin toxicity (i.e., nystagmus, sedation, lethargy). Serum levels may be monitored and the dosage of phenytoin may need to be reduced.

Isoniazid. Disulfiram alters the metabolism of isoniazid. Perform a baseline assessment of the patient's degree of alertness (e.g., orientation to name, place, time) and of coordination before initiating therapy. Make regularly scheduled subsequent mental status evaluations and compare findings. Report development of alterations.

Metronidazole. Concurrent administration of disulfiram and metronidazole may result in psychotic episodes and confusional states. Concurrent therapy is not recommended.

Benzodiazepines. Disulfiram inhibits the metabolism of specific benzodiazepines (i.e., chlordiazepoxide, diazepam, clorazepate, halazepam, flurazepam, quazepam, estrazolam). When benzodiazepine therapy is indicated, use oxazepam, alprazolam, temazepam, or lorazepam because of a different metabolic pathway not inhibited by disulfiram.

Caffeine. The cardiovascular and CNS stimulant effects of caffeine may be increased by disulfiram. If tachycardia or nervousness is noted, cut back on the consumption of caffeine-containing products such as coffee.

donepezil (don ep' ih zil)

▸ ARICEPT (air' ih sept)

Actions

Donepezil is an acetylcholinesterase inhibitor that allows acetylcholine to accumulate at cholinergic synapses, causing a prolonged and exaggerated cholinergic effect.

Uses

Although the causes are unknown, Alzheimer's disease is characterized by a loss of cholinergic neurons in the CNS, resulting in memory loss and cognitive deficits (dementia). Donepezil is used in mild to moderate dementia to enhance cholinergic function. Donepezil's function diminishes with ongoing loss of cholinergic neurons. Donepezil does not prevent or slow the neurodegeneration of Alzheimer's disease.

Therapeutic Outcomes

The primary therapeutic outcome expected from donepezil therapy is improved cognitive skills (e.g., word recall, naming objects, language, word finding, improved ability to do tasks).

Nursing Process for Donepezil

Premedication Assessment

1. Obtain baseline assessments of presenting symptoms.
2. Record baseline pulse, respirations, and blood pressure.
3. Assess for and record any gastric symptoms present before initiation of therapy.

Planning

Availability. PO: 5 and 10 mg tablets; 5 and 10 mg orally-disintegrating tablets.

Implementation

Dosage and Administration. *Adult:* PO: Initial dose: 5 mg daily at bedtime. After 4 to 6 weeks of therapy, dosage may be increased to 10 mg daily to assess therapeutic benefit. Donepezil may be taken with or without food.

The orally disintegrating tablets may be helpful in patients who have difficulty swallowing. Allow to dissolve on the tongue and follow with a glass of water.

Evaluation

Side Effects to Expect

Nausea, Vomiting, Dyspepsia, Diarrhea. These are natural extensions of the pharmacologic effects of cholinergic agents. Dosage may need to be reduced if the patient has difficulty with these adverse effects. Symptoms are less common with lower doses and tend to subside after 2 to 3 weeks of therapy. Gradually increasing the dose may help avoid these complications.

Side Effects to Report

Bradycardia. Cholinergic agents cause a slowing of the heart. Notify the health care provider if the heart rate is regularly less than 60 beats per minute.

Drug Interactions

Drugs That Enhance Therapeutic and Toxic Effects. Ketoconazole and quinidine may inhibit the metabolism of donepezil. Monitor closely for enhancement of adverse effects.

Drugs That Reduce Therapeutic Effects. Carbamazepine, dexamethasone, phenobarbital, phenytoin, and rifampin increase the metabolism of donepezil reducing its therapeutic effects. The dose of donepezil may need to be increased or the patient switched to another medicine to treat Alzheimer's disease.

Anticholinergic Agents. As a cholinergic agent, donepezil has the potential to reduce the activity of anticholinergic agents (e.g., benztropine, diphenhydramine, orphenadrine, procyclidine, trihexyphenidyl).

Succinylcholine-Type Muscle Relaxants, Cholinergic Agents. As a cholinesterase inhibitor, donepezil is likely to exaggerate the actions of depolarizing muscle relaxants (e.g., succinylcholine) during anesthesia and enhance the pharmacologic activity of cholinergic agents such as bethanechol.

lactulose (lak′ tu los)
▶ CEPHULAC (sef′ u lak)

Actions

Lactulose is a sugar that acidifies the colon, thus preventing the absorption of ammonia. It also acts as a stool softener by increasing the osmotic pressure and pulling water into the colon.

Uses

Elevated ammonia levels are thought to be a cause of portosystemic (hepatic) encephalopathy and coma. Lactulose is used to reduce formation of ammonia in the gut. Lactulose also may be used as a laxative. Use with caution in patients with diabetes mellitus. Lactulose syrup contains small amounts of free lactose, galactose, and other sugars.

Therapeutic Outcomes

The primary therapeutic outcomes expected from lactulose therapy are:

- Improved orientation to surroundings
- A gentle laxative effect with formed stool

Nursing Process for Lactulose

Premedication Assessment

1. Obtain baseline assessments of presenting symptoms.
2. Assess for and record any gastric symptoms present before initiating therapy.
3. Perform a baseline mental status examination (e.g., orientation to time, place, and date).
4. Obtain baseline laboratory studies ordered (e.g., electrolytes and serum ammonia levels).
5. Record temperature, pulse, respirations, blood pressure, and hydration status.

Planning

Availability. PO: 10 g of lactulose per 15 mL of syrup; crystals for reconstitution: 10-g and 20-g containers.

Implementation

Dosage and Administration. *Adult:* Laxative: PO: Initially 15 to 30 mL daily. Increase to 60 mL daily if necessary. Administer with fruit juice, water, or milk to make the syrup more palatable. It may take 24 to 48 hours to produce a normal bowel movement. Portosystemic encephalopathy: PO: Initially 30 to 45 mL every hour for rapid laxation. Once the laxative effect is achieved, the dosage is reduced to 30 to 45 mL three or four times daily. Adjust the dosage to produce two or three soft, formed stools daily. Rectal: Mix 300 mL of syrup with 700 mL of water or normal saline. Instill rectally every 4 to 6 hours with a rectal balloon catheter. Instruct the patient to attempt to retain for 30 to 60 minutes. Do not use soapsuds or cleansing enemas.

Evaluation

Side Effects to Expect

Belching, Abdominal Distention, Flatulence. These are common adverse effects frequently observed in the early stages of therapy and will resolve with continued therapy, but dosage reduction may be necessary. Diarrhea is a sign of overdosage and is corrected by dosage reduction.

Side Effects to Report

Electrolyte Imbalance, Dehydration. These effects may result from diarrhea. The electrolytes most commonly altered are potassium (K^+) and chloride (Cl^-). Hypokalemia is most likely to occur.

Many symptoms associated with altered fluid and electrolyte balance are subtle and resemble general symptoms of drug toxicity or the disease process itself.

Gather data relative to changes in the patient's mental status (e.g., alertness, orientation, confusion), muscle strength, muscle cramps, tremors, nausea, and general appearance (drowsy, anxious, and lethargic).

Always check the electrolyte reports for early indications of electrolyte imbalance.

Keep accurate records of input and output, daily weights, and vital signs.

Patients on long-term lactulose therapy (6 months or longer) should have serum potassium and chloride levels measured periodically.

Drug Interactions

Laxatives. Do not administer with other laxatives. Diarrhea makes it difficult to adjust to a proper dosage of lactulose.

Antibiotics. Antibiotic therapy may destroy too much of the bacteria in the colon necessary for lactulose to work. Monitor patients closely for reduced lactulose activity when concurrent antibiotic therapy is prescribed.

memantine (mem′ an teen)
▶ NAMENDA (nam en′ dah)

Actions

Memantine is an *N*-methyl-D-aspartate (NDMA) receptor inhibitor.

Uses

Although the causes are unknown, one of the neurochemical characteristics of Alzheimer's disease is persistent activation of NDMA receptors in the CNS. Memantine blocks these receptors and is used alone or in combination with an acetylcholinesterase inhibitor in the treatment of moderate to severe Alzheimer's dementia. Patients taking memantine show improvement in cognitive function and behavioral symptoms and a slower decline in activities of daily living, but memantine does not prevent or slow the neurodegeneration of Alzheimer's disease.

Therapeutic Outcomes

The primary therapeutic outcome expected from memantine therapy is improved cognitive skills (e.g., word recall, naming objects, language, word finding, improved ability to do tasks).

Nursing Process for Memantine

Premedication Assessment

1. Obtain baseline assessments of presenting symptoms.
2. Record baseline pulse, respirations, and blood pressure.

Planning

Availability. PO: 5 and 10 mg tablets.

Implementation

Dosage and Administration. *Adult:* PO: 5 mg once daily. The dose should be increased in 5-mg increments to 10 mg daily, 15 mg daily and 20 mg daily. The minimal interval between dose increases is 1 week. Memantine can be taken with or without food.

Evaluation

Side Effects to Expect and Report

Headache, Dizziness, Akathisia, Insomnia, Restlessness, Increased Motor Activity, Excitement and Agitation. Many of these symptoms decline with continued therapy and can be reduced with a longer dosage titration. Dosage may need to be reduced if the patient has difficulty with these adverse effects.

Drug Interactions

Acetazolamide, Sodium Bicarbonate. Medicines that alkalinize the pH of the urine will reduce excretion of memantine. Severe medical conditions such as renal tubular acidosis and severe urinary tract infections also may cause alkalization of the urine with potential toxicity of memantine.

probenecid (pro ben' eh sid)

Actions

Uricosuric agents act on the tubules of the kidneys to enhance the excretion of uric acid. Probenecid promotes renal excretion of a number of substances, including uric acid. It inhibits the reabsorption of urate in the kidney, which results in reduction of uric acid in the blood.

Uses

Probenecid is used to treat hyperuricemia and chronic gouty arthritis. It is not effective in acute attacks of gout and is not an analgesic.

Therapeutic Outcomes

The primary therapeutic outcome expected with probenecid therapy is prevention of acute attacks of gouty arthritis.

Nursing Process for Probenecid

Premedication Assessment

1. Inquire about time of onset of the last gout attack; do not administer medication during or within 2 to 3 weeks of an acute attack.
2. Assess for and record any gastrointestinal complaints before initiating drug therapy.
3. Ask about any history of blood dyscrasias or kidney stones; if present, withhold drug and contact a health care provider.
4. Obtain baseline blood studies as requested (e.g., uric acid level, and serum creatinine) to assess appropriateness and to monitor response to therapy.

Planning

Availability. PO: 500 mg tablets.

Implementation

NOTE: Do not start probenecid therapy during an acute attack of gout; wait 2 to 3 weeks.

Contraindication. Do NOT administer to patients with histories of blood dyscrasias or uric acid kidney stones.

Dosage and Administration. *Adult:* PO: Initially 250 mg twice daily for 1 week, then 500 mg twice daily. The dosage may be increased by 500 mg every few weeks to a maximum of 2 to 3 g daily. Administer with food or milk to diminish gastric irritation.

Maintain fluid intake at 2 to 3 L daily.

Do not administer to patients with a creatinine clearance of less than 40 mL per minute or a BUN greater than 40 mg/100 mL.

Evaluation

Side Effects to Expect

Acute Gout Attacks. Patients should be told that the incidence of gout attacks may increase for the first few months of therapy and should continue therapy without changing the dosage during the attacks.

Side Effects to Report

Nausea, Anorexia, Vomiting. Use with caution in patients with history of peptic ulcer disease. Individuals who experience symptoms of ulcers and are yet undiagnosed should be encouraged to report gastrointestinal symptoms if they increase in intensity or frequency. Always report bright red blood in vomitus, "coffee ground" vomitus, or dark tarry stools.

Hives, Pruritus, Rash. These are signs of hypersensitivity. Notify the health care provider. Therapy may have to be discontinued.

Drug Interactions

Oral Hypoglycemic Agents. Monitor for hypoglycemia (e.g., headache, weakness, decreased coordination, general apprehension, diaphoresis, hunger, blurred or double vision). The dosage of the hypoglycemic agent may need to be reduced. Notify the health care provider if any of these symptoms appear.

Acyclovir, Famciclovir, Valacyclovir, Zidovudine, Dapsone, Indomethacin, Sulfinpyrazone, Rifampin, Sulfonamides, Naproxen, Penicillins, Cephalosporins, Methotrexate, and Clofibrate. Probenecid blocks the renal excretion of these agents. See individual drugs listed for side effects to report that may indicate development of toxicity.

Salicylates. Although occasional use of aspirin will not interfere with the effectiveness of probenecid, regular use of aspirin or aspirin-containing products should be discouraged. If analgesia is required, suggest acetaminophen.

Antineoplastic Agents. Probenecid is not recommended for increased uric acid levels caused by antineoplastic therapy because of the potential development of renal uric acid stones.

Clinitest. This drug may produce false-positive Clinitest results. Use Clinistix to measure urine glucose.

tacrine (tack' rhin)
COGNEX (cohg' nehx)

Actions

Tacrine is an acetylcholinesterase inhibitor that allows acetylcholine to accumulate at cholinergic synapses, causing a prolonged and exaggerated cholinergic effect.

Uses

Although the causes are unknown, Alzheimer's disease is characterized by a loss of cholinergic neurons in the CNS, resulting in memory loss and cognitive deficits (dementia). Tacrine is used in mild to moderate dementia to enhance cholinergic function.

Therapeutic Outcomes

The primary therapeutic outcome expected from tacrine therapy is improved cognitive skills (e.g., word recall, naming objects, language, word finding, improved ability to do tasks).

Nursing Process for Tacrine

Premedication Assessment

1. Obtain baseline assessments of presenting symptoms.
2. Record baseline pulse, respirations, and blood pressure.
3. Assess for and record any gastric symptoms or abnormal liver function present before initiating therapy.
4. Obtain baseline laboratory studies ordered (e.g., liver function tests).

Planning

Availability. PO: 10, 20, 30, and 40 mg tablets.

Implementation

Dosage and Administration. *Adult:* PO: 10 mg four times daily between meals and at bedtime. After at least 6 weeks, increase the dose to 20 mg four times daily. At 6-week intervals the dosage can be increased to a maximum of 40 mg four times daily.

Serum ALT levels should be measured to assess for the development of hepatotoxicity. The risk of hepatotoxicity is greatest in the first 12 weeks of tacrine treatment. Serum ALT levels should be monitored every other week during the first 16 weeks of therapy; thereafter, ALT serum concentrations can be monitored monthly. The manufacturer recommends specific guidelines on adjustment of treatment based on ALT levels.

Evaluation

Side Effects to Expect

Nausea, Vomiting, Dyspepsia, Diarrhea. These are natural extensions of the pharmacologic effects of cholinergic agents. Dosage may need to be reduced if the patient has difficulty with these adverse effects.

Side Effects to Report

Hepatotoxicity. The symptoms of hepatotoxicity are anorexia, nausea, vomiting, jaundice, hepatomegaly, splenomegaly, and abnormal liver function tests (e.g., elevated bilirubin, AST, ALT, GGT, alkaline phosphatase, prothrombin time). Stress the importance of returning for routine laboratory studies.

Rash, Fever, Jaundice. The health care provider should be notified immediately if the patient develops a rash, fever, or jaundice. These are indications of hypersensitivity or hepatotoxicity. The manufacturer recommends that tacrine be permanently discontinued.

Bradycardia. Cholinergic agents cause a slowing of the heart. Notify the health care provider if the heart rate is regularly less than 60 beats per minute.

Drug Interactions

Theophylline. Tacrine inhibits the metabolism of theophylline, substantially elevating theophylline serum levels and creating the potential for toxicity. Theophylline dosage adjustment is usually necessary.

Cimetidine. Cimetidine inhibits the metabolism of tacrine, substantially elevating tacrine serum levels and creating the potential for toxicity. Tacrine dosage adjustment is usually necessary.

Anticholinergic Agents. As a cholinergic agent, tacrine has the potential to reduce the activity of anticholinergic agents (e.g., benztropine, diphenhydramine, orphenadrine, procyclidine, trihexyphenidyl).

Succinylcholine-Type Muscle Relaxants. As a cholinesterase inhibitor, tacrine is likely to exaggerate the actions of depolarizing muscle relaxants (e.g., succinylcholine) during anesthesia.

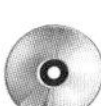

Go to your Companion CD-ROM for Appendices, an Audio Glossary, animations, Drug Dosage Calculators, customizable Patient Self-Assessment forms, and Review Questions for the NCLEX® Examination.

evolve Be sure to visit the companion Evolve site at http://evolve.elsevier.com/Clayton for WebLinks and additional online resources.

Bibliography

Online Resources

http://books.nap.edu/books/0309085373/html/index.html Institute of Medicine, Food and Nutrition Board: Dietary Reference Intakes for energy, carbohydrate, fiber, fat, fatty acids, cholesterol, protein, and amino acids (macronutrients) (2002).

http://cpmcnet.columbia.edu/dept/partnership Legato M: Men, women and medicine: what difference does sex make? Partnership for Women's Health at Columbia, Columbia University, New York, 2001.

http://fermat.nap.edu/books/0309085373/html/108.html National Academies Press, Dietary Reference Intakes for Energy, Carbohydrate, Fiber, Fat, Fatty Acids, Cholesterol, Protein, and Amino Acids (Macronutrients). (2005) Food and Nutrition Board (FNB), Institute of Medicine (IOM). PP. 107, 185.

http://oas.samhsa.gov/nsduh.htm#NSDUHinfo U.S. Department of Health and Human Services, Substance Abuse and Mental Health Services Administration, 2004, National Survey on Drug Use and Health (NSDUH).

www.acc.org/clinical/guidelines/failure//index.pdf Hunt SA, Abraham WT, Chin MH, et al: ACC/AHA 2005 guideline update for the diagnosis and management of chronic heart failure in the adult: A report of the American College of Cardiology/American Heart Association Task Force on Practice Guidelines (Writing Committee to Update the 2001 Guidelines for the Evaluation and Management of Heart Failure). American College of Cardiology Website.

www.americanheart.org American College of Cardiology/American Heart Association Task Force on Practice Guidelines for the Management of Patients with Chronic Stable Angina, Nov. 2002.

www.bardaccess.com/cathlink_20.html Bard Access Systems: Cath-Link 20 infusion port.

www.baxter.com/doctors/iv_therapies/education/ivtherapy_CE/Basics_One Basic Infiltration Scale.

www.cancer.org Cancer Facts and Figures—2005, American Cancer Society.

www.cdc.gov/brfss Centers for Disease Control and Prevention: Behavioral risk factor surveillance system survey data, Atlanta, 2005, U.S. Department of Health and Human Services.

www.cdc.gov/diabetes/pubs/estimates.htm Centers for Disease Control and Prevention. National diabetes fact sheet.

www.cdc.gov/nchs/fastats/deaths.htm Centers for Disease Control and Prevention. National Center for Health Statistics. Death—leading causes.

www.cdc.gov/nip/recs/child-schedule.htm Centers for Disease Control and Prevention: *Recommended childhood and adolescent immunization schedule.* Atlanta, 2006, U.S. Department of Health and Human Services.

www.cordem.org/wellness.htm Council of Emergency Medicine Residency Directors: Chemical dependency issues in emergency medicine residency programs, Lansing, MI. McNamara RM, Bouzoukis JK, Perina DG: Chemical dependency issues in emergency medicine residency programs.

www.guideline.gov National Guideline Clearinghouse: Management of labor.

www.ins1.org Infusion Nurses Society promotes excellence in infusion nursing through standards, education, advocacy, and outcomes research.

www.nhlbi.gov/guidelines/asthma National Institutes of Health: Guidelines for the diagnosis and management of asthma. National Asthma Education Program Expert Panel Report 2, 1997; DHHS publication No. 97-4051A. Update on selected topics 2002 (Update of the NAEPP Expert Panel Report 2, NIH Publication No. 97-4051), July, 2002.

www.oldwayspt.org/Oldways Food and nutritional think tank.

www.samhsa.gov/oas/nhsda/2k1nhsda U.S. Department of Health and Human Services, Substance Abuse and Mental Health Services Administration, 2001 National Household Survey on Drug Abuse (NHSDA).

www.surgeongeneral.gov/library/mentalhealth Mental Health: A report of the surgeon general, 1999.

www.venousaccess.com This site describes all types of vascular access, is current, and well referenced.

Publications

Abrams P, Cardozo L, Fall M, et al: The standardisation of terminology of lower urinary tract function: Report for the Standardisation Sub-committee of the International Continence Society. *Neurourol Urodynam* 21:167, 2002.

American Academy of Pediatrics: Controversies concerning vitamin K and the newborn, *Pediatrics* 112:191, 2003.

American Academy of Pediatrics: The transfer of drugs and other chemicals into human milk, *Pediatrics* 108(3):776, 2001.

American Diabetes Association: Clinical practice recommendations 2003, *Diabetes Care* 26(suppl 1), 2003.

American Diabetes Association: Standards of medical care in diabetes 2005, *Diabetes Care* 28 (suppl 1), 2005.

American Diabetes Association: Standards of medical care in diabetes 2005, *Diabetes Care* 29 (suppl 1), 2006.

American Pain Society: *Principles of analgesic use in the treatment of acute pain and cancer pain,* ed 5, Glenview, Ill., 2003, American Pain Society.

American Psychiatric Association: *Diagnostic and statistical manual of mental disorders,* ed 4, Text revision, Washington, DC, 2000, American Psychiatric Association.

Aruffo S, Grey S: Think you have a compliance problem? Think again, *Case Manager* (March/April):43, 2005.

Babcock DE, Miller MA: *Client education, theory and practice,* St Louis, 1994, Mosby.

Baldwin JN, Thibault ED: Substance abuse by pharmacists: stopping the insanity, *J Am Pharm Assoc* 41:373, 2001.

Beers H: Explicit criteria for determining potentially inappropriate medication use by the elderly, *Arch Intern Med* 57:1531, 1997.

Bickley LS, Szilagyi PG: *Bates' guide to physical examination and history taking,* ed 9, Philadelphia, 2006, Lippincott.

Billups NF: *American drug index,* ed 50, St Louis, 2006, Facts and Comparisons.

Bobak I et al: *Maternity nursing,* ed 4, St Louis, 1995, Mosby.

Boyce JM, Pittet D: Guideline for hand hygiene in health-care settings, *Am J Infect Control* 30(8):S1, 2002.

Brock GB, Lue TF: Drug-induced male sexual dysfunction: an update, *Drug Safety* 8(6):414, 1993.

Brown KM, Thomas DQ, Kotecki JE: *Physical activity and health: an interactive approach,* Boston, 2003, Jones and Bartlett.

Carpenito-Moyet LJ: *Nursing diagnosis: application to clinical practice,* ed 10, Philadelphia, 2004, Lippincott Williams & Wilkins.

Center for Substance Abuse Prevention: Curriculum Modules on Alcohol and Other Drug Problems for Schools of Social Work. In Centers for Disease Control and Prevention (CDC): *Behavioral risk factor surveillance system survey data*, Atlanta, 2003, U.S. Department of Health and Human Services, Centers for Disease Control and Prevention.

Centers for Disease Control and Prevention: Sexually transmitted diseases treatment guidelines 2002, *MMWR Morb Mortal Wkly Rep* 51(No. RR-6), 2002.

Clayton BD, Brown BK: Nausea and vomiting. In Helms RA, et al (eds.): *Textbook of therapeutics, drug and disease management,* ed 8, Philadelphia, 2006, Lippincott Williams & Wilkins.

Colodny L, Spillane J: Toward increased reporting of adverse drug reactions, *Hosp Pharm* 34(10):1179, 1999.

Commission on Classification and Terminology of the International League Against Epilepsy: proposal for revised classification of epilepsies and epileptic syndromes, *Epilepsia* 30:389, 1989.

Covington TR: Birth of a drug: the US drug development and approval process, *Facts Compar Drug News,* 11:73, 1992.

Criteria Committee of the New York Heart Association: *Nomenclature and criteria for diagnosis of diseases of the heart and great vessels,* ed 9, Boston, 1994, Little, Brown.

Davis CM: Affective education for the health profession, *Phys Ther* 6(11):1587, 1981.

DiPiro JT et al: *Pharmacotherapy, a pathophysiologic approach,* ed 6, New York, 2005, McGraw-Hill.

Dopheide JA, Stimmel GL: Sleep disorders. In Koda-Kimble MA, Young LY (eds.): *Applied therapeutics,* ed 8, Philadelphia, 2005, Lippincott Williams & Wilkins.

Dracup K, Dunbar SB, Baker DW: Rethinking heart failure, *Am J Nurs,* July, 23-27, 1995.

Ewing JA: Detecting alcoholism: the CAGE questionnaire, *JAMA* 252:1905, 1984.

Expert Panel on Detection, Evaluation, and Treatment of High Blood Cholesterol in Adults: *Third Report of the National Cholesterol Education Program (NCEP),* Bethesda, Md., NIH Publication No. 02-5215, Sept 2002, National Heart, Lung, and Blood Institute, National Institutes of Health.

Ganong WF: *Review of medical physiology,* ed 22, New York, 2005, McGraw-Hill.

Goldman L, Bennett JC (eds.): *Cecil's textbook of medicine,* ed 22, Philadelphia, 2004, Saunders.

Gurvitz JH, Rochon P: Improving the quality of medication use in elderly patients: a not-so-simple prescription, *Arch Intern Med* 162:1670, 2002.

Gurwitz JH et al: Incidence of preventability of adverse drug events in nursing homes, *Am J Med* 109:87, 2000.

Guyton AC: *Textbook of medical physiology,* ed 11, Philadelphia, 2006, Saunders.

Hardman JG, Limbird LL (eds.): *Goodman & Gilman's the pharmacological basic of therapeutics,* ed 11, New York, 2006, McGraw-Hill.

Hatcher RA et al: *Contraceptive technology,* ed 18, New York, 2004, Ardent Media.

Helms RA, et al (eds.): *Textbook of therapeutics, drug and disease management,* ed 8, Philadelphia, 2006, Lippincott Williams & Wilkins.

Herberg P: Theoretical foundations of transcultural nursing. In Boyle SJ, Andrews MM (eds.): *Transcultural concepts in nursing care,* Boston, 1989, Scott, Foresman.

Hockenberry M et al: *Wong's nursing care of infants and children,* ed 7, St Louis, 2003, Mosby.

Ignatavicius DD, Workman ML *Medical-surgical nursing: critical thinking for collaborative care,* ed 5, Philadelphia, 2006, Saunders.

Infusion Nurses Society: Infusion nursing standards of practice, Philadelphia, 2006, Lippincott Williams & Wilkins.

Institute of Medicine, Food and Nutrition Board: *Dietary reference intakes: a risk assessment model for establishing upper intake levels of nutrients,* Washington, DC, 1998, National Academy Press.

James VE: Niacin: the need for monitoring, *US Pharmacist,* February, 51-60, 1995.

Jarvis C: *Physical examination & health assessment,* ed 4, St Louis, 2004, Saunders.

Jefferson LV, Laraia, MT: Chemically mediated responses and substance-related disorders. In Stuart GW, Laraia MT (eds.): *Principles and practice of psychiatric nursing,* ed 8, St Louis, 2005, Mosby.

Johnson MD, Heriza TJ, St Dennis C: How to spot illicit drug abuse in your patients, *PostGrad Med* 106:199, 1999.

Joint National Committee on Detection, Evaluation and Treatment of High Blood Pressure: *The seventh report of the National Committee on Detection, Evaluation and Treatment of High Blood Pressure (JNC 7),* Bethesda, MD, NIH Publication, 03-5233, May, 2003, National Institutes of Health.

Kaluger G, Kaluger MF: *Human development: the span of life,* ed 3, St Louis, 1984, Mosby.

Karceski S, Morrell M, Carpenter D: The expert consensus guideline series: treatment of epilepsy, *Epilepsy Behav* 2:A1, 2001.

Kaskutas LA, Bond J, Humphreys K: Social networks as mediators of the effects of Alcoholics Anonymous, *Addiction* 97:891, 2002.

Kee JL: *Laboratory and diagnostic tests with nursing implications,* ed 7, Upper Saddle River, NJ, 206, Prentice Hall Health.

Keltner NL et al: *Psychiatric nursing,* ed 4, St Louis, 2003, Mosby.

Kirby RR et al: *Clinical anesthesia practice,* ed 2, Philadelphia, 2002, Saunders.

Klein-Schwartz W, Isetts BJ: Patient assessment and consultation. In *Handbook of non-prescription drugs,* ed 12, Washington, DC, 2000, American Pharmaceutical Association.

Knopp RH: Drug treatment of lipid disorders, *N Engl J Med* 341:498, 1999.

Koda-Kimble MA, Young LY (eds.): *Applied therapeutics,* ed 8, Philadelphia, 2005, Lippincott, Williams & Wilkins.

Koeneman KS, Mulhall JP, Goldstein I: Sexual health for the man at midlife: in-office workup, *Geriatrics* 52(Sept):76, 1997.

Kosten TR, O'Connor PG: Management of drug and alcohol withdrawal, *N Engl J Med* 348:1786, 2003.

Lasser KE et al: Timing of new black box warnings and withdrawal for prescription medications, *JAMA* 287:2215, 2002.

Laudet AB, Savage R, Mahmood D: Pathways to long-term recovery: a preliminary investigation, *J Psychoactive Drugs* 34:305, 2002.

Lazarou J, Pomerance B, Corey P: Incidence of adverse drug reactions in hospitalized patients: a meta-analysis of prospective studies, *JAMA* 279:1200, 1998.

Leininger M: *Transcultural nursing: concepts, theories, research, and practice,* ed 3, New York, 2002, McGraw-Hill.

LeMone P, Burke KM: *Medical-surgical nursing: critical thinking in client care,* ed 3, Upper Saddle River, NJ, 2004, Prentice Hall Health.

Lewis S, Heitkemper MM, Dirksen SR: *Medical-surgical nursing: assessment and management of clinical problems,* ed 6, St Louis, 2004, Mosby.

Lowdermilk DL, Perry SE, Bobak IM: *Maternity and women's health care,* ed 8, St Louis, 2004, Mosby.

Mayhew SL, Thorn D: Enteral nutrition support: an overview, *Am Pharm* NS35(2):47, 1995.

McCance KL, Huether SE: *Pathophysiology: the biologic basis for disease in adults and children,* ed 6, St Louis, 2006, Mosby.

McEvoy G (ed.): *AHFS drug information,* Bethesda, Md., 2006, American Society of Health System Pharmacists.

McPherson TL, Hersch PK: Brief substance use screening instruments for primary care settings: a review, *J Substance Abuse Treat* 18:193, 2000.

McRae AL, Brady KT, Sonne SC: Alcohol and substance abuse, *Med Clin N Am* 85(3):779, 2001.

Medical Letter, New Rochelle, NY, 2006, The Medical Letter.

Meiner SE, Lueckenotte AG: *Gerontologic nursing,* ed 3, St Louis, 2006, Mosby.

Melzack R: The McGill pain questionnaire: major properties and scoring methods, *Pain* 1:277, 1975.

Merskey H (ed.): IASP Committee on taxonomy: classification of chronic pain: descriptions of chronic pain syndromes and definitions of pain terms, *Pain* 3:S28, 1986.

Miller LG, Murray WJ: *Herbal medicinals: a clinician's guide,* New York, 1998, Haworth.

Moore N et al: Frequency and cost of serious adverse drug reactions in a department of general medicine, *Br J Clin Pharmacol* 45(3):301, 1998.

Mosby's drug consult, St Louis, 2006, Mosby.

Mullahy CM: The challenge of noncompliance for case managers, *Case Manager* (March/April):52, 2005.

National High Blood Pressure Education Program's Coordinating Committee: Primary prevention of hypertension, clinical and public health advisory from the National High Blood Pressure Education Program, *JAMA* 288:1882, 2002.

National Institutes of Health: Consensus development panel on impotence, *JAMA* 270:83, 1993.

North American Nursing Diagnosis Association: *Nursing diagnoses: definitions & classification,* 2005-2006, Philadelphia, NANDA International.

Novak K: *Drug facts and comparisons,* St Louis, 2006, Facts and Comparisons.

Nutt JG, Wooten GF: Diagnosis and initial management of Parkinson's disease, *N Engl J Med* 353:1021, 2005.

O'Donnell JT: Vitamins, minerals and nutritional supplements, *J Pharm Pract* 9(5):342, 1996.

Olanow CW, Watts RL, Koller WC: An algorithm (decision tree) for the management of Parkinson's disease (2001): treatment guidelines, *Neurology* 56(11):S5, 84, 2001.

Olsson S: The role of the WHO programme on international drug monitoring in coordinating worldwide drug safety efforts, *Drug Safety* 19(1):1, 1998.

Pagana KD, Pagana TJ: *Mosby's manual of diagnostic and laboratory tests*, ed 3, St Louis, 2006, Mosby.

Pal S: *Self-care and nonprescription pharmacotherapy.* In *Handbook of non-prescription drugs*, ed 14, Washington, DC, 2004, American Pharmacists Association.

Parker RB, Patterson JH, Johnson JA: Heart Failure. In DiPiro JP, et al (eds.): *Pharmacotherapy: a pathophysiologic approach*, ed 6, New York, 2005, McGraw-Hill.

Physicians' desk reference, ed 59, Montvale, NJ, 2006, Thomson PDR.

Plaut M, Vanentine MD: Allergic rhinitis, *N Engl J Med* 353:1934, 2005.

Potter PA, Perry AG: *Fundamentals of nursing,* ed 6, St Louis, 2004, Mosby.

Prochaska J, DiClemente C: Towards a comprehensive model of change. In Miller W, Heather N (eds.): *Training addictive behaviors: a process of change*, New York, 1986, Plenum.

Reid WH: Recognizing and dealing with impaired clinicians, Part I: recognition and reporting, *J Med Pract Manag* 17:97, 2001.

Reid WH: Recognizing and dealing with impaired clinicians, Part II: treatment options, *J Med Prac Manag* 17:145, 2001.

Repchinsky C (ed.): *Compendium of pharmaceuticals and specialties,* ed 41, Ottawa, 2006, Canadian Pharmacists Association.

Repchinsky C (ed.): *Compendium of self-care products 2002-2003,* Ottawa, 2003, Canadian Pharmacists Association.

Repchinsky C (ed.): *Patient self-care: helping patients make therapeutic choices,* Ottawa, 2002, Canadian Pharmacists Association.

Skidmore-Roth L: *Mosby's handbook of herbs & natural supplements,* ed 3, St Louis, 2006, Mosby.

Soldin OP, Soldin SJ: Review: therapeutic drug monitoring in pediatrics, *Ther Drug Monit* 24:1, 2002.

Sonis ST et al: Perspectives on cancer therapy-induced mucosal injury: pathogenesis, measurement, epidemiology, and consequences for patients. *Cancer* 100 (suppl 9):1995, 2004.

Sprague RL, Kalachnik JE: Reliability, validity and a total score cutoff for the Dyskinesia Identification System: Condensed User Scale (DISCUS) with mentally ill and mentally retarded populations, *Psychopharm Bull* 27(1):51, 1991.

Sweetman SC (ed.): *Martindale: the complete drug reference,* ed 34, London, 2005, Pharmaceutical Press.

Therapeutic Research Faculty: *Natural medicines comprehensive database,* ed 6, Stockton, CA, 2004, Therapeutic Research Faculty.

Therapeutic uses of herbs, part 2, *Pharm Lett* 98(2):1, 1998.

Therapeutic uses of herbs, *Pharm Lett* 97(4):1, 1997.

Tice AA, Parry D: Medications that require hepatic monitoring, *Hosp Pharm* 38(4):456, 2001.

Trissel LA: *Handbook on injectable drugs,* ed 13, Bethesda, Md., 2005, American Society of Health-System Pharmacists.

Tyler VE: What pharmacists should know about herbal remedies, *J Am Pharm Assoc* NS36(1):29, 1996.

US Pharmacopeia 29/National Formulary 24, Rockville, Md., 2006, US Pharmacopeial Convention.

USP DI-2005, ed 25, Greenwood Village, Colo., 2005, Thomson Micromedex.

USP dictionary of USAN and international drug names, Rockville, Md., 2005, US Pharmacopeial Convention.

Van De Graaff KM, Fox SI: *Concepts of human anatomy and physiology,* ed 3, Dubuque, Iowa, 1992, Brown.

Vlasnik JJ, Aliotta SL, DeLor B: Evidence-based assessment and intervention strategies to increase adherence to prescribed medication plans, *Case Manager* (March/April):55, 2005.

Vlasnik JJ, Aliotta SL, DeLor B: Medication adherence: factors influencing compliance with prescribed medication plans, *Case Manager* (March/April):48, 2005.

Volpicelli JR: Alcohol abuse and alcoholism: an overview, *J Clin Psychiatry,* 62(suppl 20): 4, 2001.

Willett WC: *Eat, drink, and be healthy* by the president and fellows of Harvard College. Reprinted by permission of Free Press/Simon & Schuster, Inc. © 2001, 2005.

Williams AS: Adaptive diabetes education for visually impaired persons: teaching nonvisual diabetes self-care, *J Home Health Care Pract* 4:62, 1992.

Williams SR: *Basic nutrition and diet therapy,* ed 12, St Louis, 2005, Mosby.

Williamson JS, Wyandt CM: Herbal therapies: the facts and the fiction, *Drug Topics* August 7:78, 1997.

Zhan C et al: Potentially inappropriate medication use in the community-dwelling elderly, *JAMA* 286(22):2823, 2001.

Illustration Credits

Chapter 2

2-2, From Levine RR, Walsh CT: *Pharmacology: drug actions and reactions,* ed 6, London, 2000, Parthenon.

Chapter 4

4-2, 4-3, From Carpenito-Moyet LJ: *Nursing diagnosis application to clinical practice,* ed 10, Philadelphia, 2004, Lippincott.

Chapter 7

7-2, From Potter PA, Perry AG: *Fundamentals of nursing,* ed 6, St Louis, 2005, Mosby; courtesy Baptist Hospital, Pensacola, Fla., and The Center for Case Management, South Natick, Mass.; **7-3,** from Potter PA, Perry AG: *Fundamentals of nursing,* ed 6, St Louis, 2005, Mosby; **7-5, A,** from Potter PA, Perry AG: *Fundamentals of nursing,* ed 6, St Louis, 2005, Mosby; Courtesy St. Mary's Health Center, St. Louis; **7-5, B, 7-6, 7-7, B,** courtesy of Creighton University Medical Center, Omaha, Neb.; **7-9,** from McKenry LM, Salerno E: *Mosby's pharmacology in nursing,* ed 21, St Louis, 2001, Mosby; **7-12,** courtesy of University Hospital, The University of Nebraska Medical Center; © Board of Regents of the University of Nebraska, Lincoln, Neb.

Chapter 8

8-4, Courtesy of CIBA Pharmaceutical Co., Summit, NJ; **8-6,** courtesy Oscar H. Allison, Jr.; **8-11,** from Rick Brady, Riva, Md.; **8-12,** from Potter PA, Perry AG: *Fundamentals of nursing,* ed 6, St Louis, 2005, Mosby.

Chapter 9

9-1, Courtesy of Oscar H. Allison, Jr.; **9-4, 9-6, 9-10, 9-11, 9-20,** courtesy of Chuck Dresner; **9-5,** copyright © 2003 McKesson Corporation and/or one of its subsidiaries. All rights reserved; **9-12,** from Potter PA, Perry AG: *Fundamentals of nursing,* ed 6, St Louis, 2005, Mosby; **9-14,** courtesy of Robert Manchester, RPh.

Chapter 10

10-4, 10-15 A, Courtesy of Baxter Healthcare Corp. All rights reserved; **10-9,** from Potter PA, Perry AG: *Basic nursing: theory and practice,* ed 5, St Louis, 2001, Mosby; **10-10,** copyright Eli Lilly and Co. All rights reserved. Used with permission; **10-11,** courtesy of Dey, Inc. **10-15, B,** courtesy of ICU Medical, Inc.; **10-16, 10-17, 10-18,** copyright © 2001 Becton, Dickinson and Co.

Chapter 12

12-2, A, From Perry AG, Potter PA: *Clinical nursing skills and techniques,* ed 6, St Louis, 2005, Mosby; **12-2, B,** from Otto SE: Pocket guide to intravenous therapy, ed 4, St Louis, 2001, Mosby; **12-3,** courtesy of *http://narang.com/scalpvein.html;* **12-5,** courtesy Chuck Dresner; **12-6,** from Potter PA, Perry AG: *Basic nursing: theory and practice,* ed 5, St Louis, 2001, Mosby; **12-7,** available from *www.bardaccess.com/cathlink_20.html.* Courtesy of CR Bard, Inc.; **12-10, 12-11,** redrawn from Williams PL et al (eds.): *Gray's anatomy,* ed 37, New York, 1989, Churchill Livingstone; **12-12,** redrawn from Hankins J et al: *Infusion therapy in clinical practice,* ed 2, Philadelphia, 2001, Saunders; **12-15, 12-16,** courtesy of Baxter Healthcare Corp. All rights reserved; **12-17,** courtesy of Bruce Clayton; **12-19,** from Infusion Nurses Society: Infusion nursing standards of practice, *JIN* (suppl.) 23:65, 2000; **12-20,** available from *www.baxter.com/doctors/ iv_therapies/education/ivtherapy_CE/Basics_One/Basic.*

Chapter 15

15-2, Modified from Olanow CW, et al: An algorithm for the management of Parkinson's disease: treatment guidelines, *Neurology* 56(11):84, 2001.

Chapter 20

20-1, Developed by McCaffery M, Pasero C, Paice JA. From McCaffery M, Pasero C: *Pain: clinical manual,* ed 2, St Louis, 1999, Mosby; **20-2,** World Health Organization, 2005. Available at *www.who.int/cancer/palliative/painladder/en;* **20-3,** from Hockenberry MJ, et al: *Wong's essentials of pediatric nursing,* ed 7, St Louis, 2005, Mosby; **20-4,** from Melzack R: The McGill Pain Questionnaire: major properties and scoring methods, *Pain* 1:277, 1975; **20-5,** illustration from Ignatavicius DD, Workman ML: *Medical-surgical nursing: critical thinking for collaborative care,* Philadelphia, 2006, Saunders; Simple Descriptive Pain Distress Scale, 0-10 Numeric Pain Distress Scale, and Visual Analog Scale redrawn from Acute Pain Management Guideline Panel. [1992]. *Acute pain management: Operative or medical procedures and trauma. Clinical practice guideline.* AHCPR Pub. No. 92-0032. Rockville, Md.: Agency for Health Care Policy and Research, Public Health Service, U.S. Department of Health and Human Services; Pain Relief Visual Analog Scale redrawn from Fishman B, et al. The Memorial Pain Assessment Card: A valid instrument for the evaluation of cancer pain. *Cancer,* 60[5], 1151-1158, 1987; Percent Relief Scale redrawn from the Brief Pain Inventory. Pain Research Group. Department of Neurology, University of Wisconsin-Madison.

Chapter 21

21-1, Centers for Disease Control and Prevention [CDC]. *Behavioral Risk Factor Surveillance System Survey Data,* Atlanta, Ga: U.S. Department of Health and Human Services, Centers for Disease Control and Prevention, 2004.

Chapter 23

23-1 and 23-2, From US Department of Health and Human Services: *The Sixth Report of the Joint National Committee on Detection, Evaluation, and Treatment of High Blood Pressure (JNC-VI),* Washington DC, 1997, National Institutes of Health.

Chapter 24

24-1, Modified from Phipps WJ, et al.: *Medical-surgical nursing: health and illness perspectives,* ed 7, St Louis, 2003, Mosby.

Chapter 28

28-2, From Hunt SA, et al: ACC/AHA 2005 guideline update for the diagnosis and management of chronic heart failure in the adult: A report of the American College of Cardiology/ American Heart Association Task Force on Practice Guidelines [Writing Committee to Update the 2001 Guidelines for the Evaluation and Management of Heart Failure]. *J Am Coll Cardiol* 2005; 46:1116-1143.

Chapter 31

31-1, DesignPointe Communications/Atlanta; **31-2,** From Clark JB, et al: *Pharmacological basis of nursing practice,* ed 3, St Louis, 1982, Mosby–Year Book; **31-3,** Modified from National Institutes of Health, National Heart, Lung and Blood Institute: Expert Panel Report: guidelines for the diagnosis and management of asthma, update on selected topics—2002 (update of the NAEPP Expert Panel Report 2 [NIH publication no. 97-4051A]), Washington, DC, 1997, NIH/NHLBI.

Chapter 34

34-1, Adapted from Clayton BD, Brown BK: Nausea and vomiting. In Helms RA, et al., eds.: *Textbook of therapeutics: Drug and disease management,* Philadelphia, 2006, Lippincott Williams & Wilkins.

Chapter 36

36-3, From The Expert Committee on the Diagnosis and Classification of Diabetes Mellitus: Report of the Expert Committee on the Diagnosis and Classification of Diabetes Mellitus, *Diabetes Care,* 26 (Suppl 1): S7, 2003.

Chapter 44

44-1, From American Cancer Society, 2005.

Chapter 47

47-1, From U.S. Department of Agriculture, Center for Nutrition Policy and Promotion, April 2005; **47-2,** from Brown KM, et al: Physical activity and health: an interactive approach, Sudbury, Mass., 2002, Jones and Bartlett. Reprinted with permission; **47-3,** From Willett WC: *Eat, Drink, and Be Healthy.* © 2001, 2005 by the President and Fellows of Harvard College. Reprinted by permission of Free Press/Simon & Schuster, Inc.

Chapter 48

48-1, A, Used with permission from *ConsumerLab.com;* **B,** used with permission from NSF International; **C,** used with permission from The USP.

Chapter 49

49-1, The Twelve Steps are reprinted with permission of Alcoholics Anonymous World Services, Inc. (AAWS). Permission to reprint the Twelve Steps does not mean that AAWS has reviewed or approved the contents of this publication, or that AAWS necessarily agrees with the views expressed herein. AA is a program of recovery from alcoholism *only;* use of the Twelve Steps in connection with programs and activities patterned after AA but which address other problems or in any other non-AA context, does not imply otherwise; **49-2,** from Stuart GW, Laraia MT: *Principles and practice of psychiatric nursing,* ed 7, St. Louis, 2001, Mosby; **49-3,** modified from Prochaska J, DiClemente C: Towards a comprehensive model of change. In Miller W, Heather N, (eds.): *Treating addictive behaviors: a process of change,* New York, 1986, Plenum.

Index

G

H

N

O

Q

R

T

U

ANSWERS TO **MATH REVIEW AND CONTENT REVIEW** QUESTIONS

Chapter 1

CONTENT REVIEW QUESTIONS

1. 1
2. 1
3. 2

Chapter 2

CONTENT REVIEW QUESTIONS

1. 4
2. 2
3. 3

Chapter 3

CONTENT REVIEW QUESTIONS

1. 4
2. 2
3. 3

Chapter 4

CONTENT REVIEW QUESTIONS

1. 2
2. 3
3. 1
4. 4

Chapter 5

CONTENT REVIEW QUESTIONS

1. 2
2. 2,3,4
3. 3

Chapter 7

CONTENT REVIEW QUESTIONS

1. 3
2. 4
3. 1
4. 3
5. 1
6. 2
7. 1

Chapter 8

CONTENT REVIEW QUESTIONS

1. 3
2. 4
3. 1
4. 2
5. 3

Chapter 9

CONTENT REVIEW QUESTIONS

1. 3
2. 4
3. 3
4. 4

Chapter 10

CONTENT REVIEW QUESTIONS

1. 2
2. 3
3. 4

Chapter 11

CONTENT REVIEW QUESTIONS

1. 2
2. 1
3. 1
4. 4
5. 4

Chapter 12

CONTENT REVIEW QUESTIONS

1. 1
2. 1
3. 2
4. 4
5. 4
6. 4
7. 4

Chapter 13

MATH REVIEW QUESTIONS

1. 16 mL
2. $1\frac{1}{2}$ tablets
3. 0.4 mg; 1 mL

CONTENT REVIEW QUESTIONS

1. 2
2. 3

Chapter 14

MATH REVIEW QUESTIONS

1. 2 tablets of 0.25 mg. General rule, when two dosages are available, give the least number of tablets to accurately fill the prescribed amount.
2. 4 mL of 500 mg/5 mL syrup or 8 mL of 250 mg/5 mL chloral hydrate. Neither of capsules, 250 mg or 500 mg can be given to accurately prepare the ordered dose.
3. Safe dosage range is between 6 to 9 mg, therefore prescribed amount of 7.5 mg is reasonable.

CONTENT REVIEW QUESTIONS

1. 1
2. 2
3. 2
4. 3

Chapter 15

MATH REVIEW QUESTIONS

1. 1 tablet per dose of 25/100 strength
2. 1 tablet, 250 mg per dose of 250 mg strength
3. $\frac{1}{2}$ tablet of 2.5 mg strength per dose

CONTENT REVIEW QUESTIONS

1. 3
2. 3
3. 4
4. 1

Chapter 16

MATH REVIEW QUESTIONS

1. 0.8 mL
2. 400 mg/dose
3. 0.75 mL

CONTENT REVIEW QUESTIONS

1. 1
2. 1
3. 3
4. 1,2,3
5. 1,2,4

Chapter 17

MATH REVIEW QUESTIONS

1. 2 tablets
2. Dosage available: 25, 50, and 75 mg tablets. Most likely 50 mg dispensed for this order. The 100 mg dose prescribed would require 2 tablets (50 mg strength).

CONTENT REVIEW QUESTIONS

1. 3
2. 3
3. 1
4. 1
5. 3

Chapter 18

MATH REVIEW QUESTIONS

1. 6.25 mL
2. 2 tablets
3. 0.6 mL of 20 mg/mL or 1.2 mL of 10 mg/mL. Use either available concentration.

CONTENT REVIEW QUESTIONS

1. 4
2. 3

Chapter 19

MATH REVIEW QUESTIONS

1. Orders need clarification. What is the route of administration? What form of drug is to be used? Available in 50 mg tablets; 30 and 100 mg capsules; suspension 30 and 125 mg/5 mL and in 50 mg/mL injectable forms. Give 100 mg Dilantin capsules three times per day and at hs if PO route is used. Schedule: 8:00 AM, 1:00 PM, 6:00 PM, 10:00 PM (hs).
2. Using an oral syringe, measure 2.5 mL of Tegretol suspension to administer 50 mg. Give PO approximately every 6 hours.
3. Yes, this is a reasonable order. Valproic acid (Depakene) is only available in oral forms. At 15 mg/kg/24 hr, and 110 lb (50 kg), this means a total daily dose of 750 mg/24 hour or 250 mg tid. Depakene syrup is available 250 mg/5 mL. Give 5 mL, three times per day at 7:00 AM, 2:00 PM, and 10:00 PM. (The later dose would maintain more consistent blood level.)

CONTENT REVIEW QUESTIONS

1. 1
2. 3
3. 1
4. 2
5. 4

Chapter 20

MATH REVIEW QUESTIONS

1. 2 tablets
2. 3.8 mL
3. Give 1 mL, 15 mg/mL morphine
4. Does not say PO; clarify order. Also, is this drug required qid or is it better on a q4h PRN basis?

CONTENT REVIEW QUESTIONS

1. 4
2. 2
3. 1
4. 1
5. 2
6. 3
7. 1
8. 1

Chapter 21

MATH REVIEW QUESTIONS

1. 2 tablets
2. ½ tablet
3. 0.4 mL
4. 2 mL

CONTENT REVIEW QUESTIONS

1. 1
2. 4
3. 1,2,4
4. 1,3

Chapter 22

MATH REVIEW QUESTIONS

1. 3 tablets, 4500 mg
2. 4 tablets
3. 2 tablets; 80 mg

CONTENT REVIEW QUESTIONS

1. 3
2. 1
3. 2
4. 4
5. 2
6. 1
7. 1,2,4

Chapter 23

MATH REVIEW QUESTIONS

1. Call pharmacy and ask that 0.3 mg tablets be provided. Would only need 2 tablets of 0.3 mg administered twice daily. Otherwise, 1 tablet of 0.2 mg strength and 1 tablet of 0.1 mg strength or 3 tablets of 0.1 mg strength could be administered twice daily.
2.
3.
4.
5.

CONTENT REVIEW QUESTIONS

1. 3
2. 3
3. 2
4. 3
5. 3
6. 1
7. 2

Chapter 24

MATH REVIEW QUESTIONS

1. 4 tablets; 2.4 g in 24 hours
2. 4 capsules
3. 4 mL

CONTENT REVIEW QUESTIONS

1. 2
2. 2
3. 3
4. 1
5. 1,3,4
6. 3

Chapter 25

MATH REVIEW QUESTIONS

1. 2 tablets. Sublingual administration: puncture capsule with needle and squeeze medication under the tongue.
2. 1 capsule; [missing answer here]
3. 2 mL

CONTENT REVIEW QUESTIONS

1. 2
2. 1
3. 3
4. 4
5. 1
6. 2
7. 3

Chapter 26

MATH REVIEW QUESTIONS

1. 400 mg dose × 4 days requires 4 tablets; the next 5 days require 10 tablets.
2. 2 capsules

CONTENT REVIEW QUESTIONS

1. 2
2. 1
3. 2
4. 3
5. 1,2
6. 3
7. 1

Chapter 27

MATH REVIEW QUESTIONS

1. 0.2 mL
2. 2.7 mL/hr; 2400 units have already infused; 4 mL/hr
3. 28 tablets

CONTENT REVIEW QUESTIONS

1. 2
2. 1
3. 3
4. 4
5. 1
6. 2
7. 4

Chapter 28

MATH REVIEW QUESTIONS

1. 75 kg; 450 mcg or 0.45 mg; digoxin may be administered undiluted, or each 1 mL may be diluted in 4 mL sterile water. IV dose should be given slowly over at least 5 minutes. Give with caution with hypertension because IV administration may elevate blood pressure. It is compatible with normal saline, dextrose 5%, or lactat ... nger's solution.
2. 0.5 mL of 0.25 m...
3. 1 tablet of 0.25 mg an... 0.125 mg, *or* 3 tablets of 0.125 m...

CONTENT REVIEW QUESTIONS

1. 3
2. 3
3. 1
4. 2
5. 4
6. 3
7. 3

Chapter 29

MATH REVIEW QUESTIONS

1. 100 mL/hr
2. 2 tablets
3. 4 mL

CONTENT REVIEW QUESTIONS

1. 2
2. 2
3. 2
4. 3
5. 1
6. 1,2,3,4
7. 3

Chapter 30

CONTENT REVIEW QUESTIONS

1. 3
2. 1
3. 3
4. 3
5. 4
6. 1
7. 2

Chapter 31

MATH REVIEW QUESTIONS

1. 9.4 mL or 2.7 tsp using equivalent 4 mL/tsp or 1.8 tsp using equivalent 5 mL/tsp
2. 0.25 mL
3. 87.95 = 88 mg/*individual dose*; 8.8 mL/*individual dose*

CONTENT REVIEW QUESTIONS

1. 3
2. 2
3. 2
4. 2
5. 3
6. 2
7. 2
8. 3

Chapter 32

CONTENT REVIEW QUESTIONS

1. 4
2. 3
3. 1,2,4
4. 1,2,3
5. 2
6. 1
7. 4

Chapter 33

MATH REVIEW QUESTIONS

1. 300 mL/hr
2. 0.875 = 0.88 mL

CONTENT REVIEW QUESTIONS

1. 1
2. 3
3. 4
4. 1
5. 2
6. 1
7. 3

Chapter 34

MATH REVIEW QUESTIONS

... kg; 9.2 mg of ondansetron;
...r
...L